MEDICAL
MICROBIOLOGY

THIRD EDITION

SECTION EDITORS

JOHNNY W. PETERSON, PhD
Section: Bacteriology
Professor, Department of Microbiology, University of Texas Medical Branch at Galveston, Galveston, Texas

CHARLES PATRICK DAVIS, MD, PhD
Section: Bacteriology
Associate Professor, Departments of Microbiology and Surgery, University of Texas Medical Branch at Galveston, Galveston, Texas

THOMAS ALBRECHT, PhD
Section: Virology
Professor, Department of Microbiology, University of Texas Medical Branch at Galveston, Galveston, Texas

FERDINANDO DIANZANI, MD
Section: Virology
Professor and Chairman, Institute of Virology, University of Rome Medical School, Rome, Italy; Adjunct Professor, Department of Microbiology, University of Texas Medical Branch at Galveston, Galveston, Texas

SAMUEL BARON, MD
Section: Virology
Professor and Chairman, Department of Microbiology, and Professor, Department of Internal Medicine, University of Texas Medical Branch at Galveston, Galveston, Texas

MICHAEL R. MCGINNIS, PhD
Section: Mycology
Professor and Vice Chairman, Department of Pathology, University of Texas Medical Branch at Galveston, Galveston, Texas

LEROY J. OLSON, PhD
Section: Parasitology
Professor, Department of Microbiology, University of Texas Medical Branch at Galveston, Galveston, Texas

ROBERT B. COUCH, MD
Section: Introduction to Infectious Diseases
Professor and Chairman, Department of Microbiology and Immunology; Professor and Chief, Division of Infectious Diseases, Department of Medicine, Baylor College of Medicine, Houston, Texas

MEDICAL MICROBIOLOGY

THIRD EDITION

Edited by

SAMUEL BARON, MD

Professor and Chairman
Department of Microbiology
Professor
Department of Internal Medicine
University of Texas Medical Branch at Galveston
Galveston, Texas

Associate Editor
PAULA M. JENNINGS

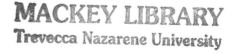

CHURCHILL LIVINGSTONE
New York, London, Edinburgh, Melbourne, Tokyo

Library of Congress Cataloging-in-Publication Data

Medical microbiology / edited by Samuel Baron. — 3rd ed.
     p. cm.
    Includes bibliographical references and index.
    ISBN 0-443-08671-0
    1. Medical microbiology. I. Baron, Samuel, date.
    [DNLM: 1. Microbiology. QW 4 M486]
QR46.M467 1991
616'.01—dc20
DNLM/DLC
for Library of Congress   91-10750
                      CIP

Distributed in the United Kingdom by Churchill Livingstone, Robert Stevenson House, 1–3 Baxter's Place, Leith Walk, Edinburgh EH1 3AF, and by associated companies, branches, and representatives throughout the world.

Chapters 3, 5, 51, 54, 55, 61, 62, 75, 76, 83, and 84 were prepared by U.S. government employees and are not subject to copyright.

Accurate indications, adverse reactions, and dosage schedules for drugs are provided in this book, but it is possible that they may change. The reader is urged to review the package information data of the manufacturers of the medications mentioned.

The Publishers have made every effort to trace the copyright holders for borrowed material. If they have inadvertently overlooked any, they will be pleased to make the necessary arrangements at the first opportunity.

Acquisitions Editor: *Debra Rapaport*
Copy Editor: *David Terry*
Cover Designer: *Paul Moran*
Book Designer: *Gloria Brown*
Production Supervisor: *Christina Hippeli*
Indexer: *Irving Conde Tullar*

Printed in the United States of America

First published in 1991   7 6 5 4 3 2 1

CONSULTING EDITORS

PREMKUMAR CHRISTADOSS, MD
Associate Professor, Department of Microbiology,
University of Texas Medical Branch at
Galveston, Galveston, Texas

LAWRENCE DREYFUS, PhD
Assistant Professor, Department of Microbiology,
University of Texas Medical Branch at
Galveston, Galveston, Texas

DAVID W. NIESEL, PhD
Associate Professor, Department of Microbiology,
University of Texas Medical Branch at Galveston,
Galveston, Texas

FRANK C. SCHMALSTIEG, JR., MD, PhD
Professor, Departments of Pediatrics and Human
Biological Chemistry and Genetics, University of Texas
Medical Branch at Galveston, Galveston, Texas

DEVELOPMENTAL EDITOR
MARGOT OTWAY

ENGLISH EDITOR
MARDELLE SUSMAN

EDITORIAL ASSISTANTS
RHONDA C. PEAKE
JULIE B. FOWLER
LOUESE McKERLIE

SCIENTIFIC ILLUSTRATOR
STEVE SCHUENKE

CONTRIBUTORS

THOMAS ALBRECHT, PhD
Professor, Department of Microbiology, University of Texas Medical Branch at Galveston, Galveston, Texas

MICHELLE J. ALFA, PhD
Assistant Professor, Department of Medical Microbiology, University of Manitoba Faculty of Medicine; Assistant Director, Department of Medical Microbiology, St. Boniface General Hospital, Winnipeg, Manitoba, Canada

G. G. ALTON, DVMS
Former Senior Principal Research Scientist, C.S.I.R.O. Animal Health Research Laboratory, Commonwealth Scientific and Industrial Research Organization, Parkville, Australia

RAZA ALY, PhD
Professor, Department of Dermatology, University of California, San Francisco, School of Medicine, San Francisco, California

SAMUEL BARON, MD
Professor and Chairman, Department of Microbiology, and Professor, Department of Internal Medicine, University of Texas Medical Branch at Galveston, Galveston, Texas

DERRICK BAXBY, PhD, MRCPath
Senior Lecturer, Department of Medical Microbiology, Liverpool University; Honorary Microbiologist, Royal Liverpool Hospital, Liverpool, England

YECHIEL BECKER, PhD
Professor, Department of Molecular Virology, Faculty of Medicine, Hebrew University of Jerusalem, Jerusalem, Israel

NEIL R. BLACKLOW, MD
Richard M. Haidack Distinguished Professor in Medicine, Molecular Genetics and Microbiology, and Chairman, Department of Medicine, University of Massachusetts Medical School, Worcester, Massachusetts

MARTIN J. BLASER, MD
Addison B. Scoville Professor, Department of Medicine; Professor and Director, Division of Infectious Diseases, Department of Microbiology and Immunology, Vanderbilt University School of Medicine; Staff Physician, Department of Veterans Affairs Medical Center, Nashville, Tennessee

ISTVAN BOLDOGH, DMB, PhD, DMSc
Associate Professor Designate, Department of Microbiology, University of Texas Medical Branch at Galveston, Galveston, Texas

PHILIP S. BRACHMAN, MD
Professor, Department of Public Health, Emory University School of Public Health, Atlanta, Georgia

DONALD J. BRENNER, MS, PhD

Chief, Meningitis and Special Pathogens Laboratory Section, Meningitis and Special Pathogens Branch, Divsion of Bacterial and Mycotic Diseases, Centers for Disease Control, Atlanta, Georgia

JANET S. BUTEL, PhD

Professor and Head, Division of Molecular Virology, Baylor College of Medicine, Houston, Texas

GILBERT A. CASTRO, PhD

Professor, Department of Physiology and Cell Biology, University of Texas Medical School at Houston, Houston, Texas

JAN CERNY, MD, PhD

Professor and Chairman, Department of Microbiology and Immunology, University of Maryland School of Medicine, Baltimore, Maryland

JAY O. COHEN, PhD

Former Microbiologist, Center for Infectious Diseases, Centers for Disease Control, Atlanta, Georgia

GARRY T. COLE, PhD

Professor, Department of Botany, University of Texas, Austin, Texas

FRANK M. COLLINS, PhD, DSc

Member, Trudeau Institute Inc., Saranac Lake, New York

ROBERT B. COUCH, MD

Professor and Chairman, Department of Microbiology and Immunology; Professor and Chief, Division of Infectious Diseases, Department of Medicine, Baylor Colege of Medicine, Houston, Texas

JOHN P. CRAIG, MD

Professor, Department of Microbiology and Immunology, State University of New York Health Science Center at Brooklyn College of Medicine, Brooklyn, New York

JOHN H. CROSS, PhD

Professor, Division of Tropical Public Health, Department of Preventive Medicine and Biometrics, Uniformed Services University of the Health Sciences F. Edward Hébert School of Medicine , Bethesda, Maryland

CHARLES PATRICK DAVIS, MD, PhD

Associate Professor, Departments of Microbiology and Surgery, University of Texas Medical Branch at Galveston, Galveston, Texas

ERIK DE CLERCQ, MD, PhD

Professor of Microbiology and Biochemistry and Chairman, Department of Microbiology, Rega Institute for Medical Research, Katholieke Universiteit Leuven, Leuven, Belgium

FERDINANDO DIANZANI, MD

Professor and Chairman, Institute of Virology, University of Rome Medical School, Rome, Italy; Adjunct Professor, Department of Microbiology, University of Texas Medical Branch at Galveston, Galveston, Texas

DENNIS M. DIXON, PhD

Associate Professor, Department of Pathology and Laboratory Medicine, Albany Medical College; Associate Director, Center for Laboratories and Research, New York State Department of Health, Albany, New York

WALTER DOERFLER, MD

Professor and Director, Institute of Genetics, University of Cologne, Cologne, Federal Republic of Germany

J. P. DUBEY, MVSc, PhD

Microbiologist, Zoonotic Disease Laboratory, Livestock and Poultry Sciences Institute, United States Department of Agriculture, Beltsville, Maryland

GISELA ENDERS, MD

Professor and Honorary Professor for Clinical Virology, Department of Virology, Faculty for Human Medicine, Philipps University, Marburg; Honorary Professor, Faculty for Virology and Microbiology, University of Hohemheim; Head, Institut für Medizinische Virologies und Infektionsepidemiologie, Stuttgart, Federal Republic of Germany

DOLORES G. EVANS, PhD

Research Associate Professor, Department of Medicine, Baylor College of Medicine; Chief, Mucosal Immunity Laboratory, Digestive Disease Section, Veterans Affairs Medical Center, Houston, Texas

DOYLE J. EVANS, JR., PhD

Research Associate Professor, Department of Medicine, Baylor College of Medicine; Chief, Bacterial Enteropathogens Laboratory, Digestive Disease Section, Veterans Affairs Medical Center, Houston, Texas

ADAM EWERT, PhD

Professor, Department of Microbiology, University of Texas Medical Branch at Galveston, Galveston, Texas

ANTHONY S. FAUCI, MD

Director, National Institute of Allergy and Infectious Diseases, National Institutes of Health, Bethesda, Maryland

FRANK FENNER, MD

Professor Emeritus, John Curtin School of Medical Research, Australian National University, Canberra, Australia

SYDNEY M. FINEGOLD, MD

Professor, Departments of Microbiology and Immunology and of Medicine, University of California, Los Angeles, UCLA School of Medicine Los Angeles; Associate Chief of Staff, Research and Development, Veterans Affairs Medical Center, West Los Angeles, California

HORST FINGER, MD

Director, Institut für Hygiene und Laboratorium Medizin, Staedtische Krankenanstalten, Krefeld, Federal Republic of Germany

RICHARD A. FINKELSTEIN, PhD

Curators' Professor, Millsap Distinguished Professor, and Chairman, Department of Molecular Microbiology and Immunology, University of Missouri — Columbia School of Medicine, Columbia, Missouri

DANIEL B. FISHBEIN, MD

Medical Epidemiologist, Division of Viral and Rickettsial Diseases, Viral and Rickettsial Zoonoses Branch, Center for Infectious Diseases, Centers for Disease Control, Atlanta, Georgia

THOMAS J. FITZGERALD, PhD

Professor, Department of Microbiology and Immunology, University of Minnesota—Duluth School of Medicine, Duluth, Minnesota

W. ROBERT FLEISCHMANN, JR., PhD

Professor, Department of Microbiology, University of Texas Medical Branch at Galveston, Galveston, Texas

MICHAEL FONS, PhD

J. W. McLaughlin Fellow, Department of Microbiology, University of Texas Medical Branch at Galveston, Galveston, Texas

SAMUEL B. FORMAL, PhD

Chief, Division of Enteric Infections, Walter Reed Army Institute of Research, Washington, DC

J. R. L. FORSYTH, MD

Director, Micobiological Diagnostic Unit, University of Melbourne, Melbourne, Australia

MARY ANN GERENCSER, PhD

Research Associate, Department of Microbiology and Immunology, West Virginia University School of Medicine, Morgantown, West Virginia

RALPH A. GIANNELLA, MD

Professor, Department of Medicine, University of Cincinnati College of Medicine; Director, Division of Digestive Diseases, Veterans Affairs Medical Center, Cincinnati, Ohio

CLARENCE J. GIBBS, JR., PhD

Deputy Chief, Laboratory of Central Nervous System Studies, National Institute of Neurological and Communicative Disorders and Stroke, National Institutes of Health, Bethesda, Maryland

ARMOND S. GOLDMAN, MD

Professor, Departments of Pediatrics, Microbiology, Human Biological Chemistry and Genetics, and Pathology, University of Texas Medical Branch at Galveston, Galveston, Texas

SHERWOOD L. GORBACH, MD

Professor, Department of Community Health and Medicine, Tufts University School of Medicine, Boston, Massachusetts

M. NEAL GUENTZEL, PhD

Professor, Division of Life Sciences, University of Texas at San Antonio; Professor, Department of Microbiology, University of Texas Medical School at San Antonio, San Antonio, Texas

THOMAS L. HALE, MD

Research Scientist, Division of Enteric Infections, Walter Reed Army Institute of Research, Washington, DC

DEBORAH J. HENDERSON, RN

Special Assistant to the Director, Center for Biologics Evaluation and Research, Food and Drug Administration, Bethesda, Maryland

DAVID J. HENTGES, PhD

Professor and Chairman, Department of Microbiology, Texas Tech University Health Sciences Center School of Medicine, Lubbock, Texas

DONALD HEYNEMAN, PhD

Professor of Parasitology, Department of Epidemiology and Biostatistics, University of California, San Francisco, School of Medicine, San Francisco, California; Chair, Joint Medical Program, and Associate Dean, Health and Medical Sciences, University of California, Berkeley, California

HERBERT HOF, MD

Professor, Institute of Medical Microbiology and Hygiene, Faculty of Clinical Medicine, University of Heidelberg; Director, Institute of Medical Microbiology and Hygiene of the Municipal Hospital, Mannheim, Federal Republic of Germany

STEPHEN L. HOFFMAN, MD, DTMH

Director, Malaria Program, Naval Medical Research Institute, Bethesda, Maryland

RANDALL K. HOLMES, MD, PhD

Associate Dean for Academic Affairs, and Chairman, Department of Microbiology, Uniformed Services University of the Health Sciences F. Edward Hébert School of Medicine, Bethesda, Maryland

WALTER T. HUGHES, MD

Professor, Department of Pediatrics, University of Tennessee, Memphis, College of Medicine; Chairman, Department of Infectious Diseases, St. Jude Children's Research Hospital, Memphis, Tennessee

BARBARA H. IGLEWSKI, PhD

Professor and Chair, Department of Microbiology and Immunology, University of Rochester School of Medicine and Dentistry, Rochester, New York

MICHAEL G. JOBLING, PhD

Postdoctoral Fellow, Department of Microbiology, Uniformed Services University of the Health Sciences F. Edward Hébert School of Medicine, Bethesda, Maryland

RICHARD T. JOHNSON, MD

Professor and Director, Departments of Neurology and Microbiology and Neuroscience, The Johns Hopkins University School of Medicine; Neurologist-in-Chief, Johns Hopkins Hospital, Baltimore, Maryland

RUSSELL C. JOHNSON, PhD

Professor, Department of Microbiology, University of Minnesota Medical School—Minneapolis, Minneapolis, Minnesota

PETER JURTSHUK, JR., PhD

Professor, Department of Biology, College of Natural Science and Mathematics, University of Houston, Houston, Texas

ALBERT Z. KAPIKIAN, MD

Head, Epidemiology Section, Laboratory of Infectious Diseases, National Institute of Allergy and Infectious Diseases, National Institutes of Health, Bethesda, Maryland

DORIS S. KELSEY, MD

Associate Professor, Department of Pediatrics, Bowman Gray School of Medicine of Wake Forest University, Winston-Salem, North Carolina

GERALD T. KEUSCH, MD

Chief, Division of Geographic Medicine, Department of Medicine, Tufts University School of Medicine, Boston, Massachusetts

KWANG-SHIN KIM, PhD

Associate Professor, Department of Microbiology, New York University School of Medicine, New York, New York

GARY R. KLIMPEL, PhD

Professor, Department of Microbiology, University of Texas Medical Branch at Galveston, Galveston, Texas

GEORGE S. KOBAYASHI, PhD

Professor, Departments of Medicine and Medical Microbiology, Washington University School of Medicine; Associate Director, Diagnostic Microbiology Laboratory, Banes Hospital, St. Louis, Missouri

CHIEN LIU, MD
Professor, Departments of Pediatrics and Medicine, and Director, Division of Infectious Diseases, University of Kansas Medical Center School of Medicine, Kansas City, Kansas

WALTER J. LOESCHE, DMD, PhD
Professor, Department of Dentistry, University of Michigan School of Dentistry; Professor, Department of Microbiology, University of Michigan School of Medicine, Ann Arbor, Michigan

JOAN C. M. MACNAB, PhD
Senior Scientist, Medical Research Council Virology Unit; Honorary Lecturer, University of Glasgow, Glasgow, Scotland

JON T. MADER, MD
Professor, Division of Infectious Diseases, Department of Internal Medicine; Member, Marine Biomedical Institute, and Chief, Division of Marine Medicine, University of Texas Medical Branch at Galveston, Galveston, Texas

AUGUSTO JULIO MARTINEZ, MD
Professor, Department of Pathology, University of Pittsburgh School of Medicine; Neuropathologist, Presbyterian University Hospital and Montefiore University Hospital, Pittsburgh, Pennsylvania

CARL F. T. MATTERN, MD
Visiting Associate Professor, Department of Obstetrics and Gynecology, The Johns Hopkins University School of Medicine, Baltimore, Maryland

MICHAEL R. McGINNIS, PhD
Professor and Vice-Chairman, Department of Pathology, University of Texas Medical Branch at Galveston, Galveston, Texas

DAVID N. McMURRAY, PhD
Associate Professor and Interim Head, Department of Medical Microbiology and Immunology, Texas A & M University College of Medicine, College Station, Texas

ERNEST A. MEYER, ScD
Professor, Department of Microbiology and Immunology, Oregon Health Sciences University School of Medicine, Portland, Oregon

HARRY M. MEYER, JR., MD
President, Medical Research Division, American Cyanamid, Inc., Pearl River, New York

MARK MIDDLEBROOKS, MD
Fellow, Division of Infectious Diseases, Department of Medicine, University of Alabama School of Medicine, Birmingham, Alabama

STEPHEN A. MORSE, PhD
Adjunct Professor, Department of Microbiology and Immunology, Emory University School of Medicine; Director, Division of Sexually Transmitted Diseases Laboratory Research, Center for Infectious Diseases, Centers for Disease Control, Atlanta, Georgia

JOHN R. MURPHY, PhD
Chief, Section of Biomolecular Medicine, Department of Medicine, University Hospital, Boston, Massachusetts

DANIEL M. MUSHER, MD
Professor, Departments of Medicine and Microbiology and Immunology, Baylor College of Medicine; Chief, Infectious Diseases Section, Veterans Administration Hospital, Houston, Texas

HAROLD C. NEU, MD
Professor, Departments of Medicine and Pharmacology, Columbia University College of Physicians and Surgeons, New York, New York

MARY C. O'CONNOR, MD
Assistant Director, Department of Infectious Disease and Epidemiology, Trinity Lutheran Hospital, Kansas City, Missouri

LEROY J. OLSON, PhD
Professor, Department of Microbiology, University of Texas Medical Branch at Galveston, Galveston, Texas

DAVID ONIONS, PhD, MRCVS
Professor, Department of Veterinary Pathology, The Veterinary School, University of Glasgow, Glasgow, Scotland

PAUL D. PARKMAN, MD
Former Deputy Director, Center for Drugs and Biologics, Food and Drug Administration, Bethesda, Maryland

GARY PATOU, BSC, MB, BS, MRCPath
Lecturer, Department of Medical Microbiology, University College and Middlesex School of Medicine, London, England

MARIA JEVITZ PATTERSON, MD, PhD
Professor, Departments of Microbiology and Public Health and Pediatrics and Human Development, Michigan State University Colleges of Osteopathic and Human Medicine, East Lansing, Michigan

JOHN R. PATTISON, MA, DM, FRCPath
Professor, Department of Medical Microbiology, University College and Middlesex School of Medicine, London, England

LAWRENCE L. PELLETIER, JR., MD
Professor, Department of Internal Medicine, University of Kansas Medical Center School of Medicine; Chief, Medical Service, Wichita Veterans Affairs Medical Center, Wichita, Kansas

GUILLERMO I. PEREZ-PEREZ, DRSc
Research Assistant Professor, Division of Infectious Diseases, Department of Medicine, Vanderbilt University School of Medicine, Nashville, Tennessee

JOHNNY W. PETERSON, PhD
Professor, Department of Microbiology, University of Texas Medical Branch at Galveston, Galveston, Texas

CHARLES J. PFAU, PhD
Professor, Department of Biology, Rensselaer Polytechnic Institute, Troy, New York

DAVID D. PORTER, MD
Professor, Department of Pathology, University of California, Los Angeles, UCLA School of Medicine, Los Angeles, California

ALAN S. RABSON, MD
Director, Division of Cancer Biology, Diagnosis, and Centers, National Cancer Institute, National Institutes of Health, Bethesda, Maryland

SHMUEL RAZIN, PhD
Dean, Faculty of Medicine, and Professor, Department of Medicine, The Hebrew University—Hadassah Medical School, Jerusalem, Israel

FRANCES L. REID-SANDEN, MS
Public Health Scientist, Division of Viral and Rickettsial Diseases, Viral and Rickettsial Zoonoses Branch, Center for Infectious Diseases, Centers for Disease Control, Atlanta, Georgia

LELAND S. RICKMAN, MD
Assistant Head, Division of Infectious Diseases, National Naval Medical Center, Bethesda, Maryland

BERNARD ROIZMAN, ScD
Joseph Regenstein Distinguished Service Professor of Virology, Division of Biological Sciences, Departments of Molecular Genetics and Cell Biology and Biochemistry and Molecular Biology, University of Chicago Division of Biological Sciences Pritzker School of Medicine, Chicago, Illinois

ALLAN R. RONALD, MD, FRCPC, FACP
Professor, Departments of Internal Medicine and Medical Microbiology, University of Manitoba Faculty of Medicine, Winnipeg, Manitoba, Canada

ZEDA F. ROSENBERG, ScD
Assistant to the Director, National Institute of Allergy and Infectious Diseases, National Institutes of Health, Bethesda, Maryland

PHILIP K. RUSSELL, MD
Professor, Department of International Health, School of Hygiene and Public Health, The Johns Hopkins University School of Medicine, Baltimore, Maryland

MILTON R. J. SALTON, ScD
Professor, Department of Microbiology, New York University School of Medicine, New York, New York

ALAN L. SCHMALJOHN, PhD
Microbiologist, U.S. Army Medical Research Institute of Infectious Diseases, Fort Detrick, Frederick, Maryland

JOHN RICHARD SEED, PhD
Professor, Department of Epidemiology, School of Public Health, University of North Carolina at Chapel Hill School of Medicine, Chapel Hill, North Carolina

ROBERT E. SHOPE, MD

Professor, Yale Arbovirus Research Unit, Department of Epidemiology and Public Health, Yale University School of Medicine, New Haven, Connecticut

WILLIAM A. SODEMAN, JR., MD

Professor and Chief, Division of Gastroenterology Department of Internal Medicine, Medical College of Ohio, Toledo, Ohio

PETER C. B. TURNBULL, BSc, MS, PhD

Anthrax Section, Division of Biologics, Public Health Laboratory Service Centre for Applied Microbiology and Research, Salisbury, Wiltshire, England

DAVID A. J. TYRRELL, MD, DRCP, FRS

Former Director, Medical Research Council, Common Cold Unit, Harvard Hospital, Salisbury, Wiltshire, England

DEREK WAKELIN, PhD, DSc

Professor, Department of Zoology, University of Nottingham, Nottingham, England

DAVID H. WALKER, MD

Professor and Chairman, Department of Pathology, University of Texas Medical Branch at Galveston, Galveston, Texas

WILLIAM WALLACE, MD

Fellow, Surgical Infectious Diseases, Division of Infectious Diseases, Department of Internal Medicine and the Marine Biomedical Institute, Division of Marine Medicine, University of Texas Medical Branch at Galveston, Galveston, Texas

THOMAS J. WALSH, MD

Medical Officer, Infectious Diseases Section, National Cancer Institute, National Institutes of Health, Bethesda, Maryland

KENNETH S. WARREN, MD

Professor, Department of Medicine, New York University School of Medicine; Adjunct Professor, Rockefeller University, New York, New York; Adjunct Professor, Department of Medicine, Tufts University School of Medicine, Boston, Massachusetts; Director for Science, Maxwell Communication Corporation, New York, New York

JOHN A. WASHINGTON, MD

Chairman, Department of Microbiology, Cleveland Clinic Foundation, Cleveland, Ohio

CAROL L. WELLS, PhD

Associate Professor, Department of Laboratory Medicine and Pathology, University of Minnesota Medical School—Minneapolis, Minneapolis, Minnesota

RICHARD J. WHITLEY, MD

Professor, Departments of Pediatrics, Medicine, and Microbiology, University of Alabama School of Medicine, Birmingham, Alabama

TRACY D. WILKINS, PhD

Strobants Professor of Agricultural Biotechnology and Head, Department of Anaerobic Microbiology, Virginia Polytechnic Institute and State University, Blacksburg, Virginia

WASHINGTON C. WINN, JR., MD

Professor, Department of Pathology, University of Vermont College of Medicine; Director, Clinical Microbiology Laboratory, Medical Center Hospital of Vermont, Burlington, Vermont

ROBERT G. YAEGER, PhD

Professor (retired), Department of Tropical Medicine, School of Public Health and Tropical Medicine; and Professor, Department of Medicine, School of Medicine, Tulane University, New Orleans, Louisiana

MARGUERITE YIN-MURPHY, MA, PhD, Dip Bact

Associate Professor, Department of Microbiology, National University of Singapore Faculty of Medicine; Director, WHO Collaborating Enterovirus Center, Singapore

RODRIGO A. ZELEDÓN, ScD

Professor, Escuela de Medicina Veterinaria, Programa de Investigacion en Enfermedades Tropicales (PIET), Universidad Nacional, Heredia, Costa Rica

ARIE J. ZUCKERMAN, MD, DSc, FRCP, FRCPath

Dean and Professor, Department of Microbiology, and Honorary Consultant in Medical Microbiology, Royal Free Hospital School of Medicine of the University of London; Director, WHO Collaborating Centre for Reference and Research on Viral Diseases, London, England

PREFACE

MICROBES AND HUMANITY

Microbes may be the most significant life form sharing this planet with humans because of their pervasive presence and their utilization of any available food source, including humans whose defenses may be breached. The ubiquitous presence of microbes and their astronomic numbers give rise to the many mutants that account for rapid evolutionary adaptation. This adaptability accounts for the ability of microbes to utilize an enormous range of nutritional sources. Depending on the food source, microbes may play either beneficial roles in maintaining life or undesirable roles in causing human, animal, and plant disease.

Beneficial roles of microbes include recycling of organic matter through microbe-induced decay and through digestion and nutrition in animals and humans. In addition, the natural microbial flora provides protection against more virulent microbes.

The microbes that cause infectious diseases may be virulent, although opportunistic diseases may also be caused by normally benign microbes. Opportunistic infections occur when the host defense mechanisms are impaired, when when microbes are present in large numbers, or when microbes reach vulnerable body sites. A striking example is the virus that causes AIDS by impairing the host's defenses to multiple microbes. Because death or severe impairment of an infected host compromises the survival of the infecting microbe, natural selection favors a predominance of less virulent microorganisms, except when microbial transmis-sion depends on disease manifestations (e.g., coughing and sneezing).

Understanding and employing the principles of microbiology and the molecular mechanisms of pathogenesis enable the physician and medical scientist to control an increasing number of infectious diseases.

RATIONALE

Medical Microbiology is effectively two books in one: a comprehensive textbook of microbiology and a concise review text. Each chapter opens with a General Concepts section that distills the key information in the chapter and is designed to be used as a rapid review or study guide. The chapters themselves are comprehensive yet free of unnecessary detail. Another form of overview is provided by the illustrations, which are uniform, telegraphic, and self-explanatory. The natural history of each major infectious disease, for example, is summarized in an "everyperson" figure with a consistent format.

The book is written at a level appropriate for both medical students and physicians. Medical relevance is emphasized throughout. Sections describe the clinical manifestations, diagnosis, and treatment of each infection, and the book concludes with a series of chapters that summarizes the infectious diseases in the context of the functioning organ systems.

ORGANIZATION

Medical Microbiology begins with a review of the immune system, focusing on the body's reponse to invading microorganisms. Bacteria are then covered, first with a series of chapters presenting the general concepts of bacterial microbiology and then with chapters detailing the major bacterial pathogens of humans. Similar sections cover virology, mycology, and parasitology. In each section, the introductory chapters stress the mechanisms of infection characteristic of the type of microorganism, thus providing the reader with a framework for understanding rather than memorizing the clinical behavior of the pathogens. The final section of the book, Introduction to Infectious Diseases, is arranged by organ system and provides a transition to clinical considerations.

ACKNOWLEDGMENTS

Primary acknowledgment must go to the many dedicated scientists who have discovered the principles of microbiology. The scientific literature acknowledges individual contributions, but textbooks cannot adequately pay such tribute. Albert Einstein identified this problem, commenting that although "there are plenty of well-endowed (scientists)...it strikes me as unfair to select a few of them for recognition." We are indebted to all these unnamed investigators.

On a more immediate level, the editors are grateful to all our contributing authors for their enthusiasm and cooperation and to our consulting editors for their expert and exhaustive scientific review. Input from focus groups of medical students was invaluable in developing the educational approach of this textbook. The support of the University of Texas in encouraging faculty members to participate in this effort has been outstanding. Finally, the section editors deserve particular praise. They have processed a formidable number of chapter manuscripts with dedication, attention to detail, scientific knowledge, and editorial skill.

In addition, we thank Phyllis G. Baron for providing educational guidance, and Amy L. Robinson and Sarah A. Lockner (University of Texas) and Jody L. Baron (Yale University) for organizing student focus groups. Our co-workers, especially Joyce Poast, Elaine Young, Jacqueline Lynch, Elizabeth Cook, Charlene Hoff, and Linda Roberts, deserve grateful recognition for their indispensable help.

Samuel Baron, MD

CONTENTS

SECTION II
VIROLOGY

SECTION III
MYCOLOGY

SECTION IV
PARASITOLOGY

I

BACTERIOLOGY

Bacteria are single-celled microorganisms that lack a nuclear membrane but are metabolically active and divide by binary fission. Superficially, bacteria appear to be relatively simple forms of life; in fact, they are sophisticated and highly adaptable. Many bacteria multiply at incredibly rapid rates, and different species can utilize an enormous variety of hydrocarbon substrates, including phenol, rubber, and petroleum. These organisms exist widely in both parasitic and free-living forms. Because they are ubiquitous and have a remarkable capacity to adapt to changing environments by selection of spontaneous mutants, the importance of bacteria in every field of medicine cannot be overstated.

The discipline of bacteriology evolved from the need of physicians to test and apply the germ theory of disease and from economic concerns relating to the spoilage of foods and wine. The initial advances in pathogenic bacteriology were derived from the identification and characterization of bacteria associated with specific diseases. During this period, great emphasis was placed on applying Koch's postulates to test proposed cause-and-effect relationships between bacteria and specific diseases. Today, most bacterial diseases of humans and their etiologic agents have been identified, although biologic and antigenic variants continue to evolve.

Major advances in bacteriology over the last century made possible the development of many effective vaccines (e.g., pneumococcal polysaccharide vaccine, diphtheria toxoid, and tetanus toxoid) as well as of other vaccines (e.g., cholera, typhoid, and plague vaccines) that are less effective or have side effects. Another major advance was the discovery of sulfonamides and antibiotics. These antimicrobial substances have not eradicated any bacterial diseases, but they are marvelous therapeutic tools. Their efficacy is reduced by the emergence of resistant bacteria. In reality, improvements in sanitation and water purification usually have a greater effect on the incidence of bacterial infections in a community than does the availability of antibiotics or bacterial vaccines. The adage "Cleanliness is next to godliness" is a sound medical principle.

Most diseases now known to have a bacteriologic etiology have been recognized for hundreds of years. Some were described in the writings of the ancient Chinese, centuries prior to the first descriptions of bacteria by Antony van Leeuwenhoek in 1677. There remain a few diseases (such as chronic ulcerative colitis) that are thought by some investigators to be caused by bacteria but for which no pathogen has been identified. Occasionally, a previously unrecognized disease is associated with a new group of bacteria. A recent example is legionnaire's disease, an acute respiratory infection caused by the previously unrecognized genus *Legionella*. Another example, less dramatic but of immense importance in understanding the etiology of venereal diseases, was the association of at least 50 percent of the cases of urethritis in male patients with *Ureaplasma urealyticum* and *Chlamydia trachomatis*.

Recombinant bacteria produced by genetic engineering will be enormously useful in bacteriologic research and already are being employed to manufacture scarce biomolecules needed for research and patient care. The antibiotic resistance genes that present such a problem to the physician because they are transferred readily among bacteria paradoxically have proved to be indispensable markers in performing genetic engineering. Genetic probes are useful in the rapid identification of microbial pathogens in patient specimens. Genetic recombinants of pathogenic bacteria constructed by site-directed mutagenesis continue to be indispensable in evaluating virulence mechanisms of bacterial pathogens. As more protective protein antigens are identified, cloned, and sequenced, live recombinant bacterial vaccines will be constructed that should be much better than the ones presently available.

In developed countries, 90 percent of documented infections in hospitalized patients are caused by bacteria. These cases probably reflect only a small percentage of the actual number of bacterial infections occurring in the general population, and usually represent the most severe cases. In developing countries, bacterial infections often exert a devastating effect on the health of the inhabitants, who become infected with a large variety of bacteria. Malnutrition, parasitic infections, and poor sanitation are a few of the factors contributing to the increased susceptibility of these individuals to bacterial pathogens. The World Health Organization (1990) estimates that each year, 3 million people die of tuberculosis, 0.5 million die of pertussis, and 25,000 die of typhoid. Diarrheal diseases, many of which are bacterial, are the second leading cause of death in the world (after cardiovascular diseases), killing 5 million people annually.

Many bacterial diseases can be viewed as a failure of the bacterium to adapt, since a well-adapted parasite ideally thrives in its host without causing significant damage. Relatively nonvirulent (i.e., well-adapted) microorganisms can cause disease under special conditions—for example, if they are present in unusually large numbers, if the host's defenses are impaired, or if anaerobic conditions exist. This textbook emphasizes only bacteria that have medical relevance. These pathogenic bacteria constitute only a small proportion of the total bacterial population; many nonpathogens are beneficial to humans and participate in essential processes such as nitrogen fixation, waste disposal, food production, drug preparation, and environmental bioremediation.

In recent years, medical scientists have concentrated on the study of pathogenic mechanisms and host defenses. Understanding host-parasite relationships involving specific pathogens requires familiarity with the fundamental characteristics of the parasite, the host, and their interactions. Therefore, the first third of this section deals with the basic concepts of the immune response, bacterial structure, taxonomy, metabolism, and genetics. Subsequent chapters emphasize normal relationships among bacteria on external surfaces; mechanisms by which microorganisms damage the host; host defense mechanisms; source and distribution of pathogens (epidemiology); principles of diagnosis; and mechanisms of action of antimicrobial drugs. These chapters provide the basis for the chapters devoted to specific bacterial pathogens and the diseases they cause. The bacteria in these chapters are grouped on the basis of physical, chemical, and biologic characteristics. These similarities do not necessarily indicate either that the bacteria are closely related or that their diseases are similar; widely divergent diseases may be caused by bacteria in the same group.

Johnny W. Peterson
C. P. Davis

1 IMMUNOLOGY OVERVIEW

JAN CERNY
ARMOND S. GOLDMAN

GENERAL CONCEPTS

INTRODUCTION

The immune system distinguishes self from nonself **(antigen)** and thus defends against infecting agents, other foreign agents, and altered host cells that cause disease.

EVOLUTION

The immune system evolved to become more complex, specific, efficient, and regulated.

ORGAN SYSTEMS

General

Leukocytes, the principal components of the immune system, are developed and maintained in two overlapping compartments: the lymphoid and reticuloendothelial systems. All leukocytes are derived from pluripotent stem cells that are found in the bone marrow during postnatal life.

Lymphoid System

The thymus, a central lymphoid organ, instructs certain lymphocytes to differentiate into thymus-dependent (T) lymphocytes. T lymphocytes circulate through the blood and lymphatics, are long lived, and aid in recognizing foreign antigens, regulating many facets of the immune system and assisting in defense against many types of infections. In contrast, thymus-independent (B) lymphocytes do not mature in the thymus and remain principally in peripheral lymphoid organs, where they be-

come antibody (immunoglobulin)-producing cells (plasma cells).

Reticuloendothelial System

The reticuloendothelial system consists of circulating monocytes; resident macrophages in the liver, spleen, lymph nodes, thymus, submucosal tissues of the respiratory and alimentary tracts, bone marrow, and connective tissues; dendritic cells in lymph nodes; Langerhans cells in the skin; and glial cells in the central nervous system. Macrophages ingest particles (phagocytosis), marshal and influence other parts of the immune system such as T lymphocytes, and serve as one type of antigen processing-presenting cells.

IMMUNE SYSTEM CELLS

The cells of the lymphoid and reticuloendothelial system produce molecules, called **cytokines,** that activate and regulate other cells in the same systems. Those produced by lymphocytes are termed **lymphokines** (i.e., interleukins and gamma interferon), and those produced by monocytes and macrophages are termed **monokines.**

Leukocytes

Neutrophils: Neutrophils are highly adherent, motile polymorphonuclear leukocytes that are recruited rapidly from the blood into sites of microbial invasion or inflammation to ingest, kill, and digest pathogens or damaged host cells. They contain receptors for opsonins, which aid in phagocytosis. When activated, they produce microbicidal substances.

Monocytes and Macrophages: Monocytes and macrophages are mononuclear leukocytes that are highly adherent, motile, and phagocytic. In addition, activated mononuclear phagocytes participate in cellular immunity and immunogenesis (see below).

Lymphocytes

Lymphocytes are divided into T cells, B cells, and natural killer (NK) cells. T and B lymphocytes are the only cells that produce and express specific receptors for antigens.

T Lymphocytes: Mature T cells express antigen-specific T-cell receptors that are clonally segregated (i.e., one cell–one receptor specificity). Every mature T cell also expresses the CD3 molecule, which forms a complex with the T-cell receptor, and in addition either the CD4 or CD8 molecule. The T-cell receptor/CD3 complex recognizes antigens associated with major histocompatibility complex molecules on target cells.

Helper T cells (CD4$^+$) (1) aid antigen-stimulated B lymphocytes to proliferate and differentiate toward antibody-producing cells, (2) recognize the complex of foreign antigen with class II major histocompatibility molecules on B cells and on other antigen-presenting cells such as macrophages, and (3) aid effector T lymphocytes in cell-mediated immunity. Suppressor/cytotoxic T cells usually express CD8 and destroy infected cells in an antigen-specific manner that is dependent upon class I major histocompatibility molecules. These cells are also capable of suppressing both T- and B-cell responses. Cell-mediated immunity (delayed hypersensitivity) is an inflammatory reaction initiated by the recognition of specific antigens by helper T cells. Consequently, lymphokines are generated, which recruit activated macrophages to eliminate foreign antigens or altered host cells.

Natural Killer Lymphocytes (NK Cells): NK cells are circulating large granular lymphocytes that do not express CD3, T-cell receptors, or immunoglobulin, but display surface receptors (CD16) for the Fc fragment of antibody. NK cells nonspecifically kill a number of tumor and virus-infected cells. That killing is enhanced by cytokines such as interleukin-2 and gamma interferon. NK cells are also activated by microbes to produce a number of cytokines (interleukin-2, alpha and gamma interferons, and tumor necrosis factor-alpha).

B Lymphocytes: Mature B cells develop as a consequence of recombinations of immunoglobulin genes and express specific surface antibodies that are IgM monomers. B cells differentiate into antibody producing/secreting cells as a result of specific antigen binding to surface immunoglobulin, internalization of the complex, antigen processing, and expression of the processed antigen on the surface in complex with class II major histocompatibility molecules. For many antigens, T cells aid in this process. As a result of the interactions of B cells with T cells, B cells may not only proliferate and express receptors (specific antibodies), but also switch the class (isotype) of immunoglobulin that they produce. Serum antibodies of the IgM class appear within 3 to 5 days after the first exposure to an immunogen (immunizing antigen). This primary antibody response peaks in 10 days and persists for some weeks. Secondary or anamnestic responses following repeated exposures to the same antigen appear more rapidly, last longer, and are principally due to IgG. When antibodies bind to antigens, they may neutralize pathogenic features of antigens such as their toxins, facilitate their ingestion by phagocytic cells (opsonization), fix to and activate complement molecules to produce opsonins and chemoattractants (see below), or participate in antibody-dependent cell-mediated cytotoxicity (ADCC).

IMMUNOGLOBULIN SUPERGENE FAMILY

Major Histocompatibility Complex

The **major histocompatibility complex** is a cluster of >100 genes that encode certain surface protein molecules that aid in regulating the immune response. The protein products of class I and II major histocompatibility complex genes are involved in rejecting foreign tissues, binding processed antigens and presenting them to T lymphocytes, and regulating immune responses.

Immunoglobulins

Immunoglobulins (antibodies) are antigen receptors that are expressed on the surface of B cells and that are secreted by those activated cells into the circulation and other extracellular sites. An immunoglobulin molecule is a symmetric peptide consisting of two identical heavy chains and two identical light chains. Each chain is divided into a variable region that is responsible for specific antigen binding and a constant region that carries out other functions such as the binding of IgG to complement or leukocytes.

TOLERANCE AND AUTOIMMUNITY

Immune tolerance normally prevents reactions against self antigens. Much of that tolerance occurs in the thymus by the elimination or inactivation of self-reactive clones of T cells. Other mechanisms of tolerance occur extrathymically and include the activation of specific suppressor T cells. Tolerance (autoimmunity) may break down because of a genetic predisposition to immunologic dysregulation, an exposure to microbial antigens that cross-react with self antigens, or the exposure to a self antigen that normally is not seen by the immune system (such as an antigen in the eye).

THE COMPLEMENT SYSTEM

The **complement system** consists of inactive circulating glycoproteins that can be sequentially activated by antigen-antibody (IgG or IgM) complexes or bacterial products to enhance inflammation or to attack cell membranes. The system consists of the classic and alternative pathways and the membrane attack complex. After activation, a number of biologically active fragments are produced that are opsonins or chemoattractants.

ONTOGENY OF THE IMMUNE RESPONSE

Mature T and B cells appear in fetal life, but there is little activation of them until the infant is exposed to immunogens postnatally. IgM is the first type of antibody produced postnatally. IgG antibody formation to protein antigens is present at birth, but IgG antibodies to polysaccharides do not appear until 2 to 2.5 years of age.

DEFENSES AGAINST INFECTIONS

The first line of defense includes the skin, mucous membranes, protective inhibitors, and IgA antibodies produced at mucosal sites. The second line of defense consists of local factors and cells that are activated or recruited to the site of microbial invasion. These include the coagulation system, the fibrinolytic system, vasoactive peptides, the complement system, resident macrophages, and inflammatory leukocytes. The third line of defense includes expansion of populations of antigen-specific B cells and T cells, production of systemic antibodies, activation of T cells, and healing characterized by disposal of opsonized pathogens by the reticuloendothelial system and repair of the tissue.

MATERNAL IMMUNE CONTRIBUTIONS TO THE INFANT

The mother transmits immunologic agents to her offspring by two major routes: the placenta (IgG) and milk (e.g., IgA, lactoferrin, lysozyme, and leukocytes).

IMMUNE DEFICIENCY

Genetic Defects

X-linked hypogammaglobulinemia is a genetic defect in the development of B cells. Only low levels of antibodies are produced in response to infecting agents. This results in an increased susceptibility to infections by highly virulent, encapsulated respiratory bacteria. T-cell deficiency is the primary problem in severe combined (B- and T-cell) immunodeficiency. Most cases are due to an X-linked recessive defect. Patients with these diseases display few T cells, decreased T-cell functions, poor antibody formation, and an increased susceptibility to opportunistic infections such as *Pneumocystis carinii* pneumonia. An autosomal recessive defect in the formation of the common β subunit of leukocyte adherence glycoproteins results in decreased ability of leukocytes to adhere and be recruited to interstitial sites of bacterial infections. Chronic granulomatous disease, a defect characterized by a deficiency in intracellular killing by neutrophils, is usually X-linked. The disease is due to a deficiency in the production of the carrier protein for cytochrome b. Consequently, the cells are unable to produce certain reactive oxygen compounds required for intracellular killing.

Acquired Defects

Protein-calorie malnutrition is the leading cause of immune deficiency. Also, certain types of infections, such as human immunodeficiency virus infection, depress parts of the immune system.

DISEASES DUE TO THE IMMUNE RESPONSE

Examples of immune responses to infecting agents that lead to disease include circulating antigen-antibody (immune) complexes of microbial antigens bound to IgM or IgG antibodies, antibodies to microorganisms that cross-react with autoantigens, vasoactive compounds from the complement system and from the metabolism of arachidonic acid, cytokines, and delayed hypersensitivity reactions.

INTRODUCTION

This chapter introduces the ways in which the immune system distinguishes self from nonself (antigens) and defends against infecting microorganisms, other foreign agents, and altered host cells that may cause disease.

EVOLUTION OF THE IMMUNE SYSTEM

The human immune system evolved from primitive but effective defenses of simpler, more ancient animal species. These basic defenses include structural barriers; acids, bases, and other chemical agents produced at those sites; and highly phagocytic, motile scavenger cells with well-developed killing and digestive powers. As a result of the evolutionary process, the mammalian immune system has become more complex, specific, efficient, and regulated. The development of specialized recognition/regulatory proteins (antibodies, cell receptors, and cytokines) expanded the repertoire, controls, and magnitude of the protective responses. These evolutionary changes permit humans to survive in a veritable sea of microorganisms and parasites, many of which display sophisticated pathogenic mechanisms including the ability to (1) enter the body through portals such as the skin, respiratory system, and the alimentary tract, (2) utilize nutrients from those sites, (3) adhere to epithelium, (4) produce virulence factors and toxins, (5) commandeer the replicative machinery of the host cells, (6) evade the immune system, and (7) cripple the host defenses. The salient features of the human defense system that have evolved to counteract these pathogenic mechanisms will be provided in the rest of this chapter.

ORGAN SYSTEMS INVOLVED IN IMMUNOLOGY

General Organization

The production, maturation, and functions of the cells of the immune system occur to a great extent in two overlapping systems, the **lymphoid system** (consisting of cells called lymphocytes) and **reticuloendothelial system** (RES) (consisting of macrophages and related mononuclear phagocytes) (Fig. 1-1). In postnatal life, the bone marrow is the principal source of the pluripotent stem cells that produce leukocytes, which operate in host defense (Fig. 1-2). The development and role of each type of leukocyte are precisely controlled, and this control accounts for the great specificity of the defense system and the rarity of untoward immune reactions.

Lymphoid System

The lymphoid system consists of lymphocytes that circulate in the bloodstream and lymph and populate lymphoid organs, including the thymus, spleen, lymph nodes, and submucosa of the respiratory and alimentary tracts (Fig. 1-1). There are three major types of lymphocytes (T, B, and NK cells), which have distinctive surface markers and functions (Fig. 1-3 and Table 1-1).

The thymus is a central lymphoid organ and is responsible for the production of the first class of

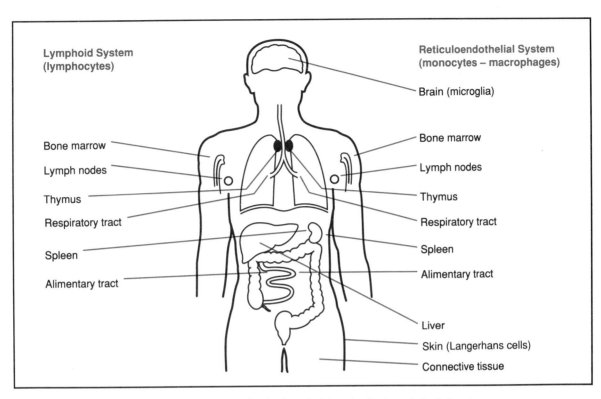

FIGURE 1-1 Major organs in the lymphoid and reticuloendothelial systems.

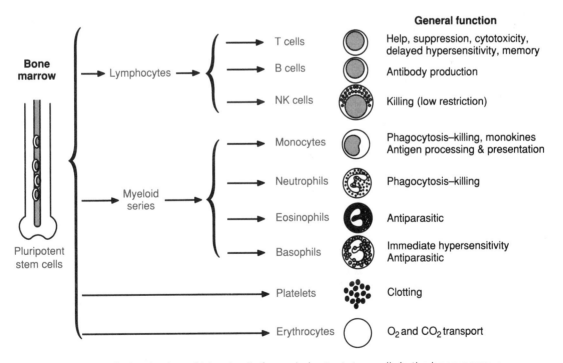

FIGURE 1-2 Production of blood cells from pluripotent stem cells in the bone marrow.

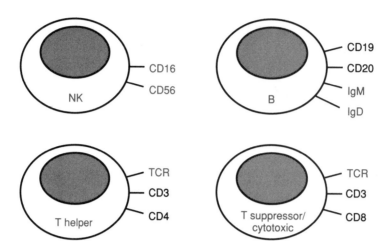

FIGURE 1-3   Principal surface markers of lymphoid populations

lymphocytes, called **thymus-dependent (T) lymphocytes.** These lymphocytes recognize foreign antigens by means of a specific surface receptor, which is related to but distinct from antibodies. Precursors of T cells enter the thymic cortex, where they proliferate and mature. Most thymic lymphocytes die. The rest mature and exit into the systemic circulation (Fig. 1-4), where they either continue to circulate or take up temporary residence in peripheral lymphoid organs (Fig. 1-5).

A second major type of lymphocytes, the **thymus-independent (B) cells** (Fig. 1-6), usually reside in peripheral lymphoid organs, where they may be stimulated to become antibody- or immunoglobulin-producing cells (plasma cells) (Fig. 1-6). The major exception, mucosal B cells, begin to develop in Peyer's patches in the lower small intestine and submucosal sites in the tracheobronchial tree, enter the circulation after local antigenic stimulation, and home to mucosal sites, where they produce the IgA that is secreted onto mucosal surfaces (see below). The third type of lymphocytes, a large granular cell that is cytotoxic, is termed a **natural killer (NK) cell.**

The circulation pathways of lymphocytes are as follows (Fig. 1-5). For example, lymphocytes enter lymph nodes either through the high endothelial venules in the paracortical regions or through af-ferent lymphatics (Fig. 1-7). B cells develop in cortical follicles that become germinal centers. The end stage of this maturational process is the formation of plasma cells, most of which reside in germinal centers and the medulla of lymph nodes, germinal centers of the spleen, the bone marrow, or submucosal sites. In contrast, T cells reside for shorter periods in paracortical regions of lymph nodes and the pericentral arteriolar regions of the spleen. After T cells leave the lymph nodes or spleen, they circulate in the blood and lymph for long periods and carry out many important functions (see below).

Reticuloendothelial System

The second major cellular system, the reticuloendothelial system (Fig. 1-1), consists of circulating monocytes and mononuclear phagocytes that reside in selected sites. These include macrophages in the liver, spleen, lymph nodes, thymus, bone marrow, connective tissues, and submucosal tissues of the respiratory and alimentary tracts; dendritic cells in lymph nodes; Langerhans cells in the skin; and glial cells in the central nervous system. Macrophages are important not only in direct defense (phagocytosis and intracellular killing) but also in marshalling other parts of the immune system, such as T lymphocytes (Table 1-1).

TABLE 1-1 Distinctive Features of Mononuclear Leukocytes

	T cells	B Cells	NK Cells	Monocyte-Macrophages
Major Function	Antigen recognition Cytotoxicity Regulation (cytokines) Cellular immunity	Antigen recognition Antibody production	Cytotoxicity Regulation (cytokines)	Phagocytosis-Killing Antigen P & P[a] Regulation
Immunologic receptors	TCR	IgM (IgD)	CD16 (for IgG)	Fc gamma (For IgG)
Other surface markers	CD3, 4, 8	CD19–21	CD56	CD11 (Mac-1)
Distribution				
Blood	++++ (ca. 75%)	++ (ca. 13%)	++ (ca. 12%)	+ (monocytes) (ca 5%)
Lymph	++++	++	++	+ (monocytes)
Peripheral lymphoid organs	++++	++++	+	++++ (macrophages)

[a] P & P, processing & presentation.

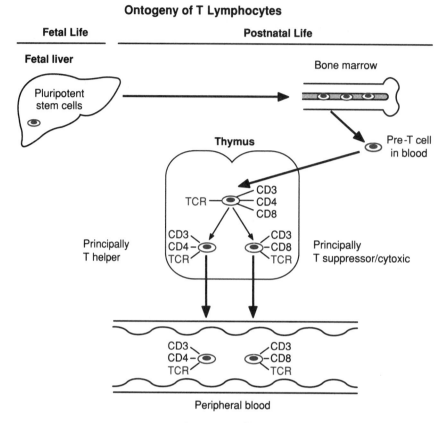

FIGURE 1-4   Ontogeny of T lymphocytes.

CELLS OF THE IMMUNE SYSTEM

The cells of the lymphoid and reticuloendothelial systems produce molecules, called **cytokines,** that act on other cells. Those produced by lymphocytes are called **lymphokines** (i.e., interleukins and gamma interferon [IFN-γ]), and those produced by monocytes and macrophages (e.g., interleukin-1 [IL-1], tumor necrosis factor-alpha [TNF-α]) are called **monokines.**

Leukocytes

Neutrophils

Neutrophils are circulating phagocytic cells that are produced from precursors (myeloid cells) in the bone marrow (Fig. 1-2). Large numbers circulate in the blood. After stimulation, mature neu-

trophils have more motility, adherence, phagocytic activity, and intracellular killing power than any other type of cell. In keeping with these features, neutrophils are rapidly recruited to sites of microbial invasion or inflammation and, once activated, ingest, kill, and digest the invading pathogen with great efficiency (Fig. 1-8). The adherence of these cells to endothelium depends in part upon integral membrane glycoproteins such as LFA-1 and Mac-1, which belong to the integrin family. These α/β heterodimers are restricted to leukocytes. Their β chains are identical, whereas the α chain of each class of protein is distinct. Other adherence molecules distinct from integrins are LAM-1 and ELAM-1.

In contrast to the transmigration of leukocytes through the intercellular junctions of endothelial

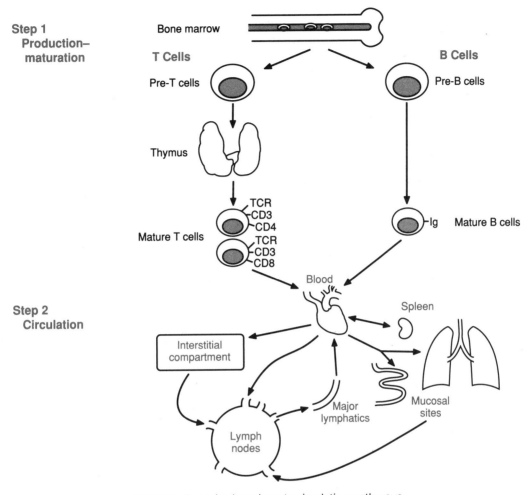

Step 1 Production–maturation

Bone marrow

T Cells

Pre-T cells

B Cells

Pre-B cells

Thymus

Mature T cells
TCR
CD3
CD4
TCR
CD3
CD8

Ig   Mature B cells

Blood

Step 2 Circulation

Spleen

Interstitial compartment

Major lymphatics

Mucosal sites

Lymph nodes

FIGURE 1-5 Major lymphocyte circulation pathways.

cells, their movement within the interstitium is largely adherence independent and is due mainly to hydraulic forces. Once neutrophils enter the interstitium, they may be further activated by chemoattractant agents liberated by invading microorganisms or produced by the host in response to injury. These chemoattractants include *N*-formylmethionyl peptides from bacteria, a proteolytic fragment of the fifth component of complement (C5a) (see the section on the complement system, below), and an inflammatory mediator leukotriene B4 produced from the metabolism of arachidonic acid.

INGESTION AND KILLING OF MICROORGANISMS **Opsonins,** which are molecules that coat the surface of foreign particles and are ligands for receptors on the surface of phagocytes, aid in the ingestion of those particles by phagocytic cells **(opsonization).** Four major types of opsonins are fibronectin (a cold-insoluble globulin); specific IgG antibodies; and active fragments of the third component of complement, C3b and C3bi. The antibodies and complement fragments facilitate the adherence of microorganisms to neutrophils by binding to specific receptors in the external membranes of the leukocytes. Mac-1 aids not only in

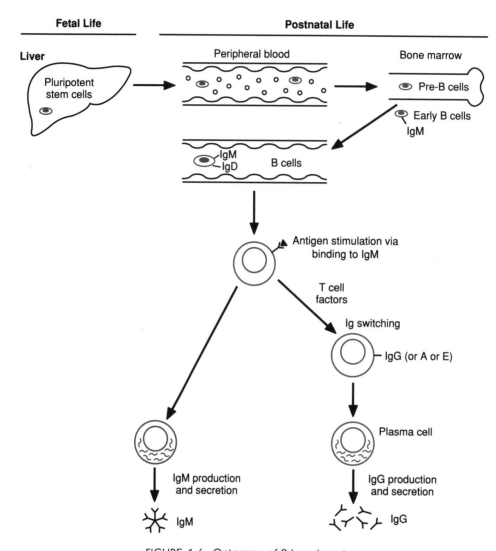

FIGURE 1-6   Ontogeny of B lymphocytes.

adherence but also in phagocytosis by its role as the C3bi receptor.

As a result of the membrane perturbation caused by foreign particles adhering to the external membrane of the phagocyte, a chain of events is initiated that culminates in the engulfment of the particle (e.g., phagocytosis or the formation of a phagosome), the fusion of the phagosome with primary (lysosomal or azurophilic) and secondary (specific) cytoplasmic granules, and the assembly of the major intracellular microbicidal system. The sequence of events is as follows. As the plasma membrane of the phagocyte invaginates, microfilaments accumulate in the nearby cytoplasm. Consequently, the invagination closes to form a phagosome. Simultaneously, a signal is transduced from the receptor-ligand complex through a guanine nucleotide-binding protein to activate phospholipase C in the plasma membrane. As a result, two secondary messengers are produced. The first, inositol triphosphate, stimulates the flux of intracellular calcium. The second, diacylglycerol, participates in the activation of protein kinase C and phospholipase A_2. Primary granules have a high

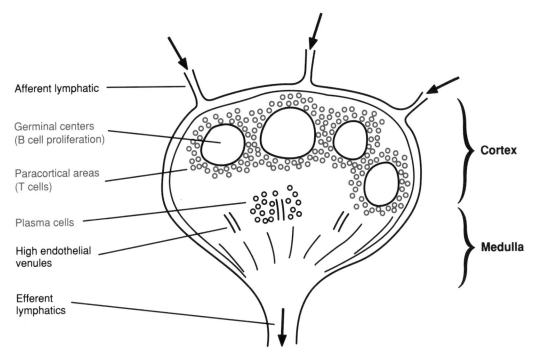

FIGURE 1-7   Lymph node: B-cell and T-cell zones.

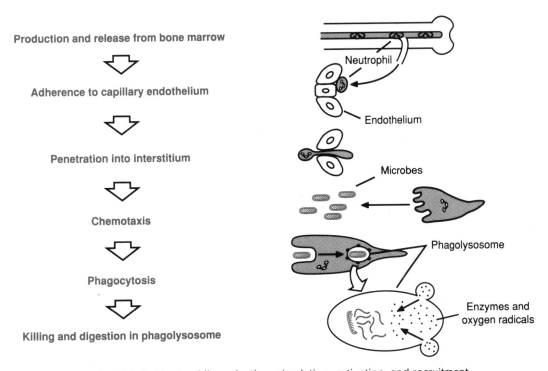

FIGURE 1-8   Neutrophil production, circulation, activation, and recruitment.

content of acid hydrolases and proteolytic enzymes that inactivate or digest microorganisms; secondary granules contain lactoferrin, gelatinase, the complement receptors CR1 and CR3, and an essential part of the intracellular killing machinery, cytochrome b_{245}.

MICROBICIDAL SUBSTANCES Once neutrophils are activated, they convert oxygen to superoxide and then to hydrogen peroxide in the presence of superoxide dismutase. The process includes the assembly of NADPH oxidase, and the up regulation of cytochrome b_{245} from membranes of specific granules. Hydrogen peroxide then reacts with chloride ions in the presence of myeloperoxidase to form chlorinated derivatives. In addition to formation of their microbicidal agents, simultaneously, primary and secondary granules extrude from the cell and attack extracellular pathogens, or if the process is excessive, host tissues.

Monocytes and Macrophages

Monocytes and **macrophages** are mononuclear leukocytes and are highly adherent, motile, and phagocytic. These properties are greatest in activated macrophages, somewhat less in unstimulated macrophages, and least in monocytes. Although some functions of these cells are similar to those of neutrophils, others are distinct. These cells are able to reside in the reticuloendothelial system for long periods. In addition, macrophages are specialized to process and present antigens to T cells in the context of class II major histocompatibility complex (MHC) molecules and to produce biologically active, pleiotropic proteins called monokines. The biologic functions of these monokines are summarized in Table 1-2. The role of monocytes and macrophages in processing and presenting antigens is dealt with in the next section. Macrophages are activated by bacterial products such as endotoxin (lipopolysaccharides), autocrine agents such as TNF-α and IL-1, or lymphokines such as IFN-γ. Activated macrophages play a prominent effector role in cellular immunity and aid in the genesis of specific immune responses.

Lymphocytes

Lymphocytes are the only cells of the immune system that intrinsically express specific receptors for antigens. They are responsible for the development and maintenance of specific immunity. The lymphocyte family is composed of three functionally distinct cell populations, T cells, B cells, and NK cells, that express specific phenotypic structures (Fig. 1-3).

T Lymphocytes

DEVELOPMENT AND MATURATION T lymphocytes originate from undifferentiated bone marrow stem cells (Fig. 1-2) that develop into precursor T cells and migrate to the thymus, where they

TABLE 1-2 Primary Functions of Selected Monokines

Function	Monokine			
	Granulocyte-Monocyte Colony-Stimulating Factor (GM-CSF)	Granulocyte CSF (G-CSF)	IL-1	TNF-α
Neutrophil production	+	+		
Neutrophil activation			+	+
Monocyte production	+		+	+
T-cell stimulation			+	+
B-cell stimulation			+	
Up-regulated MHC				+
Monocyte-macrophage activation		+	+	+
Endogenous pyrogens			+	+
Lipoprotein lipase inhibitor				+

multiply and mature (Fig. 1-4). The rate at which the thymus produces T cells is very high in childhood and declines thereafter. Mature T cells have a long life span and are responsible for much of the immunologic memory. Because of their long life and their ability to recirculate, they make up 70 to 80 percent of lymphocytes in the blood (Table 1-1).

The maturation of T cells in the thymus is characterized by a sequential appearance of certain cell surface molecules. Among the first surface molecules to appear are CD3, T-cell receptors (TCRs) (Fig. 1-9), CD4, and CD8. Thus, immature thymocytes are CD3$^+$ CD4$^+$ CD8$^+$. The TCR is initially γ/δ. During T-cell maturation, the majority of TCRs become α/β and cortical T cells lose either the CD4 or CD8 molecule to become CD3$^+$ TCR$^+$ CD4$^+$ or CD3$^+$ TCR$^+$ CD8$^+$. These mature cells migrate to the medulla of the thymus, where they exit into the systemic circulation.

The general pattern of this maturation is as follows. Lymphocytes in the thymus are exposed to various endogenous (self) proteins, particularly the products of the MHC (see below). One of the major functions of MHC molecules is to present antigens to T cells. Some nascent T cells that manifest a response against self MHC molecules are eliminated, while the remaining T cells become "educated" to recognize foreign antigens in a molecular context of self MHC. In the parlance of immunology, antigen recognition by T cells becomes "MHC restricted." That is, the mature T cell recognizes its specific antigen only if that antigen is accompanied by the correct MHC protein. TCR molecules are associated with CD3 molecules that do not have a recognition specificity but are essential for the function of the TCR (Fig. 1-9).

Two kinds of MHC genes, class I and class II (see Fig. 1-10 for their protein products) are involved in the development of T cells (see below). In the course of selective adaptation, T cells learn to recognize foreign antigens in association with protein products of either class I or II MHC genes. Class I-restricted T cells express CD8 molecules that bind to the invariant portion of class I MHC, whereas class II-restricted T cells express the CD4 molecule that reacts with class II MHC. Both CD4 and CD8 molecules participate with the foreign antigen in T-cell activation. Thus, mature T lymphocytes leaving the thymus are either CD3$^+$ TCR$^+$ CD4$^+$ or CD3$^+$ TCR$^+$ CD8$^+$.

FUNCTIONAL SUBSETS CD4 and CD8 are phenotypic features of T-cell subsets. CD4$^+$ cells are

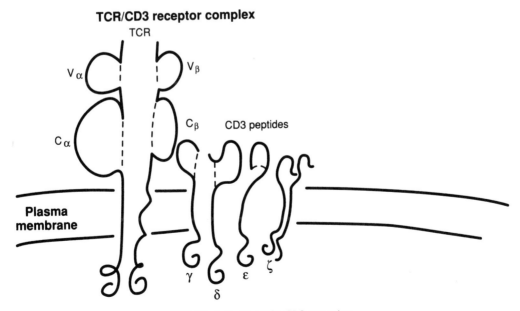

FIGURE 1-9 The TCR-CD3 complex.

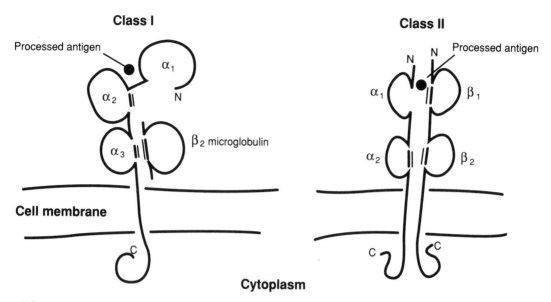

FIGURE 1-10   Structure of the MHC molecule. Sites of potential binding of processed antigen for presentation to other cells in the immune system are shown.

principally regulatory T cells, which control the functions of other lymphocytes; CD8$^+$ cells are cytotoxic/suppressor T cells, which participate in cell-mediated immunity against viruses, fungi, bacteria, and certain tumors.

Helper T (T_H) Cells. Helper T cells are CD4$^+$ lymphocytes that aid antigen-activated B cells to proliferate and differentiate into antibody-producing cells (plasma cells). The T_H cells regulate antibody responses to thymus-dependent protein antigens in the following ways. (1) First (Fig. 1-11), the protein antigen is partially digested by antigen-processing cells such as B cells, macrophages, Langerhans cells, or dendritic cells. The resultant fragments are then bound intracellularly with class II MHC protein molecules to produce a complex that is presented to the TCR of the CD4$^+$ cell. (2) The helper effect is provided by one of the following pathways. Antigen-specific T_H cells that bind the peptide fragment-class II MHC protein complex on a B cell are activated and secrete helper factors, such as interleukins, that affect the initial interacting B cell (Fib. 1-11A). Alternatively, (Fig. 1-11B1) the peptide fragment-class II MHC protein complex is presented to the T_H cell by a nonspecific accessory cell such as the macrophage, which also produces monokines. The T_H cell then

becomes activated by the antigen presentation and monokines to produce helper factors for bystander B cells.

Thymus-independent antigens such as polysaccharides do not require help from T cells (Fig. 1-11B2); however, these antigens, by activating macrophages, produce monokines such as IL-1 that in turn stimulate T_H cells to produce helper factors for bystander B cells. Which pathway is used depends on the nature and concentration of the antigen. Helper T cells also aid effector T lymphocytes (see below) in cell-mediated immunity. This process occurs according to the pathway in Figure 1-11, except that the recipient of the helper factor is an effector T cell. Some evidence suggests that T_H cells that stimulate B cells and those that stimulate T cell-mediated immunity are distinct subsets that produce different types of helper factors. In that respect, B and T cells require different lymphokines for growth and differentiation. Moreover, some T_H cells produce IFN-γ, a cytokine that activates macrophages. This process is a major aspect of cell-mediated immunity (Fig. 1-12) (see below).

Suppressor T cells. Suppressor T (T_S) cells are less well understood than the T_H subset. T_S activity may change after immunization and in various clinical

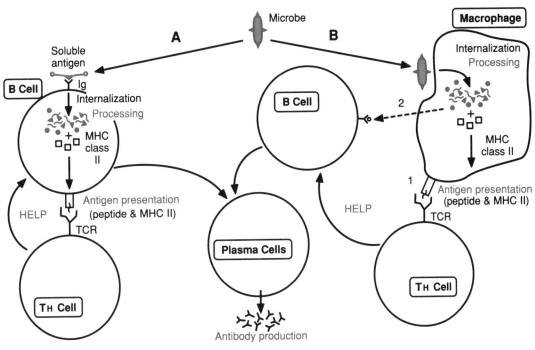

FIGURE 1-11   Antigen processing and presentation by helper T-dependent (A and B1) antigens and by helper T-independent antigens (B2).

situations. T_s lymphocytes are usually CD8+. Their MHC restriction pattern, TCR structure, and fine specificity remain controversial.

Effector cells of cell-mediated immunity. Cytotoxic T cells (CTLs) (Table 1-1) are usually CD8+ and class I MHC restricted. These cells destroy virus-infected cells in an antigen-specific manner. They develop from T cells that become stimulated when the TCR/CD3 complex reacts with a foreign antigen and MHC molecules on the surface of an in-

fected cell. Under the influence of T_H cells, effector T cells proliferate and differentiate into CTLs. The killing is virus specific and class I MHC restricted (i.e., target cells infected by a different virus or infected cells that do not express the correct MHC molecule are spared).

A special type of CTLs are alloreactive, in that they recognize and kill target cells expressing a foreign MHC molecule (i.e., cells from genetically unrelated individuals). Alloreactive CTLs are thus

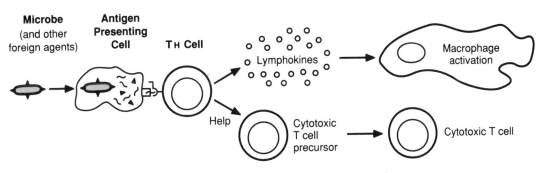

FIGURE 1-12   Genesis of cell-mediated immunity.

involved in the rejection of incompatible tissue transplants. These cells are either CD4[+] or CD8[+] and react, respectively, against class I and class II molecules.

Cells in delayed hypersensitivity. Cell-mediated antibacterial resistance **(delayed hypersensitivity)** is mediated by CD4[+] T_H cells in concert with macrophages. These are the same T_H cells that activate macrophages via the production of IFN-γ and perhaps other lymphokines.

LYMPHOKINES AND INTERLEUKINS   Lymphokines are produced primarily by T cells and modulate the activity of cells of the immune system as well as of other tissues. These proteins have multiple functions, and their preference for specific cell types is only relative (see Table 1-3 for some important lymphokines).

Natural Killer Lymphocytes

Natural killer cells (NK cells) (large granular lymphocytes) appear to be a lineage of lymphoid cells that do not express CD3, TCR, or immunoglobulin (Table 1-1 and Fig. 1-3), but display a low-affinity surface receptor for the Fc fragment of IgG (CD16; e.g., CR3). NK cells account for 10 to 15 percent of blood lymphocytes and are found in small numbers in spleen, bone marrow, liver, lung, and intestinal mucosa.

NK cells kill a number of virus-infected and tumor cells. This cytotoxicity does not depend on previous sensitization and does not require expression of MHC determinants on target cells. The cytotoxicity of NK cells is increased after exposure to cytokines such as IL-2 or IFN-γ. NK cells can also mediate ADCC via the CD16 Fc receptor. They can be activated by infecting agents to produce a number of cytokines (IL-2, IFN-γ, IFN-α, and TNF-α). Thus, NK cells may be important in regulating certain aspects of T- and B-cell activation, as well as hematopoiesis, and are believed to be important in defense against tumors and intracellular infections.

B Lymphocytes

B cells originate from pluripotent stem cells in the fetal liver and later in the bone marrow (Fig. 1-6). They are thymus-independent lymphocytes that express intrinsically produced immunoglobulins (see below) on their external membranes and differentiate into plasma cells that produce and secrete large numbers of antibody molecules (Fig. 1-6). Mature but unstimulated B cells express monomeric IgM antibodies, class II MHC molecules, the Epstein-Barr virus C3d (CR2) receptor, and mitogen (polyclonal activators) receptors on their surface (Fig. 1-13). B cells account for 10 to

TABLE 1-3   Selected Functions of Some Lymphokines

Functions	IL-2	IL-4	IL-5	IL-6	IFN-γ
Proliferation					
T cells	+	+	?		+
B cells				+	+
Differentiation					
T cells	+	?	?	+	+
B cells	+	+	+	+	+
Macrophages		+		+	+
Ig production					
IgG	+				
IgM $\xrightarrow{\text{switch}}$ IgA			+	+	
Class II MHC expression		+			
NK activation	+				+
Hematopoietic activity		+			+

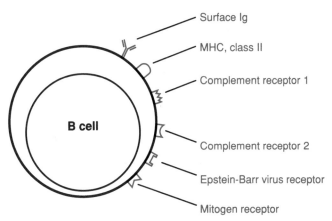

FIGURE 1-13 Surface markers on human B cells.

15 percent of blood lymphocytes. They and their progeny, antibody-producing cells, are located primarily in peripheral lymphoid organs.

B cells are characterized by their clonal organization in that each B cell expresses and produces immunoglobulin molecules of one antigen-binding specificity. Clones expressing different specificities are involved in the production of antibodies to a complex immunogen because of the multiplicity of antigenic determinants (epitopes) on the molecules. Hence, the overall antibody response is polyclonal. If the immunogen has a very limited set of epitopes, the antibody response will be oligoclonal or monoclonal.

The development of B cells from the stem cell up to the stage of mature B cells is antigen independent (Fig. 1-14). Antigen is, however, the initial trigger for B cells to transform into antibody-producing, secretory plasma cells. After antigens bind to immunoglobulins on the cell surface, the antigens are internalized and processed. This antigen-receptor interaction sends the first biochemical signal for B-cell activation. Then a fragment of the antigen is transported to the surface, where it is expressed in a complex with class II MHC molecules. This allows the B cell to interact with antigen-specific helper (CD4[+]) T cells. Consequently, lymphokine receptors are expressed on the B-cell surface and T cells are activated to produce lymphokines such IL-2, IL-4, and IL-6 (Table 1-3) that further stimulate the differentiation of B cells. In addition, certain bacterial products (generically called mitogens), such as lipopolysaccharides, activate B cells to proliferate regardless of their clonal specificity; this results in a polyclonal antibody response.

Lymphokines from helper T cells are also necessary for the class (isotype) switch that occurs in antigen-stimulated B cells. These events in B-cell differentiation are accompanied by immunoglobulin gene rearrangements (Fig. 1-14) (see below). As a result of shuffling of constant-region genes, different isotypes of immunoglobulins with the same antibody specificity are produced. The cell continues to differentiate to form plasma cells that are characterized by a lack of surface membrane immunoglobulin, but by an extensive production and secretion of antibodies of one isotype and one antibody specificity (idiotype) (see below).

IMMUNOGLOBULIN SUPERGENE FAMILY

Molecules that mediate antigen recognition and cellular interactions make up a group of structurally similar glycoproteins (Fig. 1-15) that are encoded by a family of genes that appear to have evolved from a common primordial gene. Some of the more important members of this immune supergene family are the MHC, immunoglobulins, TCR, secretory component, and certain adherence proteins such as ICAM-1. The products of

Cell type:	Antigen Independent				Antigen Induced	
	Bone Marrow		Peripheral			
	Stem cell	Pre-B cell	Immature B lymphocyte	Mature B lymphocyte	Activated B lymphocyte	Antibody-secreting cell (plasma cell)
Ig genes/ RNA:	0	Rearranged H chain genes	Rearranged H and L chain genes	Alternative splicing of H chain mRNA	1 mRNA splicing 2. Express other C_H chain genes	Change from membrane bound IgM to secreted IgM
Ig production, function:	0	Cytoplasmic μ chain only	Surface IgM; tolerance-sensitive	Surface IgM, IgD	1. Ig secretion low 2. H chain class switching	1. Ig secretion high 2. Membrane Ig decreased
Antigen reactive:	0	0	+	+	+	—
CD markers	?	CD9 |——| CD10		CD21,22 |————————|	CD23 |———|	CD38 |———|
			CD19,20 |————————————|			

FIGURE 1-14 B-lymphocyte differentiation. H and L refer to immunoglobulin (Ig) heavy and light chains, respectively.

these genes are transmembrane glycoproteins that are characterized by a common structural motif of functional domains.

Major Histocompatibility Complex

Definition

The MHC consists of a cluster of >100 genes that encode a number of biologically important molecules (Fig. 1-15). These molecules are responsible for the rejection of tissue grafts by genetically disparate individuals, as the name "histocompatibility" indicates. The physiologic functions of MHC molecules, however, transcend the terminology. These molecules aid in presenting antigens to the T lymphocytes; govern the interactions between T cells, B cells, and accessory cells; and influence the immune reactivity of an individual against foreign antigens and against self (i.e., autoimmunity). MHC genes and their protein products in all vertebrates have the same general features. Human MHC protein products are also called HLA for "human leukocyte antigens."

Structure and Genes

The two most important HLA glycoproteins are designated as class I and class II molecules (Fig. 1-10).

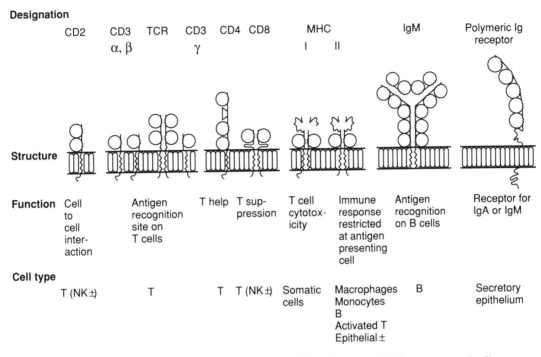

FIGURE 1-15   Representative protein products of the immunoglobulin supergene family.

CLASS I AND II MOLECULES   Class I molecules are ubiquitous on somatic cells, whereas class II molecules are restricted to macrophages, dendritic cells, Langerhans cells, B cells, activated T cells, and certain types of epithelial cells. Class I molecules have three extracellular domains (α_1, α_2, and β_1), and a cytoplasmic tail. In contrast, class II mol-

ecules have four extracellular domains (α_1, α_2, β_1, and β_2).

Class I and II HLA molecules are encoded by a cluster of genes on chromosome 6. The map (Fig. 1-16) omits a number of other genes in the cluster that are similar to class I and II but less well characterized. Three genes encode three different class I

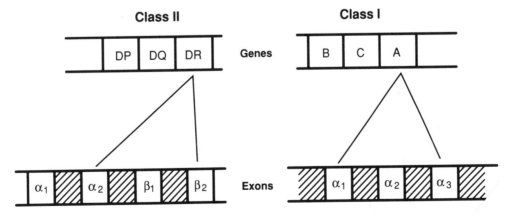

FIGURE 1-16   Genes in the MHC.

molecules: HLA-A, -B, and -C. Each gene contains three exons for the α domain: exons 1, 2, and 3. The class II cluster, HLA-D, also contains three distinct genes, DP, DQ, and DR, each of which has a separate set of exons for the α and β chains (an example for the DR gene is shown in Fig. 1-16). The HLA genes are expressed independently.

An important aspect of the HLA gene system is its polymorphism. Each gene—class I (A, B, and C) and class II (DP, DQ, and DR)—exists in different forms, or **alleles.** HLA alleles are designated by numbers and subscripts. For example, two unrelated individuals may carry class I HLA-B genes B5 and Bw41. Allelic gene products differ in one or more amino acids in the α and/or β domain(s) and are thus distinguishable by specific antibodies. Large panels of such reagents are used to type HLA haplotypes of individuals by using leukocytes that express class I and class II molecules. The genetic polymorphism of HLA genes has major implications for the function of class I and class II molecules (see below). HLA typing is used to predict the risk of certain diseases and to match donors and recipients in tissue transplantation.

Foreign antigens are taken up by various types of cells in the body, internalized, and subjected to enzymatic degradation called antigen processing. The antigenic fragments are associated with the class II molecules and transported to the cell surface. This MHC-antigen complex is recognized by the TCR on CD4$^+$ T cells. A CD4$^+$ T cell activated by an appropriate class II-antigen complex on an antigen-presenting cell, such as a macrophage, may become a helper cell for antibody or cell-mediated immune responses.

A different scenario is found for the antigens that are synthesized within the cells, such as the viral antigens in infected cells or tumor antigens. These antigens are processed and expressed in association with the class I molecule. The class I-antigen complex is recognized via the TCR by the CD8$^+$ T lymphocytes which become activated and differentiate into CTLs that destroy infected cells. The variable domains of class II MHC molecule coded by a particular allelic gene may be unable to present a given antigenic peptide and fail to present the peptide to the antigen-specific T cells.

As a result, a strong immune response to this antigen cannot be mounted. Because of the association of high and low responses to a specific antigen with particular class II alleles, MHC genes have been dubbed immune response (Ir) genes. HLA typing reveals that individuals carrying certain alleles are at high risk of developing diseases such as ankylosing spondylitis, myasthenia gravis, or type I diabetes mellitus. It is likely that this association reflects an underlying immunopathologic reaction involving class I and class II MHC molecules.

MHC genes and their products may also influence the immune repertoire of T lymphocytes. T cells interact with class I and class II molecules during their maturation in the thymus. This interaction kills immature cells whose TCRs have a high affinity for self MHC or for an MHC-self protein complex, in a process called **thymic selection.** Potentially auto-reactive T cells would be eliminated in this fashion. However, the selection process by polymorphic MHC molecules may skew the T-cell repertoire of the individual against various foreign antigens.

Immunoglobulins

Structure

Eight immunoglobulin isotypes, IgG1, IgG2, IgG3, IgG4, IgA1, IgA2, IgM, IgD, and IgE, are produced by B cells as a result of rearrangements of variable (V) genes for heavy (H) chains (V$_H$), diversity (D) genes for H chains (D$_H$), joining genes (J) for H chains (J$_H$), V genes for light (L) chains (V$_L$), J genes for L chains (J$_L$), and constant (C) region genes (see below). A four-polypeptide chain structure is found in each of these isotypes. The basic structure of immunoglobulin molecules consists of two identical L chains and two identical H chains (Fig. 1-17). The four chains are linked by disulfide bonds. Each chain is divided into two regions: the C region at the carboxy terminus and the V region at the amino terminus. The C region of an L chain consists of about 107 amino acids and has an invariant structure except for isotypic structures (κ or λ) and allotypic variants (e.g., molecular structure that is individually inherited and not species specific). The V regions of H and L chains

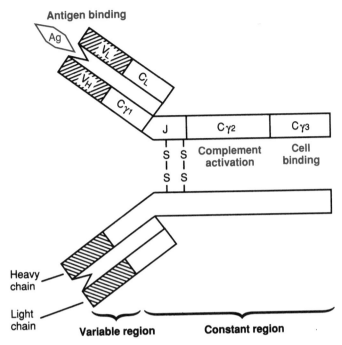

FIGURE 1-17 Structure of immunoglobulin.

display great variability in the sequence of amino acids. The V and C regions of H chains are further divided into domains characterized by folding of the polypeptide into 110-amino-acid loops. The regions of H and L chains interact to form the antigen-binding sites, whereas the C regions dictate the other functions including binding to cell surface receptors. The special properties of each immunoglobulin class are as follows (Table 1-4).

IGG IgG is a four-chain structure. The C region of the H chain consists of three domains. Interchain disulfide linkages between the $C\gamma1$ and $C\gamma2$ domains stabilize the structure and define the hinge region of the molecule. IgG is the dominant immunoglobulin in the extracellular fluids, the only immunoglobulin that is transported across the placenta, and the only immunoglobulin that is a direct opsonin.

There are four subclasses of IgG, each of which displays unique antigenic determinants on the C region of the H chains. The approximate proportion of each subclass in blood is IgG1, 70 percent; IgG2, 20 percent; IgG3, 8 percent; and IgG4, 2 percent. The antibody specificities are distributed in somewhat specific patterns in each subclass. Most neutralizing antibodies to protein toxins are found in IgG1, antibodies to polysaccharides in IgG2, and antibodies to viruses in IgG3.

IGM IgM is a pentamer of four-chain units that are bound to a separate peptide called the joining (J) chain. IgM is found principally in blood, but also occurs in external secretions. It is the most efficient binder of the C1q subunit of the first component of complement (see below) and is the first immunoglobulin to be expressed in B-cell development. Monomeric IgM is the principal antigen receptor on B cells.

IGA There are two principal molecular forms of IgA: monomers whose basic structure and numbers of domains are similar to IgG, and dimers that bind to J chains. Monomeric IgA, the second most common immunoglobulin in adult serum, is pro-

TABLE 1-4   Major Properties of Immunoglobulins[a]

Property	IgG	IgA	IgM	IgD	IgE
Molecular structure	$c_2 L_2$	$\alpha_2 L_2$ $(\alpha_2 L_2)_2$ $(\alpha_2 L_2)_2$ SC	$\mu_2 L_2$ $(\mu_2 L_2)_5$	$\delta_2 L_2$	$n_2 L_2$
Molecular mass (kDa)	150	180 210 380	900	150	195
Complement fixation	+	−	+ + +	−	−
Placental transfer	+	−	−	−	−
Body Distribution					
Blood	+++	++	+++	±	±
Interstitium	+++	++	+	±	±
External					
secretions	±	+++	++	±	±
Serum half-life (days)	20	<4	<4	<4	<4
Cell binding					
PMNs[b]	+	±	−	−	−
Macrophages	+	−	−	−	±
Basophils	±	−	−	−	+
Mast cells	±	−	−	−	+

[a] The heavy chains are c (IgG), α (IgA), μ (IgM), δ (IgD), and n (IgE). SC, Secretory component; L, light chains (j or k).

[b] PMN, Polymorphonuclear leukocytes (neutrophils).

duced primarily by plasma cells in the bone marrow, whereas dimeric IgA, the dominant immunoglobulin in external secretions, is produced by plasma cells at mucosal sites. Dimeric IgA is complexed and transported with secretory component to form secretory IgA (Fig. 1-18). Dimeric IgA binds to polymeric immunoglobulin receptors (secretory component) on the basolateral membranes of epithelial cells, and the complex is internalized and transported across the cells in an endocytic vesicle to the apical pole of the cell, where it is secreted as secretory IgA. The addition of secretory component not only facilitates the transport of dimeric IgA but also protects the molecule from proteolysis.

There are two subclasses of IgA, IgA1, and IgA2. IgA1 predominates in the blood; there is an equal distribution of the two subclasses in external secretions. IgA2 is more resistant than IgA1 to bacterial proteases.

IGD   IgD is a four-chain polypeptide structure that is similar to IgG. Although this protein is ex-

pressed along with monomeric IgM on mature B cells, only small amounts of it are found in extracellular fluids.

IGE   IgE is a four-chain polypeptide structure. Only trace amounts are found in serum. IgE binds avidly to circulating blood basophils and mast cells in the submucosa and the skin. Cell-bound IgE antibodies play a role in defense against tissue parasites and in the pathogenesis of immediate hypersensitivity by triggering the release of low-molecular-weight vasoactive compounds such as histamine, leukotrienes, and platelet-activating factor from the mast cells or basophils once they are cross-linked by antigens.

Sequence of Antibody Formation

In the primary antibody response (the first immunization), B cells are activated to form IgM antibody-producing cells. By 3 to 5 days, specific antibodies, mainly of the IgM isotype, appear in the serum and the concentration (titer) increases until a peak is reached in 10 to 14 days (Fig. 1-19). The

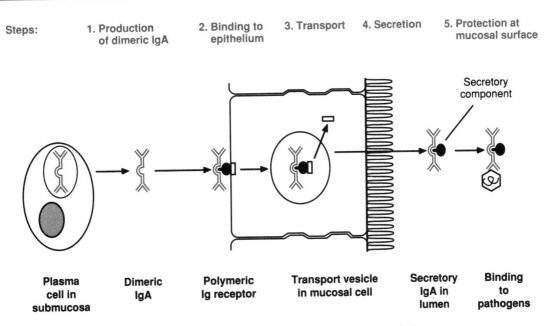

FIGURE 1-18 Assembly and secretion of secretory IgA.

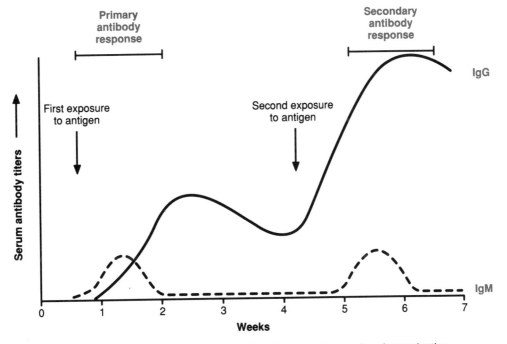

FIGURE 1-19 Isotypes of antibodies in primary and secondary immunization.

antibody titers then fall to preimmunization levels after some weeks. Upon reimmunization, there is a more rapid and extensive development of antibody-producing cells in the regional lymph node, and many of those cells have undergone isotype switch to produce IgG antibodies. As a result, the serum antibodies are primarily IgG, the antibody titers are higher and persist for much longer periods, and they have a greater affinity for antigens.

Consequences of Antibody-Antigen Binding

There are a number of important consequences of the binding of antibodies to antigens. IgM complexes are created that most efficiently activate the classic pathway of the complement system; this leads to the formation of opsonins that facilitate the removal of the complexes by the reticuloendothelial system and to other functional complement fragments. IgG binding may neutralize a toxin, opsonize a particle for ingestion by phagocytes, or activate the classic pathway of complement. Secretory IgA antibodies defend mucosal sites by binding toxins and adhering to microbial pathogens. IgE antibodies on the surface of mast cells and basophils are important in defense against parasites and the production of immediate hypersensitivity as noted above.

Genetic Basis of Antibody Diversity

As noted above, specific antibodies are generated as a consequence of immunoglobulin gene rearrangement (i.e., V, D, J, and C genes) (Fig. 1-20). The details are as follows.

VARIABLE GENES: ANTIBODY SPECIFICITY The immune system generates millions of different antibody molecules from the pool of V genes. Separate sets of V genes encode the variable domain of immunoglobulin H and L chains (i.e., V_H and V_L). The two chains are produced separately, but the mechanisms by which their diversity is achieved are similar in principle.

The L-chain gene system is simpler than the H-chain gene system. Most antibody molecules use the kappa (κ) light chain. The κ gene cluster con-

sists of ca. 300 V_L genes, ca. 4 J genes, and 1 C gene. These germ line genes form a tandem on the chromosome and are transcriptionally inactive. As the B cell matures, genes are arranged (recombined) so that one V gene is joined to a J gene, and the rearranged VJ segment, together with the C gene, is transcribed. The portion of DNA between the joined segments is deleted, and the transcripts are processed by splicing to produce the messenger RNA (mRNA) for the L chain. The λ chain is encoded by a separate cluster of V, J, and C genes, but the rearrangement and transcription are similar to that of the κ chain. Any given B cell uses only one type of L chain to produce the immunoglobulin molecule. The L chain combines with the H chain during their transport from polyribosomes to the membrane.

The H-chain gene system has a similar design, but is slightly more complex (Fig. 1-20). In addition to several hundred (but less than 1,000) V_H genes, there are more than 10 D genes and ca. 4 J genes. Furthermore, this genetic cluster has nine C genes that encode different immunoglobulin isotypes. The mature B cell (Fig. 1-14) rearranges its immunoglobulin genes, joins them, and deletes the DNA in between. The rearranged VDJ gene segment is transcribed together with the $C\mu$ and $C\delta$ genes, and this long transcript is spliced into VDJCμ and VDJCδ mRNA, resulting in the expression of IgM and IgD on the B cell surface. Both immunoglobulin molecules use the same VDJ segment and therefore possess the same immunologic specificity. The B cell is now ready to respond to a specific antigen by producing antibody.

Several major rules apply to the production of L and H chains:

1. The joining of various V, D, and J genes is entirely random ($< 1,000 \times 10 \times 4$), resulting in $\geq 50,000$ different possible combinations for VDJ$_H$ and $> 1,000$ (ca. 300×4) for VJ$_L$. Subsequent random pairing of H and L chains brings the total number of possible antibodies to $\geq 10^7$.
2. Diversity is further increased by the imprecise joining of different genetic segments.
3. Rearrangements occur on both DNA

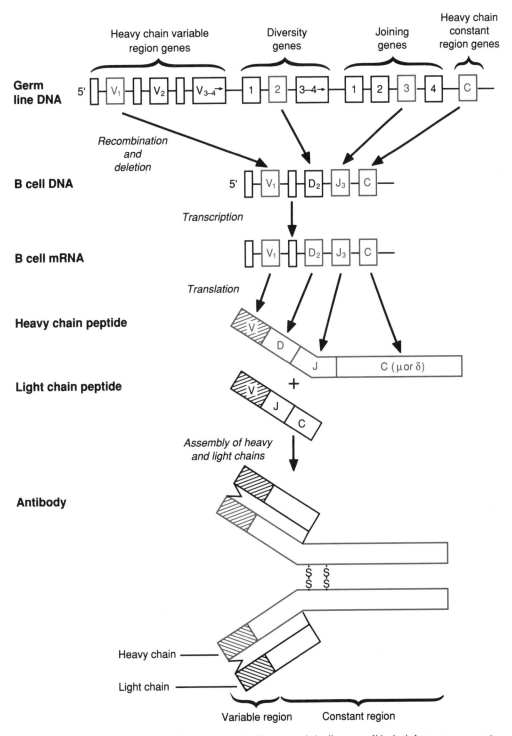

FIGURE 1-20 Mechanisms of antibody diversity: immunoglobulin gene (H-chain) rearrangement.

strands, but only one strand is transcribed (allelic exclusion).

4. Only one rearrangement occurs in the life of a B cell because of irreversible deletions in the DNA.

As a result, each mature B cell is permanently committed to one immunologic specificity that is maintained in the progeny, or clone. This constitutes the molecular basis of the clonal selection concept: each antigenic determinant triggers the response of the preexisting clone of lymphocytes bearing the specific receptor molecule. Deletion of the clone results in unresponsiveness to the antigen.

In addition to gene recombination, a mechanism exists that allows for a fine-tuning of the antibody specificity after immunization. The rearranged VDJ_H, and VJ_L genes in the B cells are uniquely susceptible to point mutagenesis by enzymes that become activated following the stimulation of the cell by the antigen. The clonal progeny of an antigen-driven B cell thus produce antibodies that may differ in one or more amino acid positions in the domains. Cells producing the mutant antibody with highest affinity for the antigen are preferentially stimulated and therefore eventually dominate the response. Antibodies produced after repeated immunization commonly have higher affinity for the antigen and contain numerous point mutations, compared with the primary antibodies produced in the primary response.

CONSTANT GENES: ANTIBODY FUNCTION   The H-chain C-region genes encode the biologic functions of immunoglobulins (Fig. 1-20). C domains enable immunoglobulins to fix complement (IgM, IgG1, IgG3), cross the placental barrier (IgG), or accumulate in mucosal secretions (secretory IgA). To accomplish these functions, B cells switch their VDJ gene from $C\mu/C\delta$, which is the original constant gene expressed in all B cells, to any other C gene. This has been termed the "isotype switch," because the C gene determines the isotype (IgM, IgG, etc.) of the antibody. The switch is accomplished by another genetic recombination, whereby the VDJ gene segment is transferred from

the $C\mu/C\delta$ junction onto another C gene downstream. Because the $C\mu$ and other interposed genes are deleted, the switch is irreversible. The new antibody maintains the same L chain and the same V_H region (encoded by VDJ), but it has new properties determined by the acquired C gene. The isotype switch mechanism appears to be promoted by specific lymphokines from T cells.

Furthermore, each antibody molecule may exist in two forms, membrane bound and secreted. Every C gene contains a 3' sequence encoding the hydrophobic cytoplasmic tail of the H chain, so that the immunoglobulin molecule produced by the B cell is inserted in the surface membrane to function as the receptor for antigen. When the B cell becomes activated and differentiates into the plasma cell, an enzyme is activated that modifies the RNA transcript. Consequently, the translated protein ends with a hydrophilic peptide and is secreted into the extracellular space.

T-Cell Receptor

The specific receptor for antigen on the T cell (TCR) (Fig. 1-9) is a heterodimer protein with motifs that are similar to immunoglobulin molecules, but whose structure is encoded by a different set of V and C genes. Moreover, T cells consist of two subsets carrying different receptors, which have been designated α/β and γ/δ.

TCR γ/δ

The γ/δ type of TCR appears early in the ontogeny of T cells. Only a minority of T cells express a heterodimer receptor consisting of γ and δ chains. These chains are encoded by very few genes, and the γ/δ repertoire is accordingly limited. The γ gene cluster consists of only seven V genes, two J genes, and four C genes. The δ genes are interspersed within the α gene locus and appear to include 10 V genes, 2 D genes, 2 J genes, and 1 C gene.

Mature γ/δ T cells appear to migrate primarily to the mucosal and cutaneous tissues. The functions of these T cells are not yet understood. Moreover, the recognition of antigen by the γ/δ T cells may not be MHC restricted.

TCR α/β

Most T lymphocytes express the α/β type of TCR. The smaller α chain is encoded in a gene cluster consisting of ca. 100 V genes, ca. 50 J genes (a surprisingly large number compared with the immunoglobulin J genes), and 1 C gene. Alpha chains of various binding specificity are generated by a random genetic recombination of one V and one J gene, which are then joined with Cα; the mechanism of this process is analogous to that used for the immunoglobulin L chain. The heavier β chain is encoded by ca. 30 V genes, 2 D genes, >10 J genes, and 2 C genes. The random joining of one of each V, D, and J genes and their rearrangement to one of the C genes is, again, similar to the process described for immunoglobulin genes. Rearranged VJCα and VDJCβ encode the α chain and β transcripts, respectively. TCR genes are rearranged as lymphocytes mature in the thymus. Mature T cells are irreversibly committed to recognize one specific antigenic epitope in complex with self MHC molecule.

The genomic organization of the α and β genes is more complicated than that of the immunoglobulin genes. Indeed, α-locus genes are interspersed with genes for the δ TCR (see below). Despite this, α and δ genes are rearranged and expressed at different times and on different lymphocytes.

The combinatorial diversity of TCR (i.e., the number of different TCRs that can be generated) is greatly increased by junctional diversity) (i.e., the variability of the junctions between different VDJ genes). New nucleotide base pairs are often added at the junction. Indeed, the junctional diversity of TCR is several orders of magnitude greater than that of an immunoglobulin gene. On the other hand, rearranged TCR genes are not subject to mutations in the way that immunoglobulin genes are. The lack of mutations appears to be related to the fact that the α/β T cells always recognize a complex of antigenic fragment with the self MHC molecule. The receptor mutation could divert the specificity toward self molecules. The α/β T cells are either CD8[+] or CD4[+], depending on their restriction to the class I or class II MHC molecule, respectively.

CD3 Complex

The TCR is noncovalently associated with a peptide complex CD3 on the lymphocyte membrane (Fig. 1-9). The CD3 complex consists of four transmembrane peptides designated γ, δ, ε, and ζ. The CD3 complex itself does not recognize the antigen and does not have variable domains. However, the CD3 complex transmits the biochemical signals that are generated by the TCR-antigen-MHC interaction on the surface and that lead to lymphocyte activation. The TCR alone is not functional. Hereditary defects in the CD3 complex structure result in T-cell malfunction.

RECOGNITION OF SELF AND IMMUNE TOLERANCE

Because the repertoire of immune specificities is vast and largely random, it is not surprising that many nascent lymphocytes possess receptors for the body's own structures. Much has been learned about the mechanisms for excluding or inactivating self-reactive lymphocytes, particularly by using the model of experimentally induced immune tolerance to foreign antigens. If an antigen is introduced into immunologically immature newborn animals, they may become unresponsive to immunization with that antigen when they reach maturity. This immunologic tolerance is characterized by the absence of both antibody- and cell-mediated responses (Figs. 1-21 and 1-22), and it is specific for the original antigen.

Subsequent experiments revealed that the induction of antigen-specific tolerance is not always restricted to immature organisms. Unresponsiveness can also be induced in adults by using relatively higher doses of soluble antigen. The induced state of unresponsiveness to the antigen is sometimes accompanied by the appearance of suppressor T cells that actively and specifically inhibit the responses of B and T cells. Recent studies also revealed that mature lymphocytes may be directly inactivated by an antigen in vitro. In that model, short exposure of lymphocytes to the antigen, either at a critical concentration or in a certain modality, leads to inactivation rather than stimulation of the cells.

Tolerance mechanisms–B cells

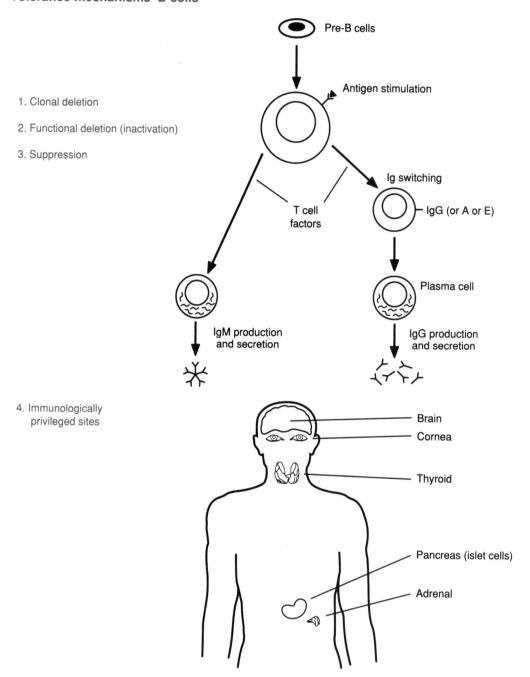

1. Clonal deletion

2. Functional deletion (inactivation)

3. Suppression

Pre-B cells

Antigen stimulation

T cell factors

Ig switching

IgG (or A or E)

Plasma cell

IgM production and secretion

IgG production and secretion

4. Immunologically privileged sites

Brain

Cornea

Thyroid

Pancreas (islet cells)

Adrenal

FIGURE 1-21   Mechanisms of immunologic tolerance: B cells.

Tolerance mechanisms–T cells

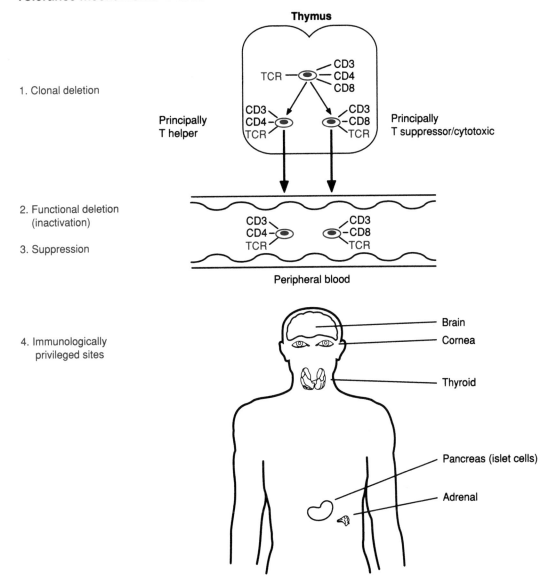

FIGURE 1-22 Mechanisms of immunologic tolerance: T cells.

Collectively, the experiments on tolerance induction demonstrate that the unresponsiveness to self probably occurs at several levels (Figs. 1-21 and 1-22). During normal development, the self-reactive lymphocyte clones may be inactivated or deleted by exposure to self macromolecules during the early stages of maturation in the thymus. The autoselection depends upon class I MHC molecules for CD8[+] T cells and class II MHC molecules for CD4[+] T cells. Cells that are not eliminated and reach their full immunologic potential may be inactivated when self molecules are presented to them at high concentrations or in a form that is tolerogenic rather than immunogenic. Also, some self-reactive lymphocytes may be suppressed by other regulatory cells.

The failure of any of the above mechanisms may result in autoimmunity. Thus, autoimmune disorders may be generated by diseases that (1) change the expression of self macromolecules or alter their presentation to immunocytes, (2) lead to the release of sequestered self antigens into the circulation or to access of immunogens to normally immunologically privileged sites, and (3) alter lymphocyte maturation and immune regulation. In addition, foreign antigens such as bacteria and viruses that cross-react with self antigens may augment any of the above mechanisms.

Certain neurotrophic agents (such as lymphocytic choriomeningitis virus) are relatively harmless unless an immune reaction takes place. In such a case an induction of tolerance may be a rational therapeutic approach.

THE COMPLEMENT SYSTEM

The complement system consists of a group of glycoproteins in the extracellular space that can be stimulated in a cascading fashion to produce biologically active fragments that either directly attack foreign substances or enhance the functions of certain types of inflammatory leukocytes. The complement system consists of two recognition-stimulation segments, the classic and alternative pathways, and a third segment, the cell membrane attack complex, which may be activated by either of the preceding pathways (Fig. 1-23).

The Classic Pathway

The classic pathway may be activated by antigen-antibody complexes of the IgG1, IgG3, or IgM isotypes by their binding to the C1q subunit of the first component of complement (Fig. 1-23). Consequently, the C1qrs subunits of C1 form an esterase that cleaves the next component, C4, into two fragments, the larger of which, C4b, binds covalently to hydroxyl or amino groups on cellular membranes. The next component, C2, after binding to C4b, is partially digested by C1s esterase to form C2b. The resultant membrane-bound complex, C4b2a, is an enzyme (C3 convertase) that cleaves C3 into two biologically active fragments, C3a and C3b.

The Alternative Pathway

The alternative pathway appears to be the more ancient in that it operates independently of anti-

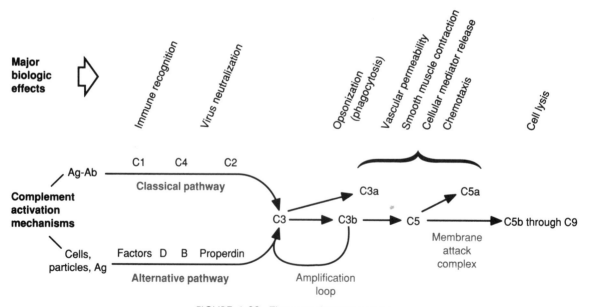

FIGURE 1-23 The complement system.

gen-antibody complexes (Fig. 1-23). The major exogenous activators of the pathway are microbial agents and their products. The major components of the pathway are the serum protein factors B, D, and P (properdin). A small amount of C3 in the fluid phase, which normally is spontaneously activated, interacts with factor B to form C3Bb, which cleaves other C3 molecules to form C3b. C3b in turn attaches to surfaces and binds factor B. The resultant C3bB is then cleaved by factor D to form C3bBb, the C3 convertase of the alternative pathway. That enzyme is distinct from the one generated from the classic pathway but serves the same purpose. This complex then is further stabilized by factor P.

The binding of C3 to factor B is prevented, particularly in the fluid phase, by a regulatory molecule, factor H. The more vigorous activation of this pathway occurs when the host is exposed to microorganisms that contain low levels of sialic acid. Under those circumstances, the binding of factor B to C3 is favored and the activation of the alternative pathway is not readily inhibited by factor H. Therefore, more C3b is generated and a positive amplification loop that produces more C3bBb (C3 convertase) is created. In contrast, sialic acid-rich encapsulated microorganisms such as *Streptococcus pneumoniae, Haemophilus influenzae,* and *Niesseria meningitidis* are incapable of activating the alternative pathway and require binding to specific IgG or IgM antibodies to activate the classic pathway and generate the C3b for phagocytosis and the formation of the membrane attack complex. The receptors for activated complement fragments are CR1, principally on phagocytic cells for C3b; CR2, principally on B cells for a fragment called C3d (receptor for EBV); and CR3 (Mac-1), on phagocytic and NK cells for inactivated C3b (C3bi) and C3d,g fragments.

The Membrane Attack Complex

As a result of the formation of C3b, C5 is cleaved into two fragments, C5b and C5a. The larger fragment, C5b, combines with C6, and the complex attaches to the cell surface, where it forms the foundation for the sequential binding of C7, C8,

and C9 (e.g., the membrane attack complex) (Fig. 1-22). C3b and its degradation product, C3bi, are opsonins. C3a and C5a are chemotaxins and anaphylotoxins, but C5a is the more potent.

ONTOGENY OF THE IMMUNE RESPONSE

There is an orderly development of the immune system during the intrauterine period. Pluripotent stem cells appear first in the yolk sac, then in the fetal liver, and finally the bone marrow. Neutrophils, monocytes, and macrophages are produced during fetal life but do not mature until after birth. An epithelial thymus appears during the first few fetal weeks and then becomes populated with lymphocytes (the intrathymic development of T cells is described earlier in this chapter). Mature T and B cells appear in the blood soon thereafter, but most are not activated. Biologically active agents such as lymphokines and antibodies are mostly not produced until after birth, when the infant is exposed to immunogens.

Neonates have as many B and T cells in the peripheral blood as adults, but the populations of these cells in the peripheral lymphoid organs are not well developed because of the paucity of prenatal antigenic stimuli. As antigen stimulation occurs, the T- and B-cell zones of the peripheral lymphoid organs are progressively populated and the products of these stimulated cells, such as antibodies, begin to appear. The sequence of immunoglobulin production is the same as the pattern found with primary-secondary immunization: IgM followed by IgG and IgA. IgG antibodies to polysaccharides are not produced, however, until the child is 2 to 2.5 years old. Secretory component is produced at birth, but the main immunoglobulin in external secretions in the first few weeks of postnatal life is IgM. Afterwards, IgA becomes the dominant immunoglobulin at mucosal sites, although IgM is also secreted.

DEFENSES AGAINST INFECTIONS

The first line of defense against most potential pathogens is the skin and mucous membranes. In addition to anatomic barriers, certain protective biochemical agents are produced at mucosal sites. These include simple chemicals, such as acids and bases, and macromolecular proteins including lysozyme, lactoferrin, secretory IgA antibodies, and interferons. The genesis of secretory IgA antibodies is as follows (Fig. 1-18). Under the influence of IL-5 and IL-6, B cells bearing surface IgM in Peyer's patches and in the submucosa of the tracheobronchial tree switch to IgA-bearing cells. When the surface antibodies of these altered cells combine with a specific antigen, the cells are stimulated to migrate through afferent lymphatics to the regional lymph nodes and then through efferent lymphatics into the vascular circulation. They then home to submucosal sites in the upper small intestine or to the respiratory system, where they differentiate into plasma cells that secrete large amounts of specific dimeric IgA antibodies and are transported across epithelial cells to the lumen by secretory component, as described above. The resultant secretory IgA is particularly well suited to mucosal sites since it is more resistant than other types of immunoglobulins to the digestive processes of the alimentary tract.

The second line of defense consists of local factors and cells that are activated or recruited to the site of microbial invasion. These local elements include the coagulation system, the fibrinolytic system, kallikrein, the complement system, resident macrophages, and elicited inflammatory cells.

If the pathogen is able to overcome the first two lines of defense, systemic responses are marshalled to prevent further invasion and damage. This third line of defense includes intracellular killing by circulating phagocytes, stimulation of monokine production, interleukin production by T cells, production of circulating antibodies by plasma cells in regional lymph nodes and the spleen, intravascular activation of the complement system, and phagocytosis of opsonized pathogens by cells of the reticuloendothelial system. Cytotoxic mechanisms directed against ingested microbes or infected cells are important in defense (Table 1-5).

Unless the microbial inoculum is overwhelming or unusually virulent or the host defenses are compromised, the infection should be contained and finally obliterated via a combination of local and systemic responses. At the same time, local fibroblasts and epithelial cells proliferate, the tissue becomes more vascularized, and the debris are removed by local tissue phagocytes. The inflammatory reaction abates, and the tissue heals.

MATERNAL IMMUNE CONTRIBUTIONS TO THE INFANT

The mother transmits immune agents to her offspring both through the placenta and in milk. Large quantities of IgG are transmitted via the placenta, whereas the other isotypes are not. Consequently, the concentration of IgG in umbilical cord blood is somewhat higher than in adults, and the levels of other isotypes are exceptionally low. Some factors are also transmitted via amniotic fluid, but little is known about their functions.

TABLE 1-5   Selected Types of Immune-Mediated Cytotoxicity

Killing Pathway[a]	Targets	Mechanisms	Recognition Process
Intraphagocytic	Bacteria Fungi	Toxic O radicals	Antibody and/or complement
Complement	Enveloped microbes Opsonized cells	Enzymatic digestion of cell surfaces	Antibody (classic); nonantibody (alternate)
NK cells	Tumor cells Infected cells	Complement-like	Nonantibody Antibody
T lymphocytes	Tumor cells Infected cells	?	Specific antigen plus MHC molecules

[a] In addition there are cytolytic cytokines, i.e., TNF-α, TNF-β, and IFN-γ.

An array of host resistance factors are transmitted to the infant in human milk; these include leukocytes, secretory IgA, lactoferrin, lysozyme, and oligosaccharides and glycoconjugates that are receptor analogs for microbial adhesions and toxins. These factors are designed to act at mucosal sites and to protect by noninflammatory mechanisms. Since the endogenous production of these agents is incompletely developed in early infancy, and since they are scarce in cow's milk and other substitute feedings, it is not surprising that breast-feeding increases resistance to gastrointestinal and respiratory infections.

IMMUNE DEFICIENCY

Much of the basic information concerning the development and function of the immune system has been learned from investigations of inherited, congenital, and acquired defects of the system. Examples of the principal defects that have led to an elucidation of the immune system are as follows.

Genetic Defects

In most patients with **X-linked hypogammaglobulinemia** disease there is a genetic defect in the development of B cells from pre-B cells in the bone marrow. Although the primary defect is not known, there is some evidence that the D and J genes required for immunoglobulin synthesis cannot be joined. Consequently, the numbers of B cells, germinal centers, and plasma cells are severely reduced and specific antibodies are produced only at very low levels. The rest of the immune system is normal. Affected individuals are unusually susceptible to infection by virulent encapsulated respiratory bacteria and enteroviruses. These patients benefit greatly from intravenous infusions of human IgG.

An abnormal gene on the X chromosome is responsible for most cases of **severe combined immunodeficiency (SCID).** In addition, an autonomal recessive defect in the formation of adenine deaminase, a defect in the formation of CD3, a defect in the post-TCR/CD3 signaling, and deficiency in the formation of IL-2 have been reported to cause this disease. Patients display few T lymphocytes, decreased T cell functions, poor antibody formation, and variable numbers of B cells and serum concentrations of immunoglobulins. As a consequence of the deficiencies in T cells, patients are very susceptible to opportunistic pathogens including *Candida albicans, Salmonella* species, *Pneumocystis carinii,* cytomegalovirus, and varicella virus. Many patients with severe combined immunodeficiency have been treated successfully with bone marrow transplants to supply normal stem cells.

Two major intrinsic defects in the function of phagocytic cells have been recognized. The first is an autosomal recessive defect in the formation of the common β subunit of the family of adherence glycoproteins. The deficiency interferes with the ability of these leukocytes to adhere to the surface of endothelial cells. Consequently, the motility of these cells on two-dimensional surfaces is impaired. Thus this defect results in bacterial infections in interstitial sites such as the skin or periodontium.

The second, **chronic granulomatous disease,** was the first recognized genetic defect of the function of phagocytic cells. The disease is X-linked in most affected patients. In those cases, the gene for the carrier protein for cytochrome b is abnormal. Consequently, the carrier protein is not produced and the cytochrome is dysfunctional. As a result the phagocytes are unable to produce toxic oxygen compounds, such as hydrogen peroxide, which are required for intracellular killing. Phagocytic cells in these patients are unable to kill catalase-positive microorganisms such as *C albicans, Escherichia coli,* and *Serratia* species because the microbial agents do not supply the oxygen substrates that are required for intracellular killing. In contrast, their cells kill catalase-negative microorganisms since those microorganisms bring hydrogen peroxide into the phagolysosome for intracellular killing.

Acquired defects. Protein-calorie malnutrition is the leading cause of immune deficiency worldwide. Protein-calorie malnutrition leads principally to a profound deficiency in the production and function of T cells, rendering the victim susceptible to many of the opportunistic infections that occur in genetic T-cell deficiencies. Certain types of infections temporarily depress parts of the immune system. For example, many acute viral infections suppress cellular immunity for several days to a few weeks, and serious bacterial infections inhibit the ability of neutrophils to respond to chemotactic agents. Thus, malnutrition and infection interact to inhibit the immune response.

Of far more concern in developed as well as developing countries is the growing epidemic of acquired immune deficiency syndrome (AIDS) due to human immunodeficiency virus (HIV) (see Ch. 62). This virus infects mainly CD4$^+$ T cells and macrophages. It binds to the CD4 surface antigen on T cells and probably a similar moiety on macrophages. Infected cells are destroyed. Since CD4$^+$ T cells are essential for the genesis of cellular immunity and for orchestrating the functioning of many other parts of the immune system, a deficiency in these T cells increases the patient's susceptibility to opportunistic infections.

DISEASE DUE TO THE IMMUNE RESPONSE

Five major types of immune responses to infecting agents may lead to disease. (1) Circulating immune complexes formed from microbial antigens such as hepatitis B virus bound to IgM or IgG antibodies may deposit in skin, synovia, or glomeruli and elicit inflammation by activating the classical pathway of complement. (2) Invading microorganisms may give rise to antibodies that cross-react with autoantigens. For example, antibodies produced against group A β-hemolytic streptococci in patients with rheumatic fever often react against sarcolemmal antigens in the cardiac muscle. (3) Vasoactive compounds may be released into local tissues or the systemic circulation because of activation of the alternative pathway of complement by sialic acid-poor bacteria such as *Salmonella* species. (4) Cytokines such as TNF-α, IL-1, and IFN-γ released during infection from stimulated macrophages and T lymphocytes may lead to fever,

dysregulate nutritional pathways, and contribute to the vascular instability seen in sepsis. (5) Finally, delayed hypersensitivity reactions that damage surrounding tissues occur in indolent infections such as tuberculosis.

REFERENCES

Coleman DL: Regulation of macrophage phagocytosis. Eur J Clin Microbiol 5:1, 1986

Fowlkes BJ, Pardoll DM: Molecular and cellular events of T cell development. Adv Immunol 44:207, 1989

Goldman AS, Goldblum RM: Human milk: immunologic-nutritional relationships. Ann NY Acad Sci 587:236, 1990

Hunkapiller T, Hood L: Diversity of the immunoglobulin gene superfamily. Adv Immunol 44:1, 1989

Jelinek DF, Lipsky PE: Regulation of human B lymphocyte activation, proliferation, and differentiation. Adv Immunol 40:1, 1987

Lerner RA: Antibodies of predetermined specificity in biology and medicine. Adv Immunol 36:1, 1984

Mestecky J, Czerkinsky C, Russell MW et al: Induction and molecular properties of secretory and serum IgA antibodies specific for environmental antigens. Ann Allergy 49:54, 1987

Nossal GJ: Immunologic tolerance: collaboration between antigen and lymphokines. Science 245:147, 1989

Rosen FS, Wedgwood RJ, Eibe M et al: Primary immunodeficiency diseases. Report of a World Health Organization. Clin Immunol Immunopathol 40:166, 1986

Schmalstieg FC: Leukocyte adherence defect. Pediatr Infect Dis J 7:867, 1988

Striebich CC, Miceli RM, Schulze DH et al: Antigen-binding repertoire and Ig H chain gene usage among B cell hybridomas from normal and autoimmune mice. J Immunol 144:1857, 1990

Vitetta ES, Fernandez BR, Myers CD, Sanders VM: Cellular interactions in the humoral immune response. Adv Immunol 45:1, 1989

Williams LW, Burks AW, Steele RW: Complement: function and clinical relevance. Ann Allergy 60:293, 1988

2 STRUCTURE

MILTON R. J. SALTON
KWANG-SHIN KIM

GENERAL CONCEPTS

Gross Morphology

Bacteria have characteristic shapes (cocci, rods, spirals, etc.) and often occur in characteristic aggregates (pairs, chains, tetrads, clusters, etc.). These traits are usually typical for a genus and are diagnostically useful.

Cell Structure

Prokaryotes have a *nucleoid* (nuclear body) rather than an enveloped nucleus and lack membrane-bound cytoplasmic organelles. The plasma membrane in prokaryotes performs many of the functions carried out by membranous organelles in eukaryotes. Multiplication is by binary fission.

Surface Structures

Flagella: The *flagella* of motile bacteria differ in structure from eukaryotic flagella. A basal body anchored in the plasma membrane and cell wall gives rise to a cylindrical protein filament. The flagellum moves by whirling about its long axis. The number and arrangement of flagella on the cell are diagnostically useful.

Pili (Fimbriae): *Pili* are slender, hairlike, proteinaceous appendages on the surface of many (particularly Gram-negative) bacteria. They are important in adhesion to host surfaces.

Capsules: Some bacteria form a thick outer *capsule* of high-molecular-weight, viscous polysaccharide gel; others have more amorphous *slime layers*. Capsules confer resistance to phagocytosis.

Important Chemical Components of Surface Structures

Cell Wall Peptidoglycans: Both Gram-positive and Gram-negative bacteria possess cell wall peptidoglycans, which confer the characteristic cell shape and provide the cell with mechanical protection. Peptidoglycans are unique to prokaryotic organisms and consist of a glycan backbone of muramic acid and glucosamine (both *N*-acetylated), and peptide chains highly cross-linked with bridges in Gram-positive bacteria (e.g., *Staphylococcus aureus*) or partially cross-linked in Gram-negative bacteria (e.g., *Escherichia coli*). The cross-linking transpeptidase enzymes are some of the targets for β-lactam antibiotics.

Teichoic Acids: Teichoic acids are polyol phosphate polymers bearing a strong negative charge. They are covalently linked to the peptidoglycan in some Gram-positive bacteria. They are strongly antigenic, but are generally absent in Gram-negative bacteria.

Lipopolysaccharides: One of the major components of the outer membrane of Gram-negative bacteria is lipopolysaccharide (endotoxin, O somatic antigen), a complex molecule consisting of a lipid A anchor, a polysaccharide core, and chains of carbohydrates. Sugars in the polysaccharide chains confer serologic specificity.

Wall-Less Forms: Two groups of bacteria devoid of cell wall peptidoglycans are the *Mycoplasma* species, which possess a surface membrane structure, and the L-forms that arise from either Gram-positive or Gram-negative bacterial cells that have lost their ability to produce the peptidoglycan structures.

Cytoplasmic Structures

Plasma Membrane: The bacterial plasma membrane is composed primarily of protein and phospholipid (about 3 : 1). It performs many functions, including transport, biosynthesis, and energy transduction.

Organelles: The bacterial cytoplasm is densely packed with 70S ribosomes. Other granules represent metabolic reserves (e.g., poly-β-hydroxybutyrate, polysaccharide, polymetaphosphate, and metachromatic granules).

Endospores: Bacillus and *Clostridium* species can produce *endospores:* heat-resistant, dehydrated resting cells that are formed intracellularly and contain a genome and all essential metabolic machinery. The endospore is encased in a complex protective spore coat.

INTRODUCTION

All bacteria, both pathogenic and saprophytic, are unicellular organisms that reproduce by binary fission. Most bacteria are capable of independent metabolic existence and growth, but some are obligately intracellular organisms. Bacterial cells are extremely small and are most conveniently measured in microns (10^{-6} m). They range in size from large cells such as *Bacillus anthracis* (1.0 to 1.3 μm $\times$ 3 to 10 μm) to very small cells such as *Pasteurella tularensis* (0.2 $\times$ 0.2 to 0.7 μm) Mycoplasmas (atypical pneumonia group) are even smaller, measuring 0.1 to 0.2 μm in diameter. Bacteria therefore have a surface-to-volume ratio that is very high: about 100,000.

Bacteria have characteristic shapes. The common microscopic morphologies are **cocci** (round or ellipsoidal cells, such as *Staphylococcus aureus* or *Streptococcus* respectively); **rods,** such as *Bacillus* and *Clostridium* species; long, filamentous branched cells, such as *Actinomyces* species; and comma-shaped and spiral cells, such as *Vibrio cholerae* and *Treponema pallidum*, respectively. The arrangement of cells is also typical of various species or groups of bacteria (Fig. 2-1). Some rods or cocci characteristically grow in chains; some, such as *Staphylococcus aureus,* form grapelike clusters of spherical cells; some round cocci form cubic packets. Bacterial cells of other species grow separately. The microscopic appearance is therefore valuable in classification and diagnosis. The higher resolving power of the electron microscope not only magnifies the typical shape of a bacterial cell but also clearly resolves its prokaryotic organization (Fig. 2-2).

THE NUCLEOID

Prokaryotic and eukaryotic cells were initially distinguished on the basis of structure: the prokaryotic **nucleoid**—the equivalent of the eukaryotic nucleus—is structurally simpler than the true eukaryotic nucleus, which has a complex mitotic apparatus and surrounding nuclear membrane. As the electron micrograph in Fig. 2-2 shows, the bacterial nucleoid, which contains the DNA fibrils, lacks a limiting membrane. Under the light microscope, the nucleoid of the bacterial cell can be visualized with the aid of Feulgen staining, which stains DNA. Gentle lysis can be used to isolate the nucleoid of most bacterial cells. The DNA is then seen to be a single, continuous, "giant" circular molecule with a molecular weight of approxi-

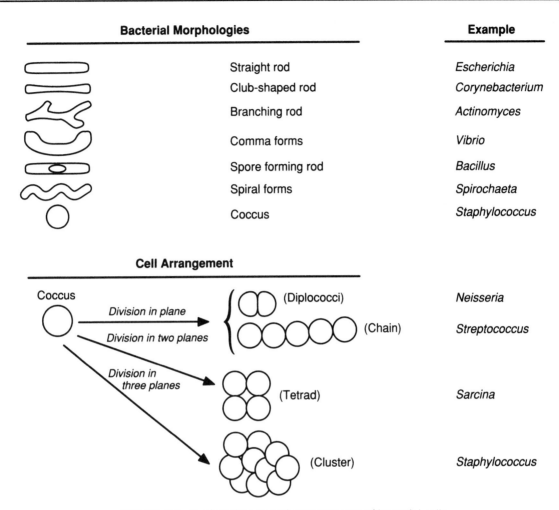

Bacterial Morphologies | **Example**

Shape	Example
Straight rod	*Escherichia*
Club-shaped rod	*Corynebacterium*
Branching rod	*Actinomyces*
Comma forms	*Vibrio*
Spore forming rod	*Bacillus*
Spiral forms	*Spirochaeta*
Coccus	*Staphylococcus*

Cell Arrangement

Coccus

Division in plane → (Diplococci) — *Neisseria*

Division in two planes → (Chain) — *Streptococcus*

Division in three planes → (Tetrad) — *Sarcina*

(Cluster) — *Staphylococcus*

FIGURE 2-1 Typical shapes and arrangements of bacterial cells.

mately 3×10^9 (see Ch. 5). The unfolded nuclear DNA would be about 1 mm long (compared with an average length of 1 to 2 μm for bacterial cells). The bacterial nucleoid, then, is a structure containing a single chromosome. The number of copies of this chromosome in a cell depends on the stage of the cell cycle (chromosome replication, cell enlargement, chromosome segregation, etc). Although the mechanism of segregation of the two sister chromosomes following replication is not fully understood, all of the models proposed require that the chromosome be permanently attached to the cell membrane throughout the various stages of the cell cycle.

Bacterial chromatin does not contain basic histone proteins, but low-molecular-weight polyamines and magnesium ions may fulfill a function similar to that of eukaryotic histones. Despite the differences between prokaryotic and eukaryotic DNA, prokaryotic DNA from cells infected with bacteriophage λ, when visualized by electron microscopy, has a beaded, condensed appearance not unlike that of eukaryotic chromatin.

SURFACE APPENDAGES

Two types of surface appendage can be recognized on certain bacterial species: the **flagella,** which are

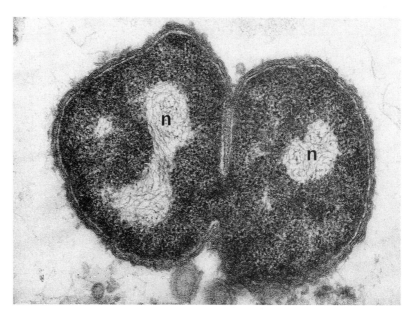

FIGURE 2-2 Electron micrograph of a thin section of *Neisseria gonorrhoeae* showing the organizational features of prokaryotic cells. Note the electron-transparent nuclear region (n) packed with DNA fibrils, the dense distribution of ribosomal particles in the cytoplasm, and the absence of intracellular membranous organelles.

organs of locomotion, and **pili** (Latin *hairs*), which are also known as **fimbriae** (Latin *fringes*). Flagella occur on both Gram-positive and Gram-negative bacteria, and their presence can be useful in identification. For example, they are found on many species of bacilli but rarely on cocci. In contrast, pili occur almost exclusively on Gram-negative bacteria and are found on only a few Gram-positive organisms (e.g., *Corynebacterium renale* and *Streptococcus pyogenes*).

Some bacteria have both flagella and pili. The electron micrograph in Fig. 2-3 shows the characteristic wavy appearance of flagella and two types of pili on the surface of *Escherichia coli*.

Flagella

Structurally, bacterial flagella are long (3 to 12 μm), filamentous surface appendages about 12 to 30 nm in diameter. The protein subunits of a flagellum are assembled to form a cylindrical structure with a hollow core. A flagellum consists of three parts: (1) the long **filament,** which lies exter-

nal to the cell surface; (2) the **hook** structure at the end of the filament; and (3) the **basal body,** to which the hook is anchored and which imparts motion to the flagellum. The basal body traverses the outer wall and membrane structures. It consists of a rod and one or two pairs of discs. The thrust that propels the bacterial cell is provided by counterclockwise rotation of the basal body, which causes the helically twisted filament to whirl. The movement of the basal body is driven by a proton motive force rather than by ATP directly. The ability of bacteria to swim by means of the propellerlike action of the flagella provides them with the mechanical means to perform *chemotaxis* (movement in response to attractant and repellent substances in the environment). Response to chemical stimuli involves a sophisticated sensory system of receptors that are located in the cell surface and/or periplasm and that transmit information to methyl-accepting chemotaxis proteins that control the flagellar motor. Genetic studies have revealed the existence of mutants with altered biochemical pathways for flagellar motility and chemotaxis.

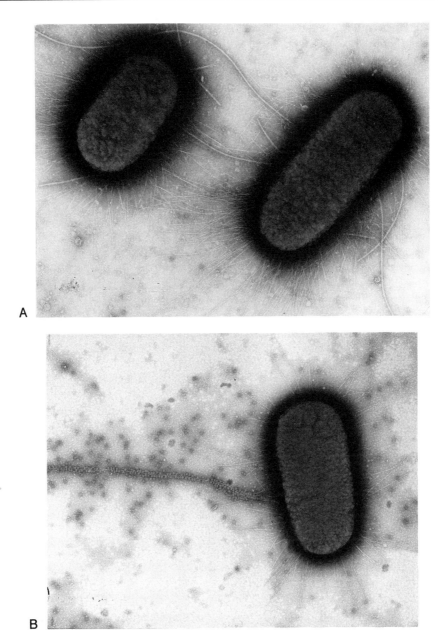

FIGURE 2-3   *(A)* Electron micrograph of negatively stained *E coli* showing wavy flagella and numerous short, thinner, and more rigid hairlike structures, the pili. *(B)* The long sex pilus can be distinguished from the shorter common pili by mixing *E coli* cells with a male bacteriophage that binds specifically to sex pili.

Chemically, flagella are constructed of a class of proteins called **flagellins.** The hook and basal-body structures consist of numerous proteins. Mutations affecting any of these gene products may result in loss or impairment of motility. Flagellins are immunogenic and constitute a group of protein antigens called the **H antigens,** which are characteristic of a given species, strain, or variant of an organism. The species specificity of the flagellins reflects differences in the primary structures of the proteins.

The number and distribution of flagella on the bacterial surface are characteristic for a given species and hence are useful in identifying and classifying bacteria. Figure 2-4 illustrates typical arrangements of flagella on or around the bacterial surface. For example, *V cholerae* has a single flagellum at one pole of the cell (i.e., it is **monotrichous**), whereas *Proteus vulgaris* and *E coli* have many flagella distributed over the entire cell surface (i.e., they are **peritrichous**). The flagella of a peritrichous bacterium must aggregate as a posterior bundle to propel the cell in a forward direction.

Flagella can be sheared from the cell surface without affecting the viability of the cell. The cell then becomes temporarily nonmotile. In time it synthesizes new flagella and regains motility. The protein synthesis inhibitor chloramphenicol, however, blocks regeneration of flagella.

Pili

The terms *pili* and *fimbriae* are usually used interchangeably to describe the thin, hairlike appendages on the surface of many Gram-negative (and a few Gram-positive) bacteria. Pili are more rigid in appearance than flagella (Fig. 2-3). In some organisms, such as *Shigella* species and *E coli,* pili are distributed profusely over the cell surface, with as many as 200 per cell. As is easily recognized in strains of *E coli,* pili can come in two types: short, abundant **common pili,** and a small number (one to six) of very long pili known as **sex pili.** Sex pili can be distinguished by their ability to bind male-specific bacteriophages (the sex pilus acts as a specific receptor for these bacteriophages) (Fig. 2-3B). The sex pili attach male to female bacteria during conjugation.

Pili in many enteric bacteria confer adhesive properties on the bacterial cells, enabling them to adhere to various epithelial surfaces, to red blood cells (causing hemagglutination), and to surfaces

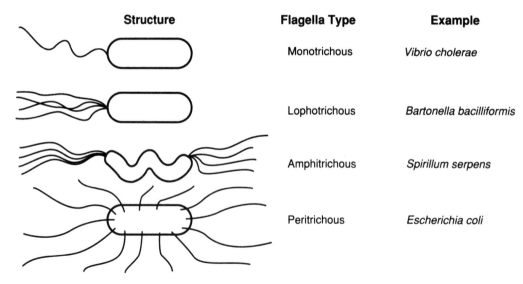

Structure	Flagella Type	Example
	Monotrichous	*Vibrio cholerae*
	Lophotrichous	*Bartonella bacilliformis*
	Amphitrichous	*Spirillum serpens*
	Peritrichous	*Escherichia coli*

FIGURE 2-4 Typical arrangements of bacterial flagella.

of yeast and fungal cells. These adhesive properties of piliated cells play an important role in bacterial colonization of epithelial surfaces and are therefore referred to as **colonization factors.** The common pili found on *E coli* exhibit a sugar specificity analogous to that of phytohemagglutinins and lectins, in that adhesion and hemagglutinating capacities of the organism are inhibited specifically by mannose. Organisms possessing this type of hemagglutination are called **mannose-sensitive** organisms. Other piliated organisms, such as gonococci, are adhesive and hemagglutinating, but are insensitive to the inhibitory effects of mannose.

SURFACE LAYERS

The surface layers of the bacterial cell have been identified by various techniques: light microscopy and staining; electron microscopy of thin-sectioned, freeze-fractured, and negatively stained cells; and isolation and biochemical characterization of individual morphologic components of the cell. The principal surface layers are capsules and loose slime, the cell wall of Gram-positive bacteria and the complex cell envelope of Gram-negative bacteria, plasma (cytoplasmic) membranes, and mesosomal membrane vesicles, which arise from invaginations of the plasma membrane. In bacteria, the cell wall forms a rigid structure of uniform thickness around the cell and is responsible for the characteristic shape of the cell (rod, coccus, or spiral). Inside the cell wall (or rigid peptidoglycan layer) is the plasma (cytoplasmic) membrane; this is usually closely apposed to the wall layer. The topographic relationships of the cell wall and envelope layers to the plasma membrane are indicated in the thin section of a Gram-positive organism *(Micrococcus lysodeikticus)* in Figure 2-5A and in the freeze-fractured cell of a Gram-negative organism *(Bacteroides melaninogenicus)* in Figure 2-5B. The latter shows the typical fracture planes seen in most Gram-negative bacteria, which are weak cleavage planes through the outer membrane of the envelope and extensive fracture planes through the bilayer region of the underlying plasma membrane.

Capsules and Loose Slime

Some bacteria form **capsules,** which constitute the outermost layer of the bacterial cell and surround it with a relatively thick layer of viscous gel. Capsules may be up to 10 μm thick. Some organisms lack a well-defined capsule but have loose, amorphous **slime layers** external to the cell wall or cell envelope. Not all bacterial species produce capsules; however, the capsules of encapsulated pathogens are often important determinants of virulence. Encapsulated species are found among both Gram-positive and Gram-negative bacteria. In both groups, most capsules are composed of high-molecular-weight viscous polysaccharides that are retained as a thick gel outside the cell wall or envelope. The capsule of *Bacillus anthracis* (the causal agent of anthrax) is unusual in that it is composed of a γ-glutamyl polypeptide. Table 2-1 presents the various capsular substances formed by a selection of Gram-positive and Gram-negative bacteria. A plasma membrane stage is involved in the biosynthesis and assembly of the capsular substances, which are extruded or secreted through the outer wall or envelope structures. Mutational loss of enzymes involved in the biosynthesis of the capsular polysaccharides can result in the smooth-to-rough variation seen in the pneumococci.

The capsule is not essential for viability. Viability is not affected when capsular polysaccharides are removed enzymatically from the cell surface. The exact functions of capsules are not fully understood, but they do confer resistance to phagocytosis and hence provide the bacterial cell with protection against host defenses to invasion.

Cell Wall and Gram-Negative Cell Envelope

The Gram stain broadly differentiates bacteria into Gram-positive and Gram-negative groups; a few organisms are consistently Gram-variable. Gram-positive and Gram-negative organisms differ drastically in the organization of the structures outside the plasma membrane but below the capsule (Fig. 2-6): in Gram-negative organisms

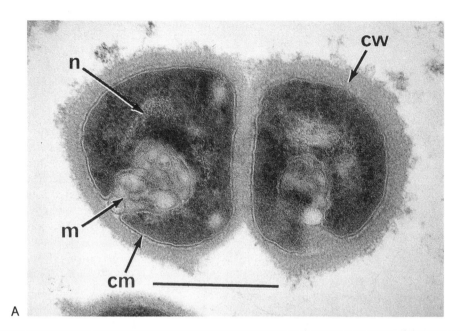

A

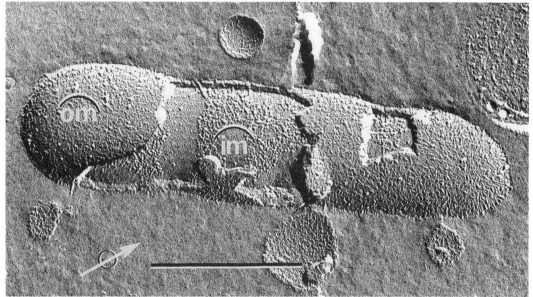

B

FIGURE 2-5 *(A)* Electron micrograph of a thin section of the Gram-positive *M lysodeikticus* showing the thick peptidoglycan cell wall (cw), underlying cytoplasmic (plasma) membrane (cm), mesome (m), and nucleus (n). *(B)* Freeze-fractured *Bacteriodes* cell showing typical major convex fracture faces through the inner (im) and outer (om) membranes. Bars = 1 µm; circled arrow in Fig. B indicates direction of shadowing.

TABLE 2-1 Nature of Capsular Substances Formed by Various Bacteria

Genus and Species	Capsular Substances
Gram-positive bacteria	
S pneumoniae	Polysaccharides: e.g., type III, glucose, glucoronic acid (cellobiuronic acid); other types, various sugars and amino sugars
Streptococcus spp	Polysaccharides: e.g., hyaluronic acid (group A), others containing amino sugars, uronic acids
B anthracis	γ-Glutamyl polypeptide
Gram-negative bacteria	
H influenzae	Polyribosephosphate
Klebsiella spp	Polysaccharides: sugars such as hexoses, fucose, uronic acids
N meningitidis	Polysaccharides: *N*-acetylmannosamine phosphate polymer (group A); sialic acid polymers (groups B and C)

these structures constitute the **cell envelope,** whereas in Gram-positive organisms they are called a **cell wall.**

Most Gram-positive bacteria have a relatively thick (about 20 to 80 nm), continuous cell wall (often called the *sacculus*), which is composed largely of peptidoglycan (also known as *mucopeptide or murein*). In thick cell walls, other cell wall polymers (such as the teichoic acids, polysaccharides, and peptidoglycolipids) are covalently attached to the peptidoglycan. In contrast, the peptidoglycan layer in Gram-negative bacteria is thin (about 5 to 10 nm thick); in *E coli*, the peptidoglycan is probably only a monolayer thick. Outside the peptidoglycan layer in the Gram-negative envelope is an outer membrane structure (about 7.5 to 10 nm thick). In most Gram-negative bacteria, this membrane structure is anchored noncovalently to lipoprotein molecules (Braun's lipoprotein), which, in turn, are covalently linked to the peptidoglycan. The lipopolysaccharides of the Gram-negative cell envelope form part of the outer leaflet of the outer membrane structure.

The organization and overall dimensions of the outer membrane of the Gram-negative cell envelope are similar to those of the plasma membrane (about 7.5 nm thick). Moreover, in Gram-negative bacteria such as *E coli*, the outer and inner membranes adhere to each other at several hundred sites (Bayer patches); these sites can break up the

continuity of the peptidoglycan layer. Table 2-2 summarizes the major classes of chemical constituents in the walls and envelopes of Gram-positive and Gram-negative bacteria.

The basic differences in surface structures of Gram-positive and Gram-negative bacteria explain the results of Gram staining. Both Gram-positive and Gram-negative bacteria take up the same amounts of crystal violet (CV) and iodine (I). The CV-I complex, however, is trapped inside the Gram-positive cell by the dehydration and reduced porosity of the thick cell wall as a result of the differential washing step with 95 percent ethanol or other solvent mixture. In contrast, the thin peptidoglycan layer and probable discontinuities at the membrane adhesion sites do not impede solvent extraction of the CV-I complex from the Gram-negative cell. The sequence of steps in the Gram stain differentiation is illustrated diagrammatically in Figure 2-7. Moreover, mechanical disruption of the cell wall of Gram-positive organisms or its enzymatic removal with lysozyme results in complete extraction of the CV-I complex and conversion to a Gram-negative reaction. Therefore, autolytic wall-degrading enzymes that cause cell wall breakage may account for Gram-negative or variable reactions in cultures of Gram-positive organisms (such as *Staphylococcus aureus, Clostridium perfringens, Corynebacterium diphtheriae,* and some *Bacillus* spp).

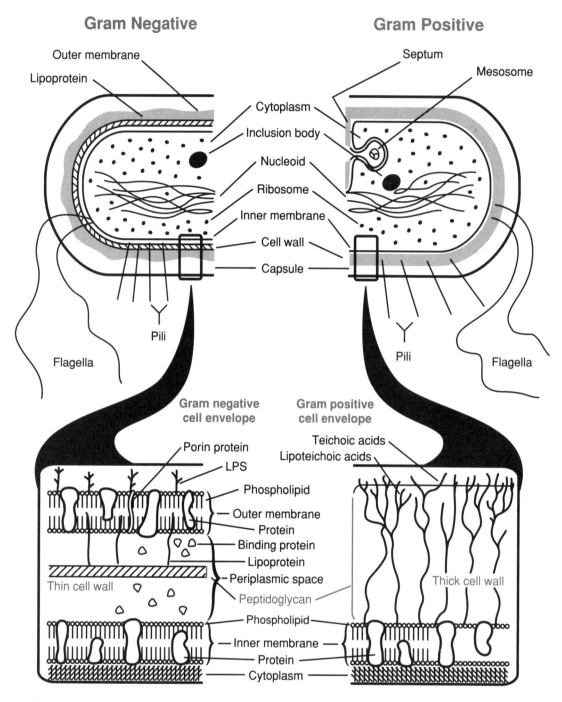

FIGURE 2-6   Comparison of the thick cell wall of Gram-positive bacteria with the comparatively thin cell wall of Gram-negative bacteria. Note the complexity of the Gram-negative cell envelope (outer membrane, its hydrophobic lipoprotein anchor; periplasmic space).

TABLE 2-2   Major Classes of Chemical Components in Bacterial Walls and Envelopes

Chemical Component	Examples
Gram-positive cell walls	
Peptidoglycan	All species
Polysaccharides	*Streptococcus* group A, B, C substances
Teichoic acid	
Ribitol	*S aureus, B subtilis, Lactobacillus* spp
Glycerol	*S epidermidis, Lactobacillus* spp
Teichuronic acids (aminogalacturonic or ami-nomannuronic acid polymers)	*B licheniformis, M lysodeikticus*
Peptidoglycolipids (muramylpeptide-polysaccharide-mycolates)	*Corynebacterium* spp, *Mycobacterium* spp, *Nocardia* spp
Glycolipids ("waxes") (polysaccharide-mycolates)	
Gram-negative envelopes	
LPS	All species
Lipoprotein	*E coli* and many enteric bacteria, *Pseudomonas aeruginosa*
Porins (Major outer membrane proteins)	*E coli, Salmonella typhimurium*
Phospholipids and proteins	All species
Peptidoglycan	Almost all species

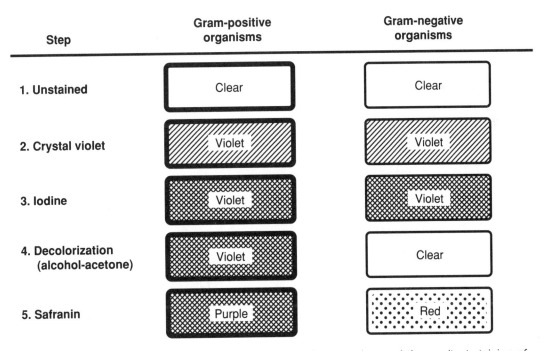

FIGURE 2-7   General sequence of steps in the Gram stain procedure and the resultant staining of Gram-positive and Gram-negative bacteria.

Peptidoglycan

Unique features of almost all prokaryotic cells (except for *Halobacterium halobium* and mycoplasmas) are cell wall peptidoglycan and the specific enzymes involved in its biosynthesis. These enzymes are target sites for inhibition of peptidoglycan synthesis by specific antibiotics. The primary chemical structures of peptidoglycans of both Gram-positive and Gram-negative bacteria have been established; they consist of a glycan backbone of repeating groups of β1,4-linked disaccharides of β1,4-*N*-acetylmuramyl-*N*-acetylglucosamine. Tetrapeptides of L-alanine-D-isoglutamic acid-L-lysine (or diaminopimelic acid)-D-alanine are linked through the carboxyl group by amide linkage of muramic acid residues of the glycan chains; the D-alanine residues are directly cross-linked to the ϵ-amino group of lysine or diaminopimelic acid on a neighboring tetrapeptide, or they are linked by a peptide bridge. In *S aureus* peptidoglycan, a glycine pentapeptide bridge links the two adjacent peptide structures. The extent of direct or peptide-bridge cross-linking varies from one peptidoglycan to another. The staphylococcal peptidoglycan is highly cross-linked, whereas that of *E coli* is much less so, and has a more open peptidoglycan mesh. The diamino acid providing the ϵ-amino group for cross-linking is lysine or diaminopimelic acid, the latter being uniformly present in Gram-negative peptidoglycans. The structure of the peptidoglycan is illustrated in Figure 2-8. A peptidoglycan with a chemical structure substantially different from that of all eubacteria has been discovered in certain archaebacteria. Instead of muramic acid, this peptidoglycan contains talosaminuronic acid and lacks the D-amino acids found in the eubacterial peptidoglycans. Interestingly, organisms containing this wall polymer (referred to as pseudomurein) are insensitive to penicillin, an inhibitor of the transpeptidases involved in peptidoglycan biosynthesis in eubacteria.

The β-1,4 glycosidic bond between *N*-acetylmuramic acid and *N*-acetylglucosamine is specifically cleaved by the bacteriolytic enzyme *lysozyme*. Widely distributed in nature, this enzyme is present in human tissues and secretions and can cause complete digestion of the peptidoglycan

Gram-negative peptidoglycan   **Gram-positive peptidoglycan**

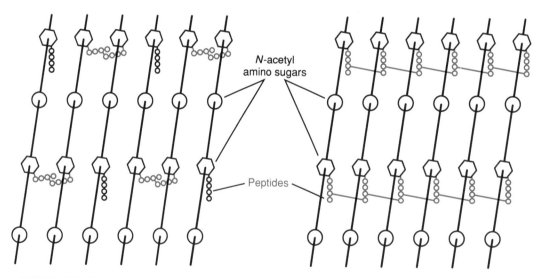

FIGURE 2-8 Diagrammatic representation of peptidoglycan structures with adjacent glycan strands cross-linked directly from the carboxyterminal D-alanine to the ϵ-amino group of an adjacent tetrapeptide or through a peptide cross bridge ⬡, *N*-acetylmuramic acid; ◯, *N*-acetylglucosamine.

walls of sensitive organisms. When lysozyme is allowed to digest the cell wall of Gram-positive bacteria suspended in an osmotic stabilizer (such as sucrose), protoplasts are formed. These protoplasts are able to survive and continue to grow on suitable media in the wall-less state. Gram-negative bacteria treated similarly produce spheroplasts, which retain much of the outer membrane structure. The dependence of bacterial shape on the peptidoglycan is shown by the transformation of rod-shaped bacteria to spherical protoplasts (*spheroplasts*) after enzymatic breakdown of the peptidoglycan. The mechanical protection afforded by the wall peptidoglycan layer is evident in the osmotic fragility of both protoplasts and spheroplasts. There are two groups of bacteria that lack the protective cell wall peptidoglycan structure, the *Mycoplasma* species, one of which causes atypical pneumonia and some genitourinary tract infections and the L-forms, which originate from Gram-positive or Gram-negative bacteria and are so designated because of their discovery and description at the Lister Institute, London. The mycoplasmas and L-forms are all Gram-negative and insensitive to penicillin and are bounded by a surface membrane structure. L-forms arising ''spontaneously'' in cultures or isolated from infections are structurally related to protoplasts and spheroplasts; all three forms (protoplasts, spheroplasts, and L-forms) revert infrequently and only under special conditions.

Teichoic Acids

Wall teichoic acids are found only in certain Gram-positive bacteria (such as staphylococci, streptococci, lactobacilli, and *Bacillus* spp); so far, they have not been found in gram-negative organisms. Teichoic acids are polyol phosphate polymers, with either ribitol or glycerol linked by phosphodiester bonds; their structures are illustrated in Figure 2-9. Substituent groups on the polyol chains can include D-alanine (ester linked), *N*-acetylglucosamine, *N*-acetylgalactosamine, and glucose; the substituent is characteristic for the teichoic acid from a particular bacterial species and can act as a specific antigenic determinant. Teichoic acids are co-

valently linked to the peptidoglycan. These highly negatively charged polymers of the bacterial wall can serve as a cation-sequestering mechanism.

Accessory Wall Polymers

In addition to the principal cell wall polymers, the walls of certain Gram-positive bacteria possess polysaccharide molecules linked to the peptidoglycan. For example, the C polysaccharide of streptococci confers group specificity. Acidic polysaccharides attached to the peptidoglycan are called *teichuronic acids*. Mycobacteria have peptidoglycolipids, glycolipids, and waxes associated with the cell wall.

Lipopolysaccharides

A characteristic feature of Gram-negative bacteria is possession of various types of complex macromolecular lipopolysaccharide (LPS). So far, only one Gram-positive organism, *Listeria monocytogenes*, has been found to contain an authentic LPS. The LPS of this bacterium and those of all Gram-negative species are also called **endotoxins,** thereby distinguishing these cell-bound, heat-stable toxins from heat-labile, protein **exotoxins** secreted into culture media. Endotoxins possess an array of powerful biologic activities and play an important role in the pathogenesis of many Gram-negative bacterial infections. In addition to causing endotoxic shock, LPS is pyrogenic, can activate macrophages and complement, is mitogenic for B lymphocytes, induces interferon production, causes tissue necrosis and tumor regression, and has adjuvant properties. The endotoxic properties of LPS reside largely in the lipid A components. Usually, the LPS molecules have three regions: the lipid A structure required for insertion in the outer leaflet of the outer membrane bilayer; a covalently attached core composed of 2-keto-3-deoxyoctonic acid (KDO), heptose, ethanolamine, *N*-acetylglucosamine, glucose, and galactose; and polysaccharide chains linked to the core. The polysaccharide chains constitute the O-antigens of the Gram-negative bacteria, and the individual monosaccharide constituents confer serologic specificity on these components. Figure 2-10 depicts the

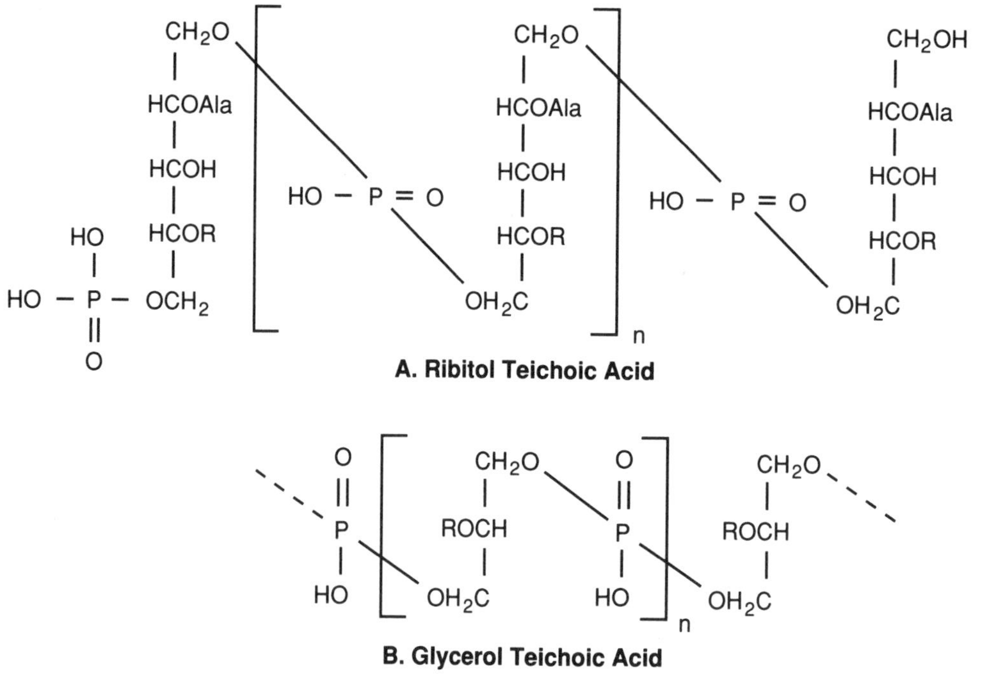

A. Ribitol Teichoic Acid

B. Glycerol Teichoic Acid

FIGURE 2-9 Structures of cell wall teichoic acids. *(A)* Ribitol teichoic acid with repeating units of 1,5-phosphodiester linkages of D-ribitol and D-alanyl ester on position 2 and glycosyl substituents (R) on position 4. The glycosyl groups may be *N*-acetylglucosaminyl (*α* or *β*) as in *S aureus* or *α*-glucosyl as in *B subtilis* W23. *(B)* Glycerol teichoic acid with 1,3-phosphodiester linkages of glycerol repeating units (1,2-linkages in some species). In the glycerol teichoic acid structure shown, the polymer may be unsubstituted (R = H) or substituted (R = D-alanyl or glycosyl).

Lipid A ———	——— Core ———	——— O Antigen
Glucosamine β-hydroxymyristate Fatty acids	Ketodeoxyoctonate Phosphoethanolamine Heptose Glucose, galactose, *N*-acetylglucosamine	Polysaccharide chains: repeating units of species-specific mono-saccharides, e.g., gal-actose, rhamnose, mannose and abequose in *S typhimurium* LPS

FIGURE 2-10 The three major, covalently linked regions that form the typical LPS.

structure of LPS. Although it has been known that lipid A is composed of β1,6-linked D-glucosamine disaccharide substituted with phosphomonester groups at positions 4' and 1, uncertainties have existed about the attachment positions of the six fatty acid acyl and KDO groups on the disaccharide. The demonstration of the structure of lipid A of LPS of a heptoseless mutant of *Salmonella typhimurium* has established that amide-linked hydroxymyristoyl and lauroxymyristoyl groups are attached to the nitrogen of the 2- and 2'-carbons, respectively, and that hydroxymyristoyl and myristoxymyristoyl groups are attached to the oxygen of the 3- and 3'-carbons of the disaccharide, respectively. Therefore, only position 6' is left for attachment of KDO units.

LPS and phospholipids help confer asymmetry to the outer membrane of the Gram-negative bacteria, with the hydrophilic polysaccharide chains outermost. Each LPS is held in the outer membrane by relatively weak cohesive forces (ionic and hydrophobic interactions) and can be dissociated from the cell surface with surface-active agents.

As in peptidoglycan biosynthesis, LPS molecules are assembled at the plasma or inner membrane. These newly formed molecules are initially inserted into the outer-inner membrane adhesion sites.

Outer Membrane of Gram-Negative Bacteria

In thin sections, the outer membranes of Gram-negative bacteria appear broadly similar to the plasma or inner membranes; however, they differ from the inner membranes and walls of Gram-positive bacteria in numerous respects. The lipid A of LPS is inserted with phospholipids to create the outer leaflet of the bilayer structure; the lipid portion of the lipoprotein and phospholipid form the inner leaflet of the outer membrane bilayer of most Gram-negative bacteria (Fig. 2-6).

In addition to these components, the outer membrane possesses several major outer membrane proteins; the most abundant is called *porin*. The assembled subunits of porin form a channel that limits the passage of hydrophilic molecules across the outer membrane barrier to those having molecular weights that are usually less than 600 to 700. Evidence also suggests that hydrophobic pathways exist across the outer membrane and are partly responsible for the differential penetration and effectiveness of certain β-lactam antibiotics (ampicillin, cephalosporins) that are active against various Gram-negative bacteria. Although the outer membranes act as a permeability barrier or molecular sieve, they do not appear to possess energy-transducing systems to drive active transport. Several outer membrane proteins, however, are involved in the specific uptake of metabolites (maltose, vitamin B_{12}, nucleosides) and iron from the medium. Thus, outer membranes of the Gram-negative bacteria provide a selective barrier to external molecules and thereby prevent the loss of metabolite-binding proteins and hydrolytic enzymes (nucleases, alkaline phosphatase) found in the periplasmic space. The periplasmic space is the region between the outer surface of the inner (plasma) membrane and the inner surface of the outer membrane (Figure 2-6). Thus, Gram-negative bacteria have a cellular compartment that has no equivalent in Gram-positive organisms. In addition to the hydrolytic enzymes, the periplasmic space holds binding proteins (proteins that specifically bind sugars, amino acids, and inorganic ions) involved in membrane transport and chemotactic receptor activities. Moreover, plasmid-encoded β-lactamases and aminoglycoside-modifying enzymes (phosphorylation or adenylation) in the periplasmic space produce antibiotic resistance by degrading or modifying an antibiotic in transit to its target sites on the membrane (penicillin-binding proteins) or on the ribosomes (aminoglycosides). These periplasmic proteins can be released by subjecting the cells to osmotic shock and after treatment with the chelating agent ethylenediaminetetraacetic acid.

INTRACELLULAR COMPONENTS

Plasma (Cytoplasmic) Membranes

Bacterial *plasma membranes*, the functional equivalents of eukaryotic plasma membranes, are referred to variously as *cytoplasmic, protoplast,* or (in

Gram-negative organisms) *inner membranes.* Similar in overall dimensions and appearance in thin sections to biomembranes from eukaryotic cells, they are composed primarily of proteins and lipids (principally phospholipids). Protein-to-lipid ratios of bacterial plasma membranes are approximately 3 : 1, close to those for mitochondrial membranes. Unlike eukaryotic cell membranes, the bacterial membrane (except for *Mycoplasma* species and certain methylotrophic bacteria) has no sterols, and bacteria lack the enzymes required for sterol biosynthesis.

Although their composition is similar to that of inner membranes of Gram-negative species, cytoplasmic membranes from Gram-positive bacteria possess a class of macromolecules not present in the Gram-negative membranes. Many Gram-positive bacterial membranes contain membrane-bound lipoteichoic acid, and species lacking this component (such as *Micrococcus* and *Sarcina* spp) contain an analogous membrane-bound succinylated lipomannan. Lipoteichoic acids are structurally similar to the cell wall glycerol teichoic acids in that they have basal polyglycerol phosphodiester 1-3 linked chains (Fig. 2-9). These chains terminate with the phosphomonoester end of the polymer, which is linked covalently to either a glycolipid or a phosphatidyl glycolipid moiety. Thus, a hydrophobic tail is provided for anchoring in the membrane lipid layers (Fig. 2-6A). As in the cell wall glycerol teichoic acid, the lipoteichoic acids can have glycosidic and D-alanyl ester substituents on the C-2 position of the glycerol.

Both membrane-bound lipoteichoic acid and membrane-bound succinylated lipomannan can be detected as antigens on the cell surface, and the glycerol-phosphate and succinylated mannan chains appear to extend through the cell wall structure (Fig. 2-6). This class of polymer has not yet been found in the cytoplasmic membranes of Gram-negative organisms. In both instances, the lipoteichoic acids and the lipomannans are negatively charged components and can sequester positively charged substances. They have been implicated in adhesion to host cells, but their functions remain to be elucidated.

Multiple functions are performed by the plasma membranes of both Gram-positive and Gram-negative bacteria. Plasma membranes are the site of active transport, respiratory chain components, energy-transducing systems, the H^+-ATPase of the proton pump (see Chapter 4), and membrane stages in the biosynthesis of phospholipids, peptidoglycan, LPS, and capsular polysaccharides. In essence, the bacterial cytoplasmic membrane is a multifunction structure that combines the mitochondrial transport and biosynthetic functions that are usually compartmentalized in discrete membranous organelles in eukaryotic cells. The plasma membrane is also the anchoring site for DNA and provides the cell with a mechanism (as yet unknown) for separation of sister chromosomes.

Mesosomes

Thin sections of Gram-positive bacteria reveal the presence of vesicular or tubular-vesicular membrane structures called **mesosomes,** which are apparently formed by an invagination of the plasma membrane. These structures are much more prominent in Gram-positive than in Gram-negative organisms. At one time, the mesosomal vesicles were thought to be equivalent to bacterial mitochondria; however, many other membrane functions have also been attributed to the mesosomes. At present, there is no satisfactory evidence to suggest that they have a unique biochemical or physiologic function. Indeed, electron-microscopic studies have suggested that the mesosomes, as usually seen in thin sections, may arise from membrane perturbation and fixation artifacts. No general agreement exists about this theory, however, and some evidence indicates that mesosomes may be related to events in the cell division cycle.

Other Intracellular Components

In addition to the nucleoid and cytoplasm (cytosol), the intracellular compartment of the bacterial cell is densely packed with ribosomes of the 70S type (Fig. 2-2). These ribonucleoprotein particles, which have a diameter of 18 nm, are not arranged on a membranous rough endoplasmic reticulum as they are in eukaryotic cells. Other granular inclusions randomly distributed in the cytoplasm of various species include metabolic reserve particles such as poly-β-hydroxybutyrate (PHB), polysaccharide and glycogenlike granules, and polymetaphosphate or metachromatic granules.

Endospores are highly heat-resistant, dehydrated resting cells formed intracellularly in members of the genera *Bacillus* and *Clostridium.* **Sporulation,** the process of forming endospores, is an unusual property of certain bacteria. The series of biochemical and morphologic changes that occur during sporulation represent true differentiation within the cycle of the bacterial cell. The process, which usually begins in the stationary phase of the vegetative cell cycle, is initiated by depletion of nutrients (usually readily utilizable sources of carbon or nitrogen, or both). The cell then undergoes a highly complex, well-defined sequence of morphologic and biochemical events that ultimately lead to the formation of mature endospores. As many as seven distinct stages have been recognized by morphologic and biochemical studies of sporulating *Bacillus* species: stage 0, vegetative cells with two chromosomes at the end of exponential growth; stage I, formation of axial chromatin filament and excretion of exoenzymes, including proteases; stage II, forespore septum formation and segregation of nuclear material into two compartments; stage III, spore protoplast formation and elevation of tricarboxylic acid and glyoxylate cycle enzyme levels; stage IV, cortex formation and refractile appearance of spore; stage V, spore coat protein formation; stage VI, spore maturation, modification of cortical peptidoglycan, uptake of dipicolinic acid (a unique endospore product) and calcium, and development of resistance to heat and organic solvents; and stage VII, final maturation and liberation of endospores from mother cells (in some species).

When newly formed, endospores appear as round, highly refractile cells within the vegetative cell wall, or **sporangium.** Some strains produce autolysins that digest the walls and liberate free endospores. The spore protoplast, or **core,** contains a complete nucleus, ribosomes, and energy-generating components that are enclosed within a modified cytoplasmic membrane. The peptidogly-

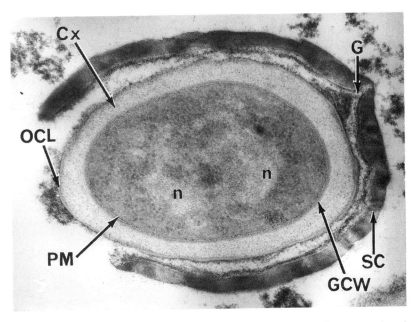

FIGURE 2-11 Electron micrograph of a thin section of a *Bacillus megaterium* spore showing the thick spore coat (SC), germinal groove (G) in the spore coat, outer cortex layer (OCL) and cortex (Cx), germinal cell wall layer (GCW), underlying spore protoplast membrane (PM), and regions where the nucleoid (n) is visible. (Courtesy of John H. Freer, University of Glasgow, Scotland.)

can spore wall surrounds the spore membrane; on germination, this wall becomes the vegetative cell wall. Surrounding the spore wall is a thick cortex that contains an unusual type of peptidoglycan, which is rapidly released on germination. A spore coat of keratinlike protein encases the spore contained within a membrane (the **exosporium**). During maturation, the spore protoplast dehydrates and the spore becomes refractile and resistant to heat, desiccation, and chemicals; these properties correlate with the cortical peptidoglycan and the presence of large amounts of calcium dipicolinate. Figure 2-11 illustrates the principal structural features of a typical endospore *(Bacillus megaterium)* on initiation of the germination process. The thin section of the spore shows the ruptured, thick spore coat and the cortex surrounding the spore protoplast with the germinal cell wall that becomes the vegetative wall on outgrowth.

REFERENCES

Costerton JW, Ingram JM, Cheng KJ: Structure and function of the cell envelope of gram-negative bacteria. Bacteriol Rev, 38:87, 1974

Di Rienzo JM, Nakamura K, Inouye M: The outer membrane proteins of gram-negative bacteria: biosynthesis, assembly, and functions. Annu Rev Biochem, 47:481, 1978

Gould GW, Hurst A (eds): The Bacterial Spore. Academic Press, San Diego, 1969

Jawetz E, Melnick JL, Adelberg EA: Medical Microbiology. Appleton & Lange, East Norwalk, CT, 1989

Rogers HJ: Bacterial Cell Structure. American Society for Microbiology, Washington, D.C., 1983

Salton MRJ, Owen P: Bacterial membrane structure. Annu Rev Microbiol, 30:451, 1976

Wright A, Tipper DJ: The outer membrane of gram-negative bacteria. p. 427. In Sokatch JR, Ornston LN (eds): The bacteria. Vol. 7. Academic Press, San Diego, 1979

3 CLASSIFICATION

DONALD J. BRENNER

GENERAL CONCEPTS

Classification

Bacteria are classified and identified to distinguish organisms and group them by criteria of interest to microbiologists or other scientists.

Nomenclature

Bacteria are named so that investigators can define them without listing their characteristics.

Species

Species are designated by biochemical and other phenotypic criteria and by DNA relatedness, which groups strains on the basis of their overall genetic similarity.

Diagnostic Identification

Bacteria are identified routinely by biochemical tests, supplemented as needed by specialized tests such as serotyping for identification of *Salmonella* and *Shigella* species. Newer molecular techniques permit species to be identified directly by gene probes, sometimes directly from the clinical specimen.

Subtyping

Because of differences in pathogenicity or the necessity to characterize a disease outbreak, strains of medical interest are often classified below the species level by serotyping, bacteriophage typing, identification of toxins or other virulence factors, characterization of plasmids, protein patterns, and enzyme typing.

New and Unusual Species

Laboratories have no difficulty identifying most bacteria. Problems develop with atypical strains and rare or newly described species. These problems are exacerbated when the strains are misidentified rather than unidentified. Therefore, laboratory personnel and physicians (at least infectious disease specialists) must be familiar with taxonomy reference texts and journals that publish papers on new species.

Role of the Clinical Laboratory

Clinical laboratories isolate, identify, and determine the antimicrobial susceptibility pattern of pathogens at the request of physicians, and interface with government public health laboratories.

INTRODUCTION

Bacteria are classified and identified to distinguish one organism from another and to group similar organisms by criteria of interest to microbiologists or to other groups of scientists. The most important level of this type of communication is the species level. A species name should mean the same thing to everyone; there can be no effective communication about bacteria if members of the same species are given different names on the basis of source of isolation, serotype, or the ability to perform a specific function, such as cause a disease or produce an antibiotic. Formerly, species were created on the basis of such criteria, which may be extremely important for clinical microbiologists and physicians but which are not a sufficient basis for establishing a species. Verification of existing species and creation of new species should involve biochemical and other phenotypic criteria as well as DNA relatedness. In *numerical* or *phenetic* approaches to classification, strains are grouped on the basis of a large number of phenotypic characteristics. DNA relatedness is used to group strains on the basis of overall genetic similarity.

Species are identified in the clinical laboratory by biochemical tests, some of which have been supplemented by serologic assessments (e.g., identification of *Salmonella* and *Shigella* species). Because of differences in pathogenicity *(Escherichia coli, Yersinia enterocolitica)* or the necessity to characterize a disease outbreak (members of the Enterobacteriaceae, *Vibrio cholerae, Clostridium, Campylobacter, Staphylococcus, Streptococcus, Pseudomonas aeruginosa)*, strains of medical interest are often classified below the species level by serology, bacteriophage typing (phage typing), or identification of toxins. Pathogenic or epidemic strains also can be classified by the presence of a specific plasmid or by their plasmid profile (the number and sizes of plasmids). Newer molecular biologic techniques have enabled researchers to identify some species (without the use of biochemical tests) by identifying a specific gene or genetic sequence, sometimes directly from the clinical specimen.

Because biochemical identification systems with computer-generated data bases are available commercially, laboratories have no difficulty in identifying typical strains of common bacteria. Problems do arise, however, when atypical strains or rare or newly described species are not in the data base. Such difficulties are compounded when the strains are misidentified rather than unidentified, and so laboratory personnel and physicians (at least infectious disease specialists) should be familiar with taxonomic reference texts and journals that publish papers on new species. In the past, bacterial nomenclature at the genus and species level changed often, and changes still occur occasionally. In addition, a species may acquire more than one name. In some cases the recognition of a new species results in a unique correlation with specific clinical problems, such as the realization that yellow strains first identified as *Enterobacter cloacae* and later shown to be a new species, *Enterobacter sakazakii*, were often responsible for neonatal meningitis. To minimize confusion, it is important to understand why these changes and synonyms exist in taxonomy.

The clinical laboratory is concerned with the rapid, sensitive, and accurate identification of pathogenic bacteria. The number and types of tests done in such a laboratory depend on its size and the population it serves. Highly specialized or rarely performed tests should be done by only state and reference laboratories. Physicians, clinical-laboratory personnel, and reference laboratory personnel must have a good working relationship if patients are to receive first-rate care. In addition, the physician and the clinical-laboratory personnel must know which diseases are reportable to state and federal health laboratories and how to report them.

DEFINITIONS
Taxonomy

Taxonomy is the science of classification. For eukaryotes, the definition of the species usually stresses the ability of similar organisms to reproduce sexually with the formation of a zygote and to produce fertile offspring. However, bacteria do not undergo sexual reproduction in the eukaryotic sense. Taxonomy involves classification, identification, and nomenclature.

Classification

Classification is the orderly arrangement of bacteria into groups. There is nothing inherently scientific about classification, and different groups of scientists may classify the same organisms differently. For example, clinical microbiologists are interested in the serotype, antimicrobial resistance pattern, and toxin and invasiveness factors in *Escherichia coli*, whereas geneticists are concerned with specific mutations and plasmids.

Identification

Identification is the practical use of a classification to isolate and distinguish certain organisms from others, to verify the authenticity or utility of a culture or a particular reaction, or to isolate and identify the organism that causes a disease or condition.

Nomenclature

Nomenclature is the means by which the characteristics of a species are defined and communicated among microbiologists. A species name should mean the same thing to all microbiologists, yet some definitions vary in different countries or microbiologic specialty groups. *Klebsiella pneumoniae* is defined differently in England than in most other parts of the world, and *Vibrio cholerae* often has been equated with a single serotype by epidemiologists and clinical microbiologists.

Species

A bacterial species is a distinct organism with certain characteristic features, or a group of organisms that resemble one another closely in the most important features of their organization. In the past, unfortunately, there was little consensus about the definition of a close resemblance, about the most important features of an organism, and about the number of features necessary to distinguish a species. Species were often defined solely by such criteria as host range, pathogenicity, ability or inability to produce gas in the fermentation of a given sugar, and rapid or delayed fermentation of sugars. Because there was no method for devising a single species definition that could be used by all researchers, criteria reflected the interests of the investigators who described a particular species. For example, bacteria that caused plant diseases were often defined by the plant from which they were isolated; also, each new *Salmonella* serotype that was discovered was given species status. These practices have been replaced by genetic criteria that can be used to define species in all groups of bacteria.

APPROACHES TO TAXONOMY

Numerical Approach

In their studies on members of the family Enterobacteriaceae, Edwards and Ewing established the following principles to characterize, classify, and identify organisms (Lennette et al., 1985):

> Classification and identification of an organism should be based on its overall morphologic and biochemical pattern. A single characteristic (pathogenicity, host range, or biochemical reaction), regardless of its importance, is not a sufficient basis for classifying or identifying an organism.

> A large and diverse strain sample must be tested to determine accurately the biochemical characteristics used to distinguish a given species.

> Atypical strains often are perfectly typical members of a given biogroup within an existing species, but sometimes they are typical members of an unrecognized new species.

In numerical taxonomy (also called computer or phenetic taxonomy), many (50 to 200) biochemical, morphologic, and cultural characteristics, as well as susceptibilities to antibiotics and inorganic compounds, are used to determine the degree of similarity between organisms. In numerical studies, investigators often calculate the *coefficient of similarity* or *percentage of similarity* between strains (where *strain* indicates a single isolate from a specimen). A dendrogram or a similarity matrix is constructed that joins individual strains into groups and places one group with other groups on the basis of their percentage of similarity. In the dendrogram in Figure 3-1, group 1 represents three *Citrobacter freundii* strains that are about 95 percent similar and join with a fourth *C freundii* strain at the level of 90 percent similarity. Group 2 is composed of three *Citrobacter diversus* strains that are 95 percent similar, and group 3 contains two *E coli* strains that are 95 percent similar, as well as a third *E coli* strain to which they are 90 percent similar. Similarity between groups 1 and 2 occurs at the 70 percent level, and group 3 is about 50 percent similar to groups 1 and 2.

Either all the characteristics in the similarity matrix are given equal weight, or certain characters may be weighted more heavily; for example, the presence of spores in *Clostridium* might be weighted more heavily than the organism's ability to use a given carbon source. A given level of similarity can be equated with relatedness at the genus, species, and, sometimes, subspecies levels. For instance, strains of a given species may cluster at a 90% similarity level, species within a given genus may cluster at the 70 percent level, and different

genera in the same family may cluster at the 50 percent or lower level (Fig. 3-1).

When this approach is the only basis for defining a species, it is difficult to know how many and which tests should be chosen; whether the tests should be weighted and, if so, how; what level of similarity should be chosen to reflect relatedness at the genus and species levels; and whether the same level of similarity applies to all groups.

Most bacteria have enough DNA to specify some 1,500 to 6,000 average-sized genes. Therefore, even a battery of 300 tests would assay only 5 to 20 percent of the genetic potential of a bacterium. Tests that are comparatively simple to conduct (such as those for carbohydrate utilization and for enzymes whose presence can be assayed colorimetrically) are performed more often than tests for structural, reproductive, and regulatory genes, whose presence is difficult to assay.

Other types of errors may occur when species are classified solely on the basis of phenotype. For example, different enzymes (specified by different genes) may catalyze the same reaction. Also, even if a metabolic gene is functional, negative reactions can occur because of the inability of the substrate to enter the cell or because of a mutation in a regulatory gene. A negative reaction also can occur if the gene is present but is not functional because of a mutation that produces an inactive protein. There is not necessarily a one-to-one correlation between a reaction and the number of genes needed to carry out that reaction. For instance, six enzymatic steps may be involved in a given pathway. If an assay for the end product is performed, a positive reaction indicates six similar enzymes, whereas a negative reaction can mean the absence or nonfunction of one to six enzymes. Fastidious strains will not cluster with nonfastidious strains from the same species. Several other strain characteristics can affect phenotypic characterization; these include growth rate, incubation temperature, salt requirement, and pH. Plasmids that carry metabolic genes can enable strains to carry out reactions that rarely, if ever, occur in plasmidless strains of the same species.

The same set of "definitive" reactions cannot be used to classify all groups of organisms, and there

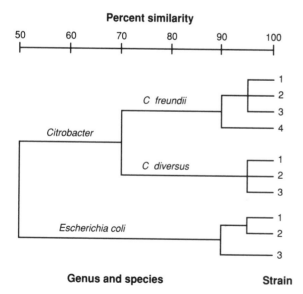

Percent similarity

FIGURE 3-1 Example of a dendrogram.

is no standard number of specific reactions that allows identification of a species. Organisms are identified on the basis of phenotype, but, from the taxonomic standpoint, definition of species solely on this basis is subject to error.

Phylogenetic Approach

The ideal means of identifying and classifying bacteria would be to compare each gene sequence in a given strain with the gene sequences for every known species. This cannot be done, but the total DNA of one organism can be compared with that of any other organism by a method called **nucleic acid hybridization** or **DNA hybridization.** This method can be used to measure the number of DNA sequences that any two organisms have in common and to estimate the percentage of divergence or unpaired nucleotide bases within DNA sequences that are related but not identical. DNA relatedness studies have been done for yeasts, viruses, bacteriophages, and many groups of bacteria.

Five factors can be used to determine DNA relatedness: genome size, guanine-plus-cytosine (G+C) content, DNA relatedness under conditions optimal for DNA reassociation, thermal stability of related DNA sequences, and DNA relatedness under conditions supraoptimal for DNA reassociation. Because it is not practical to conduct these genotypic or phylogenetic evaluations in clinical laboratories, the results of biochemical tests usually must be correlated with known phylogenetic data. For example, yellow strains of *Enterobacter cloacae* were shown by DNA relatedness, to form a separate species, *Enterobacter sakazakii*, but were not designated as such until results of practical tests were correlated with the DNA data.

Genome Size

True bacterial DNAs have genome sizes (measured as molecular weight) between 1×10^9 and 8×10^9. Genome size determinations sometimes can distinguish between groups. They were used to distinguish *Legionella pneumophila* (the legionnaire's disease bacterium) from *Rochalimaea (Rickettsia)* *quintana*. *L pneumophila* has a genome size of about 3×10^9; that of *R quintana* is about 1×10^9.

Guanine-plus-Cytosine Content

The G+C content in bacterial DNA ranges from about 25 to 75 percent. This percentage is specific, but not exclusive, for a species; two strains with a similar G+C content may or may not belong to the same species. If the G+C contents are very different, however, the strains cannot be members of the same species. Assessments of G+C content are especially useful in grouping strains for further testing.

DNA Relatedness under Conditions Optimal for DNA Reassociation

DNA relatedness is determined by allowing single-stranded DNA from one strain to reassociate with single-stranded DNA from a second strain, to form a double-stranded DNA molecule (Figure 3-2). This is a specific, temperature-dependent reaction. The optimal temperature for DNA reassociation is 25 to 30°C below the temperature at which native double-stranded DNA denatures into single strands. Many studies indicate that a bacterial species is composed of strains that are 70 to 100 percent related. In contrast, relatedness between different species is 0 to about 65 percent. It is important to emphasize that the term ''related'' does not mean ''identical'' or ''homologous.'' Similar nucleic acid sequences can reassociate.

Thermal Stability of Related DNA Sequences

Each 1 percent of unpaired nucleotide bases in a double-stranded DNA sequence causes a 1 percent decrease in the thermal stability of that DNA duplex. Therefore, a comparison between the thermal stability of a control double-stranded molecule (in which both strands of DNA are from the same organism) and that of a heteroduplex (DNA strands from two different organisms) allows assessment of divergence in related nucleotide sequences.

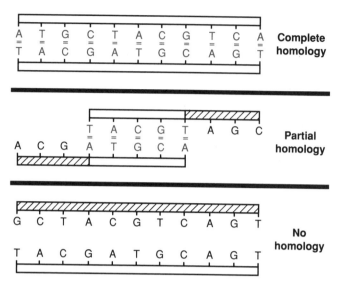

FIGURE 3-2   Diagram of DNA reassociation. DNA is composed of two purine nucleoside bases, adenine (A) and guanine (G), and two pyrimidine nucleoside bases, thymine (T) and cytosine (C). Double-stranded DNA is formed through hydrogen bonds that can occur only between the complementary bases A and T or G and C. (Top) Perfectly reassociated DNA base sequence in which all nucleosides are paired by hydrogen bonds. (Middle) Perfectly paired DNA base sequence in the center with unpaired, single-strand ends on each strand. (Bottom) None of the bases in the sequence (left to right) GCTACGTCAGTon the top strand are complementary to the sequence TACGATGCAGT in the bottom strand.

DNA Relatedness under Supraoptimal Conditions for DNA Reassociation

When the incubation temperature used for DNA reassociation is raised from 25–30°C below the renaturation temperature to only 10–15°C below the denaturation temperature, only very closely related (and therefore highly thermally stable) DNA sequences can reassociate. Strains from the same species are 60 percent or more related at these supraoptimal incubation temperatures.

Defining Species on the Basis of DNA Relatedness

Use of these five factors allows a species definition based on DNA. Thus, *E coli* can be defined as a series of strains with a G+C content of 49 to 52 moles percent, a genome molecular weight of 2.3×10^9 to 3.0×10^9, relatedness of 70 percent or more at an optimal reassociation temperature with 0 to 4 percent divergence in related sequences, and relatedness of 60 percent or more at a supraoptimal reassociation temperature. Experience with more than 300 species has produced an arbitrary phylogenetic definition of a species to which most taxonomists subscribe: "strains with approximately 70% or greater DNA-DNA relatedness and with 5°C or less divergence in related sequences." When these two criteria are met, genome size and G+C content are always similar and relatedness is almost always 60 percent or more at supraoptimal incubation temperatures. The 70 percent species relatedness rule has been ignored occasionally when the existing nomenclature is deeply ingrained, as is that for *E coli* and the four *Shigella* species. Because these organisms are all 70 percent or more related, DNA studies indicate that they should be grouped into a single species, instead of the present five species in two genera. This change has not been made because of the presumed confusion that would result.

DNA relatedness provides one species definition that can be applied equally to all organisms.
Moreover, it cannot be affected by phenotypic
variation, mutations, or the presence or absence of
metabolic or other plasmids. It measures overall
relatedness, and these factors affect only a very
small percentage of the total DNA.

Polyphasic Approach

In practice, the approach to bacterial taxonomy
should be polyphasic (Fig. 3-3). The first step is
phenotypic grouping of strains by biochemical and
antigenic reactions and any other characteristics of
interest. The phenotypic groups are then tested
for DNA relatedness to determine whether the observed phenotypic homogeneity (or heterogeneity)
is reflected by phylogenetic homogeneity or heterogeneity. The third and most important step is
reexamination of the biochemical characteristics
of the DNA relatedness groups. This allows determination of the biochemical borders of each group
and determination of reactions of diagnostic value
for the group. For identification of a given orga-

nism, the importance of specific tests is weighted
on the basis of correlation with DNA results. Occasionally, the reactions commonly used will not
distinguish completely between two distinct DNA
relatedness groups. In these cases, other biochemical tests of diagnostic value must be sought.

PHENOTYPIC CHARACTERISTICS USEFUL IN CLASSIFICATION AND IDENTIFICATION

Morphologic Characteristics

Wet-mounted and properly stained specimens can
yield a great deal of information. Simple tests can
indicate the Gram reaction of the organism;
whether it is acid fast; its motility; the arrangement
of its flagella; the presence of spores, capsules, and
inclusion bodies; and, of course, its shape. This
information often can allow identification of an
organism to the genus level, or can minimize the
possibility that it belongs to one or another group.
Colony characteristics and pigmentation are also
quite helpful. For example, colonies of several *Le-*

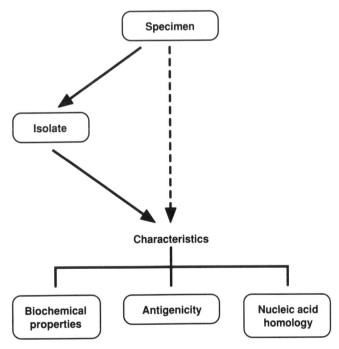

FIGURE 3-3 Bacterial identification.

gionella species autofluoresce under long-wavelength ultraviolet light, and *Proteus* species swarm on appropriate media.

Growth Characteristics

A primary distinguishing characteristic is whether an organism grows aerobically, anaerobically, facultatively (i.e., in either the presence or absence of oxygen), or microaerophilically (i.e., in the presence of a less than atmospheric partial pressure of oxygen). The proper atmospheric conditions are essential for isolating and identifying bacteria. Other important growth assessments include the incubation temperature, pH, nutrients required, and resistance to antibiotics. For example, one diarrheal disease agent, *Campylobacter jejuni*, grows well at 42°C in the presence of several antibiotics; another, *Y enterocolitica*, grows better than most other bacteria at 4°C. *Legionella, Haemophilus,* and some other pathogens require specific growth factors, whereas *E coli* and most other enterobacteria can grow on minimal media.

Antigens and Phage Susceptibility

Cell wall (O), flagellar (H), and capsular (K) antigens are used to aid in classifying certain organisms at the species level, to serotype strains of medically important species for epidemiologic purposes, or to identify serotypes of public health importance. Serotyping is also sometimes used to distinguish strains of exceptional virulence or public health importance, for example with *V cholerae* (O1 is the pandemic strain) and *E coli* (enterotoxigenic, enteroinvasive, enterohemorrhagic, and enteropathogenic serotypes).

Phage typing (determining the susceptibility pattern of an isolate to a set of specific bacteriophages) is used primarily as an aid in epidemiologic surveillance of diseases caused by *Staphylococcus aureus*, mycobacteria, *P aeruginosa, V cholerae,* and *S typhi*. Phage susceptibility also can be a valuable aid in classification and identification. For example, virtually all *Hafnia* strains are sensitive to a *Hafnia*-specific bacteriophage, and almost all clinically significant salmonellae are susceptible to *Salmonella* phage O1. Susceptibility to bacteriocins

sometimes is used as an epidemiologic strain marker.

Biochemical Characteristics

Most bacteria are identified and classified largely on the basis of their reactions in a series of biochemical tests. Some tests are used routinely for many groups of bacteria (oxidase, nitrate reduction, amino acid degrading enzymes, fermentation or utilization of carbohydrates); others are restricted to a single family, genus, or species (coagulase for staphylococci, arylsulfatase for mycobacteria, tyrosine clearing for *Proteus,* sensitivity to the vibriostatic agent O/129 for *Vibrio*).

A strong argument has been made for identifying species in the clinical laboratory. Such identification, however, depends on the number of tests done. Both the number of tests and the actual tests used vary from one group of organisms to another. Therefore, the lengths to which a laboratory should go in identifying organisms and the organisms for which it should screen must be decided in each laboratory on the basis of its function and the type of population it serves. For example, the Enteric Laboratory Section at the Centers for Disease Control (CDC) uses at least 46 tests to identify members of the Enterobacteriaceae, whereas various commercially available identification kits offer 14 to 21 tests.

CLASSIFICATION BELOW AND ABOVE THE SPECIES LEVEL

Below the Species Level

Clinical microbiologists must often distinguish strains with particular traits from other strains in the same species. Occasionally, a subspecies designation is convenient, although subspecies are not commonly used clinically. Examples of subspecies designations are six subspecies in *Salmonella enteritidis*. Salmonellae are reported clinically by serotype: *Salmonella* serotype typhi *(S typhi), Salmonella* serotype typhimurium *(S typhimurium).*

The communication needs of clinical microbiologists should be met by designations below the species level as *groups* or *types* on the basis of common serologic or biochemical reactions, phage or bacteriocin sensitivity, pathogenicity, or other characteristics. Many of these characteristics are already used and accepted: serotype, phage type, colicin type, biotype, bioserotype (a group of strains from the same species with common biochemical and serologic characteristics that set them apart from other members of the species), and pathotype (e.g., toxigenic *E coli*, invasive *E coli*, toxigenic *V cholerae*, and β-hemolytic streptococci).

Above the Species Level

In addition to species and subspecies designations, clinical microbiologists must be familiar with genera and families. A genus is a group of related species, and a family is a group of related genera.

An ideal genus would be composed of species with similar phenotypic and phylogenetic characteristics. Some phenotypically homogeneous genera approach this criterion *(Citrobacter, Yersinia,* and *Serratia)*. More often, however, the phenotypic similarity is present, but the genetic relatedness is not. *Bacillus, Clostridium, Vibrio, Campylobacter, Pseudomonas,* and *Legionella* are accepted phenotypic genera in which genetic relatedness between species is not 50 to 65 percent, but 0 to 65 percent. When phenotypic and genetic similarity are not both present, phenotypic similarity generally should be given priority in establishing genera. When organisms are identified at the bench, it is convenient to have the most phenotypically similar species in the same genus. The primary consideration for a genus is that it contain biochemically similar species that are convenient or important to consider as a group and that must be separated from one another.

The sequencing of ribosomal RNA (rRNA) genes, which have been highly conserved through evolution, allows phylogenetic comparisons to be made between species whose total DNAs are essentially unrelated. It also allows phylogenetic classification at the genus, family, and higher taxonomic levels. The rRNA sequence data are usually not used to designate genera or families unless supported by similarities in phenotypic tests.

DESIGNATION OF NEW SPECIES AND NOMENCLATURAL CHANGES

Species are named according to principles and rules of nomenclature set forth in the Bacteriological Code. Scientific names are taken from Latin or Greek. The correct name of a species or higher taxon is determined by three criteria: valid publication, legitimacy of the name with regard to the rules of nomenclature, and priority of publication (that is, it must be the first validly published name for the taxon).

To be published validly, a new species proposal must contain the species name, a description of the species, and the designation of a type strain for the species, and the name must be published in the *International Journal for Systematic Bacteriology (IJSB)*. Once proposed, a name does not go through a formal process to be accepted officially; in fact, the opposite is true—a validly published name is assumed to be correct unless and until it is challenged officially. A challenge is initiated by publishing a request for an opinion (to the Judicial Commission of the International Association of Microbiological Societies) in the *IJSB*. This occurs only in cases in which the validity of a name is questioned with respect to compliance with the rules of the Bacteriological Code. A question of classification that is based on scientific data (for example, whether a species, on the basis of its biochemical or genetic characteristics, or both, should be placed in a new genus or an existing genus) is not settled by the Judicial Commission, but by the preference and usage of the scientific community. This is why there are pairs of names such as *Citrobacter diversus/Levinea malonatica, Providencia rettgeri/Proteus rettgeri, Legionella dumoffii/Fluoribacter dumoffii,* and *Legionella micdadei/Tatlockia micdadei*. It is often necessary to be familiar with more than one name for a single organism. This is not, however, restricted to bacterial nomenclature. Multiple names exist for many antibiotics and other drugs and enzymes.

The best source of information for new species proposals and nomenclatural changes is the *IJSB*. In addition, the *Journal of Clinical Microbiology* often publishes descriptions of newly described bacteria isolated from clinical sources. Information, including biochemical reactions and sources of isolation about new organisms of clinical importance, disease outbreaks caused by newer species, and reviews of clinical significance of certain organisms may be found in the *Annals of Internal Medicine, Journal of Infectious Diseases, Clinical Microbiology Reviews,* and *Reviews of Infectious Diseases.* The data provided in these publications supplement and update *Bergey's Manual of Systematic Bacteriology,* the definitive taxonomic reference text.

ASSESSING NEWLY DESCRIBED BACTERIA

Since 1974, the number of genera in the family Enterobacteriaceae has increased from 12 to 29 and the number of species from 42 to 145, some of which have not yet been named. Similar explosions have occurred in other genera. In 1974, five species were listed in the genus *Vibrio* and four in *Campylobacter;* the genus *Legionella* was unknown. Today, there are 38 species in *Vibrio,* 16 *Campylobacter* species, and 45 species in *Legionella.* From 1980 to 1988, the total number of bacterial genera increased from 290 to 494 and the number of species from 1,693 to 2,681.

The clinical significance of the agent of legionnaire's disease was well known long before it was isolated, characterized, and classified as *Legionella pneumophila.* In most cases, little is known about the clinical significance of a new species at the time it is described. Usually, only after a species description has been published and the organism has been isolated and identified do assessments of clinical significance begin.

New species will continue to be described. Some will be pathogens, and many will be able to infect humans, especially immunocompromised, burn, postsurgical, geriatric, and acquired immune deficiency syndrome (AIDS) patients, under the right conditions (infrequent opportunistic pathogens).

ROLE OF THE CLINICAL LABORATORY

Clinical laboratories should be able to isolate, identify, and determine the antimicrobial susceptibility pattern of the vast majority of human disease

agents, so that physicians can initiate appropriate treatment as soon as possible and the source and means of transmission of outbreaks can be ascertained to control the disease and prevent its recurrence. The need to identify pathogens both quickly and cost-effectively presents a considerable challenge.

To be effective, the professional clinical laboratory staff must interact with the infectious disease staff. Laboratory scientists should make infectious disease rounds. They must keep abreast of new technology, equipment, and classification and should communicate this information to their medical colleagues. They should interpret, qualify, or explain laboratory reports. If a bacterial name is changed or a new species reported, the laboratory should provide background information, including a reference.

The clinical laboratory must be efficient. A concerted effort must be made to eliminate or minimize inappropriate and contaminated specimens, unwarranted tests, and after-hours service in the absence of an emergency. Standards for the selection, collection, and transport of specimens should be developed for both laboratory and nursing procedure manuals and reviewed periodically by a committee composed of medical, nursing, and laboratory staff.

Biochemical and Susceptibility Testing

Most laboratories today use either commercially available miniaturized biochemical test systems or automated instruments for biochemical tests and for susceptibility testing. The kits usually contain 10 to 20 tests. The test results are converted to numerical biochemical profiles that are identified by using a codebook or a computer. Most identification takes 4 to 24 hours. Also available are many biochemical test kits for which data bases are not available. These include carbon source and enzymatic tests that are not routinely used but may be valuable for a specific species and for atypical strains.

Automated instruments can be used to identify most Gram-negative fermenters and nonfermenters; most can be used for Gram-positive pathogens, but not for anaerobes. Antimicrobial susceptibility testing can be performed with this equipment by giving approximate minimum inhibitory drug concentrations. Both tasks take 4 to 24 hours. If semiautomated instruments are used, some manipulation is done by the technician, and the cultures (in miniature cards or microdilution plates) are incubated outside of the instrument. The test containers are then read rapidly by the instrument, and the identification is made automatically. Instruments are now available for identification of bacteria by cell wall fatty acid profiles generated by gas-liquid chromatography (GLC) and by protein-banding patterns generated by polyacrylamide gel electrophoresis (PAGE). Some other instruments designed to speed laboratory diagnosis of bacteria are those that detect (but do not identify) bacteria in blood cultures in 8 to 18 hours. Also available are many rapid screening systems for detecting one or a series of specific bacteria, including staphylococci, streptococci, *H influenzae, N meningitidis*, salmonellae, and chlamydiae. These screening systems are based on fluorescent antibody, agglutination, or rapid biochemical plating procedures.

It is important to diagnose pathogens presumptively before identification is completed, so that appropriate therapy can be initiated as quickly as possible. A Gram stain, spot indole test, rapid oxidase test, and spore and acid-fast stains may allow presumptive identification within minutes. Rapid enzymatic tests can render presumptive identification in 1 hour or less.

Role of the Reference Laboratory

Despite recent advances, the armamentarium of the clinical laboratory is far from complete. Few laboratories can or should conduct the specialized tests that are often essential to distinguish virulent from avirulent strains. Serotyping is done only for a few species, and phage typing only rarely. Few pathogenicity tests are performed. Not many laboratories can conduct comprehensive biochemical tests on strains that cannot be identified readily by commercially available biochemical systems. Even fewer laboratories are equipped to perform plasmid profiles, gene probes, or DNA hybridization.

These and other specialized tests for the serologic or biochemical identification of some exotic bacteria, as well as pathogenic yeasts, fungi, protozoans, and viruses, are best done in district, state, or federal reference laboratories. It is not cost-effective to keep, and control the quality of, reagents and media for tests that are seldom run or quite complex. Sensitive methods for the epidemiologic subtyping of isolates from disease outbreaks, such as electrophoretic enzyme typing, rRNA fingerprinting, whole-cell protein electrophoretic patterns, and restriction endonuclease analysis of whole-cell or plasmid DNA, are used only in reference laboratories and a few large medical centers.

Specific genetic probes are now available commercially for identifying virulence factors and many bacteria and viruses. These probes are now used mainly on isolated colonies, but gene probes will eventually allow identification by species or pathogenicity factors within 48 hours of sampling —without the need to isolate the organism. Those for *Mycoplasma* and *Legionella* are now being used directly on clinical specimens.

INTERFACING WITH PUBLIC HEALTH LABORATORIES

Hospital and local clinical laboratories interact with district, state, and federal health laboratories in several important ways (Fig. 3-4). The clinical laboratories participate in quality control and proficiency testing programs that are conducted by their state health department laboratories or by the CDC. The reference laboratories supply cultures and often reagents for use in quality control, and they conduct training programs for clinical laboratory personnel.

All types of laboratories should interact closely to provide diagnostic services and epidemic surveillance (Fig. 3-3). The primary concern of the clinical laboratory is identifying infectious disease agents and studying nosocomial and local outbreaks of disease. The local laboratory may ask the state laboratory for help in identifying an unusual organism, serotyping or phage typing various bacteria, discovering the cause or mode of transmission in a disease outbreak, or performing specialized tests not done routinely in clinical

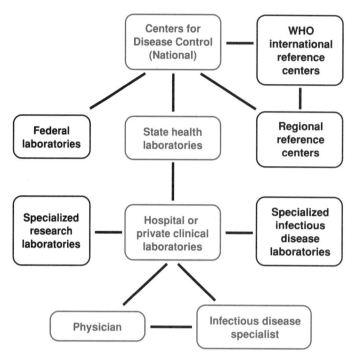

FIGURE 3-4 Pathways for laboratory identification of pathogens and information exchange.

laboratories. The local laboratory's request should be justified. Cultures should be pure and should be sent on appropriate media with pertinent clinical laboratory information, including the following: name and address of the submitting laboratory and the person to be contacted if additional information is required; culture or specimen number and type of specimen; date sent; patient name (or number), date of birth, and sex; clinical diagnosis, associated illness, date of onset, and present condition; laboratory test requested; category of agent, specific agent suspected, and any other organisms isolated; origin, source, and date of isolation of specimen; relevant epidemiologic and clinical data; treatment of patient; and previous laboratory results (biochemical or serologic tests).

These data allow the state laboratory to test the specimen properly and quickly, and they provide information about occurrences within the state. For example, a food-borne outbreak might extend to many parts of the state (or beyond its boundaries). The state laboratory can alert local physicians to the possibility of such outbreaks.

Another necessary interaction between local and state laboratories is the reporting of notifiable diseases by the local laboratory. The state laboratory makes available to local laboratories summaries of the incidence of these diseases. The state laboratories also submit the summaries to the CDC weekly (or, for some diseases, yearly), and national summaries are published weekly in the *Morbidity and Mortality Weekly Report*.

Interaction between the CDC and state and federal laboratories is very similar to that between local and state laboratories. The CDC provides quality control cultures and reagents to state laboratories, and serves as a national reference laboratory for diagnostic services and epidemiologic surveillance. The CDC participates in monitoring disease outbreaks only when invited to do so by a state health official. Local laboratories cannot send specimens or cultures directly to the CDC;

instead, they must send specimens to the state health laboratory, which, when necessary, forwards them to the CDC. The CDC reports its results back to the state laboratory, which then reports to the local laboratory.

HAZARDS OF CLINICAL LABORATORY WORK

Clinical laboratory personnel, including support and clerical employees, are subject to the risk of infection, chemical hazards, and, in some laboratories, radioactive contamination. Such risks can be prevented or minimized by a laboratory safety program.

Radiation Hazards

Personnel who work with radioactive materials should have taken a radioactivity safety course; they should wear radiation monitor badges and be aware of the methods for decontaminating hands, clothing, work surfaces, and equipment. They should wear gloves when working with radioactive compounds; when they work with high-level radiation they should use a hood and stand behind a radiation shield. Preparative radioactive work should be done in a separate room with access only by personnel who are involved directly in the work.

Chemical Hazards

Chemicals can harm laboratory personnel through inhalation or skin absorption of volatile compounds; bodily contact with acids, bases, and other harmful chemicals; or introduction of poisonous or skin-damaging liquids into the mouth. Good laboratory practices require that volatile compounds be handled only under a hood, that hazardous chemicals never be pipetted by mouth, and that anyone working with skin-damaging chemicals wear gloves and eye guards. Workers should be familiar with procedures for chemical decontamination.

Biologic Hazards

Microbiologic contamination is the greatest hazard in clinical microbiology laboratories. Laboratory infections are a danger not only to the clinical laboratory personnel but also to anyone else who enters the laboratory, including janitors, clerical and maintenance personnel, and visitors. The risk of infection is governed by the frequency and length of contact with the infectious agent, its virulence, the dose and route of administration, and the susceptibility of the host. The inherent hazard of any infectious agent is affected by factors such as the volume of infectious material used, handling of the material, effectiveness of safety containment equipment, and soundness of laboratory methods.

If possible, agents that are treated differently, such as viruses as opposed to bacteria, or *M tuberculosis* in contrast to *E coli,* should be handled in different laboratories or in different parts of the same laboratory. When the risk category of an agent is known, it should be handled in an area with appropriate containment. All specimens sent for isolation of infectious agents and all organisms sent to the laboratory for identification should be assumed to be pathogenic. A separate area should be set aside for the receipt of specimens. Personnel should be aware of the potential hazards of improperly packed, broken, or leaking packages and of the proper methods for their handling and decontamination.

To prevent infection, personnel should wear laboratory coats at all times, wash their hands at the conclusion of each exposure to pathogenic agents, be forbidden to use mouth pipetting, and not carry food or cigarettes into the laboratory. Immunization may be appropriate for employees who are exposed often to certain infectious agents, including hepatitis B, yellow fever, rabies, and polioviruses, meningococcus, *Y pestis, S typhi,* and *Francisella tularensis.*

Biosafety Levels

Infectious agents are assigned to a **biosafety level** from 1 to 4 on the basis of their virulence. The containment levels for organisms should correlate with the biosafety level assigned. Biosafety level 1 is for well-defined organisms not known to cause disease in healthy humans; it includes certain nonvirulent *E coli* strains (such as K-12) and *B subtilis.*

Containment level 1 involves standard microbiologic practices, and safety equipment is not needed.

Biosafety level 2, the minimum level for clinical laboratories, is for moderate-risk agents associated with human disease. Containment level 2 includes limited access to the work area, decontamination of all infectious wastes, use of protective gloves, and a biologic safety cabinet for use in procedures that may create aerosols. Examples of biosafety level 2 agents include nematode, protozoan, trematode, and cestode human parasites; all human fungal pathogens except *Coccidiodes immitis;* all members of the Enterobacteriaceae except *Y pestis; Bacillus anthracis;* brucellae; *Clostridium tetani; Corynebacterium diphtheriae; Haemophilus* species; leptospires; legionellae; mycobacteria other than *M tuberculosis;* pathogenic *Neisseria* species; staphylococci, streptococci, *Treponema pallidum; V cholerae;* and hepatitis and influenza viruses.

Biosafety level 3 is for agents that are associated with risk of serious or fatal aerosol infection. In containment level 3, laboratory access is controlled, special clothing is worn in the laboratory, and containment equipment is used for all work with the agent. *M tuberculosis, Coccidiodes immitis, Coxiella burnetii,* and many of the arboviruses are biosafety 3 level agents. Containment level 3 usually is recommended for work with rickettsiae, brucellae, *Y pestis,* and a wide variety of viruses, including human immunodeficiency viruses.

Biosafety level 4 indicates dangerous and novel agents that cause diseases with high fatality rates. Maximum containment and decontamination procedures are used in containment level 4, which is found in only a few reference and research laboratories. Only a few viruses (Lassa, Ebola, and Marburg viruses) are classified in biosafety level 4.

REFERENCES

Bergey's Manual of Systematic Bacteriology. Vol. 1–4. Williams & Wilkins, Baltimore, 1984–1989

Center for Infectious Diseases. Reference/Diagnostic Services. Atlanta: Centers for Disease Control

Centers for Disease Control: Morbidity and Mortality Weekly Report. Atlanta: Centers for Disease Control.

Lapage SP, et al: International Code of Nomenclature of Bacteria. 1975 revision. American Society for Microbiology, Washington, D.C., 1975

Lennette EH, et al: Manual of Clinical Microbiology 4th Ed. American Society for Microbiology, Washington, D.C., 1985

Richardson JH, Barkley WE (eds): Biosafety in Microbiological and Biomedical Laboratories. 2nd Ed. Centers for Disease Control, Atlanta, and National Institutes of Health, Bethesda, Md., 1988

Skerman VBD, McGowan V, Sneath PHA (eds): Approved lists of bacterial names. Int J Syst Bacteriol 30:225, 1980

4 BACTERIAL METABOLISM

PETER JURTSHUK, JR.

GENERAL CONCEPTS

Heterotrophic Metabolism

Heterotrophic metabolism is the biologic oxidation of organic compounds, such as glucose, to yield ATP and simpler organic (or inorganic) compounds, which are needed by the bacterial cell for biosynthetic or assimilatory reactions.

Respiration

Respiration is a type of heterotrophic metabolism that uses oxygen and in which 38 moles of ATP are derived from the oxidation of 1 mole of glucose, yielding 380,000 cal. (An additional 308,000 cal is lost as heat.)

Fermentation

In **fermentation,** another type of heterotrophic metabolism, an organic compound rather than oxygen is the terminal electron (or hydrogen) acceptor. Less energy is generated from this incomplete form of glucose oxidation, but the process supports anaerobic growth.

Krebs Cycle

The **Krebs cycle** is the oxidative process in respiration by which pyruvate (via acetyl coenzyme A) is completely decarboxylated to CO_2. The pathway yields 15 moles of ATP (150,000 calories).

Glyoxylate Cycle

The **glyoxylate cycle,** which occurs in some bacteria, is a modification of the Krebs cycle. Acetyl coenzyme A is generated directly from oxidation of fatty acids or other lipid compounds.

Electron Transport and Oxidative Phosphorylation

In the final stage of respiration, ATP is formed through a series of electron transfer reactions within the cytoplasmic membrane that drive the oxidative phosphorylation of ADP to ATP. Bacteria use various flavins, cytochrome, and non-heme iron components as well as multiple cytochrome oxidases for this process.

Mitchell Hypothesis

The **Mitchell hypothesis** explains the energy conservation in all cells on the basis of an osmotic potential caused by a proton gradient across a proton-impermeable membrane.

Bacterial Photosynthesis

Bacterial photosynthesis is a light-dependent, anaerobic mode of metabolism. Carbon dioxide is reduced to glucose, which is used for both biosynthesis and energy production. Depending on the hydrogen source used to reduce CO_2, both photolithotrophic and photoorganotrophic reactions exist in bacteria.

Autotrophy

Autotrophy is a unique form of metabolism found only in bacteria. Inorganic compounds are oxidized directly (without using sunlight) to yield energy (e.g., NH_3, NO_2,

S_2, and Fe^{2+}). This metabolic mode also requires energy for CO_2 reduction, like photosynthesis, but no lipid-mediated processes are involved. This metabolic mode has also been called **chemotrophy, chemoautotrophy,** or **chemolithotrophy.**

Anaerobic Respiration

Anaerobic respiration is another heterotrophic mode of metabolism in which a specific compound other than O_2 serves as a terminal electron acceptor. Such acceptor compounds include NO_3^-, SO_4^{2-}, fumarate, and even CO_2 for methane-producing bacteria.

The Nitrogen Cycle

The **nitrogen cycle** consists of a recycling process by which organic and inorganic nitrogen compounds are used metabolically and recycled among bacteria, plants, and animals. Important processes, including ammonification, mineralization, nitrification, denitrification, and nitrogen fixation, are carried out primarily by bacteria.

INTRODUCTION

Metabolism refers to all the biochemical reactions that occur in a cell or organism. The study of bacterial metabolism focuses on the chemical diversity of substrate oxidations and **dissimilation reactions** (reactions by which substrate molecules are broken down), which normally function in bacteria to generate energy. Also within the scope of bacterial metabolism is the study of the uptake and utilization of the inorganic or organic compounds required for growth and maintenance of a cellular steady state **(assimilation reactions).** These respective **exergonic** (energy-yielding) and **endergonic** (energy-requiring) **reactions** are catalyzed within the living bacterial cell by integrated enzyme systems, the end result being self-replication of the cell. The capability of microbial cells to live, function, and replicate in an appropriate chemical milieu (such as a bacterial culture medium) and the chemical changes that result during this transformation constitute the scope of bacterial metabolism.

The bacterial cell is a highly specialized energy transformer. Chemical energy generated by substrate oxidations is conserved by formation of high-energy compounds such as adenosine diphosphate (ADP) and adenosine triphosphate (ATP) or compounds containing the thioester bond

$$(R-\overset{\overset{\displaystyle O}{\displaystyle \|}}{C} \sim S-R),$$ such as acetyl $\sim$ *S*-coenzyme A

(acetyl $\sim$ SCoA) or succinyl $\sim$ SCoA. ADP and ATP represent adenosine monophosphate (AMP) plus one and two high-energy phosphates (AMP $\sim$ P and AMP $\sim$ P $\sim$ P, respectively); the energy is stored in these compounds as high-energy phosphate bonds. In the presence of proper enzyme systems, these compounds can be used as energy sources to synthesize the new complex organic compounds needed by the cell. All living cells must maintain steady-state biochemical reactions for the formation and use of such high-energy compounds.

Kluyver and Donker (1924 to 1926) recognized that bacterial cells, regardless of species, were in many respects similar chemically to all other living cells. For example, these investigators recognized that hydrogen transfer is a common and fundamental feature of all metabolic processes. Bacteria, like mammalian and plant cells, use ATP or the high-energy phosphate bond ($\sim$ P) as the primary chemical energy source. Bacteria also require the B-complex vitamins as functional coenzymes for many oxidation-reduction reactions needed for growth and energy transformation. An organism such as *Thiobacillus thiooxidans*, grown in a medium containing only sulfur and inorganic salts, synthesizes large amounts of thiamine, riboflavine, nicotinic acid, pantothenic acid, pyridoxine, and biotin. Therefore, Kluyver proposed the **unity theory of biochemistry** (*Die Einheit in der Biochemie*), which states that all basic enzymatic reactions supporting and maintaining life processes within cells of all organisms had more similarities than differ-

---

Chapter figures by Ms. Moon Vanko.

TABLE 4-1   Nutritional Diversity Exhibited by Physiologically Different Bacteria

Physiologic Type	Required Components for Bacterial Growth			
	Carbon Source	Nitrogen Source[a]	Energy Source	Hydrogen Source
Heterotrophic (chemoorganotrophic)	Organic	Organic or inorganic	Oxidation of organic compounds	—
Autotrophic[b] (chemolithotrophic)	CO_2	Inorganic	Oxidation of inorganic compounds	—
Photosynthetic[b]				
Photolithotrophic				
Bacterial	CO_2	Inorganic	Sunlight	H_2S or H_2
Cyanobacterial	CO_2	Inorganic	Sunlight	Photolysis of H_2O[c]
Photoorganotrophic	CO_2	Inorganic	Sunlight	Organic compounds[d]

[a] Common inorganic nitrogen sources are NO_3^- or NH_4^+ ions; nitrogen fixers can use N_2.
[b] Many phototrophs and chemotrophs are nitrogen-fixing organisms.
[c] Results in O_2 evolution (or oxygenic photosynthesis) as commonly occurs in plants.
[d] Organic acids such as formate, acetate, and succinate can serve as hydrogen donors.

ences. This concept of biochemical unity stimulated many investigators to use bacteria as model systems for studying related eukaryotic biochemical reactions that are essentially "identical" at the molecular level.

From a nutritional, or metabolic, viewpoint, three major physiologic types of bacteria exist: the **heterotrophs** (or **chemoorganotrophs**), the **autotrophs** (or **chemolithotrophs**), and the **photosynthetic bacteria** (or **phototrophs**) (Table 4-1). These are discussed below.

HETEROTROPHIC METABOLISM

Heterotrophic bacteria, which include all pathogens, obtain energy from oxidation of organic compounds. Carbohydrates (particularly glucose), lipids, and protein are the most commonly oxidized compounds. Biologic oxidation of these organic compounds by bacteria results in synthesis of ATP as the chemical energy source. This process also permits generation of simpler organic compounds (precursor molecules) needed by the bacteria cell for biosynthetic or assimilatory reactions.

The Krebs cycle intermediate compounds serve as precursor molecules (building blocks) for the energy-requiring biosynthesis of complex organic compounds in bacteria. Degradation reactions that simultaneously produce energy and generate precursor molecules for the biosynthesis of new cellular constituents are called **amphibolic.**

All heterotrophic bacteria require preformed organic compounds. These carbon- and nitrogen-containing compounds are growth substrates, which are used aerobically or anaerobically to generate reducing equivalents (e.g., reduced nicotinamide adenine dinucleotide; NADH + H[+]); these reducing equivalents in turn are chemical energy sources for all biologic oxidative and fermentative systems. Heterotrophs are the most commonly studied bacteria; they grow readily in media containing carbohydrates, proteins, or other complex nutrients such as blood. Also, growth media may be enriched by the addition of other naturally occurring compounds such as milk (to study lactic acid bacteria) or hydrocarbons (to study hydrocarbon-oxidizing organisms).

RESPIRATION

Glucose is the most common substrate used for studying heterotrophic metabolism. Most aerobic organisms oxidize glucose completely by the following reaction equation:

$$C_6H_{12}O_6 + 6O_2 \longrightarrow 6CO_2 + 6H_2O + energy$$

This equation expresses the cellular oxidation process called **respiration.** Respiration occurs within the cells of plants and animals, normally generating 38 ATP molecules (as energy) from the oxidation of 1 molecule of glucose. This yields approximately 380,000 calories (cal) per mode of glucose (ATP ≈ 10,000 cal/mole). Thermodynamically, the complete oxidation of one mole of glucose should yield approximately 688,000 cal; the energy that is not conserved biologically as chemical energy (or ATP formation) is liberated as heat (308,000 cal). Thus, the cellular respiratory process is at best about 55% efficient.

Glucose oxidation is the most commonly studied dissimilatory reaction leading to energy production or ATP synthesis. The complete oxidation of glucose may involve three fundamental biochemical pathways. The first is the **glycolytic** or Emb-den-Meyerhof-Parnas pathway (Fig. 4-1), the second is the **Krebs cycle** (also called the citric acid cycle or tricarboxylic acid cycle), and the third is the series of membrane-bound electron transport oxidations coupled to oxidative phosphorylation.

Respiration takes place when any organic compound (usually carbohydrate) is oxidized completely to CO_2 and H_2O. In aerobic respiration, molecular O_2 serves as the terminal acceptor of electrons. For anaerobic respiration, NO_3^-, SO_4^{2-}, CO_2, or fumarate can serve as terminal electron acceptors (rather than O_2), depending on the bacterium studied. The end result of the respiratory process is the complete oxidation of the organic substrate molecule, and the end products formed are primarily CO_2 and H_2O. Ammonia is formed also if protein (or amino acid) is the sub-

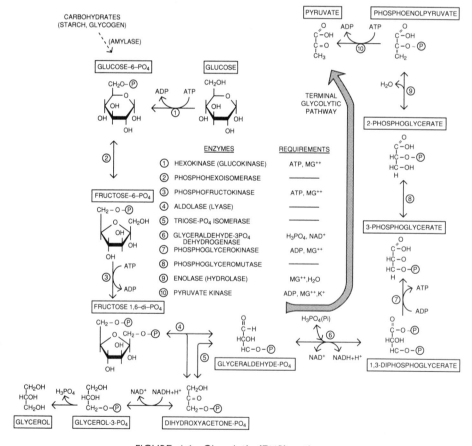

FIGURE 4-1 Glycolytic (EMP) pathway.

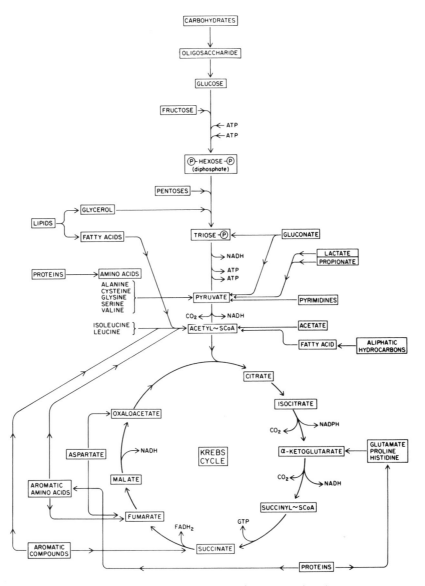

FIGURE 4-2 Heterotrophic metabolism, general pathway.

strate oxidized. The biochemical pathways normally involved in oxidation of various naturally occurring organic compounds are summarized in Figure 4-2.

Metabolically, bacteria are unlike cyanobacteria (blue-green algae) and eukaryotes in that glucose oxidation may occur by more than one pathway. In bacteria, glycolysis represents one of several pathways by which bacteria can catabolically attack glu-

cose. The glycolytic pathway is most commonly associated with anaerobic or fermentative metabolism in bacteria and yeasts. In bacteria, other minor heterofermentative pathways, such as the phosphoketolase pathway, also exist.

In addition, two other glucose-catabolizing pathways are found in bacteria: the oxidative **pentose phosphate pathway** (hexose monophosphate shunt), (Fig. 4-3) and the **Entner-Doudoroff path-**

way, which is almost exclusively found in obligate aerobic bacteria (Fig. 4-4). The highly oxidative *Azotobacter* and most *Pseudomonas* species, for example, utilize the Entner-Doudoroff pathway for glucose catabolism, because these organisms lack the enzyme phosphofructokinase and hence cannot synthesize fructose 1,6-diphosphate, a key intermediate compound in the glycolytic pathway. (Phosphofructokinase is also sensitive to molecular O_2 and does not function in obligate aerobes). Other bacteria, which lack aldolase (which splits fructose-1,6-diphosphate into two triose phosphate compounds), also cannot have a functional

glycolytic pathway. Although the Entner-Doudoroff pathway is usually associated with obligate aerobic bacteria, it is present in the facultative anaerobe *Zymomonas mobilis* (formerly *Pseudomonas lindneri*). This organism dissimilates glucose to ethanol and represents a major alcoholic fermentation reaction in a bacterium.

Glucose dissimilation also occurs by the hexose monophosphate shunt (Fig. 4-3). This oxidative pathway was discovered in tissues that actively metabolize glucose in the presence of two glycolytic pathway inhibitors (iodoacetate and fluoride). Neither inhibitor had an effect on glucose dissimila-

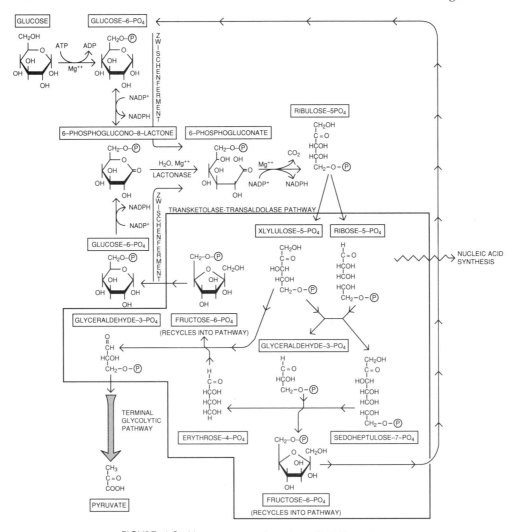

FIGURE 4-3   Hexose monophosphate (HMS) pathway.

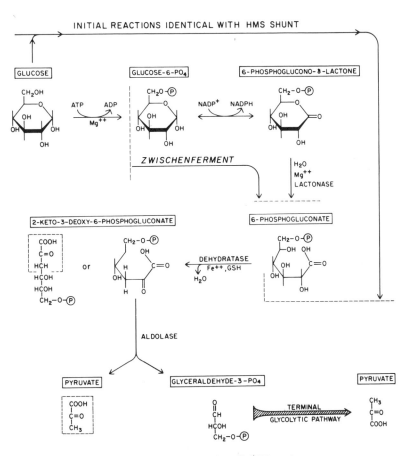

FIGURE 4-4 Entner-Doudoroff (ED) pathway.

tion, and NADPH + H$^+$ generation occurred directly from the oxidation of glucose-6-phosphate (to 6-phosphoglucono-δ-lactone) by glucose-6-phosphate dehydrogenase. The pentose phosphate pathway subsequently permits the direct oxidative decarboxylation of glucose to pentoses. The capability of this oxidative metabolic system to bypass glycolysis explains the term **shunt.**

The biochemical reactions of the **Entner-Doudoroff** pathway are a modification of the hexose monophosphate shunt, except that pentose sugars are not directly formed. The two pathways are identical up to the formation of 6-phosphogluconate (see Fig. 4-4) and then diverge. In the Entner-Doudoroff pathway, no oxidative decarboxylation of 6-phosphogluconate occurs and no pentose compound is formed. For this pathway, a new 6-carbon compound intermediate (2-keto-3-deoxy-6-phosphogluconate) is generated by the action of 6-phosphogluconate dehydratase (an Fe^{2+}- and glutathione-stimulated enzyme); this intermediate compound is then directly cleaved into the triose (pyruvate) and a triose-phosphate compound (glyceraldehyde-3-phosphate) by the 2-keto-3-deoxy-6-phosphogluconate aldolase. The glyceraldehyde-3-phosphate is further oxidized to another pyruvate molecule by the same enzyme systems that catalyze the terminal glycolytic pathway (see Fig. 4-4).

The glycolytic pathway may be the major one existing concomitantly with the minor oxidative pentose phosphate–hexose monophosphate shunt pathway; the Entner-Doudoroff pathway also may function as a major pathway with a minor hexose monophosphate shunt. A few bacteria possess only one pathway. All cyanobacteria, *Acetobacter suboxydans*, and *A xylinum* possess only the hexose monophosphate shunt pathway; *Pseudo-* *monas saccharophilia* and *Z mobilis* possess solely the Entner-Doudoroff pathway. Thus, the end products of glucose dissimilatory pathways are as follows:

Glycolytic: 1 glucose $\longrightarrow$ 2 pyruvate

Entner-Doudoroff: 1 glucose $\longrightarrow$ 1 pyruvate and glyceraldehyde-3-PO_4 $\xrightarrow{\text{Terminal glycolytic pathway}}$ 1 pyruvate

Oxidative pentose phosphate: x glucose

xCO_2

Glycolysis Recycling

Transketolase-transaldolase pathway

pentose-PO_4 + interconversion end products [hexose-PO_4], erythrose-PO_4 and [glyceraldehyde-3-PO_4]

Terminal glycolysis

Glycolytic pathway

$\downarrow$

pyruvate

The glucose dissimilation pathways used by specific microorganisms are shown in Table 4-2.

All major pathways of glucose or hexose catabolism have several metabolic features in common. First, there are the preparatory steps by which key intermediate compounds such as the triose-PO_4, glyceraldehyde-3-phosphate, and/or pyruvate are generated. The latter two compounds are almost universally required for further assimilatory or dissimilatory reactions within the cell. Second, the major source of phosphate for all reactions involving phosphorylation of glucose or other hexoses is ATP, not inorganic phosphate (Pi). Actually, chemical energy contained in ATP must be initially spent in the first step of glucose metabolism (via kinase-type enzymes) to generate glucose-6-phosphate, which initiates the reactions involving hexose catabolism. Third, NADH + H$^+$ or NADPH + H$^+$ is generated as reducing equivalents (potential energy) directly by one or more of the enzymatic reactions involved in each of these pathways.

FERMENTATION

Fermentation, another example of heterotrophic metabolism, requires an organic compound as a terminal electron (or hydrogen) acceptor. In fermentations, simple organic end products are formed from the anaerobic dissimilation of glucose (or some other compound). Energy (ATP) is generated through the dehydrogenation reactions that occur as glucose is broken down enzymatically. The simple organic end products formed from this incomplete biologic oxidation process also serve as final electron and hydrogen acceptors. On reduction, these organic end products are secreted into the medium as waste metabolites (usually alcohol or acid). The organic substrate compounds are incompletely oxidized by bacteria, yet yield sufficient energy for microbial growth. Glucose is the most common hexose used to study fermentation reactions.

In the late 1850s, Pasteur demonstrated that fermentation is a vital process associated with the growth of specific microorganisms, and that each type of fermentation can be defined by the principal organic end product formed (lactic acid, ethanol, acetic acid, or butyric acid). His studies on butyric acid fermentation led directly to the discovery of anaerobic microorganisms. Pasteur concluded that oxygen inhibited the microorganisms responsible for butyric acid fermentation because both bacterial mobility and butyric acid formation

TABLE 4-2 Glucose Dissimilation Pathways Utilized by Bacteria,
Cyanobacteria, and Yeasts

Bacteria	Glycolytic Pathway	Oxidative Pentose Phosphate Pathway	Entner-Doudoroff Pathway
Acetobacter suboxydans		Sole	
Acetobacter xylinum		Sole	
Agrobacterium spp			Major
Azotobacter vinelandii[a]			Major
Bacillus subtilis	Major	Minor	
Caulobacter spp			Major
Escherichia coli	Major	Minor	
Lactobacillus delbrueckii	Major		
Leuconostoc mesenteroides		Major	
Neisseria gonorrhoeae		Minor	Major
Neisseria meningitidis		Minor	Major
Neisseria perflava		Major	
Neisseria sicca		Major	
Pseudomonas aeruginosa[a]			Major
Pseudomonas saccharophilia			Sole
Rhizobium spp			Major
Sarcina lutea	Major	Minor	
Spirillum spp			Major
Streptococcus faecalis	Major		(Major)[b]
Streptomyces griseus	Major	Minor	
Zymomonas anaerobia			Sole
Zymomonas mobilis			Sole
All cyanobacteria		Sole	
All yeasts	Major	Minor	

[a] Most species utilize the Enter-Doudoroff pathway as major pathway.

[b] Induced by growth on gluconate.

ceased when air was bubbled into the fermentation mixture. Pasteur also introduced the terms *aerobic* and *anaerobic*. His views on fermentation are made clear from his microbiologic studies on the production of beer (from *Etudes sur la Biere*, 1876):

> In the experiments which we have described, fermentation by yeast is seen to be the direct consequence of the processes of nutrition, assimilation and life, when these are carried on without the agency of free oxygen. The heat required in the accomplishment of that work must necessarily have been borrowed from the decomposition of the fermentation matter. . . . Fermentation by yeast appears, therefore, to be essentially connected with the property possessed by this minute cellular plant of performing its respiratory functions, somehow or other, with the oxygen existing combined in sugar.

For most microbial fermentations, glucose dissimilation occurs through the glycolytic pathway (Fig. 4-1). The simple organic compound most commonly generated is pyruvate, or a compound derived enzymatically from pyruvate, such as acetaldehyde, α-acetolactate, acetyl $\sim$ SCoA, or lactyl $\sim$ SCoA (Fig. 4-5). Acetaldehyde can then be reduced by NADH + H$^+$ to ethanol, which is excreted by the cell. The end product of lactic acid fermentation, which occurs in streptococci (e.g.,

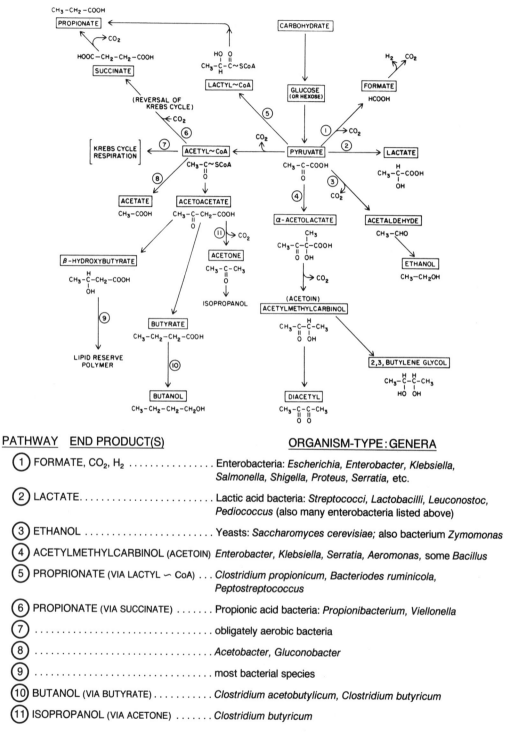

PATHWAY   END PRODUCT(S)   ORGANISM-TYPE: GENERA

(1) FORMATE, CO_2, H_2 . . . . Enterobacteria: *Escherichia, Enterobacter, Klebsiella,*
                                                    Salmonella, Shigella, Proteus, Serratia, etc.

(2) LACTATE. . . . . Lactic acid bacteria: *Streptococci, Lactobacilli, Leuconostoc,*
                                                    Pediococcus (also many enterobacteria listed above)

(3) ETHANOL . . . . Yeasts: *Saccharomyces cerevisiae;* also bacterium *Zymomonas*

(4) ACETYLMETHYLCARBINOL (ACETOIN) *Enterobacter, Klebsiella, Serratia, Aeromonas,* some *Bacillus*

(5) PROPRIONATE (VIA LACTYL ～ CoA) . . . *Clostridium propionicum, Bacteriodes ruminicola,*
                                                    Peptostreptococcus

(6) PROPIONATE (VIA SUCCINATE) . . . . Propionic acid bacteria: *Propionibacterium, Viellonella*

(7) . . . . obligately aerobic bacteria

(8) . . . . *Acetobacter, Gluconobacter*

(9) . . . . most bacterial species

(10) BUTANOL (VIA BUTYRATE) . . . . *Clostridium acetobutylicum, Clostridium butyricum*

(11) ISOPROPANOL (VIA ACETONE) . . . . *Clostridium butyricum*

FIGURE 4-5 Fermentative pathways of bacteria and the major end products formed with the organism
type carrying out the fermentation.

Streptococcus lactis) and many lactobacilli (e.g., *Lactobacillus casei, L pentosus*), is a single organic acid, lactic acid. Organisms that produce only lactic acid from glucose fermentation are **homofermenters.** Homofermentative lactic acid bacteria dissimilate glucose exclusively through the glycolytic pathway. Organisms that ferment glucose to multiple end products, such as acetic acid, ethanol, formic acid, and CO_2, are referred to as **heterofermenters.** Examples of heterofermentative bacteria include *Lactobacillus, Leuconostoc,* and *Microbacterium* species. Heterofermentative fermentations are more common among bacteria, as in the mixed-acid fermentations carried out by bacteria of the family Enterobacteriaceae (e.g., *Escherichia coli, Salmonella, Shigella,* and *Proteus* species). Many of these glucose fermenters usually produce CO_2 and H_2 with different combinations of acid end products (formate, acetate, lactate, and succinate). Other bacteria such as *Enterobacter aerogenes, Aeromonas, Serratia, Erwinia,* and *Bacillus* species also form CO_2 and H_2 as well as other neutral end products (ethanol, acetylmethylcarbinol [acetoin], and 2,3-butylene glycol). Many obligately anaerobic clostridia (e.g., *Clostridium saccharobutyricum, C thermosaccharolyticum*) and *Butyribacterium* species ferment glucose with the production of butyrate, acetate, CO_2, and H_2, whereas other *Clostridum* species (*C acetobutylicum* and *C butyricum*) also form these fermentation end products plus others (butanol, acetone, isopropanol, formate, and ethanol). Similarly, the anaerobic propionic acid bacteria (*Propionibacterium* species) and the related *Veillonella* species ferment glucose to form CO_2, propionate, acetate, and succinate. In these bacteria, propionate is formed by the partial reversal of the Krebs cycle reactions and involves a CO_2 fixation by pyruvate (the Wood-Werkman reaction) that forms oxaloacetate (a four-carbon intermediate). Oxaloacetate is then reduced to malate, fumarate, and succinate, which is decarboxylated to propionate. Propionate is also formed by another three-carbon pathway in *C propionicum, Bacteroides ruminicola,* and *Peptostreptococcus* species, involving a lactyl ~ SCoA intermediate. The obligately aerobic acetic acid bacteria (*Acetobacter* and the related *Gluconobacter* species) can also ferment glucose, producing acetate and gluconate. Figure 4-5 summarizes the pathways by which the various major fermentation end products form from the dissimilation of glucose through the common intermediate pyruvate.

For thermodynamic reasons, bacteria that rely on fermentative process for growth cannot generate as much energy as respiring cells. In respiration, 38 ATP molecules (or approximately 380,000 cal/mole) can be generated as biologically useful energy from the complete oxidation of 1 molecule of glucose (assuming 1 NAD(P)H = 3 ATP and 1 ATP → ADP + Pi = 10,000 cal/mole). Table 4-3 shows comparable bioenergetic parameters for the lactate and ethanolic fermentations by the glycolytic pathway. Although only 2 ATP molecules are generated by this glycolytic pathway, this is apparently enough energy to permit anaerobic growth of lactic acid bacteria and the ethanolic fermenting yeast, *Saccharomyces cerevisiae*. The ATP-synthesizing reactions in the glycolytic pathway (Fig. 4-1) specifically involve the substrate phosphorylation reactions catalyzed by phosphoglycerokinase and pyruvic kinase. Although all the ATP molecules available for fermentative growth are believed to be generated by these substrate phosphorylation reactions, some energy equivalents are also generated by proton extrusion reactions (acid liberation), which occur with intact membrane systems and involve the Mitchell hypothesis of energy conservation (see below) as it applies to fermentative metabolism.

KREBS CYCLE

The **Krebs cycle** (also called the *tricarboxylic acid cycle* or *citic acid cycle*) functions oxidatively in respiration and is the metabolic process by which pyruvate or acetyl ~ SCoA is completely decarboxylated to CO_2. In bacteria, this reaction occurs through acetyl ~ SCoA, which is the first product in the oxidative decarboxylation of pyruvate by pyruvate dehydrogenase. Bioenergetically, the following overall exergonic reaction occurs:

$$CH_3-\underset{\underset{O}{\|}}{C}-COOH + 5O \xrightarrow[\substack{\text{Electron transport and} \\ \text{oxidative phosphorylation}}]{\text{Krebs cycle (via } CH_3-\overset{\overset{O}{\|}}{C}-O \sim SCoA)}$$

$$3CO_2 + 2H_2O + 15ATP \ (\approx 150,000 \text{ cal/mole})$$

TABLE 4-3   Energy Obtained from Bacterial Fermentations by Substrate Phosphorylations

Fermentation	Actual Energy (cal/mole)	Theoretical Energy (cal/mole)	Efficiency (%)
Homolactic $$C_6H_{12}O_6 \xrightarrow{\text{Glycolysis}} 2CH_3-\overset{\displaystyle H}{\underset{\displaystyle OH}{C}}-COOH +$$ (Glucose) (Lactic acid)	$\approx 20,000$	57,000	35
Alcoholic $$C_6H_{12}O_6 \xrightarrow{\text{Glycolysis}} 2CH_3-\overset{\displaystyle H}{\underset{\displaystyle H}{C}}-OH + 2CO_2 +$$ (Glucose) (Ethanol)	$\approx 20,000$	58,000	34

If 2 pyruvate molecules are obtained from the dissimilation of 1 glucose molecule, then 30 ATP molecules are generated in total. The decarboxylation of pyruvate, isocitrate, and α-ketoglutarate accounts for all CO_2 molecules generated during the respiratory process. Figure 4-6 shows the enzymatic reactions in the Krebs cycle. The chemical energy conserved by the Krebs cycle is contained in the reduced compounds generated (NADH + H$^+$, NADPH + H$^+$, and succinate). The potential energy inherent in these reduced compounds is not available as ATP until the final step of respiration (electron transport and oxidative phosphorylation) occurs.

The Krebs cycle is therefore another preparatory stage in the respiratory process. If 1 molecule of pyruvate is oxidized completely to 3 molecules of CO_2, generating 15 ATP molecules, the oxidation of 1 molecule of glucose will yield as many as 38 ATP molecules, provided glucose is dissimilated by glycolysis and the Krebs cycle (further assuming that the electron transport/oxidative phosphorylation reactions are bioenergetically identical to those of eukaryotic mitochondria).

GLYOXYLATE CYCLE

In general, the Krebs cycle functions similarly in bacteria and eukaryotic systems, but major differences are found among bacteria. One difference is that in obligate aerobes, L-malate may be oxidized directly by molecular O_2 via an electron transport chain. In other bacteria, only some Krebs cycle intermediate reactions occur because α-ketoglutarate dehydrogenase is missing.

A modification of the Krebs cycle, commonly called the **glyoxylate cycle,** or **shunt** (Fig. 4-7), exists in some other bacteria. This cycle functions similarly to the Krebs cycle but lacks many of the Krebs cycle enzyme reactions. The glyoxylate cycle is primarily an oxidative pathway in which acetyl $\sim$ SCoA is generated from the oxidation, of acetate, which usually is derived from the oxidation of fatty acids. The oxidation of fatty acids to acetyl $\sim$ SCoA is carried out by the β-oxidation pathway. Pyruvate oxidation is not directly involved in the glyoxylate shunt, yet this cycle yields sufficient succinate and malate, which are required for energy production (Fig. 4-7). The glyoxylate cycle also generates other precursor compounds needed for biosynthesis (Fig. 4-7). The glyoxylate cycle was discovered as an unusual metabolic pathway during an attempt to learn how lipid (or acetate) oxidation in bacteria and plant seeds could lead to the direct biosynthesis of carbohydrates. The glyoxylate cycle converts oxaloacetate either to pyruvate and CO_2 (catalyzed by pyruvate carboxylase) or to phosphoenolpyruvate

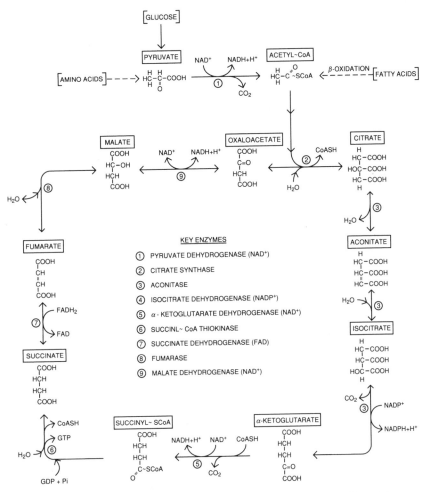

FIGURE 4-6   Krebs cycle (also tricarboxylic acid or citric acid cycle).

and CO_2 (catalyzed by the inosine triphosphate [ITP]-dependent phosphoenolpyruvate carboxylase kinase). Either triose compound can then be converted to glucose by reversal of the glycolytic pathway. The glyoxylate cycle is found in many bacteria, including *Azotobacter vinelandii* and particularly in organisms that grow well in media in which acetate and other dicarboxylic acid intermediates of the Krebs cycle are the sole carbon source. One primary function of the glyoxylate cycle is to replenish the tricarboxylic and dicarboxylic acid intermediates that are normally provided by the Krebs cycle. A pathway whose primary purpose is to replenish such intermediate compounds is called **anaplerotic.**

ELECTRON TRANSPORT AND OXIDATIVE PHOSPHORYLATION

The final stage of respiration occurs through a series of oxidation-reduction electron transfer reactions that yield the energy to drive oxidative phosphorylation; this in turn produces ATP. The enzymes involved in electron transport and oxidative phosphorylation reside on the bacterial inner (cytoplasmic) membrane. This membrane is invaginated to form structures called **respiratory vesicles, lamellar vesicles,** or **mesosomes,** which function as the bacterial equivalent of the eukaryotic mitochondrial membrane.

Respiratory electron transport chains vary

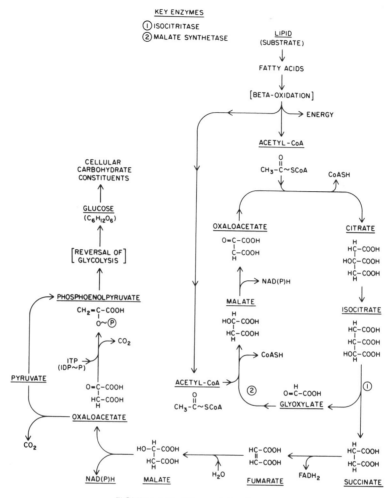

FIGURE 4-7 Glyoxylate shunt.

greatly among bacteria, and in some organisms are absent. The respiratory electron transport chain of eukaryotic mitochondria oxidizes $NADH + H^+$, $NADPH + H^+$, and succinate (as well as the coacylated fatty acids such as acetyl $\sim SCoA$). The bacterial electron transport chain also oxidizes these compounds, but it can also directly oxidize, via non-pyridine nucleotide-dependent pathways, a larger variety of reduced substrates such as lactate, malate, formate, α-glycerophosphate, H_2, and glutamate. The respiratory electron carriers in bacterial electron transport systems are more varied than in eukaryotes, and the chain is usually branched at the site(s) reacting with molecular O_2.

Some electron carriers, such as nonheme iron centers and ubiquinone (coenzyme Q), are common to both the bacterial and mammalian respiratory electron transport chains. In some bacteria, the naphthoquinones or vitamin K may be found with ubiquinone. In still other bacteria, vitamin K serves in the absence of ubiquinone. In mitochondrial respiration, only one cytochrome oxidase component is found (cytochrome $a + a_3$ oxidase). In bacteria there are multiple cytochrome oxidases, including cytochromes a, d, o, and occasionally $a + a_3$ (Fig. 4-8).

In bacteria cytochrome oxidases usually occur as combinations of $a_1 : d : o$ and $a + a_3 : o$. Bacteria also

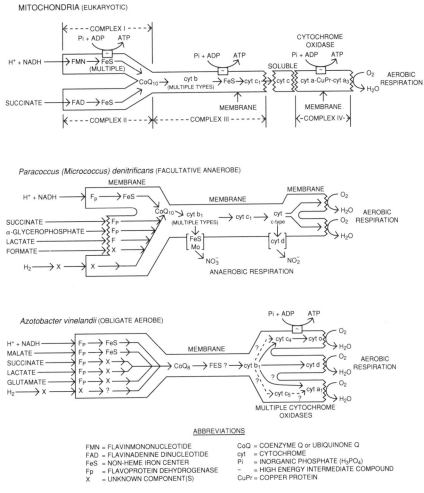

FIGURE 4-8 Respiratory electron transport chains.

possess mixed-function oxidases such as cytochromes P-450 and P-420 and cytochromes c' and $c'c'$, which also react with carbon monoxide. These diverse types of oxygen-reactive cytochromes undoubtedly have evolutionary significance. Bacteria were present before O_2 was formed; when O_2 became available as a metabolite, bacteria evolved to use it in different ways; this probably accounts for the diversity in bacterial oxygen-reactive hemoproteins.

Cytochrome oxidases in many pathogenic bacteria are studied by the bacterial oxidase reaction, which subdivides Gram-negative organisms into two major groups, oxidase positive and oxidase negative. This oxidase reaction is assayed for by using N,N,N',N'-tetramethyl-p-phenylenediamine oxidation (to Wurster's blue) or by using indophenol blue synthesis (with dimethyl-p-phenylenediamine and α-naphthol). Oxidase-positive bacteria contain integrated (cytochrome c type:oxidase) complexes, the oxidase component most frequently encountered is cytochrome o, and occasionally $a + a_3$. The cytochrome oxidase responsible for the indophenol oxidase reaction complex was isolated from membranes of *Azotobacter vinelandii*, a bacterium with the highest respiratory rate of any known cell. The cytochrome oxidase was found to be an integrated cytochrome c_4:o

complex, which was shown to be present in *Bacillus* species. These *Bacillus* strains are also highly oxidase positive, and most are found in morphologic group II.

Both bacterial and mammalian electron transfer systems can carry out electron transfer (oxidation) reactions with $NADH + H^+$, $NADPH + H^+$, and succinate. Energy generated from such membrane oxidations is conserved within the membrane and then transferred in a coupled manner to drive the formation of ATP. The electron transfer sequence is accomplished entirely by membrane-bound enzyme systems. As the electrons are transferred by a specific sequence of electron carriers, ATP is synthesized from ADP + inorganic phosphate (Pi) or phosphoric acid (H_3PO_4) (Fig. 4-8).

In respiration, the electron transfer reaction is the primary mode of generating energy; electrons ($2e^-$) from a low-redox-potential compound such as $NADH + H^+$ are sequentially transferred to a specific flavoprotein dehydrogenase or oxidoreductase (flavin mononucleotide [FMN] type for NADH or flavin adenine dinucleotide [FAD] type for succinate); this electron pair is then transferred to a nonheme iron center (FeS) and finally to a specific ubiquinone or a naphthoquinone derivative. This transfer of electrons causes a differential chemical redox potential change so that within the membrane enough chemical energy is conserved to be transferred by a coupling mechanism to a high-energy compound (e.g., ADP + Pi → ATP). ATP molecules represent the final stable high-energy intermediate compound formed.

A similar series of redox changes also occurs between ubiquinone and cytochrome *c,* but with a greater differential in the oxidation-reduction potential level, which allows for another ATP synthesis step. The final electron transfer reaction occurs at the cytochrome oxidase level between reduced cyotchrome *c* and molecular O_2; this reaction is the terminal ATP synthesis step.

MITCHELL HYPOTHESIS

A highly complex but attractive theory to explain energy conservation in biologic systems is the chemiosmotic coupling of oxidative and photosynthetic phosphorylations, commonly called the

Mitchell hypothesis. This theory attempts to explain the conservation of free energy in these processes on the basis of an osmotic potential caused by proton concentration differential (or proton gradient) across a proton-impermeable membrane. Energy is generated by the membrane-bound electron transport reactions, which in essence serve as proton pumps; energy conservation and coupling follow (an obligatory membrane phenomenon). The energy thus conserved (again within a membrane) is coupled to ATP synthesis. This would occur in all biologic cells, even in the lactic acid bacteria that lack a cytochrome-dependent electron transport chain. In this hypothesis, the membrane allows for charge separation, thus forming a proton gradient that drives all bioenergization reactions. By such means, electromotive forces can be generated by oxidation-reduction reactions that can be directly coupled to ion translocations, as in the separation of H^+ and OH^- ions in electrochemical systems. Thus, an enzyme or an electron transfer carrier on a membrane that undergoes an oxidation-reduction reaction serves as a specific conductor for OH^- (or O^{2-}), and "hydrodehydration" provides electromotive power, as it does in electrochemical cells.

The concept underlying Mitchell's hypothesis is complex, and many modifications have been proposed, but the theory's most attractive feature is that it unifies all bioenergetic conservation principles into a single concept requiring an intact membrane vesicle to function properly. Figure 4-9 shows how the Mitchell hypothesis might be used to explain energy generation, conservation, and transfer by a coupling process. The least satisfying aspect of the chemiosmotic hypothesis is the lack of understanding of how chemical energy is actually conserved within the membrane and how it is transmitted by coupling for ATP synthesis.

BACTERIAL PHOTOSYNTHESIS

Many prokaryotes (bacteria and cyanobacteria) possess phototrophic modes of metabolism (Table 4-1). The types of photosynthesis in the two groups of prokaryotes differ mainly in the type of compound that serves as the hydrogen donor in the reduction of CO_2 to glucose (Table 4-1). Photo-

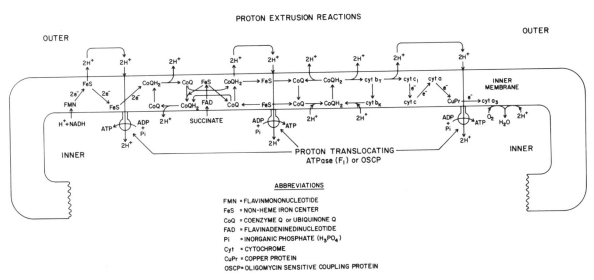

FIGURE 4-9 Mitchell hypotheses, a chemiosmotic model of energy transduction.

trophic organisms differ from heterotrophic organisms in that they utilize the glucose synthesized intracellularly for biosynthetic purposes (as in starch synthesis) or for energy production, which usually occurs through cellular respiration.

Unlike phototrophs, heterotrophs require glucose (or some other preformed organic compound) that is directly supplied as a substrate from an exogenous source. Heterotrophs cannot synthesize large concentrations of glucose from CO_2 by specifically using H_2O or (H_2S) as a hydrogen source and sunlight as energy. Plant metabolism is a classic example of photolithotrophic metabolism: plants need CO_2 and sunlight; H_2O must be provided as a hydrogen source and usually NO_3^- is the nitrogen source for protein synthesis. Organic nitrogen, supplied as fertilizer, is converted to NO_3^- in all soils by bacteria via the process of ammonification and nitrification. Although plant cells are phototrophic, they also exhibit a heterotrophic mode of metabolism in that they respire. For example, plants use classic respiration to catabolize glucose that is generated photosynthetically. Mitochondria as well as the soluble enzymes of the glycolytic pathway are required for glucose dissimilation, and these enzymes are also found in all plant cells. The soluble Calvin cycle enzymes, which are required for glucose synthesis during

photosynthesis, are also found in plant cells. It is not possible to feed a plant by pouring a glucose solution on it, but water supplied to a plant will be "photolysed" by chloroplasts in the presence of light; the hydrogen(s) generated from H_2O is used to reduce $NADP^+$ to $NADPH + H^+$. With these reduced pyridine nucleotides, CO_2 is reduced intracellularly to glucose. This metabolic process is carried out in an integrated manner by photosystems I and II ("Z" scheme) and by the **Calvin cycle pathway.** Table 4-4 summarizes the characteristics of known photosynthetic bacteria.

AUTOTROPHY

Bacteria that grow solely at the expense of inorganic compounds (mineral ions), without using sunlight as an energy source, are called **autotrophs, chemotrophs, chemoautotrophs,** or **chemolithotrophs.** Like photosynthetic organisms, all autotrophs use CO_2 as a carbon source for growth; their nitrogen comes from inorganic compounds such as NH_3, NO_3^-, or N_2 (Table 4-1). Interestingly, the energy source for such organisms is the oxidation of specific inorganic compounds. Which inorganic compound is oxidized depends on the bacteria in question (Table 4-5). Many autotrophs will not grow on media that contain organic matter, even agar.

TABLE 4-4 Characteristics Commonly Exhibited by Phototrophic Bacteria[a]

Photosynthetic Type	Characteristics	Representative Families and Genera
Purple bacteria Sulfur-type (formerly *Thiorho-daceae*), photolithotrophic bacteria	Obligate phototrophs Strict anaerobes H_2S (or H_2) serve as H source Possess S granules when H_2S used Contain bacteriochlorophyll *a* or *b*	Chromatiaceae (*Chromatium, Thiospirillum, Thiosarcina, Thiocapsa*)
Non–sulfur-type (formerly *Athiorhodaceae*), photoorganotrophic bacteria	Facultative phototrophs (have respiratory mechanism and will grow heterotrophically) Oxygen-tolerant anaerobes Most require one or more B vitamins Simple organic compounds serve as H source Contain bacteriochlorophyll *a* or *b*	Rhodospirillaceae (*Rhodopseudomonas, Rhodospirillum, Rhodomicrobium*)
Green bacteria Photolithotrophic bacteria	Obligate phototrophs Strict anaerobes Contains chlorobium chlorophyll, which is currently referred to as bacteriochlorophyll type *c* and *d* Many require vitamin B_{12} S_2 deposited extracellularly	Chlorobiaceae (*Chlorobium, Chloropseudomonas*)

[a] All are Gram negative; if motile, they exhibit polar flagellation. Most species are anaerobic, although some purple nonsulfur bacteria (family Athiorhodaceae) are facultative phototrophs and can grow as heterotrophs by using the anaerobic respiratory mode of metabolism; they are therefore oxygen tolerant. For further information, see *Bergey's Manual of Determinative Bacteriology*, 8th ed, part 1.

TABLE 4-5 Inorganic Oxidation Reactions Used by Autotrophic Bacteria as Energy Sources

Chemosynthetic Type	Inorganic Compounds Oxidized as Energy (~E) Source	Representative Families, Genera, and Species[a]	Nitrogen Cycle Reaction
NH₃ oxidizers (aerobic)	$NH_3 \longrightarrow NO_2$ $(\sim E)$ $(\sim E)$ = chemical energy or ATP produced	Nitrobacteriaceae (*Nitrosomonas, Nitrosococcus, Nitrosospira*)	Nitrification Nitrification Nitrification Nitrification
NO₂ oxidizers (aerobic)	$NO_2 \longrightarrow NO_3$ $(\sim E)$	Nitrobacteriaceae (*Nitrobacter, Nitrococcus*)	Nitrification Nitrification Nitrification
Sulfur oxidizers[b] (aerobic) Iron oxidizers (aerobic)	$S_2 \longrightarrow SO_4$ $(\sim E)$ $Fe^{2+} \longrightarrow Fe^{3+}$ $(\sim E)$ use both reactions	*Thiobacillus thiooxidans,* *Thiobacillus, ferrooxidans,* *Ferrobacillus,* *Leptothrix*	
Sulfur-compound oxidizers (anaerobic)	S_2O_3 oxidized; NO_3 reduced	*Thiobacillus denitrificans*	Denitrification

[a] All are Gram-negative species (see *Bergey's Manual of Determinative Bacteriology*, 8th ed, part 12).
[b] Strict autotrophic modes of metabolism are not present in sulfur and sulfur compound-oxidizing bacteria. For example, heterotrophic sulfur compound oxidizers are known, the aerobic species being able to oxidize $H_2S \longrightarrow S_2$, (e.g., *Beggiatoa* and *Thiothrix* species).
$(\sim E)$

Also found among the autotrophic microorganisms are the sulfur-oxidizing or sulfur-compound-oxidizing bacteria, which seldom exhibit a strictly autotrophic mode of metabolism like the obligate nitrifying bacteria (see discussion of nitrogen cycle below). The representative sulfur compounds oxidized by such bacteria are H_2S, S_2, and S_2O_3. Among the sulfur bacteria are two very interesting organisms; *Thiobacillus ferrooxidans*, which gets its energy for autotrophic growth by oxidizing elemental sulfur or ferrous iron, and *T denitrificans*, which gets its energy by oxidizing S_2O_3 anaerobically, using NO_3^- as the sole terminal electron acceptor. *T denitrificans* reduces NO_3^- to molecular N_2, which is liberated as a gas; this biologic process is called **denitrification.**

All autotrophic bacteria must assimilate CO_2, which is reduced to glucose from which organic cellular matter is synthesized. The energy for this biosynthetic process is derived from the oxidation of inorganic compounds discussed in the previous paragraph. Note that all autotrophic and phototrophic bacteria possess essentially the same organic cellular constituents found in heterotrophic bacteria; from a nutritional viewpoint, however, the autotrophic mode of metabolism is unique, occurring only in bacteria.

ANAEROBIC RESPIRATION

Some bacteria exhibit a unique mode of respiration called **anaerobic respiration.** These heterotrophic bacteria that will not grow anaerobically unless a specific chemical component, which serves as a terminal electron acceptor, is added to the medium. Among these electron acceptors are NO_3^-, SO_4^{2-}, the organic compound fumarate, and CO_2. Bacteria requiring one of these compounds for anaerobic growth are said to be **anaerobic respirers.**

A large group of anaerobic respirers are the **nitrate reducers** (Table 4-2). The nitrate reducers are predominantly heterotrophic bacteria that possess a complex electron transport system(s) allowing the NO_3^- ion to serve anaerobically as a terminal acceptor of electrons ($NO_3^- \xrightarrow{2e^-} NO_2^-$; $NO_3^- \xrightarrow{5e^-} N_2$; or $NO_3^- \xrightarrow{8e^-} NH_3$). The organic compounds that serve as specific electron donors for these three known nitrate reduction processes are shown in Table 4-6. The nitrate reductase activity is common in bacteria and is routinely used in the simple nitrate reductase test to identify bacteria (see *Bergey's Manual of Determinative Bacteriology*, 8th ed.).

$$4AH_2 + HNO_3 \xrightarrow{\text{Nitrate reduction}} 4A + NH_3 + 3H_2O + \text{energy}$$

(AH_2 = organic substrate, which serves as electron donor)

A second group of anaerobic respirers, the sulfate reducers, utilizes SO_4^{2-} ion in similar fashion

TABLE 4-6   Nitrate Reducers

Physiologic Types of Nitrate Reductases	Electron Donor(s)	Representative Organisms
Respiratory ($NO_3^- \rightarrow NO_2^-$)	Formate NADH	*Escherichia coli* *Klebsiella aerogenes*
Denitrifying ($NO_3^- \rightarrow N_2$)	NADH Pyruvate NADH, succinate	*Pseudomonas aeroginosa* *Clostridium perfringens* *Paracoccus denitrificans*
Assimilatory ($NO_3^- \rightarrow NH_3$)	Lactate H_2, formate NADH, succinate NADH NADH, lactate, glycerol-phosphate	*Staphylococcus aureus* *Vibrio succinogenes* *Bacillus stearothermophilus* *Enterobacter aerogenes* *Escherichia coli*

$(SO_4{}^{2-} \xrightarrow{8e^-} H_2S)$:

$$4AH_2 + H_2SO_4 \xrightarrow{\text{Sulfate reduction}}$$
$$4A + H_2S + 4H_2O + \text{energy}$$

The third group, the fumarate respirers, are anaerobic bacteria that require exogenous $HOOC—CH{=}CH—COOH$ for growth. Fumarate is reduced to succinate ($HOOC—CH_2—CH_2—COOH$), which is secreted as a by-product.

$$AH_2 + HOOC—\overset{\overset{H}{|}}{C}{=}\overset{\overset{H}{|}}{C}—COOH \xrightarrow{\text{Fumarate reduction}}$$
$$A + HOOC—CH_2—CH_2—COOH + \text{energy}$$

Organisms of still another specialized group of anaerobic respirers, the **methanogens,** produce methane gas ($CO_2 \xrightarrow{8e^-} CH_4$) as a metabolic end product of microbial growth. H_2 gas is the growth substrate; CO_2 is the terminal electron acceptor.

$$4H_2 + CO_2 \xrightarrow{\text{CO}_2 \text{ reduction}} CH_4 + 2H_2O + \text{energy}$$

The methanogens are among the most anaerobic bacteria known, being very sensitive to small concentrations of molecular O_2. They are also archaebacteria, which typically live in unusual and deleterious environments.

All of the above anaerobic respirers obtain chemical energy for growth by using these anaerobic energy-yielding oxidation reactions.

THE NITROGEN CYCLE

Nowhere can the total metabolic potential of bacteria and their diverse chemical-transforming capabilities be more fully appreciated than in the geochemical cycling of the element nitrogen. All the basic chemical elements (S, O, P, C, and H) required to sustain living organisms have geochemical cycles similar to the nitrogen cycle.

The nitrogen cycle is an ideal demonstration of the ecologic interdependence of bacteria, plants, and animals. Nitrogen is recycled when organisms use one form of nitrogen for growth and excrete another nitrogenous compound as a waste prod-

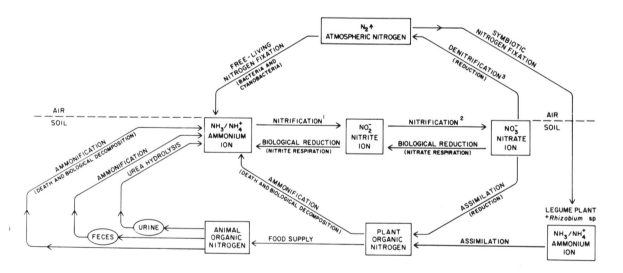

[1] Carried out primarily by chemoautotrophes of the genus *Nitrosomonas*

[2] Carried out by chemoautotrophes of the genus *Nitrobacter*

[3] Carried out by denitrifying bacteria, a property exhibited by some heterotrophic bacteria

FIGURE 4-10   The nitrogen cycle.

uct. This waste product is in turn utilized by another type of organism as a growth or energy substrate. Figure 4-10 shows the nitrogen cycle.

When the specific breakdown of organic nitrogenous compounds occurs, that is, when proteins are degraded to amino acids (proteolysis) and then to inorganic NH_3 by heterotrophic bacteria, the process is called **ammonification.** This is an essential step in the nitrogen cycle. At death, the organic constituents of the tissues and cells decompose biologically to inorganic constituents by a process called **mineralization;** these inorganic end products can then serve as nutrients for other life forms. The NH_3 liberated in turn serves as a utilizable nitrogen source for many other bacteria. The breakdown of feces and urine also occurs by ammonification.

The other important biologic processes in the nitrogen cycle include **nitrification** (the conversion of NH_3 to NO_3 by autotrophes in the soil; **denitrification** (the anaerobic conversion of NO_3 to N_2 gas) carried out by many heterotrophs); and **nitrogen fixation** (N_2 to NH_3 and cell protein). The latter is a very specialized prokaryotic process called **diazotrophy,** carried out by both free-living bacteria (such as *Azotobacter, Derxia, Beijeringeia,* and *Azomona* species) and symbionts (such as *Rhizobium* species) in conjunction with legume plants (such as soybeans, peas, clover, and bluebonnets). All plant life relies heavily on NO_3^- as a nitrogen source, and most animal life relies on plant life for nutrients.

REFERENCES

Buchanan RE, Gibbons NE (eds): Bergey's Manual of Determinative Bacteriology. 8th Ed. Williams & Wilkins, Baltimore, 1974

Green DE: A critique of the chemosmotic model of energy coupling. Proc Natl Acad Sci USA, 78:2249, 1981

Haddock BA, Hamilton WA (eds): Microbial energetics. 27th Symposium of the Society of General Microbiology. Cambridge University Press, Cambridge, 1977

Hempfling WP: Microbial Respiration. Benchman Papers in Microbiology no. 13. Downden, Hutchinson and Ross, Stroudsburg, Pa, 1979

Hill R: The biochemists' green mansions: the photosynthetic electron-transport chain in plants. In Campbell PN, Greville CD (eds): Essays in Biochemistry. Vol. 1. Academic Press, New York, 1965

Jurtshuk P, Jr, Liu JK: Cytochrome oxidase and analyses of *Bacillus* strains: existence of oxidase-positive species. Int J Syst Bacterol 33:887, 1983

Jurtshuk P, Jr, Mueller TJ, Acord WC: Bacterial terminal oxidases. Crit Rev Microbiol, 3:359, 1975

Jurtshuk P, Jr, Mueller TJ, Wong TY: Isolation and purification of the cytochrome oxidase of *Azotobacter vinelandii.* Biochim Biophys Acta 637:374, 1981

Jurtshuk P, Jr, Yang TY: Oxygen reactive hemoprotein components in bacterial respiratory systems. In Knowles CJ (ed): Diversity of Bacterial Respiratory Systems. Vol. 1. CRC Press, Boca Raton, FL, 1980

Kamp AF, La Riviere JWM, Verhoeven W (eds): Jan Albert Kluyver: His Life and Work. Interscience, New York, 1959

Kluyver JA, Van Niel CB: The microbe's contribution to biology. Harvard University Press, Cambridge, MA, 1956

Kornberg HL: The role and maintenance of the tricarboxylic acid cycle in *Escherichia coli.* In Goodwin TW (ed): British Biochemistry Past and Present. Biochemistry Society Symposium no. 30. Academic Press, London, 1970

Lemberg R, Barrett J: Bacterial cytochromes and cytochrome oxidases. In Lemberg R, Barrett J: Cytochromes. Academic Press, New York, 1973

Mandelstam J, McQuillen K, Dawes I (eds): Biochemistry of Bacterial Growth. 3rd Ed. Blackwell, Oxford, 1982

O'Leary WM: The chemistry and metabolism of microbial lipids. World Publishing Co, Cleveland, 1967

Schlegel HG, Bowier B (eds): Autotrophic Bacteria. Science Tech, Madison, WI, 1989

Thauer RK, Jungermann K, Decker K: Energy conservation in chemotrophic anaerobic bacteria. Bacteriol Rev 41:100, 1977

Thimann KV: The Life of Bacteria. 2nd Ed. Macmillan, New York, 1966

5 GENETICS

RANDALL K. HOLMES
MICHAEL G. JOBLING

GENERAL CONCEPTS

Genetic Information in Microbes

Genetic information in bacteria and many viruses is encoded in DNA, but some viruses use RNA. Replication of the genome is essential for inheritance of genetically determined traits. Gene expression usually involves transcription of DNA into messenger RNA (mRNA) and translation of mRNA into protein.

Genome Organization

The bacterial **chromosome** is a circular molecule of DNA that functions as a self-replicating genetic element **(replicon).** Extrachromosomal genetic elements such as plasmids and bacteriophages are nonessential replicons, which often determine resistance to antimicrobial agents, production of virulence factors, or other functions. The chromosome replicates semiconservatively; each DNA strand serves as a template for synthesis of its complementary strand.

Mutation and Selection

The complete set of genetic determinants of an organism constitutes its **genotype,** and the observable characteristics constitute its **phenotype. Mutations** are heritable changes in genotype that can occur spontaneously or be induced by chemical or physical treatments. The genotype and phenotype of organisms selected as reference strains constitute the **wild type,** and progeny with mutations are called **mutants. Selective media** distinguish between wild type and mutant strains based on

growth; **differential media** distinguish between them based on other phenotypic properties.

Exchange of Genetic Information

Genetic exchanges among bacteria occur by several mechanisms. In **transformation,** the recipient bacterium takes up extracellular donor DNA. In **transduction,** donor DNA packaged in a bacteriophage infects the recipient bacterium. In **conjugation,** the donor bacterium transfers DNA to the recipient by mating. **Recombination** is the rearrangement of donor and recipient genomes to form new, hybrid genomes. **Transposons** are mobile DNA segments that move from place to place within or between genomes.

Recombinant DNA and Gene Cloning

Gene cloning is the incorporation of a foreign gene into a vector to produce a recombinant DNA molecule that replicates and expresses the foreign gene in a recipient cell. Cloned genes are detected by the phenotypes they determine or by their nucleotide sequences. Recombinant DNA and gene cloning are essential tools for research in molecular microbiology and medicine. They have many medical applications, including development of new vaccines, drugs, diagnostic tests, and therapeutic methods.

Regulation of Gene Expression

Expression of genes in microbes is often regulated by intracellular or environmental conditions. Regulation can affect any step in gene expression, including transcription initiation or termination, translation, or activity of gene products. An **operon** is a set of genes that is transcribed as a single unit and expressed coordinately. **Specific regulation** induces or represses a particular gene or operon. **Global regulation** affects a set of operons, which constitute a **regulon.** All operons in the regulon are coordinately controlled by the same regulatory mechanism.

GENETIC INFORMATION IN MICROBES

The genetic material of bacteria and plasmids is DNA. Bacterial viruses (bacteriophages) have DNA or RNA as genetic material. The two essential functions of genetic material are **replication** and **expression.** Genetic material must replicate accurately so that progeny inherit all of the specific genetic determinants (the **genotype**) of the parental organism. Expression of specific genetic material under a particular set of growth conditions determines the observable characteristics **(phenotype)** of the organism. Bacteria have few structural or developmental features that can be observed easily, but they have a vast array of biochemical capabilities and patterns of susceptibility to antimicrobial agents or bacteriophages. These latter characteristics are often chosen as the inherited traits to be analyzed in studies of bacterial genetics.

Nucleic Acid Structure

Nucleic acids are large polymers consisting of repeating nucleotide units (Fig. 5-1). Each nucleotide contains one phosphate group, one pentose or deoxypentose sugar, and one purine or pyrimidine base. In DNA the sugar is D-2-deoxyribose; in RNA the sugar is D-ribose. In DNA the purine bases are adenine (A) and guanine (G) and the pyrimidine bases are thymine (T) and cytosine (C). In RNA, uracil (U) replaces thymine. Chemically modified purine and pyrimidine bases are found in some bacteria and bacteriophages. The repeating structure of polynucleotides involves alternating sugar and phosphate residues, with phosphodiester bonds linking the 3′-hydroxyl group of one nu-

cleotide sugar to the 5′-hydroxyl group of the adjacent nucleotide sugar. These asymmetric phosphodiester linkages define the polarity of the polynucleotide chain. A purine or pyrimidine base is linked at the 1′-carbon atom of each sugar resi-

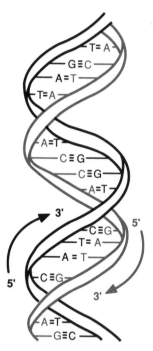

FIGURE 5-1   Double-helical structure of DNA. The backbone of each polynucleotide strand consists of alternating phosphate and deoxyribose residues linked by phosphodiester bonds, and the strands have opposite polarities (arrows). The purine and pyrimidine bases of each strand are linked to the complementary bases on the other strand by hydrogen bonds. The double helix has a diameter of 2 nm. Each full turn contains 10 nucleotide pairs and is 3.4 nm long.

due and projects from the repeating sugar-phosphate backbone. Double-stranded DNA is helical, and the two strands in the helix are antiparallel. The double helix is stabilized by hydrogen bonds between purine and pyrimidine bases on the opposite strands. At each position, A on one strand pairs via two hydrogen bonds with T on the opposite strand, or G pairs via three hydrogen bonds with C. The two strands of double-helical DNA are, therefore, complementary. Because of complementarity, double-stranded DNA contains equimolar amounts of purines (A + G) and pyrimidines (T + C), with A equal to T and G equal to C, but the mole fraction of G + C in DNA varies widely among different bacteria. Information in nucleic acids is encoded by the ordered sequence of nucleotides along the polynucleotide chain, and in double-stranded DNA the sequence of each strand determines what the sequence of the complementary strand must be. The extent of sequence homology between DNAs from different microorganisms is the most stringent criterion for determining how closely they are related.

DNA Replication

During replication of the bacterial genome, each strand in double-helical DNA serves as a template for synthesis of a new complementary strand. Each daughter double-stranded DNA molecular thus contains one old polynucleotide strand and one newly synthesized strand. This type of DNA replication is called **semiconservative.** Replication of chromosomal DNA in bacteria occurs at intracellular sites associated with the plasma membrane. When bacteria divide by binary fission after completing DNA replication, the membrane-associated DNA molecules are partitioned into each of the daughter cells. These characteristics of DNA replication during bacterial growth fulfill the requirements of the genetic material to be reproduced accurately and to be inherited by each daughter cell at the time of cell division.

Gene Expression

Genetic information encoded in DNA is expressed by synthesis of specific RNAs and proteins, and information flows from DNA to RNA to protein.

The DNA-directed synthesis of RNA is called **transcription.** Because the strands of double-helical DNA are antiparallel and complementary, only one of the two DNA strands can serve as the template for synthesis of a specific mRNA molecule. **Ribosomal RNAs (rRNAs)** and **transfer RNAs (tRNAs)** are components of the apparatus for protein synthesis, and they function in the production of many different proteins. **Messenger RNAs (mRNAs)** transmit information from DNA, and each mRNA in bacteria functions as the template for synthesis of one or more specific proteins. The process by which the nucleotide sequence of an mRNA molecule determines the primary amino acid sequence of a protein is called **translation.** A **gene** is a DNA sequence that encodes a protein, rRNA, or tRNA molecule (gene product). **Complementation tests** are used to determine whether independently isolated mutations associated with similar phenotypes affect the same or different genes.

The **genetic code** determines how the nucleotides in mRNA specify the amino acids in a polypeptide. Because there are only four different nucleotides in mRNA (U, A, C, and G), single nucleotides do not contain enough information to specify uniquely all 20 amino acids. In dinucleotides only 16 (4 × 4) arrangements of the four nucleotides are possible. However, in trinucleotides 64 (4 × 4 × 4) arrangements are possible. Therefore, trinucleotides, unlike single nucleotides and dinucleotides, can provide at least one unique sequence corresponding to each of the 20 amino acids. The "universal" genetic code used by most organisms (Table 5-1) is a triplet code in which 61 of the 64 possible trinucleotides **(codons)** encode specific amino acids and any of the three remaining codons results in termination of translation. The chain-terminating codons are called amber (UAG), ochre (UAA), and opal (UGA). They are also called **nonsense codons** because they do not specify any amino acids. The genetic code is described as **degenerate,** because several codons are used for some amino acids, and as **nonoverlapping,** because adjacent codons do not share any common nucleotides. Exceptions to the "universal" code include the use of UGA as a tryptophan codon in some *Mycoplasma* species and in mito-

TABLE 5-1   The Genetic Code[a]

First Nucleotide of Codon	Second Nucleotide of Codon				Third Nucleotide of Codon
	U	C	A	G	
U	Phe	Ser	Tyr	Cys	U
	Phe	Ser	Tyr	Cys	C
	Leu	Ser	Termination	Termination	A
	Leu	Ser	Termination	Trp	G
C	Leu	Pro	His	Arg	U
	Leu	Pro	His	Arg	C
	Leu	Pro	His	Arg	A
	Leu	Pro	His	Arg	G
A	Ile	Thr	Asn	Ser	U
	Ile	Thr	Asn	Ser	C
	Ile	Thr	Lys	Arg	A
	Met	Thr	Lys	Arg	G
G	Val	Ala	Asp	Gly	U
	Val	Ala	Asp	Gly	C
	Val	Ala	Glu	Gly	A
	Val	Ala	Glu	Gly	C

[a] Abbreviations: Ala, alanine; Arg, arginine; Asn, asparagine; Asp, aspartic acid; Cys, cysteine; Gln, glutamine; Glu, glutamic acid; Gly, glycine; His, histidine; Ile, isoleucine; Leu, leucine; Lys, lysine; Met, methionine; Phe, phenylalanine; Pro, proline; Ser, serine; Thr, threonine; Try, tyrosine; Trp, tryptophan; Val, valine.

chondrial DNA and a few additional codon differences in mitochondrial DNAs from yeasts, *Drosophila* species, and mammals. Translation of mRNA is usually initiated at an AUG codon for methionine, and adjacent codons are translated sequentially as the mRNA is read in the 5′-to-3′ direction. The corresponding polypeptide chain is assembled beginning at its amino terminus and proceeding toward its carboxy terminus. The sequence of amino acids in the polypeptide is therefore colinear with the sequence of nucleotides in the mRNA and the corresponding gene. Specific enzymatic reactions involved in DNA, RNA, and protein synthesis are beyond the scope of this chapter.

Expression of genetic determinants in bacteria involves the unidirectional flow of information from DNA to RNA to protein. In bacteriophages, either DNA or RNA can serve as genetic material. During infection of bacteria by RNA bacteriophages, RNA molecules serve as templates for RNA replication and as mRNAs. Studies with the retrovirus group of animal viruses reveal that DNA molecules can be synthesized from RNA templates by enzymes designated as RNA-dependent DNA polymerases (**reverse transcriptases**). This reversal of the usual direction for flow of genetic information, from RNA to DNA instead of from DNA to RNA, is an important mechanism for enabling information from retroviruses to be encoded in DNA and to become incorporated into the genomes of animal cells.

GENOME ORGANIZATION

DNA molecules that replicate as discrete genetic units in bacteria are called **replicons.** In some *Escherichia coli* strains, the chromosome is the only replicon present in the cell. Other bacterial strains have additional replicons, such as plasmids and bacteriophages.

Chromosomal DNA

Bacterial genomes vary in size from about 0.4×10^9 to 8.6×10^9 daltons (Da). The amount of DNA in the genome determines the maximum amount of information that it can encode. The **chromosome** of the common intestinal bacterium *E coli* is a single, circular molecular of double-stranded DNA of 3×10^9 (Da) (4,500 kilobase pairs [kbp]), accounting for about 2 to 3 percent of the dry weight of the cell. The *E coli* genome is about 0.1 percent of the size of the human genome and is sufficient to code for several thousand polypeptides of average size.

The chromosome of *E coli* has a contour length of approximately 1.35 mm, several hundred times longer than the bacterial cell, but the DNA is supercoiled and tightly packaged in the bacterial nucleoid. Chromosomal replication starts at a specific chromosomal site called the **origin** and proceeds bidirectionally until the process is completed (Fig. 5-2). Replication of the entire chromosome requires about 40 min, which exceeds the shortest division time for this bacterium. Cell division is coupled with completion of chromosomal replication, but in rapidly growing bacteria a new round of chromosomal replication begins before an earlier round is completed. Thus, the chromosome in rapidly growing bacteria is replicating at more than one point. The replication of chromosomal DNA in bacteria is complex and involves many different proteins.

Plasmids

Plasmids are replicons that are maintained as discrete, extrachromosomal genetic elements in bacteria. They are much smaller than the bacterial chromosome, varying from less than 5 to more than 100 kbp, and usually encode traits that are not essential for bacterial viability. Most plasmids are supercoiled, circular, double-stranded DNA molecules, but linear plasmids have been demonstrated in *Borrelia* and *Streptomyces* species. Closely related plasmids demonstrate **incompatibility;** they cannot be stably maintained in the same bacterial host. Classification of plasmids is based on incompatibility or on the use of specific DNA probes in hybridization tests to identify nucleotide

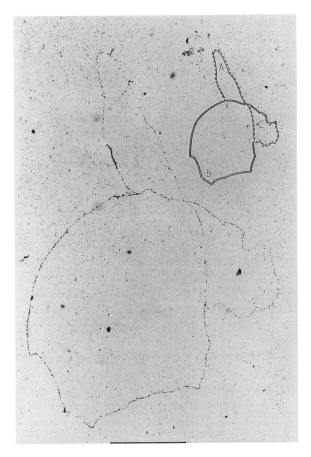

FIGURE 5-2 Autoradiograph of intact replicating chromosome of *E coli*. Bacteria were radioactively labeled with tritiated thymidine for approximately two generations. The sketch diagrams the geometry of replication. The circular chromosome replicates at two forks, X and Y. The segments of chromosome represented by double lines had completed two replications in presence of tritiated thymidine, whereas the segments represented by a solid line and a dotted line had replicated only once in the presence of tritiated thymidine. Bar, 100 μm. (From Cairns JP: The chromosome of *Escherichia coli*. Cold Spring Harbor Symp Quant Biol 28:44, 1963, with permission.)

sequences that are characteristic of specific plasmid replicons. Some hybrid plasmids contain more than one replicon. **Conjugative plasmids** code for functions that promote transfer of the plasmid from the donor bacterium to other recipient bacteria, but **nonconjugative plasmids** do not. Conjugative plasmids that also promote transfer of the bacterial chromosome from the donor bacterium to other recipient bacteria are called **fertility plasmids;** they are discussed below. The average number of a given plasmid per bacterial chromosome is called its **copy number.** Large plasmids (> 40 kbp) are often conjugative, have small copy numbers (one to several per chromosome), code for all functions required for their replication, and partition themselves among daughter cells during cell division in a manner similar to the bacterial chromosome. Plasmids smaller than 7.5 kbp usually are nonconjugative, have high copy numbers (typically 10 or more per chromosome), rely on their bacterial host to provide some functions required for replication, and are distributed randomly between daughter cells at division.

Many plasmids control medically important properties of pathogenic bacteria, including resistance to one or several antibiotics, production of toxins, and synthesis of cell surface structures required for adherence or colonization. Plasmids that determine resistance to antibiotics are often called **R plasmids** (or **R factors**). Representative toxins encoded by plasmids include heat-labile and heat-stable enterotoxins of *E coli,* exfoliative toxin of *Staphylococcus aureus,* and tetanus toxin of *Clostridium tetani.* Some plasmids are **cryptic** (i.e., they have no recognizable effects on the bacterial cells that harbor them). Comparing plasmid profiles is a useful method for assessing possible relatedness of individual clinical isolates of a particular bacterial species for epidemiologic studies. The role of plasmids in the evolution of resistance to antibiotics is discussed below.

Bacteriophages

Bacteriophages (bacterial viruses, phages) are infectious agents that replicate as obligate intracellular parasites in bacteria. Extracellular phage particles are metabolically inert and consist principally of proteins plus nucleic acid (DNA or RNA, but not both). The proteins of the phage particle form a protective shell **(capsid)** surrounding the tightly packaged nucleic acid genome. Phage genomes vary in size from approximately 2 to 200 kilobases (kb) per strand of nucleic acid and consist of double-stranded DNA, single-stranded DNA, or RNA. Phage genomes, like plasmids, encode functions required for replication in bacteria, but unlike plasmids they also encode capsid proteins and nonstructural proteins required for phage assembly. Several morphologically distinct types of phage have been described, including polyhedral, filamentous, and complex phages. Complex phages have polyhedral heads to which tails and sometimes other appendages (tail plates, tail fibers, etc.) are attached.

A single cycle of phage growth is shown in Figure 5-3. Infection is initiated by **adsorption** of phage to specific receptors on the surface of susceptible host bacteria. The capsids remain at the cell surface, and the DNA or RNA genomes enter the target cells **(penetration).** Because infectivity of genomic DNA or RNA is much lower than that of mature virus, there is a period immediately after infection called the **eclipse period** during which intracellular infectious phage cannot be detected. The infecting phage RNA or DNA is replicated to produce many new copies of the phage genome, and phage-specific proteins are produced. For most phages **assembly** of progeny occurs in the cytoplasm and **release** of the progeny occurs by cell lysis. In contrast, filamentous phages are formed at the cell envelope and released without killing the host cells. The eclipse period ends when intracellular infectious progeny appear. The **latent period** is the interval from infection until extracellular progeny appear, and the **rise period** is the interval from the end of the latent period until all phage are extracellular. The average number of phage particles produced by each infected cell (the **burst size**) is characteristic for each virus and often ranges between 50 and several hundred. For discussions of the structure, multiplication, and classification of animal viruses, see Chapters 41 and 42.

Phages are classified into two major groups: **virulent** and **temperate.** Growth of virulent phages in susceptible bacteria destroys the host cells. Infection of susceptible bacteria by temperate phages can have either of two outcomes: **lytic growth** or **lysogeny.** Lytic growth of temperate and virulent

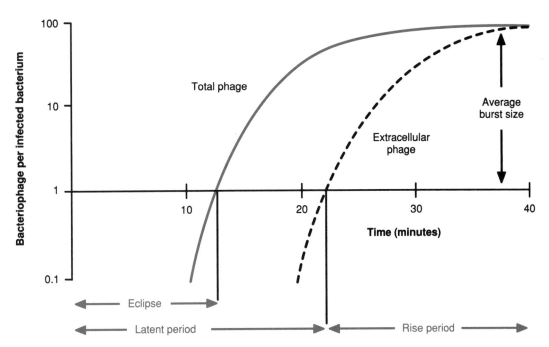

FIGURE 5-3 One-step growth of bacteriophage. A culture of susceptible bacteria was synchronously infected with bacteriophage added at time zero at a low multiplicity of infection. Unabsorbed phage was inactivated shortly thereafter by addition of antiphage antiserum, and the culture was then diluted to prevent further activity of the antiserum. Samples were taken at intervals for phage assays. Total phage (intracellular plus extracellular) was determined by testing the sample after treating it to disrupt infected bacteria, and extracellular phage was determined by testing supernatant after removal of bacteria by centrifugation or ultrafiltration. Phage titers are expressed as the number of phage per infected bacterial cell.

bacteriophages is similar, leading to production of phage progeny and death of the host bacteria. Lysogeny is a specific type of latent viral infection in which the phage genome replicates as a **prophage** in the bacterial cell. In most lysogenic bacteria the genes required for lytic phage development are not expressed, and infectious phage is not produced. Furthermore, the lysogenic cells are immune to superinfection by the virus that they harbor as a prophage. The physical state of the prophage is not identical for all temperate viruses. For example, the prophage of bacteriophage lambda (λ) in *E coli* is integrated into the bacterial chromosome at a specific site and replicates as part of the bacterial chromosome, whereas the prophage of bacteriophage P1 in *E coli* replicates as an extrachromosomal plasmid.

Lytic phage growth occurs spontaneously in a small fraction of lysogenic cells, and a few extracellular phages are present in cultures of lysogenic bacteria. For some lysogenic bacteria, synchronous **induction** of lytic phage development occurs in the entire population of lysogenic bacteria when they are treated with agents that damage DNA, such as ultraviolet light or mitomycin C. The loss of prophage from a lysogenic bacterium, converting it to the nonlysogenic state and restoring susceptibility to infection by the phage that was originally present as prophage, is called **curing.**

Some temperate phages contain genes for bacterial characteristics that are unrelated to lytic phage development or the lysogenic state, and expression of such genes is called **phage conversion** (or **lysogenic conversion**). Examples of phage conversion that are important for microbial virulence include production of diphtheria toxin by *Corynebacterium diphtheriae,* erythrogenic toxin by *Streptococcus pyogenes* (group A β-hemolytic streptococci), botulinum toxin by *Clostridium botulinum,* and Shiga-like toxins by *E coli*. In each of these examples the gene that encodes the bacterial toxin is present in a temperate phage genome. The specificity of O antigens in *Salmonella* can also be controlled by phage conversion. **Phage typing** is the testing of strains of a particular bacterial species for susceptibility to specific bacteriophages. The patterns of susceptibility to the set of typing phages provide information about the possible relatedness of individual clinical isolates. Such information is particularly useful for epidemiologic investigations.

MUTATION AND SELECTION

Mutations are heritable changes in the genome. Spontaneous mutations in individual bacteria are rare. Some mutations cause changes in phenotypic characteristics; the occurrence of such mutations can be inferred from the effects they produce. In microbial genetics, specific reference organisms are designated as **wild-type strains,** and descendants that have mutations in their genomes are called **mutants.** Therefore, mutants are characterized by the inherited differences between them and their ancestral wild-type strains. Variant forms of a specific genetic determinant are called **alleles.** Genotypic symbols are lowercase, italicized abbreviations that specify individual genes, with a (+) superscript indicating the wild-type allele. Phenotypic symbols have the first letter capitalized and are not italicized, to distinguish them from genotypic symbols. For example, the genotypic symbol for the ability to produce β-galactosidase, required to ferment lactose, is *lacZ+* and mutants that cannot produce β-galactosidase are *lacZ*. The lactose-fermenting phenotype is designated Lac+, and inability to ferment lactose is indicated by Lac−.

Detection of Mutant Phenotypes

Selective and **differential media** are helpful for isolating bacterial mutants. Some selective media permit particular mutants to grow, but do not allow the wild-type strains to grow. Rare mutants can be isolated by using such selective media. Differential media permit wild-type and mutant bacteria to grow and form colonies that differ in appearance. Detection of rare mutants on differential media is limited by the total number of colonies that can be observed. Consider a wild-type strain of *E coli* that is susceptible to the antibiotic streptomycin (phenotype Str^s) and can utilize lactose as the sole source of carbon (phenotype Lac+). Spontaneously occurring streptomycin-resistant (Str^r) mutants are rare and are usually found at frequencies of less than 1 per 10^9 bacteria in cultures of wild-type *E coli*. Nevertheless, Str^r mutants can be isolated easily by using selective media containing streptomycin, because the wild-type Str^s bacteria are killed. Isolation of lactose-negative (phenotype Lac−) mutants of *E coli* poses a different problem. On minimal media with lactose as the sole source of carbon, Lac+ strains will grow, but Lac− mutants cannot grow. On differential media such as MacConkey-lactose agar or eosin-methylene blue-lactose agar, Lac+ and Lac− strains can be distinguished by their color, but spontaneous Lac− mutants are too rare to be isolated easily. Selective media for Lac− mutants can be made by incorporating chemical analogs of lactose that are converted into toxic metabolites by Lac+ bacteria but not by Lac− mutants. The Lac− mutants can then grow on such media, but the Lac+ bacteria are killed.

Mutations that inactivate essential genes in haploid organisms are usually lethal, but such mutations can be studied if their expression can be controlled by manipulation of experimental conditions. For example, a mutation that increases the thermolability of an essential gene product may prevent bacterial growth at 42°C, although the mutant bacterium can still grow at 25°C. Conversely, cold-sensitive mutants express the mutant phenotype at low temperature, but not at high temperature. Temperature-sensitive and cold-sensitive mutations are examples of **conditional mutations,** as are suppressible mutations described later in this chapter. A **conditional-lethal** phenotype indicates that the mutant gene is essential for viability.

Spontaneous and Induced Mutations

The **mutation rate** in bacteria is determined by the accuracy of DNA replication, the occurrence of damage to DNA, and the effectiveness of mechanisms for repair of damaged DNA. For a particular bacterial strain under defined growth conditions, the mutation rate for any specific gene is constant and is expressed as the probability of mutation per cell division. In a population of bacteria grown from a small inoculum, the proportion of mutants usually increases progressively as the size of the bacterial population increases.

Mutations in bacteria can occur spontaneously and independently of the experimental methods used to detect them. This principle was first demonstrated by the **fluctuation test** (Fig. 5-4). The numbers of phage-resistant mutants of *E coli* in replicate cultures grown from small inocula were measured and compared with those in multiple samples taken from a single culture. If mutations to phage resistance occurred only after exposure to phage, the variability in numbers of mutants between cultures should be similar under both sets of conditions. In contrast, if the mutations occurred spontaneously before exposure of the bacteria to phage, the numbers of mutants should be more variable in the independently grown cultures, because differences in the size of the bacterial population when the first mutant appeared

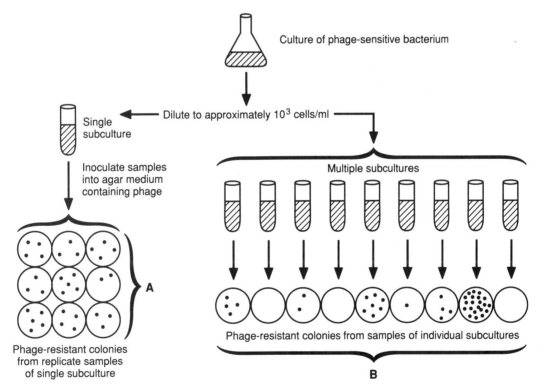

FIGURE 5-4 The fluctuation test. Differences in numbers of colonies of phage-resistant mutants in replicate samples from a single subculture *(A)* are small and reflect only expected fluctuations due to sampling errors. In contrast, numbers of phage-resistant colonies in samples from individual subcultures *(B)* are more variable and reflect both sampling errors and the independent origins of mutants in individual subcultures. Sizes of clonal populations of mutants in each culture reflect numbers of generations of growth between the times when mutations occurred and the time of sampling.

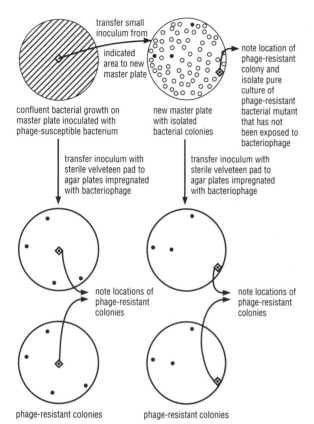

note location of phage-resistant colony and isolate pure culture of phage-resistant bacterial mutant that has not been exposed to bacteriophage

confluent bacterial growth on master plate inoculated with phage-susceptible bacterium

new master plate with isolated bacterial colonies

transfer inoculum with sterile velveteen pad to agar plates impregnated with bacteriophage

transfer inoculum with sterile velveteen pad to agar plates impregnated with bacteriophage

note locations of phage-resistant colonies

note locations of phage-resistant colonies

phage-resistant colonies

phage-resistant colonies

FIGURE 5-5   Detection of preexisting bacterial mutants by replica plating. The master plate was heavily inoculated with sample from pure cultures of phage-susceptible bacteria. After incubation, bacteria from the master plate were transferred by replica plating to duplicate agar plates impregnated with bacteriophage. Phage-susceptible bacteria were killed by the bacteriophage. Colonies of phage-resistant bacteria appeared at identical positions on duplicate plates, indicating that phage-resistant bacteria had been transferred to each replica plate from the corresponding locations on the master plate. Bacterial inocula selected from appropriate locations on the master plate contained a higher proportion of phage-resistant mutants than did the original bacterial culture. By repeating these procedures several times, it was possible to isolate pure cultures of phage-resistant bacterial mutants that had never been exposed to bacteriophage.

would contribute to the observed variability. The data indicated that the mutations to phage resistance in *E coli* occurred spontaneously with constant probability per cell division.

Replica plating confirmed that mutations in bacteria can occur spontaneously, without exposure of bacteria to selective agents (Fig. 5-5). For replica plating, a flat, sterile, velveteen surface is used to pick up an inoculum from the surface of an agar master plate and transfer samples to other agar plates. In this manner, samples of the bacterial population from the master plate are transferred to the replica plates without distorting their spatial arrangement. If the replica plates contain selective medium and the master plates do not, the positions of selected mutant colonies on the replica plates can be noted, and bacteria that were not exposed to the selective conditions can be isolated from the same positions on the master plate. Mutants of *E coli* resistant to bacteriophage T1 or to streptomycin have been isolated in this way, without exposing the wild-type bacteria to the bacteriophage or the antibiotic.

Both environmental and genetic factors affect mutation rates. Exposure of bacteria to **mutagenic agents** causes mutation rates to increase, sometimes by several orders of magnitude. Many chemical and physical agents, including X-rays and ultraviolet light, have mutagenic activity. Chemicals that are carcinogenic for animals are often mutagenic for bacteria or can be converted by animal tissues to metabolites that are mutagenic for bacteria. Standardized tests for mutagenicity in bacteria are used as screening procedures to identify environmental agents that may be carcinogenic in humans. **Mutator genes** in bacteria cause an increase in spontaneous mutation rates for a wide variety of other genes. The overall mutation rate —the probability that a mutation will occur somewhere in the bacterial genome per cell division— is relatively constant for a variety of organisms with genomes of different sizes and appears to be a significant factor in determining the fitness of a bacterial strain for survival in nature. Most mutations are deleterious or neutral, and the risk of adverse mutations for individual bacteria must be

TABLE 5-2   Classification of Mutations

Change in DNA	Effect on Polypeptide Structure	Effect on Polypeptide Function	Comments
Nucleotide substitution	1. None	1. None	1. Silent mutation (no phenotypic change)
	2. Amino acid substitution	2. Variable	2. Missense mutation (usually CRM$^+$)^a
	3. Premature termination	3. Usually lost	3. Nonsense mutations (CRM$^-$ or CRM$^+$); extragenic suppression common
Microdeletion or microinsertion	Frameshift mutation	Usually lost	Intragenic suppression common
Large insertions	Altered	Usually lost	See section on transposons
Large deletions	Altered	Usually lost	No reversion

^{a} CRM, Cross-reacting material. Mutant polypeptides are CRM$^+$ if they share antigenic determinants with the corresponding wild-type polypeptides.

balanced against the positive value of mutability as a mechanism for adaptation of bacterial populations to changing environmental conditions.

Molecular Basis of Mutations

Mutations are classified on the basis of structural changes that occur in DNA (Table 5-2). Some mutations are localized within short segments of DNA (e.g., nucleotide substitutions, microdeletions, and microinsertions). Other mutations involve large regions of DNA and include deletions, insertions, or rearrangements of segments of DNA.

When a **nucleotide substitution** occurs in a region of DNA that codes for a polypeptide, one of the three nucleotides within a single codon of a corresponding mRNA molecule will be changed. **Silent mutations** cause no change in polypeptide structure or function, because one codon in mRNA is changed to another for the same amino acid. Other substitutions cause one amino acid to be replaced by another at the specific position within the polypeptide corresponding to the altered codon. Mutations that result in replacement of one amino acid for another within a polypeptide chain are called **missense mutations.** The effects of amino acid replacements on the function of a polypeptide gene product vary and depend on the

location and the identity of the amino acid replacement. Mutant polypeptides containing amino acid replacements usually share antigenic determinants with the wild-type polypeptide and often have some residual biologic activity. Mutations that result in failure to produce a detectable gene product are called **nonsense mutations.** Nucleotide substitutions in DNA can create chain-terminating codons within a coding sequence of mRNA, resulting in production of an amino-terminal fragment of the normal polypeptide when the mutant mRNA is translated. Mutations that produce premature chain termination often result in complete loss of activity of the gene product.

Because of the triplet nature of the genetic code, the consequences of mutations caused by **insertions** or **deletions** of small numbers of nucleotides (microinsertions, microdeletions) depend on both the number and sequence of nucleotides involved. Deletion or addition of multiples of three nucleotide pairs does not affect the reading frame, but causes deletion or addition of appropriate numbers of amino acids at one site within the polypeptide. If a new chain-terminating codon is introduced, premature chain termination occurs within the polypeptide. In contrast, addition or deletion of other numbers of nucleotide pairs alters the reading frame for the entire segment of mRNA from the mutation to the distal end of the gene. Therefore, **frameshift mutations** are likely to cause drastic changes in the structure and activity of polypeptide gene products, and they are often classified as nonsense mutations.

Complementation Tests

To determine whether mutations are located in the same gene or different genes, **complementation tests** are performed with partially diploid bacterial strains (Fig. 5-6). Two copies of the region of the bacterial chromosome harboring a mutation are present in the same bacterium, with each copy containing a different mutation (mutations are in the *trans* arrangement). A wild-type phenotype indicates that the mutations are in different genes. This phenomenon is called **complementation.** If a mutant phenotype is observed, a control experi-

ment should be performed with the mutations in the *cis* arrangement to exclude the possibility that the wild-type alleles cannot be expressed normally in a partially diploid bacterial strain. Complementation tests were originally called *"cis-trans"* tests, and the term **cistron** is still used as a synonym for gene. Complementation tests can be performed and interpreted even if the specific biochemical functions of the gene products are unknown.

As an example, consider the use of complementation test to characterize two independently derived Lac⁻ mutants of *E coli*. The biochemical pathway for utilization of lactose requires β-galactoside permease (genotypic symbol *lacY*) to transport lactose into the bacterial cell and β-galactosidase (genotypic symbol *lacZ*) to convert lactose into D-glucose and D-galactose. Mutants that lack β-galactoside permease or β-galactosidase cannot utilize lactose for growth. If the mutations in both

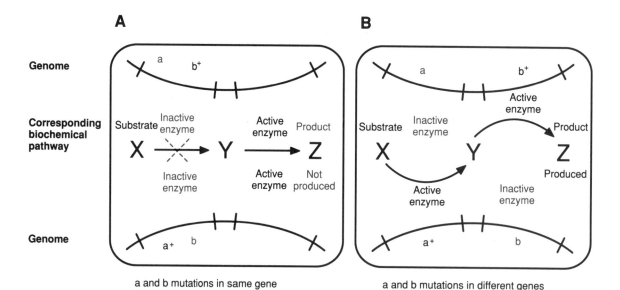

FIGURE 5-6 Complementation as a method to test for functional gene products. Two mutants, a and b, with similar phenotypes (inability to convert substrate X to product Z) were isolated. The wild-type alleles are a⁺ and b⁺. Partially diploid heterozygous strains were tested to determine whether mutations a and b are in the same structural gene (cistron) and inactivated the same gene products. *(A)* If a and b are in the same structural gene neither the a⁺b nor the ab⁺ allele codes for an active enzyme, substrate X cannot be utilized, the mutant phenotype is expressed, and no complementation occurs. *(B)* If a and b are in different cistrons the a⁺ and b⁺ alleles encode active enzymes, substrate X is converted to product Z, the wild-type phenotype is expressed, and complementation occurs.

Lac⁻ mutants inactivated the same protein (e.g., β-galactoside), a partial diploid strain containing the *lacZ* genes from both mutants in the *trans* arrangement would be unable to utilize lactose. In contrast, if the genotypes of the two mutants were *lacZ⁺ lacY* and *lacZ lacY⁺*, the partially diploid bacterium would produce active β-galactosidase from the *lacZ⁺* determinant and active β-galactoside permease from the *lacY⁺* determinant. Complementation would occur, and the partially diploid strain would utilize lactose.

Reversion and Suppression

Mutations that convert the phenotype from wild type to mutant are called **forward mutations,** and mutations that change the phenotype from mutant back to wild type are called **reverse mutations (reversions).** Bacterial strains that contain reverse mutations are called **revertants.** Analysis of mutations that cause phenotypic reversion yields useful information. Reverse mutations that restore the exact nucleotide sequence of the wild-type DNA are true reversions. True revertants are identical to wild-type strains both genotypically and phenotypically. Reverse mutations that do not restore the exact nucleotide sequence of the wild-type DNA are called **suppressor mutations (suppressors).** Some revertants that harbor suppressor mutations are phenotypically indistinguishable from wild-type strains. Other revertants, called **pseudorevertants,** can be distinguished phenotypically from wild-type strains, for example, by subtle differences in the characteristics of an enzymatic activity that has been regained (such as specific activity, substrate specificity, kinetic constants, or susceptibility to thermal or chemical inactivation). Recognition of pseudorevertant phenotypes suggests the presence of suppressor mutations.

Suppressor mutations can be intragenic or extragenic. **Intragenic suppressors** are located in the same gene as the forward mutations that they suppress. The possible locations and nature of intragenic suppressors are determined by the original forward mutation and by the relationships between the primary structure of the gene product and its biologic activity. **Extragenic suppressors** are located in different genes from mutations

whose effects they suppress. The ability of extragenic suppressors to suppress a variety of independent mutations can be tested. Some extragenic suppressors are specific for particular genes, some are specific for particular codons, and some have other specificity patterns. Extragenic suppressors that reverse the phenotypic effects of specific chain-terminating codons have been well characterized and found to alter the structure of specific tRNAs. A particular suppressor tRNA can permit a specific chain-terminating codon to be translated, resulting in incorporation of a specific amino acid into the nascent polypeptide at the position corresponding to the chain-terminating codon. In a bacterium that has a chain-terminating mutation and an appropriate extragenic suppressor, translation of the mRNA containing the mutant codon can lead either to premature chain termination or to formation of a suppressed full-length polypeptide. The biologic activity of the suppressed full-length polypeptide depends both on the amount of protein made and on the functional consequences of the specific amino acid replacement determined by the suppressor tRNA.

EXCHANGE OF GENETIC INFORMATION

The biologic significance of **sexuality** in microorganisms is to increase the probability that rare, independent mutations will occur together in a single microbe and be subjected to natural selection. Genetic interactions between microbes enable their genomes to evolve much more rapidly than by mutation alone. Representative phenomena of medical importance that involve exchanges of genetic information or genomic rearrangements include the rapid emergence and dissemination of antibiotic resistance plasmids, flagellar phase variation in *Salmonella* species, and antigenic variation of surface antigens in *Neisseria* and *Borrelia* species.

Sexual processes in bacteria involve transfer of genetic information from a donor to a recipient and result in either substitution of donor alleles for recipient alleles or addition of donor genetic elements to the recipient genome. **Transformation,**

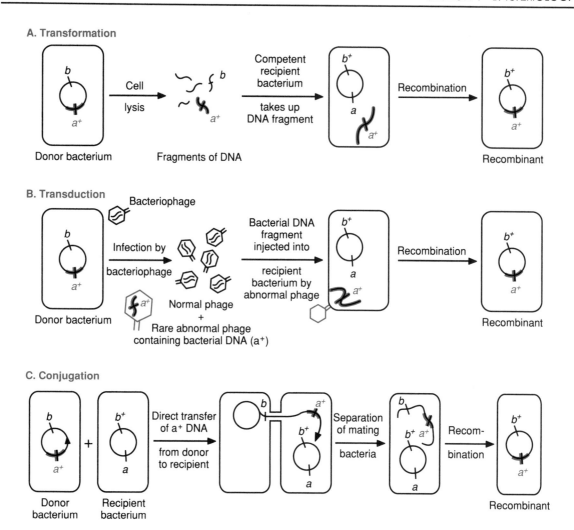

FIGURE 5-7 Exchange of genetic information in bacteria by transformation, transduction, and conjugation. *(A)* In transformation, fragments of DNA released from donor bacteria are taken up by competent recipient bacteria. *(B)* In transduction, abnormal bacteriophage particles containing DNA from donor bacteria inject their DNA into recipient bacteria. *(C)* Conjugation occurs by formation of cytoplasmic connections between donor and recipient bacteria, with direct transfer of donor DNA into the recipient cells. In all three cases, recombination between donor and recipient DNA molecules is required for formation of stable recombinant genomes. In each case, the a^+ allele from the donor strain replaces the a allele from the recipient strain.

transduction, and **conjugation** are sexual processes that use different mechanisms to introduce donor DNA into recipient bacteria (Fig. 5-7). Because donor DNA cannot persist in the recipient bacterium unless it is part of a replicon, **recombination** between donor and recipient genomes is often required to produce stable, hybrid progeny.

Recombination is most likely to occur when the donor and recipient bacteria are from the same or closely related species.

For a recombinant to be detected, its phenotype must be different from both parental phenotypes. Growth or cell division may be required before the recombinant phenotype is expressed. Delay in expression of a recombinant phenotype until a haploid recombinant genome has segregated is called the **segregation lag,** and delay until synthesis of products encoded by donor genes has occurred is called the **phenotypic lag.** Testing for **linkage** (nonrandom reassortment of parental alleles in recombinant progeny) is possible when the parental bacteria have different alleles for several genes. The donor allele of an unselected gene is more likely to be present in recombinants if it is linked to the selected donor gene than if it is not. Quantita-

tive analysis of linkage permits construction of **genetic maps.** The genome of *E coli* is circular (Fig. 5-8), as determined by both genetic linkage and direct biochemical analysis of chromosomal DNA, and the genetic map is colinear with the **physical map** of the chromosomal DNA. Genetic and physical mapping are also used to analyze extrachromosomal replicons such as bacteriophages and plasmids.

Many bacteria have **restriction systems,** consisting of **modifying enzymes** that methylate ade-

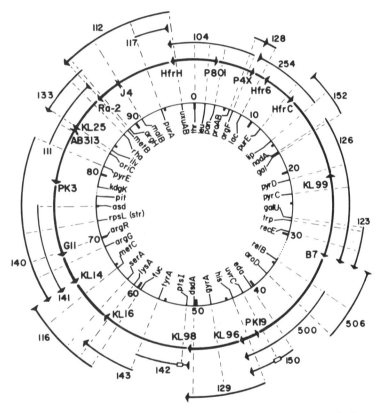

FIGURE 5-8 Circular genetic map of *E coli*. Positions of representative genes are indicated on the inner circle. The distances between genes are calibrated in minutes, based on times required for transfer during conjugation. The position of the threonine *(thr)* locus is arbitrarily designated as 0 minutes. On the next circle, symbols and arrowheads identify specific Hfr donor strains of *E coli* and their characteristics. For each Hfr strain, the point of the arrowhead is the origin for chromosomal transfer; oriented transfer of the chromosome during conjugation proceeds from the point of the arrowhead. F′ plasmids are identified by numbers, and the fragment of the *E coli* chromosome present in each F′ plasmid is represented by an arc corresponding to a specific segment of the circular genetic map. (From Bachmann BJ, Low KB: Linkage map of *Escherichia coli* K-12, edition 6. Microbiol Rev 44:31, 1980, with permission.)

nine or cytosine residues at specific sequences in their own DNA and corresponding **restriction endonucleases** that cleave foreign DNA that is incorrectly modified at the same target sequences. Such restriction systems, which probably evolved to protect bacteria against invasion by phages or plasmids, are an important barrier to genetic exchanges between different bacterial strains or species.

Transformation

In **transformation,** pieces of DNA released from donor bacteria are taken up directly from the extracellular environment by recipient bacteria. Recombination occurs between single molecules of transforming DNA and the chromosomes of recipient bacteria. To be active in transformation, DNA molecules must be large (at least 500 nucleotides). Transforming activity is destroyed rapidly by treating DNA with deoxyribonuclease (DNase). Molecules of transforming DNA correspond to very small fragments of the bacterial chromosome. Co-transformation of genes is unlikely, therefore, unless they are so closely linked that they can be encoded on a single DNA fragment. Transformation was discovered in *Streptococcus pneumoniae* and occurs in other bacterial genera including *Haemophilus, Neisseria, Bacillus,* and *Staphylococcus.* The ability of bacteria to take up extracellular DNA and to become transformed, called **competence,** varies with the physiologic state of the bacteria. Many bacteria that are not usually competent can be made to take up DNA by laboratory manipulations such as calcium shock or exposure to a high-voltage electrical pulse (electroporation). In some bacteria (including *Haemophilus* and *Neisseria* species) DNA uptake depends on the presence of specific oligonucleotide sequences in the transforming DNA, but in others (including *S pneumoniae*) DNA uptake is not sequence specific. Competent bacteria may also take up intact bacteriophage DNA **(transfection)** or plasmid DNA, which can then replicate as extrachromosomal genetic elements in the recipient bacteria. In contrast, a piece of chromosomal DNA from a donor bacterium usually cannot replicate in the recipient bacterium unless it becomes part of a replicon by recombination.

Historically, characterization of "transforming principle" from *S pneumoniae* provided the first direct evidence that DNA is the genetic material of bacteria.

Transduction

In **transduction,** bacteriophages function as vectors to introduce DNA from donor bacteria into recipient bacteria by infection. For some phages, called **generalized transducing phages,** a small fraction of the virions produced during lytic growth are aberrant and contain a random fragment of the bacterial genome instead of phage DNA. Each individual transducing phage carries a different set of closely linked genes, representing a small segment of the bacterial genome that is comparable in size to the phage genome. Transduction mediated by populations of such phages is called **generalized transduction,** because each part of the bacterial genome has approximately the same probability of being transferred from donor to recipient bacteria. When a generalized transducing phage infects a recipient cell, the transferred donor genes are expressed. **Abortive transduction** refers to the transient expression of one or more donor genes without formation of recombinant progeny, whereas **complete transduction** is characterized by production of stable recombinants that inherit donor genes and retain the ability to express them. In abortive transduction the donor DNA fragment does not replicate, and among the progeny of the original transductant only one bacterium contains the donor DNA fragment; in all other progeny the donor gene products become progressively diluted after each generation of bacterial growth until the donor phenotype can no longer be expressed. On selective medium upon which only bacteria with the donor phenotype can grow, abortive transductants produce minute colonies that can be distinguished easily from colonies of stable transductants. The frequency of abortive transduction is typically 1 to 2 orders of magnitude greater than the frequency of generalized transduction, indicating that most cells infected by generalized transducing phages do not produce recombinant progeny.

Specialized transduction differs from generalized transduction in several ways. It is mediated only by specific temperate phages, and only a few specific donor genes can be transferred to recipient bacteria. **Specialized transducing phages** are formed only when lysogenic donor bacteria enter the lytic cycle and release phage progeny. The specialized transducing phages are rare recombinants, which lack part of the normal phage genome and contain part of the bacterial chromosome located adjacent to the prophage attachment site. Many specialized transducing phages are defective and cannot complete the lytic cycle of phage growth in infected cells unless helper phages are present to provide missing phage functions. Specialized transduction results from lysogenization of the recipient bacterium by the specialized transducing phage and expression of the donor genes. Phage conversion and specialized transduction are essentially similar, except that the origin of the converting genes is unknown.

Conjugation

In **conjugation,** direct contact between the donor and recipient bacteria leads to establishment of a cytoplasmic bridge between them and transfer of part or all of the donor genome to the recipient. Donor ability is determined by specific conjugative plasmids called **fertility plasmids (F plasmids)** or sex plasmids.

The F plasmid (also called F factor) of *E coli* is the prototype for fertility plasmids in Gram-negative bacteria. Strains of *E coli* with an extrachromosomal F plasmid are called F^+ and function as donors, whereas strains that lack the F plasmid are F^- and behave as recipients. The conjugative functions of the F plasmid are specified by a cluster of at least 25 transfer (*tra*) genes, which determine expression of **F pili,** synthesis and transfer of DNA during mating, interference with the ability of F^+ bacteria to serve as recipients, and other functions. Each F^+ bacterium has 1 to 3 F pili that bind to a specific outer membrane protein (the *ompA* gene product) on recipient bacteria to initiate mating. An intracellular cytoplasmic bridge is formed, and one strand of the F-plasmid DNA is transferred from donor to recipient, beginning at a unique

origin and progressing in the 5′-to-3′ direction. The transferred strand is converted to circular double-stranded F-plasmid DNA in the recipient bacterium, and a new strand is synthesized in the donor to replace the transferred strand. Both of the exconjugant bacteria are F^+, and the F plasmid can therefore spread by infection among genetically compatible populations of bacteria. In addition to their role in conjugation, F pili function as receptors for donor-specific (male-specific) phages.

The F plasmid in *E coli* can exist as an extrachromosomal genetic element or be integrated into the bacterial chromosome (Fig. 5-9). Because the F plasmid and the bacterial chromosome are both circular DNA molecules, reciprocal recombination between them produces a larger DNA circle consisting of F-plasmid DNA inserted linearly into the chromosome. *Escherichia coli* contains multiple copies of several different genetic elements called **insertion sequences** (see the section on transposons for more detail) at various locations in its chromosome and in the F plasmid. Homologous recombination between insertion sequences in the chromosome and the F plasmid leads to preferential integration of the F plasmid at chromosomal sites where insertion sequences are located. The chromosomal sites where insertion sequences are found vary, however, among strains of *E coli*.

An *E coli* strain with an integrated F plasmid retains its ability to function as a donor in conjugal matings. Because donor strains with integrated F factors can transfer chromosomal genes to recipients with high efficiency, they are called **Hfr** (high-frequency recombination) strains. Transfer of single-stranded DNA from an Hfr donor to a recipient begins from the origin within the F plasmid and proceeds as described above, except that the transferred DNA is the hybrid replicon consisting of F plasmid integrated into the bacterial chromosome. Transfer of this entire replicon, including the bacterial chromosome, requires approximately 100 minutes. The identity of the first chromosomal gene to be transferred and the polarity of chromosomal transfer are determined by the site of integration of the F plasmid and its orientation with respect to the bacterial chromosome. Because the mating bacteria usually separate spontane-

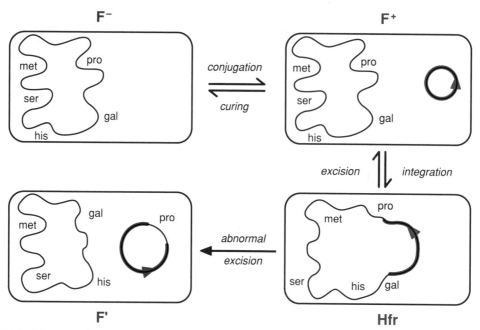

FIGURE 5-9   Role of the F plasmid in determining donor and recipient states of *E coli*. The F plasmid is representative of specific conjugative plasmids that control donor ability in *E coli*. F⁻ strains lack the F plasmid and are genetic recipients. F⁺ strains contain the F plasmid, express F pili, and are genetic donors. The F plasmid can become integrated into the bacterial chromosome at various locations to produce Hfr (high-frequency recombination) donor strains. Abnormal excision of the F plasmid can result in formation of F′ plasmids that contain segments of the bacterial chromosome. The arrowhead in the F plasmid defines the origin for transfer of DNA during conjugation.

ously before the entire chromosome is transferred, conjugation usually transfers only a fragment of the donor chromosome into the recipient. The probability that a donor gene will enter the recipient bacterium during conjugation decreases, therefore, as its distance from the F origin (and therefore the time of its transfer) increases. Mating cells can also be broken apart experimentally by strong shearing forces in a mechanical blender; this is called **interrupted mating.** Formation of recombinant progeny requires recombination between the transferred donor DNA and the genome of the recipient bacterium. Analysis of progeny from matings that are interrupted after different intervals demonstrates which chromosomal genes are transferred first by particular donor strains, the sequential times of entry for genes that are transferred subsequently, and the progressively

lower probability that genes transferred later will appear in recombinant progeny. The circularity of the *E coli* genetic map was originally deduced from the overlapping, circularly permuted groups of linked genes that were transferred early by individual donor strains in which the F factor was integrated at different chromosomal locations.

In matings between F⁺ and F⁻ bacteria, only the F plasmid is transferred with high efficiency to recipients. Chromosomal genes are transferred with very low efficiency, and it is the spontaneous Hfr mutants in F⁺ populations that mediate transfer of donor chromosomal genes. In matings between Hfr and F⁻ strains, the segment of the F plasmid containing the *tra* region is transferred last, after the entire bacterial chromosome has been transferred. Most recombinants from matings between Hfr and F⁻ cells fail to inherit the entire set of F plasmid genes and are phenotypically F⁻. In matings between F⁺ and F⁻ strains, the F plasmid spreads rapidly throughout the bacterial population and most recombinants are F⁺.

Integrated F plasmids in Hfr strains can sometimes be excised from the bacterial chromosome. If excision precisely reverses the integration process, F⁺ cells are produced. On rare occasions, however, excision occurs by recombinations involving insertion sequences or other sites on the bacterial chromosome that are some distance away from the original integration site. In such cases, segments of the bacterial chromosome can become incorporated into hybrid F plasmids that are called **F′ plasmids** (Fig. 5-9). By similar processes, segments of the bacterial chromosome can sometimes become incorporated into R plasmids to produce hybrid **R′ plasmids.** Conjugative R′ plasmids can function as fertility plasmids because they can integrate into the bacterial chromosome by homologous recombination and mediate transfer of chromosomal genes during matings with recipient bacteria. F′ plasmids, R′ plasmids, specialized transducing phages, and recombinant plasmids or phages constructed by gene cloning (described below) are hybrid replicons that can include segments of the bacterial chromosome. Therefore, any of these genetic elements can be used to construct the partially diploid bacterial strains that are required for complementation tests and other purposes.

Conjugation also occurs in Gram-positive bacteria. Gram-positive donor bacteria produce adhesins that cause them to aggregate with recipient cells, but sex pili are not involved. In some *Streptococcus* species, recipient bacteria produce extracellular sex pheromones that cause the donor phenotype to be expressed by bacteria that harbor an appropriate conjugative plasmid, and the conjugative plasmid prevents the donor cells from producing the corresponding pheromone.

Recombination

Recombination involves breakage and joining of parental DNA molecules to form hybrid, recombinant molecules. Several distinct kinds of recombination have been identified; they depend on different features of the participating genomes and require the activities of different gene products. Specific enzymes that act on DNA (e.g., exonucleases, endonucleases, polymerases, and ligases) participate in recombination. Detailed discussion of the biochemical events in recombination is beyond the scope of this chapter.

Generalized recombination involves donor and recipient DNA molecules that have homologous nucleotide sequences. Reciprocal exchanges can occur between any homologous donor and recipient sites. In *E coli*, the product of the *recA* gene is essential for generalized recombination, but other gene products also participate.

Site-specific recombination involves reciprocal exchanges only between specific sites in donor and recipient DNA molecules. The *recA* gene product is not required for site-specific recombination. Integration of the temperate bacteriophage λ into the chromosome of *E coli* is a well-studied example of site-specific recombination (Fig. 5-10). The specific attachment *(att)* sites on the *E coli* chromosome and λ phage DNA have a common core sequence of 15 nucleotides, within which reciprocal recombination occurs, flanked by adjacent sequences that are not homologous in the phage and bacterial genomes. In phage λ the product of the *int* gene (integrase) is required for the site-specific integration event in lysogenization; the products of the *int* and *xis* (excisionase) genes are both needed for the complementary site-specific excision event that occurs during induction of lytic-phage development in lysogenic cells.

Illegitimate recombination is the term used to describe nonhomologous, aberrant recombination events such as those involved in formation of specialized transducing phages. The mechanisms of illegitimate recombination are unknown.

Transposons

Transposons are segments of DNA that can move from one site in a DNA molecule to other target sites in the same or a different DNA molecule. The process is called **transposition** and occurs by a mechanism that is independent of generalized re-

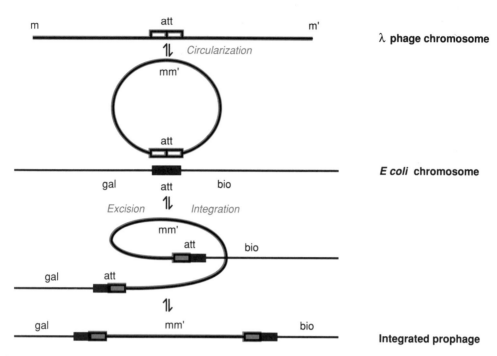

FIGURE 5-10 Integration and excision of bacteriophage λ as examples of site-specific recombination. The *gal* and *bio* operons, which respectively determine utilization of galactose and biosynthesis of biotin, are located adjacent to the bacterial attachment site *(att)*. In an infected *E coli* cell the λ DNA becomes circular by joining ends *m* and *m'*, and site-specific recombination between phage and bacterial *att* sites results in insertion of the λ genome into the bacterial chromosome. The arrangement of the prophage DNA (*m* and *m'* located internally) is therefore a circular permutation of λ virion DNA (*m* and *m'* located terminally).

combination. Transposons are important genetic elements because they cause mutations, mediate genomic rearrangements, function as portable regions of genetic homology, and acquire new genes and contribute to their dissemination within bacterial populations. Insertion of a transposon often interrupts the linear sequence of a gene and inactivates it. Transposons are important in causing deletions, duplications, and inversions of DNA segments as well as fusions between replicons. They are not self-replicating genetic elements, however, and they must integrate into other replicons to be maintained stably in bacterial genomes.

Most transposons share a number of common features. Each transposon encodes the functions necessary for its transposition, including a transposase enzyme that interacts with specific se-

quences at the ends of the transposon. During transposition, a short sequence of target DNA is duplicated and the transposon is inserted between the directly repeated target sequences. The length of this short duplication varies, but is characteristic for each transposon. The duplication is presumed to involve asymmetric cleavage of DNA at the target site, followed by synthesis of new complementary strands corresponding to the region between the cleavage sites. Some transposons insert into almost any target sequence, whereas others have relatively stringent target specificity. Two types of transposition are recognized. Excision of the transposon from a donor site followed by its insertion into a target site is called **nonreplicative transposition.** If the transposon at a donor site is replicated and a copy is inserted into the target site, however, the process is called **replicative transposition.** Replicative transposition can involve formation of a **cointegrate,** a single circular DNA molecule consisting of two replicons joined with copies of the transposon in an alternating sequence. **Resolution** of the cointegrate into its component replicons is often accomplished by a transposon-encoded resolvase that catalyzes site-specific recombination between the transposons. Generalized recombination between homologous transposons can also lead to the formation or resolution of cointegrates. Transposition differs from site-specific recombination by duplicating a segment of the target sequence and by using a variety of different target sequences for a single donor sequence.

Most transposons in bacteria can be separated into three major classes (Fig. 5-11). **Insertion sequences** and related **composite transposons** make up the first class. Insertion sequences are simplest in structure and encode only the functions needed for transposition. The known insertion sequences vary in length from approximately 780 to 1,500 nucleotide pairs, have short (15 to 25 bp) inverted repeats at their ends, and are not closely related to each other. The DNA between the inverted terminal repeats contains one (or, rarely, two) transposase gene and does not encode a resolvase. Complex transposons vary in length from about 2,000 to more than 40,000 nucleotide pairs and contain insertion sequences (or closely related sequences) at each end, usually as inverted repeats. The entire complex element can transpose as a unit. The DNA between the terminal insertion sequences of complex transposons encodes multiple functions that are not essential for transposition. In medically important bacteria, genes that determine the production of adherence antigens, toxins, or other virulence factors or that specify resistance to one or more antibiotics are often located in complex transposons. Well-known examples of complex transposons are Tn5 and Tn10, which determine resistance to kanamycin and tetracycline, respectively. The complex transposons probably evolve by transposition of homologous insertion sequences to nearby sites within a DNA molecule.

The second class of transposons consists of the highly homologous TnA family. These transposons have longer (35 to 40 bp) terminal inverted repeats than the complex transposons described above, but they lack terminal insertion sequences. All members of the family encode both transposase and resolvase functions. Well-known examples from the TnA transposon family include the ampicillin resistance transposon Tn3 and Tn1000 (the gamma-delta transposon) found in the F plasmid. The TnA family has an important place in the history of medical microbiology. The development of high-level resistance to ampicillin in *Haemophilus influenzae* and *Neisseria gonorrhoeae* during the 1970s, which severely limited the usefulness of ampicillin for treatment of gonorrhea and *Haemophilus* infections in areas where such strains became prevalent, was caused by dissemination of ampicillin resistance determinants from TnA transposons in plasmids in members of the Enterobacteriaceae to plasmids in *Haemophilus* and *Neisseria* species.

The third class of transposons consists of bacteriophage Mu and related temperate phages. The entire phage genome functions as a transposon, and replication of the phage DNA during vegetative growth occurs by replicative transposition. Prophage integration can occur at many different sites in the bacterial chromosome and often causes mutations. For this reason Mu and related phages are sometimes called **mutator phages.**

Some roles of transposons in bacterial evolution are illustrated by considering enteric Gram-negative bacteria and the structure of their plasmids. Bacteria collected during the preantibiotic era contained many plasmids, but they usually lacked resistance determinants. Many of the R plasmids from current clinical isolates belong to the same incompatibility groups as plasmids found previously, but they also determine resistance to multiple antibiotics. The close relationships between their replicons provide strong evidence that the R plasmids evolved from the older plasmids by acquisition of resistance determinants. Some of the multiple-antibiotic-resistant plasmids have individual transposons with several resistance determinants; others have multiple resistance transposons

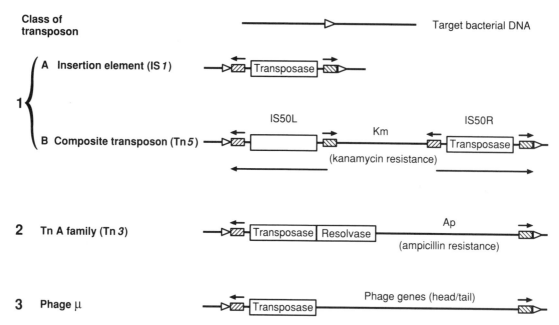

FIGURE 5-11 Features of representative transposons integrated into the bacterial chromosome. (1A) IS1 insertion sequence has a transposase gene flanked by inverted terminal repeats (hatched bars with arrows). The IS1 element is flanked by copies of the target site (open arrowheads) with the same orientation. (1B) Composite transposon Tn5 consists of the kanamycin resistance determinant flanked by inverted copies of the IS50 insertion element. (2) Transposon TnA contains the ampicillin resistance determinant, transposase, and resolvase genes between terminal inverted repeats (hatched bars with arrows), flanked by direct repeats of target site (open arrowheads). (3) Phage μ encodes a transposase that catalyzes recombination between the ends of μ DNA and target DNA. Direct repeats of the target site (open arrowheads) flank the integrated μ genome. Phage μ DNA is longer than the μ prophage and contains chromosomal sequences at both ends, reflecting the process by which prophage μ is excised and packaged.

located at separate sites; and still others contain complex hybrid resistance transposons formed by integration of one transposon into another. The stepwise acquisition of resistance determinants can lead to the formation of composite transposons that encode multiple resistance determinants. Therapeutic use of antibiotics and their incorporation into animal feeds provide selective advantages for bacteria with R plasmids, whereas conjugation, transformation, and transfection provide means for dissemination of R plasmids within and between bacterial species. After a plasmid carrying a transposon is introduced into a new bacterial host, the transposon and its determinants can jump into the chromosome or indigenous plasmids of the new host. Therefore, stability of the mobilizing plasmid in a new bacterial host is not essential for persistence of genetic determinants located on a transposon.

RECOMBINANT DNA AND GENE CLONING

Many methods are available to make hybrid DNA molecules in vitro (**recombinant DNA**) and to characterize them. Such methods include isolating specific genes in hybrid replicons, determining their nucleotide sequences, and creating mutations at designated locations **(site-directed muta-genesis).** A **clone** is a population of organisms or molecules derived by asexual reproduction from a single ancestor. **Gene cloning** is the process of incorporating foreign genes into hybrid DNA replicons. Cloned genes can be expressed in appropriate host cells, and the phenotypes that they determine can be analyzed. Some key concepts underlying representative methods are summarized here.

The first step in gene cloning is to make fragments of the donor DNA by mechanical or enzymatic methods. Certain restriction endonucleases, designated as class II, are particularly useful for preparing defined fragments of DNA molecules. They cleave both strands of double-stranded DNA molecules at specific, palindromic sequences **(restriction sites)** that usually vary from four to eight nucleotides in length, and the resulting DNA fragments are called **restriction fragments.** Some restriction endonucleases cleave at coincident sites to create blunt-ended DNA fragments, and others cut at staggered positions in the complementary strands to create DNA fragments with short, com-

plementary, single-stranded 5' or 3' ends (Table 5-3). The random probability that n adjacent nucleotides in a DNA strand will correspond to a specific restriction site is approximately $1/4^n$. Sites for enzymes that recognize unique 4-, 6-, or 8-nucleotide targets are likely to occur about once in every 256, 4,096, or 65,536 nucleotides, respectively. By choosing appropriate restriction enzymes, specific DNA molecules including bacterial chromosomes, plasmids, and phage genomes can be digested into sets of restriction fragments that have appropriate sizes for specific applications. A **restriction map** identifies the positions of target sites for specific restriction endonucleases in a DNA molecule. Restriction maps are available for many cloned DNA fragments, plasmids, and phage genomes, as well as for the entire chromosome of *E coli* and several other bacteria (as well as some yeasts).

The second step in gene cloning is to create hybrid replicons consisting of donor DNA fragments and a **cloning vector** (Fig. 5-12). Cloning vectors are small plasmid or phage replicons that have one or more restriction sites into which foreign DNA

TABLE 5-3 Specificities of Representative Class II Restriction Endonucleases

| Enzyme | Isolated from | Recognition Site[a] | | End Structure of Restriction Fragment |
		Length (bp)	Sequence (5'-3')	
*Sau*3A	*Staphylococcus aureus*	4	↓ GATC	4-base 5' extension
*Nla*III	*Neisseria lactamica*	4	↓ CATG	4-base 3' extension
*Dpn*I	*Diplococcus pneumoniae*	4	↓ GATC	Blunt
*Ssp*I	*Sphaerotilus natans*	6	↓ AATATT	Blunt
*Pst*I	*Providencia stuartii*	6	↓ CTGCAG	4-base 3' extension
*Eco*RI	*Escherichia coli*	6	↓ GAATTC	4-base 5' extension
*Cla*I	*Caryophanon latum*	6	↓ ATCGAT	2-base 5' extension
*Not*I	*Nocardia otitidis-caviarum*	8	↓ GCGGCCGC	4-base 5' extension

[a] Each recognition site in double-stranded DNA is a palindrome, and the 5'-to-3' sequence is identical for each of the antiparallel strands. Both strands are cleaved at the site indicated by the vertical arrow.

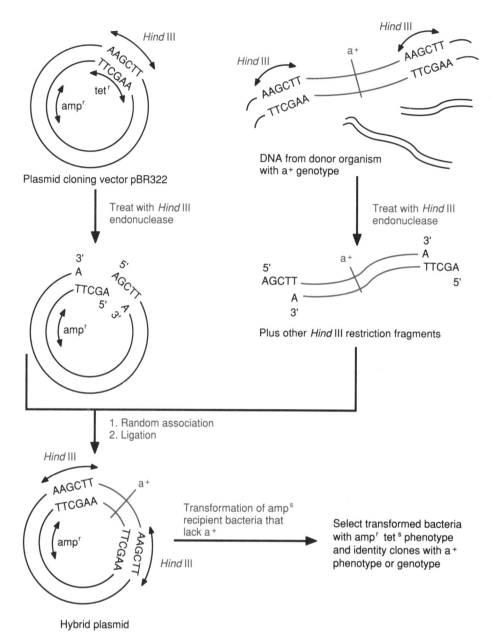

FIGURE 5-12 A typical gene cloning experiment. The plasmid cloning vector pBR322 carries genes for resistance to ampicillin (amp^r) and tetracycline (tet^r) and has only one HindIII restriction site (located within the tet^r locus). HindIII is used to treat samples of DNA from plasmid pBR322 and from a donor organism with the gene a^+ to be cloned. Provided HindIII restriction sites are located adjacent to (but not within) a^+ in donor DNA, a restriction fragment carrying a^+ can be generated from donor DNA. Hybrid plasmids are then formed by random association and ligation of the HindIII-treated donor and vector DNA fragments. The hybrid plasmids will be tet^s because the donor DNA fragments are inserted within the tet^r locus. After transformation of amp^s- recipient bacteria that also lack a^+, transconjugants with hybrid plasmids can be selected by their Amp^r Tet^s phenotypes. Strains in which the a^+ gene is present can then be identified by expression of a^+ or by testing for the polynucleotide sequence corresponding to a^+.

can be inserted. Hybrid replicons are reproduced by using DNA ligase to join the restricted vector DNA with donor DNA fragments that have compatible ends; alternatively, synthetic oligonucleotides are used as linkers to create compatibility between donor and vector DNA molecules with different ends. Ligating a vector to a heterogeneous set of DNA fragments from a donor genome is called **shotgun cloning,** and the collection of recombinant DNA molecules that contains the various fragments is called a **genomic library.** If a specific DNA fragment is available, it can be incorporated into a recombinant replicon by **direct cloning** into an appropriate vector. A wide variety of vectors are available for special purposes. Examples include **cosmids,** which are plasmid vectors that can be packaged into λ phage capsids, and **phagemids,** which are plasmid-phage hybrid replicons that can exist either as plasmids or as single-stranded DNA phages under different experimental conditions. Cosmids are useful for cloning large fragments of DNA, and phagemids are useful for recovering the cloned DNA at a later time in single-stranded form. Other specialized vectors detect promoters, transcription termination signals, or other regulatory elements within foreign DNA inserts or, conversely, provide promoters from which transcription of cloned genes can be initiated.

The final steps in gene cloning are to introduce hybrid replicons into appropriate recipient cells and test them for expression of donor genes of interest. Prokaryotic cells (including bacteria) or eukaryotic cells (including yeast, animal, and plant cells) can be used as recipients, but they differ with respect to their permissiveness for specific replicons, the transcriptional signals that they recognize, and the posttranslational modifications of protein structure that they can accomplish. Recombinant DNA molecules produced in vitro can be introduced directly into recipient cells by transformation or transfection. In addition, clones in cosmid or phage vectors can be packaged into phage coats and introduced into susceptible recipient cells by transduction. By using specialized vectors **(shuttle vectors)** that can replicate in multiple cell types, genes from any organism can be cloned

and manipulated in a convenient bacterial system and subsequently reintroduced into cells of the original organism for analysis in their natural environment.

Many methods are available to identify bacteria that contain recombinant DNA molecules. Most cloning vectors have genes for traits that can be positively selected, such as resistance to antibiotics. Furthermore, it is often possible to introduce foreign DNA into the cloning vector at a site that inactivates a nonessential, but easily recognizable, vector function. If both of these conditions are fulfilled, bacteria that contain recombinant molecules can be selected and distinguished easily from bacteria that contain only the vector. Bacteria in a genomic library that contain a particular cloned gene can be identified by using biochemical or immunologic methods to test for the desired gene product. Alternatively, the cloned gene of interest can be detected directly by using nucleic acid hybridization methods, provided that a specific DNA or RNA probe is available. Because insertion of foreign DNA into a cloning vector at an appropriate site does not inactivate its ability to replicate in appropriate recipient cells, hybrid replicons of interest can be amplified by replication and the recombinant DNA molecules or their gene products can be purified and studied. The ability to purify specific DNA molecules made it feasible to develop enzymatic and chemical methods for determining their nucleotide sequences, and current methods for introducing mutations at defined sites in cloned genes are based on knowing their restriction maps or nucleotide sequences.

Recombinant DNA methods make it feasible to clone specific DNA fragments from any source into vectors that can be studied in well-characterized bacteria, in eukaryotic cells, or in vitro. Applications of DNA cloning are emerging in all fields of biology and medicine. In medical genetics, such applications range from the prenatal diagnosis of inherited human diseases to the characterization of oncogenes and their roles in carcinogenesis. Pharmaceutical applications include large-scale production, from cloned human genes, of biologic products with therapeutic value, such as polypeptide hormones, interleukins, and enzymes. Applications in public health and laboratory medicine include development of vaccines to prevent specific infections and probes to diagnose specific infections by nucleic acid hybridization or polymerase chain reaction. The latter process uses oligonucleotide primers and DNA polymerase to amplify specific target DNA sequences during multiple cycles of synthesis in vitro, making it possible to detect rare target DNA sequences in clinical specimens with great sensitivity.

REGULATION OF GENE EXPRESSION

The phenotypic properties of bacteria are determined by their genotypes and growth conditions. For bacteria in pure culture, changes in growth conditions often result in predictable physiologic adaptations in all members of the population. Typically, essential gene products are made in amounts that permit fastest growth in the given environment, and products required under special circumstances are made only when they are needed.

Physiologic adaptations are often associated with changes in metabolic activities. The flow of metabolites through particular biochemical pathways is controlled both by regulating the synthesis of specific enzymes and by altering the activities of existing enzymes. Mechanisms that regulate the expression of genes by affecting synthesis of specific gene products are discussed here.

Specific regulation involves a gene or group of genes involved in a particular metabolic process. **Induction** and **repression** enable bacteria to regulate production of specific gene products in response to appropriate signals. Generally, catabolic enzymes are induced when the substrate for the pathway is present in the growth medium and biosynthetic enzymes are repressed by the product of the pathway. Enzymes that participate in a single biochemical pathway often occupy adjacent positions on the bacterial chromosome and are coordinately induced or repressed. They form an **operon,** a group of contiguous genes that is transcribed as a single unit and translated to produce the corresponding gene products. Organization into an operon is an important strategy for coordinately regulating the expression of genes in bacteria. Operons that can be induced or repressed are controlled by binding of specific **regulatory proteins** to particular nucleotide sequences that function as **regulatory sites** within the operon.

Global regulation simultaneously alters the expression of a group of genes and operons, collectively called a **regulon,** that are controlled by the same regulatory signal. Global regulation determines responses of bacteria to basic nutrients such as carbon, nitrogen, or phosphate; reactions to stresses such as DNA damage or heat shock; and synthesis by pathogens of specific virulence factors during growth in their host animals.

The amount of a specific protein in a bacterial cell can vary from none to many thousands of molecules. This wide range is often determined by the combined action of several regulatory mechanisms that affect the expression of the corresponding structural gene. Regulation is achieved by determining how often a gene is transcribed into functional mRNA, how efficiently the mRNA is translated into protein, how rapidly the mRNA is degraded, how rapidly the protein product turns over, and whether the activity of the protein product can be altered by allosteric effects or covalent modifications.

mRNAs as Transcriptional Units

Gene expression begins when DNA-dependent RNA polymerase (RNA polymerase) catalyzes the transcription of specific mRNA from one strand of a DNA template. Binding of RNA polymerase to DNA occurs at specific sites called **promoters,** and transcription begins adjacent to the promoter. Strong promoters can interact efficiently with RNA polymerase and initiate transcription at a high rate; weak promoters initiate transcription at low rates. In either case, mRNA is synthesized from its 5′ end toward its 3′ end at an approximately constant rate until the RNA polymerase recognizes another specific site called a **terminator.** RNA polymerase then dissociates from the template, and transcription of the mRNA is completed.

Individual mRNA molecules may code for one or more polypeptides. Transcription of an operon produces a **polycistronic mRNA** that codes for several polypeptides. Translation of polycistronic mRNAs leads to coordinate synthesis of the encoded polypeptides, but each polypeptide is synthesized as a separate molecule. A specific **ribosome-binding site** is located just upstream from the start of each coding sequence on the mRNA molecule.

mRNAs in bacteria are degraded rapidly, with an average half-life of several minutes, in contrast to tRNAs and rRNAs, which are much more stable. Although mRNAs represent about half of the newly synthesized RNA, they represent only a small fraction of the total RNA. Their short half-life has important consequences for gene expression. If the synthesis of a specific mRNA is prevented, production of the corresponding polypeptides declines rapidly.

Gene expression is controlled by regulating one or more of the steps in the pathway from the DNA template to the active gene product. Simultaneous regulation at several levels permits greater control over gene expression than would be possible with a single regulatory mechanism. The most common way to regulate gene expression in bacteria is to control the production of specific mRNAs. Since the rate of elongation of an RNA molecule is approximately constant, the major factors that control mRNA synthesis are the rate of initiation and the probability that a full-length transcript will be produced.

Regulation of Transcription Initiation

Some mRNAs in bacteria are synthesized at constant rates, resulting in **constitutive** production of the encoded polypeptides. The amounts of specific mRNAs and polypeptides produced from different constitutive genes vary greatly, however, and often reflect differences in strength of the promoters for those genes.

Transcription of many operons is regulated in response to changing environmental conditions. The promoters determine the maximum rate of transcription initiation for such operons, but regu-

latory proteins participate in controlling transcription. Nucleotide sequences in operons to which specific regulatory proteins bind are called **regulatory sites** or **operators.** Operators and promoters are located close together within operons and may have overlapping DNA sequences. The binding of regulatory proteins to operators can either increase (positive regulation) or decrease (negative regulation) the frequency of transcription initiation. Proteins that function as negative regulators are usually called **repressors.** Because regulatory proteins can diffuse through the cytoplasm, the structural genes for regulatory proteins do not have to be linked to the target operons.

The ability to sense the presence or absence of specific compounds and change the rates of synthesis of appropriate gene products is central to the control of gene expression. Regulatory proteins offer one solution to this problem of stimulus-response coupling. Many regulatory proteins are bifunctional and bind not only to appropriate operators but also to specific **effectors,** which are small molecules such as particular sugars, amino acids, and other metabolites. Furthermore, regulatory proteins are **allosteric** (i.e., they can exist in different conformations that exhibit different binding affinities for their cognate operators and effectors). A sufficient concentration of effector favors formation of the regulatory protein-effector complex, which has either high or low affinity for the operator in any specific case. In negatively regulated systems the effector functions as a **corepressor** if the regulatory protein-effector complex is the active repressor, and the effector functions as an **inducer** and causes derepression if the free regulatory protein is the active repressor. Conversely, in positively regulated systems, the effector stimulates expression of the operon if the regulatory protein-effector complex is the positive regulator and inhibits expression of the operon if the free regulatory protein is the positive regulator.

The lactose *(lac)* operon of *E coli* is an example of an inducible, negatively regulated operon (Fig. 5-13). The *lacI* gene codes for a repressor that binds to the *lac* operator and prevents transcription from the *lac* promoter. The structural gene

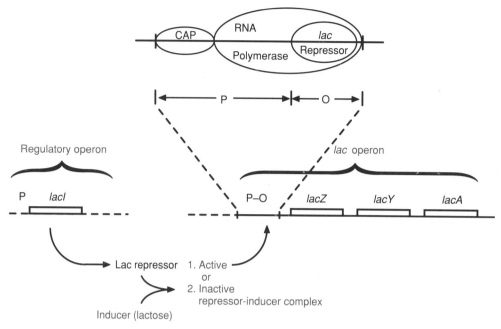

FIGURE 5-13   Regulation of the *lac* operon in *E coli*. Structural genes *lacZ, lacY,* and *lacA* code for β-galactosidase, β-galactoside permease, and β-galactoside transacetylase, respectively. The physiologic role of *lacA* is unknown. The *lac* repressor is the product of the *lacI* gene in a separate regulatory operon. Transcription of mRNA encoding *lacZ, lacY,* and *lacA* is negatively regulated. Binding of the Lac repressor to operator *lacO* prevents initiation of transcription at promoter *lacP*. Inducer binds to the Lac repressor and inactivates it. Catabolite activator protein (CAP) forms a complex with cAMP, and binding of the complex to a site immediately adjacent to the *lac* promoter stimulates transcription of the *lac* operon by RNA polymerase. An expanded diagram of the *lac* operator-promoter region shows the binding sites for CAP, RNA polymerase, and *lac* repressor.

for this repressor is separate from the *lac* operon, and the repressor is synthesized constitutively at a low rate. When inducer binds to the *lac* repressor, the complex cannot bind to the operator and cannot prevent binding of the RNA polymerase to the promoter. If other conditions are favorable, the *lac* operon is expressed, resulting in synthesis of β-galactosidase, β-galactoside permease, and β-galactoside transacetylase. The *lac* operon can be induced by lactose or by structurally related compounds such as isopropyl-β-D-thiogalactoside (IPTG). IPTG is called a **gratuitous inducer** because it induces the *lac* operon, but it is not a substrate for β-galactosidase. Negative regulation also occurs in many biosynthetic operons in *E coli*. In

such operons a product of the biosynthetic pathway functions as the effector for the negative regulatory system.

The arabinose *(ara)* operon in *E coli* is both positively and negatively regulated. In the presence of arabinose the regulatory protein stimulates transcription of the *ara* operon. In the absence of arabinose, however, the regulatory protein represses the *ara* operon.

Operons are often controlled by more than one mechanism. When *E coli* is grown in a medium containing glucose and an alternative carbon source such as lactose or arabinose, induction of the *lac* or *ara* operon and utilization of the lactose or arabinose are delayed until the glucose has been consumed. This phenomenon is called **diauxic growth.** The failure to induce the *lac* or *ara* operon in the presence of glucose is an example of **catabolite repression.** The *lac* and *ara* operons are positively regulated by cyclic-3′,5′-adenosine monophosphate (cAMP) and the catabolite gene activator (CAP) protein (the product of the *crp* gene). The cAMP-CAP complex interacts with CAP-binding sites in the regulatory regions of some operons, including the *lac* and *ara* operons, and stimulates transcription from the corresponding promoters. The level of intracellular cAMP in *E coli* is high during growth in the absence of glucose and low during growth in the presence of glucose. Catabolite repression is due, therefore, to lack of activation of cAMP-dependent operons when the bacteria are grown in the presence of glucose or certain other rapidly metabolizable carbon sources.

Regulation of Transcription Termination

Attenuation is a mechanism for regulating operons by terminating the transcription of mRNA prematurely. Attenuation is common in biosynthetic operons, including the tryptophan *(trp)*, histidine *(his)*, threonine *(thr)*, isoleucine-valine *(ilv)*, and phenylalanine *(phe)* operons. The *trp* operon in *E coli* is controlled by both repression and attenuation. In the presence of excess tryptophan, initiation of transcription from the *trp* promoter is repressed. In addition, however, transcripts that are initiated from the *trp* promoter are usually terminated before any of the structural genes of the *trp* operon are transcribed. The concentration of intracellular tryptophan required to maintain repression exceeds that needed for attenuation. Such dual control enables the cell to fine-tune the expression of the *trp* operon in response to decreasing concentrations of tryptophan.

The secondary structure of mRNA is important in attenuation. All mRNAs have a **leader sequence** between the transcriptional start site and the beginning of the coding sequence for the first structural gene. For amino acid biosynthetic operons

that are subject to attenuation, the mRNA leader sequence has two distinctive features. It encodes a short peptide containing the amino acid produced by the regulated pathway, and it can form alternative, mutually incompatible double-stranded RNA structures that participate in regulatory events. For example, the peptide encoded by the *trp* mRNA leader sequence contains two adjacent tryptophan residues, and the peptide encoded by the *his* mRNA leader sequence has a series of seven consecutive histidine residues. Figure 5-14 shows the *trp* operon and illustrates alternative secondary structures in the leader sequence of *trp* mRNA. There are three possible secondary structures for this region, the pause site (segments 1 and 2), the antiterminator (segments 2 and 3), and the attenuator (segments 3 and 4). Segment 1 of the pause site overlaps the coding region for the *trpL* peptide. Which secondary structures are formed depends on the efficiency of translation of the *trpL* peptide. When segments 1 and 2 are transcribed, they immediately anneal and cause the RNA polymerase to pause temporarily. Subsequent initiation of translation of the *trpL* peptide disrupts the pause site and allows RNA polymerase to continue transcription. If tryptophan is present, transcription of segments 3 and 4 and formation of the attenuator structure occur while the ribosome is blocking segment 2, causing the RNA polymerase to terminate transcription. If tryptophan is deficient, however, tryptophanyl-tRNA is also deficient, and the ribosome stalls at the tryptophan codons in segment 1. This allows segment 2 to anneal with newly synthesized segment 3 to form the antiterminator, thereby making segment 3 unavailable to anneal with segment 4. Formation of the attenuator is therefore prevented, and the RNA polymerase transcribes the entire *trp* operon. In this manner depletion of tryptophan (actually the supply of tryptophanyl-tRNA) is coupled to regulation of transcription of the biosynthetic operon for tryptophan.

In *E coli* transcription and translation are functionally coupled. Nonsense mutations that cause premature termination of translation often cause decreased transcription of more distal genes in the

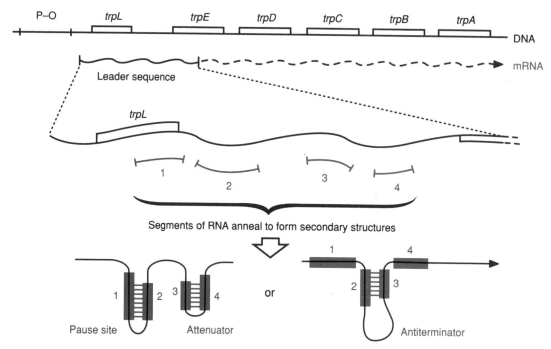

FIGURE 5-14   Regulation of the *trp* operon in *E coli*. The *trp* operon contains the five structural genes *trpE, trpD, trpC, trpB,* and *trpA,* which encode enzymes that catalyze the last reactions in tryptophan formation. Transcription initiation is controlled at the promoter–operator *(P–O)* locus, and signals within the *trp* mRNA leader sequence control termination of transcription by attenuation. The leader sequence of *trp* mRNA is expanded to show locations of the *trpL* coding sequence, the complementary segments 1, 2, 3, and 4, and their possible alternative secondary structures, which function as pause site (1–2) and attenuator (3–4) or antiterminator (2–3).

same operon. This phenomenon is called **polarity.** Ribosomes usually initiate translation of a growing mRNA molecule prior to completion of transcription, and such translation masks sites that would otherwise cause the RNA polymerase to terminate transcription. Premature termination of translation by a nonsense codon dissociates the ribosomes from the mRNA and enables RNA polymerase to interact with the unmasked transcription termination sites.

In some biologic systems, including phage λ, *antitermination* is used as a positive regulatory mechanism to control gene expression. Immediately after infection of *E coli* by λ, RNA polymerase binds to two promoters in λ DNA and initiates divergent primary transcripts, which terminate at specific sites on the λ genome. A protein encoded by one of the primary transcripts interacts with RNA polymerase and enables it to continue transcription through the primary termination sites, thereby expressing a second set of λ genes. One of the products encoded by a secondary transcript blocks termination of another mRNA, and activates expression of a third set of genes. Antitermination has a key role, therefore, in controlling the cascade of gene expression during lytic growth of phage λ. It is also involved in the regulation of *E coli* rRNA operons.

Regulation of Translation

The **ribosome-binding site** on mRNA is complementary to a sequence at the 3′ end of 16S rRNA. Interaction between these sequences facilitates formation of the initiation complex for protein synthesis. Both the extent of homology with 16S rRNA and the spacing of the ribosome-binding site from the initiation codon affect the efficiency of translation initiation. Codon usage in mRNA also influences translation efficiency. mRNAs for proteins that are required in large amounts tend to use codons that are translated by the most abundant species of tRNA, and the converse is also true.

Translational control is important for regulation of synthesis of ribosomal proteins. Production of ribosomes involves a high metabolic cost for bacteria, and at high growth rates ribosomes can constitute nearly one-half of the cell weight. Most ribosomal proteins and rRNAs are found assembled into ribosomes, and the pool of free ribosomal subunits is very small. The genes for ribosomal proteins are organized into several operons. Certain of the free ribosomal proteins directly inhibit the translation of the polycistronic mRNAs that encode them, thereby ensuring that synthesis of ribosomal proteins is balanced with the requirement for their utilization.

Regulons and Signal-Transducing Proteins

A **regulon** is a group of genes or operons controlled by a common regulator. There are several advantages to placing different operons under the control of the same regulator. It enables the sensing of a single stimulus to be coupled to expression of a large number of genes that may be needed for an appropriate response, and it eliminates the requirement for the coordinately regulated genes to be linked on the bacterial chromosome. The stimulus to which the regulon responds can be an intracellular component or an environmental signal. Individual operons may also be subject to regulation by several different mechanisms and expressed under conditions that differ from those affecting the whole regulon.

More than 20 different regulons have been identified in *E coli*. Specific examples of regulons that respond to intracellular components include the cAMP-CAP regulon described above and the regulons controlled by the **stringent response** and

the **SOS response.** When ribosomes encounter uncharged tRNA molecules during protein synthesis, the stringent response is activated and results in prompt cessation of rRNA synthesis. A novel nucleotide called guanosine-3'-diphosphate-5'-diphosphate (ppGpp) accumulates during amino acid starvation. The ppGpp produced by idling ribosomes appears to be a mediator of the stringent response, but the precise mechanism that causes inhibition of rRNA synthesis is unknown. The SOS response is associated with damage to DNA and involves induction of several repair pathways. The product of the *recA* gene detects the inhibition of DNA synthesis and initiates events leading to proteolytic cleavage and inactivation of the repressor for the SOS pathway, encoded by the *lexA* gene.

Some regulons are induced by specific environmental stimuli, such as nutrient limitation or osmotic stress. Typically, bacteria sense such environmental conditions by two-component systems. The first component is a membrane-spanning protein with extracellular and intracellular domains. Its extracellular domain detects the environmental stimulus, and its cytoplasmic domain transmits the signal. The second component is a bifunctional cytoplasmic protein. It has a receiver domain that interacts with the transmitter module of the first component, as well as an effector domain that controls expression of the corresponding regulon. The transmitter and receiver modules of the two-component regulatory systems from a wide variety of regulons are genetically related and share amino acid homology. The signal-detecting and effector domains of the proteins from different regulons vary, however, and determine the signal that is detected and the operons that are activated or repressed in response to that signal.

Global regulation is important in the physiology of pathogenic bacteria. For example, *Vibrio cholerae* and *Bordetella pertussis* express many of their virulence determinants under the control of signal-transducing systems that are related to the two-component systems described above. The expression of proteins needed for the invasive phenotype is controlled by temperature in *Shigella* species. *Yersinia enterocolitica* senses the concentration of calcium ions and couples it to expression of genes that are appropriate for an intracellular or extracellular environment. In host tissues the concentration of free iron is extremely low, and most pathogenic bacteria have high-affinity iron transport systems that are induced under low-iron conditions. The synthesis of diphtheria toxin by *Corynebacterium diphtheriae,* Shiga toxin by *Shigella dysenteriae,* exotoxin A by *Pseudomonas aeruginosa,* and other specific proteins by many pathogenic bacteria is induced under conditions of iron-limited growth. These examples illustrate how environmental factors can regulate the expression of virulence genes in pathogenic bacteria.

REFERENCES

Berg D, Howe MM (eds): Mobile DNA. American Society for Microbiology, Washington, DC, 1989

Calendar R (ed): The Bacteriophages. Plenum Press, New York, 1988

DiRita VJ, Mekalanos JJ: Genetic control of bacterial virulence. Annu Rev Genet 23:455, 1989

Freifelder D: Microbial Genetics. Jones & Barlett, Boston, 1987

Kingsman AJ, Chater KF, Kingsman SM (eds): Transposition. Forty-Third Symposium of the Society for General Microbiology. Cambridge University Press, Cambridge, 1988

Kohara Y, Adiyama K, Isono K: The physical map of the whole *E. coli* chromosome: application of a new strategy for rapid analysis and sorting of a large genomic library. Cell 40:495, 1987

Miller JF, Mekalanos JJ, Falkow S: Coordinate regulation and sensory transduction in the control of bacterial virulence. Science 243:916, 1989

Neidhardt FC, Ingraham JL, Low KB et al (eds): *Escherichia coli* and *Salmonella typhimurium:* cellular and molecular biology. American Society for Microbiology, Washington, DC, 1987

Sambrook J, Fritsch EF, Maniatis T: Molecular cloning: a laboratory manual. 2nd Ed. Cold Spring Harbor Laboratory, Cold Spring Harbor, NY, 1989

Watson JD, Hopkins NH, Roberts JW et al: Molecular biology of the gene. 4th Ed. Benjamin/Cummings, Menlo Park, CA, 1987

6 NORMAL FLORA

CHARLES PATRICK DAVIS

GENERAL CONCEPTS

Significance of the Normal Flora

The normal flora influences the anatomy, physiology, susceptibility to pathogens, and morbidity of the host organism.

Skin Flora

The varied environment of the skin results in locally dense or sparse populations, with Gram-positive organisms (e.g., staphylococci, micrococci, diphtheroids) usually predominating.

Oral and Upper Respiratory Tract Flora

A varied microbial flora is found in the oral cavity, and streptococcal anaerobes inhabit the gingival crevice. The pharynx can be a point of entry and initial colonization for *Neisseria*, *Bordetella*, *Corynebacterium*, and *Streptococcus* spp.

Gastrointestinal Tract Flora

Organisms in the stomach are usually transient, and their populations are kept low (10^3 to 10^6/g of contents) by acidity. *Campylobacter (Helicobacter)* is a potential stomach pathogen. In normal hosts the duodenal flora is sparse (0 to 10^3/g of contents). The ileum contains a moderate mixed flora (10^6 to 10^8/g of contents). The flora of the large bowel is dense (10^9 to 10^{11}/g of con-

tents) and is almost entirely anaerobic. These organisms participate in bile acid conversion and in the production of vitamin K and ammonia in the large bowel and can also cause intestinal abscesses and peritonitis.

Urogenital Flora

The vaginal flora undergoes succession, changing with the age of the individual, the vaginal pH, and hormone levels. Transient organisms (e.g., *Candida* spp) frequently cause vaginitis. The distal urethra contains a sparse mixed flora; these organisms are present in urine specimens (10^4/ml) unless a clean-catch, midstream specimen is obtained.

Conjunctival Flora

The conjunctiva harbors few or no organisms. *Haemophilus* and *Staphylococcus* are among the genera most often detected.

Host Infection

Many elements of the normal flora may act as opportunistic pathogens, especially in hosts rendered susceptible by rheumatic heart disease, immunosuppression, radiation therapy, chemotherapy, perforated mucous membranes, etc. The flora of the gingival crevice causes dental caries in about 80 percent of the population.

INTRODUCTION

A diverse microbial flora is associated with the skin and mucous membranes of every human being from shortly after birth until death. The human body, which contains about 10^{13} cells, routinely harbors about 10^{14} bacteria (Fig. 6-1). This bacterial population constitutes the *normal microbial flora*. The normal microbial flora is relatively stable, with specific genera populating various body regions during particular periods in an individual's life. Microorganisms of the normal flora may aid the host (by competing for microenvironments more effectively than such pathogens as *Sal-*

monella spp or by producing nutrients the host can use), may harm the host (by causing dental caries, abscesses, or other infectious diseases), or may exist as commensals (inhabiting the host for long periods without causing detectable harm or benefit). Even though most elements of the normal microbial flora inhabiting the human skin, nails, eyes, oropharynx, genitalia, and gastrointestinal tract are harmless in healthy individuals, these organisms frequently cause disease in compromised hosts. Viruses and parasites are not considered members of the normal microbial flora by most investigators because they are not commensals and do not aid the host.

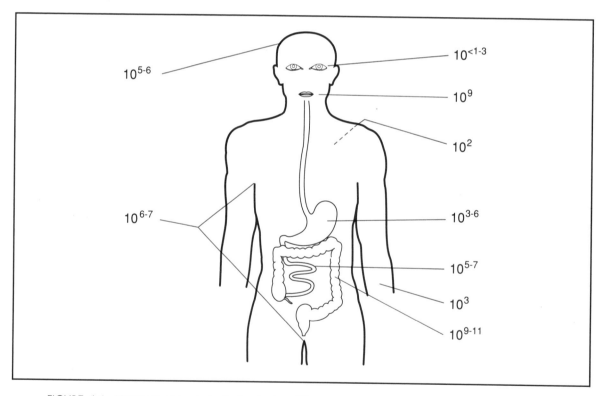

FIGURE 6-1   Numbers of bacteria that colonize different parts of the body. Numbers represent the number of organisms per gram of homogenized tissue or fluid or per square centimeter of skin surface.

SIGNIFICANCE OF THE NORMAL FLORA

The fact that the normal flora substantially influences the well-being of the host was not well understood until germ-free animals became available. Germ-free animals were obtained by cesarian section and maintained in special isolators; this allowed the investigator to raise them in an environment free from detectable viruses, bacteria, and other organisms. Two interesting observations were made about animals raised under germ-free conditions. First, the germ-free animals lived almost twice as long as their conventionally maintained counterparts, and second, the major causes of death were different in the two groups. Infection often caused death in conventional animals, but intestinal atonia frequently killed germ-free animals. Other investigations showed that germ-free animals have anatomic, physiologic, and im-

munologic features not shared with conventional animals. For example, in germ-free animals, the alimentary lamina propria is underdeveloped, little or no immunoglobulin is present in sera or secretions, intestinal motility is reduced, and the intestinal epithelial cell renewal rate is approximately one-half that of normal animals (4 rather than 2 days).

Although the foregoing indicates that bacterial flora may be undesirable, studies with antibiotic-treated animals suggest that the flora protects individuals from pathogens. Investigators have used streptomycin to reduce the normal flora and have then infected animals with streptomycin-resistant *Salmonella*. Normally, about 10^6 organisms are needed to establish a gastrointestinal infection, but in streptomycin-treated animals whose flora is altered, fewer than 10 organisms were needed to cause infectious disease. Further studies suggested that fermentation products (acetic and butyric

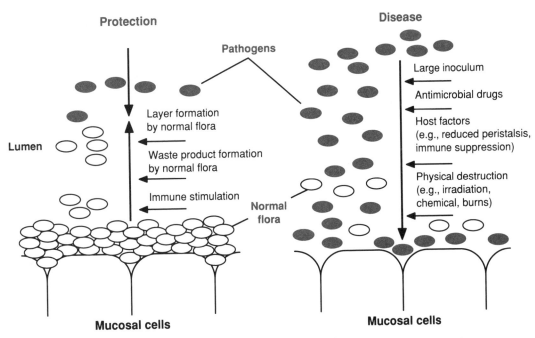

FIGURE 6-2 Mechanisms by which the normal flora competes with invading pathogens.

acids) produced by the normal flora inhibited *Salmonella* growth in the gastrointestinal tract. Figure 6-2 shows some of the factors that are important in the competition between the normal flora and bacterial pathogens.

The normal flora in humans usually develops in an orderly sequence, or *succession,* after birth, leading to the stable populations of bacteria that make up the normal adult flora. The main factor determining the composition of the normal flora in a body region is the nature of the local environment, which is determined by pH, temperature, redox potential, and oxygen, water, and nutrient levels. Other factors such as peristalsis, saliva, lysozyme, and secretion of immunoglobulins also play roles in flora control. The local environment is like a concerto in which one principal instrument usually dominates. For example, an infant begins to contact organisms as it moves through the birth canal. A Gram-positive population (bifidobacteria and lactobacilli) predominates in the gastrointestinal tract early in life if the infant is breast-fed. This bacterial population is reduced and displaced somewhat by a Gram-negative flora (Enterobacteriaceae) when the baby is bottle-fed. The type of liquid diet provided to the infant is the principal instrument of this flora control; immunoglobulins and, perhaps, other elements in breast milk may also be important.

What, then, is the significance of the normal flora? Animal and some human studies suggest that the flora influences human anatomy, physiology, lifespan, and, ultimately, cause of death. Although the causal relationship of flora to death and disease in humans is accepted, other roles of the human microflora need further study.

NORMAL FLORA OF SKIN

Skin provides good examples of various microenvironments. Skin regions have been compared to geographic regions of Earth: the desert of the forearm, the cool woods of the scalp, and the tropical forest of the armpit. The composition of the dermal microflora varies from site to site according to the character of the microenvironment. A different bacterial flora characterizes each of three regions of skin: (1) axilla, perineum, and toe webs; (2) hand, face, and trunk; and (3) upper arms and legs. Skin sites with partial occlusion (axilla, perineum, and toe webs) harbor more microorganisms than do less occluded areas (legs, arms, and trunk). These quantitative differences may relate to increased amount of moisture, higher body temperature, and greater concentrations of skin surface lipids. The axilla, perineum, and toe webs are more frequently colonized by Gram-negative bacilli than are drier areas of the skin.

The number of bacteria on an individual's skin remains relatively constant; bacterial survival and the extent of colonization probably depend partly on the exposure of skin to a particular environment and partly on the innate and species-specific bactericidal activity in skin. Also, a high degree of specificity is involved in the adherence of bacteria to epithelial surfaces. Not all bacteria attach to skin; staphylococci, which are the major element of the nasal flora, possess a distinct advantage over viridans streptococci in colonizing the nasal mucosa. Conversely, viridans streptococci are not seen in large numbers on the skin or in the nose but dominate the oral flora.

The microbiology literature is inconsistent about the density of bacteria on the skin; one reason for this is the variety of methods used to collect skin bacteria. The scrub method yields the highest and most accurate counts for a given skin area. Most microorganisms live in the superficial layers of the stratum corneum and in the upper parts of the hair follicles. Some bacteria, however, reside in the deeper areas of the hair follicles and are beyond the reach of ordinary disinfection procedures. These bacteria are a reservoir for recolonization after the surface bacteria are removed.

Staphylococcus epidermidis

S epidermidis is a major inhabitant of the skin, and in some areas it makes up more than 90 percent of the resident aerobic flora. *S epidermidis* is divided into four biotypes on the basis of variable acid production from carbohydrates. *S epidermidis* biotype I is the main type found on the skin and frequently causes infection after the insertion of a ventriculoatrial shunt in the treatment of hydrocephalus.

Staphylococcus aureus

The nose and perineum are the most common sites for *S aureus*, which is present in 10 percent to more than 40 percent of normal adults. *S aureus* is prevalent (67 percent) on vulvar skin. Its occurrence in the nasal passages varies with age, being greater in the newborn, less in adults. *S aureus* is extremely common (80 to 100 percent) on the skin of patients with certain dermatologic diseases such as atopic dermatitis, but the reason for this finding is unclear.

Micrococci

Micrococci are not as common as staphylococci and diphtheroids; however, they are frequently present on normal skin. *Micrococcus luteus (Sarcina luteus)*, the predominant species, usually accounts for 20 to 80 percent of the micrococci isolated from the skin. Micrococci and staphylococci can be distinguished by several key tests, for example, glucose utilization: micrococci utilize glucose oxidatively, whereas staphylococci utilize it both oxidatively and fermentatively.

Diphtheroids (Coryneforms)

The term *diphtheroid* denotes a wide range of bacteria belonging to the genus *Corynebacterium*. Classification of diphtheroids remains unsatisfactory; for convenience, cutaneous diphtheroids have been categorized into the following four groups: lipophilic or nonlipophilic diphtheroids; anaerobic diphtheroids; diphtheroids producing porphyrins (coral red fluorescence when viewed under ultraviolet light); and those that possess some keratinolytic enzymes and are associated with trichomycosis axillaris (infection of axillary hair). Lipophilic diphtheroids are extremely common in the axilla, whereas nonlipophilic strains are found more commonly on glabrous skin.

Anaerobic diphtheroids are most common in areas rich in sebaceous glands. Although the name *Corynebacterium acnes* was originally used to describe skin anaerobic diphtheroids, these are now classified as *Propionibacterium acnes (C acnes)* and *P granulosum (C granulosum)*. *P acnes* is seen eight times more frequently than *P granulosum* in acne lesions and is probably involved in acne pathogenesis. Children younger than 10 years are rarely colonized with *P acnes*. The appearance of this organism on the skin is probably related to the onset of secretion of sebum (a semifluid substance composed of fatty acids and epithelial debris secreted from sebaceous glands) at puberty. *P avidum*, the third species of cutaneous anaerobic diphtheroids, is rare in acne lesions and is more often isolated from the axilla.

Streptococci

Streptococci, especially β-hemolytic streptococci, are rarely seen on normal skin. The paucity of β-hemolytic streptococci on the skin is attributed at least in part to the presence of lipids on the skin, as these lipids are lethal to streptococci. Other groups of streptococci, such as α-hemolytic streptococci, exist primarily in the mouth, from where they may, in rare instances, spread to the skin.

Gram-Negative Bacilli

Gram-negative bacteria make up a small proportion of the skin flora. In view of their extraordinary numbers in the gut and in the natural environment, their scarcity on skin is striking. They are seen in moist intertriginous areas, such as the toe webs and axilla, and not on dry skin. Desiccation is the major factor preventing the multiplication of Gram-negative bacteria on intact skin. *Enterobacter, Klebsiella, Escherichia coli,* and *Proteus* spp are the predominant Gram-negative organisms. *Acinetobacter* spp (formerly *Mima-Herellia*) occurs on the skin of normal individuals and, like other Gram-negative bacteria, is more common in the moist intertriginous areas.

Nail Flora

The microbiology of a normal nail is generally similar to that of the skin. Dust particles and other extraneous materials may get trapped under the nail, depending on what the nail contacts. In addition to resident skin flora, these dust particles may carry fungi and bacilli. *Aspergillus, Penicillium,*

Cladosporium, and *Mucor* are the major types of fungi found under the nail.

ORAL AND UPPER RESPIRATORY TRACT FLORA

The oral flora is involved in dental caries and periodontal disease, which affect about 80 percent of the population in the Western world. The oral flora, its interactions with the host, and its response to environmental factors are thoroughly discussed in Chapter 99. Anaerobes in the oral flora are responsible for many of the brain, face, and lung infections that are frequently manifested by abscess formation.

The pharynx and trachea contain primarily those bacterial genera found in the normal oral cavity (for example, α- and β-hemolytic streptococci); however, anaerobes, staphylococci, neisseriae, diphtheroids, and others are also present. Potentially pathogenic organisms such as *Haemophilus*, mycoplasmas, and pneumococci may also be found in the pharynx. Anaerobic organisms also are reported frequently. The upper respiratory tract is so often the site of initial colonization by pathogens *(Neisseria meningitidis, C diphtheriae, Bordetella pertussis,* and many others) that it could be considered the first region of attack for such organisms. In contrast, the lower respiratory tract (small bronchi and alveoli) is usually sterile, because particles the size of bacteria do not readily reach it. If bacteria do reach these regions, they encounter host defense mechanisms, such as alveolar macrophages, that are not present in the pharynx.

GASTROINTESTINAL TRACT FLORA

The stomach is a relatively hostile environment for bacteria. It contains bacteria swallowed with the food and those dislodged from the mouth. Acidity lowers the bacterial count, which is highest (approximately 10^3 to 10^6 organisms/g of contents) after meals and lowest (frequently undetectable) after digestion. Some *Campylobacter* species can colonize the stomach and are associated with type B gastritis and peptic ulcer disease. Aspirates of duodenal or jejunal fluid contain approximately

10^3 organisms/ml in most individuals. Most of the bacteria cultured (streptococci, lactobacilli, enterobacteria, bacteroides) are thought to be transients. Levels of 10^5 to 10^7 bacteria/ml in such aspirates usually indicate an abnormality in the digestive system (for example, achlorhydria or malabsorption syndrome). Rapid peristalsis and the presence of bile may explain in part the paucity of organisms in the upper gastrointestinal tract. Further along the jejunum and into the ileum, bacterial populations begin to increase, and at the ileocecal junction they reach levels of 10^6 to 10^8 organisms/ml, with streptococci, lactobacilli, enterobacteria, bacteroides, and bifidobacteria predominating.

Concentrations of 10^9 to 10^{11} bacteria/g of contents are frequently found in human colon and feces. This flora includes a bewildering array of bacteria (more than 400 species have been identified); nonetheless, 95 to 99.9 percent belong to anaerobic genera such as *Bacteroides, Bifidobacterium, Eubacterium,* anaerobic streptococci *(Peptococcus* and *Peptostreptococcus),* and *Clostridium.* In this highly anaerobic region of the intestine, these genera proliferate, occupy most available niches, and produce metabolic waste products such as acetic, butyric, and lactic acids. The strict anaerobic conditions, physical exclusion (as occurs in animal studies), and bacterial waste products are factors that inhibit the growth of other bacteria in the large bowel.

Although the normal flora can inhibit pathogens, many of its members can produce disease in humans. Anaerobes in the intestinal tract are the primary agents of intra-abdominal abscesses and peritonitis. Bowel perforations produced by appendicitis, cancer, infarction, surgery, or gunshot wounds almost always seed the peritoneal cavity and adjacent organs with the normal flora. Anaerobes can also cause problems within the gastrointestinal lumen. Treatment with antibiotics may allow certain elements to become predominant and cause disease. For example, *Clostridium difficile,* which can remain viable in a patient undergoing antimicrobial therapy, may produce a pseudomembranous colitis. Other intestinal pathologic conditions or surgery can cause bacterial overgrowth in the upper small intestine. Anaerobic bacteria can then deconjugate bile acids in this region and bind available vitamin B$_{12}$ so that the vitamin and fats are malabsorbed. In these situations, the patient usually has been compromised in some way; therefore, the infection caused by the normal intestinal flora is secondary to another problem.

More information is available on the animal than the human microflora. Research on animals has revealed that unusual filamentous microorganisms attach to ileal epithelial cells and modify host membranes with few or no harmful effects. Microorganisms have been observed in thick layers on gastrointestinal surfaces (Fig. 6-3) and in the crypts of Lieberkühn. Other studies indicate that the immune response can be modulated by the intestinal flora. Studies of the role of the intestinal flora in biosynthesis of vitamin K and other host-utilizable products, conversion of bile acids (perhaps to cocarcinogens), and ammonia production (which can play a role in hepatic coma) show the dual role of

the microbial flora in influencing the health of the host. More basic studies of the human bowel flora are necessary to define their effect on humans.

UROGENITAL FLORA

The type of bacterial flora found in the vagina depends on the age, pH, and hormonal levels of the host. *Lactobacillus* spp predominate in female infants (vaginal pH approximately 5) during the first month of life. Glycogen secretion seems to cease from about 1 month of age to puberty. During this time, diphtheroids, *S epidermidis*, streptococci, and *E coli* predominate at a higher pH (approximately 7). At puberty, glycogen secretion resumes, the pH drops, and women acquire an adult flora in which *L acidophilus*, corynebacteria, peptococci, peptostreptococci, staphylococci, streptococci, and bacteroides predominate. After menopause, pH again rises, less glycogen is secreted, and the flora returns to that found in prepubescent girls. Yeasts *(Torulopsis* and *Candida)*

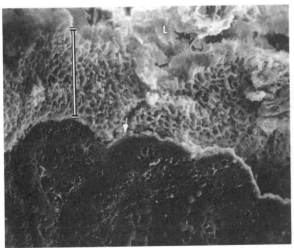
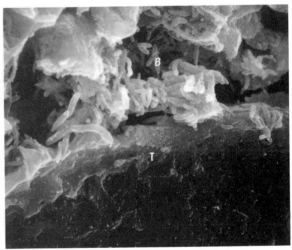

A   B

FIGURE 6-3   *(A)* Scanning electron micrograph of a cross-section of rat colonic mucosa. The bar indicates the thick layer of bacteria between the mucosal surface and the lumen (L). (X 262.) *(B)* Higher magnification of the area indicated by the arrow in Fig. A, showing a mass of bacteria (B) immediately adjacent to colonized intestinal tissue (T). (X 2,624.) (Fig. B from Davis CP: Preservation of bacteria and their microenvironmental association in the rat by freezing. Appl Environ Microbiol 31:310, 1976, with permission.)

are occasionally found in the vagina (10 to 30 percent of women); these sometimes increase and cause vaginitis.

In the anterior urethra of humans, *S epidermidis, S faecalis,* and diphtheroids are found frequently; *E coli, Proteus,* and *Neisseria* (nonpathogenic species) are reported occasionally (10 to 30 percent). Because of the normal flora in the urethra, care must be taken in clinically interpreting urine cultures; urine samples may contain these organisms at a level of 10^4/ml if a midstream (clean-catch) specimen is not obtained.

CONJUNCTIVAL FLORA

The conjunctival flora is sparse. Approximately 17 to 49 percent of culture samples are negative. Lysozyme, secreted in tears, may play a role in controlling the bacteria by interfering with their cell wall formation. When positive samples show bacteria, corynebacteria, neisseriae, and moraxellae are

cultured. Staphylococci and streptococci are also present, and recent reports indicate that *Haemophilus parainfluenzae* is present in 25 percent of conjunctival samples.

HOST INFECTION BY ELEMENTS OF THE NORMAL FLORA

This chapter has briefly described the normal human flora; however, it has not discussed the pathogenic mechanisms of various genera or the clinical syndromes in which they are involved. Although such material is presented in other chapters, note that a breach in mucosal surfaces often result in infection of the host by members of the normal flora. Caries, periodontal disease, abscesses, foul-smelling discharges, and endocarditis are hallmarks of infections with members of the normal human flora (Fig. 6-4). In addition, impairment of the host (for example, those with heart

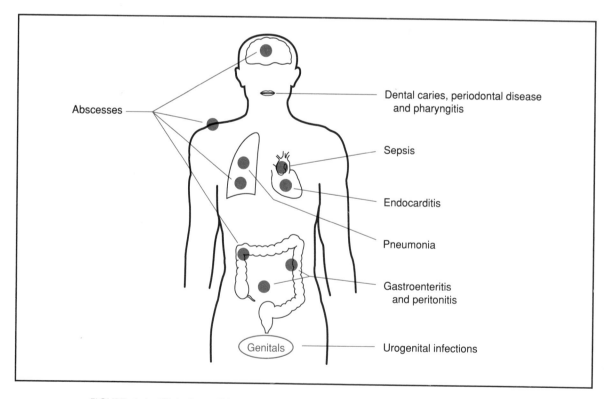

FIGURE 6-4 Clinical conditions that may be caused by members of the normal flora.

failure or leukemia) or host defenses (due to immunosuppression, chemotherapy, or irradiation) may result in failure of the normal flora to suppress transient pathogens or may cause members of the normal flora to invade the host themselves. In either situation, the host may die.

REFERENCES

Bitton G, Marshall KC: Adsorption of Microorganisms to Surfaces. John Wiley & Sons, New York, 1980

Draser BS, Hill MJ: Human Intestinal Flora. Academic Press, London, 1974

Freter R, Brickner J, Botney M, et al: Survival and implantation of *Escherichia coli* in the intestinal tract. Infect Immun 39:686, 1983

Hentges DJ, Stein AJ, Casey SW, Que JU: Protective role of intestinal flora against *Pseudomonas aeruginosa* in mice: influence of antibiotics on colonization resistance. Infect Immun 47:118, 1985

Herthelius M, Gorbach SL, Möllby R, et al: Elimination of vaginal colonization with *Escherichia coli* by administration of indigenous flora. Infect Immun 57:2447, 1989

Maibach H, Aly R: Skin Microbiology: Relevance to Clinical Infection. Springer-Verlag, New York, 1981

Marples MJ: Life in the skin. Sci Am 220:108, 1969

Savage DC: Microbial ecology of the gastrointestinal tract. Annu Rev Microbiol 31:107, 1977

7 BACTERIAL PATHOGENESIS

JOHNNY W. PETERSON

GENERAL CONCEPTS

Host Susceptibility

Resistance to bacterial infections is enhanced by phagocytic cells and an intact immune system. Initial resistance is due to nonspecific mechanisms. Specific immunity develops over time. Susceptibility to some infections is higher in the very young and the very old and in immunosuppressed patients.

Bacterial Infectivity

Bacterial infectivity results from a disturbance in the balance between bacterial virulence and host resistance. The "objective" of bacteria is to multiply rather than to cause disease; it is in the best interest of the bacteria not to kill the host.

Genetic and Molecular Basis for Virulence

Bacterial virulence factors may be encoded on chromosomal, plasmid, transposon, or temperate bacteriophage DNA; virulence factors on plasmids or temperate bacteriophage DNA may integrate into the bacterial chromosome.

Host-Mediated Pathogenesis

In certain infections (e.g., tuberculosis), tissue damage results from the toxic mediators released by lymphoid cells rather than from bacterial toxins.

Intracellular Growth

Some bacteria (e.g., *Rickettsia* species), can grow only within eukaryotic cells, whereas others (e.g., *Salmonella* species) invade cells but do not require them for growth. Most pathogenic bacteria multiply in tissue fluids and not in host cells.

Virulence Factors

Virulence factors are factors that help bacteria to (1) invade the host, (2) cause disease, and (3) evade host defenses. The following are types of virulence factors.

Adherence Factors: Many pathogenic bacteria colonize mucosal sites by using *pili* (fimbriae) to adhere to cells.

Invasion Factors: Surface components that allow the bacterium to invade host cells can be encoded on plasmids, but more often are on the chromosome.

Capsules: Many bacteria are surrounded by **capsules** that protect them from opsonization and phagocytosis.

Endotoxins: The lipopolysaccharide **endotoxins** on Gram-negative bacteria cause fever, changes in blood pressure, inflammation, lethal shock, and many other toxic events.

Exotoxins: **Exotoxins** include several types of protein toxins and enzymes produced and/or secreted from pathogenic bacteria. Major categories include **cytotoxins, neurotoxins,** and **enterotoxins.**

Siderophores: **Siderophores** are iron-binding factors that allow some bacteria to compete with the host for iron, which is bound to hemoglobin, transferrin, and lactoferrin.

INTRODUCTION

Infection is the invasion of the host by microorganisms, which then multiply in close association with the host's tissues. Infection is distinguished from **disease,** a morbid process that does not necessarily involve infection (diabetes, for example, is a disease with no known causative agent). Bacteria can cause a multitude of different infections, ranging in severity from inapparent to fulminating. Table 7-1 lists these types of infections.

The capacity of a bacterium to cause disease reflects its relative **pathogenicity.** On this basis, bacteria can be organized into three major groups. When isolated from a patient, *frank pathogens* are considered to be probable agents of disease (e.g., when the cause of diarrheal disease is identified by the laboratory isolation of *Salmonella* spp from feces). *Opportunistic pathogens* are those isolated from patients whose host defense mechanisms have been compromised. They may be the agents of disease (e.g., in patients who have been predisposed to urinary tract infections with *Escherichia coli* by catheterization). Finally, some bacteria, such as *Lactobacillus acidophilus,* are considered to

TABLE 7-1   Types of Bacterial Infections

Type of Infection	Description	Examples
Inapparent (subclinical)	No detectable clinical symptoms of infection	Asymptomic gonorrhea in women and men
Dormant (latent)	Carrier state	Typhoid carrier
Accidental	Zoonosis or environmental or inadvertent exposures	Anthrax, cryptococcal infection, and laboratory exposure, respectively
Opportunistic	Infection caused by normal flora or transient bacteria when normal host defenses are compromised	*Serratia* or *Candida* infection of the genitourinary tract
Primary	Clinically apparent invasion and multiplication of microbes in body tissues, causing local tissue injury	*Shigella* dysentery
Secondary	Microbial invasion subsequent to primary infection	Bacterial pneumonia following viral lung infection
Mixed	Two or more microbes infecting the same tissue	Anaerobic abscess (*E coli* and *Bacteroides fragilis*)
Acute	Rapid onset (hours or days); brief duration (days or weeks)	Diphtheria
Chronic	Prolonged duration (months or years)	Mycobacterial diseases (tuberculosis and leprosy)
Localized	Confined to a small area or to an organ	Staphylococcal boil
Generalized	Disseminated to many body regions	Gram-negative bacteremia (gonococcemia)
Pyogenic	Pus-forming	Staphylococcal and streptococcal infection
Retrograde	Microbes ascending in a duct or tube against the flow of secretions or excretions	*E coli* urinary tract infection
Fulminant	Infections that occur suddenly and intensely	Airborne *Yersinia pestis* (pneumonic plague)

be *nonpathogens,* because they rarely or never cause human disease. Their categorization as nonpathogens may change, however, because of the adaptability of bacteria and the detrimental effect of modern radiation therapy, chemotherapy, and immunotherapy on resistance mechanisms. In fact, some bacteria previously considered to be nonpathogens are now known to cause disease. *Serratia marcescens,* for example, causes pneumonia, urinary tract infections, and bacteremia in compromised hosts.

Virulence is the measure of the pathogenicity of an organism. The degree of virulence is related directly to the ability of the organism to cause disease despite host resistance mechanisms; it is affected by numerous variables such as the number of infecting bacteria, route of entry into the body, specific and nonspecific host defense mechanisms, and virulence factors of the bacterium. Virulence can be measured experimentally by determining the number of bacteria required to cause animal death, illness, or lesions in a defined period after the bacteria are administered by a designated route. Consequently, calculations of a lethal dose affecting 50 percent of a population of animals (LD_{50}) or an effective dose causing a disease symptom in 50 percent of a population of animals (ED_{50}) are useful in comparing the relative virulence of different bacteria.

Pathogenesis refers both to the mechanism of infection and to the mechanism by which disease develops. The purpose of this chapter is to provide an overview of the many bacterial virulence factors and, where possible, to indicate how they interact with host defense mechanisms and to describe their role in the pathogenesis of disease. It should be understood that the pathogenic mechanisms of many bacterial diseases are poorly understood, while those of others have been probed at the molecular level. The relative importance of an infectious disease to the health of humans and animals does not always coincide with the depth of our understanding of its pathogenesis. This information is best acquired by reading each of the ensuing chapters on specific bacterial diseases, infectious disease texts, and public health bulletins.

HOST SUSCEPTIBILITY

Susceptibility to bacterial infections depends on the physiologic and immunologic condition of the host and on the virulence of the bacteria. Before specific antibodies or immune T cells are formed in response to invading bacterial pathogens, the "nonspecific" mechanisms of host resistance (such as polymorphonuclear neutrophils and macrophage clearance) must defend the host against the microbes. Development of effective specific immunity (such as an antibody response to the bacterium) may require several weeks (Fig. 7-1). The normal bacterial flora of the skin and mucosal surfaces also serves to protect the host against colonization by bacterial pathogens. In most healthy individuals, bacteria from the normal flora that occasionally penetrate the body (e.g., during tooth extraction or routine brushing of teeth) are cleared by the host's cellular and humoral mechanisms. In contrast, individuals with defective immune responses are prone to frequent, recurrent infections with even the least virulent bacteria. The best-known example of such susceptibility is acquired immune deficiency syndrome (AIDS), in which the $CD4^+$ helper lymphocytes are progressively decimated by human immunodeficiency virus (HIV). However, resistance mechanisms can be altered by many other processes. For example, aging often weakens both nonspecific and specific defense systems so that they can no longer effectively combat the challenge of bacteria from the environment. Infants are also especially susceptible to certain pathogens (such as group B streptococci because their immune systems are not yet fully developed and cannot mount a protective immune response to important bacterial antigens. In addition, some individuals have genetic defects of the complement system or cellular defenses (e.g., inability of polymorphonuclear neutrophils to kill bacteria). Finally, a patient may develop granulocytopenia as a result of a predisposing disease, such as cancer, or immunosuppressive chemotherapy for organ transplants or cancer.

Host resistance can be compromised by trauma and by some underlying diseases. An individual

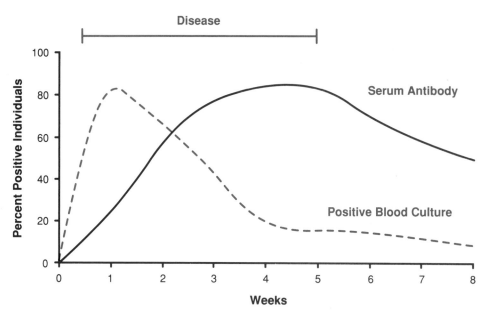

FIGURE 7-1 Serum antibody response to *Salmonella typhi* during typhoid fever and its relationship to septicemia.

becomes susceptible to infection with a variety of bacteria if the skin or mucosa is breached, particularly in the case of severe wounds such as burns or contaminated surgical wounds. Cystic fibrosis patients, who have poor ciliary function and consequently cannot clear mucus efficiently from the respiratory tract, are abnormally susceptible to infection with mucoid strains of *Pseudomonas aeruginosa,* resulting in serious respiratory distress. Ascending urinary tract infections with *Escherichia coli* are common in women and are particularly troublesome in patients with urinary tract obstructions. A variety of routine medical procedures, such as tracheal intubation and catheterization of blood vessels and the urethra, increase the risk of bacterial infection. The plastic devices used in these procedures are readily colonized by bacteria from the skin, which migrate along the outside of the tube to infect deeper tissues or enter the bloodstream. Because of this problem, it is standard practice to change catheters frequently (e.g.,

every 72 hours for peripheral intravenous catheters).

Many drugs have been developed to treat bacterial infections. Antimicrobial agents are most effective, however, when the infection is also being fought by healthy phagocytic and immune defenses. Some reasons for this situation are the poor diffusion of antibiotics into certain sites (such as the prostate gland), the ability of many bacteria to multiply or survive inside cells (where many antimicrobial agents have little or no effect), the bacteriostatic rather than bactericidal action of some drugs, and the ability of some organisms to develop resistance to multiple antibiotics.

Many bacterial pathogens are transmitted to the host by a **vector,** usually an arthropod. For example, Rocky Mountain spotted fever and Lyme disease are both vectored by ticks, and bubonic plague is spread by fleas. Susceptibility to these diseases depends partly on the host's contact with the vector.

PATHOGENIC MECHANISMS

Bacterial Infectivity

Factors that are produced by a microorganism and evoke disease are called **virulence factors.** Examples are toxins, surface coats that inhibit phagocytosis, and surface receptors that bind to host cells. Most frank (as opposed to opportunistic) bacterial pathogens have evolved specific virulence factors that allow them to multiply in their host or vector without being killed or expelled by the host's defenses. Many virulence factors are produced only by specific virulent strains of a microorganism. For example, only certain strains of *E coli* secrete diarrhea-causing enterotoxins.

Virulence factors should never be considered independently of the host's defenses; the clinical course of a disease often depends on the interaction of virulence factors with the host's response. An infection begins when the balance between bacterial pathogenicity and host resistance is upset. In essence, we live in an environment that favors the microbe, simply because the growth rate of bacteria far exceeds that of most eukaryotic cells. Furthermore, bacteria are much more versatile than eukaryotic cells in substrate utilization and biosynthesis. The high mutation rate of bacteria combined with their short generation time results in rapid selection of the best-adapted strains and species. In general, bacteria are much more resistant to toxic components in the environment than eukaryotes, particularly when the major barriers of eukaryotes (skin and mucous membranes) are breached.

From a practical standpoint, bacteria can be said to have a single objective: to reproduce. Only a few of the vast number of bacterial species in the environment consistently cause disease in a given host. From a teleologic standpoint, it is not in the best interest of the pathogen to kill the host, because in most cases the death of the host means the death of the pathogen. The most highly evolved or adapted pathogens are the ones that acquire the necessary nutritional substances for growth and dissemination with the smallest expenditure of energy and least damage to the host. For example, *Rickettsia*

akari, the etiologic agent of rickettsialpox, causes a mild, self-limited infection consisting of headache, fever, and a papulovesicular rash. Other members of the rickettsial group, such as *R rickettsii*, the agent of Rocky Mountain spotted fever, elicit more severe, life-threatening infections. Some bacteria that are poorly adapted to the host synthesize virulence factors (e.g., tetanus and diphtheria toxin) so potent that they threaten the life of the host.

Genetic and Molecular Basis for Virulence

Virulence factors in bacteria may be encoded on chromosomal DNA, bacteriophage DNA, plasmids, or transposons in either plasmids or the bacterial chromosome (Fig. 7-2; Table 7-2). For example, the capacity of *Shigella* species to invade cells is a property encoded in part on a 140-megadalton plasmid. Similarly, the heat-labile enterotoxin (LTI) of *E coli* is plasmid encoded, whereas the heat-labile toxin (LTII) is encoded on the chromosome. Other virulence factors are acquired by bacteria following infection by a particular bacteriophage, which integrates its genome into the bacterial chromosome by the process of lysogeny (Fig. 7-2). Temperate bacteriophages often serve as the basis of toxin production in pathogenic bacteria. Examples include diphtheria toxin production by *Corynebacterium diphtheriae*, erythrogenic toxin formation by *Streptococcus pyogenes*, Shiga-like toxin synthesis by *E coli*, and production of botulinum toxin (types C and D) by *Clostridium botulinum*. Other virulence factors are encoded on the bacterial chromosome (e.g., cholera toxin, *Salmonella* enterotoxin, and *Yersinia* invasion factors). Often, no information about the source or purpose of bacterial virulence genes is available.

The transfer of genes for antibiotic resistance among bacteria is a significant medical problem, although none of these properties actually confers increased virulence to the bacterium. Rather, they provide the opportunity for resistant bacteria to proliferate and express other virulence factors in patients who are being treated with an inappropri-

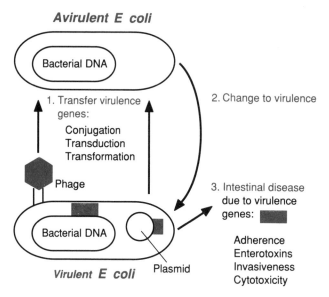

FIGURE 7-2   Mechanisms of acquiring bacterial virulence genes.

TABLE 7-2   Genetic Basis for Virulence of Selected Bacterial Pathogens

Gene(s) Encoded on	Bacterial Pathogen	Virulence Factor
Chromosome	*Vibrio cholerae*	Enterotoxin
	Salmonella typhimurium	Enterotoxin, invasion factors
	Shigella spp	Enterotoxin, invasion factors
	Aeromonas hydrophila	Enterotoxin, aerolysin
	Pseudomonas aeruginosa	Exotoxin A
	Staphylococcus aureus	Enterotoxin B
	Yersinia enterocolitica	Invasion factors
	Yersinia pseudotuberculosis	Invasion factors
	Escherichia coli	Enterotoxin (LTII)
Plasmid	*Shigella* spp	Invasion factors
	Escherichia coli	Invasion factors, colonization factor, and enterotoxin (LTI)
	Staphylococcus aureus	Exfoliative toxin
	Bacillus anthracis	Anthrax toxin
Bacteriophage	*Corynebacterium diphtheriae*	Diphtheria toxin
	Streptococcus pyogenes	Erythrogenic toxin
	Escherichia coli	Shiga-like enterotoxin
	Clostridium botulinum	Botulinum toxin (C,D)
Transposons[a]	*Escherichia coli*	Enterotoxins (STA and STB), iron acquisition, hemolysin

[a] Transposable genetic elements located on plasmids that often insert into the chromosome.

ate antibiotic. Resistance factors are discussed fully in Chapter 5.

An intriguing question regarding most bacterial protein toxins is the purpose they serve for the bacteriophage or the bacterium carrying them. Several bacterial toxins are enzymes. For example, cholera toxin, diphtheria toxin, *Pseudomonas* exotoxin A, and pertussis toxin all are NAD glycohydrolases that also act as ADP-ribosyltransferases. The toxic effect of these bacterial enzymes on the host is integral to the pathogenesis of the bacterial infections, but the function of the enzymes for the bacteria is not known. Of all the protein toxins synthesized by pathogenic bacteria, there are few instances in which the function of the protein to the bacterium is known. It would be unlikely for the bacterium or infecting bacteriophage to expend the energy necessary to synthesize these relatively high-molecular-weight and complex molecules if they offered it no advantage. Frequently the toxicity of these substances is "unintentional" as far as the bacteria are concerned, considering that the primary goal of the microorganisms is to acquire nutrients and reproduce rather than to harm the host.

Host-Mediated Pathogenesis

The pathogenesis of many bacterial infections cannot be separated from the host immune response, for much of the tissue damage is caused by the host response rather than by bacterial factors. Classic examples of host response-mediated pathogenesis are seen in diseases such as Gram-negative bacterial sepsis, tuberculosis, and tuberculoid leprosy. The tissue damage in these infections is caused by toxic factors released from the lymphocytes, macrophages, and polymorphonuclear neutrophils infiltrating the site of infection (Fig. 7-3). Often the host response is so intense that host tissues are destroyed, allowing resistant bacteria to proliferate. In lepromatous leprosy, in contrast, the absence of a cellular response to *Mycobacterium leprae* allows the bacteria to multiply to such large num-

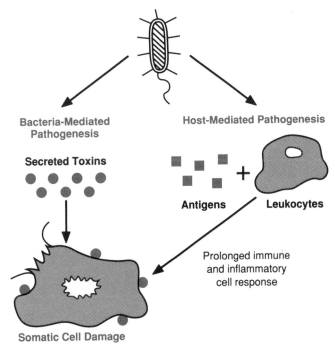

FIGURE 7-3 Generalized mechanisms of bacterial pathogenesis: bacteria-induced toxicity or host-mediated damage.

bers in the skin that they become tightly packed and replace healthy tissue. The molecular basis for this specific immune anergy is poorly understood.

Intracellular Growth

In general, bacteria that can enter and survive within eukaryotic cells are shielded from humoral antibodies and can be eliminated only by a cellular immune response. However, these bacteria must possess specialized mechanisms to protect them from the harsh effects of the lysosomal enzymes encountered within the cell (see Ch. 1). Pathogenic bacteria can be grouped into three categories on the basis of their invasive properties for eukaryotic cells (Fig. 7-4; Table 7-3). Although some bacteria (e.g., *Rickettsia*, *Coxiella*, and *Chlamydia*) grow only inside host cells, others (e.g., *Salmonella*, *Shigella*, and *Yersinia*) are facultative intracellular pathogens, invading cells when it gives them a selective advantage in the host.

Some bacteria survive the intracellular milieu by producing phospholipases to dissolve the phago-

TABLE 7-3   Intracellular or Extracellular Growth Preference Relative to Eukaryotic Cells

Category	Bacterial Pathogen
Obligate intracellular	*Rickettsia* spp *Coxiella burnetii* *Chlamydia* spp
Facultative intracellular	*Salmonella* spp *Shigella* spp *Legionella pneumophila* Invasive *Escherichia coli* *Neisseria* spp *Mycobacterium* spp *Listeria monocytogenes* *Bordetella pertussis*
Predominantly extracellular	*Mycoplasma* spp *Pseudomonas aeruginosa* Enterotoxigenic *Escherichia coli* *Vibrio cholerae* *Staphylococcus aureus* *Streptococcus pyogenes* *Haemophilus influenzae* *Bacillus anthracis*

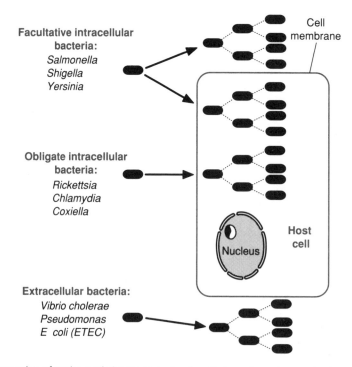

FIGURE 7-4   Examples of pathogenic bacteria, indicating their preferred growth phase within the host. (ETEC: enterotoxigenic *E coli*.)

cytic vesicle surrounding them. This appears to be the case for *R rickettsii,* which destroys the phagosomal membrane with which the lysosomes fuse. *Legionella pneumophila,* which prefers the intracellular environment of macrophages for growth, appears to induce its own uptake and blocks lysosomal fusion by undefined mechanisms. Other bacteria have evolved to the point that they prefer the low-pH environment within the lysosomal granules, as may be the case for *Coxiella burnetii,* a highly resistant member of the rickettsial group. *Salmonella* and *Mycobacterium* species also appear to be very resistant to intracellular killing by phagocytic cells, but their mechanisms of resistance are not yet fully understood. Certainly, the capacity of bacteria to survive and multiply within host cells has great impact on the pathogenesis of the respective infections.

Most bacterial pathogens do not invade cells, proliferating instead in the extracellular environment enriched by body fluids. Some of these bacteria (e.g., *V cholerae* and *Bordetella pertussis*) do not even penetrate body tissues, but, rather, adhere to epithelial surfaces and cause disease by secreting potent protein toxins. Although bacteria such as *E coli* and *P aeruginosa* are termed noninvasive, they frequently spread rapidly to various tissues once they gain access to the body. All bacteria could at some point be considered intracellular once they become ingested by polymorphonuclear neutrophils and macrophages, but these organisms are not renowned for their capacity to survive the intracellular environment or to induce their own uptake by most host cells.

Specific Virulence Factors

The virulence factors of bacteria can be divided into a number of functional types. These are discussed in the following sections.

Adherence and Colonization Factors

To cause infection, many bacteria must first adhere to a mucosal surface. For example, the alimentary tract mucosa is continually cleaned by the release of mucus from goblet cells and by the peristaltic flow of the gut contents over the epithelium. Similarly, ciliated cells in the respiratory tract sweep mucus and bacteria upward. In addition, the turnover of epithelial cells at these surfaces is fairly rapid. The intestinal epithelial cell monolayer is continually replenished, and the cells are pushed from the crypts to the villar tips in about 48 hours. To establish an infection at such a site, a bacterium must adhere to the epithelium and multiply before the mucus and extruded epithelial cells are swept away. To accomplish this, bacteria have evolved attachment mechanisms, such as pili (fimbriae), that recognize and attach the bacteria to cells (see Ch. 2). **Colonization factors** (as they are often called) are produced by numerous bacterial pathogens and constitute an important part of the pathogenic mechanism of these bacteria. Some examples of piliated, adherent bacterial pathogens are *V cholerae, E coli, Salmonella* spp, *N gonorrheae, N meningitidis,* and *Streptococcus pyogenes.*

Invasion Factors

Mechanisms that enable a bacterium to invade eukaryotic cells facilitate entry at mucosal surfaces. Some of these invasive bacteria (such as *Rickettsia* and *Chlamydia* species) are obligate intracellular pathogens, but most are facultative intracellular pathogens (Fig. 7-4). The specific bacterial surface factors that mediate invasion are not known in most instances, and often, multiple gene products are involved. Some *Shigella* invasion factors are encoded on a 140 megadalton plasmid, which, when conjugated into *E coli,* gives these noninvasive bacteria the capacity to invade cells. A similar invasion gene encoding adherence factors has recently been identified in *Yersinia pseudotuberculosis.* The mechanisms of invasion of *Salmonella, Rickettsia,* and *Chlamydia* species are not well known.

Capsules and Other Surface Components

Bacteria have evolved numerous structural and metabolic virulence factors that enhance their survival rate in the host. Capsule formation has long been recognized as a protective mechanism for bacteria (see Ch. 2). Encapsulated strains of many bacteria (e.g., pneumococci) are more virulent and more resistant to phagocytosis and intracellular killing than are nonencapsulated strains. Organisms that cause bacteremia (e.g., *Pseudomonas*) are less sensitive than many other bacteria to killing by fresh human serum containing complement components, and are called serum resistant. Serum resistance may be related to the amount and composition of capsular antigens as well as to the structure of the lipopolysaccharide. The relationship between surface structure and virulence is important also in *Borrelia* infections. As the bacteria encounter an increasing specific immune response from the host, the bacterial surface antigens are altered by mutation, and the progeny, which are no longer recognized by the immune response, express renewed virulence. *Salmonella typhi* and some of the paratyphoid organisms carry a surface antigen, the *Vi antigen*, thought to enhance virulence. This antigen is composed of a polymer of galactosamine and uronic acid in 1,4-linkage. Its role in virulence has not been defined, but antibody to it is protective.

Some bacteria and parasites have the ability to survive and multiply inside phagocytic cells. A classic example is *Mycobacterium tuberculosis*, whose survival seems to depend on the structure and composition of its cell surface. The parasite *Toxoplasma gondii* has the remarkable ability to block the fusion of lysosomes with the phagocytic vacuole. The hydrolytic enzymes contained in the lysosomes are unable, therefore, to contribute to the destruction of the parasite. The mechanisms by which bacteria such as *Legionella pneumophila*, *Brucella abortus*, and *Listeria monocytogenes* remain unharmed inside phagocytes are not understood.

Endotoxins

Endotoxins are toxic lipopolysaccharide components of the outer membrane of Gram-negative bacteria (see Ch. 2). Endotoxins exert profound biologic effects on the host, and may be lethal. They must be removed from all medical supplies destined for injection or use during surgical procedures. The term **endotoxin** was coined in 1893 by Pfeiffer to distinguish the class of toxic substances released after lysis of bacteria from the toxic substances (exotoxins) secreted by bacteria. Few, if any, other microbial products have been as extensively studied as bacterial endotoxins. Per-

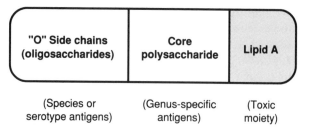

"O" Side chains (oligosaccharides)	Core polysaccharide	Lipid A
(Species or serotype antigens)	(Genus-specific antigens)	(Toxic moiety)

FIGURE 7-5   Basic structure of endotoxin (lipopolysaccharide) from Gram-negative bacteria.

haps it is appropriate that a molecule with such important biologic effects on the host, and one produced by so many bacterial pathogens, should be the subject of intense investigation.

STRUCTURE OF ENDOTOXIN   Figure 7-5 illustrates the basic structure of endotoxin. Endotoxin is a molecular complex of lipid and polysaccharide; hence, the alternate name **lipopolysaccharide.** The complex is secured to the outer membrane by ionic and hydrophobic forces, and its strong negative charge is neutralized by Ca^{2+} and Mg^{2+} ions.

The structure of endotoxin molecules from *Salmonella* spp and *E coli* is known in detail. Enough data on endotoxin from other Gram-negative organisms have been gathered to reveal a common pattern with genus and species diversity. Although all endotoxin molecules are similar in chemical structure and biologic activity, some diversity has evolved. Purified endotoxin appears as large aggregates. The molecular complex can be divided into three regions (Fig. 7-5): (1) the O-specific chains, which consist of a variety of repeating oligosaccharide residues, (2) the core polysaccharide that forms the backbone of the macromolecule, and (3) lipid A, composed usually of a glucosamine disaccharide with attached long-chain fatty acids. The polysaccharide portions are responsible for antigenic diversity, whereas the lipid A moiety confers toxicity. Dissociation of the complex has revealed that the polysaccharide is important in solubilizing the toxic lipid A component and can be replaced by bovine serum albumin.

Members of the family Enterobacteriaceae exhibit O-specific chains of various lengths, whereas *N gonorrhoeae*, *N meningitidis*, and *B pertussis* contain only core polysaccharide and lipid A. Some investigators working on the latter forms of endotoxin prefer to call them lipooligosaccharide to emphasize the chemical difference from the endotoxin of the enteric bacilli. Nevertheless, the biologic activities of all endotoxin preparations are essentially the same, with some being more potent than others.

BIOLOGIC ACTIVITY OF ENDOTOXIN The biologic effects of endotoxin have been extensively studied. Purified lipid A (conjugated to bovine serum albumin) and endotoxin elicit the same biologic responses. Table 7-4 lists some of the biologic effects of endotoxin. The more pertinent toxic effects include pyrogenicity, leukopenia followed by leukocytosis, complement activation, depression in blood pressure, mitogenicity, induction of prostaglandin synthesis, and hypothermia. These events can culminate in sepsis and lethal shock. However, it should be noted from Table 7-4 that not all effects of endotoxin are necessarily detrimental; several induce responses potentially bene-

ficial to the host, assuming the stimulation is not excessive. These include

1. mitogenic effects on B lymphocytes that increase resistance to viral and bacterial infections
2. induction of gamma interferon production by T lymphocytes, which may enhance the antiviral state, promote rejection of tumor cells, and activate macrophages and natural killer cells
3. activation of the complement cascade with the formation of C3a and C5a
4. induction of the formation of interleukin-1 by macrophages and interleukin-2 and other mediators by T lymphocytes.

Current research focuses on exploiting some of the potential beneficial effects of endotoxin derivatives and holds promise for development of future treatment regimens for stimulating the immune response.

Endotoxin, which largely accumulates in the liver following injection of a sublethal dose by the intravenous route, can be devastating because of its ability to affect a variety of cell and host proteins. Küpffer cells, granulocytes, macrophages, platelets, and lymphocytes all have cell receptors on their surface for endotoxin. The extent of involvement of each cell type probably depends on the level of endotoxin exposure. The effects of endotoxin on such a wide variety of host cells result in a complex array of host responses that can culminate in the serious condition **gram-negative sepsis,** which often leads to shock and death. The effects of endotoxin on host cells are known to stimulate prostaglandin synthesis and to activate the kallikrein system, the kinin system, the complement cascade via the alternative pathway, the clotting system, and the fibrinolytic pathways. When these normal host systems are activated and operate out of control, it is not surprising that endotoxin can be lethal. Although it is difficult to comprehend the mechanisms of all the cell responses and the myriad sequelae of the cell mediators released rather indiscriminately in the host following exposure to endotoxin, it does seem clear that the host cellular response to endotoxin, rather than a

TABLE 7-4 Multiple Biologic Activities Exhibited by Free Lipid A Component of Endotoxin

Pyrogenicity
Leukopenia, leukocytosis
Complement activation
Depression of blood pressure
Hageman factor activation
Platelet activation
Induction of plasminogen activator
Bone marrow necrosis
Hypothermia in mice
Lethal toxicity in mice
Shwartzman reaction
Induction of prostaglandin synthesis
Limulus lysate gelation
*Induction of nonspecific resistance to infection
*Induction of endotoxin tolerance
*Adjuvant activity
*Mitogenic activity for lymphocytes
*Macrophage activation
*Induction of interferon synthesis
*Induction of tumor necrosis factor synthesis

* Potentially beneficial stimulatory effects of endotoxin in low doses.

direct toxic effect of endotoxin, plays the major role in causing tissue damage (Fig. 7-3).

DETECTION OF ENDOTOXIN IN MEDICAL SOLUTIONS

Endotoxin is omnipresent in the environment. It is found in most deionized-water lines in hospitals and laboratories, for example, and affects virtually every biologic assay system ever examined. It tends to be a scapegoat for all biologic problems encountered in the laboratory, and, many times, this reputation is deserved. Because of its pyrogenic and destructive properties, extreme care must be taken to avoid exposing patients to medical solutions containing endotoxin. Even though all supplies should be sterile, solutions for intravenous administration can become contaminated with endotoxin-containing bacteria after sterilization as a result of improper handling. Furthermore, water used in the preparation of such solutions must be filtered through ion exchange resins to remove endotoxin, because it is not removed by either autoclave sterilization or filtration through bacterial membrane filters. If endotoxin-containing solutions were used in such medical procedures as renal dialysis, heart bypass machines, blood transfusions, or surgical lavage, the patient would suffer immediate fever accompanied by a rapid and possibly lethal drop in blood pressure.

Solutions for human or veterinary use are prepared under carefully controlled conditions to ensure sterility and the removal of endotoxin. Representative samples of every manufacturing batch are checked for endotoxin by one of two procedures: the *Limulus* lysate test or the rabbit pyrogenicity test. The rabbit pyrogenicity test is based on the exquisite sensitivity of rabbits to the pyrogenic effects of endotoxin. A sample of the solution to be tested usually is injected intravenously into the ear veins of adult rabbits while the rectal temperature of the animal is monitored. Careful monitoring of the temperature responses provides a sensitive and reliable indicator of the presence of endotoxin and, importantly, one measure of the safety of the solution for use in patients.

The *Limulus* lysate test is more common and less expensive. This test, which is based on the ability of endotoxin to induce gelation of lysates of amebo-cyte cells of the horseshoe crab *Limulus polyphemus,* is simple, fast, and sensitive (about 1 ng/ml). It is so sensitive, however, that trace quantities of endotoxin in regular deionized water often obscure the results. It can be used for rapid detection of certain Gram-negative infections (e.g., of cerebrospinal fluid); however, blood contains inhibitors that prevent gelation. Test kits are commercially available. The amebocyte is the sole phagocytic immune cell of the horseshoe crab, and the gelation reaction is believed to be involved in sequestering invading Gram-negative bacteria.

Exotoxins

Exotoxins, unlike the lipopolysaccharide endotoxin, are protein toxins released from viable bacteria. They form a class of poisons that is among the most potent, per unit weight, of all toxic substances. Most are heat labile. Unlike endotoxin, which is a structural component of all Gram-negative cells, exotoxins are produced by some members of both Gram-positive and Gram-negative genera. The functions of these exotoxins for the bacteria are usually unknown. In contrast to the extensive systemic and immune-system effects of endotoxin on the host, the site of action of most exotoxins is more localized and is confined to particular cell types or cell receptors. Tetanus toxin, for example, affects only internuncial neurons. In general, exotoxins are excellent antigens that elicit specific antibodies called **antitoxins.** The antitoxin can react with the exotoxin and neutralize it, whereas antibody to endotoxin reacts with the lipopolysaccharide complex but has little effect on the biologic activity of the complex, except under special conditions.

Exotoxins can be grouped into several categories (e.g., neurotoxins, cytotoxins, and enterotoxins) based on their biologic effect on host cells. **Neurotoxins** are best exemplified by the toxins produced by *Clostridium* spp, for example, the botulinum toxin formed by *C botulinum.* This potent neurotoxin acts on motor neurons by preventing the release of acetylcholine at the myoneural junctions, thereby preventing muscle excitation and producing flaccid paralysis. The **cytotoxins** constitute a larger, more heterogeneous grouping with a wide array of host cell specificities and toxic manifestations. One cytotoxin is diphtheria toxin, which is produced by *Corynebacterium diphtheriae*. This cytotoxin inhibits protein synthesis in many cell types by catalyzing the ADP-ribosylation of elongation factor II, which blocks elongation of the growing peptide chain.

Enterotoxins stimulate hypersecretion of water and electrolytes from the intestinal epithelium and thus produce watery diarrhea. Some enterotoxins also disturb normal smooth muscle contraction, causing abdominal cramping and decreased transit time for water absorption in the intestine. Enterotoxigenic *E coli* and *V cholerae* produce diarrhea after attaching to the intestinal mucosa, where they elaborate enterotoxins. Neither pathogen invades the body in substantial numbers, except in the case of *E coli* species that have acquired an invasion plasmid. Importantly, cholera toxin and *E coli* heat-labile enterotoxins I and II cause ADP-ribosylation of cell proteins in a manner similar to diphtheria toxin, except that the primary target is the regulatory protein ($G_{s\alpha}$) of adenylate cyclase, resulting in increased levels of cyclic 3′,5′-adenosine monophosphate (cAMP) (see Ch. 25). In contrast, the organisms responsible for shigellosis (*Shigella dysenteriae*, *S boydii*, *S flexneri*, and *S sonnei*) penetrate the mucosal surface of the colon and terminal ileum to proliferate and cause ulcerations that bleed into the intestinal lumen. Despite causing extensive ulceration of the mucosa, the pathogens rarely enter the bloodstream. The Shiga enterotoxin produced by *Shigella* species and the Shiga-like enterotoxin elaborated by many isolates of *E coli* inhibit protein synthesis in eukaryotic cells. It is not clear how this cytotoxic enterotoxin causes hypersecretion of water and electrolytes from the intestinal epithelium. These enterotoxins differ from those secreted by *V cholerae* and *E coli* in that the Shiga toxins are cytotoxic whereas the cholera toxin-like enterotoxins are not. The latter enterotoxins cause no structural damage to cells, and are described as **cytotonic**. The ensuing inflammatory response to the invading bacteria and/or their toxins appears to activate neurologic control mechanisms (e.g., prostaglandins, serotonin) that normally regulate water and electrolyte transport.

Siderophores

Both animals and bacteria require iron for metabolism and growth, and the control of this limited resource is often used as a tactic in the conflict between pathogen and host. Animals have evolved mechanisms of "withholding" iron from tissue fluids in an attempt to limit the growth of invading bacteria. Although blood is a rich source of iron, this iron is not readily available to bacteria since it is not free in solution. Most of the iron in blood is bound either to hemoglobin in erythrocytes or to transferrin in plasma. Similarly, the iron in milk and other secretions (e.g., tears, saliva, bronchial mucus, bile, and gastrointestinal fluid) is bound to lactoferrin.

Bacteria have evolved elaborate mechanisms to extract the iron from host proteins (Fig. 7-6). **Siderophores** are substances produced by many bacteria (and some plants) to capture iron from the host. The absence of iron triggers transcription of the genes coding for the enzymes that synthesize siderophores, as well as for a set of surface protein receptors that recognize siderophores carrying bound iron. The binding constants of the siderophores for iron are so high that even iron bound to transferrin and lactoferrin is confiscated and taken up by the bacterial cells. An example of a bacterial siderophore is enterochelin, which is produced by *Salmonella* species. Classic experiments have demonstrated that *Salmonella* mutants that have lost the capacity to synthesize enterochelin lose virulence in an assay of lethality in mice. Injection of purified enterochelin along with the *Salmonella* mutants restores virulence to the bacteria. Therefore, siderophore production by many pathogenic bacteria is considered an important virulence mechanism.

EPILOGUE

Many factors determine the outcome of the bacterium-host relationship. The host must live in an environment filled with a diverse population of microorganisms. Because of the magnitude of the infectious-disease problem, we strive to understand the natural immune mechanisms of the host so that future improvements in resistance to bacte-

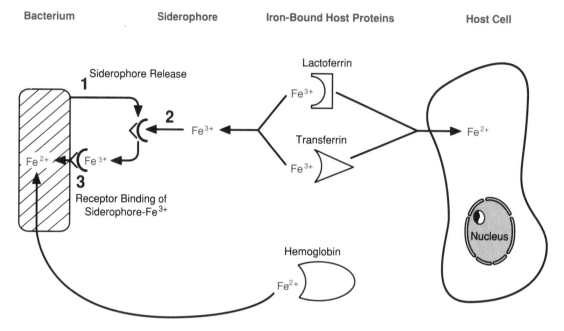

Bacterium   **Siderophore**   **Iron-Bound Host Proteins**   **Host Cell**

FIGURE 7-6 Competition between host cells and bacterial pathogens for iron, illustrating the importance of siderophores. Since free iron is scarce in tissue fluids and blood, bacterial siderophores compete effectively for Fe^{3+} bound to lactoferrin and transferrin.

rial infections may be possible. Similarly, massive research efforts are being expended to identify and characterize the virulence factors of pathogenic bacteria and hence allow us to interrupt the pathogenic mechanisms of virulent bacteria. The availability of an array of antibiotics and vaccines has provided the medical profession with powerful tools to control or cure many infections. Unfortunately, these drugs and vaccines have eliminated no bacterial disease from the human or animal populations, and bacterial infections remain a serious medical problem.

REFERENCES

Berry LJ: Bacterial toxins. Crit Rev Toxicol 5:239, 1977

Eisenstein TK, Actor P, Friedman H: Host Defenses to Intracellular Pathogens. Plenum Publishing Co, New York, 1983

Finlay BB, Falkow S: Common themes in microbial pathogenicity. Microbiol Rev 53:210, 1989

Foster TJ: Plasmid-determined resistance to antimicrobial drugs and toxic metal ions in bacteria. Microbiol Rev 47:361, 1983

Hardegree MC, Tu AT (eds): Handbook of Natural Toxins. Vol. 4: Bacterial Toxins. Marcel Dekker, New York, 1988

Iglewski BH, Clark VL (eds): Molecular Basis of Bacterial Pathogenesis. Vol. XI of The Bacteria: A Treatise on Structure and Function. Academic Press, Orlando, FL, 1990

Lüderitz O, Galanos C: Endotoxins of gram negativebacteria. p. 307. In Dorner F, Drews J (eds): Pharmacology of Bacterial Toxins. International Encyclopedia of Pharmacology and Therapeutics, Section 119. Pergamon, Elmsford, NY, 1986

Mims CA: The Pathogenesis of Infectious Disease. Academic Press, London, 1976

Payne SM: Iron and virulence in the family Enterobacteriaceae. Crit Rev Microbiol 16:81, 1988

Sack, RB: Human diarrheal disease caused by enterotoxigenic *Escherichia coli*. Annu Rev Microbiol 29:333, 1975

Smith H: Microbial surfaces in relation to pathogenicity. Bacteriol Rev 41:475, 1977

Smith H, Turner JJ (eds): The Molecular Basis of Pathogenicity. Verlag Chemie, Deerfield Beach, FL, 1980

Weinberg ED: Iron withholding: a defense against infection and neoplasia. Physiol Rev 64:65, 1984

8 SPECIFIC ACQUIRED IMMUNITY

JOHN P. CRAIG

GENERAL CONCEPTS

Defense Mechanisms

Specific acquired immunity against bacterial infections is mediated by antibodies (immunoglobulins in serum and other body fluids) and/or by cellular immune mechanisms. Resistance to most bacterial infections involves both mechanisms.

Biologic Basis of Acquired Resistance

Specific immunity starts with the stimulation of clones of B or T lymphocytes by antigenic components or products of bacteria. As in all immune mechanisms, the major features are specificity and memory.

Measurement of Resistance

Resistance to infection can be detected and measured only by observing differences in disease or death rates between immune and nonimmune animals following live microbial challenge.

Antibody-Mediated Resistance Mechanisms

Antibodies (IgG, IgA, and IgM) are most effective against bacterial infections in which secreted exotoxins or bacterial surface antigens are the major virulence factors. Important surface antigens include components of bacterial capsules and adherence pili (fimbriae).

Cell-Mediated Resistance Mechanisms

Cell-mediated immunity is most effective against infections in which bacteria multiply within phagocytic cells, chiefly macrophages. T lymphocytes represent the specific component of cell-mediated immunity, whereas macrophages, which can be activated by lymphokines produced by these T lymphocytes, represent the nonspecific component of this mechanism. This activation of macrophages enhances their power to kill intracellular bacteria.

Acquired Resistance to Infectious Disease

In most bacterial infections, humoral (immunoglobulin-mediated) and cell-mediated immune responses collaborate to provide the total specific acquired resistance against the microbe.

Artificial Immunization

Vaccines attempt to mimic nature by inducing either antibody- or cell-mediated resistance or both. The major kinds of vaccines are detoxified exotoxins (toxoids); whole, killed microorganisms; living nonpathogenic (attenuated) variants of pathogenic microorganisms; and purified virulence factors, such as capsular polysaccharides.

147

INTRODUCTION

Bacterial infections, like all infections, are usually followed by a state of specific acquired resistance to reinfection by the same microorganism. This specific acquired resistance is one facet of the host immune response to the foreign antigens present in the infecting microbe.

In bacterial infections, both humoral (antibody-mediated) and cellular immune responses (see Ch. 1) may be important in acquired resistance. Bacteria vary greatly in their growth rates, mechanisms of pathogenesis, and preferred sites of multiplication within the host. Some produce acute diseases, whereas others cause chronic infections associated with prolonged survival and multiplication of organisms within phagocytic cells. Therefore, the nature and effectiveness of the immune response to bacterial infections vary greatly, depending on the properties of the infecting bacterium and its location within the host.

BIOLOGIC BASIS OF ACQUIRED RESISTANCE

Acquired specific resistance is initiated by the stimulation and expansion of lymphocyte clones that can respond to specific antigens in the infecting microbe (see Ch. 1). Expansion of specific populations of B or T lymphocytes mediates resistance. B lymphocytes mature into plasma cells that synthesize and secrete immunoglobulins, the mediators of humoral immunity. T lymphocytes play a major role in cell-mediated immune mechanisms and as helper cells in some B-cell-mediated responses. One or both of these immune responses is involved in the increased resistance that occurs after natural infection or artificial exposure to microbial antigens (vaccination).

Antibody-mediated and cell-mediated immune responses have in common the features of specificity and memory. Memory results from the persistence of increased populations of specifically primed, antigen-reactive lymphocytes following exposure to antigen. These cells respond quickly to subsequent exposure to the same antigen by vigorous differentiation and population expansion. This cellular response leads to more rapid and greater antibody production or cell-mediated reactivity or both.

MEASUREMENT OF RESISTANCE

A method for measuring resistance is required to determine changes in specific immune resistance and to distinguish specific resistance from preexisting innate and nonspecific resistance. Resistance can be measured only by observing the differences in morbidity and mortality between immune and nonimmune animals following live microbial challenge. Although in vitro measurement of antibody and cell-mediated immunity may sometimes correlate with resistance, such measurements can never substitute fully for in vivo challenge of the whole animal. In vitro measurements do not necessarily correlate with protection against disease, because some in vitro assays measure activities of antibodies or lymphocytes that may not be protective in vivo.

ANTIBODY-MEDIATED RESISTANCE MECHANISMS

Antibody-mediated immunity in bacterial infections may be directed against antigenic toxic products (**antitoxic immunity**) or against antigens on the bacterial surface (**antibacterial immunity**). Antitoxic immunity resembles antibody-mediated antiviral immunity in that the combination of antibody with the toxin antigen prevents attachment or entry of the toxin into target cells. This process is called **toxin neutralization.**

Antitoxin may be circulating IgG or secretory IgA (sIgA), but only circulating IgG antitoxins have been clearly shown to protect against bacterial toxins in human disease. Bacterial infections in which the major manifestations of disease are caused by highly potent, secreted toxic proteins (exotoxins) are called **toxinoses;** diphtheria, tetanus, botulism, scarlet fever, and cholera are examples. Specific antitoxins can be effective in conferring resistance if they can combine with the exotoxin and neutralize it before it combines with specific receptors on target cell membranes. Once exotoxins have attached to and entered susceptible cells, antitoxin is ineffective. Therefore, in diseases in which exotoxin must be distributed by the blood from the site of synthesis to the target cell (diphtheria, tetanus, botulism, and scarlet fever), humoral antitoxic immunity is relatively effective because antitoxin can neutralize the toxin before it binds to target cell membranes. In cholera, on the other hand, exotoxin is produced by bacteria adhering to the luminal surfaces of small intestinal epithelial cells, which are also the target cells for the toxin. The toxin does not enter the bloodstream, and in humans, serum antitoxin has not been shown to be protective. It is not clear whether IgA antitoxin effectively protects against cholera in humans, but because the distance from the toxin source to its target is so short, successful neutralization of the toxin, even by local secretory antitoxin, may prove difficult.

Antibody directed against bacterial surface antigens may enhance phagocytosis by combining with surface or capsular antigens, inhibit attachment of bacterial to cell surfaces by combining with bacterial surface structures such as pili (fimbriae), inhibit bacterial motility by combining with flagellar antigens, or promote complement-mediated bacteriolysis. Precipitation of bacterial macromolecules and agglutination of whole bacterial cells probably do not increase resistance in vivo, even though serum from a resistant host may readily exhibit these reactions in vitro. The relative roles in vivo of opsonin-mediated phagocytic killing and opsonin-mediated but complement-dependent bacteriolysis are difficult to discern. A recent important study has shown, however, that inherited deficiency in the properdin component of the alternative complement pathway was associated with a predisposition to the development of meningococcal disease. Therefore, although the development of specific IgM and IgG is clearly an essential part of specific acquired immunity to meningococci, the complement system is also important as a cooperating, nonspecific mediator of host resistance to infection with neisseriae and other bacteria (see Ch. 1).

In infections with organisms that possess polysaccharide capsules, such as *Neisseria meningitidis, Streptococcus pneumoniae,* and *Haemophilus influenzae,* specific acquired resistance is attributed mainly to anticapsular antibodies, which alter the bacterial surface and thereby render the microbe more susceptible to phagocytosis and intracellular killing by granulocytes. This process is called **opsonization,** and the antibodies are called **opsonins.** Figure 8-1 shows the reciprocal relationship between the incidence of meningococcal infection and the titer of antibody specific for capsular polysaccharide in the general population. A vaccine composed of type-specific capsular polysaccharide is highly effective in preventing disease caused by meningococci of the same capsular type. Very recent field trials of a capsular polysaccharide vaccine against typhoid fever indicate that even in a predominantly intracellular infection, opsonins against a surface antigen may afford more protection than expected (see below).

Secretory IgA antibody directed against surface structures may inhibit adherence of bacteria to mucosal surfaces and prevent colonization, which is a necessary step in the pathogenesis of several bacterial infections. For example, antibodies against pili appear to confer resistance against infections with enterotoxigenic strains of *Escherichia coli* that cause diarrhea. Also, secretory IgA may function in resistance against gonococcal infections of the genitourinary tract mucosa.

Antibody-mediated immunity is judged to be important in resistance only if passive transfer of serum from an immune animal specifically protects a nonimmune animal against live bacterial challenge. Studies of passive transfer usually are done in animals. A few studies in human volunteers have assessed the value of passive immunoprophylaxis against naturally occurring disease. For certain viral infections (e.g., poliomyelitis and hepatitis A), controlled human studies have shown

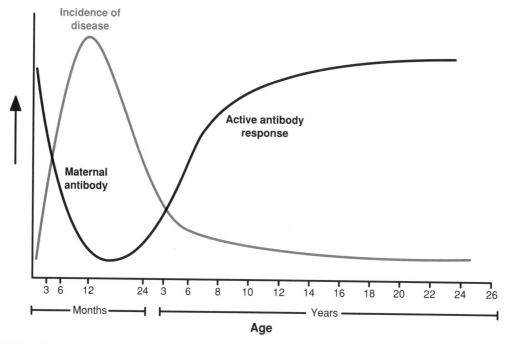

FIGURE 8-1   Relationship between age-specific incidence of meningococcal disease in the United States and prevalence of serum bactericidal activity against a pathogenic strain of *N meningitidis*. The antibody curve depicts the percentage of sera with an anti-meningococcal bactericidal titer of 1:4 or greater. (Modified from Goldschneider I, Gotschlich EC, Artenstein MS: Humoral immunity to the meningococcus. I. The role of humoral antibodies. J Exp Med 129:1307, 1969, with permission.)

that injection of serum containing specific antibody does indeed afford protection, but similar human studies have not been done for bacterial infections. The successful use of tetanus antitoxin as a routine immunoprophylactic measure for patients with wounds strongly suggests that antitoxin alone is sufficient to prevent tetanus in humans; for ethical reasons, adequately controlled studies have not been performed.

CELL-MEDIATED RESISTANCE MECHANISMS

In some bacterial infections, particularly those characterized by intracellular survival and multiplication of the microbe in mononuclear phagocytes, cell-mediated immunity may be the major factor in resistance. As noted above, this immunity involves stimulation and expansion of specific clones of T cells following initial exposure to spe-

cific microbial antigens for which they possess preexisting receptors. Sensitized T lymphocytes respond to a second exposure of the original antigens by producing lymphokines. One of these lymphokines, **macrophage-activating factor (MAF),** increases the capacity of macrophages to destroy ingested bacteria. This enhanced capacity for intraphagocytic killing is independent of antibody and is probably the major mechanism of acquired specific resistance in infections with pathogens such as brucellae, tubercle bacilli, listeriae, *Francisella tularensis*, and *Legionella pneumophila*. These intracellular bacteria, as well as certain bacterial components such as endotoxin (lipopolysaccharide), can also induce T cells to produce interferons (immune or gamma interferon), which can nonspecifically enhance intracellular killing of bacteria, protozoa, and viruses by macrophages.

The cell in the term "cell-mediated immunity" refers to the immunologically committed T lymphocyte and not to the macrophage, which is the ultimate executor in the cell-mediated immune response. In cell-mediated immunity, although the lymphocyte response is antigen specific, the increase in bactericidal activity of macrophages is nonspecific, since it is effective against a variety of unrelated organisms. Cell-mediated resistance declines after recovery from infection, but it can be recalled by reexposure of the residual population of immunologically committed lymphocytes to the antigens of the originally infecting microbe. Cell-mediated immunity of this type may be conferred on normal animals by the transfer of lymphocytes from actively immunized animals. Bactericidal activity of the macrophages of the recipient increases following exposure to the specific antigen.

Infections that elicit cell-mediated immunity usually also elicit a state of delayed hypersensitivity, which can be demonstrated by either intracutaneous injection or topical application of antigen. Delayed hypersensitivity is manifested as an area of erythema (redness) and induration (firm swelling) in the skin; this is caused by edema accompanied by a localized infiltration of mononuclear cells at the site of antigen deposition. Reactions of delayed hypersensitivity reach a peak 24 to 48 hours after the sensitized host is exposed to antigen. A positive tuberculin test (Mantoux test) is an example of this kind of response. Like cell-mediated immunity, delayed hypersensitivity can be transferred by lymphocytes. Delayed hypersensitivity is mediated by **migration inhibition factor (MIF),** a lymphokine that is produced with other lymphokines, such as macrophage-activating factor, when microbial antigens interact with immunologically committed lymphocytes. By inhibiting macrophage migration, migration inhibition factor promotes accumulation of macrophages in areas of higher antigen concentration. This series of events is the basis for skin reactions of delayed hypersensitivity, as in the positive tuberculin test. The precise relationship between delayed hypersensitivity and enhanced cellular immunity is not known. Both phenomena are mediated by immunologically committed T lymphocytes, but they do not always increase and decrease together.

In many infections, delayed hypersensitivity is associated with tissue destruction. Intense accumulations of mononuclear cells at sites of high antigen concentration in tissues may lead to a marked disturbance of function and even to tissue death. The classic example of the harmful effect of delayed hypersensitivity is seen in tuberculosis. Sensitivity to the antigens of *Mycobacterium tuberculosis* may be followed by caseation necrosis (death of host tissue that produces a homogeneous mass of cheeselike consistency and appearance). Therefore, although cell-mediated immunity and delayed hypersensitivity are associated with increased resistance to exogenous challenge with living bacteria, they are also associated with tissue destruction during the natural course of disease.

ACQUIRED RESISTANCE TO INFECTIOUS DISEASE

In different bacterial diseases, humoral and cell-mediated immune responses contribute in different proportions to specific acquired resistance. Antibody is usually decisive in controlling infections in which the bacteria remain chiefly extracellular and those in which exotoxins are major pathogenic factors. Cell-mediated immunity appears to be more important in infections in which organisms multiply chiefly in macrophages and therefore remain inaccessible to antibody. In these infections, resistance ultimately depends on heightened intraphagocytic killing, which results from the interaction of specific antigen with immunologically committed lymphocytes and is independent of antibody.

Figure 8-2 illustrates the synergistic activity of humoral and cell-mediated immunity. Antibody-coated *Salmonella typhimurium* undergoes moderate intracellular killing when engulfed by normal macrophages. In comparison, when *S typhimurium* is phagocytosed by macrophages activated by the product [macrophage-activating factor] of the interaction between *S typhimurium* antigen and immunologically committed T lymphocytes, intracellular killing is accelerated and enhanced.

In most infections, more than one mechanism of acquired immunity develops during the course of disease. The synergistic effect of this mosaic of mechanisms constitutes the specific acquired resistance displayed by the host when rechallenged

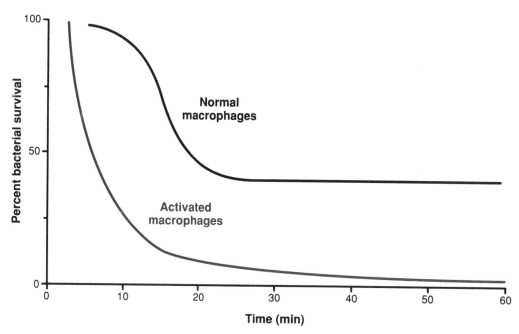

FIGURE 8-2 In vitro experiment with opsonized *Salmonella typhimurium* showing that activated macrophages exhibit a faster onset of killing and greater bactericidal capability than do normal macrophages. (Modified from Mackaness GB: Cell-mediated immunity to infection. Hosp Pract 5:73, 1970, with permission.)

with a given microbe. The relative influence of each mechanism involved probably varies from individual to individual, depending upon the host's unique immune response to the microbial antigens. Therefore, although the above generalizations usually are valid, it must be emphasized that each kind of infection in each host species, and even in each individual of a species, must be evaluated separately.

ARTIFICIAL IMMUNIZATION

Having observed the natural acquisition of resistance after recovery from smallpox, the ancient Chinese became the first to attempt artificial immunization by inoculation of scab material from patients with mild smallpox (variolation). The danger of inducing severe disease was recognized, and the price paid was often high. Many centuries later, Edward Jenner's recognition that inoculation (vaccination) with material taken from lesions of cowpox, a mild disease related to smallpox,

could protect humans against smallpox led to artificial immunization with attenuated or killed microbial vaccines.

Jenner's vaccine is the most successful artificial immunizing agent to be developed to date. As a result of a concerted worldwide vaccination campaign, the last reported case of smallpox occurred in 1978, and the World Health Organization has declared the disease eradicated. Whether the smallpox virus has indeed disappeared as a natural human parasite remains to be seen, but the achievement is unique. Eradication of smallpox by vaccination was possible because the disease was limited to humans, only one antigenic type of virus existed, and persistent infection following recovery did not occur.

The term **vaccine** (derived from "vaccinia," the Latin name for cowpox) originally referred only to smallpox vaccine. Today, however, the term vaccine can be properly applied to any **active immunizing agent,** including those composed of whole bacteria or viruses, living or killed, as well as bacterial components or products or their detoxified toxins (toxoids).

In a few bacterial and viral infections, **passive immunization** is attempted by injecting antibody-containing serum or purified immunoglobulins from animals or human volunteers who have previously been actively immunized. Such passive immunizing agents are called antisera or antitoxins.

Table 8-1 lists the major immunizing agents in current use against human bacterial infections. Antisera may be used as immunoprophylactic agents if they are given before exposure to prevent disease or as immunotherapeutic agents if used in the treatment of disease. The active immunizing agents (vaccines) are, of course, always used as prophylactic agents.

Although no bacterial diseases are likely to be eradicated by vaccination in the near future, a few of the vaccines listed in Table 8-1 have contributed significantly to the reduction in morbidity and mortality from these diseases. Bacterial infections will be difficult to eradicate by vaccination because many bacteria (1) persist in animal reservoirs or in the environment, (2) can colonize the immunized human host and are a source of infection for others, and (3) have multiple antigenic types. It has been difficult to develop bacterial vaccines because some organisms cannot be cultivated in vitro (e.g., *Treponema pallidum,* the agent of syphilis) or, when grown in vitro, may not produce the appropriate antigenic components that evoke protective immunity (e.g., *Bordetella pertussis,* the agent of whooping cough). Moreover, in many bacterial infections it is not clear which antigens are responsible for the resistance that follows recovery from natural disease and which route of administration would be most successful in stimulating this resistance.

Infections in which bacteria multiply exclusively on mucosal surfaces of the respiratory, intestinal, or genitourinary tract pose a particularly difficult problem in vaccine development. In such infections, adherence to the host cell luminal membrane is essential to pathogenesis. Adherent organisms can deliver toxic products to cell surface receptor molecules more efficiently and thus can make microbial antigens more available to the initiators of the secretory immune system than can organisms free in the lumen. Adherence may be mediated by specialized pili, as in enterotoxigenic *E coli* and gonococci, or by less clearly defined mechanisms. Also, adherence may involve multiple mechanisms acting in sequence or in concert (e.g., multiple *E coli* pilus types with different binding specificities on a single organism).

Secretory IgA directed against adherence factors protects the host by preventing the chain of events initiated by adhesion. Because attachment is the first step in invasion of mucosal cells, secretory IgA that inhibits attachment can be the major anti-invasive immune mechanism in infection in which pathogenesis is associated mainly with intracytoplasmic multiplication, such as shigellosis and diarrhea caused by enteroinvasive *E coli.*

Circulating IgA, IgG, and IgM are of little value in protecting against infections of mucosal surfaces. As an example, cholera toxoid, which evokes impressive levels of circulating IgG antitoxin, did not protect against cholera in controlled field trials. The available evidence now suggests that secretory IgA directed against adherence factors or toxins, and present in the appropriate mucosal secretions, is probably necessary to provide specific acquired resistance against these surface pathogens. This kind of immunoglobulin probably can be raised to protective levels only by exposing the appropriate mucosal surface to the relevant antigen *in the proper molecular form.* Therefore, antigen forms that may be capable of evoking protecting antibody when introduced to macrophages in the tissues (as by injection) may not be recognized by the M (membrane) cells of the Peyer's patches of the ileum when the same antigen is applied to the mucosa. Homing of secretory IgA-producing cells to the site of antigen exposure has also been shown to occur. These findings emphasize the importance of selecting the proper antigen form and site of delivery in the development of vaccines against surface infections.

Systemic infections, in which the microbe or its toxins must pass through tissues containing antibodies or sensitized lymphocytes to reach their sites of multiplication or toxic activity, do not

TABLE 8-1 Major Immunizing Agents Used Against Bacterial Infections of Humans

General Category	Disease	Agent	Comments
Passive immunization (antisera)	Diphtheria	Antitoxin (usually horse serum)	Used chiefly in treatment of diphtheria, effectiveness uncertain
	Tetanus	Antitoxin (horse serum or human tetanus immune globulin)	Used both for immunoprophylaxis (effective) and for treatment of tetanus (effectiveness uncertain)
	Botulism	Polyvalent antitoxin against several serotypes of Clostridium botulinum toxin	Used chiefly for treatment of botulism; probably effective if given early
Active immunization (vaccines)	Diphtheria	Toxoid (formalin-detoxified toxin of Coryne bacterium diphtheriae)	Widely used, effective, long-lasting
	Tetanus	Toxoid (formalin-detoxified toxin of Clostridium tetani)	Widely used, effective, long-lasting
	Pertussis	Killed Bordetella pertussis whole-cell vaccine	Widely used in children under 6 years of age; effective
	Typhoid fever	Killed Salmonella typhi whole-cell vaccine	Moderately effective against low challenge doses
		Living attenuated oral vaccine (galactose epimerase-deficient mutant of S typhi)	Moderately effective against low challenge doses
	Cholera	Killed Vibrio cholerae whole-cell vaccine	Moderate, short-lived effectiveness
	Plague	Killed Yersinia pestis whole-cell vaccine	Moderate, short-lived effectiveness
	Tuberculosis	Living attenuated strain of Mycobacterium bovis (BCG)	Moderate, long-lasting effectiveness but used only in high-risk groups
	Pneumococcal pneumonia	Polyvalent capsular polysaccharide vaccine prepared from 23 serotypes of Streptococcus pneumoniae	Effective in high-risk groups
	Meningococcal infections	Types A and C capsular polysaccharides from Neisseria meningitidis	Effective in high-risk groups
	Typhus fever	Killed Rickettsia prowazekii whole-cell vaccine	Moderately effective
	Rocky Mountain spotted fever	Killed Rickettsia rickettsii whole-cell vaccine	Moderately effective; used only for special high-risk groups

present the same obstacles to vaccine development.

Typhoid fever provides a good example of an infection in which it is still not clear which of the organism's multiple antigens plays the most important protective role in nature, or which immune mechanism (hormonal or cellular) is most important in affording protection.

A parenterally injected, killed, whole-cell typhoid vaccine has been given to millions of subjects over the past century, with variable success. Most well-controlled field trials showed that 50 to 75 percent protection could be achieved. However, because whole organisms containing numerous antigens were used, it has never been clear which components were evoking protection. Because the disease is associated with massive intracellular multiplication of bacteria within the mononuclear phagocytes of the reticuloendothelial system, it has been thought most likely that cell-mediated immunity played the major role in protection.

A mutant strain of *Salmonella typhi,* deficient in the enzyme galactose epimerase, was recently introduced as a living, oral vaccine against typhoid fever. This strain probably undergoes one or two divisions in the recipient's intestine, but the exact site of this limited multiplication and the other prerequisites for conferring immunity are not known. Nevertheless, this vaccine has also afforded moderate to high protection against typhoid fever in controlled field trials. It evokes both cell-mediated immunity and specific antibodies that could serve as opsonins. Again, the relative contributions of these two mechanisms to the acquisition of resistance are not yet clear, but animal studies suggest that both are necessary to achieve maximal protection.

Even more recently, however, a parenteral typhoid vaccine composed of one of the purified capsular polysaccharides of *S typhi,* known as the Vi antigen (from "virulence"), has proven to be as protective as either of the two previous vaccines. Experience with other bacterial capsular polysaccharides (e.g., pneumococcal and meningococcal polysaccharides) indicates that these antigens evoke predominantly a serum IgM response, with

very little or no cell-mediated immunity. Therefore, the observation that a predominantly intracellular infection such as typhoid fever can be prevented by evoking humoral immunity against the Vi antigen is very important. First, it shows that cell-mediated immunity is not always the major protective mechanism in infections in which the organism multiplies chiefly in cells of the reticuloendothelial system (cf. tuberculosis). It also suggests that when bacteremia is a major mechanism of spread throughout the tissues of the host, opsonins, which enhance phagocytic and/or bacteriolytic killing, may be the major mediators of specific acquired immunity. This may be true even though a major pathogenic mechanism may be the development and overexpression of cell-mediated immunity. Future studies with these three kinds of typhoid fever vaccines may help us differentiate more clearly between antigens that evoke protective immune mechanisms and those that evoke primarily destructive mechanisms.

Smallpox vaccine was developed before the biologic mechanisms of specific immunity were known. This emphasizes the fact that the methods needed for measuring resistance are completely independent of an understanding of the mechanism by which that resistance is acquired and expressed. However, a better understanding of these immune mechanisms will greatly improve our chances of developing vaccines that can provide protection more nearly approaching that conferred in natural disease.

REFERENCES

Collins FM: Vaccines and cell-mediated immunity. Bacteriol Rev 38:371, 1974

Goldschneider I, Gotschlich EC, Artenstein MS: Human immunity to the meningococcus. I. The role of humoral antibodies. J Exp Med 129:1307, 1969

Klugman KP, Koornhof HJ, Schneerson R et al: Protective activity of Vi capsular polysaccharide vaccine against typhoid fever. Lancet 2:1165, 1987

Lurie MB: Resistance to Tuberculosis. Harvard University Press, Boston, 1964

McNabb PC, Tomasi TB: Host defense mechanisms at mucosal surfaces. Annu Rev Microbiol 35:477, 1983

Robbins JB, Schneerson R: Polysaccharide-protein conjugates: a new generation of vaccines. J Infect Dis 161:821, 1990

Sjoholm AG, Kuijper EJ, Tijssen CC et al: Dysfunctional properdin in a Dutch family with meningococcal disease. N Engl J Med 319:48, 1988

Wahdan MH, Sérié C, Cerisier Y et al: A controlled field trial of live *Salmonella typhi* strain Ty21a oral vaccine against typhoid: three year results. J Infect Dis 145:292, 1982

Wilson GS, Miles AA, Parker MT (ed): Topley and Wilson's Principles of Bacteriology, Virology and Immunity. Vol 1. 7th Ed. Williams & Wilkins, Baltimore, 1983

9

EPIDEMIOLOGY

PHILIP S. BRACHMAN

GENERAL CONCEPTS

Definitions

Epidemiology is the study of the determinants, occurrence, and distribution of health and disease in a defined population. *Infection* is the replication of organisms in host tissue, which may cause disease. A **carrier** is an individual with no overt disease who harbors infectious organisms. **Dissemination** is the spread of the organism in the environment.

Chain of Infection

There are three major links in disease occurrence: the etiologic agent, the method of transmission (by contact, by a common vehicle, or via air or a vector), and the host.

Epidemiologic Methods

Epidemiologic studies may be (1) descriptive, organizing data by time, place, and person; (2) analytic, incorporating a case-control or cohort study; or (3) experimental. Epidemiology utilizes an organized approach to problem solving by: (1) confirming the existence of an epidemic and verifying the diagnosis; (2) developing a case definition and collating data on cases; (3) analyzing data by time, place, and person; (4) developing a hypothesis; (5) conducting further studies if necessary; (6) developing and implementing control and prevention measures; (7) preparing and distributing a public report; and (8) evaluating control and preventive measures.

INTRODUCTION

This chapter reviews the general concepts of epidemiology, which is the study of the determinants, occurrence, distribution, and control of health and disease in a defined population. Epidemiology is a descriptive science and includes the determination of rates, that is, the quantification of disease occurrence within a specific population. The most commonly studied rate is the **attack rate:** the number of cases of the disease divided by the population among whom the cases have occurred. Epidemiology can accurately describe a disease and many factors concerning its occurrence before its cause is identified. For example, Snow described many aspects of the epidemiology of cholera in the late 1840s, fully 30 years before Koch described the bacillus and Semmelweis described puerperal fever in detail in 1861 and recommended appropriate control and prevention measures a number of years before the streptococcal agent was fully described. One goal of epidemiologic studies is to define the parameters of a disease, including risk factors, in order to develop the most effective measures for control. This chapter includes a discussion of the chain of infection, the three main epidemiologic methods, and how to investigate an epidemic (Table 9-1).

Proper interpretation of disease-specific epidemiologic data requires information concerning past as well as present occurrence of the disease. An increase in the number of reported cases of a disease that is normal and expected, representing a seasonal pattern of change in host susceptibility, does not constitute an epidemic. Therefore, the regular collection, collation, analysis, and reporting of data concerning the occurrence of a disease is important to properly interpret short-term changes in occurrence.

A sensitive and specific surveillance program is important for the proper interpretation of disease occurrence data. Almost every country has a national disease surveillance program that regularly collects data on selected diseases. The quality of these programs varies, but, generally, useful data are collected that are important in developing control and prevention measures. There is an international agreement that the occurrence of four diseases—cholera, plague, smallpox (now eradicated), and yellow fever—will be reported to the World Health Organization in Geneva, Switzerland. In the United States, the Centers for Disease Control (CDC), the U.S. Public Health Service,

and the state health officers of all 50 states have agreed to report the occurrence of 44 diseases weekly and of another 10 diseases annually from the states to the CDC. Many states have regulations or laws that mandate reporting of these diseases and often also of other diseases of specific interest to the state health department.

The methods of case reporting vary within each state. **Passive reporting** is one of the main methods. In such a case, physicians or personnel in clinics or hospitals report occurrences of relevant diseases by telephone, postcard, or reporting form, usually at weekly intervals. In some instances, the report may be initiated by the public health or clinical laboratory where the etiologic agent is identified. Some diseases, such as human rabies, must be reported by telephone as soon as diagnosed. In an **active surveillance program,** the health authority regularly initiates the request for reporting. The local health department may call all or some health care providers at regular intervals to inquire about the occurrence of a disease or diseases. The active system may be used during an epidemic or if accurate data concerning all cases of a disease are desired.

The health care provider usually makes the initial passive report to a local authority, such as a city or county health department. This unit collates its data and sends a report to the next highest health department level, usually the state health department.

The number of cases of each reportable disease are presented weekly, via computer linkage, by the state health department to the CDC. Data are analyzed at each level to develop needed information to assist public health authorities in disease control and prevention. For some diseases, such as hepatitis, the CDC requests preparation of a separate case reporting form containing more specific details.

In addition, the CDC prepares and distributes routine reports summarizing and interpreting the analyses and providing information on epidemics and other appropriate public health matters. Most states and some county health departments also prepare and distribute their own surveillance re-

TABLE 9-1 Epidemiologic Methods and Investigation

Descriptive	Analytic	Experimental
Time	Case-control	Manipulate
Secular	Cohort	cause and
Periodic		note effect.
Seasonal		
Epidemic		
Place		
Person		

ports. The CDC publishes *Morbidity and Mortality Weekly Report*, which is available for a small fee from the Massachusetts Medical Society. The CDC also prepares more detailed surveillance reports for specific diseases, as well as an annual summary report, all of which can also be obtained through the Massachusetts Medical Society.

Infection is the replication of organisms in the tissue of a host; when defined in terms of infection, **disease** is overt clinical manifestation. In an inapparent (subclinical) infection, an immune response can occur without overt clinical disease. A **carrier** (colonized individual) is a person in whom organisms are present and may be multiplying, but who shows no clinical response to their presence. The carrier state may be permanent, with the organism always present; intermittent, with the organism present for various periods; or temporary, with carriage for only a brief period. **Dissemination** is the movement of an infectious agent from a source individual directly into the environment; when infection results from dissemination, the source individual is referred to as a **dangerous disseminator.**

Infectiousness is the transmission of organisms from a source, or **reservoir** (see below), to a susceptible individual. A human may be infective during the preclinical, clinical, postclinical, or recovery phase of an illness. The **incubation period** is the interval in the preclinical period between the time at which the causative agent first infects the host and the onset of clinical symptoms; during this time the agent is replicating. Transmission is most likely during the incubation period for some diseases such as measles; in other diseases such as shigellosis, transmission occurs during the clinical period. The individual may be infective during the convalescent phase or may become an asymptomatic carrier and remain infective for a prolonged period, as do approximately 5% of persons with typhoid fever.

The spectrum of occurrence of disease in a defined population includes **sporadic** (occasional occurrence); **endemic** (regular, continuing occurrence); **epidemic** (significantly increased occurrence); and **pandemic** (epidemic occurrence in multiple countries).

CHAIN OF INFECTION

The **chain of infection** includes the three factors that lead to infection: the etiologic agent, the method of transmission, and the host (Fig. 9-1). These links should be characterized before control and prevention measures are proposed. Environmental factors that may influence disease occurrence also must be evaluated.

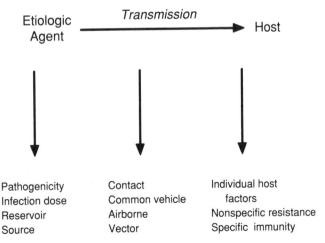

FIGURE 9-1 Summary of important aspects involved in the chain of any infection.

Etiologic Agent

The **etiologic agent** may be any microorganism that can cause infection. The pathogenicity of an agent is its ability to cause disease; pathogenicity is further characterized by describing the organism's virulence and invasiveness of the organism. **Virulence** refers to the severity of infection, which can be expressed by describing the morbidity (incidence of disease) and mortality (death rate) of the infection. An example of a highly virulent organism is *Yersinia pestis,* the agent of plague, which almost always causes severe disease in the susceptible host.

The **invasiveness** of an organism refers to its ability to invade tissue. *Vibrio cholerae* organisms are noninvasive, causing symptoms by releasing into the intestinal canal an exotoxin that acts on the tissues. In contrast, *Shigella* organisms in the intestinal canal are invasive and migrate into the tissue.

No microorganism is assuredly avirulent. An organism may have very low virulence, but if the host is highly susceptible, as when therapeutically immunosuppressed, infection with that organism may cause disease. For example, the poliomyelitis virus used in oral polio vaccine is highly attenuated and thus has low virulence, but in some highly susceptible individuals it may cause paralytic disease.

Other factors should be considered in describing the agent. The **infecting dose** (the number of organisms necessary to cause disease) varies according to the organism, method of transmission, site of entrance of the organism into the host, host defenses, and host species. Another agent factor is **specificity;** some agents (for example, *Salmonella typhimurium*) can infect a broad range of hosts; others have a narrow range of hosts. *S typhi,* for example, infects only humans. Other agent factors include antigenic composition, which can vary within a species (as in influenza virus or *Streptococcus* species); antibiotic sensitivity; resistance transfer plasmids (see Ch. 5); and enzyme production.

The **reservoir** of an organism is the site where it resides, metabolizes, and multiplies. The **source** of the organism is the site from which it is transmitted to a susceptible host, either directly or indirectly through an intermediary object. The reservoir and source can be different; for example, the reservoir for *S typhi* could be the gallbladder of an infected individual, but the source for transmission might be food contaminated by the carrier. The reservoir and source can also be the same, as in an individual who is a permanent nasal carrier of *S aureus* and who disseminates organisms from this site. The distinction can be important when considering where to apply control measures.

Method of Transmission

The method of transmission is the means by which the agent goes from the source to the host. The four major methods of transmission are by contact, by common vehicle, by air or via a vector.

In **contact transmission** the agent is spread directly, indirectly, or by airborne droplets. Direct contact transmission takes place when organisms are transmitted directly from the source to the susceptible host without involving an intermediate object; this is also referred to as person-to-person transmission. An example is the transmission of hepatitis A virus from one individual to another by hand contact. Indirect transmission occurs when the organisms are transmitted from a source, either animate or inanimate, to a host by means of an inanimate object. An example is transmission of *Pseudomonas* organisms from one individual to another by means of a shaving brush. Droplet spread refers to organisms that travel through the air very short distances, that is, less than 3 feet from a source to a host. Therefore, the organisms are not airborne in the true sense. An example of a disease that may be spread by droplets is measles.

Common-vehicle transmission refers to agents transmitted by a common inanimate vehicle, with multiple cases resulting from such exposure. This category includes diseases in which food or water as well as drugs and parenteral fluids are the vehicles of infection. Examples include food-borne salmonellosis, waterborne shigellosis, and bacteremia resulting from use of intravenous fluids contaminated with a Gram-negative organism.

The third method of transmission, **airborne transmission,** refers to infection spread by droplet nuclei or dust. To be truly airborne, the particles should travel more than 3 feet through the air from the source to the host. Droplet nuclei are the residue from the evaporation of fluid from droplets, are light enough to be transmitted more than 3 feet from the source, and may remain airborne for prolonged periods. Tuberculosis is primarily an airborne disease; the source may be a coughing patient who creates aerosols of droplet nuclei that contain tubercle bacilli. Infectious agents may be contained in dust particles, which may become resuspended and transmitted to hosts. An example occurred in an outbreak of salmonellosis in a newborn nursery in which *Salmonella*-contaminated dust in a vacuum cleaner bag was resuspended when the equipment was used repeatedly, resulting in infections among the newborns.

The fourth method of transmission is **vector borne** transmission, in which arthropods are the vectors. Vector transmission may be external or internal. External, or mechanical, transmission occurs when organisms are carried mechanically on the vector (for example, *Salmonella* organisms that contaminate the legs of flies). Internal transmission occurs when the organisms are carried within the vector. If the pathogen is not changed by its carriage within the vector, the carriage is called **harborage** (as when a flea ingests plague bacilli from an infected individual or animal and contaminates a susceptible host when it feeds again; the organism is not changed while in the flea). The other form of internal transmission is called **biologic**. In this form, the organism is changed biologically during its passage through the vector (for example, malaria parasites in the mosquito vector).

An infectious agent may be transmitted by more than one route. For example, *Salmonella* may be transmitted by a common vehicle (food) or by contact spread (human carrier). *Francisella tularensis* may be transmitted by any of the four routes.

Host

The third link in the chain of infection is the host. The organism may enter the host through the skin, mucous membranes, lungs, gastrointestinal tract, or genitourinary tract, and it may enter fetuses through the placenta. The resulting disease often reflects the point of entrance, but not always: meningococci that enter the host through the mucous membranes may nonetheless cause meningitis. Development of disease in a host reflects agent characteristics (see above) and is influenced by host defense mechanisms, which may be nonspecific or specific.

Nonspecific defense mechanisms include the skin, mucous membranes, secretions, excretions, enzymes, the inflammatory response, genetic factors, hormones, nutrition, behavioral patterns, and the presence of other diseases. Specific defense mechanisms or immunity may be natural, resulting from exposure to the infectious agent, or artificial, resulting from active or passive immunization (see Ch. 8).

The environment can affect any link in the chain of infection. Temperature can assist or inhibit multiplication of organisms at their reservoir; air velocity can assist the airborne movement of droplet nuclei; low humidity can damage mucous membranes; and ultraviolet radiation can kill the microorganisms. In any investigation of disease, it is important to evaluate the effect of environmental factors. At times, environmental control measures are instituted more on emotional grounds than on the basis of epidemiologic fact. It should be apparent that the occurrence of disease results from the interaction of many factors (Table 9-2). Some of these factors are outlined here.

EPIDEMIOLOGIC METHODS

The three major epidemiologic techniques are **descriptive, analytic,** and **experimental.** Although all three can be used in investigating the occurrence of disease, the method used most is descriptive epidemiology. Once the basic epidemiology of a disease has been described, specific analytic methods can be used to study the disease further, and a specific experimental approach can be developed to test a hypothesis.

Descriptive Epidemiology

In descriptive epidemiology, data that describe the occurrence of the disease are collected by various methods from all relevant sources. The data are

TABLE 9-2   General Factors That Influence the Occurrence of Infectious Disease

Pathogenic Agent

    Growth characteristics
    Stability
    Ability to form spores
    Possession of antibiotic resistance plasmids
    Expression of antigens
    Enzyme production
    Pathogenicity—ability to induce disease
        Virulence—influencing disease severity, morbidity, and mortality
        Invasiveness
    Dose
    Reservoir
    Source
    Mode of dissemination
    Host specificity

Disease Transmission

    Contact
        Direct
        Indirect
        Droplets
    Common vehicle
        Food
        Water
        Medication
        Solution
    Airborne
        Droplet nuclei
        Dust
        Skin squames
    Vector-borne—arthropods
        External
        Internal—harborage, true biologic transmission

Host

    Incubation period
    Nonspecific defense mechanisms
        Age
        Sex
        Skin
        Secretions
        Cough
        Ciliary function
        Peristalsis
        Inflammation
        Nutrition
        Genetic factors
        Hormones
        Personal education
        Personal hygiene
        Behavior patterns
        Chronic disease
    Specific defense mechanisms (immunity)
        Natural
            Active—apparent, inapparent
            Passive—transplacental antibody
        Artificial
            Active—vaccine, toxoid
            Passive—immune serum globulin

Environment

    Temperature
    Rainfall
    Humidity
    Radiation
    Air currents

---

then collated by time, place, and person. Four time trends are considered in describing the epidemiologic data. The **secular trend** describes the occurrence of disease over a prolonged period, usually years; it is influenced by the degree of immunity in the population and possibly nonspecific measures such as improved socioeconomic and nutritional levels among the population. For example, the secular trend of tetanus in the United States since 1920 shows a gradual and steady decline.

The second time trend is the **periodic trend**. A temporary modification in the overall secular trend, the periodic trend usually indicates a change in the antigenic characteristics of the disease agent. For example, the change in antigenic structure of the prevalent influenza A virus every 2 to 3 years results in periodic increases in the occurrence of clinical influenza caused by lack of natural immunity among the population. Additionally, a lowering of the overall immunity of a population or a segment thereof (known as **herd immunity**) can result in an increase in the occurrence of the disease. This can be seen with some immunizable diseases when periodic decreases occur in the level of immunization in a defined population. This may then result in an increase in the number of cases, with a subsequent rise in the overall level of herd immunity.

The third time trend is the **seasonal trend.** This trend reflects seasonal changes in disease occurrence following changes in environmental conditions that enhance the ability of the agent to replicate or be transmitted. For example, food-borne disease outbreaks occur more frequently in the summer, when temperatures favor multiplication of bacteria. This trend becomes evident when the occurrence of salmonellosis is examined on a monthly basis (Fig. 9-2).

The fourth time trend is the **epidemic occurrence** of disease. An epidemic is a sudden increase in occurrence due to prevalent factors that support transmission.

A description of epidemiologic data by place must consider three different sites: where the individual was when disease occurred; where the individual was when he or she became infected from the vehicle; and where the vehicle became infected with the etiologic agent. Therefore, in an outbreak

of food poisoning, the host may become clinically ill at home from food eaten in a restaurant. The vehicle may have been undercooked chicken, which became infected on a poultry farm. These differences are important to consider in attempting to prevent additional cases.

The third focus of descriptive epidemiology is the infected person. All pertinent characteristics should be noted: age, sex, occupation, personal habits, socioeconomic status, immunization history, presence of underlying disease, and other data.

Once the descriptive epidemiologic data have been analyzed, the features of the epidemic should be clear enough that additional areas for investigation are apparent.

Analytic Epidemiology

The second epidemiologic method is analytic epidemiology, which analyzes disease determinants for possible causal relations. The two main analytic methods are the **case-control** (or **case-comparison) method** and the **cohort method.** The case-

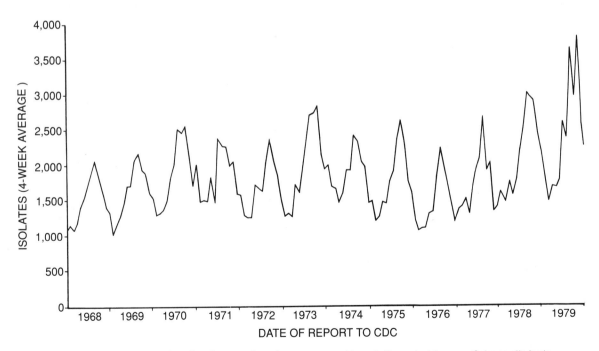

FIGURE 9-2   An example of a disease showing a seasonal trend. Reported human *Salmonella* isolations, by 4-week average, in the United States from 1968 to 1980.

control method starts with the effect (disease) and retrospectively investigates the cause that led to the effect. The case group consists of individuals with the disease; a comparison group has members similar to those of the case group except for absence of the disease. These two groups are then compared to determine differences that would explain the occurrence of the disease. An example of a case-control study is selecting individuals with meningococcal meningitis and a comparison group matched for age, sex, socioeconomic status, and residence, but without the disease, to see what factors may have influenced the occurrence in the group that developed disease.

The second analytic approach is the cohort method, which prospectively studies two populations: one that has had contact with the suspected causal factor under study and a similar group that has had no contact with the factor. When both groups are observed, the effect of the factor should become apparent. An example of a cohort approach is to observe two similar groups of people, one composed of individuals who received blood transfusions and the other of persons who did not. The occurrence of hepatitis prospectively in both groups permits one to make an association between blood transfusions and hepatitis; that is, if the transfused blood was contaminated with hepatitis B virus, the recipient cohort should have a higher incidence of hepatitis than the nontransfused cohort.

The case-control approach is relatively easy to conduct, can be completed in a shorter period than the cohort approach, and is inexpensive and reproducible; however, bias may be introduced in selecting the two groups, it may be difficult to exclude subclinical cases from the comparison group, and a patient's recall of past events may be faulty. The advantages of a cohort study are the accuracy of collected data and the ability to make a direct estimate of the disease risk resulting from factor contact; however, cohort studies take longer and are more expensive to conduct.

Another analytic method is the cross-sectional study, in which a population is surveyed over a limited period to determine the relationship between a disease and variables that may influence its occurrence.

Experimental Epidemiology

The third epidemiologic method is the experimental approach. A hypothesis is developed and an experimental model is constructed in which one or more selected factors are manipulated. The effect of the manipulation will either confirm or disprove the hypothesis. An example is the evaluation of the effect of a new drug on a disease. A group of people with the disease is identified, and some members are randomly selected to receive the drug. If the only difference between the two is use of the drug, the clinical differences between the groups should reflect the effectiveness of the drug.

EPIDEMIC INVESTIGATION

An **epidemic investigation** describes the factors relevant to an outbreak of disease; once the circumstances related to the occurrence of disease are defined, appropriate control and prevention measures can be identified. In an epidemic investigation, data are collected, collated according to time, place, and person, and analyzed and inferences are drawn.

In the investigation, the first action should be to confirm the existence of the epidemic by discussing the occurrence of the disease with physicians or others who have seen or reported cases after examining patients and reviewing laboratory and hospital records. These diagnoses should then be verified. A case definition should be developed to differentiate patients who represent actual cases, those who represent suspected or presumptive cases, and those who should be omitted from further study. Additional cases may be sought or additional patient data obtained, and a rough case count made.

This initial phase consists basically of collecting data, which then must be organized according to time, place, and person. The population at risk should be identified and a hypothesis developed concerning the occurrence of the disease. If appropriate, specimens should be collected and transported to the laboratory. More specific studies may be indicated. Additional data from these studies should be analyzed and the hypothesis confirmed or altered. After analysis, control and prevention measures should be developed and, as far as possible, implemented. A report containing this information should be prepared and distributed to those involved in investigating the outbreak and in implementing control and/or prevention measures. Continued surveillance activities may be appropriate to evaluate the effectiveness of the control and prevention measures.

In the United States, the CDC assists state health departments by providing epidemiologic and laboratory support services on request. Its assistance supports disease investigations and diagnostic laboratory activities and includes various training programs conducted in the states and at the CDC. A close working relationship exists between the CDC and state health departments. Additionally, physicians frequently consult with CDC personnel on a variety of health-related problems and attend public health training programs.

The use of epidemiology to characterize a disease before its etiology has been identified is exemplified by the initial studies of acquired immune deficiency syndrome (AIDS). The first cases came to the attention of the CDC when an increase was observed in requests for pentamidine for treatment of *Pneumocystis carinii* pneumonia. This initiated specific surveillance activities and epidemiologic studies that provided important information about this newly diagnosed disease.

Initial symptoms include fever, loss of appetite, weight loss, extreme fatigue, and enlargement of lymph nodes. A severe immune deficiency then develops, which appears to be associated with opportunistic infections. These infections include *P carinii* pneumonia, diagnosed in 52 percent of cases; Kaposi sarcoma in 26 percent of cases; and both *P carinii* pneumonia and Kaposi sarcoma in 7 percent of cases. The remaining 15 percent of AIDS patients have other parasitic, fungal, bacterial, or viral infections associated with immunodeficiencies. Among the first 2,640 cases reported to the CDC, there were 1,092 deaths, a case-fatality rate of 41 percent. Approximately 95 percent of the cases were male; 70 percent were 20 to 49 years of age at the time of diagnosis. Approximately 40 percent of the cases were reported from New York City, 12 percent from San Francisco, 8 percent from Los Angeles, and the remainder from 32 other states. Cases were reported from at least 16 other countries. Among the 90 percent of patients who were categorized according to possible risk factors, those at highest risk were homosexuals or bisexuals (70 percent), intravenous drug abusers (17 percent), Haitian entrants into the United States (9.5 percent), and persons with hemophilia (1 percent).

Analysis of these initial data, collected before the etiologic agent of AIDS was identified, supported the hypothesis that transmission occurred primarily by sexual contact, receipt of contaminated blood or blood products, or contact with contaminated intravenous needles. Spread through casual contact did not seem likely. The epidemiologic data indicated that AIDS was an infectious disease. It has now been determined that AIDS results from infection with a retrovirus of the human T cell leukemia/lymphoma virus family, which has been designated human immunodeficiency virus type 1 (HIV-1).

REFERENCES

Benenson A: Control of Communicable Disease in Man. 15th Ed., American Public Health Association, Washington, DC, 1990

Bennett JV, Brachman PS: Hospital Infections. 2nd Ed., Little, Brown, Boston, 1986

Evans AS, Brachman PS: Bacteriol Infections of Humans. Epidemiology and Control. 2nd Ed. Plenum New York, 1991

Fox JP, Hall CE, Elveback LR: Epidemiology, Man and Disease. Macmillan, New York, 1970

Hennekens CH, Buring JE: Epidemiology in Medicine. Little, Brown, Boston, 1987

Langmuir AD: The surveillance of communicable diseases of national importance. N Engl J Med 268:182, 1963

Lilienfeld AM: Foundations of Epidemiology. Oxford University Press, New York, 1980

MacMahon B, Pugh TF: Epidemiology Principles and Methods. Little, Brown, Boston, 1970

Mandell GL, Douglas RG, Jr, Bennett JE: Principles and Practice of Infectious Diseases. 3rd Ed. Churchill Livingstone, New York, 1990

Smith DM, Haupt BJ: Hospital discharge data used as feedback in planning research and education for primary care. Public Health Rep 98:457, 1983

World Health Organization: The surveillance of communicable diseases. WHO Chron 22:439, 1968

10 PRINCIPLES OF DIAGNOSIS

JOHN A. WASHINGTON

GENERAL CONCEPTS

Manifestations of Infection

The clinical presentation of an infectious disease reflects the interaction between the host and the microorganism. This interaction is affected by the host immune status and microbial virulence factors. Signs and symptoms vary according to the site and severity of infection. Diagnosis requires a composite of information, including history, physical examination, radiographic findings, and laboratory data.

Microbial Causes of Infection

Infections may be caused by bacteria, viruses, fungi, and parasites. The pathogen may be **exogenous** (acquired from environmental or animal sources or from other persons) or **endogenous** (from the normal flora).

Specimen Selection, Collection, and Processing

Specimens are selected on the basis of signs and symptoms, should be representative of the disease process, and should be collected before administration of antimicrobial agents. The specimen size and the rapidity of transport to the laboratory influence the test results.

Microbiologic Examination

Direct Examination and Techniques: **Direct examination** of specimens reveals gross pathology. **Microscopy** may identify microorganisms. Immunofluorescence, immunoperoxidase staining, and other **immunoassays** may detect specific microbial antigens. **Genetic probes** identify genus- or species-specific DNA or RNA sequences.

Culture: Isolation of infectious agents frequently requires specialized media. **Nonselective** (noninhibitory) **media** permit the growth of many microorganisms. **Selective media** contain inhibitory substances that permit the isolation of specific types of microorganisms.

Microbial Identification: Colony and cellular morphology may permit preliminary identification. Growth characteristics under various conditions, utilization of carbohydrates and other substrates, enzymatic activity, immunoassays, and genetic probes are also used.

Serodiagnosis: A high or rising titer of antibody may suggest or confirm a diagnosis.

Antimicrobial Susceptibility: Microorganisms, particularly bacteria, are tested in vitro to determine whether they are susceptible to antimicrobial agents.

INTRODUCTION

Some infectious diseases are distinctive enough to be identified clinically. Most pathogens, however, can cause a wide spectrum of clinical syndromes in humans. Conversely, a single clinical syndrome may result from infection with any one of many pathogens. Influenza virus infection, for example, causes a wide variety of respiratory syndromes that cannot be distinguished clinically from those caused by streptococci, mycoplasmas, or more than 100 other viruses.

Most often, therefore, it is necessary to use microbiologic laboratory methods to identify a specific etiologic agent. **Diagnostic medical microbiology** is the discipline that identifies etiologic agents of disease. The job of the clinical microbiology laboratory is to test specimens from patients for microorganisms that are, or may be, a cause of the illness and to provide information (when appropriate) about the in vitro activity of antimicrobial drugs against the microorganisms identified (Fig. 10-1).

The staff of a clinical microbiology laboratory should be qualified to advise the physician as well as process specimens. The physician should supply salient information on the patient, such as age and sex, tentative diagnosis or details of the clinical syndrome, date of onset, possibly significant exposures, prior antibiotic therapy, immunologic status, and underlying conditions. The clinical microbiologist participates in decisions regarding the microbiologic diagnostic studies to be performed, the type and timing of specimens to be collected, and the conditions for their transportation and storage. Above all, the clinical microbiology laboratory, whenever appropriate, should provide an interpretation of laboratory results.

MANIFESTATIONS OF INFECTION

The manifestations of an infection depend on many factors, including the site of acquisition or entry of the microorganism; organ or system tro-

pisms of the microorganism; microbial virulence; the age, sex, and immunologic status of the patient; underlying diseases or conditions; and the presence of implanted prosthetic devices or materials. The signs and symptoms of infection may be localized, or they may be systemic, with fever, chills, and hypotension. In some instances the manifestations of an infection are sufficiently characteristic to suggest the diagnosis; however, they are often nonspecific.

MICROBIAL CAUSES OF INFECTION

Infections may be caused by bacteria (including mycobacteria, chlamydiae, mycoplasmas, and rickettsiae), viruses, fungi, or parasites. Infection may be **endogenous** or **exogenous**. In endogenous infections, the microorganism (usually a bacterium) is a component of the patient's indigenous flora. Endogenous infections can occur when the microorganism is aspirated from the upper to the lower respiratory tract or when it penetrates the skin or mucosal barrier as a result of trauma or surgery. In contrast, in exogenous infections, the microorganism is acquired from the environment (e.g., from soil or water) or from another person or an animal. Although it is important to establish the cause of an infection, the differential diagnosis is based on a careful history, physical examination, and appropriate radiographic and laboratory studies, including the selection of appropriate specimens for microbiologic examination. Results of the history, physical examination, and radiographic and laboratory studies allow the physician to request tests for the microorganisms most likely to cause the infection.

SPECIMEN SELECTION, COLLECTION, AND PROCESSING

Specimens selected for microbiologic examination should reflect the disease process and be collected in sufficient quantity to allow complete microbio-

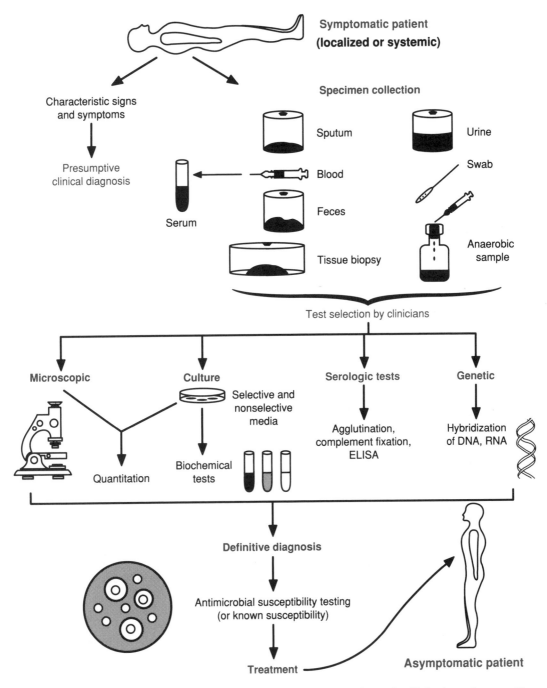

FIGURE 10-1 Laboratory procedures used in confirming a clinical diagnosis of infectious disease with a bacterial etiology.

logic examination. The number of microorganisms per milliliter of a body fluid or per gram of tissue is highly variable, ranging from less than 1 to 10^8 or 10^{10} colony-forming units (CFU). Swabs, although popular for specimen collection, frequently yield too small a specimen for accurate microbiologic examination and should be used only to collect material from the skin and mucous membranes.

Because skin and mucous membranes have a large and diverse indigenous flora, every effort must be made to minimize specimen contamination during collection. Contamination may be avoided by various means. The skin can be disinfected before aspirating or incising a lesion. Alternatively, the contaminated area may be bypassed altogether. Examples of such approaches are transtracheal puncture with aspiration of lower respiratory secretions or suprapubic bladder puncture with aspiration of urine. It is often impossible to collect an uncontaminated specimen, and decontamination procedures, cultures on selective media, or quantitative cultures must be used (see above).

Specimens collected by invasive techniques, particularly those obtained intraoperatively, require special attention. Enough tissue must be obtained for both histopathologic and microbiologic examination. Histopathologic examination is used to distinguish neoplastic from inflammatory lesions and acute from chronic inflammations. The type of inflammation present can guide the type of microbiologic examination performed. If, for example, a caseous granuloma is observed histopathologically, microbiologic examination should include cultures for mycobacteria and fungi. The surgeon should obtain several samples for examination from a single large lesion or from each of several smaller lesions. If an abscess is found, the surgeon should collect several milliliters of pus, as well as a portion of the wall of the abscess, for microbiologic examination. Swabs should be kept out of the operating room.

If possible, specimens should be collected before the administration of antibiotics. Above all, close communication between the clinician and the microbiologist is essential to ensure that appropriate specimens are selected and collected and that they are appropriately examined.

MICROBIOLOGIC EXAMINATION

Direct Examination

Direct examination of specimens frequently provides the most rapid indication of microbial infection. A variety of microscopic, immunologic, and hybridization techniques have been developed for rapid diagnosis (Table 10-1).

Sensitivity and Specificity

The *sensitivity* of a technique usually depends on the number of microorganisms in the specimen. Its *specificity* depends on how morphologically unique a specific microorganism appears microscopically or how specific the antibody or genetic probe is for that genus or species. For example, the sensitivity of Gram stains is such that the observation of two bacteria per oil immersion field ($\times$ 1,000) of a Gram-stained smear of uncentrifuged urine is equivalent to the presence of $\geq 10^5$ CFU/ml of urine. The sensitivity of the Gram-stained smear for detecting Gram-negative coccobacilli in cerebrospinal fluid from children with *Haemophilus influenzae* meningitis is approximately 75 percent because in some patients the number of colony-forming units per milliliter of cerebrospinal fluid is less than 10^4. At least 10^4 CFU of tubercle bacilli per milliliter of sputum must be present to be detected by an acid-fast smear of decontaminated and concentrated sputum.

An increase in the sensitivity of a test is often accompanied by a decrease in specificity. For example, examination of a Gram-stained smear of sputum from a patient with pneumococcal pneumonia is highly sensitive but also highly nonspecific if the criterion for defining a positive test is the presence of any Gram-positive cocci. If, however, a positive test is defined as the presence of a preponderance of Gram-positive, lancet-shaped diplococci, the test becomes highly specific but has a sensitivity of only about 50 percent. Similar

TABLE 10-1   Rapid Tests Commonly Used To Detect Microorganisms in Specimens

Specimen	Test	Application
Blood	Giemsa	Plasmodia, microfilarie
	EIA	Hepatitis A and B virus
Cerebrospinal fluid	Gram stain	Bacteria
	LA; COA	*Haemophilus influenzae, Neisseria meningitidis*
	India ink wet mount or LA	*Streptococcus pneumoniae, Cryptococcus neoformans*
Wound exudates, pus	Gram stain	Bacteria
Respiratory secretions	Gram stain	Bacteria
	Acid-fast stain	Mycobacteria, nocardiae
	IFA or genetic probe	*Legionella* species
	KOH wet mount	Fungi
	Gomori methenamine silver stain	Fungi, *Pneumocystis* species
	FA, EIA	Respiratory syncytial virus
Urine	Gram stain	Bacteria
Urethral or cervical scrapings or exudates	Gram stain, EIA	*Neisseria gonorrhoeae*
	IFA, EIA, or genetic probe	*Chlamydia trachomatis,* papillomaviruses
Genital ulcer	FA, EIA, or genetic probe	Herpes simplex virus
Feces	Methylene blue stain	Leukocytes
	Eosin wet mount, trichrome stain	Parasites
	EM, LA, EIA	Rotaviruses
	EIA	Adenoviruses

Abbreviations: COA, coagglutination; EIA, enzyme immunoassay; IFA, immunofluorescent antibody; KOH, potassium hydroxide; LA, latex agglutination.

problems related to the number of microorganisms present affect the sensitivity of immunoassays and genetic probes for bacteria, chlamydiae, and viruses. In some instances, the sensitivity of direct examination tests can be improved by collecting a better specimen. For example, the sensitivity of fluorescent antibody stain for *Chlamydia trachomatis* is higher when cervical material is obtained with a cytobrush than with a swab. The sensitivity may also be affected by the stage of the disease at which the specimen is collected. For example, the detection of herpes simplex virus by immunofluorescence, immunoassay, or culture is highest when specimens from lesions in the vesicular stage of infection are examined. Finally, sensitivity may be improved through the use of an enrichment or enhancement step in which microbial

or genetic replication occurs to the point at which a detection method can be applied.

Techniques

For microscopic examination it is sufficient to have a compound binocular microscope equipped with low-power (10X), high-power (40X), and oil immersion (100X) achromatic objectives, 10 X widefield oculars, a mechanical stage, a substage condenser, and a good light source. For examination of wet-mount preparations, a darkfield condenser or condenser and objectives for phase contrast increases image contrast. An exciter barrier filter, darkfield condenser, and ultraviolet light source are required for fluorescence microscopy.

For immunologic detection of microbial antigens, **latex particle agglutination, coagglutination,** and **enzyme-linked immunosorbent assay (ELISA)** are the most frequently used techniques in the clinical laboratory. Antibody to a specific antigen is bound to latex particles or to a heat-killed and treated protein A-rich strain of *Staphylococcus aureus* to produce agglutination (Fig. 10-2). There are several approaches to ELISA; the one most frequently used for the detection of microbial antigens uses an antigen-specific antibody that is fixed to a solid phase, which may be a latex or metal bead or the inside surface of a well in a plastic tray. Antigen present in the specimen binds to the antibody as in Fig. 10-2. The test is then completed by adding a second antigen-specific antibody bound to an enzyme that can react with a substrate to produce a colored product. The initial antigen-antibody complex forms in a manner similar to

that shown in Figure 10-2. When the enzyme-conjugated antibody is added, it binds to previously unbound antigenic sites, and the antigen is, in effect, sandwiched between the solid phase and the enzyme-conjugated antibody. The reaction is completed by adding the enzyme substrate.

Genetic probes are based on the detection of unique nucleotide sequences with the DNA or RNA of a microorganism. Once such a unique nucleotide sequence, which may represent a portion of a virulence gene or of chromosomal DNA, is found, it is isolated and inserted into a cloning vector (plasmid), which is then transformed into *Escherichia coli* to produce multiple copies of the probe. The sequence is then reisolated from plasmids and labeled with an isotope or substrate for diagnostic use. Hybridization of the sequence with a complementary sequence of DNA or RNA fol-

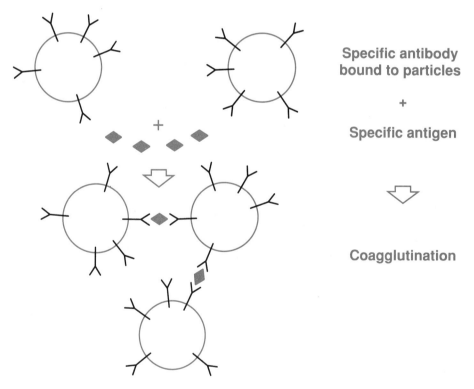

Specific antibody
bound to particles

+

Specific antigen

Coagglutination

FIGURE 10-2 Agglutination test in which inert particles (latex beads or heat-killed *S aureus* Cowan 1 strain with protein A) are coated with antibody to any of a variety of antigens and then used to detect the antigen in specimens or in isolated bacteria.

lows cleavage of the double-stranded DNA of the microorganism in the specimen.

Culture

In many instances, the cause of an infection is confirmed by isolating and culturing microorganism either in artificial media or in a living host. Bacteria (including mycobacteria and mycoplasmas) and fungi are cultured in either liquid (broth) or solid (agar) artificial media. Liquid media provide greater sensitivity for the isolation of small numbers of microorganisms; however, identification of mixed cultures growing in liquid media requires subculture onto solid media so that isolated colonies can be processed separately for identification. Growth in liquid media also cannot ordinarily be quantitated. Solid media, although somewhat less sensitive than liquid media, provide isolated colonies that can be quantified if necessary and identified. Some genera and species can be recognized on the basis of their colony morphologies.

In some instances one can take advantage of differential carbohydrate fermentation capabilities of microorganisms by incorporating one or more carbohydrates in the medium along with a suitable pH indicator. Such media are called **differential media** (e.g., eosin methylene blue or MacConkey agar) and are commonly used to isolate enteric bacilli. Different genera of the Enterobacteriaceae can then be presumptively identified by the color as well as the morphology of colonies.

Culture media can also be made **selective** by incorporating compounds such as antimicrobial agents that inhibit the indigenous flora while permitting growth of specific microorganisms resistant to these inhibitors. One such example is Thayer-Martin medium, which is used to isolate *Neisseria gonorrhoeae*. This medium contains vancomycin to inhibit Gram-positive bacteria, colistin to inhibit most Gram-negative bacilli, trimethoprim-sulfamethoxazole to inhibit *Proteus* species and other species that are not inhibited by colistin, and nystatin or anisomycin to inhibit fungi. The pathogenic *Neisseria* species, *N gonorrhoeae* and *N meningitidis*, are ordinarily resistant to the concentrations of these antimicrobial agents in the medium.

The number of bacteria in specimens may be used to define the presence of infection. For example, there may be small numbers ($\leq 10^3$ CFU/ml) of bacteria in clean-catch, midstream urine specimens from normal, healthy women; with a few exceptions, these represent bacteria that are indigenous to the urethra and periurethral region. Infection of the bladder (cystitis) or kidney (pyelone-phritis) is usually accompanied by bacteriuria of about $\geq 10^4$ CFU/ml. For this reason, **quantitative cultures** (Fig. 10-3) of urine must always be performed. For most other specimens a semiquantitative streak method (Fig. 10-3) over the agar surface is sufficient. For quantitative cultures, a specific volume of specimen is spread over the agar surface and the number of colonies per milliliter is estimated. For semiquantitative cultures, an unquantitated amount of specimen is applied to the agar and diluted by being streaked out from the inoculation site with a sterile bacteriologic loop (Fig. 10-3). The amount of growth on the agar is then reported semiquantitatively as many, moderate, or few (or 3+, 2+, or 1+), depending on how far out from the inoculum site colonies appear. An organism that grows in all streaked areas would be reported as 3+.

Chlamydiae and viruses are cultured in cell culture systems, but virus isolation occasionally requires inoculation into animals, such as suckling mice, rabbits, guinea pigs, hamsters, or primates. Rickettsiae may be isolated with some difficulty and at some hazard to laboratory workers in animals or embryonated eggs. For this reason, rickettsial infection is usually diagnosed serologically. Some viruses, such as the hepatitis viruses, cannot be isolated in cell culture systems, so that diagnosis of hepatitis virus infection is based on the detection of hepatitis virus antigens or antibodies.

Cultures are generally incubated at 35 to 37°C in an atmosphere consisting of air, air supplemented with carbon dioxide (3 to 10 percent), reduced oxygen (microaerophilic conditions), or no oxygen (anaerobic conditions), depending upon requirements of the microorganism. Since clinical

Culture Plate Methods

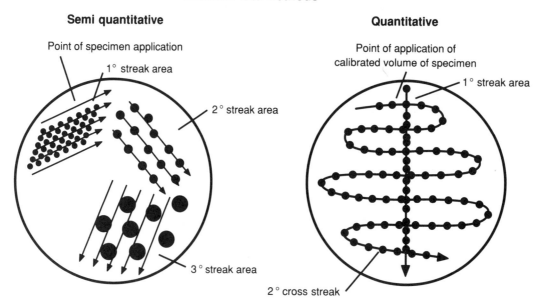

FIGURE 10-3   Quantitative versus semiquantitative culture, revealing the number of bacteria in specimens.

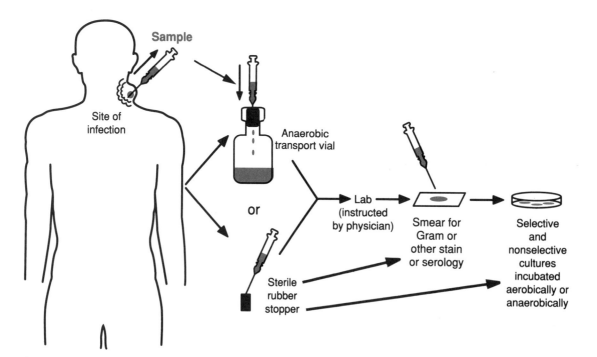

FIGURE 10-4   General procedure for collecting and processing specimens for aerobic and/or anaerobic bacterial culture.

specimens from bacterial infections often contain aerobic, facultative anaerobic, and anaerobic bacteria, such specimens are usually inoculated into a variety of general-purpose, differential, and selective media, which are then incubated under aerobic and anaerobic conditions (Fig. 10-4).

The duration of incubation of cultures also varies with the growth characteristics of the microorganism. Most aerobic and anaerobic bacteria will grow overnight, whereas some mycobacteria require as many as 6 to 8 weeks.

MICROBIAL IDENTIFICATION

Microbial growth in cultures is demonstrated by the appearance of turbidity, gas formation, or discrete colonies in broth; colonies on agar; cytopathic effects or inclusions in cell cultures; or detection of genus- or species-specific antigens or nucleotide sequences in the culture medium or cell culture system.

Identification of bacteria (including mycobacteria) is based on growth characteristics (such as the time required for growth to appear or the atmosphere in which growth occurs), colony and microscopic morphology, and biochemical, physiologic, and, in some instances, antigenic or nucleotide sequence characteristics. The selection and number of tests for bacterial identification depend upon the category of bacteria present (aerobe versus anaerobe, Gram-positive versus Gram-negative, cocci versus bacilli) and the expertise of the microbiologist examining the culture. Gram-positive cocci that grow in air with or without added CO_2 may be identified by a relatively small number of tests (see Fig. 12-4). The identification of most Gram-negative bacilli is far more complex and often requires panels of 20 tests for determining biochemical and physiologic characteristics. The identification of filamentous fungi is based almost entirely on growth characteristics and colony and microscopic morphology. Identification of viruses is usually based on characteristic cytopathic effects in different cell cultures or on the detection of virus- or species-specific antigens or nucleotide sequences.

Interpretation of Culture Results

Some microorganisms, such as *Shigella dysenteriae, Mycobacterium tuberculosis, Coccidioides immitis,* and influenza virus, are always considered clinically significant. Others that ordinarily are harmless components of the indigenous flora of the skin and mucous membranes or that are common in the environment may or may not be clinically significant, depending on the specimen source from which they are isolated. For example, coagulase-negative staphylococci are normal inhabitants of the skin and the upper respiratory tract (i.e., of the nares, oral cavity, and pharynx). Therefore, their isolation from superficial ulcers, wounds, and sputum cannot usually be interpreted as clinically significant. They do, however, commonly cause infections associated with intravascular devices and implanted prosthetic materials. However, because intravascular devices penetrate the skin and since cultures of an implanted prosthetic device can be made only after incision, the role of coagulase-negative staphylococci in causing infection can usually be surmised only when the microorganism is isolated in large numbers from the surface of an intravascular device, from each of several sites surrounding an implanted prosthetic device, or, in the case of prosthetic valve endocarditis, from several separately collected blood samples. Another example, *Aspergillus fumigatus,* is widely distributed in nature, the hospital environment, and upper respiratory tract of healthy people but may cause fatal pulmonary infections in leukemia patients or in those who have undergone bone marrow transplantation. The isolation of *A fumigatus* from respiratory secretions is a nonspecific finding, and a definitive diagnosis of invasive aspergillosis requires histologic evidence of tissue invasion.

Physicians must also consider that the composition of microbial species on the skin and mucous membranes may be altered by disease, administration of antibiotics, endotracheal or gastric intubation, and the hospital environment. For example, potentially pathogenic bacteria can often be cultured from the pharynx of seriously ill, debilitated patients in the intensive care unit, but may not cause infection.

SERODIAGNOSIS

Infection may be diagnosed by an antibody response to the infecting microorganism. This approach is especially useful when the suspected microbial agent either cannot be isolated in culture by any known method or can be isolated in culture only with great difficulty. The diagnosis of hepatitis virus and Epstein-Barr virus infections can be made only serologically, since neither can be isolated in any known cell culture system. Although human immunodeficiency virus type 1 (HIV-1) can be isolated in cell cultures, the technique is demanding and requires special containment facilities. HIV-1 infection is usually diagnosed by detection of antibodies to the virus.

The disadvantage of serology as a diagnostic tool is that there is usually a lag between the onset of infection and the development of antibodies to the infecting microorganism. Although IgM antibodies may appear relatively rapidly, it is usually necessary to obtain acute- and convalescent-phase serum samples to look for a rising titer of IgG antibodies to the suspected pathogen. In some instances the presence of a high antibody titer when the patient is initially seen is diagnostic; often, however, the high titer may reflect a past infection, and the current infection may have an entirely different cause. Another limitation on the use of serology as a diagnostic tool is that immunosuppressed patients may be unable to mount an antibody response.

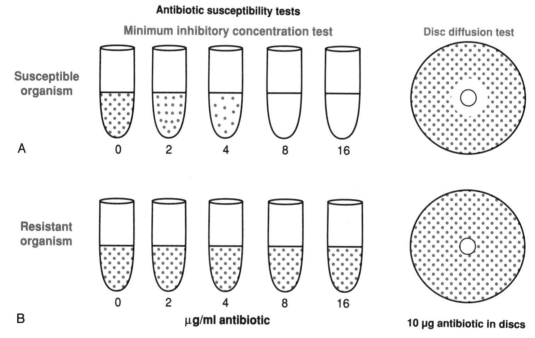

FIGURE 10-5 Two methods for performing antibiotic susceptibility tests. *(A)* Disc diffusion method. *(B)* Minimum inhibitory concentration (MIC) method. In the example shown, the same microorganism is tested by both methods against the same antibiotic. The MIC of the antibiotic for the susceptible microorganism is 8 πg/ml. The corresponding disc diffusion test shows a zone of inhibition surrounding the disk. In the second sample, a resistant microorganism is not inhibited by the highest antibiotic concentration tested (MIC > 16 πg/ml) and there is no zone of inhibition surrounding the disc. The diameter of the zone of inhibition is inversely related to the MIC.

ANTIMICROBIAL SUSCEPTIBILITY

The responsibility of the microbiology laboratory includes not only microbial detection and isolation but also the determination of microbial susceptibility to antimicrobial agents. Many bacteria, in particular, have unpredictable susceptibilities to antimicrobial agents, and their susceptibilities can be measured in vitro to help guide the selection of the most appropriate antimicrobial agent.

Antimicrobial susceptibility tests are performed by either disc diffusion or a dilution method. In the former, a standardized suspension of a particular microorganism is inoculated onto an agar surface to which paper discs containing various antimicrobial agents are applied. Following overnight incubation, any zone diameters of inhibition about the discs are measured and the results are reported as indicating susceptibility or resistance of the microorganism to each antimicrobial agent tested. An alternative method is to dilute on a $\log_2$ scale each antimicrobial agent in broth to provide a range of concentrations and to inoculate each tube or, if a microplate is used, each well containing the antimicrobial agent in broth with a standardized suspension of the microorganism to be tested. The lowest concentration of antimicrobial agent that inhibits the growth of the microorganism is the minimal inhibitory concentration (MIC). The MIC and the zone diameter of inhibition are inversely correlated (Fig. 10-5). In other words, the more susceptible the microorganism is to the antimicrobial agent, the lower the MIC and the larger the zone of inhibition. Conversely, the more resistant the microorganism, the higher the MIC and the smaller the zone of inhibition.

The term **susceptible** means that the microorganism is inhibited by a concentration of antimicrobial agent that can be attained in blood with the normally recommended dose of the antimicrobial agent and implies that an infection caused by this microorganism may be appropriately treated with the antimicrobial agent. The term **resistant** indicates that the microorganism is resistant to concentrations of the antimicrobial agent that can be attained with normal doses and implies that an infection caused by this microorganism could not be successfully treated with this antimicrobial agent.

REFERENCES

Finegold SM, Baron EJ (eds): Bailey and Scott's Diagnostic Microbiology. 7th Ed. CV Mosby, St. Louis, 1986

Koneman EW, Allen SD, Dowell VR, Jr, et al (eds): Atlas and Textbook of Diagnostic Microbiology. 3rd Ed. JB Lippincott, Philadelphia, 1988

Kunin CM: Detection, Prevention and Management of Urinary Tract Infections. 4th ed. Lea & Febiger, Philadelphia, 1987

Lennette EH, Balows A, Hausler WJ, Jr, Shadomy HJ (eds): Manual of Clinical Microbiology. 4th ed. American Society for Microbiology, Washington, DC, 1985

Pennington JE (ed): Respiratory Infections: Diagnosis and Management. 2nd ed. Raven Press, New York, 1989

Tenover FC: Diagnostic deoxyribonucleic probes for infectious diseases. Clin Microbiol Rev 1:82, 1988

Washington JA II: Bacteria, fungi, and parasites. p. 160. In Mandell GL, Douglas RG, Jr, Bennett JE (eds): Principles and Practice of Infectious Diseases. 3rd Ed. Churchill Livingstone, New York, 1990

11

ANTIMICROBIAL CHEMOTHERAPY

HAROLD C. NEU

GENERAL CONCEPTS

Basis of Antimicrobial Action

Various antimicrobial agents act by interfering with (1) cell wall synthesis, (2) plasma membrane integrity, (3) nucleic acid synthesis, (4) ribosomal function, and (5) folate synthesis.

Action of Specific Agents

Cell wall synthesis is inhibited by *β-lactams* such as penicillins and cephalosporins, which inhibit peptidoglycan polymerization, and by *vancomycin,* which combines with cell wall substrates. *Polymyxins* disrupt the plasma membrane, causing leakage. The plasma membrane sterols of fungi are attacked by *polyenes (amphotericin)* and *imidazoles. Quinolones* bind to bacterial DNA gyrase, blocking DNA replication. *Nitroimidazoles* damage DNA. *Rifampin* blocks RNA synthesis by binding to DNA-directed RNA polymerase. *Aminoglycosides, tetracycline, chloramphenicol, erythromycin,* and *clindamycin* all interfere with ribosome function. *Sulfonamides* and *trimetho-*prim block the synthesis of the folate needed for DNA replication.

Bacterial Resistance

Bacteria can evolve resistance to antibiotics. Resistance factors can be encoded on plasmids or on the chromosome. Resistance may involve decreased entry of the drug, changes in the receptor (target) of the drug, or metabolic inactivation of the drug.

Effects of Combination Therapy

Combinations of antibiotics may act *synergistically*—producing an effect stronger than the sum of the effects of the two drugs alone — or *antagonistically,* if one agent inhibits the effect of the other.

Adverse Effects of Antimicrobial Agents

Many antibiotics are toxic to the host. Alterations of the normal intestinal flora caused by antibiotics may result in diarrhea or in superinfection with opportunistic pathogens.

INTRODUCTION

The earliest evidence of successful chemotherapy is from ancient Peru, where the Indians used bark from the cinchona tree to treat malaria. Other substances were used in ancient China, and we now know that many of the poultices used by primitive peoples contained antibacterial and antifungal substances. Modern chemotherapy has been dated to the work of Paul Ehrlich in Germany, who sought systematically to discover effective agents to treat trypanosomiasis and syphilis. He discovered *p*-rosaniline, which has antitrypanosomal effects, and arsphenamine, which is effective against syphilis. Ehrlich postulated that it would be possible to find chemicals that were selectively toxic for parasites but not toxic to humans. This idea has been called the "magic bullet" concept. It had little success until the 1930s, when Gerhard Domagk discovered the protective effects of prontosil, the forerunner of sulfonamide. Ironically, penicillin G was discovered fortuitously in 1929 by Fleming, who did not initially appreciate the magnitude of his discovery. In 1939 Florey and colleagues at Oxford University again isolated penicillin. In 1944 Waksman isolated streptomycin and subsequently found agents such as chloramphenicol, tetracyclines, and erythromycin in soil samples. By the 1960s, improvements in fermentation techniques and advances in medicinal chemistry per-

mitted the synthesis of many new chemotherapeutic agents by molecular modification of existing compounds. Progress in the development of novel antibacterial agents has been great, but the development of effective, nontoxic antifungal and antiviral agents has been slow. Amphotericin B, isolated in the 1950s, remains the most effective antifungal agent. Nucleoside analogs such as acyclovir have proved effective in the chemotherapy of selected viral infections.

BIOCHEMICAL BASIS OF ANTIMICROBIAL ACTION

Bacterial cells grow and divide, replicating repeatedly to reach the large numbers present during an infection or on the surfaces of the body. To grow and divide, organisms must synthesize or take up many types of biomolecules. Antimicrobial agents interfere with specific processes that are essential for growth and/or division (Fig. 11-1). They can be separated into groups such as inhibitors of bacterial and fungal cell walls, inhibitors of cytoplasmic

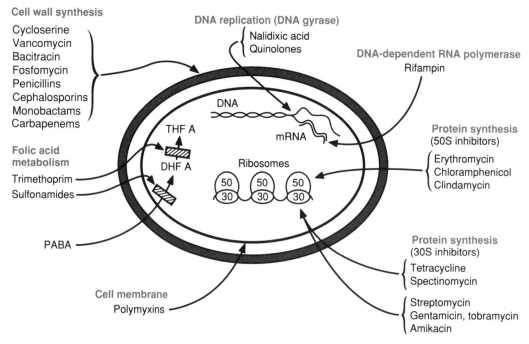

FIGURE 11-1   Sites of action of different antimicrobial agents. PABA, paraminobenzoic acid; DHFA, dihydrofolic acid; THFA, tetrahydrofolic acid.

TABLE 11-1   Mechanisms of Action of Antimicrobial Agents

Inhibitors of Bacterial Cell Wall Synthesis

    Drugs that inhibit biosynthetic enzymes
        Fosfomycin
        Cycloserine
    Drugs that combine with carrier molecules
        Bacitracin
    Drugs that combine with cell wall substrates
        Vancomycin
    Drugs that inhibit polymerization and attachment of
      new peptidoglycan to cell wall
        Penicillins
        Cephalosporins
        Carbapenems
        Monobactams

Inhibitors of Cytoplasmic Membranes

    Drugs that disorganize the cytoplasmic membrane
        Tyrocidins
        Polymyxins
    Drugs that produce pores in membranes
        Gramicidins
    Drugs that alter sterol structure of fungi
        Polyenes (amphotericin)
        Imidazoles (ketoconazole)

Inhibitors of Nucleic Acid Synthesis

    Inhibitors of nucleotide metabolism
        Adenosine arabinoside (viruses)
        Acyclovir (viruses)
        Flucytosine (fungi)
    Agents that impair DNA template function: interca-
      lating agents
        Chloroquine (parasites)
    Inhibitors of DNA replication
        Quinolones
        Nitroimidazoles
    Inhibitors of RNA polymerase
        Rifampin

Inhibitors of Ribosome Function

    Inhibitors of 30S units
        Streptomycin
        Kanamycin, gentamicin, amikacin
        Spectinomycin
        Tetracyclines
    Inhibitors of 50S units
        Chloramphenicol
        Clindamycin
        Erythromycin
        Fusidic acid

Inhibitors of Folate Metabolism

    Inhibitor of pteroic acid synthetase
        Sulfonamides
    Inhibitor of dihydrofolate reductase
        Trimethoprim

---

membranes, inhibitors of nucleic acid synthesis, and inhibitors of ribosome function (Table 11-1). Antimicrobial agents may be either **bactericidal,** killing the target bacterium or fungus, or **bacteriostatic,** inhibiting its growth. Bactericidal agents are more effective, but bacteriostatic agents can be extremely beneficial since they permit the normal defenses of the host to destroy the microorganisms.

INHIBITION OF BACTERIAL CELL WALL SYNTHESIS

As noted in earlier chapters, bacteria are classified as Gram-positive and Gram-negative organisms on the basis of staining characteristics. Gram-positive bacterial cell walls contain peptidoglycan and teichoic or teichuronic acid, and the bacterium may or may not be surrounded by a protein or polysac-

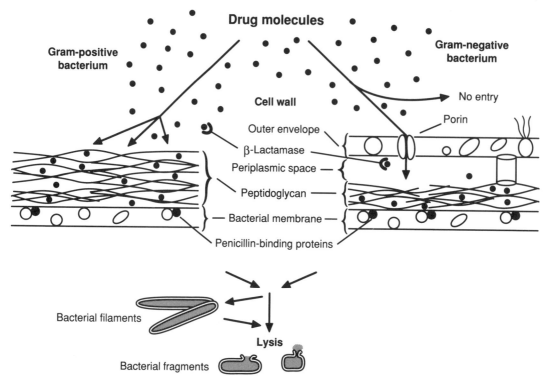

FIGURE 11-2 Outer wall of Gram-positive and Gram-negative species and detail of porin channels of Gram-negative bacteria. Antimicrobial agents diffuse easily through the loose outer wall of Gram-positive bacteria, but must go through the narrow channels of the Gram-negative species.

charide envelope. Gram-negative bacterial cell walls contain peptidoglycan, lipopolysaccharide, lipoprotein, phospholipid, and protein (Fig. 11-2). The critical attack site of anti-cell-wall agents is the peptidoglycan layer. This layer is essential for the survival of bacteria in hypotonic environments; loss or damage of this layer destroys the rigidity of the bacterial cell wall, resulting in death.

Peptidoglycan synthesis occurs in three stages. The first stage takes place in the cytoplasm, where the low-molecular-weight precursors UDP-GlcAc and UDP-MurNAc-L-Ala-D-Glu-*meso*-Dap-D-Ala-D-Ala are synthesized. A number of antimicrobial agents interfere with these early steps in cell wall biosynthesis. UTP and *N*-acetylglucosamine α-1-P are converted to UDP-*N*-acetylglucosamine, which is subsequently converted by the enzyme phosphoenolpyruvate : UDP-GlcNAc-3-enol-pyruvyltrans-

ferase. **Fosfomycins** block this transfer by a direct nucleophilic attack on the enzyme. Because mammalian enzymes such as enolase, pyruvate kinase, carboxykinases, and the shikimate enolases are not inhibited by these compounds, fosfomycins have no effect on the host. Three amino acids are added to the muramyl peptide to yield a tripeptide to which two more amino acids will be linked. The dipeptide D-alanyl-D-alanine is synthesized from two molecules of D-alanine by the enzyme D-alanyl-D-alanine synthetase. D-Alanine is produced from L-alanine by an alanine racemase. **Cycloserine** inhibits both alanine racemase and D-alanyl-D-alanine synthetase owing to the structural similarity of cycloserine and D-alanine and to the fact that cycloserine actually binds to the enzymes better than the D-alanine.

The second stage of cell wall synthesis is catalyzed by membrane-bound enzymes. The nonnucleotide portion of the precursor molecules previously made are transferred sequentially to a carrier in the cytoplasmic membrane. This carrier is a phosphorylated undecaprenyl alcohol. The lipid carrier functions as a point of attachment to the membrane for the precursors and allows for transport of the subunits across the hydrophobic interior of the cytoplasmic membrane to the outside surface. **Bacitracin** is a peptide antibiotic that specifically interacts with the pyrophosphate derivate of the undecaprenyl alcohol, preventing further transfer of the muramylpentapeptide from the precursor nucleotide to the nascent peptidoglycan.

The third stage of cell wall synthesis involves polymerization of the subunits and the attachment of nascent peptidoglycan to the cell wall. Polymerization occurs by transfer of the new peptidoglycan chain from its carrier in the membrane to the nonreducing N-acetylglucosamine of the new saccharide-peptide that is attached to the membrane. The new peptidoglycan is attached to preexisting cell wall peptidoglycan by a transpeptidase reaction that involves peptide chains in both polymers, one of which must possess a D-alanyl-D-alanine terminus. It is believed that the transpeptidase enzyme cleaves the peptide bond between two D-alanyl residues in the pentapeptide and become acylated via the carbonyl group of the penultimate D-alanine residue. This final reaction is inhibited by β-**lactam antibiotics.** These antibiotics contain a critical four-membered ring, which undergoes an acylation reaction with the transpeptidases that cross-link the polymers mentioned above. The β-lactam antibiotics are the **penicillins** (penams), **cephalosporins** (including oxacephems and cephamycins), **penems, thienamycins** (carbapenems), and **aztreonam** (monobactams) (Fig. 11-3). The enzymes involved in this final process of cell wall formation are called **penicillin-binding proteins,** since they were discovered by labeling with radioactive penicillin G. The enzymes are different in Gram-positive and Gram-negative bacteria and in anaerobic species. Differences in the penicillin-binding proteins explain, to some ex-

tent, differences in antibacterial activity of the β-lactam antibiotics. The penicillin-binding protein to which a particular β-lactam antibiotic binds affects the morphologic response of the bacterium to the agent. For example, some antibiotics bind to a penicillin-binding protein that is involved in forming the septum between dividing cells; as a result, the bacteria continue to grow into long filaments, which eventually die. Binding to another penicillin-binding protein results in rapid lysis of a bacterium because the wall bulges and the bacterium bursts. β-Lactams such as **mecillinam** (an amidino penicillin) do not bind to the penicillin-binding proteins of Gram-positive bacteria and therefore do not affect these bacteria. Aztreonam binds only to Gram-negative penicillin-binding proteins and does not inhibit Gram-positive or anaerobic species.

Vancomycin interferes with cell wall synthesis by combining with substrates essential for cell wall formation. Because vancomycin is a high-molecular-weight polypeptide (Fig. 11-4), it cannot cross the cytoplasmic membrane and cannot pass through the complex outer wall of Gram-negative bacteria. It binds to the D-alanyl-D-alanine termini of growing peptidoglycan attached to the undecaprenyl pyrophosphate and prevents interaction of muramidases with the glycan chain.

ANTIBIOTICS THAT AFFECT THE FUNCTION OF CYTOPLASMIC MEMBRANES

Bacterial Cytoplasmic Membranes

Biologic membranes are composed basically of lipid, protein, and lipoprotein. The cytoplasmic membrane acts as a diffusion barrier for water, ions, nutrients, and transport systems. Most workers now believe that membranes are a lipid matrix with globular proteins randomly distributed to penetrate through the lipid bilayer. A number of antimicrobial agents can cause disorganization of the membrane. These agents can be divided into cationic, anionic, and neutral agents. The best-known compounds are **polymyxin B** and co-

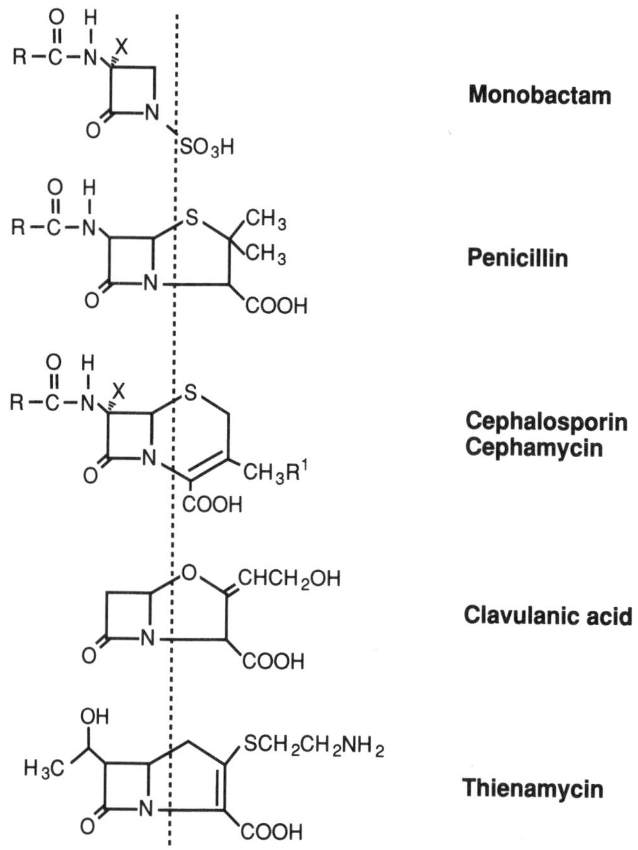

FIGURE 11-3 Basic structures of β-lactam antibiotics. Penicillins and cephalosporins/cephamycins are widely used to inhibit both Gram-positive and Gram-negative bacilli. Monobactams inhibit only aerobic Gram-negative bacilli, clavulanic acid acts as a β-lactamase inhibitor, and thienamycin inhibits a wide range of aerobic and anaerobic species. R and R^1 represent various carbon groups. X can be either hydrogen or a methoxy group.

listemethate **(polymyxin E).** These high-molecular-weight octapeptides inhibit Gram-negative bacteria that have negatively charged lipids at the surface. Since the activity of the polymyxins is antagonized by Mg^{2+} and Ca^{2+}, they probably competitively displace Mg^{2+} or Ca^{2+} from the negatively charged phosphate groups on membrane lipids. Basically, polymyxins disorganize membrane permeability so that nucleic acids and cations leak out and the cell dies. The polymyxins are of virtually no use as systemic agents since they bind to various ligands in body tissues and are potent toxins for the kidney and nervous system. **Gramicidins** are also membrane-active antibiotics that appear to act by producing aqueous pores in the membranes. They also are used only topically.

Fungal Membranes

Fungal membranes contain sterols, whereas bacterial membranes do not. The **polyene antibiotics,** which apparently act by binding to membrane sterols, contain a rigid hydrophobic center and a flexible hydrophilic section. Structurally, polyenes are tightly packed rods held in rigid extension by the polyene portion. They interact with fungal cells to produce a membrane-polyene complex that alters the membrane permeability, resulting in in-

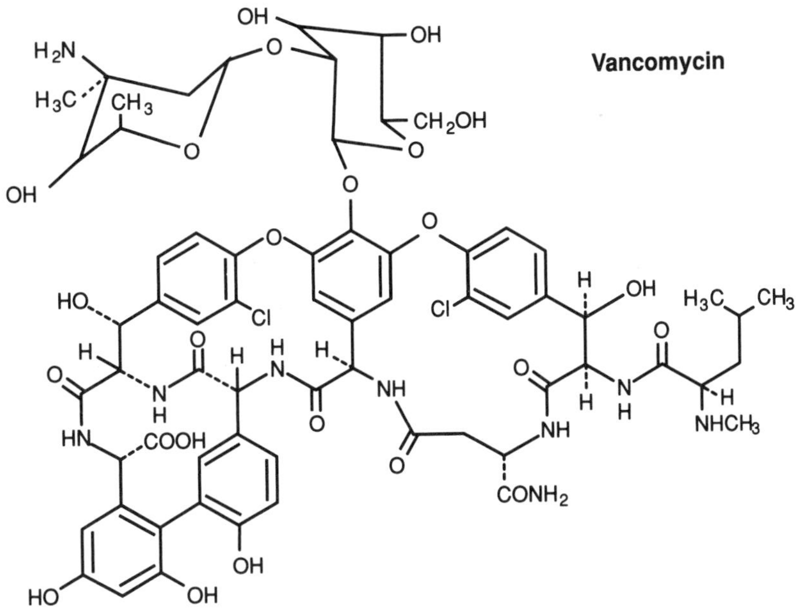

Vancomycin

FIGURE 11-4 Structure of vancomycin.

ternal acidification of the fungus with exchange of K+ and sugars; loss of phosphate esters, organic acids, nucleotides; and eventual leakage of cell protein. In effect, the polyene makes a pore in the fungal membrane and the contents of the fungus leak out. Prokaryotic cells neither bind to nor are inhibited by polyenes. Although numerous polyene antibiotics have been isolated, only **amphotericin B** is used systemically (Fig. 11-5). Nystatin is used as a topical agent and primaricin as an ophthalmic preparation.

A number of other agents interfere with the syn-

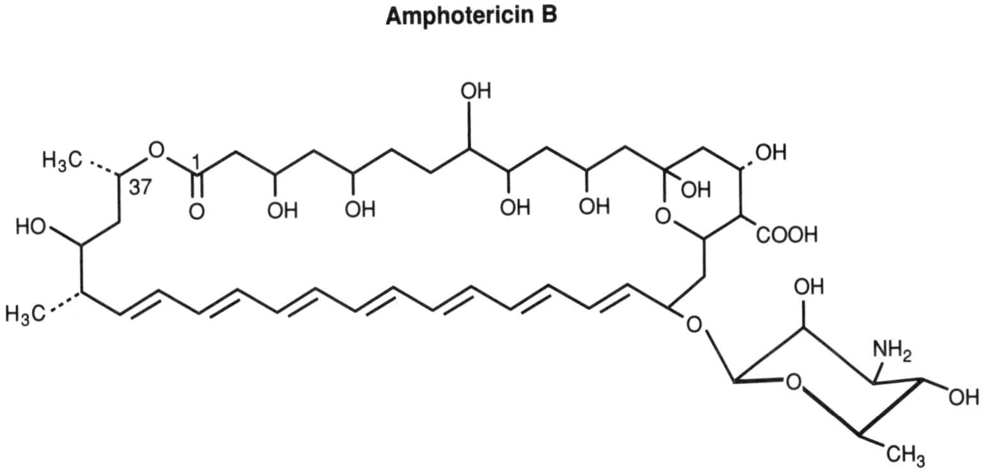

Amphotericin B

FIGURE 11-5 Structure of amphotericin B.

thesis of fungal lipid membranes. These agents belong to a class of compounds referred to as **imidazoles**: miconazole, ketoconazole, clotrimazole, and fluconazole. These compounds inhibit the incorporation of subunits into ergosterol and may also directly damage the membrane.

ANTIBIOTICS THAT INHIBIT NUCLEIC ACID SYNTHESIS

Antimicrobial agents can interfere with nucleic acid synthesis at several different levels. They can inhibit nucleotide synthesis or interconversion; they can prevent DNA from functioning as a proper template; and they can interfere with the polymerases involved in the replication and transcription of DNA.

Interference with Nucleotide Synthesis

A large number of agents interfere with purine and pyrimidine synthesis or with the interconversion or utilization of nucleotides. Other agents act as nucleotide analogs that are incorporated into polynucleotides.

Flucytosine (5-fluorocytosine) is an antifungal agent that inhibits yeast species. It is converted in the fungal cell to 5-fluorouracil, which inhibits thymidylate synthetase resulting in a deficit of thymine nucleotides and impaired DNA synthesis. **Adenosine arabinoside** inhibits viruses. It is phosphorylated in virus-infected cells and acts as a competitive analog of dATP, inhibiting the incorporation of dATP into DNA. **Acyclovir** is a nucleoside analog that, after being converted to a triphosphate, inhibits the thymidine kinase and DNA polymerase of herpesviruses. **Zidovudine** (AZT) inhibits human immunodeficiency virus (HIV) replication by interfering with viral RNA-dependent DNA polymerase (reverse transcriptase).

Agents That Impair the Template Function of DNA

A number of substances bind to DNA by intercalation. None of them is useful as an antibacterial agent; however, chloroquine and miracil D (lucanthone) inhibit plasmodia and schistosomes, respectively. These agents are thought to intercalate into the DNA and thereby to inhibit further nucleic acid synthesis. Acridine dyes such as proflavine act by this intercalation mechanism, but because they are toxic and carcinogenic in mammals they cannot be used as antibacterial agents.

Rifampin

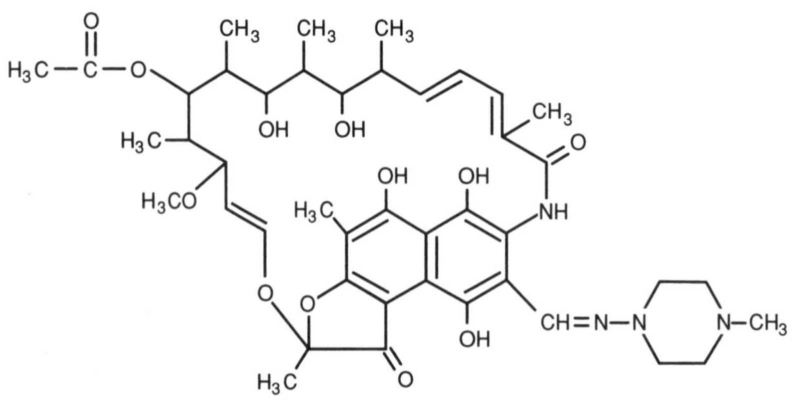

FIGURE 11-6 Structure of rifampin, which inhibits the DNA-directed RNA polymerase.

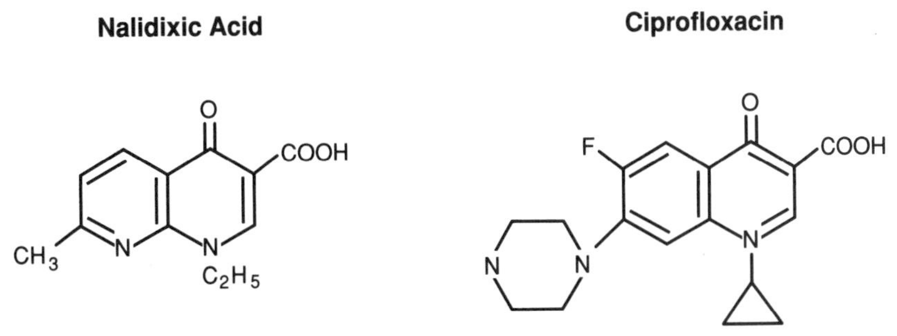

Nalidixic Acid   **Ciprofloxacin**

FIGURE 11-7   Structures of quinolone antibiotics. Nalidixic acid inhibits only aerobic Gram-negative species. In ciprofloxacin, the fluorine provides Gram-positive activity, the piperazine group increases activity against members of the *Enterobacteriaceae,* and the piperazine and cylopropyl groups give activity against *Pseudomonas* species.

Inhibition of DNA-Directed DNA Polymerase

Rifamycins are a class of antibiotics that inhibit DNA-directed RNA polymerase (Fig. 11-6). Polypeptide chains in RNA polymerase attach to a factor that confers specificity for the recognition of promoter sites that initiate transcription of the DNA. Rifampin binds noncovalently but strongly to a subunit of RNA polymerase and interferes specifically with the initiation process. However, it has no effect once polymerization has begun.

Inhibition of DNA Replication

DNA gyrase unwinds the negative supercoiling in the closed-circular duplex DNA of bacteria and is essential for replication of circular chromosomes. It is also involved in breakage and reunion of DNA strands. DNA gyrase consists of two components A and B, with the A subunit more abundant. **Quinolones** such as nalidixic acid (Fig. 11-7) bind to the A component of DNA gyrase of Gram-negative bacteria and inhibit its action. The new fluorinated quinolones such as ciprofloxacin and norfloxacin also bind to DNA gyrase and inhibit Gram-positive as well as Gram-negative organisms. The DNA gyrase B subunit can be inhibited by agents such as novobicin and coumermycin, but neither of these is used clinically.

Nitroimidazoles such as metronidazole inhibit anaerobic bacteria and protozoa. The nitro group of the nitrosohydroxyl amino moiety is reduced by an electron transport protein in anaerobic bacteria (Fig. 11-8). The reduced drug causes strand breaks in the DNA. Mammalian cells are unharmed because they lack enzymes to reduce the nitro group of these agents.

ANTIMICROBIAL INHIBITORS OF RIBOSOME FUNCTION

The basic structure and function of ribosomes are presented in Fig. 11-1. A number of antibacterial agents act by inhibiting ribosome function. Bacterial ribosomes contain two subunits, the 50S and 30S subunits, and it is possible to localize the action of antibiotics to one or both subunits. It is also possible to isolate the specific ribosomal proteins to which an agent binds and to isolate bacterial mutants that lack a specific ribosomal protein and therefore show resistance to a particular agent.

Aminoglycosides act by binding to specific ribosomal subunits. Aminoglycosides are complex sugars connected in glycosidic linkage (Fig. 11-9). They differ both in the molecular nucleus, which can be streptidine or 2-deoxystreptidine, and in the aminohexoses linked to the nucleus. Essential to the activity of these agents are free NH_4 and OH groups by which aminoglycosides bind to specific ribosomal proteins. **Streptomycin,** the first amino-

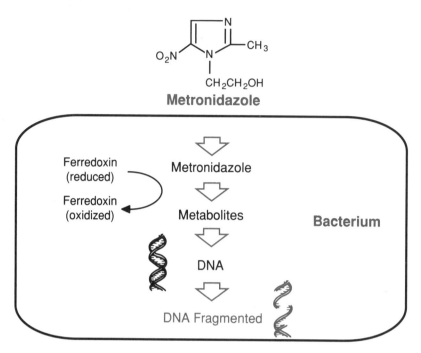

FIGURE 11-8 Structure of metronidazole and its mechanism of action. Metronidazole enters an aerobic bacterium, where, via the electron transport protein ferredoxin, it is reduced. The drug then binds to DNA, and DNA breakage occurs.

glycoside studied, was a useful tool in elucidating protein synthesis. However, it is rarely used clinically today except to treat tuberculosis, and its mode of action differs to some extent from that of the other clinically useful aminoglycosides, which are 2-deoxystreptidine derivatives such as **gentamicin, tobramycin,** and **amikacin.** Streptomycin binds to a specific S12 protein in the 30S ribosomal subunit (Fig. 11-10) and causes the ribosome to misread the genetic code. Other aminoglycosides bind not only to the S12 protein of the 30S ribosome, but also to some extent to the L6 protein of the 50S ribosome. This latter binding is quite important in terms of the resistance of bacteria to aminoglycosides. Indeed, the aminoglycoside-type drugs can combine with other binding sites on 30S ribosomes, and they kill bacteria by inducing the formation of aberrant, nonfunctional complexes as well as by causing misreading (Fig. 11-11).

Spectinomycin is an aminocylitol antibiotic that is closely related to the aminoglycosides. It binds to a different protein in the ribosome and is bacteriostatic but not bactericidal. It is used to treat penicillin-resistant gonorrhea.

Other agents that bind to 30S ribosomes are the **tetracyclines** (Fig. 11-12). These agents appear to inhibit the binding of aminoacyl-tRNA into the A site of the bacterial ribosome. Tetracycline binding is transient, so these agents are bacteriostatic. Nonetheless, they inhibit a wide variety of bacteria, chlamydias, and mycoplasmas and are extremely useful antibiotics.

There are three important classes of drugs that inhibit the 50S ribosomal subunit. **Chloramphenicol** (Fig. 11-13) is a bacteriostatic agent that inhibits both Gram-positive and Gram-negative bacteria. It inhibits peptide bond formation by binding to a peptidyltransferase enzyme on the 50S ribosome. **Macrolides** are large lactone ring compounds that bind to 50S ribosomes and appear to impair a peptidyltransferase reaction or

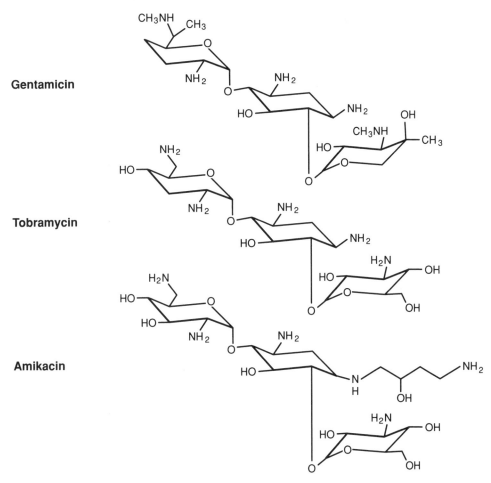

FIGURE 11-9   Structures of three aminoglycoside antibiotics used clinically. Critical aspects of the molecules are the amino and hydroxy groups that bind to proteins in the ribosomes.

translocation, or both. The most important macrolide is **erythromycin,** which inhibits Gram-positive species and a few Gram-negative species such as *Haemophilus, Mycoplasma, Chlamydia,* and *Legionella.* **Lincinoids,** of which the most important is **clindamycin,** have a similar site of activity (Fig. 11-14). Both macrolides and lincinoids are generally bacteriostatic, inhibiting only the formation of new peptide chains.

DRUGS THAT INHIBIT OTHER BIOCHEMICAL TARGETS

Both **trimethoprim** and the **sulfanomides** interfere with folate metabolism in the bacterial cell by competitively blocking the biosynthesis of tetrahydrofolate, which acts as a carrier of one-carbon fragments and is necessary for the ultimate synthesis of DNA, RNA, and bacterial cell wall proteins (Fig. 11-15). Unlike mammals, bacteria and protozoan parasites usually lack a transport system to take up preformed folic acid from their environment. Most of these organisms must synthesize folates, although some are capable of using exogenous thymidine, circumventing the need for folate metabolism.

Sulfonamides competitively block the conversion of pteridine and *p*-aminobenzoic acid (PABA) to dihydrofolic acid by the enzyme pteridine syn-

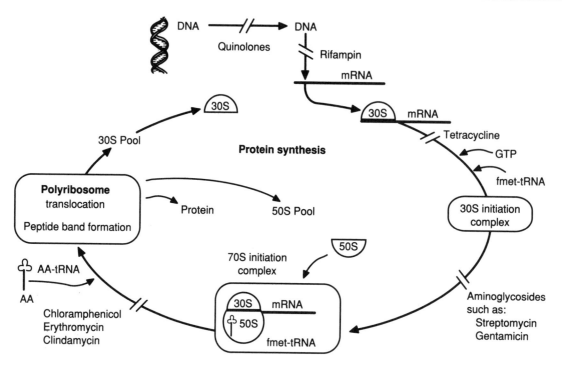

FIGURE 11-10   Diagrammatic representation of inhibition sites of protein biosynthesis by various antibiotics that bind to the 30S and 50S ribosomes.

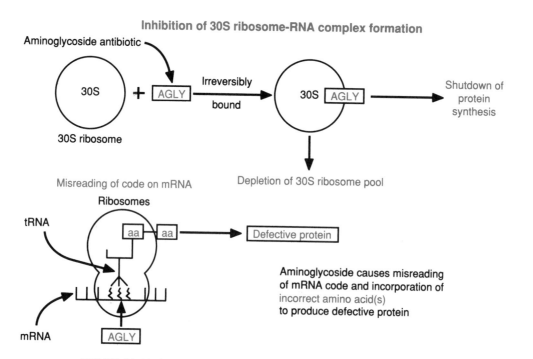

FIGURE 11-11   Inhibition of protein biosynthesis by aminoglycosides.

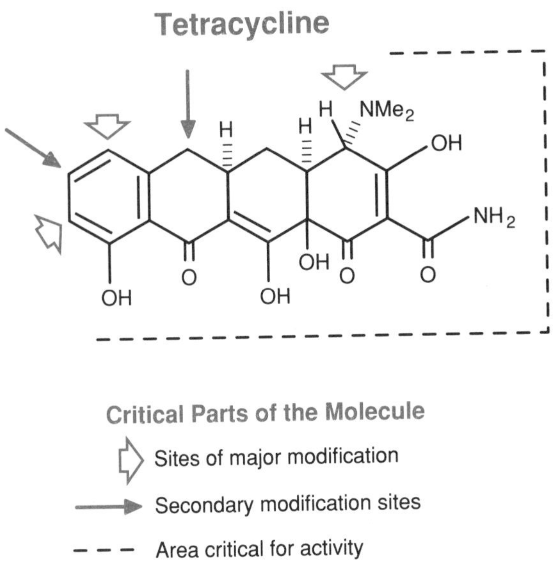

Tetracycline

Critical Parts of the Molecule

⇨ Sites of major modification

→ Secondary modification sites

− − − Area critical for activity

FIGURE 11-12 Structure of tetracycline showing the area critical for activity and major and minor points of modification.

thetase. Sulfonamides have a greater affinity than p-aminobenzoic acid for pteridine synthetase. Trimethoprim has a tremendous affinity for bacterial dihydrofolate reductase (10,000 to 100,000 times higher than for the mammalian enzyme); when bound to this enzyme, it inhibits the synthesis of tetrahydrofolate.

ANTIBACTERIAL AGENTS THAT AFFECT MYCOBACTERIA

Isoniazid is a nicotinamide derivative that inhibits mycobacteria. Its precise mode of action is not known, but it affects the synthesis of lipids, nucleic acids, and the mycolic acid of the cell walls of these species. **Ethambutol** is also an antimycobacterial agent whose mechanism of action is unknown. It is mycostatic, whereas isoniazid is mycocidal. The other antituberculosis drugs, **rifampin** and **streptomycin,** affect mycobacteria in the same manner that they inhibit bacteria. **Pyrazinamide** is a synthetic analog of nicotinamide. It is bactericidal, but its exact mechanism is unknown.

BACTERIAL RESISTANCE

Bacteria have proved adept at developing resistance to new antimicrobial agents. There are a number of ways in which bacteria can become resistant (Table 11-2). Most of the early studies of bacterial resistance focused on single-step mutational events of chromosomal origin. Resistance to the early sulfonamides, for example, was the result of a single amino acid change in the enzyme pteridine synthetase that caused sulfonamides to bind less well than p-aminobenzoic acid. Similarly, a single-step mutation that altered a ribosomal protein conferred resistance to streptomycin. In the late 1950s, Japanese workers found that enteric bacteria such as *Shigella dysenteriae* had become resistant not only to sulfonamides but also to the tetracyclines and chloramphenicol. This resistance was due not to a chromosomal change, but rather to the presence of extrachromosomal DNA that was transmissible. This type of resistance is called **plasmid resistance.**

Resistance-conferring plasmids are present in virtually all bacteria (Table 11-3). For example, resistance to ampicillin appeared in *Haemophilus influenzae* in 1974 and in *Neisseria gonorrhoeae* in 1976. In the last several years, organisms such as

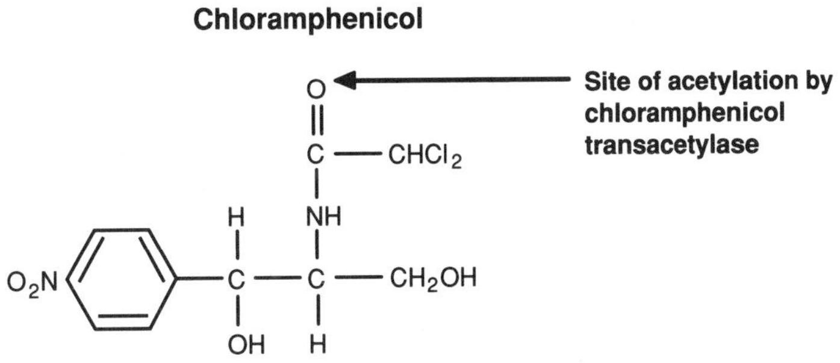

Chloramphenicol

FIGURE 11-13 Structure of chloramphenicol.

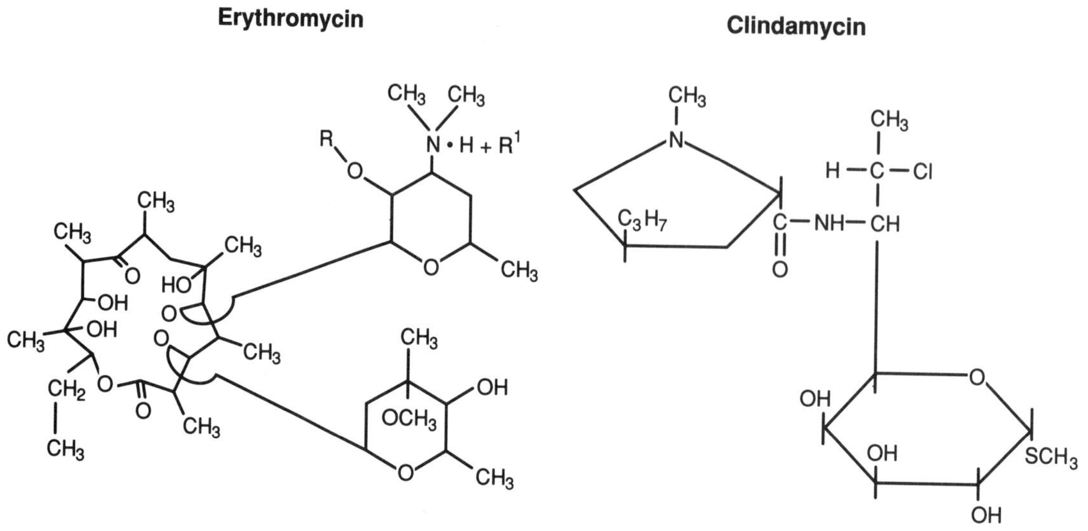

Erythromycin   **Clindamycin**

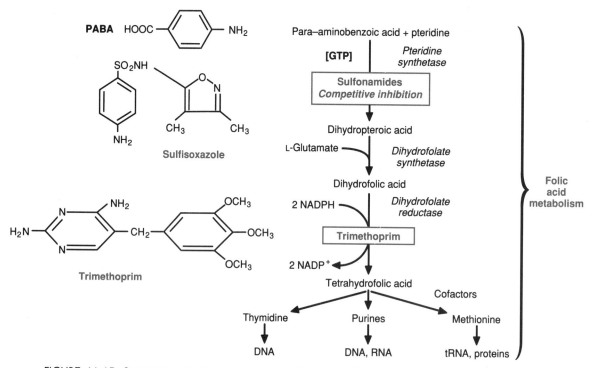

FIGURE 11-14 Structures of erythromycin (prototype of macrolide) and clindamycin. Although extremely different in structure, both compounds inhibit protein synthesis by binding to 50S ribosome.

FIGURE 11-15 Structures of sulfonamide and trimethoprim with sites of inhibition of folic acid metabolism.

TABLE 11-2   Mechanisms of Resistance

Alteration of target
    Modification to insensitivity to inhibitor
    Reduction in physiologic importance of target
    Synthesis of new target enzyme that duplicates
       function of inhibited target
Prevention of access to target
    Efflux of more drug than enters cell
    Failure of modified drug to enter cell
Inactivation of agent
    Destruction of the agent
    Modification of the agent so it fails to bind to target
Failure to convert an inactive precursor agent to its active form

enterococci have been shown to contain plasmids that confer resistance to drugs such as ampicillin and aminoglycosides.

Bacteria also contain **transposons,** which can insert into plasmids and also into the chromosome (see Ch. 5). Transposon-mediated resistance to most of the major antibiotics has been found in the past few years.

Antimicrobial agents exert a strong selective pressure on the development of both chromosomal and plasmid-mediated resistance, as discussed below. Administration of an antibiotic destroys the susceptible bacteria in a population, but may permit resistant ones to proliferate. From an epidemiologic viewpoint, plasmid-mediated resistance is the most important type, since it is transmissible, is usually highly stable, confers resistance to many different classes of antibiotics simultaneously, and often is associated with other characteristics that enable a microorganism to colonize and invade a susceptible host.

TABLE 11-3   R-Plasmid-Mediated Resistance

Antibiotic	Mechanism	Organisms
Penicillin, ampicillin, carbenicillin, etc.	β-Lactamase hydrolysis	Staphylococci, enterococci (rare), Enterobacteriaceae, pseudomonads, bacteroides
Oxacillin, methicillin, etc.	β-Lactamase hydrolysis	Enterobacteriaceae, pseudomonads
Cephalosporins	β-Lactamase	Staphylococci, Enterobacteriaceae, pseudomonads, bacteroides
Chloramphenicol	Acetylation	Staphylococci, enterococci, streptococci, Enterobacteriaceae, pseudomonads
Tetracyclines	Permeability block	Staphylococci, enterococci, streptococci, Enterobacteriaceae, pseudomonads, bacteroides

Aminoglycosides
  Streptomycin
  Neomycin
  Kanamycin
  Gentamicin
  Tobramycin
  Amikacin
	Acetylation
	Phosphorylation
	Adenylation (alters binding to ribosomes and uptake of drug)
		Staphylococci, enterococci, Enterobacteriaceae, pseudomonads

Macrolides-Lincinoids
  Erythromycin
  Clindamycin
	Altered 23S RNA	Staphylococci, enterococci, streptococci, bacteroides

Trimethoprim	Altered dihydrofolate reductase	Staphylococci, Enterobacteriaceae
Sulfonamides	Altered tetrahydropteroic synthetase	Staphylococci, enterococci, streptococci, Enterobacteriaceae, pseudomonads
Fosfomycin	Altered glucose transport system	Staphylococci, Enterobacteriaceae
Vancomycin	New protein	Enterococci, staphylococci

Mechanisms of Resistance

The basic mechanisms by which a microorganism can resist an antimicrobial agent are (1) to alter the receptor for the drug (the molecule on which it exerts its effect); (2) to decrease the amount of drug that reaches the receptor by altering entry or increasing removal of the drug; (3) to destroy or inactivate the drug; and (4) to develop resistant metabolic pathways. Bacteria can possess one or all of these mechanisms simultaneously.

Resistance Due to Altered Receptors

β-LACTAMS RESISTANCE   The ability to analyze changes in receptors for β-lactams by competition experiments in which [^{14}C]penicillin is inhibited from binding to penicillin-binding proteins has explained a number of cases of bacterial resistance to penicillins and cephalosporins. In 1977, *Streptococcus pneumoniae* strains resistant to penicillin G were encountered in South Africa. Plasmids were not the cause of the resistance. Penicillin-resistant *S pneumoniae* cells have altered penicillin-binding proteins, which bind penicillin less well. Resistance of *S pneumoniae* to penicillin has been increasing, and there are now relatively resistant isolates (minimal inhibitory concentration [MIC], 0.1 to 1μg/ml) in many parts of the world.

Altered penicillin-binding proteins also explain the resistance of some *Staphylococcus aureus* strains to β-lactamase-stable penicillins (the so-called methicillin-resistant strains). The β-lactams induce synthesis of a new penicillin-binding protein, PBP2a, which does not bind any β-lactam. The β-lactam resistance of coagulase-negative staphylococci is also the result of altered penicillin-binding proteins. Staphylococcal organisms resistant to methicillin are resistant to all penicillins, cephalosporins, and carbapenems.

The resistance of group D streptococci to β-lactam antibiotics appears to be the result of lower affinity of the penicillin-binding proteins for the penicillins. Enterococci are resistant to all cephalosporins because of failure to bind to the penicillin-binding proteins. One Gram-negative species for which resistance to β-lactam antibiotics can be correlated with diminished affinity of the target enzymes is *N gonorrhoeae*.

MACROLIDE-LINCOMYCIN RESISTANCE   Macrolide-lincomycin resistance in clinical isolates of staphylococci and streptococci has been recognized for several decades. The resistance is due to methylation of two adenine nucleotides in the 23S component of 50S RNA. This resistance is plasmid mediated, and the resistance is present on transposons. Resistance results from induction of an enzyme that is normally repressed. The methylated RNA binds macrolide-lincomycin-type drugs less well than unmethylated RNA does. Induction of resistance varies by species, and in most Gram-positive species erythromycin is a more effective inducer of resistance than is clindamycin. The plasmids that mediate macrolide-lincomycin resistance in streptococci and staphylococci have extensive structural similarity, indicating that these plasmids readily pass between these species.

RIFAMPIN RESISTANCE   The resistance of bacteria to rifampin is caused by an alteration of one amino acid in DNA-directed RNA polymerase, which results in reduced binding of rifampin. The degree of resistance is related to the degree to which the enzyme is changed, but does not correlate strictly with enzyme inhibition. This form of resistance occurs at a low level in any population of bacteria, so that resistance develops by natural selection during a course of therapy. Naturally resistant organisms are more common among members of the Enterobacteriaceae, explaining why agents of urinary tract infections rapidly became resistant to rifampin. The resistance of *Neisseria meningitidis* to rifampin appeared in closed military settings in which rifampin has been used for prophylaxis.

SULFONAMIDE-TRIMETHOPRIM RESISTANCE
Sulfonamide can be rendered ineffective by altered or new dihydropteroic synthetase that has poor affinity for sulfonamides and preferentially binds *p*-aminobenzoic acid. Sulfonamide resistance of this type can result from a point mutation or from acquisition of a plasmid that causes synthesis of the new enzyme. A most serious resistance problem is an increase in resistance to trimethoprim. This plasmid- and transposon-mediated resistance is due to production of an altered dihy-

drofolate reductase that has markedly reduced affinity for trimethoprim.

QUINOLONE RESISTANCE   Resistance of bacteria to older quinolone antibiotics such as nalidixic acid, cinoxacin, and oxalinic acid appears to be due either to an altered DNA gyrase or, in some bacteria, to failure of entry of the agent. This resistance is not plasmid mediated, but results from a mutation or from selection of resistant strains from the bacterial population. Resistance to the new fluorinated carboxy quinolones such as norfloxacin, enoxacin, and ciprofloxacin may be caused by an altered DNA gyrase A unit or by altered porins in the wall of the bacteria.

Resistance Due to Decreased Entry of a Drug

TETRACYCLINE RESISTANCE   The uptake of tetracycline by members of the Enterobacteriaceae is biphasic. In an initial energy-independent rapid phase, tetracycline binds to cell surface layers and passes by diffusion through the outer layers of the cell. In the second, energy-dependent phase, tetracycline crosses the cytoplasmic membrane, probably by means of a proton-motive force. The precise transport system has not been identified.

Tetracycline resistance is common in both Gram-positive and Gram-negative bacteria. In most cases it is plasmid encoded and inducible; however, chromosomal, constitutive resistance is found in some organisms such as *Proteus* species. Many plasmid-encoded specified tetracycline resistance determinants have been found in enteric bacteria. The most common of these determinants, TetB, is also present in *H influenzae*. Tetracycline resistance in *Staphylococcus aureus* is due primarily to small multicopy plasmids; chromosomal resistance is rare. Tetracycline resistance is found on nonconjugative plasmids in *Streptococcus faecalis* and on the chromosome of *S pneumoniae, S agalactiae* (group B streptococci), and oral streptococci. *Clostridium* species such as *C difficile* harbor chromosomal genes for tetracycline resistance.

Basically, tetracycline resistance is due to a decrease in the levels of drug accumulation. Decreased uptake and increased efflux both probably

participate: resistant bacteria bind less tetracycline, and the tetracycline they do accumulate is lost by an energy-dependent process when they are in a drug-free milieu.

Plasmid resistance to tetracyclines can be partially overcome in Gram-positive species by modifying the tetracycline nucleus. Hence, achievable concentrations of minocycline and doxycycline, in particular, will inhibit some tetracycline-resistant streptococci, such as *S pneumoniae*, and some *S aureus* strains. Molecular modification has not been successful in overcoming the tetracycline resistance of members of the Enterobacteriaceae or *Pseudomonas* or most *Bacteroides* species.

Tetracycline resistance is a major concern because it is located on plasmids near insertion sites, and these plasmids readily acquire other genetic information to enlarge the spectrum of resistance. The widespread use of tetracycline in animal feeds may be a factor in the extensive, worldwide resistance of members of the Enterobacteriaceae, particularly enteric species such as *Salmonella*, to tetracyclines and subsequently to many other drugs. Not only can tetracycline resistance move among members of the Enterobacteriaceae on plasmids, but plasmids mediating tetracycline resistance have moved between *S aureus, S epidermidis, S pyogenes, S pneumoniae*, and *S faecalis*.

FOSFOMYCIN RESISTANCE   Fosfomycin and fosmidomycin, which inhibit cell wall synthesis, enter bacteria by means of a glycerol-phosphate or glucose-6-phosphate transport system. Gram-positive bacteria in which the glucose-6-phosphate transport system is poorly developed do not take up these drugs in concentrations adequate to inhibit the cell wall synthesis. This resistance usually is chromosomal. The resistance of Gram-negative bacteria to these agents is related primarily to the presence in the population of some bacteria that can function without the transport system. Plasmids and transposons that transfer resistance to fosfomycin have been found in bacteria such as *Serratia marcescens*.

AMINOGLYCOSIDE RESISTANCE   In the most important form of aminoglycoside resistance, the compound is modified outside the cell and resistance is due partly to poor uptake of the altered compound. Also, all aminoglycosides have free amino and hydroxy groups that are essential for binding to ribosomal proteins. A number of enzymes can acetylate the amino groups and phosphorylate or adenylate the hydroxyl groups (Fig. 11-9). Other forms of resistance, such as altered binding site on 30S ribosomes, are much less common.

In members of the Enterobacteriaceae and in *Pseudomonas* species, the aminoglycosides pass through the cell wall via channels designed to admit cationic molecules to the periplasmic space. These channels, called **porin channels,** are lined by the porin protein. Aminoglycosides are then translocated across the cell membrane by an energy-dependent proton-motive force and, in the cytoplasm, bind to ribosomes located just below the membrane. Aminoglycosides bind only to ribosomes actively engaged in protein synthesis. Binding to the ribosomes induces a protein involved in the uptake of the aminoglycosides.

Bacteria may contain in the periplasmic space enzymes that acetylate, phosphorylate, or adenylate aminoglycosides to various degrees. It is not clear whether the enzymes are free in the periplasmic space or bound to the cytoplasmic membrane. The modified aminoglycosides do not bind well to ribosomes, and hence uptake is poor or absent (Fig. 11-16).

Aminoglycoside-modifying enzymes have been found in Gram-positive species such as *S aureus, S faecalis, S pyogenes,* and *S pneumoniae.* These enzymes are particularly prevalent in members of the Enterobacteriaceae and *P aeruginosa.* Many of the genes for aminoglycoside-modifying enzymes are carried on transposons.

Anaerobic organisms such as *Bacteroides* species are resistant to aminoglycosides because they lack an oxygen-dependent transport system to move the drugs across the cytoplasmic membrane. Although most resistance of *S aureus* to aminoglycosides is due to aminoglycoside-modifying enzymes, small-colony variants of staphylococci also show resistance, which may be due to a defect in adenylate cyclase or in cyclic adenosine 5′-monophosphate (cAMP)-binding proteins such that cells with a reduced growth rate do not transport aminoglycosides into the cytoplasm. Some members of the Enterobacteriaceae and *P aeruginosa* appear to be resistant because of altered porin channels, since these bacteria do not take up any drug and do not have aminoglycoside-inactivating enzymes.

Resistance Due to Destruction or Inactivation of a Drug

CHORAMPHENICOL RESISTANCE　Many Gram-positive and Gram-negative bacteria, including some recently discovered *H influenzae* strains, are resistant to chloramphenicol because they possess the enzyme chloramphenicol transacetylate, which acetylates hydroxyl groups on the chloramphenicol structure. This enzyme, unlike the aminoglycoside-inactivating enzymes and β-lactamases, is an intracellular enzyme of higher molecular weight and subunit structure. Acetylated chloramphenicol binds less well to the 50S ribosome.

β-LACTAM RESISTANCE　The best-known mechanism of bacterial resistance is the resistance to β-lactams, which is mediated by penicillinase enzymes. Resistance of *E coli* to penicillin was recognized in 1940, before sufficient penicillin was made to be clinically useful. In the 1940s, resistance of staphylococci was shown to be due to a penicillinase. As these enzymes also attack other β-lactam compounds such as cephalosporins, carbapenems, and monobactams, they would be more appropriately designated β-lactamases. The most important activity of these enzymes is alteration of the β-lactam nucleus (Fig. 11-17). β-Lactamases are widely distributed in nature and are usually classified on the basis of the principal compounds they destroy (e.g., as penicillinases or cephalosporinases) (Fig. 11-18). β-Lactamases may be chromosomally or plasmid mediated, and they may be constitutive or inducible.

In Gram-positive species, β-lactamases are primarily exoenzymes; that is, they are excreted into the milieu around the bacteria. Virtually all hospital isolates of staphylococci, both *S aureus* and *S epidermidis,* have β-lactamases, and 50 to 80 percent of community-acquired staphylococcal iso-

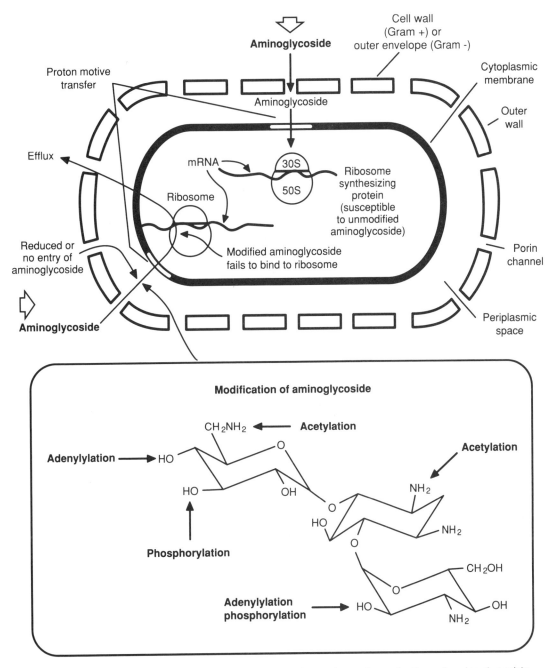

FIGURE 11-16 Diagrammatic representations of transfer and transfer reduction of aminoglycoside across the bacterial cell wall. If it is modified by acetylation, adenylation, or phosphorylation (see box), the drug will not bind to ribosomes and will leave the bacterial cell.

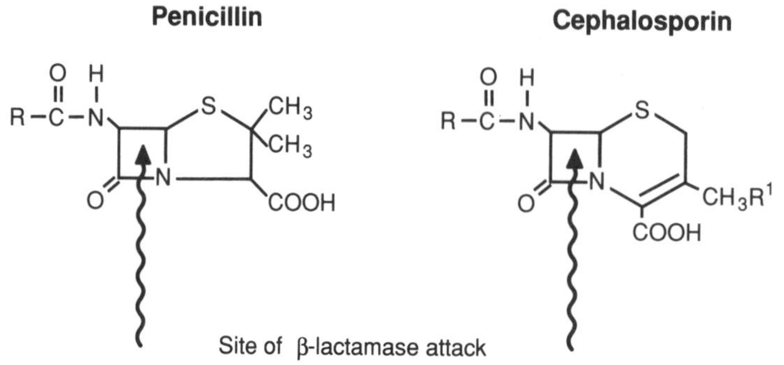

Penicillin   **Cephalosporin**

Site of β-lactamase attack

FIGURE 11-17   Site of *β*-lactamase attack in penicillins and cephalosporins.

lates produce *β*-lactamases. In Gram-negative species, both aerobic and anaerobic, *β*-lactamases are contained in the periplasmic space, thus effectively protecting the penicillin-binding proteins.

Resistance of staphylococci to *β*-lactams was soon overcome with the antistaphylococcal peni-

cillins and the cephalosporins. Some strains of *S aureus* produce more *β*-lactamase constitutively and can destroy some of the cephalosporins.

In 1974, *H influenzae* was shown to possess a plasmid-mediated *β*-lactamase. At present 10 to 35 percent of *H influenzae* strains in the United States

β-Lactamases and Their Distribution in Nature

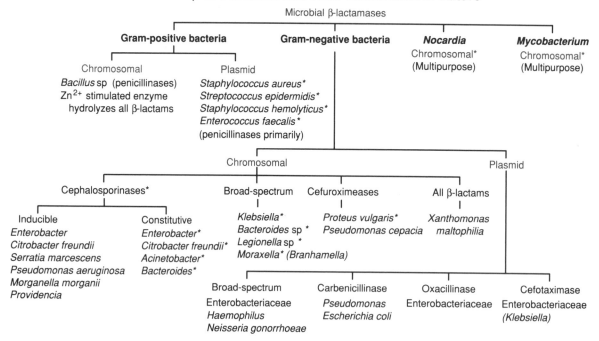

*Inhibited by clavulanate, sulbactam

FIGURE 11-18   *β*-Lactamases found in bacteria and their classification and synthesis, whether chromosomally or plasmid mediated.

produce β-lactamases. The TnA transposon has become more widespread, and the resistance of *Haemophilus* species to penicillin G and ampicillin seems to be increasing yearly. The *Haemophilus* β-lactamase is the same structurally as the enzyme found in *E coli, Salmonella, Shigella,* and *N gonorrhoeae.* The enzyme has generally been called the TEM enzyme after the initials of the Greek girl from whom an *E coli* strain containing a plasmid β-lactamase was first isolated. These enzymes are also called Richmond-Sykes class IIIa enzymes from a classification proposed by Richmond and Sykes in 1973. By far the most common plasmid β-lactamase found in nature is TEM-1, which accounts for 75 to 80 percent of plasmid-mediated β-lactamase resistance worldwide. Recently new β-lactamases have been found that hydrolyze compounds such as inomethoxy cephalosporin, which were not destroyed by other plasmid β-lactamases. The new β-lactamases have an altered amino acid composition, which permits binding to the cephalosporin and subsequent hydrolysis. How common these new enzymes will become is unknown.

Chromosomally mediated β-lactamases are present in many *Enterobacter, Citrobacter, Proteus-Providencia,* and *Pseudomonas* species. All *Klebsiella* species possess a β-lactamase, which acts primarily as a penicillinase and is chromosomally mediated. Constitutively produced β-lactamase are also present in many anaerobic species.

Table 11-3 lists the major β-lactamases of clinical importance. β-Lactamases vary in their ability to destroy penicillins and cephalosporins. β-Lactamase activity is only one component of the β-lactam resistance of Gram-negative bacteria, since resistance to β-lactams is a combination of decreased entry, β-lactamase stability, and affinity of the compounds for penicillin-binding proteins.

Synthesis of Resistant Metabolic Pathway

No synthesis of a new type of cell wall resistant to β-lactams has occurred, but some bacteria, particularly some streptococci, lack the hydrolytic enzymes necessary for forming a new cell wall, and so β-lactams do not lyse these bacteria. An altered hydrolytic system thus converts a bactericidal antibiotic into a bacteriostatic agent. Whether such resistance occurs in Gram-negative species is not clear.

Some thymidine-requiring streptococci are not inhibited by trimethoprim and sulfonamides and so are not killed by these agents. These organisms are a rare cause of urinary tract infections. Other bacteria produce adequate deoxyribosylthymine 5′-monophosphate (dTMP) by alternative methods and, as a result, survive exposure to these folate inhibitors.

Certain *Candida* or *Cryptococcus* yeasts are resistant to flucytosine because they cannot convert it to its active component, fluorouracil. Other fungi can resist the polyenes and imidazoles because they synthesize membrane components by different metabolic mechanisms.

COMBINATIONS OF ANTIMICROBIAL AGENTS

Antibiotics are frequently used in combination for the following reasons: (1) to treat a life-threatening infection; (2) to prevent emergence of bacterial resistance; (3) to treat mixed infections of aerobic and anaerobic bacteria; (4) to enhance antibacterial activity (**synergy**); and (5) to use lower doses of a toxic drug. Combined treatment is reasonable when the precise agents of a serious infection are unknown. Use of two or more drugs to prevent the emergence of resistance is effective for tuberculosis and for therapy of some chronic infections. The use of combinations to achieve synergy is more complicated. Synergy occurs when a combination of two drugs causes inhibition or killing when used at a fourfold-lower concentration than that of either component drug used separately (Fig. 11-19). However, indifference or antagonism may occur instead. **Indifference** means that the combined action is the same as with either component; **antagonism** refers to a reduction in the activity of one or both components in the presence of the other (Fig. 11-19).

Important examples of bacterial synergy include (1) combinations of anti-cell wall agents with aminoglycosides, (2) use of β-lactamase inhibitors with

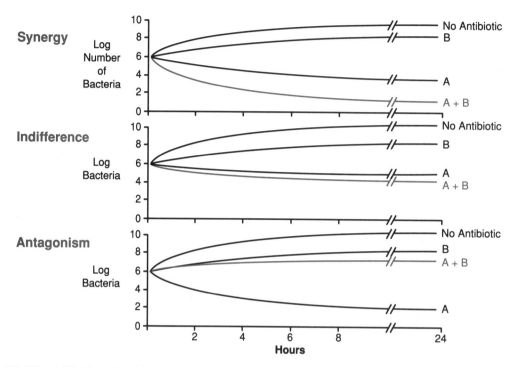

FIGURE 11-19   Example of how two antibiotics (A and B) may interact with synergy, indifference, or antagonism.

β-lactamase-susceptible antibiotics, and (3) combinations of drugs that act on sequential steps in bacterial metabolic or synthetic pathways. Examples of synergy that have proved clinically important are the combination of penicillin and streptomycin to treat *Enterococcus faecalis* endocarditis and the combination of carbenicillin and gentamicin to treat *P aeruginosa* infections. Recently the β-lactamase inhibitor clavulanic acid or sulbactam has been combined with amino penicillins to inhibit *S aureus*, *Klebsiella pneumoniae*, *H influenzae*, and anaerobic organisms such as *Bacteroides* species, all of which are resistant to amoxicillin or ampicillin when they contain β-lactamases. The combination of sulfamethoxazole and trimethoprim attacks two parts of the folic acid cycle and synergistically inhibits many bacteria. Finally, combinations of two penicillins that affect different stages of cell wall synthesis in Gram-negative bacteria are synergistic. This is true for the combination of mecillinam (amdinocillin), which binds to PBP2 of bacteria,

and penicillins or cephalosporins, which bind to PBP 1b or 3.

Antagonism can occur when a bacteriostatic agent is combined with a bactericidal agent. The classic example has been the combination of chlortetracycline and penicillin in treatment of pneumococcal meningitis. This effect has not been explained from a molecular standpoint, and tetracyclines and penicillins or cephalosporins are used to treat mixed infections such as pelvic inflammatory disease due to *N gonorrhoeae* and *Chlamydia*. Some β-lactam antibiotics can induce β-lactamases that inactivate other β-lactams, and antagonism can be shown in the test tube, but the relevance for clinical infections is not established.

TOXICOLOGY OF ANTIMICROBIAL AGENTS

Antimicrobial agents can be directly toxic, can interact with other drugs to increase their toxicity, or can alter microbial flora to cause infection by organisms that are normally saprophytic. Allergic reactions can be caused by any agent, but penicillins can produce either immediate, IgE-mediated, or delayed hypersensitivity reactions. Cutaneous reactions have been reported with every class of antimicrobial agent. Hematologic reactions can range from the life-threatening blood dyscrasias that occurs in 1 in 60,000 individuals who receive chloramphenicol to hemolytic anemia due to sulfonamides in individuals who lack the enzyme glucose-6-phosphate dehydrogenase. Depression of blood platelet activity has occurred with many agents. By altering the gastrointestinal flora, almost all antibiotics can cause overgrowth of *Clostridicum difficile,* which produces a toxin that causes diarrhea and even pseudomembranous colitis. Alteration of intestinal flora by antibiotics can also result in overgrowth of *Candida* in the mouth, vagina, or gastrointestinal tract. Since a number of antibiotics are metabolized in the liver, damage to the liver can occur. This has been of particular concern with isoniazid, which is used to treat tuberculosis. Damage to the kidneys can follow the use of aminoglycosides. Neurologic toxicity is fortunately fairly uncommon, but the aminoglycosides can damage the auditory or vestibular apparatus if the dosage is not closely monitored.

Bacteria continue to evolve new mechanisms of resistance to old and to new antimicrobial agents. Some bacteria such as *P aeruginosa* are particularly adept at utilizing a number of different mechanisms simultaneously to become resistant to agents in virtually every class and those with such diverse sites of action as cell wall, protein biosynthesis, or DNA and RNA synthesis. Progress in medicine will keep patients alive who have nosocomial infections with resistant pathogens.

MECHANISM TO REDUCE BACTERIAL RESISTANCE

Proper selection of new antibiotics will be a major force in slowing the development of antimicrobial resistance. Proper hygiene practices will reduce

TABLE 11-4 Mechanisms To Reduce Antibiotic Resistance

1. Control, reduce, or cycle antibiotic usage
2. Improve hygiene in hospitals and among hospital personnel and reduce movement of patients to eliminate the dissemination of resistant organisms within hospitals
3. Discover or develop new antibiotics
4. Modify existing antibiotics chemically to produce compounds inert to known mechanisms of resistance
5. Develop inhibitors of antibiotic-modifying enzymes
6. Define agents that would "cure" resistance plasmids

plasmid transfer and the establishment of multiple drug-resistant bacteria in the hospital and will delay the appearance of such species in the community. Table 11-4 lists a number of mechanisms to prevent bacterial resistance. The health care provider must be continually alert to the appearance of antibiotic resistance within the hospital and community.

REFERENCES

Bryan LE: General mechanisms of resistance to antibiotics. J Antimicrob Chemother 22(Suppl A):1, 1982

Gale EF, Cundliffe E, Reynolds PE et al: The Molecular Basis of Antibiotic Action. 2nd Ed. John Wiley & Sons, New York, 1981

Kucers A, Bennett N: The use of antibiotics. 4th Ed. JB Lippincott, Philadelphia, 1985

Lorian V (ed): Antibiotics in Laboratory Medicine. 3rd Ed. Williams & Wilkins, Baltimore, 1991

Neu HC (ed): Update on antibiotics. I. Med Clin N Am 71:1051, 1987

Neu HC (ed): Update on antibiotics. II. Med Clin N Am 72:555, 1988

Norrby SR, Bergan T, Holm SE et al (eds): Evaluation of new beta-lactam antibiotics. Rev Infect Dis 8(Suppl 3):S235, 1986

Waxman DJ, Strominger JL: Beta-lactam antibiotics: biochemical modes of action. p. 210. In Morin RB, Gorman M (eds): Chemistry and Biology of Beta-Lactam Antibiotics. Academic Press, San Diego, 1982

Wolfson JS, Hooper DC (eds): Quinolone Antimicrobial Agents. American Society for Microbiology, Washington, 1989

12

STAPHYLOCOCCUS

JAY O. COHEN

GENERAL CONCEPTS

Clinical Manifestations

Staphylococcus infections take several forms: (1) *S aureus* may infect any organ, usually causing a small, focal lesion (e.g., a boil or a stye). *S aureus* may alternatively cause bacteremia, septicemia, deep-wound infections, endocarditis, pneumonia, and/or osteomyelitis. (2) *S epidermidis* is a skin commensal and may cause bacteremia or endocarditis. (3) *S saprophyticus* is found in urinary tract infections, especially in girls. (4) *S intermedius* occurs in infections of dogs and other animals. (5) *S capitis, S warner, S haemolyticus, S saccharolyticus,* and other new species occur mostly in the environment and in the normal flora and are only occasionally pathogenic.

Structure

Staphylococci are Gram-positive cocci 1 μm in diameter. They form clumps.

Classification and Antigenic Types

S aureus and *S intermedius* are coagulase positive; other staphylococci are coagulase negative. Staphylococci are salt tolerant, grow on nutrient agar, and are often hemolytic. Group- and type-specific antigens occur.

Pathogenesis

S aureus colonizes the nasal passages and axillae; *S epidermidis* colonizes the skin. Staphylococci may invade the host when defenses break down. *S aureus* produces

toxins and enzymes that contribute to pathogenicity. Enterotoxins cause food poisoning. Other toxins are responsible for the scalded skin syndrome and the toxic shock syndrome.

Host Defenses

Both naturally occurring and stimulated antibodies are produced. Bacterial protein A reacts with IgG at the Fc fragment. Protein A influences immunity and may interfere with the complement system.

Epidemiology

Epidemic strains of *S aureus* are found especially in hospitals. Phage typing and other markers are used to identify epidemic strains.

Diagnosis

The diagnosis is based on a Gram strain showing Gram-positive cocci in clumps from broth. Coagulase-positive cultures are *S aureus* or *S intermedius. S aureus* is protein A positive. Repeated isolation of a similar type of *S epidermidis* is helpful in the diagnosis of bacteremia.

Control

Patients and staff carrying epidemic strains should be isolated from noninfected persons. Phage typing should be used to identify strains. Hospital nursery employees should wash hands before handling each baby. Eradication of epidemic strains is impossible because of the close association of staphylococci with humans and animals.

Treatment

Infections are treated with penicillinase-resistant antibiotics such as methicillin and vancomycin.

INTRODUCTION

Bacteria in the genus *Staphylococcus* are opportunistic pathogens of humans and some other mammals. Traditionally, they are divided into two groups on the basis of their ability to clot blood plasma (the **coagulase reaction**). The **coagulase-positive** staphylococci constitute the species *S aureus.* The **coagulase-negative** staphylococci are basically saprophytes, even though they occasionally cause infections. These staphylococci were originally referred to as *S epidermidis,* but since then have been further differentiated according to biochemical characteristics and cell wall chemistry.

The staphylococci form a variety of extracellular substances, some of which are correlated with virulence. The overall virulence of a strain probably results from the cumulative effect of several of these substances during infection. Antibodies are effective in neutralizing the staphylococcal toxins and enzymes, but both antibiotics and surgical drainage are often necessary to cure abscesses, large boils, and wound infections.

CLINICAL MANIFESTATIONS

Coagulase-positive staphylococci are notorious for causing boils, furuncles, styes, infantile impetigo, and other superficial skin infections in humans (Figs. 12-1 and 12-2). They may cause more serious infections in persons debilitated by chronic illness, traumatic injury, burns, or immunosuppression. These infections include staphylococcal pneumonia, deep abscesses (Fig. 12-3), osteomyelitis, acute endocarditis, phlebitis, mastitis, and meningitis. *S aureus* has been isolated from infections of all organs of the body.

The introduction of antibiotics and the long hospitalization of chronically ill persons have resulted in a dramatic change in the host-parasite relationship of humans and staphylococci. Chronically ill, debilitated patients such as burn and cancer victims often suffer severe infections caused by *S aureus* strains that are resistant to many commonly used antibiotics. Similarly, mastitis (udder infection) in dairy cattle, which in the days before antibiotics was caused mainly by group B and C streptococci, now is caused mainly by penicillin-resistant coagulase-positive staphylococci.

STRUCTURE

Staphylococci are Gram-positive cocci about 0.5 to 1.0 μm in diameter. They grow in clusters, pairs, and, occasionally, short chains. The clusters arise because staphylococci divide in two planes. The configuration of the cocci helps one to distinguish micrococci and staphylococci from streptococci, which usually grow in chains. Observations must be made on cultures grown in broth, because streptococci grown on solid medium may appear in clumps. Several fields should be examined before deciding whether clumps or chains predominate.

The catalase test is also important, as it distinguishes the streptococci, which are catalase negative, from other Gram-positive cocci. The test can be performed by flooding an agar slant or broth culture with several drops of 3% hydrogen peroxide. Catalase positive cultures bubble at once. The test should be done on a duplicate culture because peroxide is bactericidal, but it should not be done on blood agar plates because the blood itself may produce bubbles.

CLASSIFICATION AND ANTIGENIC TYPES

Traditionally, the staphylococci have been divided into two groups according to their ability to clot

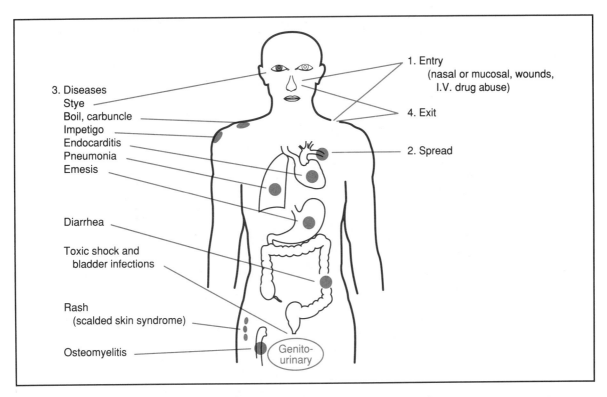

FIGURE 12-1 Pathogenesis of staphylococcal infections.

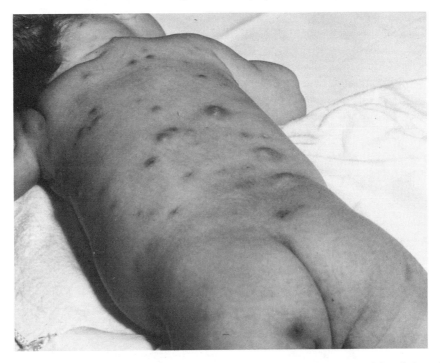

FIGURE 12-2 Widespread staphylococcal furunculosis in an infant. (Photograph by Centers for Disease Control. From Shulman JA, Nahmias AJ: Staphylococcal infections: clinical aspects. p. 461. In Cohen JO (ed): The Staphylococci. John Wiley & Sons, New York, 1972, with permission.)

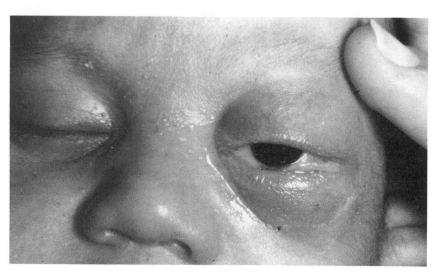

FIGURE 12-3 Child with thrombosis of the cavernous sinus (venous space in dura mater), a serious complication of staphylococcal skin infection. (Photograph by Centers for Disease Control. From Shulman JA, Nahmias AJ: Staphylococcal infections: clinical aspects. p. 462. In Cohen JO (ed): The Staphylococci. John Wiley & Sons, New York, 1972, with permission.)

blood plasma (the coagulase reaction). **Coagulase-positive staphylococci** are members of the species *S aureus*. They are considered to be opportunistic pathogens in humans and some other mammals. The **coagulase-negative staphylococci** are considered to be saprophytes, even though they are occasionally responsible for infections. Recently, the coagulase-positive strains have been subdivided according to the animal host, kind of plasma coagulated, serotype, and bacteriophage type.

Antigens

S aureus strains have group-specific and type-specific antigens. More than 90 percent of *S aureus* strains have protein A at the surface. This antigen is not found on coagulase-negative staphylococci and has not been reported in any other microbial species. Protein A reacts with the IgGs of humans, mice, rabbits, and other mammals. The reaction occurs through the Fc fragment of the IgG molecule and thus is different from the usual antibody reaction. The ability to react does not appear to require antigenic stimulation. Protein A reactions

have been observed by serum gel precipitation, fluorescent-antibody, and slide agglutination tests. The amounts of reactive immunoglobulin and the intensities of the reactions differ from animal to animal.

The ability of *S aureus* to attract IgG antibodies that attach at the Fc portion is the basis for various serologic tests for both soluble and dispersed insoluble antigens, as this characteristic makes possible a process called **coagglutination,** in which the IgG-coated *S aureus* agglutinates in the presence of antigen. The IgG used in these tests is from specific antisera against the antigen being measured. A quantitative measurement of antigen can be obtained by preparing serial dilutions. The specific antibody-combining sites are free to react with antigen, even though the other end of the molecule is attached to the staphylococcal cell. Combination with the antigen causes the staphylococci to agglutinate, thus providing a useful test to detect numerous antigens (see Fig. 10-2).

Another surface antigen that is group specific for *S aureus* is a specific ribitol teichoic acid known as polysaccharide A. An α-linked glucosyl glycerol teichoic acid has been identified in coagulase-negative staphylococci and named polysaccharide B. The teichoic acids can be identified and distinguished by serum-gel diffusion tests.

In addition to the group-specific antigens of staphylococci, type-specific antigens have been used for serotyping *S aureus*. Staphylococci have usually been further differentiated by **phage typing**, in which strains are distinguished by the pattern of susceptibility to lysis by specific bacteriophages.

Toxins

S aureus strains have been shown to release several toxins into the environment (Table 12-1). However, no one strain produces all of the toxins; most of the toxins can be specifically identified by serum-gel precipitation. They also can be identified by a neutralization test, that is, by counteracting the toxic effects with specific antiserum.

Hemolysins

Hemolysins cause red blood cells to lyse, and they act against cell membranes with some degree of specificity. α-Hemolysin is most active against rabbit erythrocytes. It is found in almost all human strains of staphylococci and in most animal strains.

β-Hemolysin (a sphingomyelinase) is much more active against sheep erythrocytes than against human or rabbit erythrocytes. This toxin is found in 88 percent of *S aureus* animal strains, but in only 10 percent of human *S aureus* strains. Two other weaker hemolysins, δ and ϵ, are found in both human and animal strains.

Leukocidin

Many strains of *S aureus* produce leukocidins, which are toxins that kill leukocytes and macrophages. The Panton-Valentine leukocidin is the only toxin that attacks leukocytes but no other cells. Woodin has shown that this leukocidin is composed of two separate proteins, both of which are required for a strong antileukocytic effect. The two components have been separated on carboxymethyl cellulose and are recognized as nonidentical antigens in serum-gel precipitations when diffused against rabbit immune serum.

Enterotoxins

Some *S aureus* strains release enterotoxins into foods. When the food is eaten, the enterotoxins cause a form of food poisoning. Usually the food is contaminated with large numbers of staphylococci. Vomiting and sometimes diarrhea occur

TABLE 12-1 Extracellular Substances Formed by Staphylococci

Toxins and Enzymes	Action
Hemolysins	Causes lysis of erythrocytes
α-Toxin	Most active against rabbit erythrocytes
β-Hemolysin	Most active against sheep erythrocytes
δ-Hemolysin	Weak hemolysin
ϵ-Hemolysin	Weak hemolysin
Leukocidin	Lethal toxicity for leukocytes and macrophages
Enterotoxins (serologically distinct types, A–E)	Intestinal fluid secretion
Exfoliative (epidermolytic) toxins	Dermonecrosis
Toxic shock syndrome toxin	Pyrogenic toxin perhaps leading to death
Coagulase	Clot formation
Fibrinolysin (staphylokinase)	Fibrin clots dissolved
DNase (nuclease)	Hydrolysis of the 5′ phosphodiester bond of DNA
Lipases (lipase, esterase, and phosphatidase)	Lipid hydrolysis
Hyaluronidase	Hydrolyzes hyaluronic acid in tissues

within a few hours after ingestion of food. Most people recover after 24 hours. The several serologically distinct staphylococcal enterotoxins (A, B, C, C_1, C_2, D, and E) are resistant to the proteolytic enzymes of the digestive tract, although they are simple, single-chain, globular proteins. The known enterotoxins, A to E, can be identified by serologic tests such as serum-gel diffusion and radioimmunoassay. At present, only a few laboratories have the capability to identify these toxins routinely. When the toxin in a food cannot be identified, epidemiologic evidence of staphylococcal food poisoning usually shows large numbers of staphylococci in samples of the food eaten by most of the sick persons.

Scalded Skin Syndrome (Exfoliative or Epidermolytic) Toxins

S aureus strains, particularly some of those of bacteriophage group II, cause a type of childhood impetigo called the **scalded skin syndrome,** in which the outer layers of the epidermis peel off, revealing "scalded" skin. Recently, two of these toxins were demonstrated in bacteriophage group II strains, one plasmid encoded and the other inherited chromosomally. The two toxins are distinct immunologically.

A case of toxic epidermal necrolysis due to *S aureus* has been described in an infant who developed toxic shock syndrome and died. It is important to distinguish this syndrome from staphylococcal scalded skin syndrome, which usually is self-limiting.

Toxic Shock Syndrome Toxin

In 1980, a new disease was observed that affects young women when they are menstruating. The symptoms of the disease resemble those reported by Todd and Fishaut (1978), who isolated a new toxin from cultures of the staphylococci from skin infections. The new disease was called **toxic shock syndrome (TSS).** Shortly thereafter, TSS cases were reported in which severe symptoms and some deaths occurred. Unlike the earlier subjects, these women did not have skin infections or other overt

signs of infection. However, most of the women affected were menstruating at the onset of TSS and almost all had used tampons. Seventy-three deaths in 941 cases were reported to the Centers for Disease Control (CDC). Accordingly, TSS must be counted as an important disease because of the severity of its symptoms. On the other hand, the disease is relatively rare when one considers the millions of women at risk and the small percentage who show symptoms. A few cases of TSS have been reported in men and nonmenstruating women; however, these patients usually had overt staphylococcal infections.

Recent work, done independently in two different laboratories, has resulted in the isolation and identification of an exotoxin that was present in all strains of staphylococci isolated from patients with TSS. The toxin is pyrogenic in rabbits but does not lead to the rash seen in humans. The capacity to identify the toxin enhances the ability to study the epidemiology and toxicology of this new disease. The toxin is now called **TSS toxin 1 (TSST 1).**

Extracellular Enzymes

In addition to known toxins of *S aureus*, enzymes are produced by staphylococci that diffuse from the cells and are active on extracellular substrates (Table 1). Some of these have been considered to be pathogenicity factors primarily because they are often found in the more virulent strains of staphylococci.

Coagulase

Aside from its taxonomic importance in delineating potentially pathogenic strains, coagulase has been assigned a pathogenic role in infections by some investigators. This role in infections is debatable because of the frequency with which humans and animals carry coagulase-positive staphylococci without apparent harm. If coagulase is a factor in infections, it does not appear to be involved in the early stages of disease. Some authors have distinguished between two different molecular forms of coagulase, as the substrate of one is human plasma and that of the other is bovine plasma. Some strains produce both forms of coagulase simultaneously, and each form is active on its substrate in the presence or absence of the other.

Fibrinolysin (Staphylokinase)

About 95 percent of coagulase-positive staphylococci from humans produce fibrinolysin, an enzyme that dissolves fibrin clots. Only 9 percent of 115 animal strains tested made fibrinolysin. This difference is important in distinguishing animal and human strains. Fibrinolysin is not an important pathogenicity factor. An enzyme similar to fibrinolysin from group A streptococci has been purified and used in human medicine to help debride wounds in which fibrin is part of the lesion.

DNase (Nuclease)

S aureus strains produce a thermostable, calcium-activated enzyme called deoxyribonuclease (DNase). The enzyme hydrolyzes the 5' phosphodiester bond and thereby differs in action from pancreatic DNase and some other phosphodiesterases. The ability to produce this DNase is a property of virulent staphylococci, but the contribution of DNase to virulence in microorganisms is not well understood.

Lipases

Staphylococci produce several lipid-hydrolyzing enzymes. Lipolysis probably depends on three enzymes—lipase, esterase, and phosphatidase. About 99.5 percent of human strains of *S aureus* are lipolytic, as are 30 percent of coagulase-negative strains. One of the tests used to demonstrate lipases involves the ability of some strains of staphylococci to break down egg yolk, usually in an agar medium. The relationship between egg yolk positivity and potential pathogenicity has been a subject of much controversy; some reports indicate that possession of egg-yolk-lysing factor delineates more pathogenic strains, and other reports make the opposite inference, that the egg-yolk-negative strains are more capable of spreading and setting up systemic infections. These contrary opinions still exist, and the argument has not been resolved.

Hyaluronidase

Hyaluronidase hydrolyzes hyaluronic acid of human and animal tissues. Duran-Reynolds in 1929 described this activity as the **spreading factor** and showed that such enzymes could enhance the spread of viral or microbial infections in animals. Modern researchers use the term **hyaluronic lyases** for these factors. Abramson and Friedman in 1964 demonstrated the presence of four multiple molecular forms of this enzyme. Its pathogenicity is not well known, but it does tend to be found in coagulase positive strains that produce pathogenicity factors such as fibrinolysin, DNase, lipases, and protease.

PATHOGENESIS

Some of the staphylococcal products described above correlate with virulence. Overall virulence probably results from the cumulative effect of several of these substances during infection. Antibodies are effective in neutralizing the toxic effects of the staphylococcal toxins and enzymes, but both antibiotics and surgical drainage are often necessary to cure abscesses, large boils, and wound infections.

The staphylococci are often viewed as microorganisms on their way to a commensal, nonpathogenic relationship with humans. All coagulase-negative staphylococci, except perhaps *S saprophyticus,* are considered noninvasive and only occasionally pathogenic. *S epidermidis* is found on normal human skin. Coagulase-positive staphylococci (the *S aureus* strains) appear to be carried naturally in the anterior nares and in the axillae, although they are occasionally isolated from skin. The use of antibiotics in hospitals has allowed populations of antibiotic-resistant bacteria to develop; these bacteria are often carried by hospital personnel and patients. Specific strains of *S aureus* causing hospital epidemics in nurseries and in surgical and burn wards have been detected by phage typing, serotyping, determining antibiotic resistance patterns (antibiograms), and performing plasmid analysis.

Pigeons, dogs, and other animals carry coagulase-positive staphylococci peculiar to the host animal. Dogs often carry *S intermedius,* a coagulase-positive form that does not produce protein A. Although these animals occasionally become infected with staphylococci, the relationship appears to be often commensal.

The pathogenesis of *S aureus* infections is not well understood. Many factors found in *S aureus* strains, but not in coagulase-negative strains, are considered virulence factors; these include heat-resistant DNase, coagulase, α-hemolysin, leukocidin, and protein A. Strains isolated during serious infections have more of these factors than do strains from carriers, but little is known about the role of these factors in initiating infections or about the interactions that may allow staphylococci to invade the host. All strains capable of producing enterotoxin do not necessarily cause food poisoning. The strain must also be capable of growing well in a specific food, and it must produce significant amounts of toxin.

Therefore, the staphylococci are enigmatic. They can be isolated from the human flora, but their presence may not be significant; however, isolation from a deep abscess, pleural fluid, bone, spinal fluid, superficial abscess, or blood indicates serious infection. Before an infection is considered to be serious, large numbers of staphylococci should be isolated and identified, except in blood specimens, in which any bacteria isolated are significant.

HOST DEFENSES

S aureus appears to have been associated with humans for a long time. Both parasite and host have developed factors against each other and even against the defense factors. Human serum contains a heat-labile opsonin that facilitates the phagocytosis of staphylococci. Some *S aureus* strains can live inside the leukocyte and eventually kill it. Some strains produce a capsule that makes them refractory to phagocytosis. Humans can make antibody to these capsules and thereby promote opsonization of these virulent strains for phagocytosis.

Several examples of interaction between *S aureus* and its hosts have been reported. Staphylo-

coccal protein A can attract IgG antibodies to the staphylococcal surfaces without regard to the specificity of the antibodies. This attraction apparently does not lead to opsonization of, or injury to, the staphylococci. This reaction may also block complement-mediated bactericidal mechanisms by binding the Fc portion of IgG and masking complement receptor sites on the staphylococcus-specific immunoglobulin.

For each of the staphylococcal protein pathogenicity factors, such as toxins and enzymes, specific antibodies can be evoked in humans to inactivate the factor. Even before antibiotic therapy is introduced into the struggle, the host and bacterium engage in a complex tug-of-war.

Antibody defenses against *S aureus* can be arbitrarily divided into four categories: (1) naturally occurring antibodies and antibodylike activities; (2) group antibodies, found in adult humans, against a common staphylococcal antigen (teichoic acid or peptidoglycan); (3) specific antibodies evoked in response to vaccines or infections, perhaps against only a few strains; and (4) antibodies against staphylococcal toxins. The interplay between these factors and cell-mediated immunity leading to recovery from infections is not understood. Despite the development of significant immunologic responses, antibiotics and surgical drainage usually are necessary to cure abscesses, large boils, and wound infections.

EPIDEMIOLOGY

Although serious infections have been observed since the beginning of modern bacteriology, the epidemiology of *S aureus* infections has changed dramatically since penicillin and other antibiotics were introduced. Almost all *S aureus* strains were at first sensitive to penicillin. By the mid-1950s, however, hospital strains of staphylococci were invariably resistant to penicillin and often to several other antibiotics as well. By the 1970s, most community-acquired staphylococcal infections were due to penicillinase-producing staphylococci. Penicillin resistance was shown to be caused by production of a β-lactamase (penicillinase) enzyme that inactivates penicillin. Epidemics caused by certain virulent strains of *S aureus* occurred in hospital nurseries, burn wards, and surgical wards; severe illnesses and some deaths resulted. Antibiotic resistance, especially penicillin resistance, can be transferred genetically from one *S aureus* cell to another on a plasmid introduced into the new strain by a bacteriophage in a process called **transduction.**

The staphylococci are still responsible for serious infections, but hospital epidemics are less common, probably because synthetic penicillins have been introduced that are resistant to penicillinase and are therefore effective against penicillin-resistant bacteria. New procedures to prevent cross-infection in hospital nurseries are credited with the decline of serious outbreaks in these areas. Methicillin-resistant staphylococci have been reported in hospitals in Europe and the United States. The mechanism of resistance is not enzymatic. The strains have not been epidemic, but the possibility of serious hospital infections remains. Changes in staphylococcal disease over the years have been caused by the introduction of new antibiotics and by the placement of most debilitated patients in hospitals.

DIAGNOSIS

Isolation and Identification

The presence of staphylococci in a lesion might first be suspected after examination of a direct Gram stain of a specimen. (Because of the small numbers of staphylococci present in blood, they are more likely to be detected by culture than by Gram stain). With the Gram stain, only the presence of Gram-positive cocci can be detected. Specific early identification can be achieved by direct fluorescent antibody staining with anti-staphylococcal serum.

The organism usually is isolated by streaking material from a swab onto solid media such as blood agar, tryptic soy agar, or heart infusion agar. Specimens likely to be highly contaminated with other microorganisms can be plated on selective media, such as mannitol salt agar, which contains 7.5 percent sodium chloride, or potassium tellurite agar. A Gram stain should be made of the isolated organism and tests run for catalase and coagulase production. The staphylococci are distinguished from other Gram-positive cocci by the tests shown in Fig. 12-4. Other tests are useful in confirming a diagnosis of *S aureus,* specifically one that demonstrates heat-stable DNase and another that tests sensitivity to lysostaphin (an extracellular peptidase made by a coagulase-negative staphylococcus); *S aureus* is readily lysed by 50 μg of lysostaphin per ml; most coagulase-negative staphylococci are resistant to this level of lysostaphin, but higher levels lyse these staphylococci. Micrococci are completely refractory to lysostaphin. A test that demonstrates protein A on the cells or in the broth supernatants or both confirms identification of *S aureus.*

Isolation of coagulase-negative staphylococci from the skin is not considered medically significant, because they are part of the normal microbial flora. However, these organisms, especially *S epidermidis*, have been implicated as the cause of subacute endocarditis. Therefore, isolation of coagulase-negative staphylococci from blood is important. A test should be set up to observe the ability of the isolate to ferment glucose anaerobically.

All staphylococci are capable of anaerobic growth with fermentation of glucose, but micrococci are not. *Micrococcus* strains are seldom the primary pathogens in specimens isolated during infections. The micrococci are considered chance contaminants in a blood sample, unless they have been isolated repeatedly. All members of the genus *Micrococcus* are coagulase negative and contain 57 to 75 moles percent guanine plus cytosine, whereas staphylococci contain between 30 and 40 moles percent. This is an important taxonomic difference, but only research laboratories have the capability to perform the test.

A single isolation of coagulase-negative cocci from a blood culture may result from chance contamination; repeated isolation usually indicates an infection. If several consecutive isolates have the same biotype, phage type, or antibiogram or are identical by some other valid marker system, infection rather than chance contamination is probable.

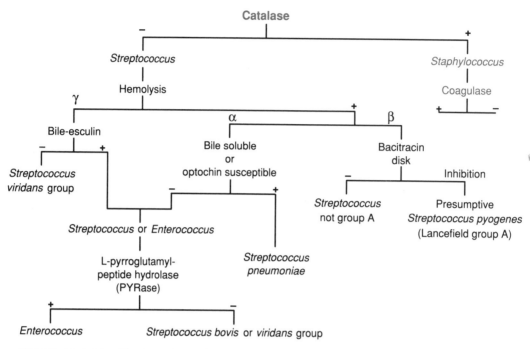

FIGURE 12-4   Identification scheme for distinguishing the several genera of Gram-positive cocci.

Phage Typing

S aureus organisms are ubiquitous on humans and in the environment. In epidemics, however, a single virulent strain is often at fault. Determining the source and extent of the epidemic requires knowledge of the type as well as the species. This knowledge is usually gained by phage typing, which is based on different lytic patterns obtained when different strains of bacteriophage are dropped on agar plates previously seeded with the test cultures of *S aureus*. After a period of incubation, usually at 30°C, the plate is examined for areas of lysis. In the international basic set of 24 bacteriophages, each bacteriophage has been assigned an Arabic numeral. Thus, if a culture is lysed by bacteriophages 80 and 81, its bacteriophage type is 80/81. The bacteriophages used have been carefully selected for this purpose, that is, for specificity coupled with the ability to lyse a reasonable proportion of strains. Phage typing is usually done in a reference laboratory such as that of a state public health department.

Serotyping

Methods for serotyping staphylococci were developed before phage typing. At first, the staphylococci could not be divided into enough different types by the antisera available. Recent research has resulted in successful systems of typing to identify multiple factors. The validity of serotyping and phage typing has been demonstrated by comparative studies. Despite these successes, phage typing is usually preferred because it is more readily available, is easier to perform, and can be carried out under international standards. The use of both methods for the same group of isolates results in better differentiation of the strains.

CONTROL

Infections

Because staphylococci are part of the normal flora, they cannot be eliminated from humans. It is probable that in past generations, most people were infected primarily by their own staphylococci.

Today, however, many staphylococcal infections are produced by hospital strains of staphylococci, which have caused epidemics in nurseries, burn wards, and surgical wards.

The circumstances that resulted in the development of reservoirs of antibiotic-resistant *S aureus* in hospitals have been complex; often, the procedures to limit the spread of hospital staphylococci and to combat epidemics also have been complex. When development of new antibiotics did not offer security against epidemics in the nursery, innovative measures were taken to prevent colonization with epidemic strains. One such measure was to implant penicillin-sensitive *S aureus* 502A in the nose and on the umbilical cord of each newborn. Although this technique was successful, other procedures for preventing cross-infections between babies and the introduction of synthetic penicillins were primarily responsible for reducing the threat of epidemics in nurseries. Isolation equipment, designed like the isolators used in germ-free animal research, has limited opportunities for staphylococci and other pathogens to contaminate burn patients.

Food Poisoning

S aureus enterotoxins remain the most common cause of food poisoning. Recent research has led to development of better diagnostic procedures for identifying the staphylococcal enterotoxins. Today, when an outbreak occurs because a commercially produced food is contaminated by a food handler, it is possible to determine which lots of food contain enterotoxin. In addition, recently developed procedures for preparing food for large groups of people reduce opportunities for bacterial contamination.

TREATMENT

Patients with staphylococcal infections are usually treated with antibiotics and by surgical drainage. In emergencies, when antibiotic sensitivity information is not yet available, a synthetic penicillin that is resistant to penicillinase (methicillin, nafcillin, or oxacillin) is chosen. When penicillin allergy precludes the use of penicillin derivatives, appropriate second-line antibiotics are cephalosporins, vancomycin, gentamicin, rifampin, or clindamycin. The new cephalosporins include cephaloridine, cefuroxime, cephelexin, cefotaxime, ceftizoxine, cefuzonam, and cefotetan. When time permits, therapy should be based on the results of antibiotic sensitivity testing. A literature search for antibiotics used in the treatment of staphylococcal infections in 1988 indicated that reports mentioned at least 71 different compounds. Some *S aureus* strains from the community are penicillin sensitive; in such cases, maintaining an adequate level of penicillin for 7 days or more is the treatment of choice.

FUTURE TRENDS

The future of staphylococcal diseases is hard to predict because staphylococci are so intimately associated with humans and their environment. In other animals, a true commensal relationship frequently exists between *S aureus* and the host. Factors that enhance immunity in chronically ill and immune-deficient persons reinforce the possibility of a commensal relationship, but the continued introduction of new antibiotics tends to prolong the existing situation, in which antibiotic-resistant staphylococci predominate in hospitals. However, whether the staphylococci exist as commensals or as serious pathogens, or both, they no doubt will continue to be intimately associated with humankind.

REFERENCES

Chesney PJ, Jaucian R-MC, McDonald RA et al: Exfoliative dermatitis in an infant. Association with enterotoxin F-producing staphylococci. Am J Dis Child 137:899, 1983

Christensen P, Kahlmeter G, Jonsson S, Kronvall K: New method for the serological grouping of streptococci with specific antibodies adsorbed to protein A-containing staphylococci. Infect Immun 7:881, 1973

Cohen JO (ed): The Staphylococci. John Wiley & Sons, New York, 1972

Cohen JO: Serological typing of staphylococci for epidemiological studies. Ann NY Acad Sci 236:485, 1974

Cohen JO, Smith PB: Serological typing of *Staphylococ-*

cus aureus. II. Typing by slide agglutination and comparison with phage typing. J Bacteriol 88:1364, 1964

Kloos WE: Natural populations of the genus *Staphylococcus.* Annu Rev Microbiol 34:559, 1980

Kloos WE, Schleifer KH: Simplified scheme for routine identification of human *Staphylococcus* species. J Clin Microbiol 1:82, 1975

Oeding P, Digranes A: Classification of coagulase-negative staphylococci in the diagnostic laboratory. Acta Pathol Microbiol Scand Sect B 85:136, 1977

Shinefield HR, Ribbles JC, Boris M, et al: Bacterial interference between strains of *S aureus.* Ann NY Acad Sci 236:444, 1974

Todd J, Fishaut M: Toxic-shock syndrome associated with phage-group-1 staphylococci. Lancet 2:1116, 1978

Tyson W, Wensley DF, Anderson JD et al: Atypical staphylococcal toxic shock syndrome: two fatal cases. Pediatr Infect Dis J 8:642, 1989

Woodin AM: Assay of the two components of staphylococcal leukocidin and their antibodies. J Pathol Bacteriol 81:63, 1961

13 *STREPTOCOCCUS*

MARIA JEVITZ PATTERSON

GENERAL CONCEPTS

STREPTOCOCCUS PYOGENES, OTHER STREPTOCOCCI, AND *ENTEROCOCCUS*

Clinical Manifestations

Acute ***Streptococcus pyogenes*** infections may take the form of pharyngitis, scarlet fever (rash), impetigo, cellulitis, or erysipelas. Patients may also develop immune-mediated sequelae such as acute rheumatic fever and acute glomerulonephritis. *S agalactiae* may cause meningitis, neonatal sepsis, and pneumonia in neonates; adults may experience vaginitis, puerperal fever, urinary tract infection, skin infection, and endocarditis. **Viridans streptococci** can cause endocarditis, and ***Enterococcus*** is associated with urinary tract and biliary tract infections. **Anaerobic streptococci** participate in mixed infections of the abdomen, pelvis, brain, and lungs.

Structure

Streptococci are Gram-positive, nonmotile, nonspore-forming, catalase-negative cocci that occur in pairs or chains. Older cultures may lose Gram-positive character. Most streptococci are facultative anaerobes, and some are obligate (strict) anaerobes. Most require enriched media (blood agar). Group A streptococci have a hyaluronic acid capsule.

Classification and Antigenic Types

Streptococci are classified on the basis of colony morphology, hemolysis, biochemical reactions, and (most definitively) serologic specificity. They are divided into three groups by the type of hemolysis on blood agar: β hemolytic (clear, complete lysis of red cells), α hemolytic (incomplete, green hemolysis), and γ hemolytic (no hemolysis). Serologic grouping is based on antigenic differences in cell wall carbohydrates (groups A to V), in cell wall pili-associated protein, and in the polysaccharide capsule in group B streptococci.

Pathogenesis

Streptococci are members of the normal flora. Virulence factors of group A streptococci include (1) M protein and lipoteichoic acid for attachment; (2) a hyaluronic acid capsule that inhibits phyagocytosis; (3) other extracellular products, such as erythrogenic toxin, which causes the rash of scarlet fever; and (4) streptokinase, streptodornase (DNase B), and streptolysins. Some strains are nephritogenic. Immune-mediated sequelae do not reflect dissemination of bacteria. Non-group A strains have no defined virulence factors.

Host Defenses

Antibody to M protein gives type-specific immunity to group A streptococci. Antibody to erythrogenic toxin prevents the rash of scarlet fever. Cell-mediated immunity is important in the pathogenesis of acute rheumatic fever. Maternal IgG protects the neonate against group B streptococci.

Epidemiology

Group A β-hemolytic streptococci are spread by respiratory secretions and fomites. The incidence of both respiratory and skin infections peaks in childhood. Infection

215

can be transmitted by asymptomatic carriers. Acute rheumatic fever is most common among the poor; susceptibility may be partly genetic. Group B streptococci are common in the normal vaginal flora and occasionally cause invasive neonatal infection.

Diagnosis

Diagnosis is based on cultures from clinical specimens. Serologic methods can detect group A or B antigen; definitive antigen identification is by the precipitin test. Bacitracin sensitivity presumptively differentiates group A from other β-hemolytic streptococci (B, C, G); group B streptococci typically show hippurate hydrolysis; group D is differentiated from other viridans streptococci by bile solubility and optochin sensitivity. Acute glomerulonephritis and acute rheumatic fever are identified by anti-streptococcal antibody titers. In addition, acute rheumatic fever is diagnosed by clinical criteria.

Control

Prompt penicillin treatment of streptococcal pharyngitis precludes an antibody response and therefore prevents glomerulonephritis and acute rheumatic fever. Vaccines are under development.

STREPTOCOCCUS PNEUMONIAE

Clinical Manifestations

S pneumoniae causes pneumonia, meningitis, and sometimes occult bacteremia.

Structure

Pneumococci are lancet-shaped, catalase-negative, capsule-forming, α-hemolytic cocci or diplococci. Autolysis is enhanced by adding bile salts.

Classification and Antigenic Types

There are more than 85 antigenic types of S pneumoniae, which are determined by capsule antigens. There is no Lancefield group antigen.

Pathogenesis

S pneumoniae is a normal member of the respiratory tract flora; invasion results in pneumonia. The only virulence factor is the polysaccharide capsule, which protects the bacterium against phagocytosis.

Host Defenses

Protection against infection depends on a normal mucociliary barrier and intact phagocytic and T-independent immune responses. Type-specific anti-capsule antibody is protective.

Epidemiology

Pneumococcal pneumonia is most common in elderly, debilitated, or immunosuppressed individuals. The disease often sets in after a preceding viral infection damages the respiratory ciliated epithelium; incidence therefore peaks in the winter.

Diagnosis

Diagnosis is based on a sputum Gram stain and culture; blood or cerebrospinal fluid may also be cultured. Capsular antigen can be detected serologically. Pneumococci are distinguished from viridans streptococci by the quellung (capsular swelling) reaction, bile solubility, and optochin inhibition.

Control

Treatment is usually with penicillin. Strains resistant to multiple antibiotics, including tetracycline and sometimes penicillin, are emerging. A vaccine is available.

INTRODUCTION

The genus *Streptococcus*, a heterogeneous group of Gram-positive bacteria, has broad significance in medicine and industry. Various streptococci are important ecologically as part of the normal microbial flora of animals and humans; some can also cause subacute, acute, or chronic diseases. Among the significant human diseases attributable to streptococci are scarlet fever, rheumatic heart disease, glomerulonephritis, and pneumococcal pneumonia. Streptococci are essential in industrial and dairy processes and as indicators of pollution.

The nomenclature for streptococci, especially the nomenclature in medical use, has been based largely on serogroup identification of cell wall components rather than on species names. For several decades, interest has focused on two major species that cause severe infections: *S pyogenes* (group A streptococci) and *S pneumoniae* (pneumococci). Recently, two members have been assigned a new genus, the group D enterococcal species (which account for 98% of human enterococcal infections) are now *Enterococcus faecalis* and *E faecium*.

In recent years, increasing attention has been given to other streptococcal species, partly because innovations in serogrouping methods have led to advances in understanding the pathogenetic and epidemiologic significance of these species. A variety of cell-associated and extracellular products are produced by streptococci, but their relationship to pathogenesis has not been defined. Some of the other medically important streptococci are *S agalactiae* (group B), an etiologic agent of neonatal disease; *E faecalis* (group D), a major cause of endocarditis; and *S mutans* and *S sanguis* (viridans group), which are involved in dental caries. These and other streptococci of medical importance are listed in Table 13-1 by serogroup designation, normal ecologic niche, and associated disease(s).

TABLE 13-1   Medically Important Streptococci

Type species	Lancefield serogroup	Normal habitat	Significant human disease
S pyogenes	A	Humans	Acute pharyngitis and others
S agalactiae	B	Cattle, humans	Neonatal meningitis and sepsis and infections in adults
S equisimilis	C	Wide human and animal distribution	Endocarditis, bacteremia, pneumonia, meningitis, mild upper respiratory infection
E faecalis *S bovis* (nonenterococcus)	D	Human and animal intestinal tracts, dairy products	Biliary or urinary tract infection, endocarditis, bacteremia
S anginosus	F, G[a]	Humans, animals	Subcutaneous or organ abscesses, endocarditis, mild upper respiratory infection
S sanguis[b]	H	Humans	Endocarditis, caries
S salivarius	K	Humans	Endocarditis, caries
None	O	Humans	Endocarditis
S suis	R	Swine	Meningitis
"Viridans" *S mitis, S mutans*[c]	None identified	Humans	Caries, endocarditis
Anaerobic or microaerophilic	None identified	Wide human and animal distribution	Brain and pulmonary abscesses, gynecologic infections
S pneumoniae	None identified	Humans	Lobar pneumonia and others

[a] Strains of the *S anginosus* group (*S constallatus, S intermedius, S milleri*, minute strains) may possess antigens of groups A, C, F, or G, or no identifiable Lancefield group antigen.

[b] A disparate grouping undergoing further definition.

[c] Other viridans streptococci (*S sanguis, S salivarius, S milleri, S bovis, and S faecalis*) have identified group antigen(s); nutritionally variant streptococci may be included in this diverse category.

CLINICAL MANIFESTATIONS

In humans, streptococci cause disease chiefly in the respiratory tract, bloodstream, and skin. Human disease is most commonly associated with group A streptococci. Acute group A streptococcal disease is most often a respiratory infection (pharyngitis or tonsillitis) or a skin infection (pyoderma). Also medically significant are the late immune sequelae, not directly attributable to dissemination of bacteria, of group A infections (rheumatic fever following respiratory infection and glomerulonephritis following respiratory or skin infection), which remain a major worldwide health concern. Much effort is being directed toward clarifying the risk and mechanisms of these sequelae and identifying rheumatogenic and nephritogenic strains. There is also a renewed interest in safe and effective streptococcal vaccines.

STRUCTURE

Both *S pyogenes* and *S pneumoniae* are Gram-positive, nonmotile, nonsporulating cocci; they usually require complex culture media. *S pyogenes* characteristically is a round to ovoid coccus 0.6 to 1.0 μm in diameter (Fig. 13-1). It divides in one plane and thus occurs in pairs or (especially in liquid media or clinical material) in chains of various lengths. *S pneumoniae* is a diplococcus, 0.5 to 1.25 μm in diameter, typically described as lancet shaped but sometimes difficult to distinguish morphologically from other streptococci. Streptococcal cultures older than the logarithmic phase, which is the most active growth period of a culture, may lose their Gram-positive staining characteristics.

Unlike *Staphylococcus*, all streptococci lack catalase. Most are facultative anaerobes, but some are obligate anaerobes. They often have a mucoid or

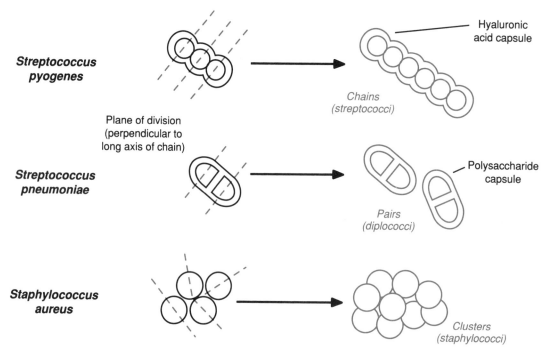

FIGURE 13-1 Morphology of the streptococci in comparison with staphylococci. Streptococci divide in a single plane and tend not to separate, causing chain formation. Capsules are antiphagocytic.

smooth colony morphology, and *S pneumoniae* colonies exhibit a central depression caused by rapid partial autolysis. As *S pneumoniae* colonies age, viability is lost during fermentative growth in the absence of catalase and peroxidase because of the accumulation of peroxide. Some group B and D streptococci produce pigment. Recently, streptococcal nutritional variants, which form satellite thiol- or pyridoxal-dependent colonies adjacent to staphylococcal colonies, have been reported. These variants do not grow on routine subculture, but have gained increasing attention as important agents of endocarditis.

CLASSIFICATION, ANTIGENIC TYPES, AND EXTRACELLULAR GROWTH PRODUCTS

Classification

The type of hemolytic reaction displayed on blood agar has long been used to classify the streptococci. *β*-**Hemolysis** is associated with complete lysis of red cells surrounding the colony, whereas *α*-**hemolysis** is a partial or "greening" hemolysis associated with partial loss of red cell hemoglobin. Nonhemolytic colonies have been termed *γ-hemolytic*. Hemolysis is affected by the species and age of red cells as well as by properties of the base medium. Use of the hemolytic reaction in classification is not completely satisfactory: some group A streptococci appear nonhemolytic; group B streptococci can manifest *α*-, *β*-, or even *γ*-hemolysis; and most *S pneumoniae* strains are *α*-hemolytic but can cause *β*-hemolysis during anaerobic incubation. The viridans group, although linked by the property of *α*-hemolysis, is actually an extremely diverse group of organisms that do not usually react with Lancefield grouping sera. The taxonomy and biochemical and genetic relationships of these organisms are currently being clarified (Table 13-1).

Antigenic Types

The cell wall structure of group A streptococci is among the most intensively studied of any bacteria (Fig. 13-2). The cell wall is composed of repeating units of *N*-acetylglucosamine and *N*-acetylmuramic acid, the standard peptidoglycan. For decades, the definitive identification of streptococci has rested on the serologic reactivity of cell wall polysaccharide antigens originally delineated by Rebecca Lancefield. Eighteen group-specific antigens were established. The group A polysaccharide is a polymer of *N*-acetylglucosamine and rhamnose. Some group antigens are shared by more than one species; no Lancefield group antigen has been identified for *S pneumoniae* or for some other *α*- or *γ*-hemolytic streptococci. Advances in serologic methods have shown that other streptococci possess several established group antigens.

The cell wall also consists of several structural proteins (Fig. 13-2). In group A streptococci, the R and T proteins may serve as epidemiologic markers, but the M proteins are clearly virulence factors associated with resistance to phagocytosis. More than 50 types of *S pyogenes* M proteins have been identified on the basis of antigenic specificity. Both the M proteins and lipoteichoic acid are supported externally to the cell wall on pili (fimbriae), and the lipoteichoic acid, in particular, appears to mediate bacterial attachment to host epithelial cells. M protein, peptidoglycan, *N*-acetylglucosamine, and group-specific carbohydrate portions of the cell wall have antigenic moieties similar in size and charge to those of mammalian muscle and connective tissue.

The capsule of *S pyogenes* is composed of hyaluronic acid, which is chemically similar to that of host connective tissue and is therefore nonantigenic. In contrast, the antigenically reactive and chemically distinct capsular polysaccharide of *S pneumoniae* allows the single species to be separated into more than 80 serotypes. The antiphagocytic *S pneumoniae* capsule is the sole virulence factor of these organisms; type 3 *S pneumoniae*, which produces copious quantities of capsular material, are the most virulent. Unencapsulated *S pneumoniae* cells are avirulent. The polysaccharide capsule in *S agalactiae* allows differentiation into types Ia, Ib, Ic, II, and III.

Finally, the cytoplasmic membrane of *S pyogenes* has antigens similar to those of human cardiac,

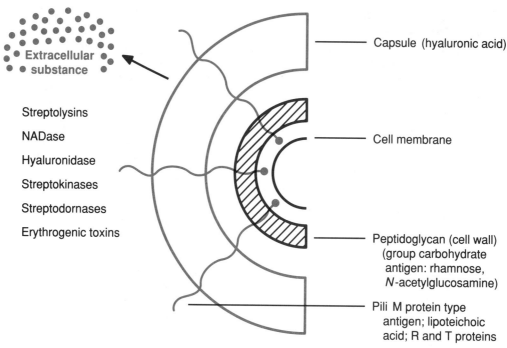

FIGURE 13-2 Cell surface structure of *S pyogenes* and extracellular substances.

skeletal, and smooth muscle, heart valve fibroblasts, and neuronal tissues.

Extracellular Growth Products

The importance of the interaction of streptococcal products with mammalian blood and tissue components is becoming widely recognized. The soluble extracellular growth products or toxins of the streptococci, especially of *S pyogenes* (Fig. 13-2), have been studied intensely. Streptolysin S is an oxygen-stable cytolysin; streptolysin O is a reversibly oxygen-labile cytolysin. Both are leukotoxic, as is NADase. Hyaluronidase (spreading factor) can digest host connective tissue hyaluronic acid as well as the organism's own capsule. Streptokinases participate in fibrin lysis. Streptodornases A to D possess deoxyribonuclease (DNase) activity; streptodornases B and D possess ribonuclease (RNase) activity as well. This large repertoire of products may be important in the pathogenesis of *S pyogenes*

by enhancing virulence; however, antibodies to these products appear not to protect the host, even though they have diagnostic importance.

When *S pyogenes* is lysogenized by certain bacteriophages, an erythrogenic exotoxin is produced that is associated with damage to small blood vessels and the rash of scarlet fever. Nonlysogenized strains are atoxic. Reemergence of these exotoxin-producing strains has been associated with toxic shock-like syndrome (see Ch. 12) and other forms of severe tissue destruction.

Virulence factors in the other streptococcal species are less well understood. In group B streptococci, carbohydrate surface antigens associated with antiphagocytosis have been identified, as has neuraminidase, which may play a role in pathogenesis. In the viridans streptococci, production of the exopolysaccharide (glycocalyx) is associated with the ability to adhere to the cardiac valves and to form vegetations on the valve leaflets.

PATHOGENESIS

S Pyogenes and S Pneumoniae Infections

Streptococci vary widely in pathogenic potential. Despite the remarkable array of cell-associated and extracellular products described above (Fig. 13-2), no clear scheme of pathogenesis has been developed. *S pneumoniae* and, to a lesser extent, *S pyogenes* are part of the normal human nasopharyngeal flora. Their numbers are usually limited by competition from the nasopharyngeal microbial ecosystem and by nonspecific host defense mechanisms, but failure of these mechanisms can result in disease. However, disease usually results from the acquisition of a new strain following alteration of the normal flora. *S pyogenes* causes inflammatory purulent lesions at the portal of entry, often the upper respiratory tract or the skin. Some strains of streptococci show a predilection for the respira-

tory tract; others prefer skin. Generally, streptococcal isolates from the pharynx and respiratory tract do not cause skin infections.

Invasion of other portions of the upper or lower respiratory tracts results in infections of the middle ear (otitis media), sinuses (sinusitis), or lungs (pneumonia). In addition, meningitis can occur by direct extension of infection from the middle ear or sinuses to the meninges or by way of bloodstream invasion from the pulmonary focus. Bacteremia can also result in infection of bones (osteomyelitis) or joints (arthritis).

S pyogenes (a group A streptococcus) is the leading cause of bacterial pharyngitis and tonsillitis (Fig. 13-3). Indeed, only group A streptococci are sought routinely in cases of pharyngitis, although groups B, C, and G are sometimes identified. *S pyogenes* infections can also result in sinusitis, otitis, mastoiditis, pneumonia, arthritis, bone infections, and, more infrequently, meningitis or endocar-

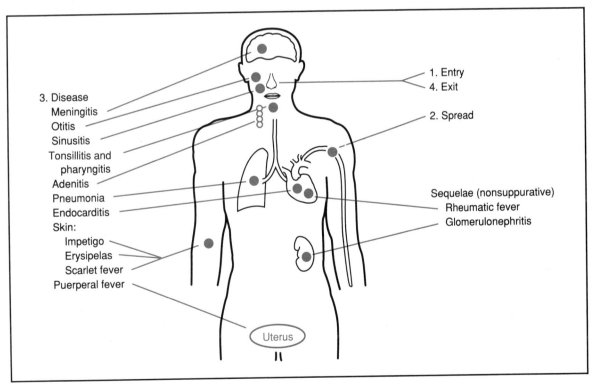

FIGURE 13-3 Pathogenesis of *S pyogenes* infections.

ditis. *S pyogenes* infections of the skin can be superficial (impetigo) or deep (cellulitis). Although scarlet fever was formerly a severe complication of streptococcal infection, it is now little more than streptococcal pharyngitis accompanied by rash. Similarly, erysipelas, a form of cellulitis accompanied by fever and systemic toxicity, is less common today.

The capsule of *S pneumoniae* renders it resistant to phagocytosis. The ability to evade this important host defense mechanism allows *S pneumoniae* to survive, multiply, and spread to various organs (Fig. 13-4). *S pneumoniae* is the leading cause of bacterial pneumonia in adults. Pleural effusion is the most common complication of *S pneumoniae* infection, and empyema (pus in the pleural space) is one of the most serious. This organism is also the most common cause of sinusitis, acute bacterial otitis media, and conjunctivitis beyond early childhood. Dissemination from a respiratory focus results in serious disease: outpatient bacteremia in children, meningitis, occasionally acute septic ar-

thritis and bone infections in patients with sickle cell disease, and, more rarely, peritonitis (especially in patients with nephrotic syndrome) or endocarditis.

Late Sequelae

Infection with *S pyogenes* (but not *S pneumoniae*) can give rise to serious late sequelae: acute rheumatic fever and acute glomerulonephritis. These sequelae begin 1 to 3 weeks after the acute illness, a latency period consistent with an immune-mediated rather than pathogen-disseminated etiology. Whether all *S pyogenes* strains are rheumatogenic is still controversial; however, clearly not all are nephritogenic. These differences in pathogenic potential are not yet understood.

Acute rheumatic fever is a sequela only of pharyngeal infections, but acute glomerulonephritis can follow infections of the pharynx or the skin. Although there is no adequate explanation for the precise pathogenesis of acute rheumatic fever or

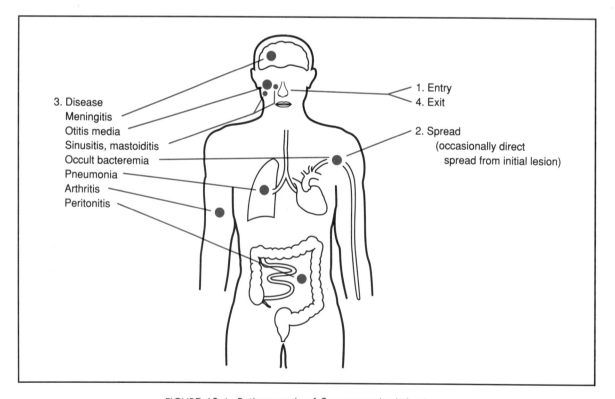

FIGURE 13-4 Pathogenesis of *S pneumoniae* infections.

for its absence after streptococcal pyoderma, an abnormal or enhanced immune response seems essential. Also, persistence of the organism, due perhaps in part to the greater avidity with which it adheres to host pharyngeal cells, is associated with an increased likelihood of rheumatic fever. Acute glomerulonephritis results from deposition of antigen-antibody-complement complexes on the basement membrane of kidney glomeruli. The antigen may be streptococcal in origin, or it may be a host tissue species with antigenic determinants similar to those of streptococcal antigen (cross-reactive epitopes for endocardium, sarcolemma, and vascular smooth muscle). In the United States, the incidence of acute rheumatic fever had decreased dramatically, but several areas have reported a resurgence in cases. Acute rheumatic fever can result in permanent damage to the heart valves. Fewer than 1 percent of sporadic streptococcal pharyngitis infections result in acute rheumatic fever; however, recurrences are common, and lifelong antibiotic prophylaxis is recommended following a single case. The incidence of acute glomerulonephritis in the United States is more variable, perhaps owing to cycling of nephritogenic strains, but appears to be decreasing; recurrences are uncommon, and prophylaxis following an initial attack is unnecessary.

Other Streptococcal Species

Lancefield Group Streptococci

Streptococcal groups B, C, and G initially were recognized as animal pathogens (Table 13-1) and as part of the normal human flora. Recently, the pathogenic potential for humans of some of these non-group-A streptococci has been clarified. Group B streptococci, which cause bovine mastitis, are a leading cause of neonatal septicemia and meningitis and thus account for significant mortality. Early-onset neonatal disease is thought to be transmitted principally from the mother; late-onset meningitis is acquired horizontally, in some instances as a nosocomial infection. Recently, group B organisms also have been associated with pneumonia in elderly patients. They are part of the normal oral and vaginal flora and have also been isolated during adult urogenital infection, menin-

gitis, bacteremia, and endocarditis. Group C and G streptococci are associated with both mild and severe human disease. None of these groups has been implicated in acute rheumatic fever or acute glomerulonephritis. Group D streptococci are important agents of urinary tract infections and of infections associated with biliary tract procedures; they are also associated with disseminated infection, bacteremia, and endocarditis. In particular, *S bovis* bacteremia has been recognized more often in cases of bowel disease. Group F streptococci are associated with abscess formation and purulent disease. Group R streptococci, well-documented causes of meningitis and septicemia in pigs, also pose a serious health hazard to workers in the pork industry.

Viridans Streptococci

The biochemically and antigenically diverse group of organisms classified as viridans streptococci, as well as other nongroupable streptococci of the oral cavity, include etiologic agents of bacterial endocarditis. Dental manipulation and dental disease with the associated transient bacteremia are the most common predisposing factors in bacterial endocarditis, especially if heart valves have been damaged by previous rheumatic fever or by congenital cyanotic heart disease. *S mutans* and *S sanguis* are odontopathogens, responsible for the formation of dental plaque, the dense adhesive microbial mass that colonizes teeth and is linked to caries and other human oral disease (see Ch. 99). *S mutans* is the more cariogenic of the two species, and its virulence is directly related to its ability to synthesize glucan from fermentable carbohydrates as well as to modify glucan in promoting increased adhesiveness.

Anaerobes

Like their aerobic counterparts, anaerobic streptococci are part of the normal flora, particularly of the mouth and intestinal tract but also of the upper respiratory and genital tracts and the skin. These anaerobic organisms are linked to a wide variety of serious mixed infections of the female genital tract as well as to brain, pulmonary, and abdominal abscesses.

HOST DEFENSES

Streptococcal disease results when endogenous or exogenous streptococci circumvent the normal host defenses. *S pyogenes* and *S pneumoniae* infections usually result from exogenous secondary invasion following viral disease or disturbances in the normal bacterial flora.

In the normal host, nonspecific defense mechanisms prevent organisms from penetrating beyond the superficial epithelium of the upper respiratory tract. These mechanisms include mucociliary movement and the cough, sneeze, and epiglottal reflexes. The host phagocytic system is a second line of defense against pathogens.

Organisms can be opsonized by activation of the classical or alternative complement pathway or by specific immunoglobulin binding.

The capsules of both *S pyogenes* and *S pneumoniae* allow the organisms to evade opsonization by immunoglobulin. The hyaluronic acid outer surface of *S pyogenes* is only weakly antigenic; however, protective immunity results from the development of type-specific antibody to the M protein of the pili, which protrude from the cell wall through the capsular structure. This antibody develops after respiratory and skin infections and is persistent. Presumably, IgA in the respiratory secretions and IgG in serum are the important protective antibody classes. *S pyogenes* is rapidly killed following phagocytosis enhanced by specific antibody. Prompt, effective antibiotic treatment of streptococcal infections may preclude the development of this persistent antibody. Evidence has shown that antibody to the erythrogenic toxin involved in scarlet fever is also persistent. This is the basis of the Dick test, an in vivo skin test, rarely used today, which measures host antitoxin. The capsular polysaccharides of *S pneumoniae* are highly antigenic and type specific. Type-specific anticapsular antibodies to these T-independent antigens result in effective opsonization and host recovery. Recovery from untreated *S pneumoniae* infections clearly is due to opsonizing antibody. Even when adequate and appropriate antibiotic therapy is given, opsonizing antibody probably contributes significantly to recovery from pneumococcal disease.

The normal host is somewhat resistant to *S pneumoniae* disease, but compromised hosts of several types are highly susceptible to serious infections: alcoholics, semicomatose patients, very young and very old individuals, patients who have undergone splenectomy, and patients with underlying diseases (specifically, chronic cardiac, pulmonary, or renal disease; sickle cell anemia; leukopenia; multiple myeloma; cirrhosis; and diabetes).

Cross-reactive antigens, especially between *S pyogenes* and various mammalian tissues, help explain the autoimmune responses that develop following some infections. The level of humoral response to infection with *S pyogenes* is greater in patients with rheumatic fever than in patients with uncomplicated pharyngitis. In addition, cell-mediated immunity may play a significant role in acute rheumatic fever.

The susceptibility of neonates to group B streptococci may result from the immaturity of neonatal phagocytes, humoral immunity, or cell-mediated immunity, or from lack of passively acquired maternal antibody.

Recent evidence from the rhesus monkey animal model in dental research shows that IgG may be more important than IgA or IgM in protection against caries, probably because IgG is the antibody isotype most efficient at enhancing phagocytosis of *S mutans*. Cell-mediated immunity participates in the protective host response against caries.

EPIDEMIOLOGY

The streptococci are widely distributed in nature and frequently form part of the normal human flora (Table 13-1). Approximately 5 to 15 percent of humans carry *S pyogenes* or *S agalactiae* in the nasopharynx. *S pneumoniae* infects humans exclusively, and no reservoir is found in nature. The carrier rate of *S pneumoniae* in the normal human nasopharynx is 20 to 40 percent.

All ages, races, and sexes are susceptible to streptococcal disease. Because *S pneumoniae* is a delicate organism, sensitive to heat, cold, and drying, transmission requires close person-to-person contact. Infection is unlikely except when host resistance is reduced, as described above, or after the introduction of a more virulent strain. In the United States, pneumococcal disease is most prevalent in the winter, coinciding with increased rates of acquisition but not necessarily of carriage. Alaskan natives have higher rates of invasive pneumococcal disease than do other American populations. The reason for this is unclear. The incidence of respiratory disease attributed to *S pyogenes* peaks at about 6 years of age and then again at 13 years of age; it is highest during late winter and early spring in temperate climates. Skin infections are most common among preschool-age children and are most prevalent in late summer and early fall in temperate climates (when hot, humid weather prevails) and at all times in tropical climates. *S pyogenes* is spread by respiratory droplets or by contact with fomites used by the index individual, either patient or carrier. Skin infections often follow minor skin irritation, such as insect bites. There are occasional reports of streptococcal disease transmitted by rectal carriers, and of food-borne and vector-borne outbreaks.

The world prevalence of the serious late sequelae of *S pyogenes* infections (acute rheumatic fever and acute glomerulonephritis) has shifted from temperate to tropic climates. In particular, acute rheumatic fever had ceased to be a major health concern in the United States, despite no concomitant decline in group A streptococcal pharyngitis. These diseases particularly affect persons with a low standard of living and limited access to medical care. Since 1985, there have been scattered outbreaks of acute rheumatic fever in some regions of the United States. Temporal and geographic clustering provides further evidence for "rheumatogenic" strains. Whether ethnic or racially determined factors affect this shift is not known.

Other streptococcal groups show striking epidemiologic features. An increasing prevalence of non-group-A streptococci over group A streptococci in throats has been reported. Studies of the vaginal flora among women of childbearing age show a *S agalactiae* carrier rate of 2 to 30 percent. Transmission of the organisms to neonates of vaginally infected mothers ranges from 1 to 25 percent, but the incidence of neonates with disease (in

contrast to colonized, healthy neonates) is low. *S suis* has been linked to meningitis among meat handlers. Isolation of *S milleri* or *S bovis* from the bloodstream should raise suspicion, respectively, of visceral abscess formation and bowel disease (including colon carcinoma). In the United States, enterococci are the third most common nosocomial pathogen. The widespread usage of newer cephalosporins, which have poor activity against enterococci, means that enterococci have become clinically significant isolates.

DIAGNOSIS

Clinical

It is not usually possible to diagnose streptococcal pharyngitis or tonsillitis on clinical grounds alone. Accurate differentiation from viral pharyngitis is difficult even for the experienced clinician, and therefore the use of bacteriologic methods is essential. When documented streptococcal pharyngitis is accompanied by an erythematous punctiform rash, the diagnosis of scarlet fever can be made. Rheumatic fever is a late sequela of pharyngitis and is marked by fever, polyarthritis, and carditis. A combination of clinical and laboratory criteria (Table 13-2) is used in the diagnosis of acute rheumatic fever. The other late sequela, acute glomerulonephritis, is preceded by pharyngitis or pyoderma; is characterized by fever, blood in the urine **(hematuria)**, and edema; and is sometimes accompanied by hypertension and elevated blood urea nitrogen **(azotemia)**. Pneumococcal pneumonia is a life-threatening disease, often characterized by edema and rapid lobar consolidation.

Specimens for Direct Examination and Culture

S pyogenes is usually isolated from throat cultures. In cases of cellulitis or erysipelas thought to be caused by *S pyogenes*, aspirates obtained from the advancing edge of the lesion may be diagnostic. *S pneumoniae* is usually isolated from sputum or blood. Precise identification is based on the Gram stain and on biochemical properties, as well as on serologic characteristics when group antigens are

TABLE 13-2   Jones Diagnostic Criteria for Acute Rheumatic Fever[a]

Major	Minor
Carditis	Clinical
Polyarthritis	Fever
Erythema marginatum	Arthralgia
Subcutaneous nodules	Previous rheumatic fever
Chorea	Laboratory
	Increased erythrocyte sedimentation rate
	Increased C-reactive protein level
	ECG
	Increased PR interval

[a] In conjunction with culture or serologic evidence of recent streptococcal infection. (From American Heart Association, Jones criteria (revised) for guidance in the diagnosis of rheumatic fever. Circulation, 32:664, 1965, with permission.)

present. Table 13-3 shows biochemical tests that provide sensitive group-specific characteristics permitting presumptive identification of Gram-positive, catalase-negative cocci.

Identification

Hemolysis should not be used as a stringent criterion for identification. Bacitracin susceptibility is a widely used screening method for presumptive identification of *S pyogenes;* however, some *S pyogenes* strains (up to 10 percent) are resistant to bacitracin and some group C and G streptococci (about 3 to 5 percent) are susceptible to bacitracin. Some of the group B streptococci also may be bacitracin sensitive, but are presumptively identified by their properties of hippurate hydrolysis and positive CAMP test. *S pneumoniae* can be separated from other α-hemolytic streptococci on the basis of sensitivity to surfactants, such as bile or optochin (ethylhydrocupreine hydrochloride). These agents activate autolytic enzymes that hydrolyze peptidoglycan in the organisms.

Presumptive identification is usually not carried further. Serologic grouping has not been performed as often as it might be because of the lack of available methods and the practical constraints of time and cost; however, only serologic methods (Table 13-4) provide definitive identification of the streptococci. The Lancefield capillary precipi-

tation test is the classical serologic method. *S pneumoniae,* which lacks a demonstrable group antigen by the Lancefield test, is conventionally identified by the quellung or capsular swelling test that employs type-specific anticapsular antibody. Inspection of Gram-stained sputum remains a reliable predictor for initial antibiotic therapy in community-acquired pneumonia.

New methods for serogrouping that show sensitivity and specificity are being explored. Organisms from throat swabs, incubated for only a few hours in broth, can be examined for the presence of *S pyogenes* by the direct fluorescent antibody assay or enzyme-linked immunosorbent assay (ELISA). Additional rapid antigen detection systems for the group carbohydrate are becoming increasingly popular. However, the sensitivity of these currently available rapid tests for group A streptococcal carbohydrate does not allow exclusion of streptococcal pharyngitis without conventional throat culture. *S pneumoniae* can be identified rapidly by counterimmunoelectrophoresis, a modification of the gel precipitin method. The coagglutination test (see Ch. 12) is a more sensitive modification of the conventional direct bacterial agglutination test. The Fc portion of group-specific antibody binds to protein A of dead staphylococci, leaving the Fab portion free to react with specific streptococcal antigen. The attachment of antibody to other carrier particles in suspension

TABLE 13-3 Characteristics for the Presumptive Identification of Streptococci of Human Clinical Importance

Procedure	Results for Group:						
	A	B	D (enterococcus)	D (nonenterococcus)	Non-A, B, D	S pneumoniae	Viridans
Hemolysis[a]	β	β, α, γ	α, β, γ	α, γ, β	β, α, γ	α	α
Bacitracin sensitivity	+	−(+)[b]	−	−	−(+)	±	−
CAMP test	−	+	−	−	−	−	−
Growth at 45°C	−	−	+	+	−	−	+
Optochin sensitivity	−(+)	−(+)	−	−	−(+)	+	−
Hydrolysis of sodium hippurate	−	+	−(+)	−	−	−	−(+)
Tolerance to 6.5 percent NaCl	−	±	+	−	−	−	−
Hydrolysis of esculin in presence of 40 percent bile	−	−	+	+	−	−	−(+)
Hydrolysis of pyrrolidonyl naphthylamide	+	−	+	−	−	−	−

[a] In general order of frequency.
[b] Signs in parentheses indicate occasional result.

TABLE 13-4   Methods for Serogrouping Streptococci

Nature of Streptococcal Antigen	Techniques
Whole cells	Fluorescent antibody Direct bacterial agglutination Coagglutination with staphylococcal protein A Carrier agglutination (antibody-coated latex particles) Quellung reaction (for *S pneumoniae*)
Soluble extract	Precipitation (classical capillary or counterimmunoelectrophoresis) Coagglutination with staphylococcal protein A Carrier agglutination (antibody-coated latex particles) Enzyme-linked immunosorbent assay (ELISA) Antigen capture assays

(for example, latex) also is used. The fact that whole streptococcal cells can be used in recently developed methods circumvents the difficulties involved in extracting components that retain appropriate antigenic reactivity. These newer serogrouping methods should make it more practical to identify not only β-hemolytic isolates from the blood or normally sterile sites, but also α-hemolytic and nonhemolytic strains. Such information will expand our understanding of the importance of non-group A streptococci.

Serologic Titers

Antibodies to some of the extracellular growth products of the streptococci are not protective but can be used in diagnosis. The antistreptolysin O and anti-NADase titers are more commonly elevated after pharyngeal infections than after skin infections. In contrast, antihyaluronidase is elevated after skin infections, and anti-DNase B rises after both pharyngeal and skin infections. Titers observed during late sequelae (acute rheumatic fever and acute glomerulonephritis) reflect the site of primary infection. Although it is not as well known as the ASO test, the anti-DNase B test appears superior because high-titer antibody is detected following skin and pharyngeal infections and during the late sequelae. Those titers should be interpreted in terms of the age of the patient and geographic locale.

Although not used in diagnosis, bacteriocin production and phage typing of streptococci are employed in research and epidemiologic studies.

CONTROL

Antibiotic Treatment

Penicillin remains the drug of choice for *S pyogenes* and *S pneumoniae* infections. Unlike the other streptococci, group D enterococci are resistant to penicillins, including penicillinase-resistant penicillins such as methicillin, nafcillin, dicloxacillin, and oxacillin, and are becoming increasingly resistant to many other antibiotics. Group B streptococci are often resistant to tetracycline and kanamycin, but remain sensitive to penicillin at clinically achievable levels in blood, even though the minimal inhibitory concentrations (MICs) of penicillin for these organisms are considerably higher than for *S pyogenes*. Although the duration of penicillin therapy varies with the degree of invasiveness, streptococcal pharyngitis is generally adequately treated with 10 days of antibiotic therapy, and pneumococcal pneumonia with 7 to 14 days. If penicillin allergy occurs, an alternative drug for treating pharyngitis is erythromycin, although sporadic erythromycin and tetracycline resistance has been reported. Lifelong prophylaxis against recurrences of rheumatic fever with long-acting penicillin or erythromycin is required. Sulfonamides will not eradicate streptococci and therefore are not acceptable for treating streptococcal pharyngitis, but sulfadiazine is effective for preventing recurrent attacks of rheumatic fever. Additional prophylactic coverage before some dental and surgical procedures is necessary in the setting of rheumatic heart disease or prosthetic heart valves. Although streptococcal pharyngitis is usually a benign, self-limited disease, therapy is important to prevent rheumatic fever. There is no convincing evidence that antibiotic therapy prevents glomerulonephritis. Disconcertingly, in recent outbreaks of acute rheumatic fever some patients did not have a history of pharyngitis.

Treatment of the asymptomatic pharyngeal carrier of *S pyogenes* remains controversial, although recent evidence suggests that the carrier state involves no risk to the carrier or to others and that it is frequently difficult to eradicate, despite the exquisite sensitivity of the organism to penicillin in vitro. Similar failure of antibiotic therapy to eradicate nasopharyngeal carriage or to prevent reinfection with *S pneumoniae* also occurs. In the United States, the level of resistance of *S pneumoniae* to penicillin remains low, but isolates must be carefully monitored for evolving resistance. Treating pregnant carriers of group B streptococci, or their colonized neonates, in an effort to avoid serious neonatal disease remains controversial for several reasons: the high carrier rate documented in several parts of the country, the associated high risk of penicillin hypersensitivity, the potential increase in infections with penicillin-resistant organisms, the difficulty in effecting eradication, and the low risk of neonatal disease. Intrapartum chemoprophylaxis of group B infections is being evaluated.

Clearly, penicillin has reduced the severe morbidity and mortality associated with *S pneumoniae*. Endocarditis is uniformly fatal unless treated. Serious infections with group D enterococci often require a synergistic regimen combining penicillin or ampicillin with an aminoglycoside, although complicated urinary tract infections with enterococci can be treated with ampicillin alone. An alternative drug of choice is vancomycin, but recently vancomycin-resistant enterococci have been isolated. Nosocomial acquisition of these resistant organisms is of concern.

Antibiotic Resistance

Antibiotic resistance among the streptococci is an increasing problem. Genetic studies show that in vitro resistance can be plasmid mediated. The mechanisms involved in the in vivo genetic exchange are not clearly defined. Evidence is accumulating that oral streptococci may be the important donors of resistance plasmids. The first penicillin-resistant *S pneumoniae* isolates were reported in 1967 in Australia and in 1974 in North America. In New Guinea, where the first penicillin-resistant strains were reported in 1971, one-third of *S pneumoniae* isolates from patients with severe pneumococcal disease were resistant by 1978 and some strains resistant to erythromycin or tetracycline, as well as some multiply resistant strains, also have been reported. In South Africa, outbreaks of infection with strains of *S pneumoniae* resistant to β-lactam antibiotics (penicillins and cephalosporins) as well as to tetracycline, chloramphenicol, erythromycin, streptomycin, clindamycin, sulfonamides, and rifampin have been reported. Although antibiotic resistance among *S pneumoniae* isolates is infrequent in the United States, it should be monitored, especially in serious pneumococcal disease or in settings with particularly susceptible patients, such as debilitated children or immunocompromised individuals. No penicillin-resistant *S pyogenes* isolates have been described, although rare erythromycin-resistant strains, reported as early as 1959 and increasing in prevalence, are a significant problem in other parts of the world.

Vaccination

With the introduction of antibiotics, previously successful pneumococcal vaccines fell into disuse. However, although prompt treatment with antibiotics has reduced the serious consequences of *S pneumoniae* infections (a pre-antibiotic mortality rate of 30 percent), the disease incidence remains unchanged and attention has been redirected to vaccines for *S pneumoniae* as well as for other streptococci. Pneumococcal vaccines (containing the pneumococcal polysaccharides of the most prevalent serotypes) have been licensed in several countries, including the United States. Initial use shows them to be useful and safe, and efficacy studies are in progress. In 1983, the U.S. Food and Drug Administration licensed a vaccine containing 23 serotypes, representing coverage against nearly 89 percent of the pneumococcal isolates submitted to the Centers for Disease Control (CDC) in the 1987 to 1988 National Surveillance Study. The population target of pneumococcal vaccines includes those at high risk for serious pneumococcal disease: elderly individuals, immunocompromised patients (those with lymphoma, asplenia, myeloma, or acquired immune deficiency syndrome [AIDS]), and those with sickle cell anemia, nephrotic syndrome, or chronic cardiopulmonary disease. Vaccines for the other streptococci remain experimental.

Vaccine production for the streptococci presents several formidable problems. A large number of serotypes must be included in effective *S pyogenes* and *S pneumoniae* vaccines. Continuing surveillance to determine prevalent serotypes is necessary to ensure that the vaccine formulations remain appropriate. For *S pyogenes* vaccines, it is critical to determine rheumatogenic and nephritogenic strains to limit the required multivalency of the vaccines. Toxicity has been associated with M protein preparations, but lack of immunogenicity in highly purified preparations of antigens is still a problem. With streptococcal vaccines, the potential risk of antigenic cross-reactivity with cardiac tissue and an associated increased risk of acute rheumatic fever must be appreciated.

Passive immunity in group B streptococcal neonatal infection appears protective. Polyvalent hyperimmune gamma globulin and human monoclonal IgM antibody that reacts with multiple serotypes are undergoing efficacy studies. Active immunization of pregnant women with undegraded sialic acid-containing polysaccharide group B antigens is another important aspect of control.

The streptococci are ubiquitous, and their significance in medicine is remarkable. Exciting advances are being made in diagnosis, in understanding the mechanisms of pathogenesis, and in control of these well-known organisms. Problems with antibiotic resistance must preclude complacency in dealing with these common pathogens.

REFERENCES

Aukenthaler R et al: Group G streptococcal bacteremia: clinical study and review of the literature. Rev Infect Dis 5:196, 1983

Baker CJ: Immunization to prevent group B streptococcal disease: victories and vexations. J Infect Dis 161:917, 1990

Broome CV, Facklam RR: Epidemiology of clinically significant isolates of *Streptococcus pneumoniae* in the United States. Rev Infect Dis 3:277, 1981

Coykendall AL: Classification and identification of the viridans streptococci. Clin Microbiol Rev 2:315, 1989

Dajani AJ et al: Prevention of rheumatic fever. A statement for health professionals by the Committee on Rheumatic Fever, Endocarditis, and Kawasaki Disease of the Council on Cardiovascular Disease in the Young, the American Heart Association. Pediatr Infect Dis J 8:263, 1989

Denny FW et al: Prevention of rheumatic fever: treatment of the preceding streptococcic infection. J Am Med Assoc 143:151, 1950

Dillon HC: Post-streptococcal glomerulonephritis following pyoderma. Rev Infect Dis 1:935, 1979

Gullberg RM, Homann SR, Phair JP: Enterococcal bacteremia: analysis of 75 episodes. Rev Infect Dis 11:74, 1989

Kellogg JA, Manzella JP: Detection of group A streptococci in the laboratory or physician's office. J Am Med Assoc 255:2638, 1986

Klein RS et al: Association of *Streptococcus bovis* with carcinoma of the colon. N Engl J Med 297:800, 1977

Klugman KP: Pneumococcal resistance to antibiotics. Clin Microbiol Rev 3:171, 1990

McCarty M: An adventure in the pathogenetic maze of rheumatic fever. J Infect Dis 143:375, 1981

McGhee JR, Michalek SM: Immunobiology of dental caries: microbial aspects and local immunity. Annu Rev Microbiol 35:595, 1981

Schwartz JS: Pneumococcal vaccine: clinical efficacy and effectiveness. Ann Intern Med 96:208, 1982

Stevens DL et al: Severe group A streptococcal infections associated with a toxic shock-like syndrome and scarlet fever toxin A. N Engl J Med 321:1, 1989

Wannamaker LW: Changes and changing concepts in the biology of group A streptococci and the epidemiology of streptococcal infections. Rev Infect Dis 1:967, 1979

Ward, J: Antibiotic resistant *Streptococcus pneumoniae*: clinical and epidemiologic aspects. Rev Infect Dis 3:254, 1981

Zabriskie JB: Rheumatic fever: the interplay between host, genetics and microbe. Circulation 71:1077, 1985

14 NEISSERIA, BRANHAMELLA, MORAXELLA, AND ACINETOBACTER

STEPHEN A. MORSE

GENERAL CONCEPTS

NEISSERIA GONORRHOEAE

Clinical Manifestations

Symptomatic or asymptomatic **localized infections** include urethritis, cervicitis, proctitis, pharyngitis, and conjunctivitis. **Disseminated infections** occur either by extension to adjacent organs (pelvic inflammatory disease, epididymitis) or by bacteremic spread (skin lesions, tenosynovitis, septic arthritis, endocarditis, and meningitis).

Structure

Cells are Gram-negative cocci, usually seen in pairs with the adjacent sides flattened.

Classification and Antigenic Types

N gonorrhoeae strains are typed on the basis of their growth requirements (auxotyping) or by antigenic differences in protein I (serotyping).

Pathogenesis

Gonorrhea is usually acquired by sexual contact. Gonococci adhere to columnar epithelial cells, penetrate them, and multiply on the basement membrane. Gonococcal lipopolysaccharide stimulates the production of tumor necrosis factor, which causes cell damage. Gonococci may disseminate in the bloodstream. Strains that cause disseminated infections are usually resistant to serum complement.

Host Defenses

Infection stimulates inflammation and local immunity; however, it is not known whether the secretory immune response is protective. Serum antibodies also appear. Protection, if it exists, may be strain specific.

Epidemiology

Gonorrhea is a **sexually transmitted disease** of worldwide importance. The highest attack rate in both men and women occurs between 15 and 29 years of age. Host-related factors such as the number of sexual partners, contraceptive practices, sexual preference, and population mobility contribute to the incidence of gonorrhea.

Diagnosis

Gonorrhea cannot be diagnosed solely on clinical grounds. For men, a Gram-stained smear of urethral exudate showing intracellular Gram-negative diplococci is diagnostic. For women, and for men when a direct smear is not definitive, culturing on selective medium is required. *N gonorrhoeae* must be differentiated from other *Neisseria* species. Isolates should be examined for **antibiotic resistance.** Serologic tests are not recommended for uncomplicated infections.

Control

Recommended treatment is third-generation cephalosporin plus tetracycline. Sex partner(s) should be referred and treated. No effective vaccine yet exists. Condoms are effective in preventing gonorrhea.

NEISSERIA MENINGITIDIS
Clinical Manifestations
N meningitidis has two presentations, as **meningococcemia,** characterized by skin lesions, and as **acute bacterial meningitis.** Fulminant disease (with or without meningitis) is characterized by multisystem involvement and high mortality.

Structure
Cell morphology is identical to that of *N gonorrhoeae.* The antiphagocytic polysaccharide capsule is a prominent feature.

Classification and Antigenic Types
N meningitidis is grouped, on the basis of capsular polysaccharides, into 12 serogroups, some of which are subdivided according to the presence of outer membrane protein and lipopolysaccharide antigens.

Pathogenesis
Infection is by aspiration of infective particles, which attach to epithelial cells of the nasopharyngeal and oropharyngeal mucosa, cross the mucosal barrier, and enter the bloodstream. Blood-borne bacteria may enter the central nervous system and cause meningitis, if not cleared.

Host Defenses
Meningococci establish systemic infections only in individuals who lack serum bactericidal antibodies directed against the capsular or noncapsular antigens of the invading strain, or in patients deficient in the late-acting complement components.

Epidemiology
Asymptomatic carriage of meningococci in the nasopharynx provides a reservoir for infection but also enhances host immunity. Attack rates peak in infants 3 months to 1 year old. Meningococcal meningitis occurs both sporadically (mainly groups B and C meningococci) and in epidemics (mainly group A meningococci), with the highest incidence during late winter and early spring.

Diagnosis
Symptoms are suggestive; diagnosis is confirmed by identifying *N meningitidis* in specimens of blood, cerebrospinal fluid, and nasopharyngeal secretions collected before antibiotic administration.

Control
Penicillin is the drug of choice. Household contacts require chemoprophylaxis with rifampin. Groups A, C, AC, and ACYW135 capsular polysaccharide vaccines are available. In children under 1 year old, antibody levels decline rapidly after immunization. Routine vaccination is not recommended.

OTHER GENERA AND SPECIES
Branhamella catarrhalis is a coccus resembling *Neisseria.* It causes lower respiratory infection in adults with chronic lung disease and is a common cause of otitis media, sinusitis, and conjunctivitis in children. *Moraxella* is an oxidase-positive bacterium, sometimes mistaken for *Neisseria,* that may be isolated from eye infections and is a secondary invader in some respiratory tract infections. *Acinetobacter* species are short bacilli or coccoid bacteria that act as opportunistic pathogens. They are sometimes secondary invaders of damaged tissues.

INTRODUCTION
The family Neisseriaceae comprises the genera *Neisseria, Branhamella, Moraxella,* and *Acinetobacter.* The only significant human pathogens are *N gonorrhoeae,* the agent of gonorrhea, and *N meningitidis,* an agent of acute bacterial meningitis. *N gonorrhoeae* infections have a high prevalence and low mortality, whereas *N meningitidis* infections have a low prevalence and high mortality.

Gonococcal infections are acquired by sexual contact and usually affect the urethra in men and the cervix in women, although the infection may disseminate to a variety of tissues. The pathogenic mechanism involves the attachment of the gonococci to ciliated epithelial cells via pili (fimbriae) and the production of cytotoxic factors (endotoxin). Similarly, the lipopolysaccharide of meningococci is highly toxic, but an additional virulence factor is the antiphagocytic capsule. Both pathogens produce proteases that cleave human immunoglobulin A (IgA), and these enzymes are involved in circumventing the local host defense. Many normal individuals harbor meningococci, whereas gonococci are present only if sexual contact with an infected person has occurred. Epidemics of meningococcal meningitis occur sporadically. Gonococcal infections occur frequently and affect large numbers of sexually active people. Other species in this genus are primarily parasites on mucosal surfaces of humans and other animals. Human disease caused by these organisms usually is associated with opportunistic infections in compromised patients.

NEISSERIA GONORRHOEAE

CLINICAL MANIFESTATIONS

Gonorrheal infection is generally limited to superficial mucosal surfaces lined with columnar epithelium. The areas most frequently involved are the cervix, urethra, rectum, pharynx, and conjunctiva (Fig. 14-1). Squamous epithelium, which lines the adult vagina, is not susceptible to infection by the gonococcus. However, the prepubertal vaginal epithelium, which has not been keratinized under the influence of estrogen, may be infected. Hence, gonorrhea in young girls may present as vulvovaginitis. Mucosal infections are usually characterized by a marked local neutrophilic response (purulent discharge).

The most common symptom of uncomplicated gonorrhea is a discharge that may range from a

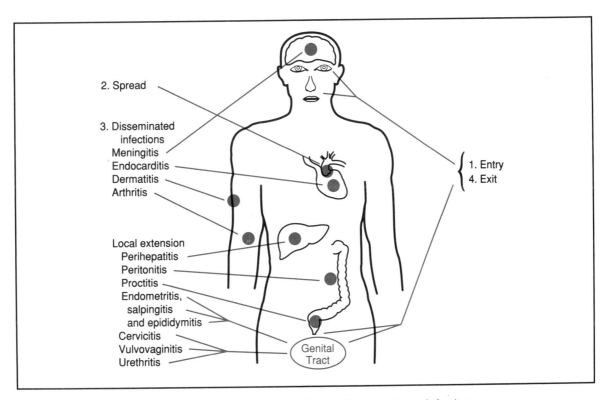

FIGURE 14-1 Clinical manifestations of *N gonorrhoeae* infection.

scanty, clear, or cloudy fluid to one that is copious and purulent. Dysuria is often present. Men with asymptomatic urethritis are an important reservoir for transmission. In addition, such men and those who ignore their symptoms are at increased risk for developing complications.

Endocervical infection is the most common form of uncomplicated gonorrhea in women. Such infections are usually characterized by vaginal discharge and sometimes by dysuria (because of coexistent urethritis). The cervical os may be erythematous and friable, with a purulent exudate. About 50 percent of women with cervical infections are asymptomatic. Local complications include abscesses in Bartholin's and Skene's glands.

Rectal infections with *N gonorrhoeae* occur in about one-third of women with cervical infection. They most often result from autoinoculation with cervical discharge and are rarely symptomatic. Rectal infections in homosexual men usually result from anal intercourse and are more often symptomatic. The symptoms and signs of gonococcal proctitis range from mild burning on defecation to itching to severe tenesmus and from mucopurulent discharge to frank blood in the stools.

Pharyngeal infections are diagnosed most often in women and homosexual men with a history of fellatio. Such infections may be a focal source of gonococcemia.

Ocular infections can have serious consequences (corneal scarring or perforation); prompt diagnosis and treatment are therefore important. Ocular infections occur must commonly in newborns who are exposed to infected secretions in the birth canal. Keratoconjunctivitis is occasionally seen in adults as a result of autoinoculation.

Disseminated gonococcal infections result from gonococcal bacteremia. Asymptomatic infections of the pharynx, urethra, or cervix often serve as focal sources for bacteremia. The most common form of disseminated gonococcal infection is the **dermatitis-arthritis syndrome.** It is characterized by fever, chills, skin lesions, and arthralgias (usually involving the hands, feet, and elbows), which are due to periarticular inflammation of the tendon sheaths. Occasionally, a patient develops a septic joint with effusion. Skin lesions may be macular, pustular, centrally necrotic, or hemorrhagic.

Rarely, disseminated gonococcal infection causes endocarditis or meningitis.

Gonococci may ascend from the endocervical canal through the endometrium to the fallopian tubes and ultimately to the pelvic peritoneum, resulting in endometritis, salpingitis, and, finally, peritonitis. Women usually present with pelvic and abdominal pain, fever, chills, and cervical motion tenderness. This complex of signs and symptoms is referred to as **pelvic inflammatory disease (PID).** This disease may also be caused by other sexually transmitted organisms (e.g., *Chlamydia trachomatis*) as well as by non-sexually transmitted bacteria that are part of the normal vaginal flora. Complications of pelvic inflammatory disease include tubo-ovarian abscesses, pelvic peritonitis, or Fitz-Hugh and Curtis syndrome, which is an inflammation of Glisson's capsule of the liver. As many as 15 percent of women with uncomplicated cervical infections may develop pelvic inflammatory disease. The disease may have serious consequences, including an increased probability of infertility and ectopic pregnancy.

STRUCTURE

Neisseria species are Gram-negative cocci, 0.6 to 1.0 μm in diameter. The organisms are usually seen in pairs with the adjacent sides flattened. Pili —hairlike filamentous appendages—extend several micrometers from the cell surface and have a role in adherence. The outer membrane is composed of proteins, phospholipids, and lipopolysaccharide (LPS). Features that distinguish gonococcal LPS from enteric LPS are the highly branched basal oligosaccharide structure and the absence of repeating O-antigen subunits. Gonococci characteristically release outer membrane fragments (blebs) during growth. These blebs contain LPS and may have a role in pathogenesis.

CLASSIFICATION AND ANTIGENIC TYPES

The gonococcus is an obligate human pathogen. It is one of two *Neisseria* species that cause significant human infections. The genus also includes several nonpathogenic species (Table 14-1), which may be part of the normal flora and therefore can be confused with *N gonorrhoeae*. Gonococcal strains can be characterized according to their nutritional requirements (**auxotyping**). A panel of monoclonal antibodies specific for epitopes on protein I have also been used to type strains. Strains exhibiting specific reaction patterns are termed **serovars.** A combined auxotype-serovar classification provides greater resolution among gonococcal isolates and is useful in epidemiologic investigations.

PATHOGENESIS

Our knowledge of the molecular basis of gonococcal pathogenesis is incomplete (Fig. 14-2). Attachment of gonococci to mucosal cells is mediated in part by pili, although nonspecific factors such as surface charge and hydrophobicity may be important. Pili undergo both phase and antigenic variation. Additional gonococcal surface antigens (e.g., protein II) are involved in attachment to host cells. Gonococci attach only to microvilli of nonciliated columnar epithelial cells; attachment to ciliated cells is not observed.

Much of our knowledge of gonococcal invasion comes from studies with tissue culture cells and human fallopian tube organ culture. After gonococci attach to the nonciliated epithelial cells of the fallopian tube, they are surrounded by the microvilli, which draw them to the surface of the mucosal cell. The gonococci appear to enter the epithelial cells by a process called **parasite-directed endocytosis.** This process seems to be initiated by microbial factors because it does not occur unless the gonococci are viable and because it involves host cells that are not normally phagocytic. An unidentified factor in serum enhances engulfment of gonococci. The process is inhibited by drugs that block the actions of the microtubule (demecolcine) and microfilament (cytochalasin B) systems. During endocytosis the membrane of the mucosal cell retracts, pinching off a membrane-bound vacuole that contains gonococci; this vacuole is rapidly transported to the base of the cell, where gonococci are released by exocytosis into the subepithelial tissue. Gonococci are not destroyed within the

phagocytic vacuole; it is not clear whether they replicate in the vacuoles.

The major porin protein of the gonococcal outer membrane, **protein I,** has been proposed as a candidate invasin (a substance that helps mediate invasion into a host cell). The insertion of protein I into neutrophils treated with f-Met-Leu-Phe (f MLP) and leukotriene B_4, inhibits degranulation but not the generation of the superoxide anion. The significance of these observations with respect to the pathogenesis of gonorrhea remains to be determined.

Gonococci can produce one or several outer membrane proteins called **proteins II.** These proteins are subject to phase variation and are usually found on cells from colonies possessing an opaque phenotype (O^+). At any one time, a gonococcus may express zero, one, or several different proteins II. Trypsinlike proteases present in cervical mucus may help select for protease-resistant transparent (O^-) colony phenotypes. O^+ colony phenotypes (protease sensitive) predominate in cultures taken during the middle portion of the menstrual cycle. Cervical proteases increase during the second half of the cycle, resulting in an increase in the O^- phenotype. The O^- colony types can be isolated from tubal as well as endocervical cultures; O^+ colony phenotypes have been isolated more often from endocervical cultures than from tubal cultures.

Protein III is an outer membrane protein found in all strains of *N gonorrhoeae*. It does not undergo phase variation and is found in a complex with protein I and LPS. It shares partial homology with a protein of *Escherichia coli*. Antibodies to this region of protein III, induced either by a neisserial infection or by colonization with *E coli*, block bactericidal antibodies directed against protein I and LPS.

LPS has a profound effect on the virulence and pathogenesis of gonorrhea. Gonococci can express several antigenic types of LPS and can alter the type of LPS they express by an as yet unknown mechanism. Gonococcal LPS produces mucosal damage in fallopian tube organ cultures and brings about the release of enzymes, such as proteases and phospholipases, that may be important in pathogenesis. More recent evidence suggests that

TABLE 14-1 Differential Characteristics of Organisms in the Genera Neisseria and Branhamella[a]

Characteristic[b]	N gonorrhoeae	N meningitidis	N lactamica	N sicca	N subflava[c]	N flavescens	N cinerea	N mucosa	B catarrhalis
Acid from									
Glucose	+	+	+	+	+	−	−	+	−
Maltose	−	+	+	+	+	−	−	+	−
Lactose	−	−	+	−	−	−	−	−	−
Fructose	−	−	−	+	V	−	−	+	−
Sucrose	−	−	−	+	V	−	−	+	−
Growth on									
TM, or MTM, or NYC, or ML medium[d]	+	+	+	−	−	−	−	−	d
Chocolate or blood agar at 22°C	−	−	V	V	V	+		+	+
Nutrient agar at 35°C	−	−	+	+	V	+	+	+	+
Polysaccharide synthesis from 5% sucrose	φ	φ	?	+[e]	d	+	−	+	−
Production of H2S	−	−	−	+	+	+	?	+	−
Presence of capsule	V	d	?	V	+	−	?	+	−
Reduction of nitrate	−	−	−	−	−	−	−	+	+
Reduction of nitrite[f]	+	d	+	+	+	+	+	+	+
Deoxyribonuclease	−	−	−	−	−	−	−	−	+
IgA1 protease	+	+	−	−	−	−	?	−	−

[a] All species contain catalase and cytochrome oxidase.

[b] +, most strains positive (≥ 90 percent); −, most strains negative (≥ 90 percent); d, some strains positive; V, character inconstant within single strain; φ, no growth on medium with 5 percent sucrose; ?, not known.

[c] New species consisting of N subflava, N flava, and N perflava.

[d] TM, Thayer-Martin medium; MTM, modified Thayer-Martin medium; NYC, New York City medium; ML, Martin-Lewis medium.

[e] N sicca forms an iodine-positive product when grown on tryptic soy agar without 5% sucrose. This reaction, which does not occur with N subflava, may be used as a differentiating characteristic.

[f] 0.001% (wt/vol) nitrite. Higher concentrations of nitrite (≥ 0.1 percent) are toxic for many species.

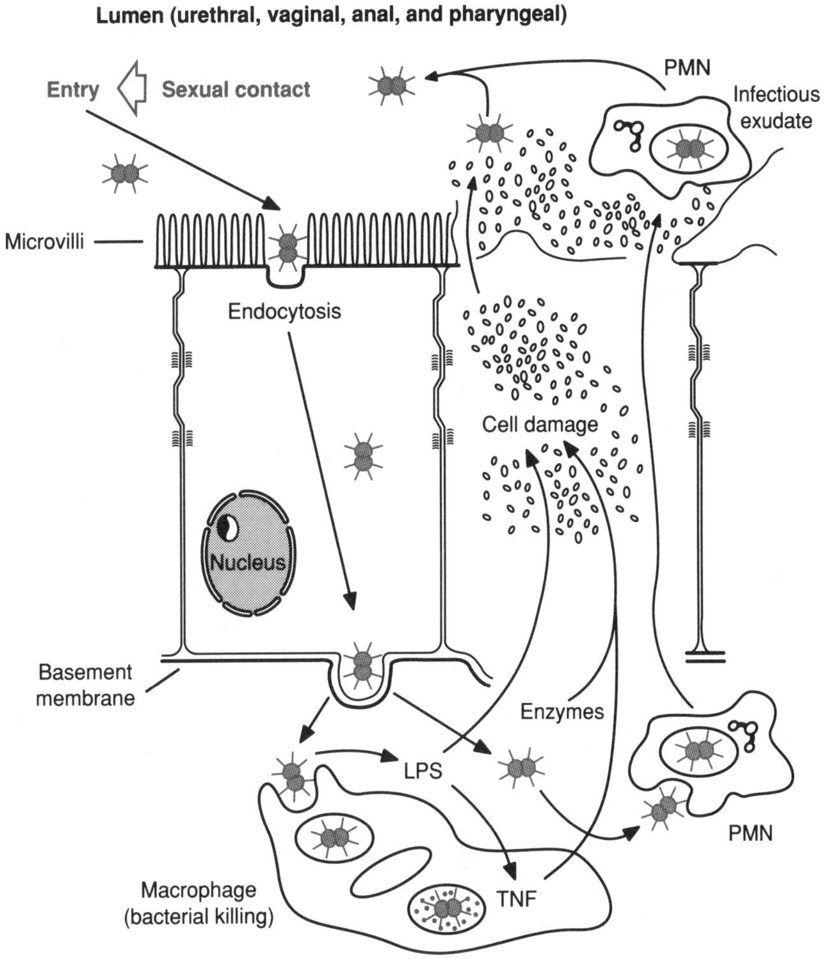

Lumen (urethral, vaginal, anal, and pharyngeal)

FIGURE 14-2   Pathogenesis of uncomplicated gonorrhea. Gonococci can invade columnar epithelial cells, although they do not invade ciliated columnar epithelium of the respiratory tract.

gonococcal LPS stimulates the production of tumor necrosis factor (TNF) in fallopian tube organ cultures; inhibition of tumor necrosis factor with specific antiserum prevents tissue damage. Thus, gonococcal LPS appears to have an indirect role in mediating tissue damage. Gonococcal LPS is also involved in the resistance of *N gonorrhoeae* to the bactericidal activity of normal human serum. Oligosaccharides containing epitopes defined by specific monoclonal antibodies are associated with a serum-resistant phenotype.

Gonococci can utilize host-derived cytidine monophospho-*N*-acetylneuraminic acid in vivo to sialylate the oligosaccharide component of its LPS, converting a serum-sensitive organism to a serum-resistant one. When such organisms are grown in vitro, their resistance to killing by normal human serum is rapidly lost. There is antigenic similarity between neisserial LPS and antigens present on human erythrocytes. This similarity to self may preclude an effective immune response to these LPS antigens.

Gonococci are highly autolytic and release peptidoglycan fragments during growth. These fragments, released by bacterial and/or host peptidoglycan hydrolases, are toxic for fallopian tube mucosa and contribute to the intense inflammatory reactions characteristic of gonococcal disease.

N gonorrhoeae is highly efficient at utilizing transferrin-bound iron for in vitro growth; many strains can also utilize lactoferrin-bound iron. Gonococci (and meningococci) bind only human transferrin. This specificity is thought to be the reason why these organisms are exclusively human pathogens. Nevertheless, the role of transferrin- and lactoferrin-bound iron in in vivo growth is unknown. Gonococci express several new proteins when grown under iron-restricted conditions similar to the conditions occurring in the host. The roles of these iron-regulated proteins in pathogenesis and in the acquisition of iron are areas of intense interest. Gonococci cannot grow anaerobically unless low concentrations of the alternative electron acceptor nitrite are present. Under these conditions they produce novel proteins. These proteins are apparently produced during an infection because antibodies are present in the serum specimens of patients with uncomplicated gonorrhea, disseminated gonococcal infection, or pelvic inflammatory disease. These data suggest that some gonococci in the host are growing under anaerobic conditions. Further studies will determine the relevance of these proteins to pathogenesis.

Strains of *N gonorrhoeae* (and *N meningitidis*) produce two distinct extracellular **IgA1 proteases,** which cleave the heavy chain of human immunoglobulin A1 (IgA1) at different points within the hinge region. Type 1 protease cleaves a prolyl-seryl peptide bond and type 2 protease cleaves a prolyl-threonyl bond in the hinge region of the heavy chain. This region is missing in human IgA2, and so this isotype is not susceptible to cleavage. Each gonococcal or meningococcal isolate elaborates only one of these two enzymes. Split products of IgA1 have been found in the genital secretions of women with gonorrhea, suggesting that the gonococcal IgA1 protease is present and active during genital infection. However, the IgA2 isotype is predominant on mucosal surfaces. Attempts to detect the enzyme in genital secretions have been unsuccessful. The gene encoding the gonococcal IgA1 protease has been cloned and insertionally inactivated. A strain lacking a functional IgA1 protease attached to and invaded human fallopian tube mucosa to the same extent as an isogenic strain with a functional IgA1 protease. Therefore, the role of this enzyme in pathogenesis remains unclear.

HOST DEFENSES

Not everyone exposed to *N gonorrhoeae* acquires the disease. This may be due to variations in the size or virulence of the inoculum, to nonspecific resistance, or to specific immunity. A 50 percent infective dose (ID_{50}) of about 1,000 organisms has been established, based on the experimental urethral inoculation of male volunteers. There is no reliable ID_{50} for women, although it is assumed to be similar.

Nonspecific factors have been implicated in natural resistance to gonococcal infection. In women, changes in the genital pH and hormones may increase resistance to infection at certain times of the menstrual cycle. Urinary solutes exhibit bactericidal and bacteriostatic activity for *N gonorrhoeae*. Factors in urine that seem to be important are pH, osmolarity, and the concentration of urea. The variability in the susceptibility of gonococcal strains to the bactericidal and bacteriostatic properties of urine is thought to be one of the reasons why some men do not develop a gonococcal infection when exposed.

Most uninfected individuals have serum antibodies that react with gonococcal antigens. These antibodies probably result from colonization or infection with various Gram-negative bacteria that possess cross-reactive antigens. These "natural" antibodies differ, both qualitatively and quantitatively, from person to person, but may be important in an individual's natural resistance to infection.

Infection with *N gonorrhoeae* stimulates both mucosal and systemic antibodies to a variety of gonococcal antigens. Mucosal antibodies are primarily IgA and IgG. In genital secretions, antibodies have been identified that react with proteins I and II, LPS, and some of the iron-regulated proteins. Vaccine trials have suggested that antipilus antibodies inhibit the pilus-mediated attachment of the homologous gonococcal strain. Complement is present in endocervical secretions, but in much lower concentrations than in blood. However, there is little evidence to support a role for a complement-mediated bactericidal defense mechanism on the genital mucosa. In general, the IgA response is brief and declines rapidly after treatment; IgG levels decline more slowly.

More information is available about the function of systemic humoral immune mechanisms in gonococcal infection. Gonococcal antigens such as pili, proteins I through III, and LPS elicit a serum antibody response during an infection. Antipilus antibody levels tend to be higher in women than in men and are related to the number of previous infections. The predominant IgG subclass that reacts with a variety of gonococcal antigens is IgG3, followed by IgG1 and IgG4. IgG2 is minimal, suggesting that polysaccharides are not important in the immune response to gonococcal infection. Anti-protein I antibodies may be bactericidal for the gonococcus. IgG that reacts with protein III blocks the bactericidal activity of antibodies directed against protein I and LPS. Genital infection with *N gonorrhoeae* stimulates a serum antibody response against the LPS of the infecting strain. Disseminated gonococcal infection results in higher levels of anti-LPS antibody than do genital infections.

Strains that cause uncomplicated genital infections usually are killed by normal human serum and are termed **serum sensitive.** This bactericidal activity is mediated by IgM and IgG that recognize sites on the LPS. Strains that cause disseminated infections are not killed by most normal human serum and are referred to as **serum resistant.** Resistance is mediated, in part, by IgA that blocks the IgG-mediated bactericidal activity of the serum. Serum specimens from convalescent patients with disseminating infections contain bactericidal IgG to the LPS of the infecting strain.

Individuals with inherited complement deficiencies have a markedly increased risk of acquiring systemic neisserial infections and are subject to recurring episodes of systemic gonococcal and meningococcal infections, indicating that the complement system is important in host defense. Gonococci activate complement by both the classic and alternative pathways. Complement activation

by gonococci leads to the formation of the C5b–9 complex (membrane attack complex) on the outer membrane. In normal human serum, similar numbers of C5b–9 complexes are deposited on serum-sensitive and serum-resistant organisms, but the membrane attack complex is not functional on serum-resistant organisms. Other complement-mediated functions, such as opsonophagocytosis and chemotaxis, are more efficient with serum-sensitive than with serum-resistant gonococci. This may be a significant factor in the pathogenesis of disseminated gonococcal infection and probably contributes to the relative lack of genital symptoms observed with this disease.

Normal human serum contains opsonic anti-protein I IgG. Antibodies to various surface-exposed antigens are also present in cervical and urethral secretions of patients with gonorrhea and probably contribute to the opsonophagocytosis of the organism. Protein II is important in gonococcus-neutrophil interactions. Gonococci possessing certain proteins II interact with neutrophils in the absence of antibodies. Once phagocytosed, gonococci are killed by both oxygen-dependent and oxygen-independent mechanisms. The survival of gonococci within neutrophils has been the subject of considerable controversy, with no clear-cut answer yet available. The opsonization and phagocytosis of gonococci are comparatively more important in mucosal infections than in protection from systemic gonococcal (and meningococcal) infections.

EPIDEMIOLOGY

The only natural host for *N gonorrhoeae* is the human. Gonorrhea is one of the most frequently reported infectious diseases in the United States. Between 1977 and 1988, the number of reported cases decreased 31.2 percent, from 1 million to 688,000 cases per year; in 1989, the number of reported cases increased 2 percent over those reported in 1988. The Centers for Disease Control (CDC) estimates that there are two unreported cases for every reported case of gonorrhea. Gonorrhea is transmitted almost exclusively by sexual contact. The highest incidence occurs between the ages of 18 and 24 years in women and 20 and 24 years in men. Persons who have multiple sex partners are at highest risk. Rates of gonorrhea are higher in males and in minority and inner-city populations.

Gonorrhea is usually contracted from a sex partner who is either asymptomatic or has only minimal symptoms. It is estimated that the efficiency of transmission after one exposure is about 35 percent from an infected woman to an uninfected man and 50 to 60 percent from an infected man to an uninfected woman. More than 90 percent of men with urethral gonorrhea will develop symptoms within 5 days; fewer than 50 percent of women with anogenital gonorrhea will do so. Women and men with asymptomatic infections are at higher risk of developing pelvic inflammatory disease and disseminated gonococcal infection.

DIAGNOSIS

Gonococcal infection produces several common clinical syndromes that have multiple causes or that mimic other conditions. Laboratory tests are often required to differentiate among the etiologic agents causing urethritis or cervicitis. The etiologic diagnosis of salpingitis and pelvic peritonitis is quite difficult because mixed infections are common and laparoscopy is required to obtain appropriate cultures. Gonococcal perihepatitis may mimic acute cholecystitis. All of the above syndromes are also caused by *Chlamydia trachomatis,* a sexually transmitted bacterium that causes more infections in the United States than *N gonorrhoeae.* The gonococcal arthritis-dermatitis syndrome must be differentiated from meningococcemia and Reiter syndrome in particular and from other causes of septic arthritis.

Customarily, the laboratory diagnosis of gonorrhea is made presumptively and then confirmed; the latter process involves identifying characteristics that distinguish *N gonorrhoeae* from other *Neisseria* spp that may be present in the specimen. Nonpathogenic *Neisseria* are normal inhabitants of the oropharynx and nasopharynx and occasionally are isolated from other sites infected by *N gonorrhoeae.* A presumptive diagnosis of gonorrhea may be made from Gram-stained smears of urethral, cervical, and rectal specimens if Gram-negative diplococci are observed within leukocytes; it is equivocal if only extracellular Gram-negative diplococci are seen and negative if no Gram-negative diplococci are seen. Gram stain diagnosis has a sensitivity and specificity of >95 percent in men with symptomatic urethritis. The specificity of Gram stain diagnosis in women is also high if the cervix is wiped clean to remove vaginal secretions before collecting the specimen; however, the sensitivity is only about 50 percent. The sensitivity and specificity of the Gram stain for rectal specimens are lower than with cervical specimens.

Specimens for the laboratory diagnosis of gonorrhea should be collected before treating the patient. Ideally, specimens should be inoculated onto appropriate media and incubated immediately after collection at 35 to 36.5°C in a CO_2-enriched atmosphere, which can be obtained by using a candle extinction jar or a CO_2 incubator. Urethral specimens are normally obtained from heterosexual men; urethral, rectal, and pharyngeal specimens are normally obtained from homosexual men; and cervical and rectal specimens are normally obtained from women. Specimens are collected with cotton, polyester, or calcium alginate swabs. When appropriate, specimens may also be obtained from the urethra and from Bartholin's and Skene's glands of infected women. Blood cultures should be performed for patients with suspected disseminated infection. Synovial fluid cultures should be performed for patients with septic arthritis.

Urethral, cervical, and pharyngeal specimens are inoculated onto selective medium such as Thayer-Martin, Martin-Lewis, or GC-Lect medium. These are complex media that contain antimicrobial and antifungal agents to inhibit the growth of unwanted organisms. Rectal specimens should be inoculated onto modified Thayer-Martin medium, which contains trimethoprim lactate to inhibit the growth and swarming of *Proteus* species. Specimens collected from normally sterile sites such as blood, synovial fluid, and conjunctivae may be inoculated onto a nonselective medium such as chocolate agar.

The combination of oxidase-positive colonies and Gram-negative diplococci provides a presumptive identification of *N gonorrhoeae*. Fluorescent-antibody staining, coagglutination, specific biochemical tests (Table 14-1), and DNA probes may be used for confirmation. Serologic tests for uncomplicated gonorrhea have not proved satisfactory.

CONTROL

There is no effective vaccine to prevent gonorrhea. Candidate vaccines consisting of pilus protein or protein I are of little benefit. The development of an effective vaccine has been hampered by the lack of a suitable animal model and the fact that an effective immune response has never been demonstrated. Condoms are effective in preventing the transmission of gonorrhea.

Contact tracing to identify source contacts (i.e., those who infected the index patient) has been useful in identifying asymptomatic individuals or those with ignored symptoms. Contact tracing has also been used to identify contacts who were exposed to the index patient and who may have become infected.

The evolution of antimicrobial resistance in *N gonorrhoeae* may ultimately affect the control of gonorrhea. Strains with multiple chromosomal resistance to penicillin, tetracycline, erythromycin, and cefoxitin have been identified in the United States and most other parts of the world. Sporadic high-level resistance to spectinomycin has also been reported.

Penicillinase-producing strains of *N gonorrhoeae* were first described in 1976. Five related β-lactamase plasmids of different sizes have been identified in these strains. The strains cause more than one-half of all gonococcal infections in parts of Africa and Asia. Their prevalence has increased dramatically in the United States since 1984 and has affected nearly every major metropolitan area.

Plasmid-mediated high-level resistance of *N gonorrhoeae* to tetracycline has recently been observed. This resistance is due to the presence of the streptococcal *tetM* determinant on a gonococcal conjugative plasmid.

The current CDC *Treatment Guidelines* recommend treatment of all gonococcal infections with antibiotic regimens effective against resistant strains. The recommended antimicrobial agent is ceftriaxone. Since a significant proportion of patients with gonorrhea are also infected with *C trachomatis*, a tetracycline or erythromycin has been added to treat this concomitant infection.

◄ *NEISSERIA MENINGITIDIS* ►

CLINICAL PRESENTATION

N meningitidis infection results from the blood-borne dissemination (meningococcemia) of the meningococcus, usually following an asymptomatic or mildly symptomatic nasopharyngeal carrier state or a mild rhinopharyngitis (Fig. 14-3). The mildest form is a transient bacteremic illness characterized by fever and malaise; symptoms resolve spontaneously in 1 to 2 days. Acute meningococcemia is more serious and is often complicated by meningitis. The manifestations of meningococcal meningitis are similar to acute bacterial meningitis caused by organisms such as *Streptococcus pneumoniae, Haemophilus influenzae,* and *E coli*. The manifestations result from both infection and increased intracranial pressure. Chills, fever, malaise, and headache are the usual manifestations of infection; headache, vomiting, and, rarely, papilledema may result from increased intracranial pressure. Signs of meningeal inflammation are also present. The onset of meningococcal meningitis may be abrupt or insidious.

Infants with meningococcal meningitis rarely display signs of meningeal irritation. Irritability and refusal to take food are typical; vomiting occurs early in the disease and may lead to dehydration. Fever is typically absent in children younger than 2 months of age. Hypothermia is more common in neonates. As the disease progresses, apneic episodes, seizures, disturbances in motor tone, and coma may develop.

In older children and adults, specific symptoms and signs are usually present, with fever and altered mental status the most consistent findings.

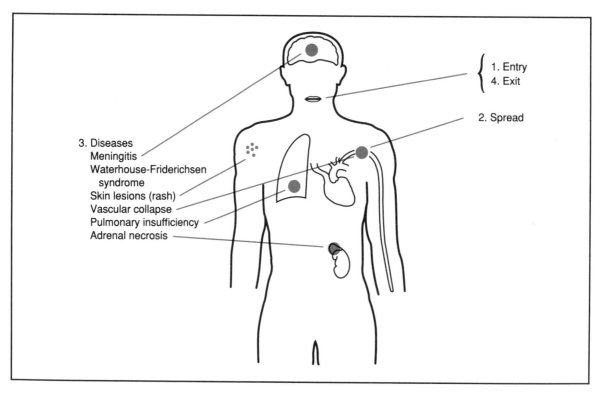

FIGURE 14-3   Clinical manifestations of *N meningitidis* infection.

Headache is an early, prominent complaint and is usually very severe. Nausea, vomiting, and photophobia are also common symptoms.

Neurologic signs are common; approximately one-third of patients have convulsions or coma when first seen by a physician. Signs of meningeal irritation such as cervical rigidity (Brudzinski sign), thoracolumnar rigidity, hamstring spasm (Kernig sign), and exaggerated reflexes are common.

Petechiae (minute hemorrhagic spots in the skin) or purpura (hemorrhages into the skin) occurs from the first to the third day of illness in 30 to 60 percent of patients with meningococcal disease, with or without meningitis. The lesions may be more prominent in areas of the skin subjected to pressure, such as the axillary folds, the belt line, or the back.

Fulminant meningococcemia (Waterhouse-Friderichsen syndrome) occurs in 5 to 15 percent of patients with meningococcal disease and has a high mortality rate. It begins abruptly with sudden high fever, chills, myalgias, weakness, nausea, vomiting, and headache. Apprehension, restlessness, and, frequently, delirium occur within the next few hours. Widespread purpuric and ecchymotic skin lesions appear suddenly. Typically, no signs of meningitis are present. Pulmonary insufficiency develops within a few hours, and many patients die within 24 hours of being hospitalized despite appropriate antibiotic therapy and intensive care.

STRUCTURE

The only distinguishing structural feature between *N meningitidis* and *N gonorrhoeae* is the presence of a polysaccharide capsule in the former. The capsule is antiphagocytic and is an important virulence factor.

CLASSIFICATION AND ANTIGENIC TYPES

Meningococcal capsular polysaccharides provide the basis for grouping these organisms. Twelve serogroups have been identified (A, B, C, H, I, K, L,

X, Y, Z, 29E, and W135). The chemical composition of these capsular polysaccharides, where known, is listed in Table 14-2. The prominent outer membrane proteins of *N meningitidis* have been designated class 1 through class 5. The class 2 and 3 proteins function as porins and are analogous to gonococcal protein I. The class 4 and 5 proteins are analogous to gonococcal protein III and proteins II, respectively. Serogroup B and C meningococci have been further subdivided on the basis of serotype determinants located on the class 2 and 3 proteins. A few serotypes are associated with most cases of meningococcal disease, whereas other serotypes within the same serogroup rarely

TABLE 14-2   Chemical Composition of *N meningitidis* Capsular Polysaccharides

Serogroup	Structural Repeating Unit[a]
Serogroup A[b] (homopolymer)	ManNAc-(1-P $\xrightarrow{\alpha}$ 6)- 3 | OAc
Serogroup B (homopolymer) Serogroup C[c] (homopolymer)	NeuNAc-(2 $\xrightarrow{\alpha}$ 8)- NeuNAc-(2 $\xrightarrow{\alpha}$ 9)- 7 8 | | OAc OAc
Serogroup H (monosaccharide-glycerol repeating unit) Serogroup I (disaccharide repeating unit)	→ 4) α-D-Gal-(1 → 2)-Gro-(3-P → → 4) α-L-GulNAcA (1 → 3)β-D-ManNAcA(1→ | 4-OAc
Serogroup K (disaccharide repeating unit)	→ 3)-β-D-ManNAcA-(1 → 4)-β-D-ManNAcA-(1→ | 4-OAc
Serogroup L (triasaccharide repeating unit)	→ 3)-β-D-GlcNAc-(1 → 3) β-D-GlcNAc-(1 → 3) α-D-GlcNAc-(1-P-
Serogroup W135 (disaccharide repeating unit) Serogroup X (homopolymer) Serogroup Y (BO)[d] (disaccharide repeating unit)	6-D-Gal(1 $\xrightarrow{\alpha}$ 4)-NeuNAc(2 $\xrightarrow{\alpha}$ 6)- GlcNAc(1-P → 4)- 6-D-Glc(1 $\xrightarrow{\alpha}$ 4)-NeuNAc(2 $\xrightarrow{\alpha}$ 6) | OAc
Serogroup Z (monosaccharide glycerol repeating unit) Serogroup 29E (disaccharide repeating unit)	D-GalNAc(1 $\xrightarrow{\alpha}$ 1′)-Gro-(3′-P $\xrightarrow{\alpha}$ 4) D-GalNAc(1 $\xrightarrow{\beta}$ 7)-KDO(2 $\xrightarrow{\alpha}$ 3)- 4,5 | OAc

[a] Gal, galactose; Glc, glucose; ManNAc, *N*-acetylmannosamine (2-acetamido-2-deoxy-D-mannose); NeuNAc, *N*-acetylneuraminic acid (sialic acid); OAc, O-acetylated; Gro, glycerol; P, phosphate; Gul-NAcA, 2-acetamido-2-deoxy-L-guluronic acid; ManNAcA, 2-acetamido-2-deoxy-mannuronic acid; GlcNAc, *N*-acetylglucosamine (2-acetamido-2-deoxy-D-glucose); GalNAc, *N*-acetylgalactosamine (2-acetamido-2-deoxy-D-galactose).

[b] Group A is substituted with O-acetyl at C-3 on about 70 percent of the ManNAc-P residues.

[c] Group C is substituted on C-7 or C-8 with 1 mole of *O*-acetyl per mole of sialic acid. One-quarter of the sialyl residues are not acetylated. Some di-O-acetylated residues (C-7 and C-8) may exist.

[d] The Y polysaccharide contains 1.3 moles of *O*-acetyl per NeuNAc residue. The most probable site for acetylation is C-3, C-4, or C-7.
[13]C nuclear magnetic resonance studies have shown that the serogroup BO polysaccharide is identical to serogroup Y, although BO contains 1.8 moles of *O*-acetyl per mole of NeuNAc.

caused disease. All known group A strains have the same protein serotype antigens in the outer membrane. Another serotyping system is based on the antigenic diversity of meningococcal LPS. The LPS types are independent of the protein serotypes, although certain combinations frequently occur together.

PATHOGENESIS

The human nasopharynx is the only known reservoir of *N meningitidis*. Meningococci are spread via respiratory droplets, and transmission requires aspiration of infective particles. Meningococci attach to the nonciliated columnar epithelial cells of the nasopharynx. Attachment is mediated by pili and possibly by other outer membrane components. Invasion of the mucosal cells occurs by a mechanism similar to that observed with gonococci. However, once internalized, meningococci remain in an apical location within the epithelial cell; the route by which they gain access to the subepithelial space remains unclear. Trimers of class 2 and 3 proteins have the ability to translocate from intact cells and insert into eukaryotic cell membranes to form voltage-dependent channels. This process may be important in invasion.

Purified meningococcal LPS is highly toxic and is as lethal for mice as the LPS from *E coli* or *Salmonella typhimurium;* however, meningococcal LPS is 5 to 10 times more effective than enteric LPS in eliciting a dermal Shwartzman reaction in rabbits. Meningococcal LPS suppresses leukotriene B_4 synthesis in human polymorphonuclear leukocytes. The loss of leukotriene B_4 deprives the leukocytes of a strong chemokinetic and chemotactic factor.

The events after bloodstream invasion are unclear. Relatively little information is known about how the meningococcus enters the central nervous system.

HOST DEFENSES

The integrity of the pharyngeal and respiratory epithelium may be important in protection from invasive disease. Chronic irritation of the mucosa due to dust or low humidity, or damage to the mucosa resulting from a concurrent viral or mycoplasmal upper respiratory infection, may be predisposing factors for invasive disease.

The presence of serum bactericidal IgG and IgM is probably the most important host factor in preventing invasive disease. These antibodies are directed against both capsular and noncapsular surface antigens. The antibodies are produced in response to colonization with carrier strains of *N meningitidis, N lactamica,* or other nonpathogenic *Neisseria* species. Protective antibodies are also stimulated by cross-reacting antigens on other bacterial species. The role of bactericidal antibodies in prevention of invasive disease explains why high attack rates are seen in infants from 6 to 9 months old, the age at which maternally acquired antibodies are being lost.

The immunity conferred by specific antibody may not be absolute. Illness has been documented in individuals with levels of antibodies considered to be protective. It has been postulated that the activity of the bactericidal antibodies might be blocked by IgA, induced by other meningococcal strains, or by cross-reacting antigens on enteric or other respiratory bacteria. Since IgA does not bind complement, it may block binding sites for the bactericidal IgG and IgM. Persons with complement deficiencies may develop meningococcemia despite protective antibody. This underscores the importance of the complement system in protection from meningococcal disease.

EPIDEMIOLOGY

The meningococcus usually inhabits the human nasopharynx without causing detectable disease. This carrier state may last for a few days to months and is important because it not only provides a reservoir for meningococcal infection but also enhances host immunity. Between 3 and 30 percent of normal individuals are carriers at any given time, yet few develop meningococcal disease. Even during epidemics of meningococcal meningitis in military recruits, when the carrier rate may reach 95 percent, the incidence of systemic disease is less than 1 percent. Meningococcal carriage rates are highest in older children and young adults, but the attack rates are higher in children, peaking at 5 years of age (group B) and 4 to 14 years of age (group C). The low incidence of disseminated disease following colonization suggests that host rather than bacterial factors play an important determining role.

Meningococcal meningitis occurs sporadically and in epidemics, with the highest incidence during late winter and early spring. Most epidemics are caused by group A strains, but small outbreaks have occurred with group B and C strains. Sporadic cases generally are caused by group B, C, and Y strains. Whenever group A strains become prevalent in the population, the incidence of meningitis increases markedly.

DIAGNOSIS

The most characteristic manifestation of meningococcemia is the skin rash, which is essential for its recognition. Petechiae are the most common type of skin lesion. Ill-defined pink macules and maculopapular lesions also occur. Lesions are sparsely distributed over the body. They tend to occur in crops and on any part of the body; however, the face is usually spared and involvement of the palms and soles is less common. The skin rash may progress from a few ill-defined lesions to a widespread eruption within a few hours.

Acute bacterial meningitis has characteristic signs and symptoms. Except in epidemic situations, it is difficult to identify the causative agent without laboratory tests.

In cases of suspected meningococcal disease, specimens of blood, cerebrospinal fluid, and nasopharyngeal secretions should be collected before administration of any antimicrobial agents and examined for the presence of *N meningitidis*. Success in isolation is reduced by prior therapy; however, the microscopic diagnosis is not significantly affected. The cerebrospinal fluid should be concentrated by centrifugation and a portion of the sediment cultured on chocolate or blood agar. The plates should be incubated in a candle jar or CO_2 incubator. The presence of oxidase-positive colonies and Gram-negative diplococci provides a presumptive identification of *N meningitidis*. Produc-

tion of acid from glucose and maltose but not sucrose, lactose, or fructose may be used for confirmation. The serologic group may be determined by a slide agglutination test, using first polyvalent and then monovalent antisera.

Nasopharyngeal specimens must be obtained from the posterior nasopharyngeal wall behind the soft palate and then should be inoculated onto a selective medium such as Thayer-Martin medium and processed as above.

Blood specimens are inoculated in 10- to 15-ml aliquots onto each of three blood bottles to give a final concentration of 10% (vol/vol). Evacuated bottles should be vented. Some strains of *N meningitidis* are inhibited by the sodium polyanetholsulfonate contained in blood culture medium. Toxicity may be overcome by the addition of gelatin. Sodium amylosulfate is not toxic for the meningococcus. Blood cultures are subcultured blindly onto chocolate or blood agar for confirmation.

Gram-stained smears of cerebrospinal fluid may be diagnostic; however, finding neisseriae in these smears is often more difficult than finding the strains that cause pneumococcal meningitis. Quellung tests may be of value.

CONTROL

Group A, C, Y, and W135 capsular polysaccharide vaccines are available and can be used to control outbreaks due to the meningococcal serogroups covered by the vaccine. The A, C, AC, and ACYW135 polysaccharide formulations are currently licensed in the United States. The polysaccharide vaccines are ineffective in young children, and the duration of protection is limited in children vaccinated at 1 to 4 years of age. Routine vaccination of the civilian population in industrialized countries is not currently recommended because the risk of infection is low and most endemic disease occurs in young children. The group B capsular polysaccharide is a homopolymer of sialic acid and is not immunogenic in humans. A group B meningococcal vaccine consisting of outer membrane protein antigens has recently been developed but is not licensed in the United States.

Meningococcal disease arises from association with infected individuals, as evidenced by the 500-

to 800-fold greater attack rate among household contacts than among the general population. Because such household members are at high risk, they require chemophrophylaxis. Sulfonamides were the chemoprophylactic agent of choice until the emergence of sulfonamide-resistant meningococci. At present, approximately 25 percent of clinical isolates of *N meningitidis* in the United States are resistant to sulfonamides; rifampin is therefore the chemoprophylactic agent of choice.

Penicillin is the drug of choice to treat meningococcemia and meningococcal meningitis. Although penicillin does not penetrate the normal blood-brain barrier, it readily penetrates the blood-brain barrier when the meninges are acutely inflamed.

BRANHAMELLA

Branhamella catarrhalis organisms are cocci that morphologically resemble *Neisseria* cells. Other relevant characteristics are presented in Table 14-1. *B catarrhalis* is a parasite of the mucous membranes of mammals. It was formerly placed in the genus *Neisseria;* however, studies of DNA base content, fatty acid composition, and genetic transformation showed that this organism did not belong in that genus. *B catarrhalis* should be considered more than a harmless commensal of the mucous membranes of humans. It is an infrequent, yet significant, cause of severe systemic infections such as pneumonia, meningitis, and endocarditis. It is an important cause of lower respiratory tract infections in adults with chronic lung disease and a common cause of otitis media, sinusitis, and conjunctivitis in otherwise healthy children and adults. *B catarrhalis* may cause clinical syndromes indistinguishable from those caused by gonococci, and so it is important to distinguish these organisms from one another. Many strains produce β-lactamase.

MORAXELLA

The genus *Moraxella* is composed of organisms that are morphologically similar to *Acinetobacter;*
however, *Moraxella* is oxidase positive and shows no serologic cross-reactivity with *Acinetobacter.* Some strains may possess pili.

Moraxella species are parasites of the mucous membranes of humans and other warm-blooded animals. Many species are nonpathogenic. *M lacunata* can be isolated from the eyes and may cause conjunctivitis in humans living under conditions of poor hygiene. *M nonliquefaciens* is found in the upper respiratory tract, especially the nose, and may be a secondary invader in respiratory infections. *M urethralis* can be isolated from urine and the female genital tract. Some strains formerly designated as *Mima polymorpha* subsp *oxidans* belong in this species. These organisms can be mistaken for *N gonorrhoeae* unless appropriate biochemical characteristics are determined. Unlike *Acinetobacter*, *Moraxella* is sensitive to penicillin.

ACINETOBACTER

Organisms of the genus *Acinetobacter* are typically short rods about 1.0 to 1.5 by 1.5 to 2.5 μm in the logarithmic phase; they are coccoid in the stationary phase. Cells occur predominantly in pairs and in short chains. Some strains possess pili.

Acinetobacter species have been somewhat difficult to classify in the past because they do not have enough unique phenotypic properties for unequivocal differentiation from other similar-looking organisms. All strains are strict aerobes. Some produce an extracellular lipase and gelatinase. Many strains isolated from humans show hemolysis on blood agar plates owing to the production of a phospholipase C.

Acinetobacter is usually associated with opportunistic infections in compromised patients. Some infections may be serious, but most are minor. Usually, isolation of these organisms is of slight clinical significance, representing only contamination or secondary invasion of damaged tissues. Strains of *Acinetobacter* are usually resistant to 5 units of penicillin; many strains are highly resistant owing to production of β-lactamase. Organisms are usually sensitive to gentamicin, tobramycin, kanamycin, polymyxin B, colistin, or the tetracyclines.

REFERENCES

Brooks GF, Donegan EA: Gonococcal Infection. Edward Arnold, London, 1985

DeVoe IW: The meningococcus and mechanisms of pathogenicity. Microbiol Rev 46:162, 1982

Holmes KK, Mardh PA, Sparling PF, Wiesner PJ et al (eds): Sexually Transmitted Diseases. 2nd Ed. McGraw-Hill, New York, 1990

Morse SA, Broome CV, Cannon J et al (eds): Perspectives on pathogenic neisseriae. Clin Microbiol Rev 2:S1, 1989

15

BACILLUS

PETER C. B. TURNBULL

GENERAL CONCEPTS

Clinical Manifestations

Anthax is caused by *Bacillus anthracis*. Humans acquire the disease directly from contact with infected herbivores or indirectly via their products. The clinical forms include (1) cutaneous anthrax (eschar with edema), from handling infected material (this accounts for more than 95 percent of cases); (2) intestinal anthrax, from eating infected meat; and (3) pulmonary anthrax, from inhaling spore-laden dust. Several other *Bacillus* spp, in particular *B cereus* and to a lesser extent *B subtilis* and *B licheniformis,* are periodically associated with bacteremia/septicemia, endocarditis, meningitis, and infections of wounds, the ears, eyes, respiratory tract, urinary tract, and gastrointestinal tract. *Bacillus cereus* causes two distinct food poisoning syndromes: a rapid-onset **emetic syndrome** characterized by nausea and vomiting, and a slower-onset **diarrheal syndrome.**

Structure and Classification

Bacillus species are rod-shaped, endospore-forming aerobic or facultatively anaerobic, Gram-positive bacteria; in some species cultures may turn Gram-negative with age. The many species of the genus exhibit a wide range of physiologic abilities that allow them to live in every natural environment. Only one endospore is formed per cell. The spores are resistant to heat, cold, radiation, desiccation, and disinfectants. *Bacillus anthracis* needs oxygen to sporulate; this constraint has important consequences for epidemiology and control.

In vivo, *B anthracis* produces a polypeptide (polyglutamic acid) capsule that protects it from phagocytosis. The genera *Bacillus* and *Clostridium* constitute the family Bacillaceae. Species are identified by using morphologic and biochemical criteria.

Pathogenesis

The virulence factors of *B anthracis* are its capsule and three-component toxin, both encoded on plasmids. *Bacillus cereus* produces numerous enzymes and aggressins. The principal virulence factors are a necrotizing enterotoxin and a potent hemolysin (cereolysin). Emetic food poisoning probably results from the release of emetic factors from specific foods by bacterial enzymes.

Host Defenses

The reasons for marked differences in susceptibility to anthrax among different animal species are not known. The protective actions of the live-spore animal vaccine or the human chemical vaccines are based on induction of humoral and cell-mediated immunity to the protective antigen component of anthrax toxin.

Epidemiology

Individuals at risk for anthrax include those in contact with infected animals or animal products. Episodes of *B cereus* food poisoning occur sporadically worldwide and result from ingestion of contaminated food in which the bacteria have multiplied to high levels under conditions of improper storage after cooking.

Diagnosis

Cutaneous anthrax is diagnosed on the basis of the characteristic papule (early) or eschar (later) with extensive surrounding edema, backed by a history of exposure to animals or their products. Diagnosis is confirmed by observation of characteristic encapsulated bacilli in polychrome methylene blue-stained smears of blood, exudate, lymph, cerebrospinal fluid, etc., and/or by culture. Other *Bacillus* infections are diagnosed following culture of the bacteria.

Control

Anthrax: Control in animals is essential for control in humans. In endemic areas, animals that die suddenly should be handled cautiously and livestock should be vaccinated annually. A human vaccine is available for individuals in high-risk occupations. Anthrax is readily treated with antibiotics (e.g., penicillin, tetracycline, chloramphenicol, gentamicin, or erythromycin).

Other Bacillus Infections: Control is by good hygiene. Treatment is with non-β-lactam antibiotics for Gram-positive bacteria. Food poisoning is controlled by adequate cooking, avoidance of recontamination of cooked food, and proper storage (efficient refrigeration).

Pharmaceutical, Agricultural, and Industrial Importance

Many of the physiologic properties and specialized metabolites of *Bacillus* species are used in the pharmaceutical, agricultural, and food industries. On the other hand, the resistance of the spores to sterilization and disinfection makes them problem contaminants in foods, medical supplies, surgical procedures, etc.

INTRODUCTION

Bacillus species are aerobic, sporulating, rod-shaped bacteria that are ubiquitous in nature. *Bacillus anthracis,* the agent of anthrax, is the only obligate *Bacillus* pathogen in vertebrates. *Bacillus larvae, B lentimorbus, B popilliae, B sphaericus,* and *B thuringiensis* are pathogens of specific groups of insects. A number of other species, in particular *B cereus,* are occasional pathogens of humans and livestock, but the large majority of *Bacillus* species are harmless saprophytes.

Anthrax has afflicted humans throughout recorded history. The fifth and sixth plagues of Egypt described in Exodus are widely believed to have been anthrax. The disease was featured in the writings of Virgil in 25 BC and was familiar in medieval times as the Black Bane. It was from studies on anthrax that Koch established his famous postulates in 1876, and vaccines against anthrax — the best known being that of Pasteur (1881) — were among the first bacterial vaccines developed.

Bacillus species are used in many medical, pharmaceutical, agricultural, and industrial processes that take advantage of their wide range of physiologic characteristics and their ability to produce a host of enzymes, antibiotics, and other metabolities. Bacitracin and polymyxin are two well-known antibiotics obtained from *Bacillus* species. Several species are used as standards in medical and pharmaceutical assays. The spores of the obligate thermophile *B stearothermophilus* are used to test heat sterilization procedures, and *B subtilis* subsp *globigii,* which is resistant to heat, chemicals, and radiation, is widely used to validate alternative sterilization and fumigation procedures. Certain *Bacillus* species are important in the natural or artificial degradation of waste products. Some *Bacillus* insect pathogens are used as the active ingredients of insecticides.

Because the spores of many *Bacillus* species are resistant to heat, radiation, disinfectants, and desiccation, they are difficult to eliminate from medical and pharmaceutical materials and are a frequent cause of contamination. *Bacillus* species are well known in the food industries as troublesome spoilage organisms.

CLINICAL MANIFESTATIONS

Although anthrax remains the best-known *Bacillus* disease, in recent years other *Bacillus* species have been increasingly implicated in a wide range of infections including abscesses, bacteremia/septicemia, wound and burn infections, ear infections, endocarditis, meningitis, ophthalmitis, osteomyelitis, peritonitis, and respiratory and urinary tract infections. Most of these occur as secondary or mixed infections or in immunodeficient or otherwise immunocompromised hosts (such as alcoholics and diabetics), but a significant proportion are primary infections in otherwise healthy individuals. Some of these infections are severe or lethal. Of the species listed in Table 15-1, most frequently implicated in these types of infection is *B cereus,* followed by *B licheniformis* and *B subtilis. Bacillus alvei, B brevis, B circulans, B coagulans, B macerans, B pumilus, B sphaericus,* and *B thuringiensis* cause occasional infections. As secondary invaders, *Bacillus* species may exacerbate preexisting infections by producing either tissue-damaging toxins or metabolites such as penicillinase that interfere with treatment.

Bacillus cereus is well known as an agent of food poisoning, and a number of other *Bacillus* species, particularly *B subtilis* and *B licheniformis,* are also incriminated periodically in this capacity.

Anthrax

Anthrax is primarily a disease of herbivores. Humans acquire it as a result of contact with infected animals or animal products. In humans the disease takes one of three forms, depending on the route of infection. **Cutaneous anthrax,** which accounts for more than 95 percent of cases worldwide, results from infection through skin lesions; **intestinal anthrax** results from ingestion of spores, usually in infected meat; and **pulmonary anthrax** results from inhalation of spores.

Cutaneous anthrax usually occurs through contamination of a cut or abrasion, although in some countries biting flies may also transmit the disease. After a 2- to 3-day incubation period, a small pimple or **papule** appears at the inoculation site. A surrounding ring of vesicles develops. Over the next few days, the central papule ulcerates, dries, and blackens to form the characteristic **eschar** (Fig. 15-1). The lesion is painless and is surrounded by marked edema that may extend for some distance. Pus and pain appear only if the lesion becomes infected by a pyogenic organism. Similarly, marked lymphangitis and fever usually point to a secondary infection. In most cases the disease remains limited to the initial lesion and resolves spontaneously. The main dangers are that a lesion on the face or neck may swell to occlude the airway or may give rise to secondary meningitis. If host defenses fail to contain the infection, however, fulminating septicemia develops. Approximately 20 percent of untreated cases of cutaneous anthrax progress to fatal septicemia. However, *B anthracis* is susceptible to penicillin and other common antibiotics, so effective treatment is almost always available.

Intestinal anthrax is analogous to cutaneous anthrax but occurs on the intestinal mucosa. As in cutaneous anthrax, the organisms almost certainly can invade the mucosa only through a preexisting lesion. Generalized disease develops when the organisms spread from the mucosal lesion to the lymphatic system. In pulmonary anthrax, inhaled spores are transported by alveolar macrophages to the mediastinal lymph nodes, where they germinate and multiply to initiate systemic disease. Gastrointestinal and pulmonary anthrax are both more dangerous than the cutaneous form because they are usually identified too late for treatment to be effective.

Herbivorous animals, the primary hosts of *B anthracis,* contract the infection by ingesting spores on forage plants; the spores are derived from soil or dust or are deposited on leaves by flies after feeding on an anthrax-infected carcass. If the spores enter a lesion in the gastrointestinal mucosa, they germinate and are taken into the bloodstream and lymphatics, finally producing **systemic anthrax,** which is usually fatal.

Symptoms prior to fulminant systemic anthrax may be absent or mild, consisting, for example, of malaise, low fever, and mild gastrointestinal symptoms in the case of gastrointestinal disease. During this phase the organism is multiplying and produc-

TABLE 15-1   Basic Characteristics for Identification
of Selected *Bacillus* Species[a]

Species[b]	Motility	Catalase Production	Parasporal Bodies	Lipid Globules in Protoplasm	Lecithovitellin Reaction	Citrate Utilization	Anaerobic Growth	V-P Reaction	pH in V-P Medium <6.0	Growth at 50°C	Growth at 65°C	Growth in 7% NaCl	Acid from AS Glucose	Acid + Gas from AS Glucose	Nitrate Reduction	Casein Hydrolysis	Starch Hydrolysis	Propionate Utilization
Morphologic group 1																		
B megaterium	+	+	−	+	−	+	−	−	v	−	−	+	+	−	v	+	+	n
B cereus	+	+	−	+	+	+	+	+	+	−	−	+	+	−	+	+	+	n
B cereus subsp *mycoides*	−	+	−	+	+	+	+	+	+	−	−	+	+	−	+	+	+	n
B anthracis	−	+	−	+	+	v	+	+	+	−	−	+	+	−	+	+	+	n
B thuringiensis	+	+	+	+	+	+	+	+	+	−	−	+	+	−	+	+	+	n
B licheniformis	+	+	−	−	−	+	+	+	v	+	−	+	+	−	+	+	+	+
B subtilis	+	+	−	−	−	+	−	+	v	+	−	+	+	−	+	+	+	−
B pumilus	+	+	−	−	−	+	−	+	+	+	−	+	+	−	−	+	−	−
B firmus	v	+	−	−	−	−	−	−	−	−	−	+	+	−	+	+	+	−
B coagulans	+	+	−	−	−	v	+	v	+	+	−	−	+	−	v	v	+	−
Morphologic group 2																		
B polymyxa	+	+	−	−	−	−	+	+	v	−	−	−	+	+	+	+	+	n
B macerans	+	+	−	−	−	v	+	−	−	+	−	−	+	+	+	−	+	n
B circulans	v	+	−	−	−	v	v	−	v	+	−	v	+	−	v	v	+	n
B stearothermophilus	+	v	−	−	−	−	−	+	+	+	+	−	+	−	v	v	+	n
B alvei	+	+	−	−	−	−	+	+	+	−	−	−	+	−	−	+	+	n
B laterosporus[c]	+	+	−	−	(+)	−	+	−	−	+	−	v	+	−	+	+	−	n
B brevis	+	+	−	−	−	v	−	−	−	+	−	−	+	−	v	+	−	n
Morphologic group 3																		
B sphaericus	+	+	−	−	−	v	−	−	−	−	−	v	−	−	−	v	−	n

[a] V-P, Voges-Proskauer; AS, ammonium salt; +, more than 85 percent of strains examined by Gordon et al. were positive; −, more than 85 percent of strains negative; v, variable; n, test not applicable; (+), under colony which must be scraped off to see positive reaction.

[b] Species grouped according to the classification scheme of Gordon et al. (see References). Morphologic group 1: sporangium not swollen by spore; spore ellipsoidal or cylindrical, central or terminal; Gram positive. Morphologic group 2: sporangium swollen by ellipsoidal spore; spore central or terminal; Gram variable. Morphologic group 3: sporangium swollen by spore; spore spherical, subterminal, or terminal; Gram variable.

[c] Sporangium and spore have characteristic canoe shape.

ing toxin in the regional lymph nodes and spleen. Breakdown of these organs, probably of the spleen in particular, releases toxin and bacilli. This causes the sudden onset of hyperacute illness with dyspnea, cyanosis, high fever, and disorientation, which progress in a few hours to shock, coma, and death. Although symptoms vary somewhat with the host species, this final acute phase is marked by a rapid buildup of bacilli in the blood. In humans, blood cultures are not always positive.

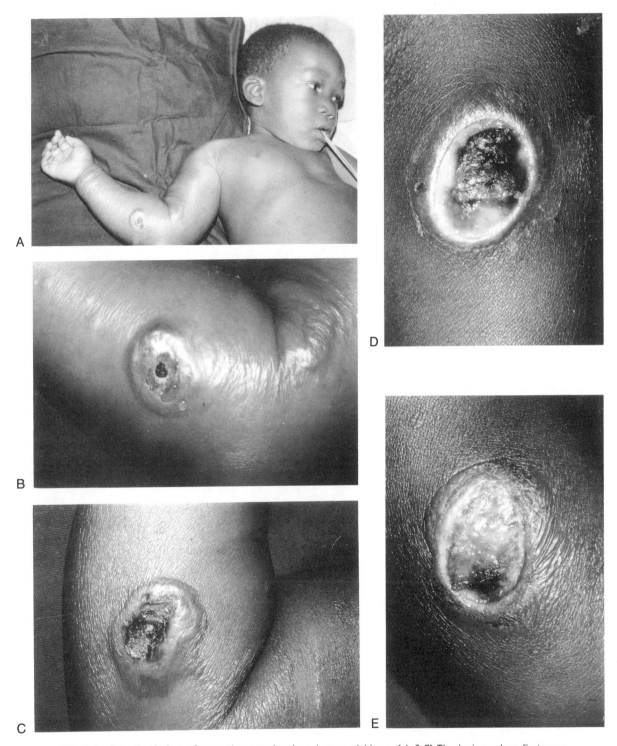

FIGURE 15-1 Evolution of an anthrax eschar in a 4-year-old boy. (*A & B*) The lesion when first seen (day 0). Note the arm swollen from the characteristic edema. (*C*) Day 6. (*D*) Day 10. (*E*) Day 15. Although penicillin treatment was begun immediately and the lesion was sterile by about 24 hours, it continued to evolve and resolve as seen. (Photographs kindly supplied by W. E. Kobuch, M.D., St. Luke's Hospital, Lupane, Bulawayo, Zimbabwe.)

Bacillus Food Poisoning

Bacillus cereus can cause two distinct types of food poisoning. The diarrheal type is characterized by diarrhea and abdominal pain occurring 8 to 16 hours after consumption of the contaminated food. It is associated with a variety of foods, including meat and vegetable dishes, sauces, pastas, desserts, and dairy products. In emetic disease, on the other hand, nausea and vomiting begin 1 to 5 hours after the contaminated food is eaten. Boiled rice that is held for prolonged periods at ambient temperature and then quick-fried before serving is the usual offender, although dairy products or other foods are occasionally responsible. The symptoms of food poisoning caused by other *Bacillus* species (*B subtilis, B licheniformis,* and others) are less well defined. Diarrhea and/or nausea occurs 1 to 14 hours after consumption of the contaminated food. A wide variety of food types have proved responsible in recorded instances.

A *Bacillus* food poisoning episode usually occurs because spores survive cooking or pasteurization and then germinate and multiply when the food is inadequately refrigerated. The symptoms of *B cereus* food poisoning are caused by a toxin or toxins produced in the food during this multiplication. Toxins have not yet been identified for other *Bacillus* species that cause food poisoning.

STRUCTURE AND CLASSIFICATION

The family Bacillaceae, consisting of rod-shaped bacteria that form endospores, has two principal subdivisions: the anaerobic spore-forming bacteria of the genus *Clostridium,* and the aerobic or facultatively anaerobic spore-forming bacteria of the genus *Bacillus,* frequently referred to as ASBs (aerobic spore bearers). *Bacillus* cultures are Gram positive when young, but in some species become Gram negative as they age.

Most *Bacillus* species are saprophytes. Table 15-1 lists the identifying characteristics of some of the species most likely to be encountered by the physician. Not only are *Bacillus* endospores resistant to hostile physical and chemical conditions, but also various species have unusual physiologic properties that enable them to survive or thrive in

harsh environments, ranging from desert sands and hot springs to Arctic soils and from fresh waters to marine sediments. The genus includes thermophilic, psychrophilic, acidophilic, alkaliphilic, halotolerant, and halophilic representatives, which are capable of growing at temperatures, pH values, and salt concentrations at which few other organisms could survive.

Figure 15-2 shows the structure of a generalized *Bacillus* endospore (details of the structure differ from species to species). One spore is produced per vegetative cell. The central **protoplast,** or **germ cell,** carries the constituents of the future vegetative cell, accompanied by dipicolinic acid, which is essential to the heat resistance of the spore. Surrounding the protoplast is a **cortex** consisting largely of peptidoglycan (murein), which is also important in the heat and radiation resistance of the spore. The inner layer, the **cortical membrane** or **protoplast wall,** becomes the cell wall of the new vegetative cell when the spore germinates. The **spore coats,** which constitute up to 50 percent of the volume of the spore, protect it from chemicals, enzymes, etc.

The events involved in sporulation of vegetative cells and in germination of spores are complex and are influenced by factors such as temperature, pH, and the availability of certain divalent cations and carbon- and nitrogen-containing compounds. Spores formed under different conditions have different stabilities and degrees of resistance to heat, radiation, chemicals, desiccation, and other hostile conditions.

PATHOGENESIS

The pathogenicity of *B anthracis* depends on two virulence factors: a poly-γ-D-glutamic acid polypeptide capsule, which protects it from phagocytosis by the defensive phagocytes of the host, and a toxin produced in the log phase of growth. This toxin consists of three proteins: **protective antigen** (PA) (82.7 kDa), **lethal factor** (LF) (90.2 kDa), and **edema factor** (EF) (88.9 kDa). Host proteases in the blood and on the eukaryotic cell surface activate protective antigen by cutting off a 20-kDa segment, exposing a binding site for lethal factor and edema factor. The activated 63-kDa protec-

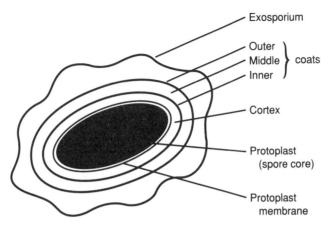

Exosporium

Outer
Middle } coats
Inner

Cortex

Protoplast
(spore core)

Protoplast
membrane

FIGURE 15-2 Cross section of a *Bacillus* spore.

tive-antigen polypeptide binds to specific receptors on the host cell surface, thereby creating a secondary binding site for which lethal factor and edema factor compete. It appears that lethal factor and edema factor enter the cell to exert their toxic effect by a mechanism analogous to that by which the A subunit of cholera toxin enters the cell (see Ch. 24), with protective antigen behaving as the B (binding) moiety (Fig. 15-3). Edema factor, which is presumed to be responsible for the characteristic edema of anthrax, is a calmodulin-dependent adenylate cyclase. (Calmodulin is the major intracellular calcium receptor in eukaryotic cells.) The only other known bacterial adenylate cyclase is produced by *Bordetella pertussis* (see Ch. 31), but the two toxins do not appear to be closely related. Lethal factor is presumed also to be an enzyme, but its mode of action is not known.

The toxin and capsule of *B anthracis* are encoded on two large plasmids called pXO1 (110 MDa) and pXO2 (60 MDa), respectively. Strains lacking either of these plasmids have greatly reduced virulence (Fig. 15-4). The attenuated live vaccine strain developed by Sterne in 1937, which is still the basis of most anthrax vaccines for livestock, lacks pXO2 and is therefore Cap$^-$ Tox$^+$. The protection afforded by such vaccines apparently is related primarily to antibodies specific for the protective antigen component of the toxin. In contrast, the attenuated vaccine strains developed by Pasteur 110 years ago were inadvertently cured of pXO1

(by subculturing at 42° to 43°C); these Pasteur strains are therefore Cap$^+$ Tox$^-$. Strains of this type do not induce protective immunity; the partial effectiveness of Pasteur's vaccines is now believed to have been due to the residual uncured (Cap$^+$ Tox$^+$) cells they contained, and this would also explain the partial virulence of these strains.

The only other *Bacillus* species for which virulence factors have been identified is *B cereus*. A 38- to 46-kDa protein complex has been shown in animal models to cause necrosis of the skin or intestinal mucosa, to induce fluid accumulation in the intestine (Fig. 15-5), and to be a lethal toxin. This protein is believed to be responsible for the necrotic and toxemic nature of severe *B cereus* infections and for the diarrheal form of food poisoning. *Bacillus cereus* also produces two hemolysins; one of these, **cereolysin** (58 kDa), is a potent necrotic and lethal toxin. Although this toxin is neutralized by serum cholesterol, it probably contributes to the pathogenesis of *B cereus* infections. Little is known about the other hemolysin at present. Phospholipases produced by *B cereus* may act as exacerbating factors by degrading host cell membranes following exposure of their phospholipid substrates in wounds or other infections. The agent responsible for the emetic type of *B cereus* food poisoning has not been clearly identified. The emesis may be induced by breakdown products resulting from the action of one or more *B cereus* enzymes on the food.

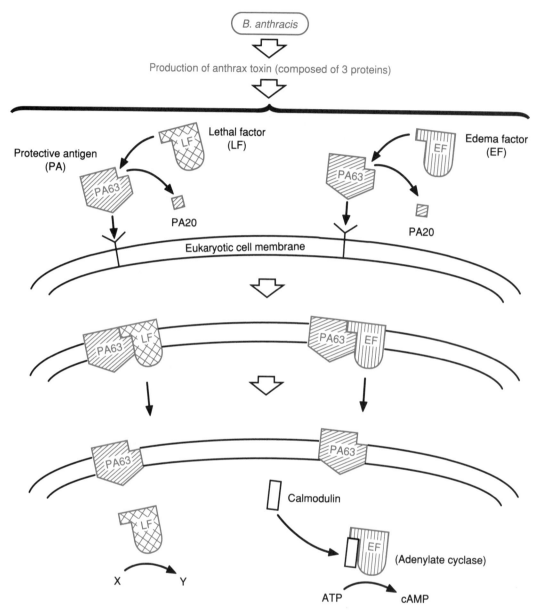

FIGURE 15-3   Mechanism of action of the anthrax toxin. The toxin is composed of three proteins. Protective antigen (PA) binds to an appropriate site on the host cell membrane. A cell surface protease cleaves off a 20-kDa piece from the protective antigen and thereby exposes a secondary binding site for which lethal factor (LF) and edema factor (EF) compete. These then pass across the cell membrane, where they carry out their intracellular actions. The edema results from increased synthesis of cyclic AMP by edema factor (adenylate cyclase), whereas lethal factor-induced lethality is caused by undefined enzymatic pathways (x → y). (Model by S. H. Leppla, Ph.D, Bacteriology Division, U.S. Army Medical Research Institute of Infectious Diseases, Fort Detrick, Frederick, MD.)

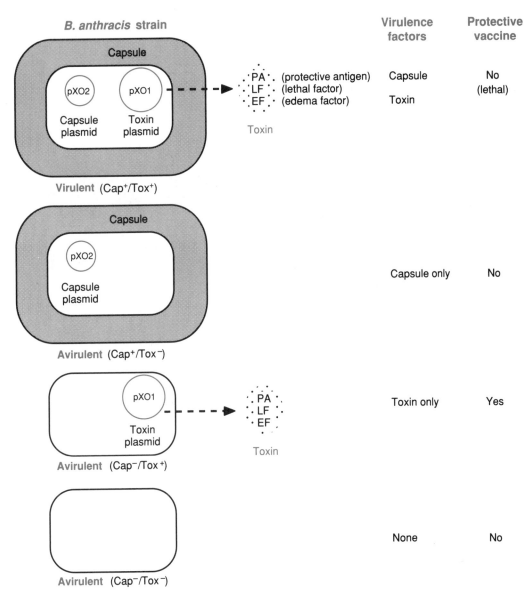

FIGURE 15-4 Genetics of virulence factor production by *B anthracis*. Plasmids pXO1 and pXO2 encode, respectively, the anthrax toxin and capsule. Curing the bacteria of pXO1 produces an encapsulated, nontoxigenic strain that is nonprotective. Curing of pXO2 produces a toxigenic nonencapsulating strain that can be used as a protective vaccine. Production of protective antigen is essential for a strain to be protective.

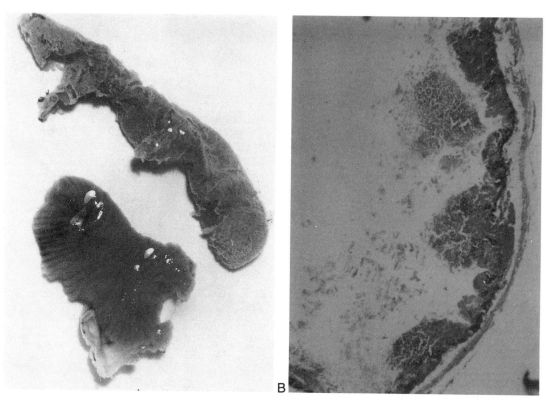

FIGURE 15-5   Necrosis of rabbit ileal mucosa 4 hours after introduction of a toxigenic cell-free culture filtrate of *B cereus*. (*A*) Gross appearance of the luminal surface of the ileum compared with a section of control ileum. (*B*) Histologic appearance of a cross-section of the toxin-exposed ileum. (From Turnbull PCB: Studies on the production of enterotoxins by *Bacillus cereus*. J Clin Pathol 29:941, 1976, with permission.)

HOST DEFENSES

Anthrax has been documented in a wide variety of warm-blooded animals. Some species, such as rats, chickens, and dogs, are quite resistant to the disease, whereas others (notably herbivores such as cattle, sheep, and horses) are very susceptible. Humans have intermediate susceptibility. The specific mechanisms of resistance in the more resistant species are not known.

Protective immunity against anthrax requires antibodies against components of anthrax toxin, primarily protective antigen. Both the noncellular human vaccines and live-spore animal vaccines confer protection by eliciting antibodies to protective antigen. The poly-γ-D-glutamic acid capsule of

B anthracis is poorly immunogenic, and antibodies to the polysaccharide and other components of the cell wall are not protective.

Nothing is known about immune responses to food poisoning or other types of infections with *Bacillus* species other than *B anthracis*. These types of infection are rare, and effective vaccines against them have not been developed.

EPIDEMIOLOGY

The ultimate reservoir of *B anthracis* is contaminated soil, in which spores remain viable for long periods. Herbivores, the primary hosts, become infected when foraging in a contaminated region. Because the organism does not depend on an animal reservoir, it cannot readily be eradicated from a region, and anthrax remains endemic in many countries. Humans become infected almost exclusively through contact with infected animals or animal products. Human anthrax is traditionally classified as either **nonindustrial** or **industrial anthrax,** depending on whether the disease is acquired directly from animals or indirectly during handling of contaminated animal products. **Nonindustrial anthrax** usually affects people who work with animals or animal carcasses, such as farmers, veterinarians, knackers, and butchers, and is almost always cutaneous. **Industrial anthrax,** acquired from handling contaminated hair, hides, wool, bone meal, or other animal products, has a higher chance of being pulmonary as a result of the inhalation of spore-laden dust.

The development of an effective animal vaccine in the 1930s, together with improved factory hygiene, introduction of procedures for sterilizing imported animal products, replacement of animal products with man-made alternatives, and the availability since the mid-1960s of a human vaccine, has resulted in a greatly reduced incidence of the disease in North America. Human anthrax is now very rare in the United States. However, major epidemics still break out in endemic countries, normally following an outbreak in livestock. Nonendemic countries must remain alert for episodes of anthrax arising from imported animal products.

DIAGNOSIS

The clinical diagnosis of anthrax is confirmed by directly visualizing or culturing the anthrax bacilli. Fresh smears of vesicular fluid, fluid from under the eschar, blood, lymph node or spleen aspirates, or (in meningitic cases) cerebrospinal fluid are stained with polychrome methylene blue (M'Fadyean's stain) and examined for the characteristic square-ended, blue-black bacilli surrounded by a pink capsule (Fig. 15-6). (It should be remembered that _B anthracis_ organisms are not invariably detected in stained blood smears of humans dying of anthrax.) Alternatively, the bacilli may be cultured from these specimens and checked for sensitivity to the anthrax gamma phage, for penicillin

sensitivity, and for capsule formation. Colonies grown overnight at $37°C$ on blood agar are gray or white, nonhemolytic, with a dry, ground-glass appearance; they are at least 3 mm in diameter and sometimes have tails (Fig. 15-7). Capsules can be seen in polychrome methylene blue-stained smears of cultures grown on nutrient agar containing 0.7 percent sodium bicarbonate and incubated overnight under CO_2 (e.g., in a candle jar); encapsulated colonies are mucoid. Alternatively, 2 ml of blood (such as commercial defibrinated horse blood) inoculated with a pinhead quantity of material from a suspected colony and incubated at $37°C$ yields readily demonstrable encapsulated bacilli in 6 hours. On occasion, it is still necessary to use mouse or guinea pig inoculation to isolate _B anthracis_. Culturing may be unsuccessful if the patient has been treated with antibiotics.

Isolation of _B anthracis_ from old specimens or from animal or environmental material being examined for public health purposes is more difficult, particularly if, as is often the case, _B cereus_ or other _Bacillus_ species are present in substantial numbers. The specimen should be examined both unheated and heated to $60°C$ to $65°C$ for 15 min with subculture to both blood or nutrient agar and specialized selective agars. It is sometimes necessary to use mouse or guinea pig inoculation to isolate _B anthracis_. Up to about 0.2 ml of the specimen (or an aqueous extract of the specimen) is injected subcutaneously into a mouse, or intramuscularly or subcutaneously in a guinea pig (more sensitive than a mouse); the encapsulated bacilli can be seen in a smear of blood aspirated from the heart of the animal at death, and the bacteria are readily observed in and isolated from this blood. If soil samples are being used, the animals should be injected 24 hours earlier with tetanus and gas gangrene antitoxin.

When a specimen from an individual not suspected clinically of having anthrax yields substantial numbers of Gram-positive bacilli, the specimen should be cultured and tested as shown in Figure 15-8 to determine the _Bacillus_ species present. The most common _Bacillus_ species may be identified by the characteristics in Table 15-1. Incrimination of a _Bacillus_ species as the cause of an infection is usually based on its presence in large numbers at

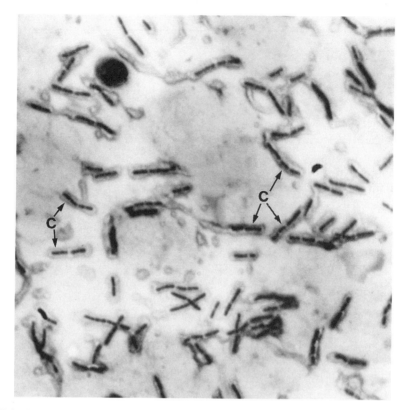

FIGURE 15-6 Blood smears from a guinea pig that died of anthrax, stained with M'Fadyean stain (polychrome methylene blue). The capsule (C) is pink around the dark-blue bacilli. Although not obvious from this photograph, anthrax bacilli frequently have square ends.

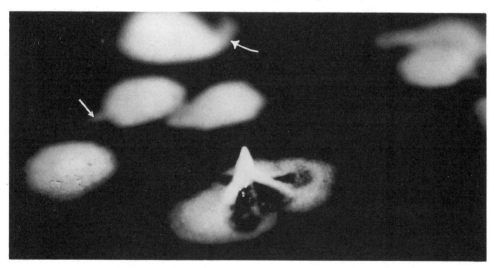

FIGURE 15-7 Colonies of *B anthracis* on a blood agar plate. Note the characteristic tackiness of colonies that allow them to be teased upright with a loop (foreground) and the characteristic tailing seen in the background (arrows). (Photograph kindly supplied by R. W. Charlton. From Turnbull PCB, Kramer JM, Melling J: *Bacillus*. p. 187. In Parker MT, Duerden BI (eds): Systematic Bacteriology. Topley and Wilson's Principles of Bacteriology, Virology and Immunity. Vol. 2. Edward Arnold, Sevenoaks, England, 1990, with permission.)

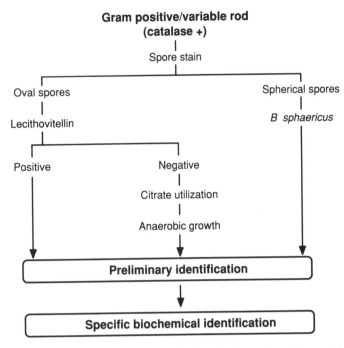

FIGURE 15-8   Flow chart for identification of principal *Bacillus* species.

the infection site, especially in the absence of other known pathogens. Since *Bacillus* species are common environmental organisms, their presence in small numbers is not generally considered significant. For this reason, the use of selective or enrichment systems for isolating clinically relevant, non-anthrax *Bacillus* species is confined to just a few situations, such as the retrospective examination of feces several days after a food poisoning incident (by which time the offending *Bacillus* organism may be present in only small numbers). It is nevertheless probably true that *Bacillus* species found in clinical specimens are dismissed as irrelevant contaminants more often than they should be.

CONTROL

To comprehend the strategies used to control anthrax, it is important to understand the cycle of infection in susceptible animals. As a susceptible animal with anthrax approaches death, its blood contains as many as 10^9 bacilli/ml (depending on the species). Necrosis of the walls of small blood vessels during the acute phase of the illness leads to

hemorrhages and to characteristic bloody exudations from the mouth, nose, and anus—a highly diagnostic sign. These exudates carry vast numbers of the bacilli, which sporulate on exposure to air and produce a heavily contaminated environmental site that is potentially capable of infecting other animals for many years.

Because sporulation of *B anthracis* requires oxygen and therefore does not occur inside a closed carcass, regulations in most countries forbid postmortem examination of animals when anthrax is suspected. The vegetative cells in the carcass are killed in a few days by the process of putrefaction. Nevertheless, in the case of livestock, legislation invariably requires that the carcass be burnt or buried in quicklime.

Livestock in endemic areas are effectively protected by yearly inoculations with a vaccine made from spores of a live attenuated strain (see above). Noncellular vaccines for human use are available for individuals in high-risk occupations. They appear to have contributed to the decline in incidence of industrial anthrax since they became available in the 1960s, but animal studies suggest that there are limitations to their ability to protect against anthrax. The human vaccine available in the United States is an aluminum hydroxide-adsorbed cell-free filtrate of a *B anthracis* culture grown to maximize the yield of protective antigen and minimize the quantities of lethal factor, edema factor, and other unwanted metabolites.

Bacillus anthracis is susceptible to penicillin and to almost all other broad-spectrum antibiotics. Because it is easily recognized, cutaneous anthrax is almost always treated early and cured. Gastrointestinal and pulmonary anthrax infections are difficult to identify before the fulminant phase and therefore carry a high mortality. In uncomplicated anthrax cases, adequate treatment consists of 500 mg of penicillin V taken orally every 6 hours for 5 days, or 600 mg (1 million units) of procaine penicillin administered intramuscularly every 12 to 24 hours for 5 days. In severe cases, 1,200 mg (2 million units) of penicillin G should be administered intravenously every 6 hours, reverting to the intramuscular regime of 600 mg every 12 to 24 hours once recovery starts. If pulmonary anthrax is suspected, continuous-drip administration is advisable. Tetracycline, chloramphenicol, gentamicin, or erythromycin may be used if the patient has penicillin hypersensitivity.

Avoidance of other types of *Bacillus* infections is largely a matter of observing proper hygiene. *Bacillus cereus* and its close relatives *B thuringiensis* and *B mycoides* produce potent β-lactamases and thus are not responsive to penicillin, ampicillin, or the cephalosporins. They are mostly resistant to trimethoprim as well. These species are generally sensitive to standard empirical treatment with an aminoglycoside combined with vancomycin and to chloramphenicol, erythromycin, tetracycline, clindamycin, and sulfonamides.

Bacillus food poisoning, like all types of food poisoning, can largely be prevented by proper food handling. Food should be cooked adequately; cooked food should not be recontaminated from uncooked food (separate utensils and cutting surfaces should be used for cooked and uncooked food); and, of particular importance, cooked food should be stored under proper refrigeration.

REFERENCES

Claus D, Berkeley RCW: Genus *Bacillus* Cohn 1872, 174[AL]. p. 1105. In Sneath PHA, Mair NS, Sharpe ME, Holt JG (eds): Bergey's Manual of Systematic Bacteriology. Vol. 2. Williams & Wilkins, Baltimore, 1986

Gordon RE, Haynes WC, Pang CH-N: The genus *Bacillus*. U.S. Department of Agriculture Agricultural Handbook no. 427. U.S. Department of Agriculture, Washington DC, 1973.

Kramer JM, Gilbert RJ: *Bacillus cereus* and other *Bacillus* species. p. 21. In Doyle MP (ed): Foodborne Bacterial Pathogens. Marcel Dekker, New York, 1989

Leppla SH: *Bacillus anthracis* calmodulin-dependent adenylate cyclase: chemical and enzymatic properties and interactions with eucaryotic cells. Adv Nucleotide and Protein Phosphoryl Res 17:189, 1984

Leppla SH, Friedlander AM, Singh Y et al: A model for anthrax toxic action at the cellular level. p. 41. In Turnbull PCB (ed): Proceedings of the International Workshop on Anthrax, 11 to 13 April 1989, Winchester, England. Salisbury Medical Bulletin no. 68, Special Supplement, 1990

Norris JR, Berkeley RCW, Logan NA et al: The genera *Bacillus* and *Sporolactobacillus*. p. 1711. In Starr MP, Stolp H, Trüper HG (eds): The Prokaryotes. A Handbook on Habitats, Isolation and Identification of Bacteria. Vol. 2. Springer-Verlag, New York, 1981

Parry JM, Turnbull PCB, Gibson JR: A Colour Atlas of *Bacillus* Species. Wolfe Medical Atlas no. 19. Wolfe Publishing, London, 1983

Turnbull PCB: Studies on the production of enterotoxins by *Bacillus cereus*. J Clin Pathol 29:941, 1976

Turnbull PCB: Anthrax. p. 364. In Smith GR, Easmon CR (eds): Bacterial Diseases. Topley and Wilson's Principles of Bacteriology, Virology and Immunity. Vol 3. Edward Arnold, Sevenoaks, England, 1990

Turnbull PCB, Kramer JM, Melling J: *Bacillus*. p. 187. In Parker MT, Duerden BI (eds): Systematic Bacteriology. Topley and Wilson's Principles of Bacteriology, Virology and Immunity. Vol. 2. Edward Arnold, Sevenoaks, England, 1990

16 MISCELLANEOUS PATHOGENIC BACTERIA

HERBERT HOF

GENERAL CONCEPTS

LISTERIA MONOCYTOGENES

This microorganism is a potential pathogen for both humans and animals. Most human cases occur in patients with debilitating disease or in prenatal or neonatal infants. Sepsis, meningitis, and disseminated abscesses occur in infected patients. Meat, vegetables, and various milk products are the most common sources of infection.

ERYSIPELOTHRIX RHUSIOPATHIAE

This species is transmitted occasionally from infected pigs to farmers or veterinarians, in whom it causes primarily inflammatory infections of the skin. Septicemia and endocarditis may develop secondarily.

PROPIONIBACTERIUM ACNES

A common inhabitant of the crypts of the skin, this species may contribute to acne.

STREPTOBACILLUS MONILIFORMIS

This species may infect individuals through the bite of infected rodents. After local ulcerative inflammation, life-threatening septicemia may develop.

CALYMMATOBACTERIUM GRANULOMATIS

This microorganism causes granuloma inguinale, a venereal disease with local tissue destruction in the genital, inguinal, and perianal region.

INTRODUCTION

The microorganisms discussed in this chapter are taxonomically unrelated. The human infections they cause are rare except in the case of *Listeria* and *Propionibacterium acnes*. Some of these infections are fatal; others tend to be self-limited. Recognition depends largely on the proper use of bacteriologic methods, which is important not only to ensure appropriate therapy but also to exclude other possible agents.

263

LISTERIA MONOCYTOGENES

CLINICAL MANIFESTATIONS

Listeriosis is a serious disease for humans, with a mortality greater than 25 percent. There are two main clinical manifestations, sepsis and meningitis (Fig. 16-1). Meningitis is often complicated by encephalitis, which is exceptional among bacterial infections. Occasionally, pyogenic infections of various organs have been found. Relapses may occur after apparent recovery.

STRUCTURE, CLASSIFICATION, AND ANTIGENIC TYPES

All *Listeria* species are small, Gram-positive rods, which are sometimes arranged in short chains. In direct smears they may be coccoid, so they can be mistaken for streptococci. Longer cells can be suggestive of corynebacteria. Flagella are produced at room temperature rather than at 37°C. Hemolysin production is an important marker for *L monocytogenes*, although it is not definitive, as *L ivanovii* and *L seeligeri* are likewise hemolytic on blood agar. Further biochemical characterization is necessary to distinguish the different *Listeria* species.

It may be desirable for epidemiologic purposes to identify a particular strain by serotyping to characterize surface antigens, such as O antigens (teichoic acids) and H antigens (proteins). The serovars 1/2a and 4b are responsible for up to 90 percent of all cases of listeriosis.

A particular property of *L monocytogenes* is the ability to multiply at low temperatures (Fig. 16-2). Bacteria therefore can accumulate in contaminated food stored in the refrigerator.

PATHOGENESIS

Listeria monocytogenes is presumably ingested with raw, contaminated food (Fig. 16-2). An invasion factor secreted by the pathogenic bacteria enables them to penetrate host cells of the epithelial lining. Since this microorganism is widely distributed, this

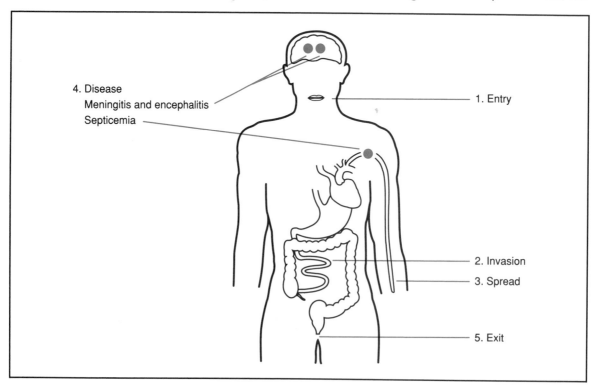

FIGURE 16-1 Pathogenesis of listeriosis.

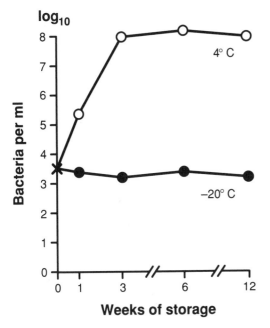

FIGURE 16-2 Multiplication of *L monocytogenes* in broth at low temperature.

event may occur rather often. Normally, the immune system eliminates the infection before it spreads. Indeed, most adults who have no history of listeriosis have T lymphocytes primed specifically by *Listeria* antigens. If the immune system is compromised, however, systemic disease may develop. *Listeria monocytogenes* multiplies not only extracellularly but also intracellularly within macrophages after phagocytosis. It therefore belongs to the large group of facultatively intracellular pathogens (Table 16-1).

Survival within the phagosomes and eventual escape into the cytoplasm are mediated by a toxin, which also acts as a hemolysin. This toxin is one of the so-called **SH-activated hemolysins,** which are produced by a number of different bacteria such as serogroup A streptococci, pneumococci, and *Clostridium perfringens.* Obviously, nature has preserved the genetic code for this bacterial product in several species, and consequently the hemolysins from these different bacteria have common biochemical, biologic, and antigenic properties. Nonhemolytic variants of *L monocytogenes* are completely avirulent, as are the nonhemolytic species *L innocua* and *L welshimeri.* Hemolysin is not the only *Listeria* virulence factor, however, since the hemolytic *Listeria* species besides *L monocytogenes* (i.e., *L seeligeri* and *L ivanovii*) possess rather limited pathogenicity.

HOST DEFENSES

Because it multiplies intracellularly, *L monocytogenes* is largely protected against humoral immune factors such as antibodies, and the effective host response is cell mediated, involving both lymphokines (especially interferon) produced by CD4+ (T-helper) cells and direct lysis of infected cells by CD8+ (cytotoxic) T lymphocytes. Both these fundamental defense mechanisms are expressed in the microenvironment of the infective foci. Histologically, these foci are organized as granulomas, characterized by a central accumulation of epithelial

TABLE 16-1 List of Some Facultative or Obligate Intracellular Microorganisms

Type of Microorganism	Agent	Disease
Bacteria	*Mycobacterium tuberculosis*	Tuberculosis
	Salmonella typhi	Typhoid fever
	Yersinia pestis	Plague
	Legionella pneumophila	Legionellosis
	Listeria monocytogenes	Listeriosis
Fungi	*Histoplasma capsulatum*	Histoplasmosis
Protozoa	*Toxoplasma gondii*	Toxoplasmosis
	Leishmania donovani	Kala azar
	Trypanosoma cruzi	Chagas disease

cells (macrophages) with irregularly shaped nuclei and large, delicately structured cytoplasm and by peripheral lymphocytes recognizable by a round nucleus and a narrow border of intensely staining cytoplasm (Fig. 16-3).

EPIDEMIOLOGY

Listeria species are found in living and nonliving matter. Various foodstuffs of vegetable and animal origin are sources of infection. Animal and human carriers also have been described. Most human cases of listeriosis develop in immunocompromised hosts: newborns, old people, cancer patients, and transplant recipients. Reports of sporadic cases of listeriosis are becoming more frequent as the number of persons at risk, especially because of immunosuppression by medical therapy, increases. Outbreaks of listeriosis are due mainly to a common source of contaminated food.

Listeriosis also may be transmitted congenitally across the placenta. The immunocompetent mother suffers at worst a brief, flulike febrile ill-ness, but the fetus, whose defense system is still immature, becomes seriously ill. Depending on the stage of gestation, the fetus is either stillborn or born with signs of congenital infection. Typically, multiple pyogenic foci are found in several organs (granulomatosis infantiseptica). The onset of listeriosis is delayed (i.e., a few days after birth) when infection is acquired during labor by bacteria colonizing the genital tract of the mother.

DIAGNOSIS

Listeria monocytogenes is implicated when monocytosis is observed in the peripheral blood as well as the cerebrospinal fluid. Early diagnosis may be obtained by finding pleocytosis with Gram-positive rods in a Gram stain of smears of the cerebrospinal fluid. Final proof is obtained by culture. Serologic tests are highly unreliable.

CONTROL

Hygienic food processing and storage may reduce the risk of listeriosis. Individuals in high-risk

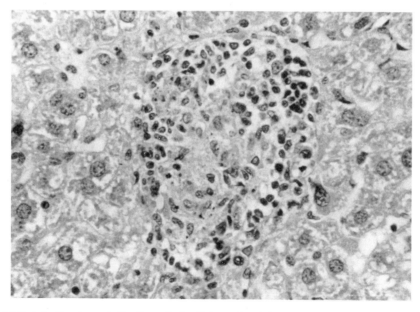

FIGURE 16-3 Infective focus in the liver of mice 7 days after infection with *L monocytogenes*. Note the granulomatous reaction characterized by central accumulation of epithelioid cells (macrophages) and the presence of some dark, round cells (lymphocytes) in the periphery.

groups (i.e., immunocompromised individuals and pregnant women) should avoid uncooked food or should at least marinate salads for a long time in a vinegar-based dressing to kill adherent bacteria.

Since a cell-mediated immune response (the most potent weapon against *L monocytogenes*) is induced only by injection of living antigen, vaccination is difficult. Even an attenuated living vaccine is dangerous for persons with impaired defenses, the proper target group. Completely avirulent live bacteria do not trigger an effective, cell-mediated immune response.

Antimicrobial agents are the mainstay of treatment. Most of the common antibiotics, except cephalosporins, are active against *L monocytogenes* in vitro. In practice, ampicillin combined with an aminoglycoside has given the best results. However, because infection occurs mainly in infirm patients and because intracellular bacteria are hardly accessible to most drugs, the cure rate is low. Furthermore, *Listeria* cells, although inhibited, are not killed by ampicillin. High doses for prolonged periods are indicated.

◄ *ERYSIPELOTHRIX RHUSIOPATHIAE* ►

CLINICAL MANIFESTATIONS

The most common human infection by *E rhusiopathiae* is **erysipeloid,** a well-defined, violet or wine-colored inflammatory lesion of the skin of the fingers or hand (Fig. 16-4). Itching is typical. Infrequently, septicemia develops, followed by various organ manifestations such as endocarditis or arthritis without fever.

STRUCTURE AND CLASSIFICATION

Erysipelothrix rhusiopathiae is a slender, Gram-positive rod similar to *L monocytogenes*. In general, *E rhusiopathiae* rods are longer, especially in rough variants. They grow on routine culture media under aerobic conditions, but preferentially in a CO_2 atmosphere. In contrast to *L monocytogenes*, they are nonmotile, nonhemolytic, and catalase negative. The production of H_2S is highly indica-

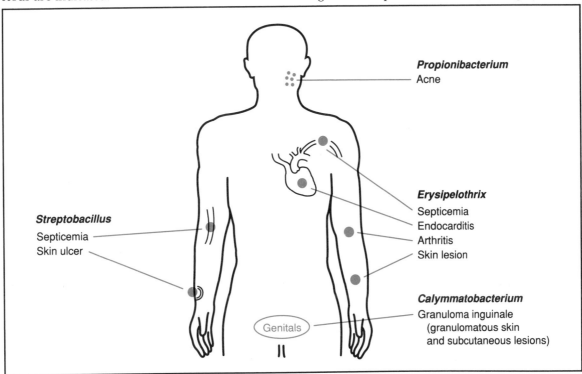

FIGURE 16-4 Disease manifestations of *E rhusiopathiae, P acnes, C granulomatis,* and *L moniliformis.*

tive, since very few other Gram-positive bacteria have this property.

PATHOGENESIS

A minor skin injury may facilitate the penetration of *E rhusiopathiae* after contact with infected material. After an incubation of 1 to 4 days the local lesion develops; spontaneous recovery occurs in 2 to 3 weeks. Septicemia has been observed without previous local lesions so that an oral infection is assumed. Endocarditis may develop in a few cases.

EPIDEMIOLOGY

Erysipelothrix rhusiopathiae is found in mammals, poultry, and fish. Individuals who have occupational exposure to such animals (i.e., farmers, veterinarians, slaughterhouse workers, and fish handlers) are at risk.

DIAGNOSIS

The typical, nonpyogenic lesions on occupationally exposed persons suggest erysipeloid. Since there is no wound, a swab is not useful. Bacteria can be cultured from a biopsy of the progressing, inflamed edge of the lesion. Blood culture is indicated in the setting of sepsis and endocarditis.

CONTROL

Penicillin is the drug of choice to treat serious infections. Since local skin infection is self-limited, therapy is not essential.

◀ PROPIONIBACTERIUM ▶ ACNES

CLINICAL MANIFESTATIONS

The pathogenic role of *Propionibacterium acnes* is still disputed. Although it is often detected in anaerobic blood cultures, it normally colonizes the skin crypts and is transported to cultures by pure chance (Fig. 16-4). Nevertheless, in compromised patients even this nonpathogenic species may induce pathologic reactions, such as endocarditis. In skin lesions *P acnes* is often found with other path-

ogenic bacteria, such as *Staphylococcus aureus* or actinomycetes, and is thought to support the damaging effect of those pathogens. It is doubtful whether *P acnes* alone is able to induce acne.

STRUCTURE AND CLASSIFICATION

The club-shaped Gram-positive rods of *P acnes* resemble the diphtheroids but, unlike the latter, are slow-growing and anaerobic, so that their presence in blood cultures is detected after about a week.

PATHOGENESIS

Propionibacterium acnes produces several metabolic products, hemolysin, and various enzymes such as lipase and neuraminidase, which are excreted into the surroundings. These metabolites may clear the way for other bacteria. Furthermore, *P acnes* degrades sebaceous matter to produce fatty acids that stimulate an inflammatory reaction.

EPIDEMIOLOGY

Propionibacterium acnes normally colonizes the deep crypts of the skin, where the availability of oxygen is reduced. The same applies to mucous membranes of the oroanal areas. They may be transported to other sites by chance.

CONTROL

Practically all common antibiotics, including penicillins, erythromycin, and tetracyclines, can be used to treat *P acnes* infections.

◀ STREPTOBACILLUS ▶ MONILIFORMIS

CLINICAL MANIFESTATIONS

Streptobacillus moniliformis causes the clinical disease called **rat bite fever.** At the site of the rodent bite, an ulcer appears; this may heal spontaneously (Fig. 16-4). Occasionally, the infection spreads to the regional lymph nodes, and bacteremia has been observed. General malaise and fever may be present after a few days. This generalized disease may be fatal. Colonization of various parts of the body, such as joints or endocardium, may lead to chronic disease accompanied by local symptoms. Rat bite fever also is caused by *Spirillum minus,* a very different bacterium (see Ch. 35).

STRUCTURE AND CLASSIFICATION

Streptobacillus moniliformis is a Gram-negative, nonmotile rod of variable length. The individual cells are not regularly shaped or stained, and thus pleomorphism is seen in smears. There is a tendency for spontaneous development of cell-wall-deficient L-forms (see Ch. 2). Consequently, growth on artificial media depends on certain additives, such as serum or ascitic fluid, which are not always present in common culture media. Growth is best under a CO_2 atmosphere.

PATHOGENESIS

Humans usually become infected with *S moniliformis* through the bite of an infected rat. Ingestion of contaminated food has rarely been incriminated as the source of infection.

HOST DEFENSES

The nonspecific resistance mechanisms in the skin and draining lymph nodes prevent dissemination. The low pH in the stomach normally guarantees that *S moniliformis* cannot survive gastric passage.

EPIDEMIOLOGY

S moniliformis belongs to the common bacterial flora of the nasopharynx of rats, from which it reaches humans directly by a rat bite or indirectly via food.

DIAGNOSIS

The coincidence of fever after a rat bite draws attention to this infection. Positive cultures can be obtained from blood or synovial fluid. Mice are highly susceptible to *S moniliformis,* exhibiting a rapid lethal infection after inoculation. Because of the existence of L-forms, special media must be used for culture, since on conventional agar plates L-form colonies hardly are visible and are likely to be overlooked.

◁ *CALYMMATOBACTERIUM GRANULOMATIS* ▷

CLINICAL PRESENTATION

C granulomatis causes **granuloma inguinale.** This infection typically is localized in the genital region (Fig. 16-4). It spreads to adjacent areas, and the regional lymph nodes also may be inflamed. Persistent granulomatous lesions tend to ulcerate, destroying skin and subcutaneous tissue.

STRUCTURE AND CLASSIFICATION

Calymmatobacterium granulomatis is a Gram-negative, nonmotile rod. The capsule that surrounds the bacterial cell appears similar to that of *Klebsiella*. Addition of egg yolk and incubation in a CO_2 atmosphere are required for growth on artificial media.

PATHOGENESIS

Calymmatobacterium granulomatis is normally present in the gut flora and may be transmitted to the genital area by autoinoculation or sexual contact. After penetrating the skin the bacteria induce an inflammatory reaction, which may lead to destruction of the infected tissue. Within the inflammatory foci *C granulomatis* is found mainly intracellularly (Table 16-1) inside tissue macrophages (Donovan bodies). This is highly typical for granuloma inguinale. Superinfection of ulcers with other pathogenic organisms is possible.

HOST DEFENSES

Antibodies against *C granulomatis* are produced during acute infection; their role in defense remains unclear. Cell-mediated defense mechanisms, expressed by a granulomatous reaction, are important in recovery.

EPIDEMIOLOGY

Granuloma inguinale occurs most frequently in people living under poor socioeconomic conditions (e.g., in the tropics). In the United States, infection of blacks is seven times more frequent than infection of whites. Transmission by sexual contacts is most common. Other sexually transmitted diseases, such as syphilis, may be associated.

DIAGNOSIS

Microscopic evidence of intracellular Gram-negative encapsulated rods in ulcerative skin wounds of the genitoinguinal region is highly indicative for granuloma inguinale. Since experience with *C granulomatis* is lacking in most laboratories, cultural diagnosis probably will fail. Eventually, the yolk sac of 5-day-old chicken embryos can be inoculated directly with the infected material.

CONTROL

Infection can be prevented by cleanliness or by avoiding sexual contacts with infected persons. Antibiotics active against intracellular bacteria, such as tetracycline or erythromycin, are effective in treatment.

REFERENCES

Davis MC: Granuloma inguinale. A clinical, histological and ultrastructural study. J Am Med Assoc 211:632, 1970

Edelson PJ: Intracellular parasites and phagocytic cells: cell biology and pathophysiology. Rev Infect Dis 4:124, 1982

Gellin BG, Broome CV: Listeriosis. J Am Med Assoc 261:1313, 1989

Hahn H, Kaufmann SHE: The role of cell-mediated immunity in bacterial infection. Rev Infect Dis 3:1221, 1981

Lal S, Nicholas C: Epidemiological and clinical features in 165 cases of granuloma inguinale. Br J Vener Dis 46:461, 1970

Rogosa M: *Streptobacillus moniliformis* and *Spirillum minus.* p. 400. In Lenette EH, Balows A, Hausler WJ Jr, Shadomy HJ (eds): Manual of Clinical Microbiology. 4th Ed. American Society for Microbiology, Washington, DC, 1985

Weaver RE: *Erysipelothrix.* p. 209. In Lenette EH, Balows A, Hausler WJ Jr, Shadomy HJ (eds): Manual of Clinical Microbiology. 4th Ed. American Society for Microbiology, Washington, DC, 1985

17 ANAEROBES: GENERAL CHARACTERISTICS

DAVID J. HENTGES

GENERAL CONCEPTS

Clinical Manifestations

Symptoms are related to the absence of oxygen from the affected area: hence, abscesses, devitalized tissue, and penetration of foreign matter lead to clinical infection.

Oxygen Toxicity

Low or undetectable levels of superoxide dismutase and catalase allow oxygen radicals to form in anaerobic bacteria and to inactivate other bacterial enzyme systems.

Pathogenic Anaerobes

Anaerobes are potentially pathogenic when displaced from normal environments (human colon, soil) and implanted in dead or dying tissue; abscesses, pneumonias, and oral and pelvic infections result.

Processing of Clinical Specimens

Anaerobic conditions are required for sample collection, culturing, and identification.

INTRODUCTION

The broad classification of bacteria as **anaerobic, aerobic,** or **facultative** is based on the types of reactions they employ to generate energy for growth and other activities. In their metabolism of energy-containing compounds, aerobes require molecular oxygen as a terminal electron acceptor and cannot grow in its absence (see Chapter 4). Anaerobes, on the other hand, cannot grow in the presence of oxygen. Oxygen is toxic for them, and they must therefore depend on other substances as electron acceptors. Their metabolism frequently is

a fermentative type in which they reduce available organic compounds to various end products such as organic acids and alcohols. The facultative organisms are the most versatile. They preferentially utilize oxygen as a terminal electron acceptor, but also can metabolize in the absence of oxygen by reducing other compounds. Much more usable energy, in the form of high-energy phosphate, is obtained when a molecule of glucose is completely catabolized to carbon dioxide and water in the presence of oxygen (38 molecules of ATP) than when it is only partially catabolized by a fermentative process in the absence of oxygen (2 molecules of ATP). The ability to utilize oxygen as a terminal electron acceptor provides organisms with an extremely efficient mechanism for generating energy. Understanding the general characteristics of **anaerobiosis** provides insight into how **anaerobic bacteria** can proliferate in damaged tissue and why special care is needed in processing clinical specimens that may contain them.

OXYGEN TOXICITY

Several studies indicate that aerobes can survive in the presence of oxygen only by virtue of an elaborate system of defenses. Without these defenses, key enzyme systems in the organisms fail to function and the organisms die. Obligate anaerobes, which live only in the absence of oxygen, do not possess the defenses that make aerobic life possible and therefore cannot survive in air.

During growth and metabolism, oxygen reduction products are generated within microorganisms and secreted into the surrounding medium. The **superoxide anion,** one oxygen reduction product, is produced by univalent reduction of oxygen:

$$O_2 \xrightarrow{e^-} O_2^-$$

It is generated during the interaction of molecular oxygen with various cellular constituents, including reduced flavins, flavoproteins, quinones, thiols, and iron-sulfur proteins. The exact process by which it causes intracellular damage is not known; however, it is capable of participating in a number of destructive reactions potentially lethal to the cell. Moreover, products of secondary reactions may amplify toxicity. For example, one hypothesis holds that the superoxide anion reacts with hydrogen peroxide in the cell:

$$O_2^- + H_2O_2 \longrightarrow OH^- + OH^{\cdot} + O_2$$

This reaction, known as the Haber-Weiss reaction, generates a free hydroxyl radical ($OH^{\cdot}$), which is the most potent biologic oxidant known. It can attack virtually any organic substance in the cell. A subsequent reaction between the superoxide anion and the hydroxyl radical produces singlet

oxygen (O_2^*), which is also damaging to the cell:

$$O_2^- + OH^{\cdot} \longrightarrow OH^- + O_2^*$$

The excited singlet oxygen molecule is very reactive. Therefore, superoxide must be removed for the cells to survive in the presence of oxygen.

Most facultative and aerobic organisms contain a high concentration of an enzyme called **superoxide dismutase.** This enzyme converts the superoxide anion into ground-state oxygen and hydrogen peroxide, thus ridding the cell of destructive superoxide anions:

$$2O_2^- + 2H^+ \xrightarrow{\text{Superoxide Dismutase}} O_2 + H_2O_2$$

The hydrogen peroxide generated in this reaction is an oxidizing agent, but it does not damage the cell as much as the superoxide anion and tends to diffuse out of the cell. Many organisms possess **catalase** or **peroxidase** or both to eliminate the H_2O_2. Catalase uses H_2O_2 as an oxidant (electron acceptor) and a reductant (electron donor) to convert peroxide into water and ground-state oxygen:

$$H_2O_2 + H_2O_2 \xrightarrow{\text{Catalase}} 2H_2O + O_2$$

Peroxidase uses a reductant other than H_2O_2:

$$H_2O_2 + H_2R \xrightarrow{\text{Peroxidase}} 2H_2O + R$$

One study showed that facultative and aerobic organisms lacking superoxide dismutase possess high levels of catalase or peroxidase. High concentrations of these enzymes may alleviate the need for superoxide dismutase, because they effectively scavenge H_2O_2 before it can react with the superoxide anion to form the more active hydroxyl radical. However, most organisms show a positive correlation between the activity of superoxide dismutase and resistance to the toxic effects of oxygen.

In another study, facultative and aerobic organisms demonstrated high levels of superoxide dismutase. The enzyme was present, generally at lower levels, in some of the anaerobes studied, but was totally absent in others. The most oxygen-sensitive anaerobes as a rule contained little or no superoxide dismutase. In addition to the activity of superoxide dismutase, the rate at which an organism takes up and reduces oxygen was determined to be a factor in oxygen tolerance. Very sensitive anaerobes, which reduced relatively large quantities of oxygen and exhibited no superoxide dismutase activity, were killed after short exposure to oxygen. More tolerant organisms reduced very little oxygen or else demonstrated high levels of superoxide dismutase activity.

The continuous spectrum of oxygen tolerance among bacteria appears to be due partly to the activities of superoxide dismutase, catalase, and peroxidase in the cell and partly to the rate at which the cell takes up oxygen (Fig. 17-1). Clearly, other factors influence tolerance: the location of protective enzymes in the cell (surface versus cytoplasm), the rate at which cells form toxic oxygen products (e.g., the hydroxyl radical or singlet oxygen), and the sensitivities of key cellular components to the toxic oxygen products.

PATHOGENIC ANAEROBES

Anaerobic bacteria are widely distributed in nature in oxygen-free habitats. Many members of the indigenous human flora are anaerobic bacteria, including spirochetes and Gram-positive and Gram-negative cocci and rods. For example, the human colon, where oxygen tension is low, contains large populations of anaerobic bacteria, exceeding 10^{11} organisms/g of colon content. Anaerobes in this region frequently outnumber facultative organisms by a factor of at least 100. Oxygen-sensitive organisms also are numerous in other areas of the body, such as the gingival crevices, tonsillar crypts, nasal folds, hair follicles, the urethra and vagina, and tooth surfaces.

Anaerobic indigenous flora components are potentially pathogenic if displaced from their normal habitat. Most anaerobic infections are endogenously acquired from members of the microflora, although *Clostridium*, found principally in the soil, also produces infections in humans. Proliferation of anaerobic bacteria in tissue depends on the absence of oxygen. Oxygen is excluded from the tis-

Anaerobic Bacteria

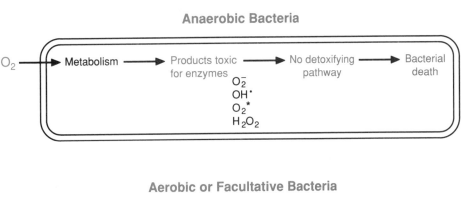

Aerobic or Facultative Bacteria

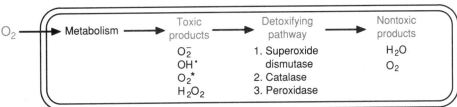

FIGURE 17-1   Effects of oxygen on aerobic, anaerobic, and facultative anaerobic bacteria.

sue when the local blood supply is impaired by trauma, obstruction, or surgical manipulation. Anaerobes multiply well in dead tissue. Multiplication of aerobic or facultative organisms in association with anaerobes in infected tissue also diminishes oxygen concentration and develops a habitat that supports growth of anaerobic bacteria.

Infections produced by anaerobic bacteria occur in all parts of the human body (Fig. 17-2). The infected tissues usually contain a mixture of several kinds of anaerobes and frequently also contain aerobic and facultative bacteria. The types of infections commonly produced by anaerobic bacteria are as follows:

1. **Intra-abdominal infections.** Abscesses, postoperative wound infections, and generalized peritonitis produced by anaerobes occur as a consequence of bowel perforation during surgery or injury.
2. **Pulmonary infections.** Anaerobic lung infections may originate in the bronchi or the blood. Aspirations from the upper respiratory tract, which contain large numbers of anaerobic bacteria, are responsible for initiating infection in the bronchi.
3. **Pelvic infections.** Anaerobic infections of the vagina and uterus sometimes occur after gynecologic surgery or in association with malignancy of pelvic organs.
4. **Brain abscesses.** Anaerobes infrequently produce meningitis, but are a common cause of brain abscesses. The infecting organisms usually originate in the upper respiratory tract.
5. **Skin and soft tissue infections.** Combinations of anaerobes, aerobes, and facultative organisms often act synergistically to produce these infections.
6. **Oral and dental infections.** These local infections frequently extend to the face and neck and sometimes to other areas of the body such as the brain.
7. **Bacteremia and endocarditis.** Anaerobic

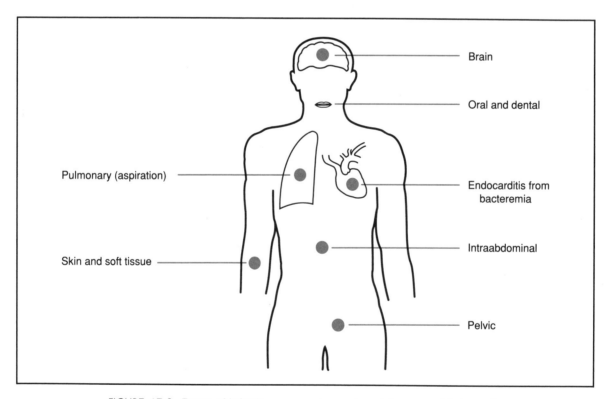

FIGURE 17-2 Types of infection commonly produced by anaerobic bacteria.

bacteremia may follow disturbance in an area of the body where an established flora or an infection exists. Endocarditis, an inflammation of the endothelial lining of the heart cavities, is occasionally caused by anaerobic bacteria, especially anaerobic streptococci.

With the exception of the clostridia, which have been studied extensively, the mechanisms by which anaerobes cause infections in humans are not well understood. *Clostridium* species produce various toxins that destroy tissue cells, and two species, *C botulinum* and *C tetani,* release the neurotoxins responsible for botulism and tetanus, respectively. Enzymes excreted by other anaerobic bacteria, including proteases, lipases, hyaluronidase, chondroitin sulfatase, and neuraminidase, may play a role in infection by causing tissue cell destruction, and β-lactamase may act as a virulence factor by inactivating antibiotics that possess a β-lactam ring, such as the penicillins and cephalosporins. In addition, the capsules surrounding some anaerobic bacteria probably interfere with phagocytosis and act as a barrier against penetration by antimicrobial agents.

PROCESSING OF CLINICAL SPECIMENS

When collecting specimens from patients for isolation and identification of anaerobic bacteria associated with infections, precautions must be taken to exclude air (Fig. 17-3). Materials for anaerobic culture are best obtained with a needle and syringe. Unless the specimen can be sent to the laboratory immediately, it is placed in an anaerobic transport tube containing oxygen-free carbon dioxide or nitrogen. The specimen is injected through the rubber stopper in the transport tube and remains in the anaerobic environment of the tube until processed in the bacteriology laboratory. If the specimen is collected with a swab, only a

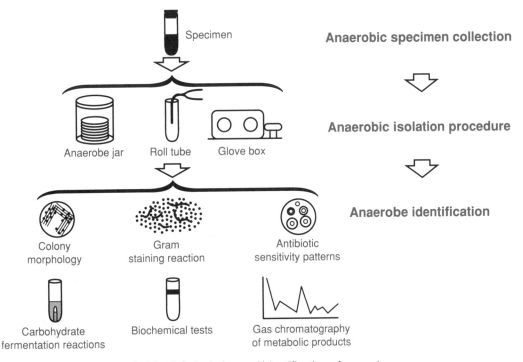

FIGURE 17-3 Isolation and identification of anaerobes.

special commercially available anaerobic swab transport system is used.

Specimens should be free of contaminating bacteria. Material from sites that are normally sterile, such as blood, spinal fluid, or pleural fluid, poses no problem provided the usual precautions are taken to decontaminate the skin properly before puncturing it to obtain the specimen. Fecal specimens, sputum specimens, or vaginal secretions cannot be cultured routinely for pathogenic anaerobes because they normally contain other anaerobic organisms. Aspirates from abscesses or the specific sites of infections must be obtained in these cases to avoid undue contamination with indigenous flora components.

Although several techniques are available for maintaining an oxygen-free environment during the processing of specimens for anaerobic culture, the **anaerobic jar** is the most common. It is a medium-sized glass or plastic jar with a tightly fitting lid containing palladium-coated alumina particles, which serve as a catalyst. It can be set up by two methods. The easiest uses a commercially available hydrogen and carbon dioxide generator envelope (GasPak) that is placed in the jar along with the culture plates. The generator is activated with water. Oxygen within the jar and the hydrogen that is generated are converted to water in the presence of the catalyst, thus producing anaerobic conditions. Carbon dioxide, which is also generated, is required for growth by some anaerobes and stimulates the growth of others. An alternative method for achieving anaerobiosis in the jar consists of evacuation and replacement. Air is evacuated from the sealed jar containing the culture plates and is replaced with an oxygen-free mixture of 80 percent nitrogen, 10 percent hydrogen, and 10 percent carbon dioxide.

More sophisticated procedures are used to isolate extremely oxygen-sensitive microorganisms that cannot be recovered by using the anaerobic jar. One, the **roll tube method,** consists of a stoppered test tube containing oxygen-free gas and a thin layer of prereduced agar medium on its inside surface. The medium in the tube is inoculated with a loop while the tube is rotated. This produces a spiral track on the agar surface. The tube is flushed with a stream of carbon dioxide to prevent entry of air while it is open during inoculation.

The **anaerobic glove box isolator** is another innovation developed for isolating anaerobic bacteria. It is essentially a large clear-vinyl chamber, with attached gloves, containing a mixture of 80 percent nitrogen, 10 percent hydrogen, and 10 percent carbon dioxide. A lock at one end of the chamber is fitted with two hatches, one leading to the outside and the other to the inside of the chamber. Specimens are placed in the lock, the outside hatch is closed, and the air in the lock is evacuated and replaced with the gas mixture. The inside hatch is then opened to introduce the specimen into the chamber. Conventional bacteriologic procedures are employed to process the specimen in the oxygen-free atmosphere.

Although these complex systems are needed to isolate anaerobic flora components, studies have shown that the anaerobic jar is adequate to recover clinically significant anaerobes. The extremely oxygen-sensitive bacteria of the microflora apparently are not associated with infectious processes.

Procedures for cultivation and identification of anaerobic bacteria are well established (Fig. 17-3). A variety of selective and nonselective media is available for cultivation of anaerobes. A reliable, nonselective medium consists of *Brucella* agar supplemented with sheep blood, hemin, cysteine, sodium carbonate, and menadione. Usual bacteriologic procedures are used to identify anaerobes. These are based on Gram-staining reactions, cellular and colony morphology, antibiotic sensitivity patterns, carbohydrate fermentation reactions, and other biochemical tests. Analysis of metabolic end products, especially organic acids, provides additional information useful in classifying these organisms.

REFERENCES

Balows A, DeHaan RM, Dowell VR, Guze LB (eds): Anaerobic Bacteria. Charles C Thomas, Springfield, IL, 1974

Finegold SM: Anaerobic Bacteria in Human Disease. Academic Press, San Diego, 1977

Finegold SM, George WL (eds): Anaerobic Infections in Humans. Academic Press, San Diego, 1989

Holdeman LV, Cato EP, Moore WEC (eds): Anaerobe Laboratory Manual. 4th Ed. Virginia Polytechnic Institute and State University Anaerobe Laboratory, Blacksburg, 1977

Lennette EH, Spaulding EH, Truant JP (eds): Manual of Clinical Microbiology. 2nd Ed. American Society for Microbiology, Washington, D.C., 1974

Morris JG: The physiology of obligate anaerobiosis. Adv Microb Physiol 12:169–246, 1975

Sutter VL, Citron DM, Finegold SM: Wadsworth Anaerobic Bacteriology Manual. 3rd Ed. CV Mosby, St. Louis, 1980

18 CLOSTRIDIA: SPORE-FORMING ANAEROBIC BACILLI

CAROL L. WELLS
TRACY D. WILKINS

GENERAL CONCEPTS

CLOSTRIDIA

Clostridia are strictly anaerobic to aerotolerant spore-forming bacilli found in soil as well as in the normal intestinal flora of humans and other animals. There are both Gram-positive and Gram-negative species, although the majority of isolates are Gram positive. Exotoxin(s) plays an important role in pathogenesis.

GAS GANGRENE AND RELATED CLOSTRIDIAL WOUND INFECTIONS

Clinical Manifestations

The severity of clostridial wound infections ranges from invasion of live tissue with systemic toxemia to relatively benign superficial contamination of already necrotic tissue.

Structure

The clostridia that cause gas gangrene are anaerobic, spore-forming bacilli, but some species (e.g., *Clostridium perfringens*) may not readily sporulate.

Classification and Antigenic Types

Clostridial wound infections are typically polymicrobial. The primary pathogens include *C perfringens, C novyi, C septicum*, and others.

Pathogenesis

Wounds are contaminated by clostridia from the environment or the normal flora. The anaerobic tissue environment facilitates the replication of clostridia and secretion of toxins.

Host Defenses

Host defenses are essentially absent. There is little, if any, innate immunity.

Epidemiology

Clostridia are ubiquitous in the soil and in the normal microbial flora of humans and other animals; clostridial wound infections are found worldwide.

Diagnosis

Diagnosis is by recognition of a characteristic lesion coupled with both Gram stains of tissue and bacterial culture.

Control

Treatment involves administration of antimicrobial agents (e.g., penicillin or chloramphenicol) coupled as necessary with tissue debridement.

TETANUS AND *CLOSTRIDIUM TETANI*

Clinical Manifestations

Tetanus is characterized by twitching of muscles around a wound and by pain in neck and jaw muscles (**trismus**) and around the wound. Patients have no fever, but sweat profusely.

279

Structure

These organisms are Gram-positive bacilli with terminal spores.

Classification and Antigenic Types

Clostridium tetani is the only species. There are no serotypes.

Pathogenesis

Clostridium tetani cells multiply and secrete exotoxins in a contaminated anaerobic wound. The spasmogenic toxin fixes to neural gangliosides and blocks glycine release, permitting contraction of antagonistic muscles.

Host Defenses

Host defenses are essentially absent. There is little, if any, innate immunity. Active immunity follows vaccination with tetanus toxoid.

Epidemiology

Clostridium tetani is ubiquitous in soil worldwide and is occasionally found in the intestinal flora of humans and other animals.

Diagnosis

Diagnosis is primarily by the clinical symptoms. The wound may not be obvious. *Clostridium tetani* is recovered from only one-third of all implicated wounds.

Control

Vaccination with tetanus toxoid is protective. Tetanus is treated with penicillin or chloramphenicol and by wound debridement. Other measures include tetanus immunoglobulin and supportive therapy.

BOTULISM AND
CLOSTRIDIUM BOTULINUM

Clinical Manifestations

Botulism may start with gastrointestinal symptoms. The cranial nerves are initially affected, followed by descending, symmetric paralysis of motor nerves, with critical involvement of the respiratory tree. Muscle paralysis may occur.

Structure, Classification, and Antigenic Types

These organisms are bacilli with oval, subterminal spores. *Clostridium botulinum* is the only species. It consists of several biochemically distinct organisms that pro-

duce botulinum toxin. There are seven types of neurotoxins, designated A, B, C, D, E, F, and G. Some are encoded on bacteriophage DNA.

Pathogenesis

There are three forms of botulism: (1) adult botulism, caused by ingestion of preformed toxin in food; (2) infant botulism, in which the organism replicates and secretes toxin in the intestinal tract; and (3) wound botulism, in which the organism replicates in the wound and secretes toxin. Toxin binds to neuromuscular junctions of parasympathetic nerves and interferes with acetylcholine release, causing paralysis.

Host Defenses

No host defenses are known.

Epidemiology

Clostridium botulinum is ubiquitous in soil worldwide. Improper canning of foods is a major cause of botulism.

Diagnosis

Diagnosis is from the clinical symptoms and laboratory tests. A finding of normal spinal fluid helps to eliminate numerous other central nervous system disorders.

Control

The best means of control is proper food handling. Treatment includes an attempt to neutralize unbound toxin. Supportive care is of primary importance.

PSEUDOMEMBRANOUS COLITIS AND
CLOSTRIDIUM DIFFICILE

Clinical Manifestations

Patients have antibiotic-associated diarrhea and pseudomembranes on colonic mucosa.

Structure, Classification, and Antigenic Types

These organisms are bacilli with large, oval, subterminal spores. *Clostridium difficile* is the only species. There are no defined serotypes. Toxigenic and nontoxigenic strains exist. The former produce toxin A (enterotoxin) and toxin B (cytotoxin).

Pathogenesis

Broad-spectrum antibiotic therapy eliminates many members of the competing normal flora, permitting intestinal overgrowth of toxigenic *C difficile*.

Host Defenses

No host defenses are known.

Epidemiology

Clostridium difficile is a component of the normal intestinal flora of a small percentage of healthy adults and a large percentage of healthy neonates. It also may be found in the environment, especially in hospitals.

Diagnosis

The presence of severe diarrhea coupled with the demonstration of organisms and/or toxin in feces, and the demonstration of pseudomembranes by colonoscopy, constitute the most reliable means of diagnosis.

Control

The antimicrobial agents of choice are metronidazole and vancomycin. Relapses can occur. Supportive therapy may be needed.

OTHER PATHOGENIC CLOSTRIDIA

Clostridium perfringens causes food poisoning and necrotizing enteritis; *C sordellii* causes endometritis; *C septicum* is correlated with the presence of cancer; *C tertium* may cause bacteremia, and *C ramosum*, although not implicated as a pathogen, is frequently isolated from clinical specimens.

INTRODUCTION

The clostridia are the best studied of all the anaerobes that infect humans. They cause a variety of human diseases, the most important of which are gas gangrene, tetanus, botulism, pseudomembranous colitis, and food poisoning. In most cases, clostridia are opportunistic pathogens; that is, one or more species establishes a nidus of infection in a particular site in a compromised host. All pathogenic clostridial species produce protein exotoxins (such as botulinum and tetanus toxins) that play an important role in pathogenesis.

Most generalizations about *Clostridium* have exceptions. The clostridia are classically anaerobic rods, but some species can become aerotolerant on subculture; a few species (*C carnis, C histolyticum,* and *C tertium*) can grow under aerobic conditions. Most species are Gram positive, but a few are Gram negative. Also, many Gram-positive species easily lose the Gram reaction, resulting in Gram-negative cultures.

The clostridia form characteristic spores, whose position is useful in species identification; however, some species do not sporulate unless exposed to exacting culture conditions. Many clostridia are transient or permanent members of the normal flora of the human skin and the gastrointestinal tracts of humans and other animals. Unlike typical members of the human bacterial flora, most clostridia also occur worldwide in the soil.

Because clostridia are ubiquitous saprophytes, many clostridia isolated from clinical specimens are accidental contaminants and are not involved in a disease process. Because these organisms are normally found on the skin, even a pure culture of clostridia isolated from the blood may have no clinical significance. In determining the importance of a clinical isolate of clostridia, the clinician should consider the frequency of isolation of the species, the presence of other microbes of pathogenic potential, and the clinical symptoms of the patient. Many clostridial infections can be controlled by antibiotic therapy (e.g., penicillin, chloramphenicol, vancomycin, or metronidazole) accompanied, in some cases, by tissue debridement. Antitoxin therapy and toxoid immunization are clearly useful in some clostridial infections, such as tetanus.

GAS GANGRENE AND RELATED CLOSTRIDIAL WOUND INFECTIONS

CLINICAL MANIFESTATIONS

Clostridial wound infections may be divided into three categories: **gas gangrene** or clostridial myonecrosis, **anaerobic cellulitis,** and **superficial contamination.** Gas gangrene can have a rapidly fatal outcome and requires prompt, often aggressive, treatment. The more common clostridial wound infections are much less acute and require much less radical treatment; however, they may share some characteristics with gas gangrene and must be included in the differential diagnosis.

Gas gangrene is an acute disease with a poor prognosis and often fatal outcome (Fig. 18-1). Initial trauma to host tissue damages muscle and impairs blood supply. This lack of oxygenation causes the oxidation-reduction potential to decrease and allows the growth of anaerobic clostridia. Initial symptoms are generalized fever and pain in the infected tissue. As the clostridia multiply, various exotoxins (including hemolysins, collagenases, proteases, and lipases) are liberated into the surrounding tissue, causing more local tissue necrosis and systemic toxemia. Infected muscle is discolored and edematous and produces a foul-smelling exudate; gas bubbles form as a result of anaerobic fermentation. As capillary permeability increases, the accumulation of fluid increases and venous return eventually is curtailed. As more tissue becomes involved, the clostridia multiply within the increasing area of dead tissue, releasing more toxins into the local tissue and into the systemic circulation. Because ischemia plays a significant role in the pathogenesis of gas gangrene, the muscle groups most frequently involved are those in the extremities that are served by one or two major blood vessels.

Clostridial septicemia, although rare, may occur in the late stages of the disease. Severe shock with massive hemolysis and renal failure is usually the ultimate cause of death. The incubation period, from the time of wounding until the establishing of gas gangrene, varies with the infecting clostridial species from 1 to 6 days, but may be as long as 6 weeks. Average incubation times for the three most prevalent infecting organisms are as follows: C perfringens, 10 to 48 hours; C septicum, 2 to 3 days; and C novyi, 5 to 6 days. Because the organisms need time to establish a nidus of infection, the time lag between wounding and the appropriate medical treatment is a significant factor in the initiation of gas gangrene.

Like gas gangrene, anaerobic cellulitis is an infection of muscle tissue, but here the infecting organisms invade only tissue that is already dead; the infection does not spread to healthy, undamaged tissue. Anaerobic cellulitis has a more gradual onset than gas gangrene and does not include the systemic toxemia associated with gas gangrene. Pain is minimal, and although only dead tissue is infected, the disease can spread along the planes between muscle groups, causing the surrounding tissue to appear more affected than it actually is. Anaerobic cellulitis may cause the formation of many gas bubbles, producing infected tissue that looks similar to the gaseous tissue of gas gangrene. Some tissue necrosis does occur, but it is caused by decreased blood supply and not invasion by the infecting organism. With adequate treatment, anaerobic cellulitis has a good prognosis.

Superficial contamination, the least serious of the clostridial wound infections, involves infection of only necrotic tissue. Usually, the patient experiences little pain and wound healing proceeds normally; however, occasionally an exudate forms and the infection interferes with wound healing. Superficial wound contamination caused by clostridia usually involves C perfringens, with staphylococci, streptococci, or both as frequent coisolates.

STRUCTURE

The clostridia that cause gas gangrene are anaerobic, spore-forming bacilli, but some species (e.g., C perfringens) may not readily sporulate.

CLASSIFICATION AND ANTIGENIC TYPES

Clostridial wound infections usually are polymicrobic because the source of wound contamina-

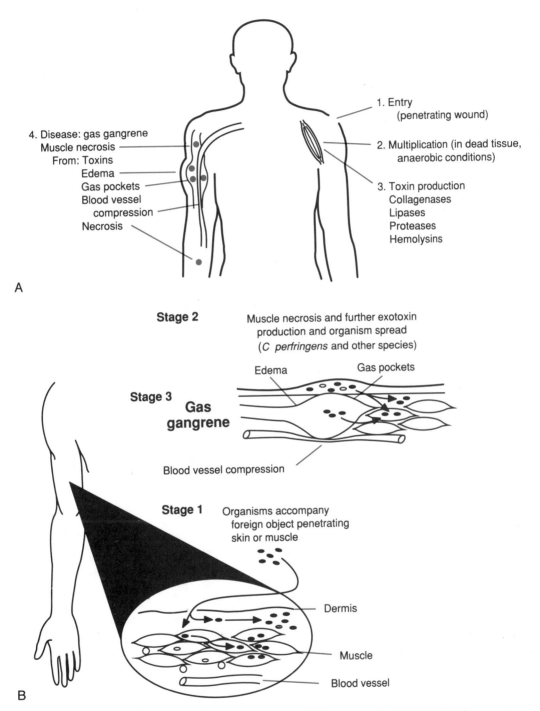

FIGURE 18-1   Pathogenesis of gas gangrene. *(A)* Macroscopic; *(B)* microscopic.

tion (feces, soil) is polymicrobic. In gas gangrene and anaerobic cellulitis, the primary pathogen can be one of various clostridial species including *C perfringens* (80 percent), *C novyi* (40 percent), *C septicum* (20 percent), and, occasionally, *C bifermentans, C histolyticum,* or *C fallax.* Other bacterial isolates include *Proteus, Bacillus, Escherichia, Bacteroides,* and *Staphylococcus.* The distinctive or unique properties of the causative agents of gas gangrene are difficult to list; morphologic characteristics and biochemical reactions vary among these species, and a reliable laboratory manual should be consulted for their proper identification. Isolation of 10^7 or more clostridia/ml of wound exudate is strong evidence for a clostridial wound infection.

The most frequently isolated pathogen, *C perfringens,* has five types, designated A, B, C, D, and E. Each of these types produces a semi-unique spectrum of protein toxins. α-Toxin (a lecithinase, also called phospholipase C) and θ-toxin (oxygen-labile hemolysin) are of primary importance in the disease pathology. α-Toxin is lethal and necrotizing, and θ-toxin may be responsible for intravascular hemolysis.

PATHOGENESIS

All clostridial wound infections occur in an anaerobic tissue environment caused by an impaired blood supply secondary to trauma, surgery, foreign bodies, or cancer. Contamination of the wound by clostridia from the external environment or from the normal flora produces the infection. The detailed pathogenesis of the disease is intimately associated with the clinical presentation as described above (Fig. 18-1).

HOST DEFENSES

Host defenses against clostridial wound infections are essentially absent. Even repeated episodes of clostridial wound infection do not produce effective immunity.

EPIDEMIOLOGY

Clostridial spores are ubiquitous in the soil, on human skin, and in the gastrointestinal tracts of humans and other animals. Therefore, the agents of clostridial wound infections are not environmentally restricted. Even operating theaters can be habitats for infecting clostridial organisms and spores. The incidence of clostridial wound infections has declined with the advance of prompt, adequate medical treatment. Historically, war casualties have had the greatest incidence of gas gangrene; however, the prompt evacuation and medical attention given U.S. casualties in the Vietnam war greatly decreased the incidence of gas gangrene in these soldiers, emphasizing the importance of prompt medical treatment.

DIAGNOSIS

Diagnosis of clostridial wound infections is based on clinical symptoms coupled with Gram stains and bacterial culture of clinical specimens. Once initiated, gas gangrene may spread and cause death within hours. By the time the typical lesions are evident, the disease usually is firmly established and the physician must treat the patient on a clinical basis without waiting for laboratory confirmation. Characteristic lesions and the presence of large numbers of Gram-positive bacilli (with or without spores) in a wound exudate provide strong presumptive evidence. Spores are rare in cultures of *C perfringens,* the most common agent. A common laboratory test for presumptive identification of *C perfringens* is the Nagler reaction, which detects the presence of α-toxin, one of the most prominent toxins produced by *C perfringens.* However, several other *Clostridium* species also have a positive Nagler reaction, so this test is not entirely specific for *C perfringens.*

Discussion of the differential diagnosis of clostridial wound infections appropriately includes streptococcal myositis, as this disease can be characterized by an edematous, necrotizing, often gaseous lesion. Like anaerobic cellulitis and superficial contamination with clostridia, streptococcal myositis is a relatively localized disease, but its later stages may include some systemic toxicity that mimics the toxemia of gas gangrene.

CONTROL

Correction of the anaerobic conditions combined with antibiotic treatment form the basis for therapy. Penicillin is the drug of choice for all clostridial wound infections; chloramphenicol is a second-choice antibiotic. Successful treatment of the less severe forms of clostridial wound infections includes local debridement and antibiotic therapy; after these measures are taken, recovery usually proceeds along a steady, positive course. Treatment of gas gangrene includes radical surgical debridement coupled with high doses of antibiotics. Blood transfusions and supportive therapy for shock and renal failure also may be indicated.

The usefulness of gas gangrene antitoxin is controversial. Some physicians maintain that the efficacy of this polyvalent antitoxin has been proved in the past, but better medical care now may have eliminated the need for its use. Others believe that because of insufficient data, antitoxin should be administered systemically as early as possible after diagnosis and that it should be injected locally into tissue that cannot be excised.

Disagreements also exist concerning the efficacy of hyperbaric oxygen therapy. Certain chelating agents such as ethylenediaminetetracetic acid (EDTA) and diethylenetriamine pentaacetic acid (DTPA) may aid in treatment of gas gangrene caused by *C perfringens* since they inhibit the activity of α-toxin (the most damaging toxin released by this organism).

Obviously, prevention of wound contamination is the single most important factor in controlling clostridial wound infections. In the past, immunization has been considered a possible preventive measure for gas gangrene. However, several factors have discouraged the use of active immunization; these include difficulty in preparing a suitable antigenic toxoid, availability of prompt wound treatment, and accessibility of effective therapeutic agents.

TETANUS AND CLOSTRIDIUM TETANI

CLINICAL MANIFESTATIONS

Tetanus is a severe disease caused by the toxin of *C tetani* (Fig. 18-2). This organism grows in wounds and secretes a toxin that invades systemically and causes spasms of voluntary muscles. The initial symptom is cramping and twitching of muscles around a wound. The patient usually has no fever but sweats profusely and begins to experience pain, especially in the area of the wound and around the neck and jaw muscles (**trismus**). Portions of the body may become extremely rigid, and **opisthotonos** (a spasm in which the head and heels are bent backward and the body bowed forward) is common. Complications include fractures, bowel impaction, intramuscular hematoma, muscle ruptures, and pulmonary, renal, and cardiac problems.

STRUCTURE

Clostridium tetani is an anaerobic Gram-positive rod that forms terminal spores, giving it a characteristic tennis racquet appearance. Some strains do not sporulate readily, and spores may not appear until day 3 or 4 of culture. Most strains are motile with peritrichous flagella; colonies often swarm on agar plates, but some strains are nonflagellated and nonmotile. The presence of *C tetani* should be suspected on isolation of a swarming rod that produces indole and has terminal spherical spores, but does not produce acid from glucose. This organism produces the toxin **tetanospasmin,** but nontoxigenic strains also exist. Tetanospasmin is responsible for tetanus. The two most susceptible animal species are horses and humans.

CLASSIFICATION AND ANTIGENIC TYPES

Clostridium tetani is the only species. There are no serotypes.

PATHOGENESIS

As with all clostridial wound infections, the initial event in tetanus is trauma to host tissue, followed by accidental contamination of the wound with *C tetani* (Fig. 18-2). Tissue damage lowers the oxidation-reduction potential and provides an environment suitable for growth. Once growth is initiated, the organism itself is not invasive and remains confined to the necrotic tissue, where the vegetative cells of *C tetani* elaborate the lethal toxin. The in-

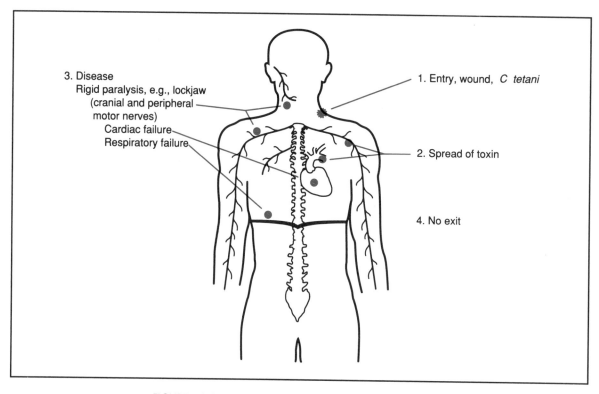

FIGURE 18-2 Pathogenesis of tetanus caused by *C tetani*.

cubation period from the time of wounding to the appearance of symptoms varies from a few days to several weeks, depending on the infectious dose and the site of the wound (the more peripheral the wound, the longer the incubation time).

Tetanus can be initiated in two different ways, resulting in either ascending or descending tetanus. In the ascending form, toxins travel along the neural route (peripheral nerves), causing a disease confined to the extremities and seen most often in inadequately immunized persons. In descending tetanus, all of the toxin cannot be absorbed by local nerve endings; therefore, it passes into the blood and lymph with subsequent absorption by all the motor nerves. The most susceptible centers are the head and neck; the first symptom is usually trismus (lockjaw), with muscle spasms descending from the neck to the trunk and limbs. As the disease progresses, the spasms increase in severity, becoming very painful and exhausting. Spasms

often are initiated by environmental stimuli that may be as insignificant as the flash of a light or the sound of a footstep.

Clostridium tetani actually produces two toxins: tetanolysin, a hemolysin that is inactivated by cholesterol and has no role in pathogenesis, and tetanospasmin, a spasmogenic toxin responsible for the classic symptoms of the disease. The spasmogenic toxin binds to gangliosides in neural tissue and blocks the release of glycine, a transmitter substance that normally prevents contraction of antagonistic muscles. Muscle spasms and convulsions result. Tetanospasmin also may act on the sympathetic nervous system, the neurocirculatory system, and the neuroendocrine system. Its potency is similar to that of *C botulinum* toxin; as little as 130 μg constitutes a lethal dose for humans. The fatality rates for untreated tetanus are 90 percent for neonates and 40 percent for adults. However, with aggressive hospital care, these fatality rates can be substantially reduced. The ultimate cause of death is usually pulmonary or cardiac failure.

HOST DEFENSES

Although there are scattered reports that tetanus antibodies can be acquired by natural, presumably enteric infection with *C tetani*, innate immunity to tetanus toxin does not typically exist. Also, one or more episodes of tetanus do not produce immunity to future attacks. There are at least two reasons for the lack of immune response: the toxin is potent, and the amount released may be too small to trigger immune mechanisms but still be large enough to cause symptoms, and, because the toxin binds firmly to neural tissue, it may not interact effectively with the immune system.

EPIDEMIOLOGY

Clostridium tetani can be isolated from the soil in almost every environment throughout the world. It can be found among the gastrointestinal flora of humans and horses. Isolation of *C tetani* from the intestinal flora of horses, coupled with the high frequency of equine tetanus, led to the erroneous assumption that the horse was the animal reservoir of *C tetani*.

Generalized outbreaks of tetanus do not occur, but certain populations can be considered at risk. Historically, wounded soldiers have had a high incidence of tetanus, but this phenomenon has declined with widespread use of immunizations. Umbilical tetanus (tetanus neonatorum) usually is a generalized, fulminating, fatal disease of neonates of unimmunized mothers who have given birth under unsanitary conditions. In the United States, intravenous drug abusers have become another population with an increasing incidence of clinical tetanus. Tetanus is rare in most developed countries (the United States has about one case per million per year). However, in some developing countries, it is still one of the leading causes of death. In developing countries, approximate mortality rates remain 85 percent for neonatal tetanus and 50 percent for nonneonatal tetanus. This is an unfortunate situation because tetanus is completely preventable with adequate immunization.

DIAGNOSIS

Diagnosis of tetanus is obvious in advanced cases; however, successful treatment depends on early diagnosis before a lethal amount of toxin becomes fixed to neural tissue. The patient should be treated on a clinical basis without waiting for laboratory data. *Clostridium tetani* can be recovered from the wound in only about one-third of the cases, and a wound is not even evident in 10 to 20 percent of cases. The clinician should be aware that toxigenic strains of *C tetani* can grow actively in the wound of an immunized person but that the presence of antitoxin antibodies prevents initiation of tetanus. Also, because tetanus is common in the soil, the mere presence of *C tetani* in a wound does not imply that the organism is actively replicating and secreting toxin.

Numerous syndromes, including rabies and meningitis, have symptoms similar to those of tetanus and must be considered in the differential diagnosis. Ingestion of strychnine (found in rat poison) can cause symptoms that closely resemble those of tetanus. Trismus can occur in encephalitis, phenothiazine reactions, and diseases involving the jaw.

CONTROL

Injections of tetanus toxoid are prophylactic. Currently, booster doses every 10 years are recommended by the Centers for Disease Control (CDC). More frequent boosters are unnecessary and may cause local reactions resembling the Arthus phenomenon, or a delayed hypersensitivity reaction. Because of their immunodeficient state, acquired immune deficiency syndrome (AIDS) patients may not respond to prophylactic injections of tetanus toxoid.

Treatment of diagnosed tetanus has a number of aspects. The offending organism must be removed by local debridement. Penicillin or chloramphenicol is usually administered to kill the bacteria, but may not be a necessary adjunct in therapy. Tetanus immunoglobulin is injected intramuscularly into different sites, including the involved extremity, in an attempt to neutralize unbound systemic toxin. This tetanus antiserum is available both as horse serum and as human serum; the horse serum preparation has the usual potential side effect of serum sickness, but the human preparation is much more expensive. Supportive measures, such as respiratory assistance and intravenous fluids, are often critical to survival. Recommended tranquilizers and sedatives to relieve muscle spasms include phenobarbital, thiopental sodium (Pentothal), and diazepam (Valium). Analgesics that will not cause respiratory depression should be used; these include codeine, meperidine (Demerol), and morphine.

In cases of clean, minor wounds, tetanus toxoid should be administered only if the patient has not had a booster dose within the past 10 years. For more serious wounds, toxoid should be administered if the patient has not had a booster dose within the past 5 years. All patients who have a reasonable potential for contracting tetanus should receive injections of tetanus immunoglobulin.

BOTULISM AND CLOSTRIDIUM BOTULINUM

CLINICAL MANIFESTATIONS

Botulism caused by the toxin of a diverse group of clostridia called *C botulinum*. This neurotoxin characteristically causes a symmetric, descending paralysis (Fig. 18-3). The symptoms of botulism can occur in both the nervous system and the alimentary tract of the patient. Therefore, many diseases enter into the differential diagnosis, including pharyngitis, gastroenteritis, intestinal obstruction, myasthenia gravis, encephalitis, muscular dystrophy, meningitis, poliomyelitis, cerebrovascular accident, Guillain-Barré syndrome, chemical food poisoning, and tick paralysis. For infant botulism, additional syndromes enter into the differential diagnosis: failure to thrive, acute infantile polyneuropathy, dehydration, and various hereditary and metabolic disorders. Infant

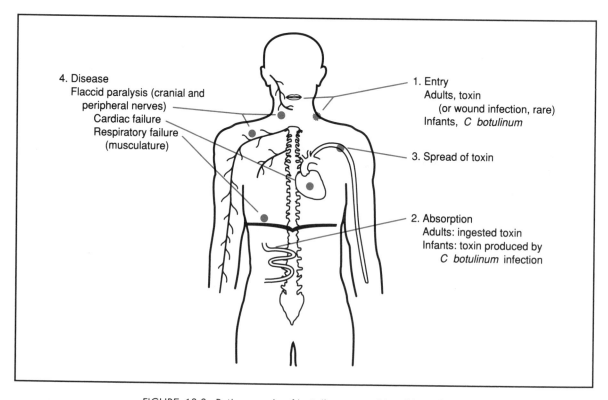

FIGURE 18-3 Pathogenesis of botulism caused by *C botulinum*.

botulism often is missed by physicians, but it always should be considered if any of the typical symptoms are present.

STRUCTURE, CLASSIFICATION, AND ANTIGENIC TYPES

Unlike most species of bacteria, which comprise strains that have a close genetic relationship and similar cultural characteristics, the "species" *C botulinum* consists of several distinct groups of organisms that have a common name solely because they produce similar toxins. The name *C botulinum* is therefore only a convenience that reflects the medical importance of the species. A strain of *C botulinum* usually produces only one of seven toxin types, designated A, B, C, D, E, F, and G. Type C and D toxins are encoded by the genetic material contained in bacteriophages that infect the bacteria. *C botulinum* strains producing types C and D toxins can be interconverted by use of specific bacteriophage. Types C and D can even be transformed into *C novyi* by curing bacteria of the botulinum phage and substituting a phage that codes for a *C novyi* toxin. To add to the confusion, a few strains of *C baratii* and *C butyricum* have recently been reported to secrete botulinum toxin. In addition, certain proteolytic strains of *C botulinum* are indistinguishable from *C sporogenes* except by toxin assay. Therefore, the production of a pharmacologically similar neurotoxin is the single distinctive property of a clostridium that places it in the botulinum "species." All the organisms that produce this toxin are anaerobic Gram-positive, peritrichous rods. Oval subterminal spores are produced in extremely variable numbers, depending on the particular isolate and on the culture medium. Culture reactions vary greatly, and the species includes highly proteolytic and nonproteolytic strains as well as saccharolytic and nonsaccharolytic strains.

Of the seven serologically distinct neurotoxins produced by *C botulinum* types A, B, E, and F are the most toxic for humans. Types C and D are most toxic for other animals. Type G is rare, with only a few reported human cases. The toxins often are released from the bacteria as inactive proteins that must be cleaved by a protease to expose the active site. These proteases may be produced by the cell itself or may be in the body fluids of the infected host. Type A toxin is the most potent poison known: ingestion of only 10^{-8} g of this toxin can kill a human. Put another way, the amount of toxin that could be held on the tip of a dissecting probe could kill 40 medical students.

PATHOGENESIS

The pathogenicity of *C botulinum* depends entirely on neurotoxin production (Fig. 18-3). In humans, these toxins cause disease in three ways: (1) the well-known form of food poisoning results from ingestion of toxin in improperly preserved food; (2) wound botulism, a rare disease, results from growth of *C botulinum* in the necrotic tissue of a wound; and (3) infant botulism is caused when the organism grows and produces toxin in the intestines of infants.

From its site of entry into the body, the toxin travels through the blood and lymphatic systems (and possibly the nervous system). It then becomes fixed to cranial and peripheral nerves, but exerts almost all of its action on the peripheral nervous system. It appears to bind to receptor sites at the neuromuscular junctions of parasympathetic nerves and prevents impulses from passing from motor nerves to parasympathetic nerves by interfering with the release of acetylcholine, the transmitter substance. The result is muscle paralysis. The cranial nerves are affected first, followed by a descending, symmetric paralysis of motor nerves. The early involvement of cranial nerves causes problems with eyesight, hearing, and speech. Double or blurred vision, dilated pupils, and slurred speech are common symptoms. Decreased saliva production causes a dryness of the mouth and throat, and swallowing may be painful. An overall weakness ensues, followed by descending paralysis with critical involvement of the respiratory tree. Death usually is caused by respiratory failure, but cardiac failure can be the primary cause. Mortality is highest for type A, followed by type E and then type B, possibly reflecting the affinities of the toxins for neural tissue: type A binds most firmly, followed by type E and then type B. Fatality rates are directly proportional to the infectious dose and inversely proportional to the incubation time of the disease.

Food Poisoning

In botulism food poisoning, the toxin is produced by the vegetative cells of *C botulinum* in contaminated food and preformed toxin then is ingested with the contaminated food. The incubation time can vary from a few hours to 10 days, but most commonly is 18 to 36 hours. Only a small, but effective, percentage of the ingested toxin is absorbed through the intestinal mucosa, the remainder being eliminated in the feces. Gastrointestinal disturbances are early symptoms of the disease in about one-third of the patients with type A or B food poisoning and in almost all of the cases involving type E toxin. These symptoms include nausea, vomiting, and abdominal pain. Diarrhea often is present, but constipation also may occur. Symptoms of toxemia then become apparent. No fever occurs in the absence of complicating infections.

Wound Botulism

The initial event in wound botulism is contamination of a wound by *C botulinum*. The organisms are not invasive and are confined to the necrotic tissue, where they replicate and elaborate the lethal neurotoxin. The incubation time varies from a few days to as long as 2 weeks. The only differences in the symptoms of wound botulism and food poisoning (in addition to a possibly longer incubation time) are that wound botulism lacks gastrointestinal symptoms and a wound exudate or a fever or both may be present. *Clostridium botulinum* may be present in a wound but create no symptoms of botulism. There have been several recent reports of wound botulism in intravenous drug abusers, who are now emerging as a population at risk.

Infant Botulism

In contrast to botulism food poisoning caused by ingestion of preformed toxin, infant botulism results from germination of spores in the gastrointestinal tract, where vegetative cells then replicate and release the botulinum toxin. This appears to be related to the composition of the intestinal flora of infants. Almost all reported cases have occurred in infants between 2 weeks and 6 months of age. In infant botulism, the usual first indication of illness, constipation, is often overlooked. The infant then becomes lethargic and sleeps more than normally. Suck and gag reflexes diminish, and dysphagia often becomes evident as drooling. Later, head control may be lost and the infant becomes flaccid. In the most severely affected babies, respiratory arrest can occur.

There are scattered reports that *C botulinum* can occasionally multiply and secrete toxin in the intestinal tracts of adults with an altered intestinal flora.

HOST DEFENSES

Host defenses against *C botulinum* are undefined. Some people can tolerate ingestion of botulinum toxin better than others. The reason for this phenomenon is obscure, but it could be due to differences in the efficiency of uptake of the toxin from the intestine or in transporting the toxin to neural tissue. An attack of botulism does not produce effective immunity. The small amount of toxin in the circulation and its affinity for neural tissue probably prevent adequate amounts of toxin from interacting with the immune system.

EPIDEMIOLOGY

Clostridium botulinum spores are found worldwide in the soil (including sea sediments) and in small numbers in the gastrointestinal tracts of some birds, fish, and mammals. In the United States, the most frequent isolate is type A, followed by B and E and occasionally F. In Europe, type B is the most frequent isolate, whereas A is comparatively rare.

Originally, botulism food poisoning was thought to be associated only with contaminated meat, especially sausage; however, it is now known that *C botulinum* can grow equally well in many types of food including vegetables, fish, fruits, and condiments. Inadequate sterilization techniques during home canning are responsible for most cases of botulism during this century. The toxin is usually produced at pH 4.8 to 8.5. However, even acidic foods such as canned tomatoes have been responsible for several recent cases of botulism food poisoning. In addition, certain culture conditions cause toxin production at pH values lower than 4.6. In general, germination of botulinum spores is favored in food kept warm under anaerobic conditions for a long period.

DIAGNOSIS

Although all forms of botulism are difficult to diagnose, prompt diagnosis and treatment are crucial to survival. Laboratory tests offer little in establishing an initial diagnosis of botulism, and accordingly, the finding of normal cerebrospinal fluid can help to eliminate many of the diseases concerned with central nervous system disorders. In infant botulism, an electromyogram pattern of brief, small-amplitude overabundant motor reaction potentials often is seen.

Confirmation of the initial diagnosis rests on demonstrating toxin in feces, serum, or vomitus. In adult botulism, serum samples rarely yield type A toxin because of the strong affinity of this toxin for neural tissue. In infant botulism, circulating toxin can occasionally be found in the serum. Fecal samples are the best specimens for detecting toxin in botulism food poisoning or in infant botulism because only a small percentage of ingested or in situ-formed toxin is absorbed through the intestinal mucosa. Toxin may be excreted for days or even weeks following botulism food poisoning. It is usually detected by its lethal effect in mice and neutralization of this effect by specific antisera. In infants, the organism can usually be cultured from the stool.

Clostridium botulinum spores exist throughout the environment; all adults have probably ingested these spores with no ill effects. Because spores can cause poisoning in infants, obvious sources should be eliminated from the infant's environment and especially the infant's diet. Honey is the only dietary ingredient that has been implicated, and honey is no longer recommended for infants under 1 year of age. Most cases are not caused by ingesting honey, however, so this will not eliminate

the disease. The other more common environmental sources of spores, such as soil and dust, are not so easily controlled. There is no evidence for infant-to-infant transmission of *C botulinum*.

CONTROL

The best way to control botulism food poisoning is to use adequate food preservation methods and to heat all canned food before eating. Because botulinum toxin is heat labile, boiling food for a few minutes will eliminate toxin contamination; however, the spores themselves are not destroyed by boiling, and proper canning procedures must be followed to kill clostridial spores.

Once a case of wound botulism or food poisoning has been diagnosed, therapy has four objectives: to eliminate the source of the toxin, to eliminate any unabsorbed toxin, to neutralize any unbound toxin with specific antitoxin, and to provide general supportive care.

Food Poisoning in Adults and Wound Botulism

In food poisoning, the unabsorbed toxin may be eliminated by stomach lavage and high enemas. Although cathartics may be used to eliminate residual toxin, they may have adverse effects in patients with bowel paralysis. In wound botulism, debridement and antibiotic therapy with penicillin are used to eliminate the offending organism. Antibiotic therapy is of questionable value in food poisoning, but is advocated by those who believe the organism can replicate in the adult intestinal tract.

For both food poisoning and wound botulism, antitoxin therapy is most effective if administered early; however, clear-cut evidence for the efficacy of antitoxin therapy exists for only type E toxin. Antitoxin is available from the CDC; trivalent ABE botulinum antitoxin is currently recommended. Unfortunately, all antitoxins are equine preparations, so a significant percentage of patients experience reactions typical of anaphylaxis and serum sickness. Therefore, before they receive antitoxin, all patients should be tested for sensitivity to horse serum. The most important aspect of treatment in botulism is close observation of the patient and availability of adequate facilities for immediate respiratory support. Respiratory failure may occur within minutes, and immediate respiratory assistance often saves the lives of patients with botulism toxemia. Owing to improvements in supportive care, the mortality rate for botulism has been dramatically reduced from approximately 60 percent (in the 1940s) to 10 percent.

All cases of botulism food poisoning should be reported immediately to local, state, or federal authorities, who will then take steps to minimize the chance of an outbreak. All persons suspected of ingesting contaminated food should be closely observed. Antitoxin should be administered both to those with overt symptoms and to those who have definitely ingested contaminated food.

Infant Botulism

Treatment for infant botulism is similar to that for adult botulism food poisoning, with a few exceptions. Oral antibiotic therapy is not indicated, because it may unpredictably alter the intestinal flora and allow accidental overgrowth of *C botulinum*. Cathartics and enemas are also potentially dangerous. The value of antitoxin therapy in infants still is disputed for the following reasons: antitoxin therapy has not been shown to have a definite therapeutic effect, and the currently available horse serum preparation has produced anaphylaxis in infants. The most significant aspect of therapy for infant botulism is supportive care. The infant should be kept under close supervision, with facilities for respiratory support immediately available. The fatality rate for infant botulism is a surprisingly low 2 percent.

◄ PSEUDOMEMBRANOUS COLITIS AND *CLOSTRIDIUM DIFFICILE* ►

CLINICAL MANIFESTATIONS

Diarrhea is accepted as a natural accompaniment of treatment with many antibiotics. Although this diarrhea usually causes only minor concern, it can

evolve into a life-threatening enterocolitis. Many antibiotics have been associated with pseudomembranous colitis, including ampicillin, cephalosporins, clindamycin, tetracyclines, and chloramphenicol. Patients treated with clindamycin have a higher incidence of the disease, but most cases are found in patients treated with other antibiotics because of the more widespread use of these agents. Occasionally, antineoplastic agents with antibacterial activity will induce pseudomembranous colitis.

The first symptoms of pseudomembranous colitis are severe abdominal pain with a watery, usually nonbloody diarrhea (Fig. 18-4). Fever, hypoalbuminemia, and leukocytosis are common. Complications may include intractable colitis, intestinal perforation, and toxic megacolon. Histologically, the colon responds to the toxin by a leukocytic infiltrate into the lamina propria and by elaboration of a mixture of fibrin, mucus, and leukocytes, which form gray, white, or yellow patches on the mucosa. These areas are called pseudomembranes, hence the common term **pseudomembranous colitis.** Pseudomembranes usually develop after 4 to 10 days of antibiotic treatment, but they may appear 1 to 2 weeks after all antibiotic therapy has stopped. Mortality varies from hospital to hospital, but may be as high as 10 percent. The ultimate cause of death often is difficult to determine, as most patients show a nonspecific deterioration over a period of weeks.

The incidence of pseudomembranous colitis has been diminishing in recent years, probably owing to early diagnosis of the disease and prompt antimicrobial therapy. In most instances, once a patient develops antibiotic-associated diarrhea, and *C difficile* and/or toxin is detected in the stool, appropriate antimicrobial therapy is begun and the symptoms are not allowed to progress to the formation of colonic pseudomembranes. Therefore, in recent years the terms "*C difficile* diarrhea" and "*C difficile*" have come to be associated with a spectrum of diseases including diarrhea and colitis in the absence of pseudomembranes, as well as pseudomembranous colitis. The common factors in all of these diseases are the presence of diarrhea associated with antibiotic therapy and the

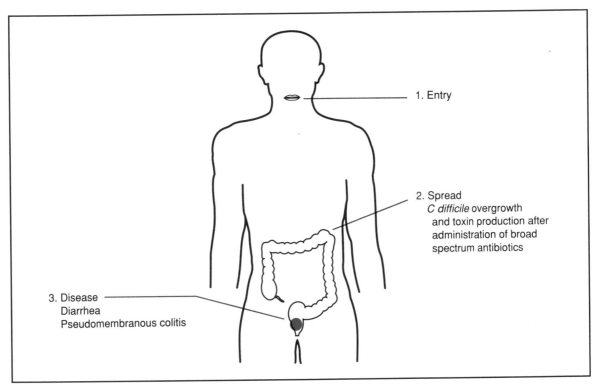

FIGURE 18-4 Pathogenesis of pseudomembranous colitis caused by *C difficile.*

recovery of *C difficile* organisms and/or toxin from the stool.

STRUCTURE, CLASSIFICATION, AND ANTIGENIC TYPES

Clostridium difficile is a slender, Gram-positive bacillus that produces large, oval, subterminal spores. It is an anaerobe, and some strains are extremely sensitive to oxygen. It is nonhemolytic and does not produce lecithinase or lipase reactions on egg yolk agar. Its proteolytic ability is weak and limited to digestion of gelatin. The products of fermentation are many and complex; they include acetic, butyric, isovaleric, valeric, isobutyric, and isocaproic acids, but only small amounts of each are produced. There are no defined serotypes.

PATHOGENESIS

Pseudomembranous colitis is caused by the growth of *C difficile* in the colon (Fig. 18-4). The organism appears unable to compete successfully in the normal colon ecosystem, but can compete when the normal flora is disturbed by antibiotics, allowing overgrowth of *C difficile*. This organism then replicates and secretes toxins; the resulting pathology is largely limited to the colon. During growth, *C difficile* produces two potent toxins. Toxin A is an enterotoxin that causes fluid accumulation in the bowel; toxin B is primarily a cytopathic agent. Both toxins kill experimental animals, and both probably are involved in the pathology of disease. Cytotoxicity tests on fecal filtrates depend on the neutralization of toxin B activity with antitoxin. Toxin A and toxin B always occur together.

HOST DEFENSES

Host defenses for pseudomembranous colitis are largely unknown. The best host defense against pseudomembranous colitis is maintenance of the stability of the normal intestinal flora.

EPIDEMIOLOGY

Clostridium difficile is a member of the normal intestinal flora of a small percentage of adults. There is some evidence that pseudomembranous colitis can be acquired as a nosocomial pathogen, and the incidence of this disease varies greatly from hospital to hospital. This seems to be due in part to contamination of hospital environments with the spores of *C difficile* and in part to different types of patient populations in various hospitals. Patients with *C difficile* diarrhea excrete large numbers of *C difficile* spores; care should be taken not to expose other patients receiving antibiotics. Healthy adults do not carry significant numbers of *C difficile* organisms, but healthy infants may have large numbers in their feces. Most studies report a high carriage rate of approximately 50 percent in neonates. The toxins also are present in these infants' stools but, for unknown reasons, appear to have no adverse effect. The same amounts of toxins are associated with disease in adults.

DIAGNOSIS

The diagnosis of pseudomembranous colitis requires demonstration of pseudomembranes by colonoscopy. *Clostridium difficile* can be isolated from the stools of almost all patients with this disease. Diagnosis of *C difficile* diarrhea or *C difficile* disease implies the presence of diarrhea associated with antibiotic therapy and the recovery of *C difficile* organisms and/or toxin from the stool. However, the isolation of toxigenic *C difficile* from patients with antibiotic-associated diarrhea is not a definitive diagnosis of *C difficile* diarrhea or *C difficile* disease, because other enteric pathogens are usually not excluded. Most cases of severe diarrhea are caused not by *C difficile*, but by other enteric pathogens such as *Campylobacter* spp, *Salmonella* spp, *Shigella* spp, and toxigenic strains of *Escherichia coli*. Moreover, antimicrobial therapy increases the likelihood of isolating *C difficile* from the fecal flora; *C difficile* is isolated from the feces of approximately 20 percent of asymptomatic hospitalized patients who are receiving antimicrobial therapy.

A good selective medium has been developed for the isolation of *C difficile* from stool. In addition, a cytotoxicity assay has been used extensively to detect the production of toxin B, which can be neutralized with specific antitoxin. The cytotoxicity test can be done directly on fecal filtrates and yields information on the amount of toxin present. This test for toxin B is time-consuming and cumbersome. There is a new rapid latex agglutination test that detects the presence of a *C difficile* antigen. However, this test is not specific because the antiserum cross-reacts with several other species of bacteria in the fecal flora. The antiserum in the latex agglutination test is also incapable of distinguishing between toxigenic and nontoxigenic strains of *C difficile*. It is therefore recommended that a positive latex agglutination test be confirmed by the demonstration of toxin B.

CONTROL

In many cases, symptoms resolve 1 to 14 days after therapy with the offending antibiotic is discontinued. Vancomycin or metronidazole are the antibiotics of choice to treat active disease. *C difficile* is susceptible to these agents, but symptoms can reappear when therapy is discontinued. Some patients have had many relapses; fecal enemas can help such patients to establish a normal flora. Constipating agents, such as atropine diphenoxylate (Lomotil) or codeine, should not be used. Supportive therapy is needed to compensate for the often severe fluid and electrolyte loss.

◄ OTHER PATHOGENIC ► CLOSTRIDIA

FOOD POISONING AND *C PERFRINGENS*

Clostridium perfringens is a major cause of food poisoning in the United States. The disease results from ingestion of a large number of organisms in contaminated food, usually meat or meat products. Food poisoning usually does not occur unless the food contains at least 10^6 to 10^7 organisms/g.

The spores are ubiquitous and, if present in food, can be triggered to germinate when the food is heated. Some heat-sensitive strains germinate without heating. After germination, the number of organisms quickly increases in warm food because the generation time can be extremely short (12 minutes) and multiplication occurs over a wide temperature range. After the organisms in contaminated food are ingested, they sporulate in the intestine and produce enterotoxin, which is part of the spore coat protein.

Clostridium perfringens type A is the usual agent, and serotyping is necessary and available for epidemiologic studies. Incubation time is 8 to 22 hours after ingestion of contaminated food, with a mean of 14 hours. Symptoms include diarrhea, cramps, and abdominal pain. Fever, nausea, and vomiting are rare, and the disease lasts only about 24 hours. The organism and its enterotoxin usually can be isolated from the feces of infected persons. The mortality rate is essentially zero, but elderly and immunocompromised patients should be closely supervised.

NECROTIZING ENTERITIS AND *C PERFRINGENS*

Necrotic enteritis in humans has not been well documented. In adults, the disease appears to result from ingesting large amounts of food contaminated with *C perfringens,* usually type C. It generally follows ingestion of a large meal, implicating bowel distension and bacterial stasis as contributing factors. The intestinal pathology varies considerably and may include sloughing of intestinal mucosa, submucosa, and mesenteric lymph nodes. Intestinal perforations occur frequently. The best-documented cases of this disease involve the natives of New Guinea, who develop necrotic enteritis ("pig-bel") after eating large quantities of improperly cooked pork that has been contaminated with the bowel contents of the animal. The course of the disease is fulminant, and the mortality rate is high. Scattered cases of necrotizing enteritis with *C perfringens* as the prominent bacterial isolate have been reported in Western countries.

In these cases, controversy exists concerning whether *C perfringens* is a primary invader, an accidental contaminant, or an opportunistic pathogen.

Some evidence suggests that acute necrotizing enterocolitis of infants may be caused by a clostridium, but definitive evidence is lacking. The theory is supported by the fact that pneumatosis cystoides intestinalis, a syndrome that can be caused by *C perfringens,* often is present in cases of acute necrotizing enterocolitis of infants. In addition, *C perfringens, C butyricum, C difficile,* and other clostridia are often isolated in cases of neonatal necrotizing enterocolitis, but a clear pathogenic role for clostridia has yet to be elucidated.

ENDOMETRITIS AND *C SORDELLII*

Clostridium sordellii is part of the normal intestinal flora of humans. It produces a potentially lethal toxin that is serologically related to the toxin of *C difficile.* There are scattered reports in the literature of *C sordellii* wound infections, most of which involve significant trauma. Recently, *C sordellii* has been implicated as the agent of fulminant, fatal endometritis in otherwise healthy women. Because specimens taken during gynecologic infections are often not adequately cultured for anaerobic bacteria, the true frequency of *C sordellii* endometritis is currently unknown.

CANCER AND *C SEPTICUM*

Clostridium septicum is a spindle-shaped rod that is motile in young cultures. The organism produces toxins designated alpha, beta, gamma, and delta; the alpha toxin is necrotizing and lethal for mice. Whether *C septicum* is a member of the normal flora or whether it takes advantage of a compromised host is uncertain. It is not strongly invasive, but has been associated with gas gangrene. Interestingly, several studies correlate *C septicum* bacteremia with the presence of cancer somewhere in the body. The most frequent association is with colorectal cancer, but association with others, including leukemia, lymphoma, and sarcoma, has also been found. In one survey of *C septicum* bacteremia, 49 of 59 patients (83 percent) had an underlying cancer and, in 28 of these cases, the portal of entry appeared to be the distal ileum or the colon. In a smaller study, seven of eight patients with *C septicum* bacteremia had gastrointestinal neoplasms. Therefore, in the absence of an overt infection, isolation of *C septicum* should alert the physician to the possible presence of a tumor, probably in the ileum or the colon. Immediate antibiotic therapy is indicated because most patients die quickly of the infection if not treated. Penicillin is the antibiotic of choice, but chloramphenicol, carbenicillin, and cephalothin also have been used successfully.

BACTEREMIA AND *C TERTIUM*

Clostridium tertium is an aerotolerant organism that is usually considered to be nonpathogenic. However, there are recent scattered reports that this organism causes bacteremia. Most cases have involved neutropenic patients, and the gastrointestinal tract appears to be the source of the infection. This organism may cause many more cases of bacteremia than is currently appreciated. Its aerotolerant nature may result in its misidentification as a *Bacillus* species.

C RAMOSUM

Little, if anything, is known about the pathogenesis of *C ramosum,* but it usually is listed with the 10 anaerobic species most frequently isolated from clinical specimens. This frequency suggests that *C ramosum* may have an as yet unrecognized pathogenic significance. It frequently is misidentified, as the Gram reaction is lost easily and spores are difficult to detect.

REFERENCES

Arnon SS: Infant botulism. Annu Rev Med 31:541, 1980

Finegold SM, George WL (eds): Anaerobic Infections in Humans. Academic Press, San Diego, 1989

Furste W: Seventh International Conference on Tetanus, Copanello (Catanzaro) Italy, 10 to 15 September 1984. J Trauma 27:99, 1986

George WL, Sutter VL, Citron D, Finegold SM: Selective and differential medium for isolation of *Clostridium difficile*. J Clin Microbiol 9:214, 1979

Hogan SF, Ireland K: Fatal, acute, spontaneous endometritis resulting from *Clostridium sordellii*. Am J Clin Pathol 91:104, 1989

Holdeman LV, Cato EP, Moore WEC (eds): Anaerobe Laboratory manual. 4th Ed. Virginia Polytechnic Institute and State University, Blacksburg, 1977

Koransky JR, Stargel MD, Dowell VR: *Clostridium septicum* bacteremia, its clinical significance. Am J Med 66:63, 1979

Lima AAM, Lyerly DM, Wilkins TD et al: Effects of *Clostridium difficile* toxins A and B in rabbit small and large intestine in vivo and on cultured cells in vitro. Infect Immun 56:582, 1988

Lyerly DM, Ball DW, Toth J, Wilkins TD: Characterization of cross-reactive proteins detected by Culturette brand rapid latex test for *Clostridium difficile*. J Clin Microbiol 26:397, 1988

Lyerly DM, Krivan HC, Wilkins TD: *Clostridium difficile:* its disease and toxins. Clin Microbiol Rev 1:1, 1988

Morbidity and Mortality Weekly Report: Tetanus — United States, 1985–1986. 36:477, 1987

Pelfry TM, Turk RP, Peoples JB, Elliott DW: Surgical aspects of *Clostridium septicum* bacteremia. Arch Surg 119:546, 1984

Richardson SA, Alcock PA, Gray G: *Clostridium difficile* and its toxin in healthy neonates. Br Med Q 287:878, 1983

Schofield F: Selective primary health care: strategies for control of disease in a developing world. XXII. Tetanus: a preventable problem. Rev Infect Dis 8:144, 1986

Schwan A: Relapsing *Clostridium difficile* enterocolitis cured by rectal infusion of homologous feces. Lancet 2:845, 1983

Smith IDS: Botulism. The Organism, Its Toxins, the Disease. Charles C Thomas, Springfield, IL, 1977

Speirs G, Warren RE, Rampling A: *Clostridium tertium* septicemia in patients with neutropenia. J Infect Dis 158:1336, 1988

Sullivan NM, Pellet S, Wilkins TD: Purification and characterization of toxins A and B of *Clostridium difficile*. Infect Immun 35:1032, 1982

19
ANAEROBIC COCCI

CAROL L. WELLS
TRACY D. WILKINS

GENERAL CONCEPTS

Clinical Manifestations
Anaerobic cocci are opportunistic pathogens that cause a variety of infections, including abscesses, gangrene, cellulitis, bacteremia, pneumonia, peritonitis, and pelvic inflammatory disease.

Structure, Classification, and Antigenic Types
The group includes both Gram-positive and Gram-negative cocci. The anaerobic cocci are physiologically diverse, including both strict anaerobes and aerotolerant species. The most significant pathogens are *Peptostreptococcus*, *Streptococcus* (both Gram positive) and *Veillonella* (Gram negative).

Pathogenesis
Infection usually results from invasion of damaged tissue by members of the normal flora. Most infections are polymicrobial, but 10 to 15 percent represent pure culture infections.

Host Defenses
Host defenses are unknown.

Epidemiology
Anaerobic cocci are part of the normal flora of the skin, the mouth, and the intestinal and genitourinary tracts. Certain species are being associated with specific types of infection.

Diagnosis
Diagnosis is by laboratory isolation of organisms from specimens collected during the infection. Because anaerobic cocci are members of the normal flora, their presence in small numbers may not be significant.

Control
Treatment includes antibiotics (penicillin, clindamycin, etc.), drainage of abscesses, and debridement.

INTRODUCTION

Anaerobic cocci cause a multitude of infections. They are part of the normal microbial flora of the skin, the mouth, and the intestinal and genitourinary tracts of healthy individuals, and act as opportunistic pathogens, participating usually in mixed infections in traumatized tissue or in compromised hosts.

CLINICAL MANIFESTATIONS

Anaerobic cocci are not involved in any single specific disease process; rather, they may be present in a great variety of infections involving all areas of the human body (Fig. 19-1). These infections may range in severity from mild skin abscesses, which disappear spontaneously after incision and drainage, to more serious infections such as brain abscess, bacteremia, necrotizing pneumonia, and septic abortion. Infection by anaerobic cocci (and by anaerobes in general) usually involves invasion of devitalized tissue by organisms that are part of the normal flora of the affected tissue or of the surrounding areas.

Brain abscess, with a mortality of 40 percent, is one of the more serious infections involving an-

aerobic cocci. Anaerobes, rather than facultative or aerobic organisms, are a major cause; the anaerobic cocci, *Bacteroides*, and *Fusobacterium* are the predominant groups isolated. Anaerobic cocci often have been isolated in pure culture from brain abscesses. Chronic otitis media or mastoiditis frequently is the primary source of the organisms that secondarily infect the brain. Pleuropulmonary infection, sinusitis, congenital heart defects, and bacterial endocarditis are other conditions predisposing to brain abscess by blood-borne metastases.

Pleuropulmonary infections involving anaerobic cocci include lung abscesses, necrotizing pneumonia, aspiration pneumonitis, and empyema. The incidence of anaerobes in these infections is 50 to 90 percent; anaerobic cocci account for about 40 percent of the anaerobic isolates. *Fusobacterium nucleatum* and *Bacteroides melaninogenicus* are often isolated together. These organisms are

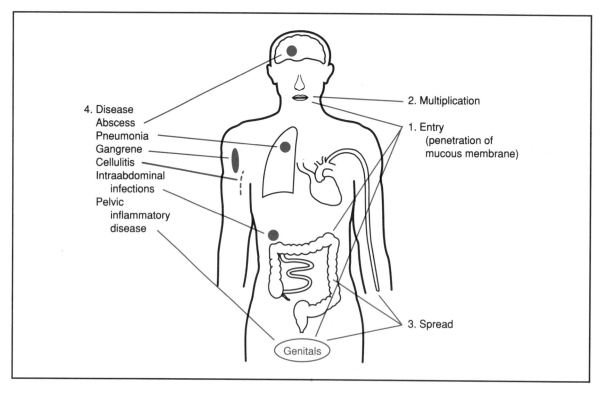

FIGURE 19-1 Pathogenesis of anaerobic cocci.

part of the normal microbial flora of the mouth and enter the lower respiratory tract as a result of aspiration, usually in association with altered consciousness. Anaerobic pleuropulmonary infections frequently develop slowly and often are chronic. The mortality rate is about 15 percent.

Anaerobic cocci are involved in several skin and soft tissue infections that may be confused with clostridial myonecrosis (gas gangrene). These severe infections include anaerobic streptococcal myonecrosis, progressive bacterial synergistic gangrene, necrotizing fasciitis, crepitant cellulitis, chronic burrowing ulcer, and synergistic necrotizing cellulitis; mortality is as high as 75 percent. These conditions are characterized by a purulent exudate; by various degrees of tissue necrosis involving the skin, fascia, and/or underlying muscles; and sometimes by systemic toxicity. The infecting organisms often produce gas. Anaerobic cocci often are isolated with other organisms in these infections. They are characteristically found with *Staphylococcus aureus* and *Streptococcus pyogenes* in progressive bacterial synergistic gangrene and also are found with Gram-negative aerobic or facultative bacilli or *Bacteroides* species, or both, in synergistic nonclostridial myonecrosis and synergistic necrotizing cellulitis. Diabetes mellitus and vascular insufficiency (often associated with trauma) are predisposing factors. Decubitus ulcers and postoperative wound infections are other soft tissue infections from which anaerobic cocci have been isolated.

Anaerobic cocci have been recognized as significant pathogens in puerperal fever and septic abortion since the early 1900s. Other infections of the female genital tract in which anaerobic cocci have been implicated are pyometra, tuboovarian abscesses, postoperative wound infections following gynecologic surgery, and pelvic inflammatory disease, often in association with gonococci. Anaerobic cocci (notably *Peptostreptococcus prevotii, P anaerobius,* and *Streptococcus intermedius*) and *B fragilis* are the most frequently isolated anaerobes from these infections. Like the anaerobic cocci associated with other infections, these organisms are part of the normal flora of the affected area or of the surrounding tissues—in this case, the vagina.

Peritonitis, intra-abdominal abscesses, and abscesses of the liver, spleen, and pancreas are types of intra-abdominal infections from which anaerobic cocci have been isolated; *P prevotii* and *P anaerobius* are the most frequently isolated species. Again, these are polymicrobic infections; concomitant isolates may be *Bacteroides, Streptococcus,* and *Escherichia coli.*

STRUCTURE, CLASSIFICATION, AND ANTIGENIC TYPES

The anaerobic cocci form a physiologically diverse group that has recently undergone significant taxonomic changes. Both Gram-negative and Gram-positive species exist. Not all anaerobic cocci require stringent anaerobic conditions; for example, strains of *S intermedius* are quite aerotolerant and may grow under reduced oxygen tension. Anaerobic cocci may be proteolytic or saccharolytic or both. They produce a variety of short-chain volatile fatty acids (e.g., acetic, propionic, butyric, caproic, and lactic acids) from the fermentation of simple sugars and amino acids. Both *P magnus* and *P anaerobius* possess species-specific cell wall antigens; in other anaerobic cocci, species-specific antigens have not yet been identified. *Peptostreptococcus* and *Streptococcus* are the most clinically important genera, with *P magnus* as the most frequent clinical isolate.

Species of anaerobic Gram-positive cocci can be difficult to distinguish, but a few biochemical tests can be helpful. *Peptostreptococcus anaerobius* is the only species susceptible to sodium polyanethol sulfonate, and *P asaccharolyticus* is the only indole-positive species. Of the butyric acid producers, *P tetradius* (formerly *Gaffkya anaerobia*) is strongly saccharolytic and urease positive, whereas *P prevotii* is weakly saccharolytic and usually urease negative. *Peptostreptococcus magnus* and *P micros* are similar biochemically and are distinguished primarily on the basis of cell size. The three prominent anaerobic *Streptococcus* species (*S intermedius, S constellatus,* and *S morbillorum*) are strongly saccharolytic and produce large amounts of lactic acid. These anaerobic streptococci are typically aerotolerant. Because the species of anaerobic Gram-positive cocci are relatively poorly defined, it is not unusual for a given isolate to be identified as simply *Streptococcus* sp or *Peptostreptococcus* sp. Other genera of anaerobic Gram-positive cocci include *Ruminococcus* and *Coprococcus,* which are considered nonpathogenic members of the fecal flora.

The three genera of anaerobic Gram-negative cocci are *Veillonella, Acidominococcus,* and *Megosphora. Veillonella parvula* is the species most frequently isolated from clinical specimens. *Veillonella* can be presumptively identified by the red fluorescence of colonies under ultraviolet light. This fluorescence is lost rapidly on exposure to oxygen.

PATHOGENESIS

Anaerobic cocci are isolated most often from a wide variety of polymicrobial infections (usually along with *Bacteroides* spp or facultative organisms or both), indicating a synergistic role in these infections. Approximately 10 to 15 percent of isolates of anaerobic cocci come from pure culture infections, thus indicating that these organisms can be significant pathogens. The anaerobic cocci represent 25 to 30 percent of all anaerobic clinical isolates; among anaerobes, they are second only to the Gram-negative anaerobic bacilli in frequency of isolation from clinical specimens. They have received little attention from microbiologists and clinicians; consequently, it is not known whether they produce toxins or capsules or have other pathogenic attributes.

HOST DEFENSES

Peptostreptococcus magnus infection (in pure culture) of hip prostheses has produced a serum antibody response; however, in most cases, specific immune responses to anaerobic cocci have not been investigated.

EPIDEMIOLOGY

Anaerobic cocci are part of the normal flora of the skin, the mouth, and the intestinal and genitourinary tracts of healthy individuals. Recently, with increasing study of the anaerobic cocci as patho-

gens, certain species are being associated with specific types of infection. As noted above, *P prevotii* and *P anaerobius* are associated with female genital tract and intra-abdominal infections. *Peptostreptococcus magnus,* the most frequently isolated anaerobic coccus, is associated most often with chronic bone and joint infections and ankle ulcers. Pure cultures of this organism are not rare; they account for 15 percent of all *P magnus* isolates. The presence of foreign bodies, such as prosthetic joints, seems to be particularly significant in *P magnus* infections. In a recent study, anaerobic cocci were isolated in 15 of 246 cases (6 percent) of monomicrobial anaerobic bacteremia in cancer patients, indicating a relatively rare but significant pathogenic potential for anaerobic cocci in this patient population. *Veillonella* and the anaerobic *Streptococcus* species are the anaerobic cocci most frequently isolated from infected human bites. These organisms are part of the normal oral flora.

DIAGNOSIS

Anaerobic infections generally occur in compromised hosts. The primary host defense deficiency in these infections is the disruption of natural barriers (such as the skin and mucous membranes). Diabetes mellitus, connective-tissue disorders, atherosclerotic disease, cancer (especially of the colon, uterus, and lung), irradiation damage, immunosuppressive treatment, and alcoholism may disrupt these natural barriers.

To establish a definite role for anaerobic cocci in infections, it is necessary to isolate the causative organism from the affected tissue or the bloodstream. Because anaerobic cocci form a significant part of the normal flora, the proper choice of specimen is critical. For example, coughed sputum, feces, and vaginal swabs, all of which could be contaminated with members of the normal microbial flora, are unacceptable.

CONTROL

Treatment of infections caused by anaerobic cocci consists of antibiotic therapy plus drainage or debridement, or both, of nectrotic tissue. In general, penicillin is the drug of choice; clindamycin or metronidazole can be used for patients allergic to penicillin. However, in vitro antimicrobial susceptibility tests have shown that some strains of anaerobic cocci are resistant to penicillin or to clindamycin. Metronidazole is typically active against most strains of anaerobic cocci; however, aerotolerant species, such as *Streptococcus* species, are uniformly resistant. Brain abscesses must be treated with an antimicrobial agent such as chloramphenicol, penicillin, or metronidazole, sufficient doses of which can cross the blood barrier. Frequently, *B fragilis,* an anaerobic Gram-negative rod, is present in infections containing anaerobic cocci; this organism produces a β-lactamase that can protect other organisms in the infection from the action of penicillin.

REFERENCES

Bourgault AM, Rosenblatt JE, Fitzgerald RH: *Peptococcus magnus:* a significant human pathogen. Ann Intern Med 93:244, 1980

Brook I, Walker RI: Pathogenicity of anaerobic gram-positive cocci. Infect Immun 45:320, 1984

Fainstein V, Elting LS, Bodey GF: Bacteremia caused by non-sporulating anaerobes in cancer patients—a 12-year experience. Medicine 3:151, 1989

Finegold SM, George WL (eds): Anaerobic Infections in Humans. Academic Press, San Diego, 1989

Holdeman, LV, Cato EP, Moore, WEC (eds): Anaerobe Laboratory Manual. 4th Ed. Virginia Polytechnic Institute and State University, Blacksburg, 1977

Lambe DW, Jr, Vroon DH, Rietz CW: Infections due to anaerobic cocci. In Balows A (ed): Anaerobic Bacteria: Role in Disease. Charles C Thomas, Springfield, IL 1974

Sutter VL, Citron DM, Finegold SM (eds): Wadsworth Anaerobic Bacteriology Manual. 4th Ed. Star Publishing Co., Belmont, CA, 1985

Tabaqchali S: Rapid techniques for the identification of anaerobic bacteria and presumptive diagnosis. Scand J Infect Dis, suppl. 35:23, 1982

Taylor AG, Finham WJ, Golding MA, Cook J: Infection of total hip prostheses by *Peptococcus magnus,* an immunofluorescence and ELISA study of two cases. J Clin Pathol 32:61, 1979

20 ANAEROBIC GRAM-NEGATIVE BACILLI

SYDNEY M. FINEGOLD

GENERAL CONCEPTS

Clinical Manifestations

Anaerobic Gram-negative bacilli are common elements of the mucous membrane flora throughout the body; they often act as secondary pathogens. They are the most common anaerobes involved in infection and include some of the most antibiotic-resistant species.

Structure, Classification, and Antigenic Types

Some are pleomorphic, whereas others have distinctive morphology. All are obligate anaerobes. The key characters for classification are motility, arrangement of flagella, and organic and volatile fatty acid metabolic end products. Antigens are not useful.

Pathogenesis

They usually invade as opportunistic pathogens through a break in the mucosa. A low redox potential favors infection. Some types produce virulence factors or interfere with host defenses (e.g., by inhibiting phagocytosis).

Host Defenses

Antibodies, complement (via both classic and alternative pathways), and cell-mediated immunity (involving both polymorphonuclear leukocytes and T lymphocytes) are important.

Epidemiology

Infections arise endogenously from the mucosal flora.

Diagnosis

Clues suggesting anaerobic infection include foul-smelling discharge, proximity of infection to mucosa, abscess formation, necrosis and gas in tissues, septic thrombophlebitis, various distinctive clinical pictures (e.g., tonsillitis with sepsis), and results of a Gram stain of clinical specimens. Collection of clinical specimens should avoid the mucosal flora, and transport must be anaerobic.

Control

Control involves (1) surgical drainage of abscesses and debridement of necrotic tissue; and (2) use of antibiotics (particularly metronidazole, imipenem, chloramphenicol, or combinations of amoxicillin, ticarcillin, or ampicillin with β-lactamase inhibitors).

INTRODUCTION

At present there are 23 genera of Gram-negative anaerobic bacilli. In most clinical infections, only the genera *Bacteroides, Porphyromonas,* and *Fusobacterium* need be considered. These genera are prevalent in the body as members of the normal flora (Fig. 20-1), constituting one-third of the total anaerobic isolates from clinical specimens, and may become involved in infections throughout the body (Fig. 20-2). Within the *Bacteroides* group, *B fragilis* is the most common pathogen, followed by *B thetaiotaomicron* and other members of the *B fragilis* group. Among the bile-sensitive *Bacteroides* species, the ones most commonly encountered clinically are *B melaninogenicus, B oris,* and *B buccae. Porphyromonas asaccharolytica* is also common. *Fusobacterium nucleatum* is the *Fusobacterium* species most often found as a pathogen, but *F necrophorum* occasionally produces serious disease. These gen-

era contain numerous other species that rarely or never infect humans.

CLINICAL MANIFESTATIONS

Gram-negative anaerobic bacilli may cause infections anywhere in the body; the most common types are pleuropulmonary, intra-abdominal, and female genital tract infections (Table 20-1). In addition, they may play a role in such diverse pathologic processes as periodontal disease and colon cancer. *Bacteroides, Porphyromonas,* and *Fusobacterium* produce enzymes (collagenase, neuraminidase, deoxyribonuclease [DNase], heparinase, and proteinases) that may play a role in pathogenesis by helping the organisms to penetrate tissues and to set up infection after surgery or other trauma. The incidence of infection by these organisms can best be reduced or eliminated by avoiding conditions that decrease the redox potential of tissues and by

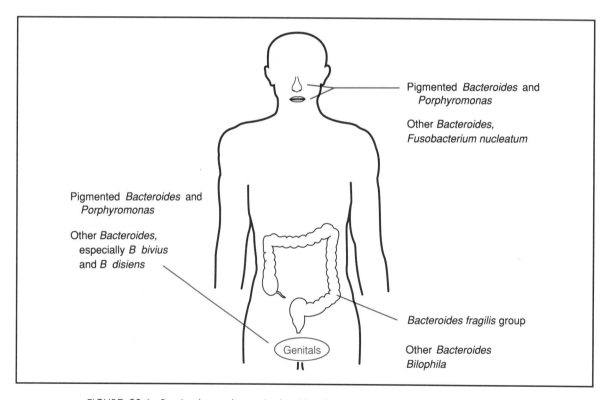

FIGURE 20-1 Predominant sites colonized by *Bacteroides* and other anaerobic bacilli.

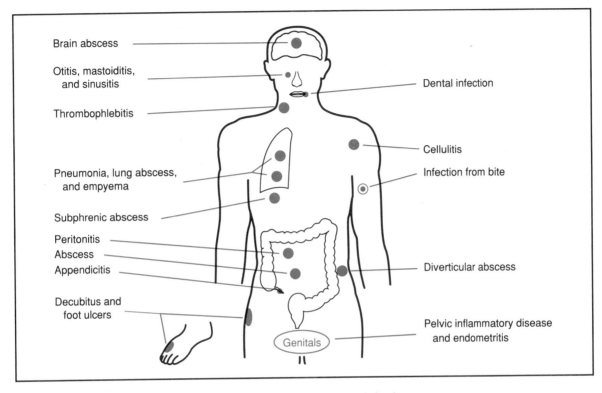

FIGURE 20-2 Sites of anaerobic infections.

TABLE 20-1 Common Syndromes of
Anaerobic Infection

Bite infections
Oral or dental infection
Aspiration pneumonia, lung abscess, empyema
Postabortion and puerperal infections
Infections following
    Bowel and gallbladder surgery
    Gynecologic surgery
Appendicitis, diverticulitis
Septicemia with
    Cancer
    Diabetes
    Corticosteroids
    "Negative" blood cultures
Septic thrombophlebitis
Gas-forming infection
Putrid infections

preventing introduction of the anaerobes into compromised host tissues.

STRUCTURE, CLASSIFICATION, AND ANTIGENIC TYPES

Bacteroides fragilis (Fig. 20-3), the most important of all anaerobes because of its frequency of occurrence in clinical infection and its resistance to antimicrobial agents, is a Gram-negative bacillus with rounded ends 0.5 to 0.8 μm in diameter and 1.5 to 4.5 μm long. Most strains are encapsulated. Vacuolization or irregular staining is common, particularly in broth media. Some pleomorphism also may be seen, particularly in broth media. By electron microscopy, the ultrastructure of *B fragilis* is similar to that of other Gram-negative bacteria. The guanine-plus-cytosine content is 42 percent. *Bacteroides melaninogenicus* and *P asaccharolytica* are short to coccoid Gram-negative rods; they pro-

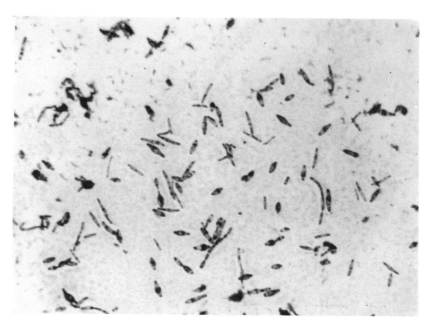

FIGURE 20-3 Microscopic morphology of *B fragilis* from broth culture. Note the irregular staining, rounded ends of bacilli, and some pleomorphism.

duce a distinctive pigment (brown to black), which is a heme derivative that colors the colony (Figs. 20-4 and 20-5); *P asaccharolytica* is encapsulated. Many strains of *B melaninogenicus* require vitamin K, or similar compounds, as well as heme. Other *Bacteroides* species are much less common.

Numerous studies of the endotoxin of Gram-negative anaerobic bacilli have determined that the *B fragilis* endotoxin contains little or no lipid A, 2-ketodeoxyoctanate, or heptose. It also lacks β-hydroxymyristic acid. This endotoxin exhibits little biologic activity in various test systems and little chemotactic activity; what activity there is is complement-mediated by the alternative pathway. Poor biologic activity of endotoxin also has been demonstrated for the closely related species *B thetaiotaomicron*, *B ovatus*, *B vulgatus*, and *B distasonis*. *Porphyromonas asaccharolytica* also does not have any β-hydroxymyristic acid, and its endotoxin is inactive biologically. *Bacteroides melaninogenicus* endotoxin contains no heptose or 2-ketodeoxyoctanate, and it and the endotoxin of *B oralis* both

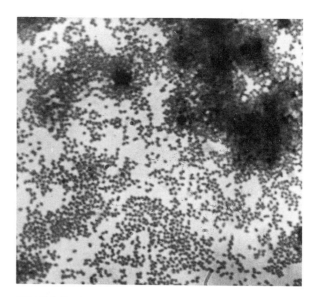

FIGURE 20-4 Microscopic morphology of *B melaninogenicus*. Organisms are tiny coccobacilli that stain regularly.

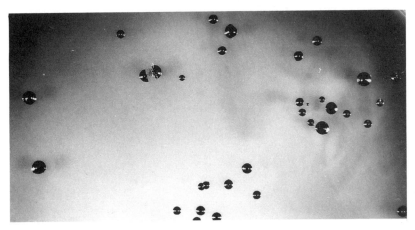

FIGURE 20-5   Colony morphology of *B melaninogenicus.* Note the jet-black pigmented colonies.

show weak biologic activity. Serologic methods have not been reliable for characterizing *Bacteroides* strains.

Members of the genus *Fusobacterium* (Figs. 20-6 and 20-7) may be spindle shaped or may have parallel sides and rounded ends. The guanine-plus-cy-

tosine content ranges from 26 to 34 percent. Cells of *F necrophorum* often are elongated or filamentous, are curved, and possess spherical enlargements and large, free, round bodies. *Fusobacterium nucleatum,* although not producing infections as serious as those caused by *F necro-*

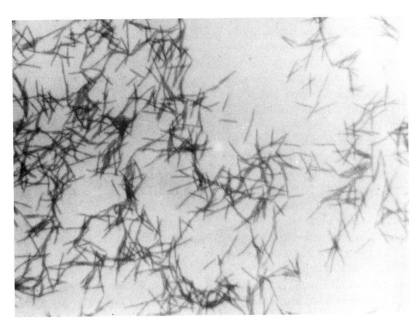

FIGURE 20-6   Microscopic morphology of *F nucleatum* from broth culture. Note the regular staining and thin, delicate bacilli with tapered ends. Organisms are sometimes found end to end.

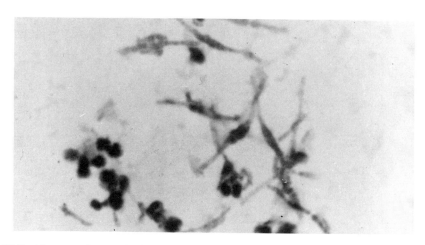

FIGURE 20-7   Microscopic morphology of *F mortiferum* from broth culture. Note the filaments with swollen central portions, large round bodies, and irregular staining.

phorum, is much more common clinically. The cells of this species are usually spindle shaped, are 5 to 10 μm long, and are often seen in pairs, end to end.

The lipopolysaccharide of *F necrophorum* is located in a multilayered external coat. The endotoxin varies from strain to strain in its content of 2-ketodeoxyoctanate and sugars. Although biologic activity varies also, many strains do show strong biologic activity, comparable to that of *Salmonella enteritidis*. The endotoxin of *F nucleatum* also is variable in its biologic activity, but often exhibits strong activity, comparable to that of *S enteritidis*.

Bacteriophages active against *B fragilis* are not uncommon. They are species specific and active against most strains. Bacteriocins also are produced by strains of *B fragilis* and *B thetaiotaomicron*. Plasmids have been found in about half the *Bacteroides* strains studied. For the most part, the biologic and clinical significance of these plasmids is not known; however, some code for resistance to such antimicrobial agents as clindamycin, erythromycin, tetracycline, chloramphenicol, ampicillin, and cephalothin. Plasmid-mediated antibiotic resistance has been transferred from strains of *B fragilis* to other strains of this species, to *B thetaiotaomicron*, and to *Escherichia coli*. Such resistance also has been transferred from *B distasonis* to *B fragilis*.

Most strains of the *B fragilis* group can deconjugate bile acids and are equally active whether the bile acid is conjugated with glycine or with taurine. Rarely, *B melaninogenicus* may deconjugate bile acids, but in general this species, *B oralis*, and *F nucleatum* are inhibited by bile acids and do not deconjugate them. *Fusobacterium necrophorum* also is active in deconjugating bile acids but is active primarily on taurine conjugates. A few strains of *Bacteroides* whose species is not known can convert primary bile acids to secondary bile acids. *Bacteroides thetaiotaomicron* can convert some lithocholic acid to its ethyl ester. Because lithocholic acid is toxic in humans and has been shown to exert tumor-promoting activity in animals, this reaction may be important. *Bacteroides fragilis* hydrolyzes the conjugated metabolites of benzpyrene. Glucuronidase produced by anaerobic Gram-negative bacilli may be of special significance in deconjugating compounds that had previously been detoxified in the liver by combination with glucuronide. There is speculation that this enzyme may be important in promoting bowel cancer. The activity of *B thetaiotaomicron*, *B distasonis*, and other members of the *B fragilis* group against plant polysaccharides, chondroitin, and mucin may be a factor in colon cancer and other disorders. Dietary fiber consists primarily of plant cell wall polysaccharides that are not digested in the stomach or small bowel.

Certain *Bacteroides* species possess distinguishing enzymes. Superoxide dismutase has been found in *B fragilis, B thetaiotaomicron, B vulgatus,* and *B ovatus.* In general, a good correlation exists between superoxide dismutase activity and oxygen tolerance. No consistent relationship has been found between catalase activity and oxygen tolerance, however. β-Lactamase activity has been demonstrated in several *Bacteroides* species; it accounts for most of the resistance to various β-lactam antibiotics, such as penicillins and cephalosporins, although other mechanisms are responsible occasionally. Urease is produced by *Bilophila wadsworthia* and by *Bacteroides ureolyticus (B corrodens).* The latter organism also produces an agarase, which accounts for pitting of the agar by the colonies. A related pitting organism, *Bacteroides gracilis,* is much more pathogenic and is relatively resistant to antimicrobial agents, as is *Bilophila.*

PATHOGENESIS

Bacteroides, Porphyromonas, and *Fusobacterium* species are prevalent in the indigenous flora on all mucosal surfaces. They may have an opportunity to penetrate tissues and then to set up infection under certain circumstances such as surgical or other trauma or when tumors arise at the mucosal surface (Table 20-2). In certain cases, such as aspiration pneumonia, anaerobic bacteria from a site of normal carriage may move into another area that is normally free of organisms and infect that site. Tissue necrosis and poor blood supply lower the oxidation-reduction potential, thus favoring the growth of anaerobes. Accordingly, vascular disease, cold, shock, trauma, surgery, foreign bodies, cancer, edema, and gas production by bacteria may significantly predispose to infection with anaerobes, as may prior infection with aerobic or facultative bacteria. Antimicrobial agents such as aminoglycosides, to which anaerobes are notably resistant, may facilitate anaerobic infection. Conditions predisposing to anaerobic infection are summarized in Table 20-2. The more aerotolerant anaerobes are more likely to survive after the normally protective mucosal barrier is broken and until conditions are satisfactory for their multipli-

TABLE 20-2   Conditions Predisposing to Anaerobic Infection

General
Diabetes
Corticosteroids
Leukopenia
Hypogammaglobulinemia
Immunosuppression
Cytotoxic drugs
Splenectomy
Collagen disease
Decreased redox potential
Tissue anoxia
Tissue destruction
Aerobic infection
Foreign body
Calcium salts
Burns
Peripheral vascular insufficiency
Specific clinical situations
Cancer
Colon, uterus, lung
Leukemia
Gastrointestinal and female pelvic surgery
Gastrointestinal trauma
Human and animal bites
Aminoglycoside therapy

cation and invasion. Once anaerobes begin to multiply, they can maintain their own reduced environment by excreting end products of fermentative metabolism. Infections involving Gram-negative anaerobic bacilli often are characterized by abscess formation and tissue destruction, as are most anaerobic infections.

Bacteroides, Porphyromonas, and *Fusobacterium* species produce enzymes that may play a role in pathogenesis. *Bacteroides melaninogenicus* is one of the few bacteria that produce collagenase, an enzyme of considerable importance. Strains of *B melaninogenicus* with high collagenolytic activity produce more acute infection when combined with an anaerobic *Vibrio* species than do strains with weak collagenolytic activity. Cell extracts of *B melaninogenicus* strains with collagenolytic activity, when given with a live *Fusobacterium* species, produce more severe lesions in rabbits than does the organism or the extract given alone. *Porphyromonas gin-*

givalis also produces collagenase and has trypsin-like activity. Neuraminidase may be important in the pathogenesis of *Bacteroides* infection. This enzyme alters neuraminic acid-containing glycoproteins of human plasma; *Bacteroides* strains isolated from clinical specimens have higher neuraminidase activity than do those isolated from stools, and strains of the *B fragilis* group have greater activity of this type than do strains of other *Bacteroides* species. Hyaluronidase is produced by many strains of the *B fragilis* group and pigmented anaerobic Gram-negative rods. DNase is also produced by *B fragilis* and may be an important factor in infection. Many *Bacteroides* species produce phosphatase. A heparinase produced by *B fragilis* strains may contribute to intravascular clotting and hence increases the dosage of heparin needed to treat septic thrombophlebitis in infections caused by this organism. The lipopolysaccharides of *B fragilis*, *B vulgatus*, and *F mortiferum* activate the Hageman factor and thereby initiate the intrinsic pathway of coagulation. Fibrinolysin is produced by many *B melaninogenicus* group strains and by a few *B fragilis* group strains. *Porphyromonas asaccharolytica* produces proteinases that render it capable of hydrolyzing gelatin, casein, coagulated protein, plasma protein, azacol, and collagen. Strains of *Bacteroides* and *P gingivalis* degrade complement factors and immunoglobulins G and M. A strain of *B melaninogenicus* produces phospholipase A.

Fusobacterium necrophorum produces a leukocidin and hemolyses erythrocytes of humans, horses, rabbits, and, much less extensively, sheep and cattle. Certain *F necrophorum* cells hemagglutinate the erythrocytes of humans, chickens, and pigeons. A bovine isolate of *F necrophorum* demonstrates phospholipase A and lysophospholipase activity. *Fusobacterium gonidiaformans* produces an appreciable inflammatory reaction when inoculated into the skin of rabbits; when injected intraperitoneally into mice, it leads to liver abscesses and occasionally death. A specific toxin has not yet been isolated.

Other factors may be involved in the continued growth and potential pathogenicity of certain anaerobes. For example, *B melaninogenicus* can inhibit the growth of certain other organisms. Also, anaerobes such as *B melaninogenicus* sometimes inhibit phagocytosis and killing of other organisms during mixed infection. Constituents of the cell envelope and cell surface may contribute to pathogenicity. The capsule of organisms such as *B fragilis* may be an important virulence factor. The mechanism by which the capsule may enhance virulence remains to be determined, but it is interesting that *B fragilis* strains adhere to rat peritoneal mesothelium better than do unencapsulated species of *Bacteroides*. Pili (fimbriae) and lectinlike adhesins may also be important in the adherence of *Bacteroides* cells to epithelial surfaces. Butyrate and succinate produced by *Bacteroides* show a cytotoxic effect.

HOST DEFENSES

Polymorphonuclear leukocytes have oxygen-dependent and oxygen-independent microbicidal systems. Components of both systems might be important in phagocytic killing of anaerobes under conditions of varying oxygen tension. Specifically, polymorphonuclear leukocytes normally kill *B fragilis* under anaerobic and aerobic conditions. Random migration of polymorphonuclear leukocytes does not differ significantly under aerobic and anaerobic conditions. The same holds true for chemotaxis in response to factors generated by immune complexes in plasma; however, chemotaxis in response to factors generated by bacteria in plasma is markedly depressed under anaerobic conditions, and products of *Bacteroides* species may suppress neutrophil chemotaxis and phagocytic killing.

Studies of host defenses indicate that other interactions may occur between the bacteria and the host cells. *Bacteroides fragilis*, one organism used in the chemotaxis study described above, is more resistant to the normal bactericidal activity of serum than are other members of the *B fragilis* group. *Fusobacterium mortiferum* is killed by serum alone or by serum plus leukocytes under aerobic and anaerobic conditions. Under anaerobic conditions, *B thetaiotaomicron* and *B fragilis* are phagocytosed and killed intracellularly by human polymorphonuclear leukocytes only in the presence of normal human serum. Similar results are obtained in an aerobic environment, except that *B fragilis* is phagocytosed and killed intracellularly to some extent in the absence of serum. There is evidence that the capsule of certain *Bacteroides* strains interferes with their phagocytosis.

Immunoglobulin and components of the classic and alternative complement pathways participate in chemotaxis, bacteriolysis, and opsonophagocytic killing of various Gram-negative anaerobic bacilli. Antibody to the capsular polysaccharide of *B fragilis* can be induced in animals by infection with encapsulated strains or by implantation of the capsular material itself along with outer membrane components that stimulate an antibody response. Such immunization of animals confers significant protection against subsequent abscess development from *B fragilis* strains. Furthermore, a study of women with acute pelvic inflammatory disease demonstrated antibody to the capsular antigen of *B fragilis* in women whose infecting flora contained *B fragilis;* the antibody was quantified by precipitin analysis. Immunodiffusion techniques have also been used on trichloroacetic acid extracts from *B fragilis* in detecting precipitating antibodies against this organism in sera of immune rabbits. Data indicate that more than one serotype exists.

Fusobacterium necrophorum persists for an extended period in the liver, where its proliferation in Küpffer cells impairs macrophage function.

There is also evidence that T cells may be involved in immunity of humans to *B fragilis,* specifically linked to early stages of abscess formation.

EPIDEMIOLOGY

All infections involving anaerobic Gram-negative bacilli arise endogenously when mucosal damage related to surgery, trauma, or disease permits tissue penetration by members of the indigenous flora. Knowledge of the composition of the indigenous flora at various sites under different circumstances permits the clinician to anticipate the likely infecting species in acute infections in different locations. The pathogenicity of various species also must be taken into account. Ecologic determinants include the oxygen sensitivity of various organisms, the ability of organisms to adhere (discussed in Chapter 7), and microbial interrelationships. These interrelationships permit one organism to supply growth factors needed by another, to provide assistance with adherence or motility to another organism, and to facilitate the production of inhibitory substances.

At birth, an infant's oral cavity usually is sterile; but by 12 months of age, *Fusobacterium* species can be cultured from 50 percent of infants and *Bacteroides* species from a smaller percentage. In the human gingival crevice area, Gram-negative anaerobic rods account for 16 to 20 percent of the total cultivable flora. *Bacteroides melaninogenicus* is seldom isolated before the age of 6 years, but by the early teens this organism can be isolated from the gingival crevice area of most individuals. In the presence of acute ulcerative gingivitis or advanced chronic periodontal disease, counts of *Fusobacterium* in saliva are higher than the usual 10^4 to $10^6/$ ml. Gram-negative anaerobic rods usually constitute 8 to 17 percent of the cultivable flora of human dental plaque. Selective localization is illustrated by the fact that *B melaninogenicus* is found routinely in the gingival crevice but is not found, or is only rarely found, on the tongue, cheek, or coronal tooth surface.

The stomach normally has few organisms and, as a rule, no anaerobic bacteria; however, in the presence of pathologic conditions such as duodenal ulcer with bleeding or obstruction, abnormal colonization with *B fragilis* may occur in the stomach. In the terminal ileum, approximately equal numbers of facultative aerobes and anaerobes are present, with *Bacteroides* being one of the major anaerobes. *Bacteroides* species are almost invariably found in the feces of adult subjects; the mean count is $10^{11}/$g. *Fusobacterium* species are found in the feces of 18 percent of adults; the mean count is $10^8/$g. *B thetaiotaomicron* and *B vulgatus* are the dominant species of *Bacteroides* encountered, followed by *B distasonis, B ovatus,* and *B fragilis.* In animal studies, *Bacteroides* protects against infection with *Salmonella* or *Shigella.*

Bacteroides and *Fusobacterium* species are common in the vaginal flora. In one quantitative study of the vaginal and cervical flora, *Bacteroides* species were recovered from half of the patients, with mean concentrations of 10^6/g of material. *Bacteroides* species recovered from the normal cervical flora of healthy women include *B oralis, B fragilis, B capillosus, B bivius, B disiens, B oris, B buccae,* and *B ureolyticus.*

Studies of the normal urethral flora are relatively limited, but various *Fusobacterium* and *Bacteroides* species have been isolated. Fusiform bacilli and *B melaninogenicus* have been found regularly on the external genitalia.

Bacteroides cells placed on the forearms of human volunteers may persist for a few hours; strains placed on laboratory benches may survive even 10 hours after exposure to air, and *Bacteroides* has been recovered from the hospital environment on occasion. Clearly, however, the source of infection with these organisms is the indigenous flora of the body, particularly of mucosal surfaces.

DIAGNOSIS

The clinical characteristics of infection with *Bacteroides* or *Fusobacterium* are primarily those seen with anaerobes in general. These characteristics include foul-smelling discharge, location of infection in proximity to mucosal surfaces, tissue necrosis, gas in tissues or discharges, association of infection with cancer, infection related to the use of aminoglycosides, septic thrombophlebitis, infection following human or animal bites, and certain distinctive clinical features. The clinical presentation of *F necrophorum* sepsis may be distinctive in that onset is characterized by sore throat and fever often accompanied by chills. A membranous tonsillitis with foul odor to the breath may be noted, and in the absence of effective therapy, bacteremia and widespread metastatic infection will occur. Black discoloration of blood-containing exudates or red fluorescence of such exudates

under ultraviolet light indicates infection with *B melaninogenicus* or *P asaccharolytica.*

A definitive diagnosis requires demonstration or isolation of the organisms responsible for the infection. Even direct Gram stain may be helpful because of the frequently unique morphology of Gram-negative anaerobic bacilli. In general, these organisms are pale staining and they may stain erratically. *Fusobacterium* cells may exhibit classic tapered ends and filamentous forms, with or without swollen areas and large round bodies. Direct gas-liquid chromatography of clinical specimens occasionally provides important clues to the presence of certain Gram-negative anaerobic bacilli. Large amounts of butyric acid in the absence of isobutyric or isovaleric acid indicate the presence of *Fusobacterium.* The presence of succinic acid and only Gram-negative rods seen on Gram stain, or of both succinic and isobutyric acid in the specimen, indicates that *Bacteroides* is present. Both direct and indirect fluorescent antibody techniques may be useful for rapid detection of *Bacteroides* and *Fusobacterium* in clinical material. False-positive reactions are sometimes a problem. Collection of clinical specimens should avoid the mucosal flora, and transport must be anaerobic. Reagents are available commercially; they will undoubtedly be improved. Use of selective and differential media may facilitate isolation and identification of different Gram-negative anaerobic bacilli. Tests for antibody development in response to the infection are not practical.

CONTROL

There are two primary guidelines in preventing anaerobic infections: avoiding conditions that reduce the redox potential of the tissues and preventing the introduction of anaerobes of the normal flora to wounds, closed cavities, or other sites prone to infection. Prophylactic antimicrobial therapy is effective in selected situations. Patients with acute leukemia who are to be treated intensively with antitumor chemotherapy may be managed with a diet low in bacterial count and with administration of an antimicrobial regimen designed to reduce significantly the total body flora, including anaerobes. Some workers have advocated using antibacterial regimens that are relatively inactive against anaerobes; as a result, anaerobes persist in the bowel and provide colonization resistance against potential aerobic or facultative pathogens. There is some disagreement on this point.

Anaerobic bacteremia following dental manipulation may be managed effectively by administering an agent such as penicillin 1 hour before the manipulation and continuing for a limited period (12 to 24 hours) afterward. The effectiveness of prophylactic antimicrobial therapy before bowel surgery is now well established. The physician may use oral neomycin plus erythromycin or oral neomycin plus tetracycline, giving the therapy for a limited time just before surgery to prevent overgrowth of other organisms. Prophylaxis also is effective before certain types of gynecologic surgery. When infection already is established but surgery is indicated (appendectomy, cholecystectomy), antimicrobial therapy just before surgery again may be helpful. Appropriate therapy of established infections such as chronic otitis media and sinusitis may prevent subsequent spread of infection that could lead to intracranial abscess. Precautions to minimize aspiration are helpful in preventing anaerobic pulmonary infection. Care must be observed in feeding feeble or confused patients and those who have difficulty swallowing. Good surgical technique minimizes the risk of postoperative infection. Minimizing injury and devitalization of tissue during surgery protects against infection. The use of closed methods of bowel resection, when feasible, decreases the likelihood of infection with members of the bowel flora.

Table 20-3 indicates the relative effectiveness of a number of drugs against Gram-negative anaerobic bacilli. Aminoglycosides such as gentamicin and amikacin are inactive against most anaerobes. The activity of erythromycin varies significantly according to the testing procedure. Erythromycin and vancomycin are not currently approved by the Food and Drug Administration for anaerobic infections. Most penicillins and cephalosporins are less active than penicillin G; unfortunately, in-

creasing numbers of anaerobes are showing resistance to penicillin, usually on the basis of β-lactamase production. Ampicillin, carbenicillin, and penicillin V are roughly comparable to penicillin G on a weight basis, but the high blood levels safely achieved with carbenicillin and similar penicillins make them effective against 80 to 95 percent of *B fragilis* strains. Cefoxitin, which is resistant to penicillinase and cephalosporinase, used to be active against 95 percent of *B fragilis* strains, but now 25 percent of strains are resistant in some centers. Similarly, 20 percent of *B fragilis* strains are now resistant to clindamycin. The third-generation cephalosporins are usually less active than cefoxitin against the *B fragilis* group. Drugs active against essentially all Gram-negative (and other) anaerobes are metronidazole, imipenem, chloramphenicol, and combinations of β-lactam drugs plus a β-lactamase inhibitor.

In addition to antimicrobial therapy, surgery is important in treating anaerobic infection. This includes drainage of abscesses, excision of necrotic tissue, relief of obstruction, and ligation or resection of infected veins. Percutaneous nonsurgical drainage may be effective in certain patients. Lung abscess, which responds well to medical therapy, is the primary exception to the rule that abscesses require surgical drainage.

Hyperbaric oxygen therapy is not useful in *Bacteroides, Porphyromonas,* or *Fusobacterium* infections. General supportive measures are, of course, important in managing any type of serious infection. Anticoagulation may be useful in patients with septic thrombophlebitis, along with appropriate antimicrobial therapy.

As noted above, the *B fragilis* group is among the most resistant of all anaerobes to antimicrobial agents. In part, this is related to β-lactamase production by *B fragilis* and related strains, but other mechanisms of resistance exist as well. *Bacteroides gracilis* is often resistant to penicillins and cephalosporins (including piperacillin and cefoxitin) and to clindamycin. *Bilophila* is also often resistant to penicillins and cephalosporins, including cefoxitin. Plasmid-mediated transferable resistance to several antimicrobial agents has been demon-

TABLE 20-3 Antimicrobial Susceptibility of Gram-Negative Anaerobic Bacilli[a]

| Pathogen | Effectiveness[b] of Antimicrobial Agent | | | | | | | Ticarcillin/ | |
	Penicillin	Chloramphenicol	Clindamycin	Erythromycin	Tetracycline	Metronidazole	Imipenem	Clavulanate[c]	Cefoxitin
B fragilis group	1	3	2–3	1–2	1–2	3	3	3	2–3
Pigmented Bacteroides and Porphyromonas spp	2–3	3	3[d]	2–3	2	3	3	3	3
F varium	2–3	3	1–2	1	2	3	2–3	3	3
Other Fusobacterium spp	4	3	3	1	3	3	3	3	3

[a] Only drugs that might be used therapeutically are included; not all these agents are routinely used clinically for anaerobic infections, and not all are approved by the Food and Drug Administration.

[b] Numbers: 4, drug of choice; 3, good activity; 2, moderate activity; 1, poor or inconsistent activity.

[c] Other combinations of β-lactam drug and a β-lactamase inhibitor are comparable.

[d] A few strains are resistant.

strated with *B fragilis* and related *Bacteroides* species. Numerous other *Bacteroides* species also produce β-lactamases. Chloramphenicol acetyltransferase has been demonstrated in *Bacteroides,* but is not generally clinically significant. Among the fusobacteria, the primary organism manifesting resistance is *F varium.* Many strains of this species are resistant to clindamycin, and a number are resistant to penicillins and cephalosporins.

REFERENCES

Finegold SM: Anaerobic Bacteria in Human Disease. Academic Press, San Diego, 1977

Finegold SM, George WL (eds): Anaerobic Infections in Humans. Academic Press, San Diego, 1989

Holdeman LV, Cato EP, Moore WEC: Anaerobe Laboratory Manual. 4th Ed. Virginia Polytechnic Institute and State University, Blacksburg, 1977

Kasper DL, Finegold SM (eds): Virulence factors of anaerobic bacteria (symposium). Rev Infect Dis 1:March–April, 1979, pp 1–400

Rosebury T: Microorganisms Indigenous to Man. McGraw-Hill, New York, 1962

Smith LDS, Williams BL: The Pathogenic Anaerobic Bacteria. 3rd Ed. Charles C Thomas, Springfield, IL, 1984

Styrt B, Gorbach SL: Recent developments in the understanding of the pathogenesis and treatment of anaerobic infections. N Engl J Med 321:240, 298, 1989

Sutter VL, Citron DM, Edelstein MAC, Finegold SM: Wadsworth Anaerobic Bacteriology Manual. 4th Ed. Star Publishing Co., Belmont, CA, 1985

21

SALMONELLA

RALPH A. GIANNELLA

GENERAL CONCEPTS

Clinical Manifestations

Salmonellosis ranges clinically from common *Salmonella* gastroenteritis (diarrhea, abdominal cramps, and fever) to enteric fevers (including typhoid fever), which are life-threatening febrile systemic illnesses. Focal infections and an asymptomatic carrier state occur.

Structure, Classification, and Antigenic Types

Salmonella species are Gram-negative, flagellated, facultatively anaerobic bacilli characterized by O, H, and Vi antigens. The genus contains more than 1,800 serovars, which current classification considers to be separate species.

Pathogenesis

Pathogenic salmonellae ingested in food invade the mucosa in the small and large intestines and produce toxins. An acute inflammatory response in the intestinal mucosa causes diarrhea and may lead to ulceration and destruction of mucosa. The bacteria can disseminate from the intestines to cause systemic disease.

Host Defenses

Both nonspecific and specific defenses are active (nonspecific defenses consist of gastric acidity, intestinal mucus, intestinal transit time, lactoferrin, and lysozyme; specific defenses consist of mucosal and systemic antibodies and genetic resistance to invasion). Various host factors affect susceptibility.

Epidemiology

Nontyphoidal salmonellosis is a worldwide disease of humans and animals. Animals are the main reservoir, and the disease is usually food borne, although it can be spread from person to person. The salmonellae that cause typhoid and other enteric fevers spread mainly from person to person via the fecal-oral route and have no significant animal reservoirs. Asymptomatic human carriers ("typhoid Marys") may spread the disease.

Diagnosis

Salmonellosis should be considered in any acute diarrheal or febrile illness without obvious cause; the diagnosis is confirmed by isolating the organisms from clinical specimens (stool or blood).

Control

Effective vaccines exist for typhoid fever but not for nontyphoidal salmonellosis. Those diseases are controlled by hygienic slaughtering practices and thorough cooking and refrigeration of food.

INTRODUCTION

Salmonellae are ubiquitous human and animal pathogens, and **salmonellosis,** a disease that affects an estimated 2 million Americans each year, is common throughout the world. Salmonellosis in humans usually takes the form of a self-limiting food poisoning (gastroenteritis), but occasionally manifests as a serious systemic infection (enteric fever), which requires prompt antibiotic treatment. In addition, salmonellosis causes substantial losses of livestock.

CLINICAL MANIFESTATIONS

Some infectious disease texts recognize three clinical forms of salmonellosis: (1) **gastroenteritis,** (2) **septicemia,** and (3) **enteric fevers.** This chapter focuses on the two extremes of the clinical spectrum—gastroenteritis and enteric fever. The septicemic form of *Salmonella* infection can be an intermediate stage of infection in which the patient is not experiencing intestinal symptoms and the bacteria cannot be isolated from fecal specimens. The severity of the infection and whether it remains localized in the intestine or disseminates to the bloodstream may depend on the resistance of the patient and the virulence of the *Salmonella* isolate.

The incubation period for *Salmonella* gastroenteritis (food poisoning) depends on the dose of bacteria. Symptoms usually begin 6 to 48 hours after ingestion of contaminated food or water and usually take the form of nausea, vomiting, and diarrhea. Myalgia and headache are common; however, the cardinal manifestation is diarrhea. Fever (38°C to 39°C) and chills are also common. At least two-thirds of patients complain of abdominal cramps. The duration of fever and diarrhea varies, but is usually 2 to 7 days.

Enteric fevers are severe systemic forms of salmonellosis. The best-studied enteric fever is **typhoid fever,** the form caused by *S typhi,* but any species of *Salmonella* may cause this type of disease. The symptoms begin after an incubation period of 10 to 14 days. Enteric fevers may be preceded by gastroenteritis, which usually resolves before the onset of the systemic disease. The symptoms of enteric fevers are nonspecific and include fever, malaise, anorexia, headache, and myalgias. Enteric fevers are severe infections and may be fatal if antibiotics are not promptly administered.

STRUCTURE, CLASSIFICATION, AND ANTIGENIC TYPES

Salmonellae are Gram-negative, flagellated, facultatively anaerobic bacilli possessing three major antigens: **H** or **flagellar antigen; O** or **somatic antigen;** and **Vi antigen** (possessed by only a few serotypes). H antigen occurs in either or both of two forms called **phase 1** and **phase 2.** The organisms tend to change from one phase to the other. O antigens occur on the surface of the outer membrane and are determined by specific sugar sequences. Vi antigen is a superficial antigen overlying the O antigen; it is present in a few serotypes, the most important being *S typhi.*

Antigenic analysis of salmonellae by using specific antisera offers clinical and epidemiologic advantages. Determination of antigenic structure permits one to identify the organisms clinically and assign them to one of nine serogroups (A through I), each containing many serovars (Table 21-1). H antigen also provides a useful epidemiologic tool with which to investigate outbreaks of salmonellosis and to determine the source of infection and the way it is spread.

As with other Gram-negative bacilli, the cell envelope of salmonellae contains a complex lipopolysaccharide (LPS) structure that is liberated on lysis of the cell and, to some extent, during culture. The lipopolysaccharide moiety may function as an endotoxin and may be important in determining the virulence of the organisms. This macromolecular endotoxin complex consists of three components: an outer O-polysaccharide coat, a middle portion (the R core), and an inner lipid A coat. Lipopolysaccharide structure is important for several reasons. First, the nature of the repeating sugar units in the outer O-polysaccharide chains is responsible for O-antigen specificity; it may also help determine the virulence of the organism. Salmonellae lacking the complete sequence of O-sugar repeat units are called **rough** because of the rough ap-

TABLE 21-1   Ecologic Classification of Salmonellae

Species	Representative Serovar(s)[a]	Reservoir (Host preferences)
S choleraesuis	One only	Animals (swine)
S typhi	One only	Humans
S enteritidis	*Paratyphi-A*	Humans
	Schottmuelleri	
	Pullorum	Animals (fowl)
	Dublin	Animals (cattle)
	Typhimurium	
	Derby	
	Enteritidis	Humans and many animals
	Heidelberg and hundreds of related serovars	

[a] It is now accepted practice to refer to the 1,800 serovars of *Salmonella* as though they constituted separate species (e.g., *S pullorum*).
(Adapted from Grady GF, Keusch GT: Pathogenesis of bacterial diarrheas. N Engl J Med 285:831, 1971, with permission.)

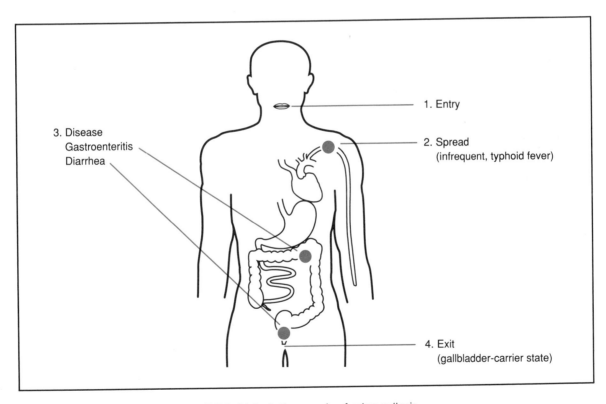

FIGURE 21-1 Pathogenesis of salmonellosis.

pearance of the colonies; they are usually avirulent or less virulent than the **smooth** strains, which possess a full complement of O-sugar repeat units. Second, antibodies directed against the R core (common enterobacterial antigen) may protect against infection by a wide variety of Gram-negative bacteria with a common core structure or may moderate their lethal effects. Third, the endotoxin component of the cell wall may be important in the pathogenesis of many Gram-negative infections. Endotoxins evoke fever; activate the serum complement, kinin, and clotting systems; depress myocardial function; and alter lymphocyte function. Circulating endotoxin may be responsible in part for many of the manifestations of septic shock that can occur in systemic infections.

PATHOGENESIS

Salmonellosis includes several syndromes (gastroenteritis, enteric fevers, septicemia, focal infections, and an asymptomatic carrier state) (Fig. 21-1). Particular serotypes show a strong propensity to produce a particular syndrome (*S typhi, S paratyphi-A,* and *S schottmuelleri* produce enteric fever; *S choleraesuis* produces septicemia or focal infections; *S typhimurium* and *S enteritidis* produce gastroenteritis); however, on occasion, any serotype can produce any of the syndromes. In general, more serious infections occur in infants, in adults over the age of 50, and in individuals with debilitating illnesses.

Most nontyphoidal salmonellae enter the body when contaminated food is ingested (Fig. 21-2). Person-to-person spread of salmonellae also occurs. To be fully pathogenic, salmonellae must possess a variety of attributes called **virulence factors.** These include (1) the ability to invade cells, (2) a complete lipopolysaccharide coat, and (3) possibly the elaboration of toxin(s). After ingestion the organisms colonize the ileum and colon, invade the intestinal epithelium, and proliferate within the epithelium and lymphoid follicles. The mechanisms by which salmonellae invade the epithelium are not well understood, but involve an initial binding to specific receptors on the epithelial cell surfaces followed by invasion; the invasion is depen-

dent on microfilaments and microtubules and probably involves endocytosis. Attachment and invasion appear to be under distinct genetic control and involve genes on both chromosomes and plasmids. These processes are delicately controlled interactions whereby the salmonellae synthesize proteins to adhere to and invade epithelial cells. The salmonellae are induced to synthesize these proteins in response to proteinaceous molecules on the surface of epithelial cells.

After invading the epithelium, the organisms spread to mesenteric lymph nodes and throughout the body via the systemic circulation; they are taken up by the reticuloendothelial cells. The reticuloendothelial system confines and controls spread of the organism; however, depending on the serotype and the effectiveness of the host defenses against that serotype, some organisms may infect the liver, spleen, gallbladder, bones, meninges, and other organs (Fig. 21-1). Fortunately, most serotypes are killed promptly in extraintestinal sites, and the most common human *Salmo-*

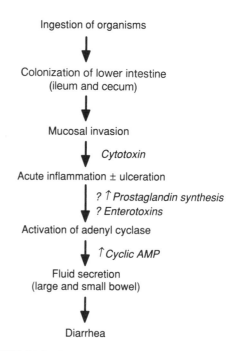

FIGURE 21-2   Scheme of the pathogenesis of *S enteritis* and diarrhea.

nella infection, gastroenteritis, remains confined to the intestine.

After invading the intestine, most salmonellae induce an acute inflammatory response, which occasionally causes ulceration. They may elaborate **cytotoxins** that inhibit protein synthesis. Whether these cytotoxins contribute to the inflammatory response or to ulceration is not known. Because of the intestinal inflammatory reaction, symptoms of inflammation such as fever, chills, abdominal pain, leukocytosis, and diarrhea are common. The stools may contain polymorphonuclear leukocytes, blood, and mucus.

Much is now known about the mechanisms of *Salmonella* gastroenteritis and diarrhea. Figures 21-2 and 21-3 summarize the pathogenesis of *Salmonella* enteritis and diarrhea. Only strains that penetrate the intestinal mucosa cause an acute inflammatory reaction and diarrhea (Fig. 21-4); the diarrhea is due to secretion of fluid and electrolytes by the small and large intestines. The mechanisms of secretion are unclear, but the secretion is not merely a manifestation of tissue destruction and ulceration. *Salmonella* penetrate intestinal epithelial cells but, unlike *Shigella* and invasive *E coli*, do not escape the phagosome. Thus, the extent of intercellular spread and ulceration of the epithelium is minimal. *Salmonella* escape from the basal side of the epithelial cells into the lamina propria. Systemic spread of the organisms can occur, giving rise to enteric fever. Invasion of the intestinal mucosa is followed by activation of mucosal adenylate cyclase; the resultant increase in cyclic adenosine 5^1-monophosphate (cAMP) induces secretion. The mechanism by which adenylate cyclase is stimulated is not understood; it may involve local production of prostaglandins or other components of the inflammatory reaction. In addition, *Salmonella* strains elaborate a choleralike toxin that may function as an enterotoxin. However, the precise role

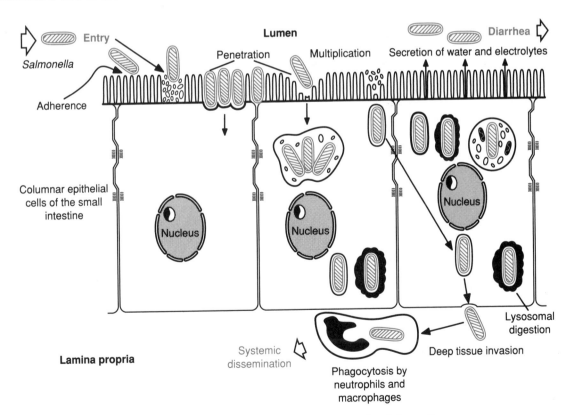

FIGURE 21-3 Invasion of intestinal mucosa by *Salmonella*.

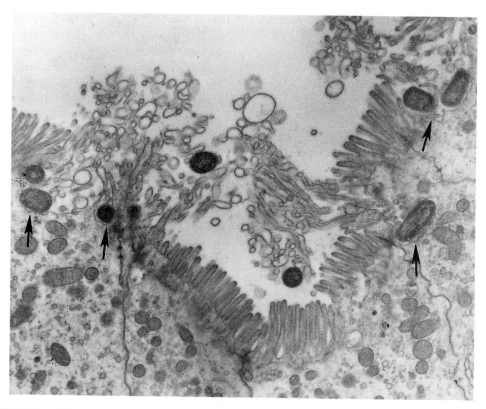

FIGURE 21-4 Electron photomicrograph demonstrating invasion of guinea pig ileal epithelial cells by *S typhimurium*. Arrows point to invading *Salmonella* organisms. (Courtesy Akio Takeuchi, Walter Reed Army Institute of Research, Washington, DC.)

TABLE 21-2   Host Defenses against Salmonellae

Host Defense	Examples of Factors
Gastric factors	Gastric acidity
	Rate of gastric emptying
Intestinal factors	Intestinal motility
	Normal intestinal flora
	Mucus
	Secretory antibodies
	Genetic resistance to invasion
Nonspecific and other factors	Nutritional state
	Lactoferrin
	Gut reticuloendothelial cells
	Lysozyme

of this exotoxin in the pathogenesis of *Salmonella* enterocolitis and diarrhea has not been established.

HOST DEFENSES

Various host defenses are important in resisting intestinal colonization and invasion by *Salmonella* (Table 21-2). Normal gastric acidity (pH < 3.5) is lethal to salmonellae. In healthy individuals, the number of ingested salmonellae is reduced in the stomach, so that fewer or no organisms enter the intestine. Normal small intestinal motility also protects the bowel by sweeping ingested salmonellae through quickly. The normal intestinal microflora protects against salmonellae, probably through anaerobes, which liberate short-chain fatty acids that are thought to be toxic to salmonellae. Alteration of the anaerobic intestinal flora by antibiotics renders the host more susceptible to salmonellosis. Secretory or mucosal antibodies also are thought to protect the intestine against salmonellae. Animal strains genetically resistant to intestinal invasion by salmonellae have been described. When these host defenses are absent or blunted, the host becomes more susceptible to salmonellosis; factors that render the host more susceptible to salmonellosis are listed in Table 21-3. The role of host defenses in salmonellosis is extremely important, and much remains to be learned.

EPIDEMIOLOGY

Contaminated food is the major mode of transmission of nontyphoidal salmonellae, because salmonellosis is a zoonosis and has an enormous animal reservoir. The most common animal reservoirs are chickens, turkeys, pigs, and cows; dozens of other domestic and wild animals also harbor these organisms. Because of the ability of salmonellae to survive in meats and animal products that are not thoroughly cooked, animal products are the main vehicle of transmission. The magnitude of the problem is demonstrated by the following recent yields of salmonellae: 41 percent of turkeys examined in California, 50 percent of chickens examined in Massachusetts, and 21 percent of commercial frozen egg whites examined in Spokane, WA.

The epidemiology of typhoid fever and other enteric fevers primarily involves person-to-person spread because these organisms lack a significant animal reservoir. Contamination with human feces is the major mode of spread, and the usual vehicle is contaminated water. Occasionally, contaminated food (usually handled by an individual who harbors *S typhi*) may be the vehicle. Plasmid fingerprinting and bacteriophage lysotyping of *Salmonella* isolates are powerful epidemiologic tools for studying outbreaks of salmonellosis and tracing the spread of the organisms in the environment.

In typhoid fever and nontyphoidal salmonellosis, two other factors have epidemiologic significance. First, an asymptomatic human carrier state exists for the agents of either form of the disease. Approximately 3 percent of persons infected with *S typhi* and 0.1 percent of those infected with nontyphoidal salmonellae become chronic carriers. The carrier state may last from many weeks to years. Thus, human as well as animal reservoirs exist. Interestingly, children rarely become chronic typhoid carriers. Second, the use of antibi-

TABLE 21-3 Factors Increasing Susceptibility to Salmonellosis

Location or Factor	Specific Condition
Stomach	Achlorhydria Gastric surgery
Intestine	Antibiotics administration Gastrointestinal surgery (?) Idiopathic inflammatory bowel disease
Hemolytic anemia	Especially sickle cell anemia and other hemoglobinopathies
Impaired systemic immunity	Carcinomatosis, leukemias, lymphomas Immunosuppressive drugs and others

otics in animal feeds and indiscriminate use of anti-biotics in humans increase antibiotic resistance in salmonellae by promoting the transfer of R factors.

DIAGNOSIS

The diagnosis of salmonellosis requires bacteriologic isolation of the organisms from appropriate clinical specimens. Laboratory identification of the genus *Salmonella* is done by biochemical tests; the serotype is confirmed by serologic testing. Feces, blood, and other specimens should be plated on several nonselective and selective agar media (blood, MacConkey, eosin-methylene blue, bismuth sulfite, *Salmonella-Shigella,* and brilliant green agars) as well as into enrichment broth such as selenite or tetrathionate. Any growth in enrichment broth is subsequently subcultured onto the various agars. The biochemical reactions of suspicious colonies are then determined on triple sugar iron agar and lysine-iron agar, and a presumptive identification is made. Recently, biochemical identification of salmonellae has been simplified by systems that permit the rapid testing of 10 to 20 biochemical parameters simultaneously. The presumptive biochemical identification of *Salmonella* then can be confirmed by antigenic analysis of O and H antigens by using polyvalent and specific antisera. Fortunately, approximately 95 percent of clinical isolates can be identified with the available group A through E typing antisera. *Salmonella* isolates then should be sent to a central or reference laboratory for more comprehensive serologic testing and confirmation.

CONTROL

Salmonellae are difficult to eradicate from the environment. However, because the major reservoir for human infection is poultry and livestock, reducing the number of salmonellae harbored in these animals would significantly reduce human exposure. In Denmark, for example, all animal feeds are treated to kill salmonellae before distribution, resulting in a marked reduction in salmonellosis. Other helpful measures include changing animal slaughtering practices to reduce cross-con-tamination of animal carcasses; protecting processed foods from contamination; providing training in hygienic practices for all food-handling personnel in slaughterhouses, food processing plants, and restaurants; cooking and refrigerating foods adequately in food processing plants, restaurants, and homes; and expanding governmental enteric disease surveillance programs.

Vaccines are available for typhoid fever and are partially effective, especially in children. No vaccines are available for nontyphoidal salmonellosis. Continued research in this area and increased understanding of the mechanisms of immunity to enteric infections are of great importance.

General salmonellosis treatment measures include replacing fluid loss by oral and intravenous routes and controlling pain, nausea, and vomiting. Specific therapy consists of antibiotic administration. Typhoid fever and enteric fevers should be treated with antibiotics; chloramphenicol is the drug of choice. Antibiotic therapy of nontyphoidal salmonellosis should be reserved for the septicemic, enteric fever, and focal infection syndromes. Antibiotics are not recommended for uncomplicated *Salmonella* gastroenteritis because they do not shorten the illness and they significantly prolong the fecal excretion of the organisms and increase the number of antibiotic-resistant strains.

REFERENCES

Black PH, Kunz LJ, Swartz MN: Salmonellosis—a review of some unusual aspects. N Engl J Med 262:811, 864, 921, 1960

Finlay RB, Falkow S: A comparison of microbial invasion strategies of Salmonella, Shigella, and Yersinia species. p. 227. In Horwitz MA (ed): Bacteria–Host Cell Interaction. Alan R. Liss, New York, 1988

Finlay RB, Heffron F, Falkow S: Epithelial cell surfaces induce Salmonella proteins required for bacterial adherence and invasion. Science 243:940, 1989

Galan JE, Curtiss R: Cloning and molecular characterization of genes whose products allow *Salmonella typhimurium* to penetrate tissue culture cells. Proc Natl Acad Sci USA 86:6383, 1989

Giannella RA: Importance of the intestinal inflammatory reaction in *Salmonella*-mediated intestinal secretion. Infect Immun 23:140, 1979

Giannella RA, Broitman SA, Zamcheck N: Influence of

gastric acidity on bacterial and parasitic enteric infections: a perspective. Ann Intern Med 78:271, 1973

Giannella RA, Formal SB, Dammin GJ et al: Pathogenesis of salmonellosis. Studies of fluid secretion, mucosal invasion, and morphologic reaction in the rabbit ileum. J Clin Invest 52:441, 1973

Giannella RA, Gots RE, Charney AN et al: Pathogenesis of Salmonella-mediated intestinal fluid secretion: activation of adenylate cyclase and inhibition by indomethacin. Gastroenterology 69:1238, 1975

Koo FCW, Peterson JW, Houston CW et al: Pathogenesis of experimental salmonellosis: inhibition of protein synthesis by cytotoxin. Infect Immun 43:93, 1984

Rubin RH, Weinstein L: Salmonellosis: Microbiologic, Pathologic and Clinical Features. Stratton Intercontinental Medical Book Corp, New York, 1977

Stephen J, Wallis TS, Starkey WG et al: Salmonellosis: in retrospect and prospect. In Evered D, Whelan J (eds): Microbial Toxins and Diarrheal Disease. CIBA Found Symp 112:175, 1985

22
SHIGELLA

THOMAS L. HALE
GERALD T. KEUSCH
SAMUEL B. FORMAL

GENERAL CONCEPTS

Clinical Manifestations

Symptoms of **shigellosis** include abdominal pain, tenesmus, watery diarrhea, and/or dysentery (multiple scanty, bloody, mucoid stools). Other signs may include abdominal tenderness, fever, vomiting, dehydration, and convulsions.

Structure, Classification and Antigenic Types

Shigellae are Gram-negative, nonmotile, facultatively anaerobic, non-spore-forming rods. Virulence genes are carried on a large plasmid. Shigellae are closely related to *Escherichia coli*, but are differentiated by their failure to ferment lactose (*S sonnei* is a late lactose fermenter) or to decarboxylate lysine. *Shigella* is divided into four serogroups with multiple serotypes: A (*S dysenteriae*, 12 serotypes), B (*S flexneri*, 6 serotypes), C (*S boydii*, 18 serotypes), and D (*S sonnei*, 1 serotype).

Pathogenesis

Infection is by ingestion (usually through fecal-oral contamination), with an incubation period of up to 4 days. Large plasmids are necessary for expression of the invasive phenotype. Organisms invade and multiply within colonic epithelial cells, spread to adjacent cells, erode the epithelium, and cause ulcers. They also synthesize toxins. **Colitis** is almost always present in the rectosigmoid area and less frequently in more proximal areas of the colon. Septicemia is rare.

Host Defenses

Nonspecific defenses include mucus secretion, interferon, and inflammation. Shigellae entering the lamina propria are phagocytosed and killed by inflammatory cells. Subsequently, antibody to lipopolysaccharide somatic antigen and plasmid-encoded proteins is produced locally and systemically. The protective role of antibody and cell-mediated immunity is unknown, but serotype-specific immunity has been demonstrated.

Epidemiology

Shigellosis is common (10 to 20 percent of enteric disease) where sanitation is poor. In developed countries, single-source, food-borne outbreaks and institutional epidemics occur sporadically.

Diagnosis

Shigellosis can be correctly diagnosed in 50 percent of patients on the basis of fresh blood in the stool, but watery, mucoid diarrhea is the only symptom of some *S sonnei* infections. Clinical diagnosis should be confirmed by cultivation and identification of cells in feces.

Control

Prevention depends on sanitation. Severe dysentery is treated with ampicillin or trimethoprim-sulfamethoxazole and oral rehydration therapy is used for acute diarrhea.

INTRODUCTION

Gram-negative, facultative anaerobes of the genus *Shigella* are the principal agents of bacillary dysentery. Dysentery differs from profuse watery diarrhea, e.g., choleraic diarrhea, in that the dysenteric stool is scant and contains blood, mucus, and inflammatory cells. However, some individuals suffering from *Shigella* infections experience moderate diarrhea instead of dysentery. Bacillary dysentery is responsible for a significant proportion of acute intestinal disease among children in developing countries and for sporadic outbreaks in developed countries. Although the molecular basis of shigellosis is complex, the initial step in pathogenesis appears to be the invasion of the colonic mucosa followed by intracellular bacterial multiplication within the cytoplasm of colonic epithelial cells. Intercellular spread of shigellae result in a focus of infection characterized by degeneration of the epithelium and by an acute inflammatory response in the lamina propria. Ulceration of the intestinal mucosa results in leakage of blood, inflammatory elements, and mucus into the intestinal lumen. Shigellosis should be suspected in any patient with mucoid stools, bloody stools, or febrile diarrhea.

CLINICAL PRESENTATION

Shigellosis has two basic clinical presentations: (1) watery diarrhea associated with vomiting and dehydration, and (2) dysentery characterized by a small volume of bloody, mucoid stools and abdominal pain (cramps and tenesmus). Estimates of the relative frequencies of these symptoms are given in Table 22-1. Diarrheal disease is most often associated with *S sonnei* infections, whereas *S flexneri* or *S dysenteriae* infections may have a prodrome of diarrhea but are usually characterized by dysentery. Human challenge studies with *S flexneri* indicate the following average incubation periods: 1.5 days for fever, 2.5 days for positive stool culture, 3.5 days for abdominal pain, 4.0 days for diarrhea, and 6 days for dysentery. These incubation periods also depend on the number of organisms ingested. The average duration of symptoms in untreated adults is 7 days, and stool cultures may remain positive for 30 days or longer.

The clinical features of shigellosis are summarized in Figure 22-1. Although the intestinal dysfunction that elicits diarrhea during *Shigella* infections is unclear, diarrhea occurs most often in patients who have proximal colitis involving the transverse color or cecum; these patients show net

TABLE 22-1   Clinical Characteristics of Shigellosis

Symptom	Approximate Percentage of Patients[a]		
	S sonnei	*S flexneri*	*S dysenteriae*
Watery diarrhea	75	30	30
Stool mucus	50	75	95
Stool blood	10	50	80
Abdominal pain	50	70	85
Vomiting	60	30	40
Fever	5	10	10

[a] Based on data from Dacca Hospital, Dacca, Bangladesh.

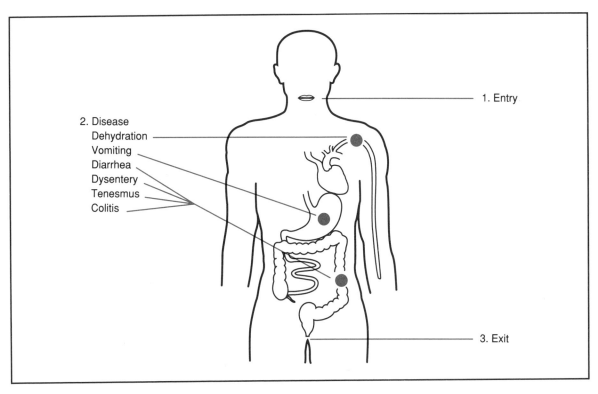

FIGURE 22-1   Pathogenesis of shigellosis in humans.

water secretion as well as impaired absorption in the inflamed colon. In patients with dysentery, colitis is usually confined to the distal colon, net water secretion is minimal, and there is slight net absorption of water in the colon. Under these conditions, the volume of stool depends largely on the ileocecal flow, and the patient exhibits the frequent, scanty stools (300 to 1,300 g/day) that characterize bloody diarrhea or dysentery.

Among the possible complications of *Shigella* infections are bacteremia, convulsions, reactive arthritis, and hemolytic-uremic syndrome. In developing countries, bacteremia usually due to *S dysenteriae* type 1, occurs in malnourished, non-breast-fed children. Bacteremia is uncommon in otherwise healthy adults. Convulsions occur in up to 25 percent of children under the age of 4 years. Youth, high fever, and a family history of seizures are risk factors for possible development of a convulsive episode. Reactive arthritis or the associated Reiter syndrome has been observed as a chronic

sequela in outbreaks involving *S flexneri,* with a reported incidence as high as 0.2 to 2.4 percent. Individuals who are positive for the HLA-B27 histocompatibility antigen have a strong predisposition for this sequela. In contrast to *S flexneri, S sonnei* is not associated with arthritic sequelae. Finally, hemolytic-uremic syndrome is a rare complication in children infected with *S dysenteriae* type 1. This syndrome is characterized by a triad of microangiopathic hemolytic anemia, thrombocytopenia, and acute renal failure.

STRUCTURE, CLASSIFICATION, AND ANTIGENIC TYPES

Organisms of the genus *Shigella* belong to the tribe Escherichia in the family Enterobacteriaceae. Shigellae are Gram-negative, nonmotile, facultatively anaerobic, non-spore-forming rods. Although *Shigella* is classified as a separate genus on the basis of pathogenicity, DNA hybridization studies indicate that *Escherichia coli* and the four *Shigella* species could be considered the same species in an evolutionary sense. *Shigella dysenteriae* (serogroup A, consisting of 12 serotypes), *S flexneri* (serogroup B, consisting of 6 serotypes), and *S boydii* (serogroup C, consisting of 18 serotypes) are very similar biochemically and are usually differentiated by serotyping of the lipopolysaccharide O-somatic antigen. *Shigella sonnei* (serogroup D, consisting of one serotype) is biochemically distinct from the other serogroups in that it expresses β-D-galactosidase and ornithine decarboxylase. Certain serotypes of *E coli,* designated enteroinvasive *E coli* (EIEC), are similar to shigellae both biochemically and in their ability to cause diarrheal disease. Some EIEC are serologically related to shigellae. For example, EIEC O124 agglutinates in *S dysenteriae* serotype 3 antiserum.

PATHOGENESIS
Pathology

The colonic lesions in shigellosis resemble those in ulcerative colitis. There is characteristic rectosigmoid involvement with differing proximal extension of erythema, edema, loss of vascular pattern, focal and petechial hemorrhages, and adherent layers of purulent exudate. Biopsied specimens from affected areas reveal edema, capillary congestion, focal hemorrhages, crypt hyperplasia, goblet cell depletion, mononuclear and polymorphonuclear cell infiltrations, shedding of epithelial cells and erythrocytes, and microulcerations. The pathogenic mechanism of bacillary dysentery is illustrated in Figures 22-2 and 22-3. Adherence, penetration, and endocytosis of shigellae can best be observed in vitro, whereas the latter stages

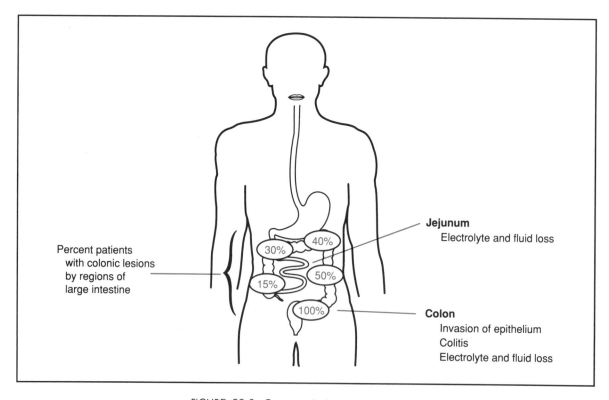

FIGURE 22-2 Gross pathology of shigellosis.

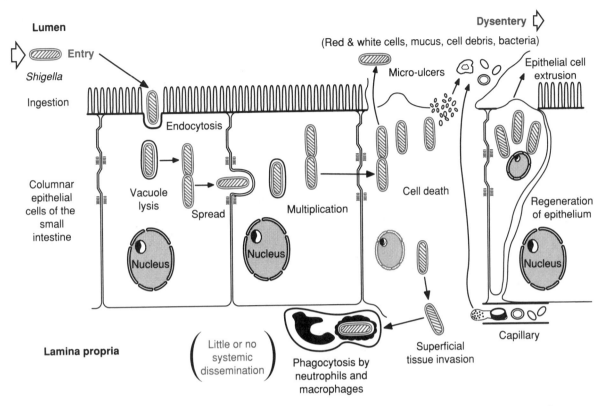

FIGURE 22-3 Histopathology of acute colitis following peroral infection with shigellae. The pathologic changes have been summarized in temporal stages as follows: penetration of the mucus layer and adherence of shigellae to enterocytes, endocytosis of bacteria (i.e., invasion) and escape from endocytic vacuoles, intracellular bacterial multiplication in the enterocyte cytoplasm, and intercellular spread of bacteria to contiguous cells followed by micro-ulceration of the mucosa. The last stage is characterized by the following: pyknotic changes in infected enterocytes, shedding of enterocytes into the lumen of the bowel, goblet cell depletion, and cellular inflammatory infiltrates in the lamina propria.

(goblet cell depletion and cellular inflammatory infiltrates) are best observed in the monkey or human mucosa. Ingested shigellae invade the colonic epithelium, grow within enterocytes, and induce cytopathic changes that result in ulceration of the mucosa. Organisms are found with decreasing frequency in luminal epithelial cells, deep crypt cells, polymorphonuclear cells, macrophages, and the lamina propria. The relative lack of free shigellae in the lamina propria indicates that organisms that traverse the basement membrane are readily eliminated by the inflammatory response. There is a distinct correlation between the quantity of bacilli present in the tissues and the intensity of this response.

Genetics of Virulence

Genetic analysis of virulence has been facilitated by the discovery that large plasmids (180 to 240 kilobases) are necessary for expression of the invasive phenotype in all *Shigella* species and in EIEC. Cultured human epithelial cells (HeLa, HEp-2, etc.) has been used as experimental models for study of the biochemical basis of virulence. In the tissue culture model, a constellation of plasmid-encoded proteins is necessary to induce cells to ingest shigellae by a process morphologically and biochemically similar to phagocytosis. These studies imply that plasmid-encoded proteins act as receptors, which bind to ligands on the plasma membrane and induce endocytosis; however, neither the plasmid-encoded receptor nor the host cell ligand has yet been identified.

Progression of Disease

After the ingestion of shigellae, the endocytic vacuoles dissipate, host cell protein synthesis and mitochondrial respiration are inhibited, and transported nutrients are incorporated into organisms multiplying freely in the cytoplasm. The biochemical basis of these processes is unclear, but it is again apparent that plasmid-encoded bacterial proteins are involved. The lysis of endocytic vacuoles has a profound effect on the pathogenesis of shigellae because it retards the spread of organisms to the lamina propria. In contrast to shigellae, *Salmonella* species remain within endocytic vacuoles, and these organisms can be transcytosed across the intact intestinal epithelium in a process which leads to colonization of lymphoid tissues and systemic spread.

The last critical stage in the pathogenesis of shigellosis is the spread of organisms to contiguous epithelial cells. This is a particularly interesting problem of cell biology since shigellae lack the flagella required for spread in agarose culture media. The tissue culture model shows that intercellular shigellae cause a localized polymerization of actin microfilaments in the cytoplasm, and this apparently provides a motive force for bacterial movement and intracellular spread. A plasmid-encoded outer membrane protein is strongly associated with microfilament polymerization, but the biochemical basis of this phenomenon is uncharacterized.

Recent provocative observations in the infected ileum of rabbits suggest that shigellae are preferentially taken up by the membranous (M) cells overlying the lymphoid follicles. The phagocytic vacuoles of the M cells lyse, and intracellular bacterial multiplication elicits ulceration of the follicular epithelium. Although it is unwise to directly extrapolate these observations to human disease, it should be noted that the diffuse lymphoid tissue of the rectosigmoid area may be a portal of mucosal invasion by shigellae.

Toxins

S dysenteriae type 1 synthesizes a potent cytotoxin **(Shiga toxin)** that also has enterotoxic activity in animal models. The role of this toxin in shigella diarrhea is unclear since *S dysenteriae* is not uniquely associated with this clinical manifestation (Table 22-1). Shiga toxin contributes to the capillary destruction and focal hemorrhages that are associated with bloody stools, but this also occurs in infections with other *Shigella* species (Table 22-1). The latter organisms synthesize **"Shiga-like" toxins,** which can be neutralized by antibody raised against Shiga toxin, but the levels of Shiga-like toxin are at least 1000-fold lower than the levels of Shiga toxin expressed by *S dysenteriae* type 1. *Shigella flexneri* and *S sonnei* also reportedly express cytotoxins that are not Shiga-like toxins (i.e., are not neutralized by Shiga antitoxin), and this cytotoxic activity is associated with fever and occult stool blood. The cytotoxic manifestation of Shiga toxin may be responsible for the prevalence of bacteremia and hemolytic-uremic syndrome in *S dysenteriac* type 1 infections, but the role of cytotoxins in *Shigella* diarrhea or dysentery has yet to be defined.

HOST DEFENSES

Since the ingestion of 10 organisms causes disease in 10 percent of volunteers and 500 organisms routinely cause disease in 50 percent of healthy adults, nonspecific host defense mechanisms are apparently ineffective in preventing primary *Shigella* infections. During the acute phase of dysentery, peristaltic motion of the bowel is increased and goblet cells evacuate copious quantities of mucus. These nonspecific reactions to colonic inflammation sweep shigellae and extruded enterocytes out of the intestinal tract and thus discourage establishment of new foci of infection. On the cellular level, primary tissue cultures (mouse embryo fibroblasts) produce beta interferon when infected with shigellae, and interferon also renders uninfected cells resistant to *Shigella* infection. In addition, natural killer (NK) lymphocytes from the blood of nonimmune individuals lyse HeLa cells infected with *S flexneri*. These in vitro observations may not accurately reflect the host response to *Shigella* infections, but they do suggest that nonspecific defense mechanisms such as interferon and natural killer cells may retard the spread of shigellae within the intestinal mucosa.

Short-term, serotype-specific immunity to reinfection occurs in rhesus monkeys and humans challenged with *S flexneri,* but safe and effective vaccines protecting against shigellosis are not yet available. The contributions of antibody and cellular factors to immunity are poorly understood. Although shigellae are basically intracellular pathogens, there are two possible stages of infection at which antibody might have some protective effect. Mucosal immunoglobulin A (IgA) neutralizing the plasmid-encoded determinants of bacterial invasion could prevent attachment or ingestion of shigellae by colonic enterocytes. Four plasmid-encoded proteins that are putative determinants of the invasive phenotype elicit strong IgG and IgA responses in the mucosa of infected monkeys. However, convalescent-phase antiserum recognizing these "invasion plasmid antigens" has not been shown to inhibit *Shigella* invasion in vitro.

Alternatively, IgA and IgG in the inflammatory transudate elicited by mucosal destruction could opsonize extracellular shigellae that reach the lamina propria. Both phagocytic killing of opsonized shigellae by polymorphonuclear leukocytes and antibody-dependent, lymphocyte-mediated bactericidal activity have been demonstrated in vitro. Since opsonizing antibody is directed against the somatic antigen, this antibody could mediate serotype-specific immunity to shigellosis.

EPIDEMIOLOGY

Shigellosis occurs only in humans and subhuman primates. The source of infection is the excreta of infected individuals or convalescent carriers. Direct spread is by the fecal-oral route, while contaminated food, flies, water, and inanimate objects can serve as vectors. Shigellosis is endemic in areas of developing countries that are overcrowded and have inadequate sanitation. In developed countries, sporadic common-source outbreaks usually involve uncooked foods, such as salads. Waterborne outbreaks usually involve semipublic water systems, such as those found at camps or trailer parks, which are inadequately protected from sewage contamination. Direct spread often occurs in institutional environments such as children's daycare centers, mental hospitals, nursing homes, and prisons. Homosexual men are also at increased risk for direct transmission of *Shigella* infections, and recurrent or recrudescent illness complicating human immunodeficiency virus infection has been observed.

DIAGNOSIS

Clinical

Any patient presenting with watery diarrhea and fever should be suspected of having shigellosis. The diarrheal stage of this infection cannot be distinguished clinically from other bacterial, viral, and protozoan infections. Nausea and vomiting can accompany the diarrhea, but these symptoms are often observed in infections with nontyphoidal salmonellae and enterotoxigenic organisms. Bloody, mucoid stools are highly indicative of shigellosis, but the differential diagnosis should include EIEC, *Salmonella enteritidis, Yersinia enterocolitica, Campylobacter* species, and especially *Entamaeba histolytica.* Although blood is common in the stools of patients with amebiasis, it is usually dark brown rather than bright red, as in *Shigella* infections. Microscopic examination of stool smears from patients with amebiasis should reveal the presence of erythrophagocytic trophozoites in the absence of polymorphonuclear leukocytes, whereas bacillary dysentery is characterized by sheets of polymorphonuclear leukocytes. Sigmoidoscopic examination of a patient experiencing acute shigellosis reveals a diffusely erythematous mucosal surface with small ulcers, whereas amebiasis is characterized by discrete ulcers without generalized inflammation.

Laboratory

Although clinical signs of shigellosis are cause for suspicion, diagnosis must depend on isolation and identification of the agent in the feces. Positive cultures are most often obtained from blood-tinged plugs of mucus in freshly passed stool specimens during the acute phase of disease. Rectal swabs may also be used to isolate shigellae, but in all cases the specimen should either be deposited in a holding medium such as buffered glycerol saline or processed rapidly by the clinical laboratory. The isolation procedure usually involves an initial streaking on differential and selective media followed by aerobic incubation to inhibit growth of the predominantly anaerobic fecal flora. Differential media, such as MacConkey agar or eosin methylene blue agar, inhibit the growth of Gram-positive organisms, but permit growth of most members of the Enterobacteriaceae. The latter organisms can be differentiated on the basis of dark-centered colonies (lactose fermenters) and colorless colonies (non-lactose fermenters that are possible *Shigella* or *Salmonella* species). Selective media, such as *Salmonella-Shigella* agar or Hektoen enteric agar, inhibit the growth of most coliforms, but allow the propagation of salmonellae and shigellae. A tube of Hajna Gram-negative broth may also be inoculated with the stool specimen and subcultured onto differential or selective agar media after 6 to 8 hours of incubation at 37°C. This procedure is usually more effective in enriching for *Salmonella* than for *Shigella*.

After overnight incubation at 37°C, non-lactose-fermenting colonies are streaked and stabbed into tubed slants of Kligler's iron agar or triple sugar iron agar medium. In these differential media, shigellae produce an alkaline slant and an acid butt with no bubbles of gas in the agar. This reaction is presumptive identification for *Shigella* species, and slide agglutination tests with antisera for serogroup and serotype confirm the identifica-

tion. Additional biochemical tests can be used to identify shigellae. For example, *S dysenteriae* can be differentiated from the other *Shigella* species by its failure to ferment mannitol.

In some instances, *E coli* biotypes closely resemble those of *Shigella* species (e.g., nonmotile, anaerogenic, late lactose fermenters), but these *E coli* strains can be differentiated by the ability to ferment mucate, to decarboxylate lysine, and to grow on sodium acetate agar. *Shigella*-like *E coli* strains often carry large plasmids that are homologous to the *Shigella* invasion plasmid, and infections with these EIEC are characterized by bloody diarrhea. Although EIEC are associated with specific somatic antigen serotypes, serologic screening of *E coli* isolates is laborious. In contrast, correct identification of *Shigella* usually poses no difficulty for the clinical laboratory, but the process does require 48 hours. The dual need for rapid and effective screening of stool specimens for enteroinvasive pathogens has encouraged the development of methods for detection of all organisms harboring invasion plasmids. These methods include the use of DNA probes hybridizing with a common plasmid fragment and an enzyme-linked immunosorbent assay (ELISA) with antiserum recognizing the plasmid-encoded proteins. Although highly accurate when used with isolated colonies, these techniques are not yet sensitive enough to detect enteroinvasive pathogens directly from fresh stool specimens.

CONTROL

As is the case with most intestinal infections, the most effective method of controlling shigellosis is to develop safe water supplies and effective means of feces disposal. Although these solutions are usually possible in developed countries, they are at best a long-range strategy for control of enteric infections in developing countries. The estimated five million annual deaths attributed to diarrheal disease in the latter countries, not to mention the major contribution to malnutrition in the survivors, require more immediate and practical approaches. In endemic areas, the most effective intervention strategy to minimize morbidity and mortality might be a comprehensive media and personal outreach program consisting of the following components: (1) educating all residents to actively avoid fecal contamination and to wash their hands after contamination, (2) encouraging mothers to breast-feed infants, (3) encouraging the use of oral rehydration therapy to offset the effects of acute diarrhea, and (4) encouraging mothers to provide convalescent nutritional care in the form of extra food for children early in recovery from diarrhea or dysentery.

Although severe dehydration is uncommon in shigellosis, the first consideration in treating diarrheal disease is correction of any hydration abnormalities that result from isotonic dehydration, metabolic acidosis, and significant potassium loss. The oral rehydration treatment developed by the World Health Organization has proven effective and safe in the treatment of acute diarrhea, provided that the patient is not vomiting or in shock and that treatment is administered before the onset of severe dehydration. Dysentery in the absence of diarrhea does not produce significant fluid loss. Opiates such as paregoric, which induce intestinal stasis, should be used only when pain, tenesmus, and anxiety are pronounced or when rectal prolapse is threatened. These drugs prolong the febrile state and extend the period of *Shigella* excretion in the stools.

With proper fluid replacement, shigellosis is generally a self-limiting disease and the decision to use antibiotics should be predicated on the severity of disease, the age of the patient, and the likelihood of further transmission. Antibiotic treatment reduces the average duration of illness from 5–7 days to 3 days; it also reduces the period of *Shigella* excretion after symptoms subside. Absorbable drugs, such as ampicillin (3 g/day for 5 days), will cure most *S flexneri* infections, but *S sonnei* is likely to be resistant to this agent. Tetracycline is also effective against *S flexneri*, but is now contraindicated in children of the age group that is most often infected. Trimethoprim (8 mg/kg/day) with sulfamethoxazole (40 mg/kg/day) will eradicate organisms quickly from the intestine, and this is the treatment of choice for ampicillin-resistant strains. Knowledge of patterns of drug resistance in the community and surveillance of resistance profiles in isolates from individual patients should determine therapeutic choices. The patient should be monitored until stools are consistently free of *Shigella*.

REFERENCES

Barada FA Jr, Guerrant RL: Sulfamethoxazole-trimethoprim versus ampicillin in treatment of acute invasive diarrhea. Antimicrob Agents Chemother 17:961, 1980

Black RE, Craun GF, Blake PA: Epidemiology of common-source outbreaks of shigellosis in the United States, 1961–1975. Am J Epidemiol 108:47, 1978

Bunning VK, Raybourne RB, Archer DL: Foodborne enterobacterial pathogens and rheumatoid disease. J Appl Bacteriol Symp Suppl:87S, 1988

Butler T, Dunn D, Dahms B et al: Causes of death and histopathological findings in fatal shigellosis. Pediatr Infect Dis J 8:767, 1989

Butler T, Speelman P, Kabir I et al: Colonic dysfunction during shigellosis. J Infect Dis 154:817, 1986

Davis H, Taylor JP, Perdue JN, Stelma GN Jr: A shigellosis outbreak traced to commercially distributed shredded lettuce. Am J Epidemiol 128:1312, 1988

DuPont HL, Hornick AT, Dawkins T et al: The response of man to virulent *Shigella flexneri* 2a. J Infect Dis 119:296, 1969

Farmer JJ III, Davis BR, Hickman-Brenner FW et al: Biochemical identification of new species and biogroups of *Enterobacteriaceae* isolated from clinical specimens. J Clin Microbiol 21:46, 1985

Rohde JE: Selective primary health care: strategies for control of disease in the developing world. XV. Acute diarrhea. Rev Infect Dis 6:840, 1984

Speelman P, Kabir I, Islam M: Distribution of colonic lesions in shigellosis: a colonoscopic study. J Infect Dis 150:899, 1984

Stoll BJ, Glass RI, Huq MI et al: Epidemiologic and clinical features of patients infected with *Shigella* who attended a diarrheal disease hospital in Bangladesh. J Infect Dis 146:177, 1982

Takeuchi A, Formal SB, Sprinz H: Experimental acute colitis in the rhesus monkey following peroral infection with *Shigella flexneri*. Am J Pathol 52:503, 1968

Taylor DN, Echeverria P, Sethabutr O et al: Clinical and microbiological features of *Shigella* and enteroinvasive *Escherichia coli* infections detected by DNA hybridization. J Clin Microbiol 26:1362, 1988

Wassef JS, Keren DF, Mailloux JL: Role of M cells in initial antigen uptake and in ulcer formation in the rabbit intestinal loop model of shigellosis. Infect Immun 57:858, 1989

Wharton M, Spiegel RA, Horan JM et al: A large outbreak of antibiotic-resistant shigellosis at a mass gathering. J Infect Dis 162:1324, 1990

23 *CAMPYLOBACTER AND HELICOBACTER*

GUILLERMO I. PEREZ-PEREZ
MARTIN J. BLASER

GENERAL CONCEPTS

CAMPYLOBACTER JEJUNI AND OTHER ENTERIC CAMPYLOBACTERS

Clinical Manifestations

Campylobacter species cause gastroenteritis with diarrhea, abdominal pain, fever, nausea, and vomiting.

Structure

Campylobacter species are Gram-negative, microaerophilic, nonfermenting, motile rods with a single polar flagellum. They are oxidase positive and grow optimally at 37°C or 42°C.

Classification and Antigenic Types

Campylobacter species have many serogroups. However, only a few serogroups account for most human isolates in a given geographic region. *C jejuni* possesses several common surface-exposed antigens, including porin protein and flagellin.

Pathogenesis

The bacteria colonize the small and large intestines, causing inflammatory diarrhea and fever. Stools contain leukocytes and blood. The role of toxins in pathogenesis is unclear.

Host Defenses

Nonspecific defenses such as gastric acidity and intestinal transit time are important. Specific immunity, involving intestinal immunoglobulin (IgA) and humoral antibodies, develops.

Epidemiology

Campylobacter jejuni and *C coli* are endemic worldwide and hyperendemic in developing countries. Infants and young adults are most often infected. Disease incidence peaks in the summer. Sporadic outbreaks are associated with contaminated animal products or water. Domestic and wild animals are the reservoirs for the organisms.

Diagnosis

Observation of darting motility in fresh fecal specimens or of vibrio forms on Gram stain permit presumptive diagnosis; definitive diagnosis is established by stool culture.

Control

Control depends on measures to prevent transmission from animal reservoirs to humans.

HELICOBACTER PYLORI AND OTHER GASTRIC *CAMPYLOBACTER*-LIKE ORGANISMS

Clinical Manifestations

Helicobacter pylori is associated with type B gastritis (antral stomach inflammation) and appears to play a role in the pathogenesis of peptic ulcer disease. It is not known whether the organisms cause acute disease.

Structure

The organism is distinguished by multiple, sheathed flagella and abundant urease.

Classification and Antigenic Types

The antigenic structures are not completely defined; strains are differentiated by restriction endonuclease analysis.

Pathogenesis

Helicobacter pylori shelters from gastric acid in the gastric mucous layer and probably is able to adhere to gastric epithelial cells. Production of urease and cytotoxin is associated with injury to the gastric epithelium.

Host Defenses

Local and systemic immune responses are universal, but the importance of these responses and of nonspecific defenses are not clear.

Epidemiology

The prevalence of infection increases with age. The source and mode of transmission are not known.

Diagnosis

Examination of gastric biopsy specimens or stained smears allows presumptive diagnosis; definitive diagnosis is made by culturing. Recently, noninvasive techniques such as the urea breath test and serologic tests have been developed to diagnose *H. pylori* infection.

Control

No therapy is universally effective; bismuth compounds are reported to reduce infection.

OTHER PATHOGENIC *CAMPYLOBACTER* SPECIES

Campylobacter fetus causes bacteremia in compromised hosts and self-limited diarrhea in previously healthy individuals. *Campylobacter cinaedi* and *C fennelliae* cause enteric and extraintestinal diseases in homosexual men and in travelers.

INTRODUCTION

Campylobacters are Gram-negative, microaerophilic bacteria that are widely distributed in the animal kingdom. They have been known as animal pathogens for almost 80 years. However, because they are fastidious and slow growing in culture, they have been recognized as human gastrointestinal pathogens only during the last 15 years. They can cause diarrheal illnesses, systemic infection, type B gastritis, and peptic ulcer disease.

   Table 23-1 lists the *Campylobacter* species known to be pathogenic for humans. *Campylobacter jejuni* and, less often, *C coli* and *C laridis* are the most common bacterial causes of acute diarrheal illness in developed countries. *Helicobacter pylori* (formerly known as *C pylori*), which was first cultured from gastric biopsy tissues in 1982, causes type B gastritis and may be associated with the pathogenesis of peptic ulcer disease. *Campylobacter fetus* subsp *fetus* occasionally causes systemic illnesses in compromised hosts.

CAMPYLOBACTER JEJUNI AND OTHER ENTERIC CAMPYLOBACTERS

CLINICAL MANIFESTATIONS

The symptoms and signs of *Campylobacter* enteritis are not distinctive enough to differentiate it from illness caused by many other enteric pathogens. Symptoms range from mild gastrointestinal distress lasting 24 hours to a fulminating or relapsing colitis that mimics ulcerative colitis or Crohn's disease (Fig. 23-1). The predominant symptoms experienced by individuals in developed countries are diarrhea, abdominal pain, fever, nausea, and vomiting. A history of grossly bloody stools is common, and many patients have at least 1 day with eight or more bowel movements; fecal leukocytes are usually present. A choleralike illness with massive watery diarrhea may also occur. Most patients re-

TABLE 23-1 *Campylobacter* and *Helicobacter* Species Associated with Clinical Manifestations of Human Infection

Enteric Group	Gastric Group
C jejuni	*H pylori*
C coli	Gastric *Campylobacter*-like organisms
C lari	
C fetus	
C upsaliensis	
C hyointestinalis	
C cryaerophila	
C cineadi	
C fennelliae	

cover within a week, but 10 to 20 percent experience relapse or a prolonged severe illness. **Toxic megacolon, pseudomembranous colitis, and massive lower gastrointestinal hemorrhage** also have been described. Mesenteric adenitis and appendicitis have been reported in children and young adults.

Among populations in developing countries, infection by *C jejuni* and closely related organisms is associated with much milder illness, without

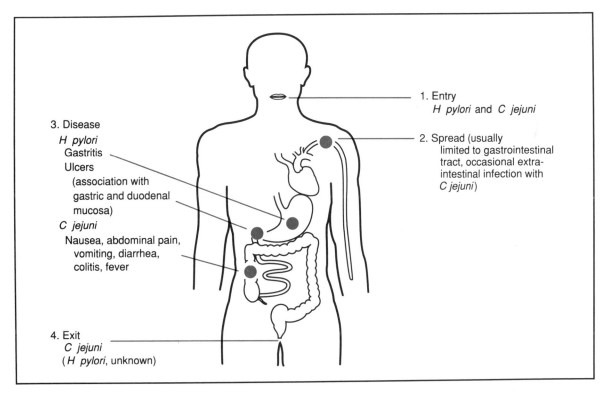

FIGURE 23-1 Pathogenesis of *Campylobacter* and *Helicobacter* infection in humans.

bloody diarrhea, fever, or fecal leukocytes. Asymptomatic infection is much more common than in the developed countries, especially in older children and adults. However, when travelers from developed countries acquire *C jejuni* infections in developing countries, the symptoms are those associated with an inflammatory process. This indicates that organisms in the developing countries are fully pathogenic.

STRUCTURE

Campylobacter jejuni, like all *Campylobacter* species, is a microaerophilic, nonfermentative, Gram-negative organism. The name *Campylobacter*, meaning "curved rod," describes the appearance of the organisms (Fig. 23-2). In young cultures, organisms are comma shaped, spiral, S shaped, or gull-winged shaped; as cultured age or are subjected to atmospheric or temperature stresses, round or coccoid forms appear.

C jejuni, which is structurally similar to other Gram-negative bacilli, is motile, with single flagella at one or both poles of the cell. The cell envelope has an inner bipolar lipoprotein cell membrane, a thin peptidoglycan layer, an outer bipolar lipoprotein layer with the lipid moiety of a lipopolysaccharide layer embedded in it, and the carbohydrate portion extending to the surface of the cell. Interspersed in the outer membrane layer are membrane proteins, some of which are exposed to the surface and are antigenic for infected hosts. Many *Campylobacter* species contain surface proteins that are external to the outer membrane. *Campylobacter* lipopolysaccharide has endotoxin activity similar to that of other Gram-negative bacteria.

All *Campylobacter* species except *H pylori* are similar in structure and appearance. The *Campylobacter* and *Helicobacter* species and subspecies may be differentiated by biochemical markers (Table 23-2).

CLASSIFICATION AND ANTIGENIC TYPES

Based on heat-labile antigens, at least 91 serogroups of both *C jejuni* and *C coli* have been de-

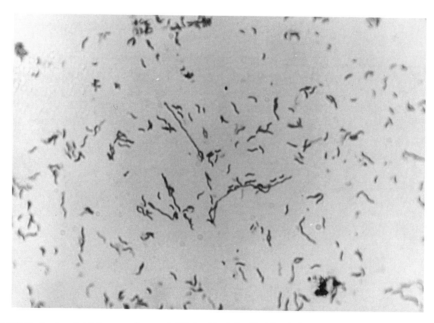

FIGURE 23-2 Forty-eight-hour culture of *C jejuni* (originally King's "related vibrios") showing typical thin, comma-, S-, or gull-winged shaped forms. In broth cultures, chained organisms may appear as elongated forms. All forms are Gram negative and motile. (× 1,000.) (Courtesy of Robert Weaver, Ph.D.)

TABLE 23-2   Differentiation of *Campylobacter* and *Helicobacter* Species Related to Human Disease

					Test				
						Growth			
Species	Catalase	H_2S	Hippurate Test	Urease Activity	25°C	37°C	42°C	Ceph[a]	NA[b]
C jejuni	+	+	+	−	−	+	+	R	S
C coli	+	+	−	−	−	+	+	R	R
C lari	+	+	−	−	−	+	+	S	S
C upsaliensis	−/w[c]	+	−	−	−	+	+	S	S
C fetus subsp *fetus*	+	v[d]	−	−	+	+	v	S	R
C cineadi	w	+	−	−	−	+	−	S	S
C fennelliae	w	+	−	−	−	+	−	S	S
H pylori	+	+	−	+	−	+	−	S	R

[a] Ceph, Cephalothin.
[b] NA, Nalidixic acid.
[c] w, Weak positive.
[d] v, Variable.

scribed. In addition, 42 and 18 different heat-stable somatic (O) antigens have been described among isolates of *C jejuni* and *C coli* organisms, respectively. Although geographic differences in the prevalence of serogroups exist, 10 O groups account for about 70 percent of human infections. Similarly, only a few serogroups account for most human isolates in any geographic region. Serotyping has been of value in numerous epidemiologic investigations.

Despite the antigenic diversity of these organisms, *C jejuni* possesses several common surface-exposed antigens, which have been used for development of serologic tests. Major antigens include the **porin protein** (M_r 45,000), **flagellin** (M_r 63,000), and a protein (M_r 30,000) of unknown function. The flagellar proteins undergo both on-off switching and antigenic phase variation.

PATHOGENESIS

As with other enteric pathogens, the attack rate of *C jejuni* enteritis varies with the ingested dose. In outbreaks of *Campylobacter* enteritis, the incubation period has ranged from 1 to 7 days, with most illness developing 2 to 4 days after infection.

Infection leads to multiplication of organisms in the intestines. Patients shed 10^6 to 10^9 *Campylobacter* cells/g of feces, concentrations similar to those shed in *Salmonella* and *Shigella* enteric infections. The sites of tissue injury include the small and large intestines, and the lesions are acute exudative and hemorrhagic inflammations.

Severely ill patients frequently have colonic involvement, consisting of inflammation of the lamina propria with neutrophils, eosinophils, and mononuclear cells. Destruction of epithelial glands with crypt abscess formation occurs in severe cases (Fig. 23-3). The pathologic lesions seen in *Campylobacter* colitis are indistinguishable from those in ulcerative colitis. Therefore, before ulcerative colitis can be diagnosed, *C jejuni* infection must be ruled out.

The mechanisms by which *C jejuni* causes illness are uncertain. Cellular infiltration in colonic biopsy specimens of patients with *Campylobacter* infections and the occasional presence of bacteremia suggest that these organisms may be invasive. That most *Campylobacter* enteritis in developed countries is associated with fever and the presence of fecal leukocytes and blood in the stool also suggests the invasive characteristics of the organisms. *Campylobacter jejuni* is invasive in vitro in chicken embryo cells and causes bacteremia in experimentally infected mice, rabbits, calves, and chickens.

Some *C jejuni* isolates elaborate cytotoxins similar to Shiga toxin, but in very low titer. Moreover, several isolates elaborate an enterotoxin similar to

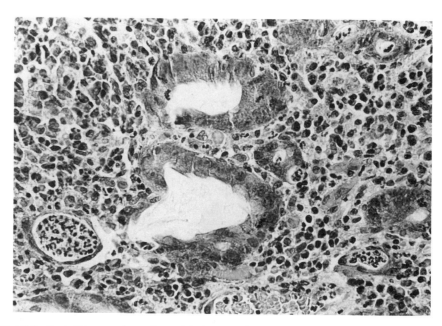

FIGURE 23-3 Rectal biopsy of a patient with *Campylobacter* colitis. There is increased cellularity of the lamina propria with neutrophils, plasma cells, and eosinophils. Glandular epithelial cells are degenerated and thinned, with loss of goblet cells. A crypt abscess is present (lower left). (Hematoxylin and eosin stain; × 250.)

cholera toxin. Enterotoxin production has been more frequently observed in isolates from developing countries, where infection by *C jejuni* has been associated with watery diarrhea. However, the clinical significance of the toxigenicity of these organisms is still unclear. *Campylobacter jejuni* may adhere in vitro to several tissue culture lines. This may be important in intestinal colonization or may enhance tissue invasion. However, the actual in vivo significance of adherence remains undefined.

HOST DEFENSES

Campylobacter jejuni and related organisms are capable of infecting healthy persons as well as immunocompromised patients. The minimal infection-causing dose of *C jejuni* is not known, although volunteers who have ingested as few as 800 organisms have become ill. *Campylobacter jejuni* can be killed by hydrochloric acid, suggesting that normal gastric acidity may be an important barrier against infection. Neutrophils often are

observed in the feces of patients infected with *C jejuni*, and colonic biopsy specimens from patients with *Campylobacter* colitis have shown marked infiltration with neutrophils, suggesting that these cells may be important in host defense. In mice, macrophages are important for clearance of bacteremia and, in vitro, *C jejuni* antigens stimulate a T-cell response.

Acutely infected persons frequently develop elevated specific serum immunoglobulin A (IgA), IgG, and IgM titers, which may persist for several weeks. Experimentally infected animals and humans manifest specific intestinal IgA production. Whether the antibody response eliminates the infection or protects against reinfection is not known. However, upon challenge with *C jejuni*, human volunteers with elevated specific serum IgA levels were likely to develop asymptomatic infection with only a brief duration of pathogen excretion. In contrast, hypogammaglobulinemic persons and those with acquired immune deficiency syndrome (AIDS) are at increased risk for severe, recurrent, or bacteremic infections. *Campylobacter jejuni* isolates are usually susceptible to complement-mediated killing by normal serum. Regardless of the exact host defense mechanisms involved, most *C jejuni* infections resolve spontaneously.

EPIDEMIOLOGY

In developed countries *C jejuni* is an important cause of diarrhea, particularly in children and young adults (Fig. 23-4). Between 3 and 14 percent of patients with diarrhea who seek medical attention are infected with *C jejuni*. Asymptomatic carriers are rare. The attack rate is highest in children less than 1 year old and gradually decreases throughout childhood. A second peak occurs in young adults (18 to 29 years old). Although *C jejuni* enteritis occurs throughout the year, the highest isolation rates occur in summer, as with other enteric pathogens.

In contrast, up to 40 percent of healthy children in developing countries may carry the organism at any time. This is an age-related phenomenon, with the highest excretion rates in very young children. Case-to-infection ratios decline with age, which probably is indicative of acquisition of immunity due to recurrent exposure.

The ultimate reservoir for *C jejuni* is the gastrointestinal tract of many wild animals and a variety of domestic animals, including food animals (cattle, sheep, poultry, swine, and goats). More than 50 percent of poultry sold in the United States is contaminated with *C jejuni*. Transmission from food sources accounts for most human infections. Rodents and pets (including dogs, cats, and birds) also may transmit infection to humans, and excreta from wild animals may contaminate water supplies. Therefore, *C jejuni* infection may be transmitted via food, water, or direct contact with infected animals; in rare cases it may be transmitted from person to person.

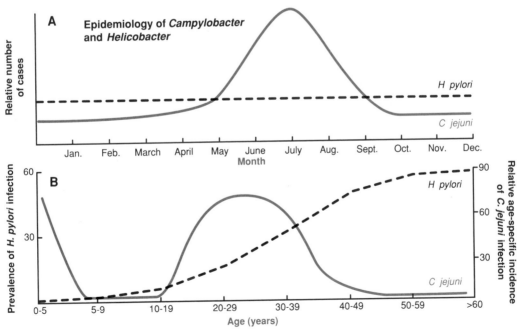

FIGURE 23-4 Comparison of the epidemiology of *C jejuni* (——) and *H pylori* (- - - -) by seasonal distribution by month (*A*) and by age (*B*) in the United States.

DIAGNOSIS

Campylobacter enteritis is hard to tell from enteritis caused by other pathogens. The presence of neutrophils or blood in the feces of patients with acute diarrheal illnesses is an important clue to *Campylobacter* infection. Darting motility in a fresh fecal specimen or characteristic vibrio forms visible after Gram staining permit a presumptive diagnosis. The Diagnosis is confirmed by isolating the organism from a fecal culture or, rarely, a blood culture (Fig. 23-5). Because of its growth requirement for a microaerobic atmosphere, special laboratory methods are needed to isolate *C jejuni*. Plating methods must be selective to inhibit the growth of competing microorganisms in the fecal flora. The traditional approach to isolating *C jejuni* has been to use media that contain antibiotics to which *C jejuni* is resistant but most members of the usual flora are susceptible. However, owing to their motility and small diameter, *Campylobacter* organisms have been isolated by filtration methods that do not use antibiotic-containing media. Use of filters (pore size, 0.6 μm) in conjunction with nonselective media improves stool culture yields of both *C jejuni* and the atypical enteric campylobacters.

Because *Campylobacter* is microaerophilic, cultures must be incubated in an environment with reduced oxygen, optimally between 5 and 10 percent. However, *C jejuni* will also grow in candle jars. The optimal temperature for growth is 42°C for *C jejuni* and 37°C for many of the other enteric camphylobacters. When selective methods are used, suspicious colonies can be readily identified by their spreading character, mucoid appearance, and grayish color. The series of biochemical reactions outlined in Table 23-2 can identify the *Campylobacter* species. Serologic methods for diagnosis are only research tools at present. Recently, a nonradioactive gene probe has become available for rapid identification of *C jejuni* and *C coli* from isolated colonies.

CONTROL

Control of *Campylobacter* enteritis depends largely on interrupting the transmission of the organism to humans from farm and domestic animals, food of animal origin, or contaminated water. Individuals can reduce the risk of *Campylobacter* infection by properly cooking and storing meat and dairy products, avoiding contaminated drinking water and unpasteurized milk, and washing their hands after contact with animals or animal products.

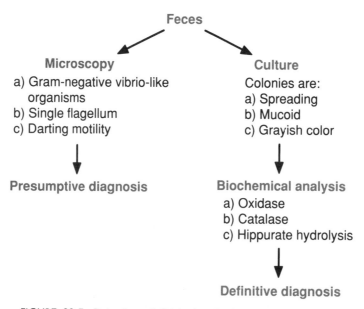

FIGURE 23-5   Detection of *C jejuni* and related enteric bacteria.

Specific treatment with antimicrobial agents appears indicated for persons with severe or prolonged symptoms. However, for mild infections the efficacy of treatment with antimicrobial agents has not yet been demonstrated. When treatment is required, erythromycin and ciprofloxacin appear to be the agents of choice.

The presence of several surface-exposed, broadly specific proteins may permit vaccine development.

HELICOBACTER PYLORI AND OTHER GASTRIC CAMPYLOBACTER-LIKE ORGANISMS

CLINICAL MANIFESTATIONS

Helicobacter pylori (sometimes called gastric *Campylobacter*-like organism, or GCLO) has repeatedly been shown to be associated with type B gastritis, which involves principally the antrum of the stomach (Fig. 23-1). Higher percentages of patients with gastritis than without gastritis harbor *H pylori*. Even though these reports have been criticized for the selected nature of the patients (most were undergoing endoscopy for upper abdominal symptoms) or observer bias, the increase in frequency of *H pylori* in the patients with gastritis is significant. In studies of asymptomatic volunteers who underwent endoscopy and biopsies of gastric mucosa, there was essentially universal correlation of *H pylori* with histologic gastritis. *Helicobacter pylori* evidently does not colonize gastric adenocarcinoma tissue, but colonizes adjacent noncancerous tissue. The relative specificity of *H pylori* for certain histologic and topographic forms of gastritis suggests that it causes gastritis rather than being merely a commensal in the stomach. The organisms are present on the luminal surface of mucus-secreting cells and within gastric pits, but usually do not invade tissue. Colonization of the affected areas of the gastric mucosa is patchy (heavily colonized areas are adjacent to those with no colonization). Organisms are generally not present over areas of intestinal metaplasia in the gastric mucosa. Essentially all patients with duodenal ulcers harbor *H pylori* in the duodenum. In duodenal ulcer disease, *H pylori* is associated with gastric metaplasia, but not with normal duodenal mucosa. This is further evidence of the specificity of the organisms for gastric-type epithelial cells. Antral gastritis is nearly always present in patients with either gastric or duodenal ulcers.

STRUCTURE

Helicobacter pylori differs genetically from other members of the genus *Campylobacter* and has been reclassified from *Campylobacter* to the separate genus *Helicobacter*. It further differs from other campylobacters in having multiple sheathed flagella (Fig. 23-6), a unique composition of fatty acids, and a smooth rather than wrinkled surface. Most campylobacters contain either unipolar or bipolar single unsheathed flagella and have a wrinkled surface. *Helicobacter pylori* organisms are small, microaerophilic, nonsporulating, Gram-negative bacteria. They are curved rods, 3.5 μm long and 0.5 to 1 μm wide, with a spiral periodicity. Unlike other campylobacters, *H pylori* produces urease and does not grown when incubated below 30°C. Growth is poor in most liquid media; either a blood or a hemin source appears essential. Growth is best on chocolate or blood agar plates after incubation for 2 to 5 days.

CLASSIFICATION AND ANTIGENIC TYPES

The antigenic nature of *H pylori* has not been completely defined. The whole-cell and outer membrane profiles of all *H pylori* isolates have major similarities and are substantially different from those of *C jejuni* and *C fetus*. However, *H pylori* does have strain-specific protein and lipopolysaccharide antigens, so it may be possible to type the organism. Simple systems for biotyping and serotyping *H pylori* are not yet available, but strains can be differentiated by restriction endonuclease analysis.

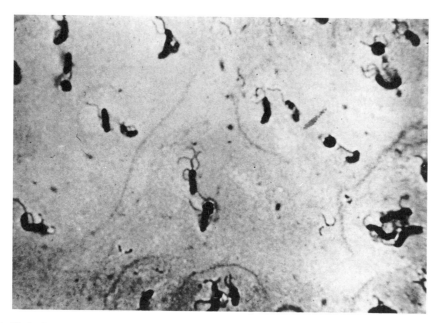

FIGURE 23-6 Seventy-two-hour culture of *H pylori* showing typical thin, comma- or S-shaped forms. All forms are Gram -negative and motile with multiple sheathed flagella. Old cultures may present coccoid forms. (× 1,000.) (Courtesy of Donna R. Morgan, Ph.D.)

PATHOGENESIS

Helicobacter pylori cells are readily killed by brief exposure to hydrochloric acid solutions with pH below 4.0. This is paradoxical for an organism whose primary residence is the gastric lumen. However, several factors may explain this phenomenon. Firstly, *H pylori* lives in the mucus layer overlaying the gastric mucosa, a niche protected against gastric acid. This mucus is relatively thick and viscous and maintains a pH gradient from approximately pH 2 adjacent to the gastric lumen to pH 7.4 immediately above the epithelial cell. Secondly, *H pylori* is among the most efficient producers of urease. An important effect of this metabolic activity is the release of ammonia, which buffers acidity. Third, *H pylori* is highly motile in even very viscous mucus. This motility may allow organisms to migrate to the most favorable pH. Finally, acute *H pylori* infection is associated with hypochlorhydria.

Inflammatory infiltrates with polymorphonuclear leukocytes, eosinophils, and an increased number of lymphocytes are observed in the epithelium and lamina propria (Fig. 23-7). The exact mechanism by which *H pylori* causes tissue injury is unknown. At present there is little evidence for direct tissue invasion by *H pylori*. Pathogenic organisms that do not invade tissue may elaborate exotoxins. A heat-labile, trypsin-sensitive extracellular product of *H pylori* that is cytotoxic to tissue culture cell lines has been described. *Helicobacter pylori* also appears to affect the gastric mucus layer in which it resides. Isolates cultured in vitro produce an extracellular protease. This proteolytic activity affects the ability of mucus to retard the diffusion of hydrogen ions. Mucus depletion over inflamed tissues is characteristic of *H pylori*-associated gastritis.

HOST DEFENSES

Although gastric acid plays an important role in protection against many enteric organisms, it is not a sufficient barrier to prevent colonization of the gastric mucosa by *H pylori*. Infected persons develop high titers of serum and local IgA and IgG antibodies to *H pylori*. Longitudinal serologic

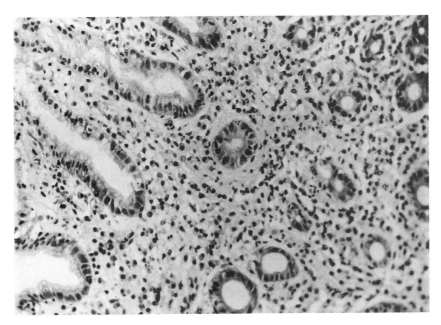

FIGURE 23-7   Antral gastric biopsy from a patient with *H pylori* gastritis. There is increased cellularity of the epithelium and lamina propria with neutrophils, eosinophils, and lymphocytes. (Hematoxylin and eosin stain, × 100.) (Courtesy of Donna R. Morgan, Ph.D.)

studies show that *H pylori* can persist despite these high antibody levels. It is not known whether these specific antibodies play any protective role, such as inhibiting adherence or promoting opsonophagocytosis. The role of cell-mediated immunity to these persistent pathogens has not been explored.

EPIDEMIOLOGY

Helicobacter pylori is found worldwide and affects persons from diverse socioeconomic strata. The prevalence of these infections, as documented by both histologic and serologic studies, rises with age, as does that of gastritis. The source and mechanism of transmission of *H pylori* are unknown. Spiral organisms are common in the mouth and the lower intestinal tract in all mammals; accordingly, these areas are potential reservoirs for *H pylori*. However, neither culture nor histologic studies have identified the organisms in sites outside the human stomach and duodenum. *Helicobacter pylori* is frequently isolated from asympto-

matic persons who have no dyspeptic or ulcer-related symptoms. There is now evidence that *H pylori* infection is more common among populations in developing areas than in more industrialized countries. Infection, defined by confirmed seropositivity, persists for years and possibly for life. If seropositivity reflects acquisition of *H pylori*, as suggested by several studies, the annual incidence in adult populations in developed countries is approximately 1 percent.

Other gastric *Campylobacter*-like organisms have now been observed in a variety of animals, including rodents, primates, and swine. Ferret isolates are clearly different from human isolates, but organisms from swine and other primates appear similar, if not identical. Human exposure to nonhuman primates is not sufficiently frequent to explain the wide prevalence of *H pylori* infection in humans. Food-borne transmission would not be unusual for an enteric pathogen, but no other environmental reservoirs of *H pylori* have been identified. Person-to-person transmission remains a possibility.

DIAGNOSIS

To date, *H pylori* has been isolated exclusively from gastric tissue or from biopsies of esophageal or duodenal tissue containing gastric metaplasia (Fig. 23-8). *Helicobacter pylori* can be presumptively identified in freshly prepared gastric biopsy smears by phase-contrast microscopy, based on the characteristic motility of the microorganisms, and by staining histologic sections from gastric biopsies with Gram (carbol fuchsin counterstain), Warthin-Starry silver, Giemsa, or acridine orange stain. Gastric *Campylobacter*-like organisms can also be seen directly in fixed tissue stained with hematoxylin and eosin. *Helicobacter pylori* infections are diagnosed by isolating the microorganism from gastric biopsy specimens, using nonselective media, such as chocolate agar, or antibiotic-containing selective media, such as those of Skirrow or Goodwin. Spiral organisms that are oxidase, catalase, and urease positive can be identified as *H pylori*. In gastric biopsies, *H pylori* can be diagnosed presumptively on the basis of the presence of preformed urease.

All of the above tests require endoscopy and biopsy. Recently, a noninvasive technique known as the urea breath test has been developed to diagnose *H pylori* infection. Infection can also be diagnosed accurately by detecting serum antibodies to *H pylori* antigens. Serologic methods will greatly facilitate diagnosis in individual patients and aid studies of the epidemiology of this newly recognized infection.

CONTROL

To date, the mechanisms of transmission and source of infection remain unknown. Therefore, control of *H pylori* infections is problematic. The role of antimicrobial therapy for treatment of this infection is uncertain at present.

OTHER PATHOGENIC
CAMPYLOBACTER
SPECIES

Campylobacter fetus subsp *fetus,* well known as an animal pathogen, may cause bacteremia and other extraintestinal infections in compromised hosts, as

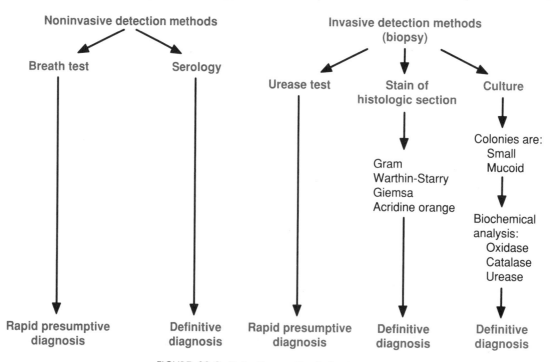

FIGURE 23-8 Detection methods for *H pylori.*

well as an uncommon self-limited diarrheal illness in previously healthy persons. Recognized complications of *C fetus* infection include meningitis, endocarditis, pneumonia, thrombophlebitis, septicemia, arthritis, and peritonitis.

Campylobacter fetus shares with most of the other *Campylobacter* species the characteristics mentioned above. However, it has some specific properties. Virtually all *C fetus* isolates from humans possess lipopolysaccharide molecules with long polysaccharide side chains. Two major serogroups, A and B, are identified. A microcapsule of high-molecular-weight, antigenically related surface array proteins has been associated with serum and phagocytosis resistance. These proteins apparently mediate serum resistance by inhibiting the binding of complement component C3b, thereby conferring to the organism a significant survival advantage.

Campylobacter cinaedi and *C fennelliae* are two newly recognized *Campylobacter* species, which have been associated with enteric and extraintestinal diseases in homosexual men and in travelers to developing countries.

REFERENCES

Blaser MJ: *Helicobacter pylori* and the pathogenesis of gastroduodenal inflammation. J Infect Dis 161:626–633, 1990.

Blaser MJ, Berkowitz ID, LaForie FM et al: *Campylobacter* enteritis: clinical and epidemiologic features. Ann Intern Med 91:179, 1979

Butzler JP, Skirrow MB: *Campylobacter* enteritis. Clin Gastroenterol 8:737, 1979

Cover TL, Blaser MJ: The pathobiology of *Campylobacter* infections in humans. Annu Rev Med 40:269, 1989

Dooley CP, Cohen H, Fitzgibbons PL et al: Prevalence of *Helicobacter pylori* infection and histologic gastritis in asymptomatic persons. N Engl J Med 321:1562, 1989

Goodwin CS, Armstrong JA, Chilvers T et al: Transfer of *Campylobacter pylori* and *Campylobacter mustelae* to *Helicobacter* gen. nov. as *Helicobacter pylori* comb. nov. and *Helicobacter mustelae* comb. nov. respectively. Int J Syst Bacteriol 39:397, 1989

Graham DY, Klein PD, Evans DJ, Jr, et al: *Campylobacter pylori* detected non-invasively by the ^{13}C-urea breath test. Lancet 1:1174, 1988

King EO: The laboratory recognition of *Vibrio fetus* and a closely related vibrio isolated from cases of human vibriosis. Ann NY Acad Sci 98:700, 1962

Penner JL: The genus *Campylobacter:* a decade of progress. Clin Microbiol Rev 1:157, 1988

Perez-Perez GI, Dworkin BM, Chodos JE, Blaser MJ: *Campylobacter pylori* antibodies in humans. Ann Intern Med 109:11, 1988

Smibert RM: Genus *Campylobacter*. p. 111. In Krieg NR, Holt HG (eds): Bergey's Manual of Systematic Bacteriology. Vol 1. Williams & Wilkins, Baltimore, 1984

Tauxe RV, Patton CM, Edmonds P et al: Illness associated with *Campylobacter laridis,* a newly recognized *Campylobacter* species. J Clin Microbiol 21:222, 1985

24 VIBRIO CHOLERAE AND OTHER PATHOGENIC VIBRIOS

RICHARD A. FINKELSTEIN

GENERAL CONCEPTS

VIBRIO CHOLERAE

Clinical Manifestations

Vibrio cholerae may cause mild or inapparent infection or **cholera,** a life-threatening secretory diarrhea characterized by voluminous, watery stools, often accompanied by vomiting and resulting in acidosis and hypovolemic shock.

Structure, Classification, and Antigenic Types

Vibrios are Gram-negative, highly motile curved rods with a single polar flagellum. They tolerate alkaline media that kill most intestinal commensals, but they are sensitive to acid. Numerous free-living vibrios are known, some potentially pathogenic. Cholera is caused by only two serotypes, **Inaba (AC)** and **Ogawa (AB),** and two biotypes, **classic** and **El Tor,** of toxigenic O group 1 *V cholerae*. These organisms may be identified by agglutination in O group 1-specific antiserum directed against the lipopolysaccharide component of the cell wall and by demonstration of their enterotoxigenicity.

Pathogenesis

Cholera is transmitted by the fecal-oral route. Vibrios are sensitive to acid, and most die in the stomach. Surviving virulent organisms may adhere to and colonize the small bowel, where they secrete the potent cholera enterotoxin (CT), **choleragen.** This toxin binds to the plasma membrane of intestinal epithelial cells and re-

leases an enzymatically active subunit that causes a rise in cyclic adenosine 5^1-monophosphate (cAMP) production. The resulting high intracellular cAMP level causes massive secretion of electrolytes and water into the intestinal lumen.

Host Defenses

Gastric acid, mucus secretion, and intestinal motility are the prime nonspecific defenses against *V cholerae*. Breast-feeding in endemic areas is important in protecting infants from disease. Disease results in effective specific immunity, involving primarily secretory immunoglobulin (IgA), as well as IgG antibodies, against vibrios, somatic antigen, outer membrane protein, and/or the enterotoxin and other products.

Epidemiology

Cholera is endemic or epidemic in areas with poor sanitation; it occurs sporadically or as limited outbreaks in developed countries. In coastal regions it may persist in shellfish and plankton. Long-term convalescent carriers are rare. Enteritis caused by the halophile *V parahaemolyticus* is associated with raw or improperly cooked seafood.

Diagnosis

The diagnosis is suggested by strikingly severe, watery diarrhea. For rapid diagnosis, a wet mount of liquid stool is examined microscopically. The characteristic

351

motility of vibrios is stopped by specific antisomatic antibody. Other methods are culture of stool or rectal swab samples on TCBS agar and other selective and nonselective media; the slide agglutination test of colonies with specific antiserum; fermentation tests (oxidase positive); and enrichment in peptone broth followed by fluorescent antibody tests, culture, or retrospective serologic diagnosis.

Control

Control by sanitation is effective but not feasible in endemic areas. A good vaccine has not yet been developed. A parenteral vaccine of whole killed bacteria has been used widely, but is relatively ineffective. An experimental oral vaccine of killed whole cells and toxin B-subunit protein is less than ideal. Living attenuated genetically engineered mutants are promising, but cause limited diarrhea as a side effect. Antibiotic prophylaxis is feasible for small groups over short periods.

OTHER *VIBRIO* INFECTIONS

Other serogroups of *V cholerae* may cause diarrheal disease and other infections but are not associated with epidemic cholera. *Vibrio parahaemolyticus* is an important cause of enteritis associated with the ingestion of raw or improperly prepared seafood. Other *Vibrio* species including *V vulnificus* can cause infections of humans and other animals including fish. *Campylobacter* species (formerly included with vibrios) can cause enteritis. *C pylori*, now known as *Helicobacter pylori*, is associated with gastric and duodenal ulcers (see Ch. 23).

INTRODUCTION

Vibrios are highly motile, Gram-negative, curved or comma-shaped rods with a single polar flagellum. Of the vibrios that are clinically significant to humans, *Vibrio cholerae* O group 1, the agent of cholera, is the most important. *Vibrio cholerae* was first isolated in pure culture by Robert Koch in 1883, although it had been seen by other investigators, including Pacini, who is credited with describing it first in Florence in 1854.

Cholera is a life-threatening secretory diarrhea induced by an enterotoxin secreted by *V cholerae*. Cholera and the cholera enterotoxin are increasingly recognized as the prototypes for a wide variety of diarrheal disease, collectively known as the **enterotoxic enteropathies;** of these, diarrhea due to enterotoxigenic strains of *Escherichia coli* (see Ch. 26) are the most important. Cholera remains a major epidemic disease. There have been seven great pandemics, the latest having started in 1961.

Other vibrios may also be clinically significant in humans, and some are known to cause diseases in domestic animals. Nonpathogenic vibrios are widely distributed in the environment, particularly in estuarine waters and seafoods. For this reason, isolation of a vibrio from a patient with diarrheal disease does not necessarily indicate an etiologic relationship.

◀ *VIBRIO CHOLERAE* ▶

CLINICAL MANIFESTATIONS

Following an incubation period of 6 to 48 hours, cholera begins with the abrupt onset of watery diarrhea (Fig. 24-1). The initial stool may exceed 1 L, and several liters of fluid may be secreted within hours, leading to hypovolemic shock. Vomiting usually accompanies the diarrheal episodes. Muscle cramps may occur as water and electrolytes are lost from body tissues. Loss of skin turgor, scaphoid abdomen, and weak pulse are characteristic of cholera. Various degrees of fluid and electrolyte loss are observed, including mild and subclinical cases. The disease runs its course in 2 to 7 days; the outcome depends upon the extent of water and electrolyte loss and the adequacy of water and electrolyte repletion therapy. Death can

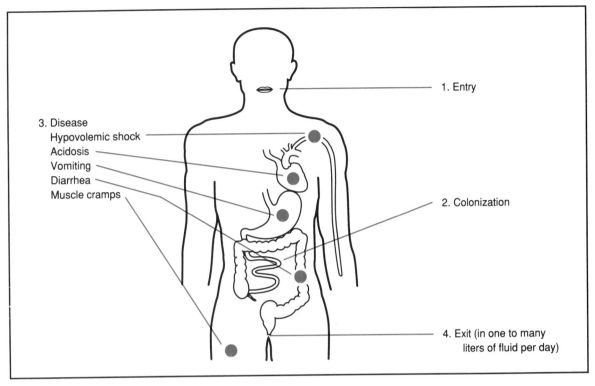

FIGURE 24-1   Pathophysiology of cholera.

occur from hypovolemic shock, metabolic acidosis, and uremia resulting from acute tubular necrosis.

STRUCTURE, CLASSIFICATION, AND ANTIGENIC TYPES

The cholera vibrios (*V cholerae* group O1) are Gram-negative, slightly curved rods whose motility depends on a single polar flagellum. Their nutritional requirements are simple. Fresh isolates are prototrophic (i.e., they grow in media containing an inorganic nitrogen source, a utilizable carbohydrate, and appropriate minerals). In adequate media, they grow rapidly with a generation time of less than 30 minutes. Although they reach higher population densities when grown with vigorous aeration, they can also grow anaerobically. Vibrios are sensitive to low pH and die rapidly in solutions below pH6; however, they are quite tolerant of alkaline conditions. This tolerance has been exploited in the choice of media used for their isolation and diagnosis.

The vibrios that cause epidemic cholera have been subdivided into two biotypes: **classic** and **El Tor.** Classic *V cholerae* was first isolated by Koch. Subsequently, in the early 1900s, some vibrios resembling *V cholerae* were isolated from Mecca-bound pilgrims at the quarantine station at El Tor that had been established to try to control cholera in the Sinai peninsula. These vibrios resembled classic *V cholerae* in many ways but caused lysis of goat or sheep erythrocytes in a test known as the Greig test. Because the pilgrims from whom they were isolated did not have cholera, these hemolytic El Tor vibrios were regarded as relatively insignificant except for the possibility of confusion with true cholera vibrios. In the 1930s, similar hemolytic vibrios were associated with relatively restricted outbreaks of diarrheal disease, called **paracholera,** in the Celebes. In 1961, cholera caused by El Tor vibrios erupted in Hong Kong and

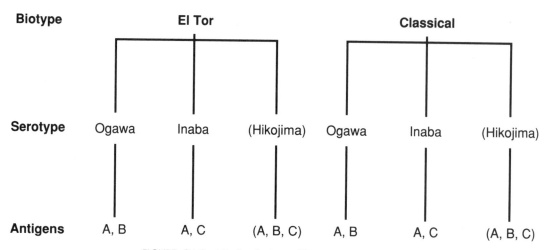

FIGURE 24-2 *Vibrio cholerae* (O group 1 antigen).

spread virtually worldwide. Although in the course of this pandemic most *V cholerae* biotype El Tor strains lost their hemolytic activity, a number of ancillary tests differentiate them from vibrios of the classic biotype.

The operational serology of the cholera vibrios, which belong in O antigen group 1 is relatively simple. Both biotypes (El Tor and classic) contain two major serotypes, **Inaba** and **Ogawa** (Fig. 24-2). These serotypes are differentiated in agglutination and vibriocidal antibody tests on the basis of their dominant heat-stable lipopolysaccharide somatic antigens. The cholera group has a common antigen, **A,** and the serotypes are differentiated by the type-specific antigens, **B (Ogawa)** and **C (Inaba).** An additional serotype, Hikojima, which has both specific antigens, is rare.

Other antigenic components of the vibrios, such as outer membrane protein antigens, have not been extensively studied. The cholera vibrios also have common flagellar antigens. Cross-reactions with *Brucella* and *Citrobacter* species have been reported. Because of DNA relatedness and other similarities, the *nonagglutinable* vibrios are now classifed as *V cholerae.* The term *nonagglutinable* is a misnomer because it implies that these vibrios are not agglutinable; in fact, they are not agglutinable in antisera against the O antigen group 1 cholera vibrios, but they are agglutinable in their own specific antisera. More than 50 serotypes are now rec-

ognized. Some strains of nonagglutinable vibrios (or non-O group 1 *V cholerae*) cause diarrheal disease by means of an enterotoxin related to the cholera enterotoxin and, perhaps, by other mechanisms, but these strains have not been associated with devastating outbreaks like those caused by the true cholera vibrios. Recently, vibrio strains that agglutinate in some O group 1 cholera diagnostic antisera but not in others have been isolated from environmental sources. Volunteer feeding experiments have shown that these atypical O group 1 vibrios are not enteropathogenic in humans. Recent studies using specific toxin gene probes indicate that the environmental isolates not only are nontoxigenic, but also do not possess any of the genetic information encoding cholera toxin, although some isolates from diarrheal stools do.

The cholera vibrios cause many distinctive reactions. They are oxidase positive. The O group 1 cholera vibrios almost always fall into the Heiberg I fermentation pattern; that is, they ferment sucrose and mannose but not arabinose, and they produce acid but not gas. *Vibrio cholerae* also possesses lysine and ornithine decarboxylase, but not arginine dihydrolase. Freshly isolated agar-grown vibrios of the El Tor biotype, in contrast to classic *V cholerae,* produce a cell-associated mannose-sensitive hemagglutinin active on chicken erythrocytes. This activity is readily detected in a rapid slide test. In addition to hemagglutination, numerous tests have been proposed to differentiate the classic and El Tor biotypes, including production of a hemolysin, sensitivity to selected bacteriophages, sensitivity to polymyxin, and the Voges-Proskauer test for acetoin. El Tor vibrios originally were defined as hemolytic. They differed in this characteristic from classic cholera vibrios; however, during the most recent pandemic, most El Tor vibrios (except for the recent isolates from Texas and Louisiana) had lost the capacity to express the hemolysin. Most El Tor vibrios are Voges-Proskauer positive and resistant to polymyxin and to bacteriophage IV, whereas classic vibrios are sensitive to them. As both biotypes cause the same disease, these characteristics have only epidemiologic significance. Strains of the El Tor biotype, however, produce less cholera enterotoxin, but appear to colonize intestinal epithelium better than vibrios of the classic variety; also, they seem somewhat more resistant to environmental factors. Thus, El Tor strains have a higher tendency to become endemic and exhibit a higher infection-to-case ratio than the classic biotype.

PATHOGENESIS

Recent studies with laboratory animal models and human volunteers have provided a detailed understanding of the pathogenesis of cholera. Initial attempts to infect healthy American volunteers with cholera vibrios revealed that the oral administration of up to 10^{11} living cholera vibrios rarely had an effect; in fact, the organisms usually could not be recovered from stools of the volunteers. After the administration of bicarbonate to neutralize gastric acidity, however, cholera diarrhea developed in most volunteers given 10^4 cholera vibrios. Therefore, gastric acidity itself is a powerful natural resistance mechanism. It also has been demonstrated that vibrios administered with food are much more likely to cause infection.

Cholera is exclusively a disease of the small bowel. To establish residence and multiply in the human small bowel (normally relatively free of bacteria because of the effective clearance mechanisms of peristalsis and mucus secretion), the cholera vibrios have one or more adherence factors that enable them to adhere to the microvilli (Fig. 24-3). Several hemagglutinins and the toxin-coregulated pili have been suggested to be involved in adherence but the actual mechanism has not been defined. The motility of the vibrios may affect virulence by enabling them to penetrate the mucus layer. They also produce mucinolytic enzymes, neuraminidase, and proteases. The growing cholera vibrios elaborate the cholera enterotoxin (CT), **choleragen,** a polymeric protein (M_r 84,000) consisting of two major domains or regions. The A region (M_r 28,000), responsible for biologic activity of the enterotoxin, is linked by noncovalent interactions with the B region (M_r 56,000), which is composed of five identical noncovalently associated peptide chains of M_r 11,500. The B region, also known as **choleragenoid,** binds the toxin to its receptors on host cell membranes. It is also the immunologically dominant portion of the holotoxin. The structural genes that encode the synthesis of CT reside on the *V cholerae* chromosome, in contrast to those for the heat-labile enterotoxins (LTs) of *E coli* (Ch. 25), which are encoded by plasmids. The amino acid sequences of these structurally, functionally, and immunologically related enterotoxins are very similar: their differences account for the differences in physiochemical behavior and the antigenic distinctions that have been noted. There are at least two antigenically related but distinct forms of cholera enterotoxin, called CT-1 and CT-2. *Vibrio cholerae* exports its enterotoxin, whereas the *E coli* LTs occur primarily in the periplasmic space. This may account for the reported differences in severity of the diarrheas caused by these organisms. Studies of adult American volunteers have shown that 5 μg of CT, administered orally with bicarbonate, causes 1 to 6 L of diarrhea; 25 μg causes more than 20 L.

Synthesis of CT and other virulence-associated factors such as toxin-coregulated pili are believed to be regulated by a transcriptional activator, Tox R, a transmembrane DNA-binding protein.

The molecular events in these diarrheal diseases involve an interaction between the enterotoxins and intestinal epithelial cell membranes (Fig. 24-4). The toxins bind through region B to a glycolipid, the G_{M1} ganglioside, which is practically ubiq-

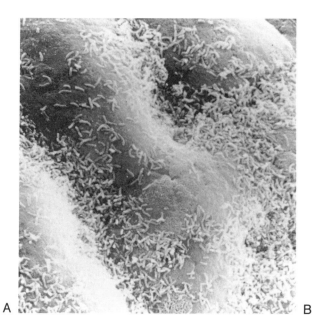

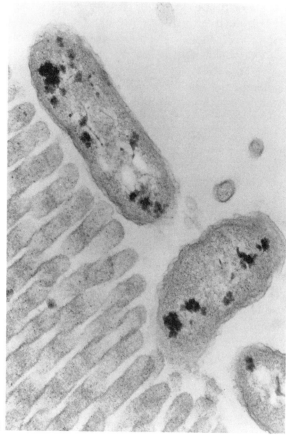

A   B

FIGURE 24-3 *Vibrio cholerae* attachment and colonization in experimental rabbit ileal loops. The events are assumed to be similar in human cholera. *(A)* Scanning electron microscopy during early infection. Curved vibrios adhering to epithelial surface. (Approximately × 4,000.) *(B)* Transmission electron microscopy of vibrios in both end-on and horizontal modes close to tips of microvilli. (From Nelson ET, Clements JD, Finkelstein RA: *Vibrio cholerae* adherence and colonization in experimental cholera: electron microscopic studies. Infect Immun 14:527, 1976, with permission.)

uitous in eukaryotic cell membranes. Following this binding, the A region, or a major portion of it known as the A_1 peptide ($M_r21,000$), penetrates the host cell and enzymatically transfers ADP-ribose from nicotinamide adenine dinucleotide (NAD) to a target protein, the guanosine 5'-triphosphate (GTP)-binding regulatory protein associated with membrane-bound adenylate cyclase. Thus, CT (and LT) resembles diphtheria toxin in causing transfer of ADP-ribose to a substrate. With diphtheria toxin, however, the substrate is elongation factor 2 and the result is cessation of host cell protein synthesis. With CT, the ADP-ribosylation reaction essentially locks adenylate cyclase in its "on mode" and leads to excessive production of cyclic adenosine 5^1-monophosphate (cAMP). Pertussis toxin, another ADP-ribosyl transferase, also increases cAMP levels, but by its effect on another G-protein, G_i (Fig. 24-5). The subsequent cAMP-mediated cascade of events has not yet been delineated, but the final effect is hypersecretion of chloride and bicarbonate followed by water, resulting in the characteristic isotonic voluminous cholera stool. In hospitalized patients,

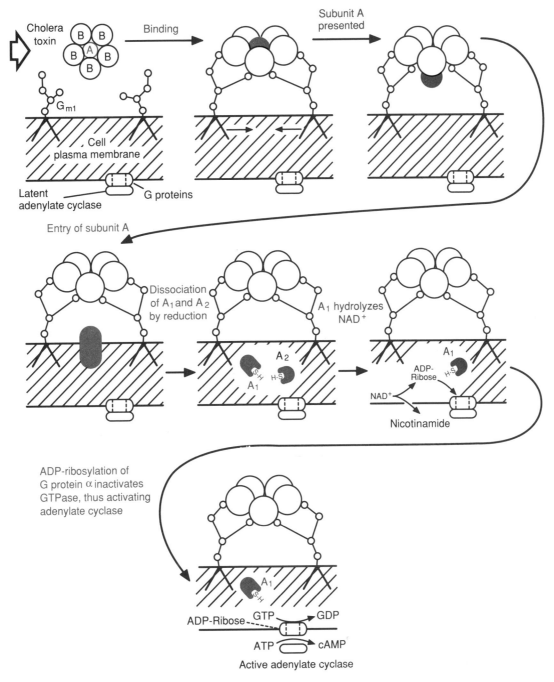

FIGURE 24-4 Mechanism of action of cholera enterotoxin. Cholera toxin approaches target cell surface. B subunits bind to oligosaccharide of G_{M1} ganglioside. Conformational alteration of holotoxin occurs, allowing the presentation of the A subunit to cell surface. The A subunit enters the cell. The disulfide bond of the A subunit is reduced by intracellular glutathione, freeing A_1 and A_2. NAD is hydrolyzed by A_1, yielding ADP-ribose and nicotinamide. One of the G proteins of adenylate cyclase is ADP-ribosylated, inhibiting the action of GTPase and locking adenylate cyclase in the "on" mode. (Modified from Fishman PH: Mechanism of action of cholera toxin: events on the cell surface. p. 85. In Field M, Fordtran JS, Schultz SG (eds): Secretory Diarrhea. Waverly Press, Baltimore, 1980, with permission.)

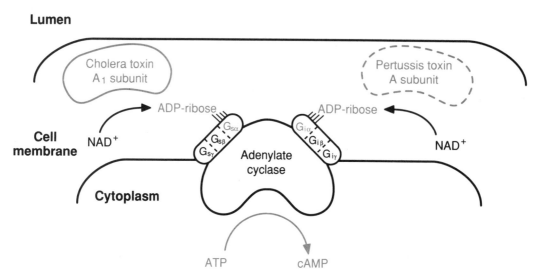

FIGURE 24-5 Comparison of activities of cholera enterotoxin (CT) with pertussis toxin (PT). The α-subunits of G_s and G_i, with GTP-binding sites, are ADP-ribosylated, respectively, by A_1 peptide of CT or by the A subunit of PT, preventing, respectively, the hydrolysis of G_s-GTP to GDP or the responsiveness of G_i to inhibitory hormones, both effectively producing increases in adenylate cyclase activity. (Modified from Gill DM, Woolkalis M: Toxins which activate adenylate cyclase. CIBA Found Symp 112:57, 1985, with permission.)

this can result in losses of 20 L or more of fluid per day. The stool of an actively purging, severely ill cholera patient can resemble rice water — the supernatant of boiled rice. Because the stool can contain 10^8 viable vibrios per ml, such a patient could shed 2×10^{12} cholera vibrios per day into the environment. Perhaps by production of CT, the cholera vibrios thus ensure their survival by increasing the likelihood of finding another human host. Recent evidence suggests that prostaglandins may also play a role in the secretory effects of cholera enterotoxin.

Various animal models have been used to investigate pathogenic mechanisms, virulence, and immunity. Ten-day-old suckling rabbits develop a fulminating diarrheal disease after intraintestinal inoculation with virulent *V cholerae* or CT. Adult rabbits are relatively resistant to colonization by cholera vibrios; however, they do respond, with characteristic outpouring of fluid, to the intraluminal inoculation of live vibrios or enterotoxin in surgically isolated ileal loops. Suckling mice are susceptible to intragastric inoculation of vibrios

and to orally administered toxin. Adult conventional mice are also susceptible to orally administered toxin, but resist colonization except in isolated intestinal loops. Interestingly, however, germ-free mice can be colonized for months with cholera vibrios. They rarely show adverse effects, although they are susceptible to cholera enterotoxin. Dogs have been used experimentally, although they are relatively refractory and require enormous inocula to elicit choleraic manifestations. Chinchillas also are susceptible to diarrhea following intraintestinal inoculation with moderate numbers of cholera vibrios. Infections initiated by extraintestinal routes of inoculation (e.g., intraperitoneal) largely reflect the toxicity of the lipopolysaccharide endotoxin. The intraperitoneal infection in mice has been used to assay the protective effect of conventional killed vibrio vaccines (no longer widely used).

Various animals, including humans, rabbits, and guinea pigs, also respond to intradermal inoculation of relatively minute amounts of CT with a characteristic delayed (maximum response at 24 hours), sustained (visible up to 1 week or more), erythematous, edematous induration associated with a localized alteration of vascular permeability. In laboratory animals, this response can be measured after injecting a protein-binding dye, such as trypan blue, that extravasates to produce a zone of bluing at the site of intracutaneous inoculation of toxin. This observation has been exploited in the assay of CT and its antibody and in the detection of other enterotoxins.

In addition, because of the broad spectrum of activity of CT on cells and tissues that it never contacts in nature, various in vitro systems can be used to assay the enterotoxin and its antibody. In each, the toxin causes a characteristically delayed, but sustained, activation of adenylate cyclase and increased production of cAMP, and it may cause additional, readily recognizable, morphologic alterations of certain cultured cell lines. The cells most widely used for this purpose are Chinese hamster ovary (CHO) cells, which elongate in response to picogram doses of the toxin, and mouse Y-1 adrenal tumor cells, which round up. Cholera toxin has become an extremely valuable experimental probe to identify other cAMP-mediated responses. It also activates adenylate cyclase in pigeon erythrocytes, a procedure that was used by D. Michael Gill to define its mode of action.

These assays and models also have been applied in the study of an expanding number of CT-related and unrelated enterotoxins. These include the LTs of *E coli*, which are structurally and immunologically similar to it and are effective in any model that is responsive to CT. The small molecular weight heat-stable enterotoxin (ST) of *E coli*, which activates guanylate cyclase, is rapidly active in the infant mouse and certain other intestinal models, and is clearly unrelated to CT. CT-related enterotoxins have been reported from certain nonagglutinable (non-O group I) *Vibrio* strains and a *Salmonella* enterotoxin was shown to be related immunologically to CT. CT-like factors from *Shigella* and *V parahaemolyticus* have thus far been demonstrated only in sensitive cell culture systems. Other enterotoxins and enterocytotoxins, which elicit cytotoxic effects on intestinal epithelial cells, also have been described from *Escherichia, Kleb-*

siella, Enterobacter, Citrobacter, Aeromonas, Pseudomonas, Shigella, V parahaemolyticus, Campylobacter, Yersinia enterocolitica, Bacillus cereus, Clostridium perfringens, C difficile, and staphylococci. *Escherichia coli,* some vibrio strains, and some other enteric bacteria produce cytotoxins that, like Shiga toxin of *Shigella dysenteriae,* act on Vero (African green monkey kidney) cells in vitro. These toxins have been called Shiga-like toxins, Shiga toxin-like toxins, Vero toxins, and Vero cytotoxins. The classic staphylococcal enterotoxins perhaps should more properly be called neurotoxins, as they affect the central nervous system rather than the gut directly to cause fluid secretion or histopathologic effects.

HOST DEFENSES

Infection with cholera vibrios results in a spectrum of responses. These range from no observed manifestations except perhaps a serologic response (the most common) to acute purging, which must be treated by hospitalization and fluid replacement therapy; this is the classic response. The reasons for these differences are not entirely clear, although it is known that individuals differ in gastric acidity and that hypochlorhydric individuals are most prone to cholera. Whether individuals differ in the availability of intestinal receptors for cholera vibrios or for their toxin has not been established. Prior immunologic experience of subjects at risk is certainly a major factor. For example, in heavily endemic regions such as Bangladesh, the attack rate is relatively low among adults in comparison with children; in neoepidemic areas, cholera is more frequent among the working adult population. Resistance is related to the presence of circulating antibody and, perhaps more importantly, local immunoglobulin A (IgA) antibody against the cholera bacteria or the cholera enterotoxin or both. Intestinal IgA antibody can prevent attachment of the vibrios to the mucosal surface and neutralize or prevent binding of the cholera enterotoxin. For reasons that are not clear, individuals of blood group O are slightly more susceptible to cholera. Breast-feeding is highly recommended as a means of increasing immunity of infants to this and other diarrheal disease agents.

Recovery from cholera probably depends on two factors: elimination of the vibrios by antibiotics or the patient's own immune response, and regeneration of the poisoned intestinal epithelial cells. Treatment with a single 200-mg dose of doxycycline has been recommended recently. As studies in volunteers demonstrated conclusively, the disease is an immunizing process; patients who have recovered from cholera are solidly immune for at least 3 years.

Cholera vaccines consisting of killed cholera bacteria administered parenterally have been used since the turn of the century; however, recent controlled field studies indicate that little, if any, effective immunity is induced in immunologically virgin populations by such vaccines, although they do stimulate preexisting immunity in the adult population in heavily endemic regions. Controlled studies have likewise shown that a cholera toxoid administered parenterally was ineffective in preventing cholera. Probably the natural disease should be simulated to induce truly effective immunity. Studies of volunteers have shown that a hypotoxigenic mutant of *V cholerae*, administered orally, did stimulate effective immunity. Recently, a mutant strain (called Texas Star-SR) has been isolated that produces the B region of the cholera enterotoxin but no A region and is thus avirulent. This mutant produces effective active immunity in laboratory animal models and in volunteers. However, despite its inability to produce complete cholera toxin, the mutant produced slight diarrhea in some of the volunteers. The results suggest that cholera vibrios may have additional mechanisms of causing intestinal malfunction in addition to the cholera enterotoxin. Perhaps the act of colonization itself is involved or other toxic factors are present. Subsequent studies in volunteers with genetically engineered Tox⁻ or A⁻B⁺ strains have indicated that they caused more severe diarrhea (although not cholera) in a larger proportion of volunteers than the Texas Star strain. If a mutant with no undesirable side effects could stimulate local production of anti-B-subunit antibodies in humans, it might also be effective against the en-

terotoxic enteropathies that depend on choleragen-related enterotoxins. Studies have established, for example, that the plasmid-mediated, *E coli* LT is structurally, immunologically, and functionally related to the cholera enterotoxin and that immunity against cholera toxin is protective against *Salmonella* in an experimental model. Laboratory studies also have shown that orally administered killed bacteria and inactivated cholera toxin or **choleragenoid** stimulate effective immunity. Combined preparations of bacterial somatic antigen and toxin antigen act synergistically in stimulating immunity in laboratory animals; that is, the combined protective effect is closer to the product than to the sum of the individual protective effects. However, a large field study evaluating such nonviable oral vaccines in Bangladesh revealed that neither the whole-cell bacterin nor the killed vibrios supplemented with the B-subunit protein of the cholera enterotoxin induced sufficient protection to justify their recommendation for public health use.

In any case, even if these vaccines were effective, the requirement for large and repeated doses would make them too expensive for use in the developing areas that are usually afflicted with epidemic cholera. Moreover, they were clearly less effective in children — the primary target population in heavily endemic areas.

EPIDEMIOLOGY

Humans apparently are the only natural host for the cholera vibrios. Cholera is acquired by the ingestion of water or food contaminated with the feces of an infected individual. Previously, the disease swept the world in six great pandemics and later receded into its ancestral home in the Indo-Pakistani subcontinent. In 1961, the El Tor biotype (a subset distinguished by physiologic characteristics) of *V cholerae*, not previously implicated in widespread epidemics, emerged from the Celebes (now Sulawesi), causing the seventh great cholera pandemic. In the course of their migration, the El Tor biotype cholera vibrios virtually replaced *V cholerae* of the classic biotype that formerly was responsible for the annual cholera epidemics in

India and East Pakistan (now Bangladesh). The pandemic that began in 1961 is now heavily seeded in Southeast Asia and in Africa. It has also invaded Europe, North America, and Japan, where the outbreaks have been relatively restricted and self-limited because of more highly developed sanitation. Several new cases were reported in Texas in 1981 and sporadic cases have since been reported in Louisiana and other Gulf Coast areas. Interestingly, after nearly 20 years of relative quiescence, *V cholerae* of the classic biotype is being isolated with increasing frequency in India and Bangladesh.

Cholera appears to exhibit three major epidemiologic patterns: **heavily endemic, neoepidemic** (newly invaded, cholera-receptive areas), and in developed countries with good sanitation, occasional **limited outbreaks**. These patterns probably depend largely on environmental factors (including sanitary and cultural aspects), the prior immune status or antigenic experience of the population at risk, and the inherent properties of the vibrios themselves, such as their resistance to gastric acidity, ability to colonize, and toxigenicity. In the heavily endemic region of the Indian subcontinent, cholera exhibits some periodicity; this may vary from year to year and seasonally, depending partly on the amount of rain and degree of flooding. Because humans are the only reservoirs, survival of the cholera vibrios during interepidemic periods probably depends on a relatively constant availability of low-level undiagnosed cases and transiently infected, asymptomatic individuals. Long-term carriers have been reported but are extremely rare. The classic case occurred in the Philippines: "cholera Dolores" harbored cholera vibrios in her gallbladder for 12 years after her initial attack in 1962. Her carrier state resolved spontaneously in 1973; no secondary cases had been associated with her well-marked strain. Recent studies, however, have suggested that cholera vibrios can persist for some time in shellfish in coastal regions of infected areas.

During epidemic periods, the incidence of infection in communities with poor sanitation is high enough to frustrate the most vigorous epidemiologic control efforts. Although transmission occurs primarily through water contaminated with human feces, infection also may be spread within households and by contaminated foods. Thus, in heavily endemic regions, adequate supplies of pure water may reduce but not eliminate the threat of cholera.

In neoepidemic cholera-receptive areas, vigorous epidemiologic measures, including rapid identification and treatment of symptomatic cases and asymptomatically infected individuals, education in sanitary practices, and interruption of vehicles of transmission (e.g., by water chlorination), may be most effective in containing the disease. In such situations, spread of cholera usually depends on traffic of infected human beings, although spread between adjacent communities can occur through bodies of water contaminated by human feces. John Snow was credited with stopping an epidemic in London, England, by the simple expedient of removing the handle of the "Broad Street pump" (a contaminated water supply) in 1854, before acceptance of the "germ theory" and before the first isolation of the "Kommabacillus" by Robert Koch.

In such developed areas as Japan, Northern Europe, and North America, cholera has been introduced repeatedly in recent years, but has not caused devastating outbreaks; however, Japan has reported secondary cases and, in 1978, the United State experienced an outbreak of about 12 cases in Louisiana. In that outbreak, sewage was infected, and infected shellfish apparently were involved. Interestingly, the hemolytic vibrio strain implicated was identical to one that caused an unexplained isolated case in Texas in 1973.

DIAGNOSIS

Rapid bacteriologic diagnosis offers relatively little clinical advantage to the patient with secretory diarrhea, because essentially the same treatment (fluid and electrolyte replacement) is employed regardless of etiology; nevertheless, rapid identification of the agent can profoundly affect the subsequent course of a potential epidemic outbreak.

Because of their rapid growth and characteristic colonial morphology, *V cholerae* can be easily isolated and identified in the bacteriology laboratory, provided, first, that the presence of cholera is suspected and, second, that suitable specific diagnostic antisera are available. The vibrios are completely inhibited or grow somewhat poorly on usual enteric diagnostic media (MacConkey agar or eosin-methylene blue agar), but they can be isolated from stool samples or rectal swabs from cholera cases on simple meat extract (nutrient) agar or bile salts agar at slightly alkaline pH values. Following observation of characteristic colonial morphology with a stereoscopic microscope using transmitted oblique illumination, microorganisms can be confirmed as cholera vibrios by a rapid slide agglutination test with specific antiserum. Classic and El Tor biotypes can be differentiated at the same time by performing a direct slide hemagglutination test with chicken erythrocytes: all freshly isolated agar-grown El Tor vibrios exhibit hemagglutination; all freshly isolated classic vibrios do not. In practice, this can be accomplished with material from patients as early as 6 hours after streaking the specimen in which the cholera vibrios usually predominate; however, to detect carriers (asymptomatically infected individuals) and to isolate cholera vibrios from food and water, enrichment procedures and selective media are recommended. Enrichment can be accomplished by inoculating alkaline (pH 8.5) peptone broth with the specimen and then streaking for isolation after an approximate 6-hour incubation period; this process both enables the rapidly growing vibrios to multiply and suppresses much of the commensal microflora. An effective selective medium is thiosulfate-citrate-bile salts-sucrose (TCBS) agar, on which the sucrose-fermenting cholera vibrios produce a distinctive yellow colony. However, the usefulness of this medium is limited because serologic testing of colonies grown on it occasionally proves difficult, and different lots vary in their productivity. This medium is also useful in isolating *V parahaemolyticus.*

The classic case of cholera, which includes profound secretory diarrhea and should evoke clinical suspicion, can be diagnosed within a few minutes in the prepared laboratory by finding rapidly motile bacteria on direct, bright-field, or dark-field microscopic examination of the liquid stool. The technician can then make a second preparation to

which a droplet of specific anti-*V cholerae* O group 1 antiserum is added. This quickly stops vibrio motility. Another rapid technique is the use of fluorescein isothiocyanate-labeled specific antiserum (fluorescent antibody technique) directly on the stool or rectal swab smear or on the culture after enrichment in alkaline peptone broth. For cultural diagnosis, both nonselective and selective (TCBS) media may be used. Although demonstration of typical agglutination essentially confirms the diagnosis, additional conventional tests such as oxidase reaction, indole reaction, sugar fermentation reactions, gelatinase, lysine, arginine, and ornithine decarboxylase reactions may be helpful. Tests for chicken cell hemagglutination, hemolysis, polymyxin sensitivity, and susceptibility to phage IV are useful in differentiating the El Tor biotype from classic *V cholerae.* Tests for toxigenesis may be indicated.

Diagnosis can be made retrospectively by confirming significant rises in specific serum antibody titers in convalescents. For this purpose, conventional agglutination tests, tests for rises in complement-dependent vibriocidal antibody, or tests for rises in antitoxic antibody can be employed. Convenient microversions of these tests have been developed. Passive hemagglutination tests and enzyme-linked immunosorption assays (ELISAs) have also been proposed.

Cultures that resemble *V cholerae* but fail to agglutinate in diagnostic antisera (nonagglutinable or non-O group 1 vibrios) present more of a problem and require additional tests such as oxidase, decarboxylases, inhibition by the vibriostatic pteridine compound 0/129, and the "string test." The string test demonstrates the property, shared by most vibrios and relatively few other genera, of forming a mucuslike string when colony material is emulsified in 0.5 percent aqueous sodium deoxycholate solution. Additional tests for enteropathogenicity and toxigenesis may be useful.

CONTROL

Treatment of cholera consists essentially of replacing fluid and electrolytes. Formerly, this was accomplished intravenously, using costly sterile pyrogen-free intravenous solutions. The patient's fluid losses were conveniently measured by the use of buckets, graduated in half-liter volumes, kept underneath an appropriate hole in an army-type cot on which the patient was resting. Antibiotics such as tetracycline, to which the vibrios are sensitive, are useful adjuncts in treatment. They shorten the period of infection with the cholera vibrios, thus reducing the continuous source of cholera enterotoxin; this results in a substantial saving of replacement fluids and a markedly briefer hospitalization. Note, however, that fluid and electrolyte replacement is all-important; patients who are adequately rehydrated and maintained will virtually always survive, and antibiotic treatment alone is not sufficient.

Recently it has been recognized that almost all cholera patients and others with similar severe secretory diarrheal disease can be maintained by fluids given orally if the solutions contain a usable energy source such as glucose. Because of this discovery, packets containing appropriate salts are distributed by such organizations as WHO and UNICEF to cholera-afflicted areas, where they are dissolved in water as needed. One such formulation, called ORS for oral rehydration salts, contains NaCl, 3.5 g; KCl, 1.5 g; NaHCO$_3$, 2.5 g; and glucose, 20.0 g. This mixture is dissolved in 1 L of water and taken orally in increments. Flavoring may be added. Improved versions of ORS, including rice-based formulations that reduce stool output and can be made at home, have been recommended. Unfortunately, this technique, which will save countless millions of lives in developing countries, has not yet been widely accepted by practicing physicians in developed countries.

The possibility of pharmacologic intervention (e.g., a pill that will stop choleraic diarrhea after it has started), has been considered. Two drugs, chlorpromazine and nicotinic acid, have been effective in experimental animals, although the precise mechanism of action has yet to be defined.

Like smallpox and typhoid, cholera—under natural circumstances—appears to affect only humans; therefore, *V cholerae* as an etiologic entity could conceivably disappear with the last human infection. Nevertheless, the spectrum of cholera-like diarrheal diseases probably will persist for some time.

Cholera is essentially a disease associated with poor sanitation. The simple application of sanitary principles—protecting drinking water and food from contamination with human feces—would go a long way toward controlling the disease; however, at present, this is not feasible in the underdeveloped areas that are afflicted with epidemic cholera or are considered to be cholera receptive. Meanwhile, development of a vaccine that would effectively prevent colonization and manifestations of cholera would be extremely helpful. As indicated above, such vaccines are presently being tested. Antibiotic or chemotherapeutic prophylaxis is feasible and may be indicated under certain circumstances. It also should be mentioned that the incidence of cholera is significantly higher in formula-fed than in breast-fed babies.

Present information indicates that *V parahaemolyticus* enteritis could be almost completely prevented by applying appropriate procedures to prevent multiplication of the organisms in contaminated seafood, such as keeping it refrigerated continually.

◄ OTHER *VIBRIO* ► INFECTIONS

Other vibrios may be clinically significant also. These include members of a poorly defined and relatively heterogeneous group of nonagglutinable or noncholera vibrios (called NAG vibrios or NCV or non-O group 1 *V cholerae*). *Vibrio parahaemolyticus,* a halophilic (salt-loving) vibrio associated with enteritis is acquired by ingestion of raw or improperly cooked seafoods. Another halophilic vibrio, which ferments lactose and for this reason was called the L + vibrio, has recently been identified as *V vulnificus*. It has been associated with wound infections as well as fatal septicemias. Other groups of vibrios, previously referred to as group F and EF-6, have recently been classified into species: *V fluvialis, V hollisae, V furnissia,* and

V damsela. Vibrio mimicus is a recently described sucrose-negative species. *Vibrio fetus,* a group of anaerobic to microaerophilic spirally curved rods associated with venereally transmitted infertility and abortion in domestic animals, is now called *Campylobacter jejuni* and is considered to belong in the family Spirillaceae rather than in the family Vibrionaceae. *Campylobacter jejuni* has been associated with dysenterylike gastroenteritis, duodenal and gastric ulcers, as well as with other types of infection, including bacteremic and central nervous system infections in humans (see Ch. 23). Another vibrolike organism, *Helicobacter pylori* (formerly known as *C pylori*) causes gastritis and predisposes to duodenal ulcers. Although some similarities in habitat and other properties occur, members of the family Vibrionaceae are separated taxonomically from members of the family Enterobacteriaceae: the oxidase test (vibrios are usually oxidase positive) is particularly useful. Other vibrios exist, and some of these may be responsible for diseases in fish and other lower animals. As vibrios are widely distributed in the environment, particularly in estuarine waters and in seafoods, reports of their isolation from patients with diarrheal disease do not necessarily always imply an etiologic relationship.

Choleralike vibrios have been reported in Maryland's Chesapeake Bay but have not been associated with any human cases despite more than 15 years of extensive surveillance. These vibrios are probably nonpathogenic nonagglutinable (non-O group 1) vibrios, or the atypical O group 1 vibrios mentioned above, which do not contain the genes for toxin production, do not colonize, and are avirulent.

Relatively little is known about the epidemiology of nonagglutinable vibrios. When sought, these vibrios have been found widely in brackish surface waters (sewers, marshes, bogs, and coastal areas), and are generally more numerous in warmer months. They appear to be free-living aquatic organisms; whether particular subsets are potential pathogens is not yet clear. Strains isolated from humans with diarrheal disease more frequently give positive responses in assays for enterotoxins or enteropathogenicity, but the pathogenic mechanism of other isolates associated with shellfish remains undefined.

An epidemiologic pattern is more evident with *V parahaemolyticus,* which is clearly part of the normal flora or coastal and estuarine waters throughout the world. Although originally recognized in Japan, *V parahaemolyticus* enteritis has been reported virtually worldwide within the last decade. Its reported frequency varies widely, partly because of inherent differences in distribution and partly because many laboratories do not use the appropriate culture medium (TCBS) to isolate these organisms. Two types of clinical syndromes, both usually self-limited, have been observed. The most common is a watery diarrhea, perhaps with associated abdominal cramps, nausea, vomiting, and fever, with a modal incubation period of 15 hours. A dysenteric syndrome with a short incubation period of 2 ½ hours also has been described. In Japan, about 24 percent of reported cases of food poisoning are attributed to *V parahaemolyticus.* The disease occurs primarily during summer, possibly reflecting the increased presence of the organism in the marine environment during those months, as well as the enhanced opportunity for it to multiply in unrefrigerated foods. It appears to be transmitted exclusively by food, primarily raw or improperly prepared seafood. As growth of this organism is inhibited at temperatures below 15° C, rapid cooling and refrigeration of seafoods that are eaten raw would vastly reduce the incidence of disease. The organisms are killed by heating to 65° C for 10 minutes; therefore, properly handled cooked seafood should present no problem. The role played in virulence and pathogenesis by the thermostable direct hemolysin, which is responsible for the positive Kanagawa phenomenon (a hemolytic reaction around colonies growing on a particular blood agar medium), is not yet fully defined. This hemolysin is clearly associated with pathogenicity, but whether it is merely an associated marker or intimately involved in the disease process awaits further research. Be this as it may, only strains that possess the Kanagawa hemolysin are considered pathogenic. In laboratory studies, the isolated hemolysin has been reported to be cytotoxic, cardiotoxic, and lethal.

REFERENCES

Blake JD, Weaver RE, Hollis DG: Diseases of humans (other than cholera) caused by vibrios. Annu Rev Microbiol, 34:341, 1980

Clemens JD, Harris JR, Sack DA et al: Field trial of oral cholera vaccines in Bangladesh: results of one year of follow-up. J Infect Dis 158:60, 1988

Finkelstein RA: Cholera. Crit Rev Microbiol 2:553, 1973

Finkelstein RA: Cholera. In Germanier R (ed): Bacterial Vaccines. Academic Press, San Diego, 1984

Finkelstein RA: Cholera, the cholera enterotoxins, and the cholera enterotoxin-related enterotoxin family. p. 85. In Owen P, Foster TS (eds): Immuno-chemical and Molecular Genetic Analysis of Bacterial Pathogens. Elsevier, Amsterdam, 1988

Finkelstein RA, Burks MF, Zupan A et al: Epitopes of the cholera family of enterotoxins. Rev Infect Dis 9:544, 1987

Gill DM: Seven toxic peptides that cross cell membranes. p. 291. In Jeljaszewicz I, Wadstrom T (eds): Bacterial Toxins and Cell Membranes. Academic Press, San Diego, 1978

Hoge CW, Watsky D, Peeler RN et al: Epidemiology and spectrum of *Vibrio* infections in a Chesapeake Bay community. J Infect Dis 160:985, 1989

Kaper JB, Moseley SL, Falkow S: Molecular characterization of environmental and nontoxigenic strains of *Vibrio cholerae*. Infect Immun 32:661, 1981

Lai C-Y: The chemistry and biology of cholera toxin. Crit Rev Biochem 9:171, 1980

Levine MM, Black RE, Clements ML et al: Evaluation in humans of attenuated *Vibrio cholerae* El Tor Ogawa strain Texas Star-SR as a live oral vaccine. Infect Immun 43:515, 1984

Levine MM, Kaper JBV, Black RE, Clements ML: New knowledge on pathogenesis of bacterial enteric infections as applied to vaccine development. Microbiol Rev 47:510, 1983

Levine MM, Kaper JP, Herrington D et al: Volunteer studies of deletion mutants of *Vibrio cholerae* O1 prepared by recombinant techniques. Infect Immun 56:161, 1988

Marchlewicz BA, Finkelstein RA: Immunologic differences among the cholera/coli family of enterotoxins. Diagn Microbiol Infect Dis 1:129, 1983

Mekalanos JJ, Swartz DJ, Pearson GDN et al: Cholera toxin genes: nucleotide sequence, deletion analysis and vaccine development. Nature (London) 306:551, 1983

Miller VL, Taylor RK, Mekalanos JJ: Cholera toxin transcriptional activator Tox R is a transmembrane DNA binding protein. Cell 48:271, 1987

Morris JG, Jr, Black RE: Cholera and other vibrioses in the United States. N Engl J Med 312:343, 1985

Moss J, Vaughn M: Activation of adenylate cyclase by choleragen. Annu Rev Biochem 48:581, 1979

Ouchterlony Ö, Holmgren J (eds): Cholera and related diarrheas; molecular aspects of a global health problem. 43rd Nobel Symposim, co-sponsored by the World Health Organization. S Karger, Basel, 1980

Peterson JW, Ochoa LG: Role of prostaglandins and cAMP in the secretory effects of cholera toxin. Science 245:857, 1989

World Health Organization: Diarrheal diseases control programme. Report of the tenth meeting of the technical advisory group (Geneva, March 13–17, 1989). WHO/D/89 32:1, 1989

van Heyningen WE, Seal JR: Cholera: The American Scientific Experience, 1947–1980. Westview Press, Boulder CO, 1983

25 ESCHERICHIA COLI IN DIARRHEAL DISEASE

DOYLE J. EVANS, JR.
DOLORES G. EVANS

GENERAL CONCEPTS

Clinical Manifestations

Depending on the virulence factors they possess, virulent *Escherichia coli* strains cause either noninflammatory diarrhea (watery diarrhea) or inflammatory diarrhea (dysentery with stools usually containing blood, mucus, and leukocytes).

Structure, Classification, and Antigenic Types

These are Gram-negative bacilli of the family Enterobacteriaceae. Virulent strains differ from nonvirulent *E coli* only in possessing genetic elements for virulence factors. Strains producing enterotoxins are called enterotoxigenic *E coli* (ETEC).

Pathogenesis

Transmission is by the fecal-oral route. Pili (fimbriae) allow the bacteria to colonize the ileal mucosa. **Cytotonic enterotoxins** (encoded on plasmid or bacteriophage DNA) induce watery diarrhea. Plasmid-encoded **invasion factors** permit invasion of the mucosa, and plasmid- or bacteriophage-encoded **cytotoxic enterotoxins** induce tissue damage; the presence of either of these factors induces a host inflammatory reaction with an influx of lymphocytes and resulting dysentery.

Host Defenses

Gastric acid and intestinal transit time are important defenses. Specific intestinal immunoglobulin A (IgA) develops and appears to be protective.

Epidemiology

Infection is common where sanitation is poor; both infants and susceptible travelers to developing countries are particularly at risk. The disease is most serious in infants.

Diagnosis

The diagnosis is suggested by the clinical picture and confirmed by stool culture. Serotyping is occasionally performed for outbreaks.

Control

Prevention depends on sanitary measures to prevent fecal-oral transmission: hand-washing and proper preparation of food; chlorination of water supplies; and sewage treatment and disposal. Parenteral or oral fluid and electrolyte replacement is used to prevent dehydration. Broad-spectrum antibiotics are used in chronic or life-threatening cases.

INTRODUCTION

Escherichia coli is a common member of the normal flora of the large intestine. As long as these bacteria do not acquire genetic elements coding for virulence factors, they remain benign commensals. Strains that acquire bacteriophage or plasmid DNA for **enterotoxins** or **invasion factors** become virulent and can cause either a plain, watery diarrhea or an inflammatory dysentery. These diseases are most familiar to Westerners as **traveler's diarrhea,** but they are also major health problems in endemic countries, particularly among infants. Three groups of *E coli* are associated with diarrheal diseases. *Escherichia coli* strains that produce enterotoxins are called **enterotoxigenic E coli (ETEC).** There are numerous types of enterotoxin. Some of these toxins are **cytotoxic,** damaging the mucosal cells, whereas others are merely **cytotonic,** inducing only the secretion of water and electrolytes. A second group of *E coli* strains have invasion factors and cause tissue destruction and inflammation resembling the effects of *Shigella.* A third group of serotypes, called **enteropathogenic E coli (EPEC),** are associated with outbreaks of diarrhea in newborn nurseries, but produce no recognizable toxins or invasion factors. Figure 25-1 presents a summary of the diseases caused by virulent *E coli.*

NONINFLAMMATORY DIARRHEAS CAUSED BY ENTEROTOXIGENIC *ESCHERICHIA COLI*

CLINICAL MANIFESTATIONS

The diarrheal disease caused by ETEC is characterized by a rapid onset of watery, nonbloody diarrhea of considerable volume, accompanied by little or no fever (Fig. 25-2). Other common symptoms are abdominal pain, malaise, nausea, and vomiting. Diarrhea and other symptoms cease spontaneously after 24 to 72 hours.

STRUCTURE, CLASSIFICATION, AND ANTIGENIC TYPES

ETEC organisms are Gram-negative, short rods not visibly different from *E coli* found in the normal flora of the human large intestine. Virulence-associated fimbriae are too small to be seen by light microscopy. All ETEC contain plasmids, but this is also not a distinguishing feature unless gene probe techniques are used to detect specific virulence-associated genes on these plasmids.

E coli organisms are serogrouped according to the presence or absence of specific heat-stable somatic antigens (O antigens) composed of polysac-

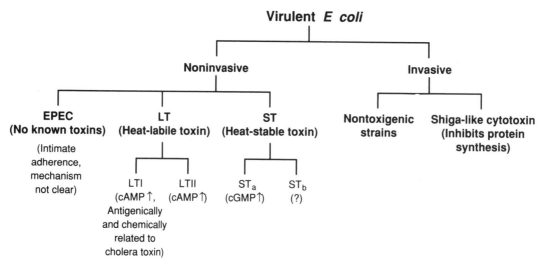

FIGURE 25-1 Virulence mechanisms of *E coli.*

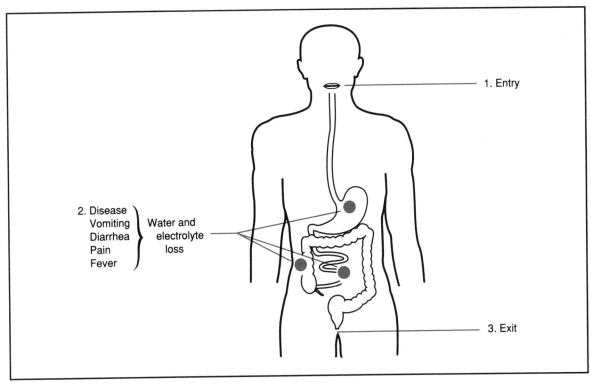

FIGURE 25-2 Pathogenesis of *E coli* diarrheal disease.

charide chains linked to the core lipopolysaccha-ride (LPS) complex common to all Gram-negative bacteria. O specificity is determined by sugar or amino-sugar composition and by the sequence of these outer polysaccharide chains. More than 170 different O-specific antigens have been defined since Kauffmann began this method of typing *E coli* in 1943. In normal **smooth strains,** which are typable, the core LPS is buried beneath the O anti-gen. Also occurring are untypable O-minus mu-tants in which the core LPS is exposed; these are called **rough strains.** There is considerable cross-reactivity among *E coli* O antigens; also, many O groups of *E coli* are cross-reactive or identical with specific O groups of *Shigella, Salmonella,* or *Kleb-siella.*

Escherichia coli serotypes are specific O-group/ H-antigen combinations. The H antigens are the flagellar antigens, of which there are at least 56 types. *Escherichia coli* isolates may be nonmotile and nonflagellated and hence H negative (H−). H typing is important for *E coli* associated with diar-rheal disease for two reasons. First, a strain causing an outbreak or epidemic can be differentiated from the normal stool flora by its unique O:H anti-genic makeup. Second, most ETEC belong to spe-cific serotypes (Table 25-1); this relationship facili-tates their identification even in isolated cases. The reason for the close association between specific serotypes and the production of plasmid-deter-mined virulence factors remains a mystery.

Most *E coli* isolates also produce heat-labile, sur-face-associated proteins antigenically unrelated to O and H. These antigens can be seen in electron micrographs as filamentous structures called pili (fimbriae), which are much thinner and usually more rigid than flagella. Commensal *E coli* strains usually produce so-called **common pili,** which are defined as a specific set of antigens. When *E coli* possessing common pili are mixed with erythro-

TABLE 25-1   Major Enterotoxigenic *E coli* Serogroups and Serotypes Grouped
According to Their Reported Colonization Factor Antigens[a]

CFA/I	CFA/II	CFA/IV	Other
O15:H11, O15:H–	O6:H16, O6:H–	O25:H42	O159:H4
O25:H42	O8:H9, O8:H–	O115:H40	
O63:H12, O63:H–	O80, O85	O148:H48	
O78:H11, O78:H12	O139	O167:H5	
O78:H-, O128ac			
O153:H12, O153:H45			

[a] Several CFAs initially identified as CFA/III have not yet been proven to be unrelated to CFA/I or CFA/IV.

cytes (the standard test uses guinea pig erythrocytes), rapid hemagglutination occurs; this hemagglutination is blocked and also reversed by millimolar concentrations of the carbohydrate mannose.

ETEC possess specialized pili, antigenically unrelated to common pili, which act as ligands to bind the bacterial cells to specific complex carbohydrate receptors on the epithelial cell surfaces of the small intestine. Since this interaction results in colonization of the intestine by ETEC, with subsequent multiplication on the gut surface, these pili are termed **colonization factor antigens** (CFAs). Most ETEC isolates produce either CFA/I, CFA/II or CFA/IV, whereas CFA/III and an undetermined number of other CFAs occur on other particular serotypes (Table 25-1). CFA-type pili play a major role in host specificity; for instance, different CFAs (e.g., K88, K99, and 987P) are produced by *E coli* that cause acute diarrhea in domestic animals.

A simple presumptive assay for CFAs on *E coli* is a test for a mannose-resistant (non-common pili) hemagglutination reaction with either human or bovine erythrocytes. However, identification must be confirmed by reaction of the bacteria with antibody directed against a specific CFA.

Genes coding for the production of CFAs reside on the ETEC virulence plasmids, usually on the same plasmids that carry the genes for one or both of the two types of *E coli* enterotoxin, **heat-labile enterotoxin** (LT) and **heat-stable enterotoxin** (ST). Most cases of ETEC diarrhea are caused by *E coli* possessing a CFA and both LT and ST; fewer

are caused by those possessing a CFA and only one toxin (usually LT); and the fewest are caused by *E coli* that lack a CFA and possess only ST.

PATHOGENESIS

Escherichia coli diarrheal disease is contacted orally by ingestion of food or water contaminated with a pathogenic strain shed by an infected person. ETEC diarrhea occurs in all age groups, but mortality is most common in infants, particularly in the most undernourished or malnourished infants in developing nations.

The pathogenesis of ETEC diarrhea involves two steps: intestinal colonization, followed by elaboration of diarrheagenic enterotoxin(s) (Fig. 25-3). ST is actually a family of toxic peptides ranging from 18 to about 50 amino acid residues in length. Those termed STa can stimulate intestinal guanylate cyclase, the enzyme that converts guanosine 5′-triphosphate (GTP) to cyclic guanosine 5′-monophosphate (cGMP). Increased intracellular cGMP inhibits intestinal fluid uptake, resulting in net fluid secretion. Those termed STb do not seem to cause diarrhea by the same mechanism. The method of choice for testing suspect *E coli* isolates for ST production involves injection of culture supernatant fluids into the stomach of infant mice and seeing whether diarrhea ensues. Specific DNA gene probes have also been developed to test isolated colonies for the presence of plasmids coding for ST and for LT.

The *E coli* LTs are antigenic proteins whose mechanism of action is similar to that of *Vibrio*

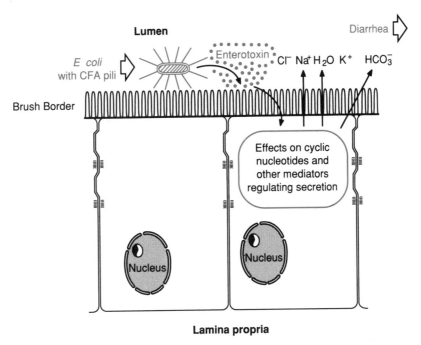

FIGURE 25-3 Cellular pathogenesis of ETEC having CFA pili.

cholerae enterotoxin. LT I shares antigenic determinants with cholera toxin, and their primary amino acid sequences are similar; LT II is different in amino acid composition from cholera toxin and is encoded by genes in the *E coli* chromosome, although its mechanism of action appears to be the same as that of LT I.

LT I is composed of two types of subunits. One type of subunit (the B subunit) binds the toxin to the target cells via a specific receptor that has been identified as G_{M1} ganglioside. The other type of subunit (the A subunit) is then activated by cleavage of a peptide bond and internalized. It then catalyzes the ADP-ribosylation (transfer of ADP-ribose from nicotinamide adenine dinucleotide [NAD]) of a regulatory subunit of membrane-bound adenylate cyclase, the enzyme that converts ATP to cAMP. This activates the adenylate cyclase, which produces excess intracellular cAMP, which leads to hypersecretion of water and electrolytes into the bowel lumen.

LT production is demonstrable by serologic methods, by testing for diarrheagenic activity in ligated rabbit intestine, and by testing for specific cAMP-mediated morphological changes in cultured Y-1 adrenal tumor cells or Chinese hamster ovary (CHO) cells.

HOST DEFENSES

As in any orally transmitted disease, the first line of defense against ETEC diarrhea is gastric acidity. Other nonspecific defenses are small-intestinal motility and a large population of normal flora in the large intestine.

Information about intestinal immunity against diarrheal disease is still somewhat superficial. However, intestinal secretory immunoglobulin (IgA) directed against surface antigens such as the CFAs and against the LTs appear to be the key to immunity from ETEC diarrhea. Passive immune

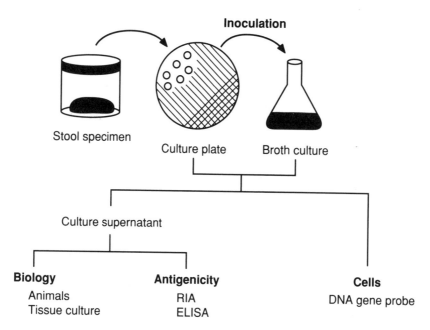

FIGURE 25-4 Laboratory methods for isolation and identification of ETEC.

protection of infants by colostral antibody is important. Human breast milk also contains nonimmunoglobulin factors (receptor-containing molecules) that can neutralize *E coli* toxins and CFAs.

EPIDEMIOLOGY

Escherichia coli diarrheal disease of all types is transmitted from person to person with no known important animal vectors. The incidence of *E coli* diarrhea is clearly related to hygiene, food processing sophistication, general sanitation, and the opportunity for contact. The geographic frequency of ETEC diarrhea is inversely proportional to the sanitation standards. Single-source outbreaks of ETEC diarrhea involving contaminated water supplies or food have been found in adults in the United States and Japan. Adults traveling from temperate climates to more tropical areas typically experience traveler's diarrhea caused by ETEC. This phenomenon is not readily explained, but contributing factors are low levels of immunity and an increased opportunity for infection.

DIAGNOSIS

ETEC diarrhea is characterized by copious watery diarrhea with little or no fever. The diarrheal stool yields a virtually pure culture of *E coli*. Since the disease is self-limiting, virulence testing of isolates and serotyping is impractical except in an outbreak situation. Confirmation is achieved by serotyping, serologic identification of a specific CFA on isolates, and demonstration of LT or ST production. Reference or research laboratories can analyze the isolates for toxin-producing capacity (Fig. 25-4).

CONTROL

Escherichia coli diarrheal disease is best controlled by preventing transmission and by stressing the importance of breast-feeding of infants, especially where ETEC is endemic. The best treatment is oral fluid and electrolyte replacement (intravenous in severe cases). Antibiotics are not recommended because this practice leads to an increased burden of antibiotic-resistant pathogenic *E coli* and of more life-threatening enteropathogens.

INFLAMMATORY DIARRHEAS CAUSED BY ENTEROINVASIVE, CYTOTOXIC, AND ENTEROPATHOGENIC *ESCHERICHIA COLI*

CLINICAL MANIFESTATIONS

Diarrhea caused by the enteroinvasive, cytotoxic, and enteropathogenic (EPEC) strains of *E coli* ranges from very mild to severe. Illness is usually protracted and accompanied by fever. Infection with a few serogroups (O157, O26) is characterized by bloody diarrhea (**hemorrhagic colitis**). Infection with the *Shigella*-like serogroups presents as bacillary dysentery (i.e., abdominal pain and scanty stool containing blood and mucus).

STRUCTURE, CLASSIFICATION, AND ANTIGENIC TYPES

As is the case with ETEC, these strains of *E coli* are not detectably different in structure from *E coli* of the normal flora. The EPEC serogroups listed in Table 25-2 were the first *E coli* groups to be recognized as causative agents of diarrhea in infants. Their status as pathogens remained controversial for decades, mainly because the same O groups can be isolated from healthy contacts in outbreaks and from healthy adults. Recent work has proven that these *E coli* serogroups do possess an antigenic adherence factor (termed **EPEC adherence factor**

[EAF]), which is plasmid mediated but nonfimbrial and is not detectable by standard serotyping techniques. Also, isolates of certain EPEC serogroups (O20, O26, O44, O112, O114) are more frequently negative for EAF.

Table 25-2 lists the *Shigella*-like enteroinvasive *E coli* serotypes (i.e., those with somatic antigens reactive with specific anti-*Shigella* typing serum). Also, like *Shigella*, these *E coli* strains are non motile and therefore H negative. These serogroups do not harbor ETEC virulence plasmids and therefore are also CFA negative.

A small but important group of EPEC includes serotypes O157:H7, O26:H11, and some O111 isolates. These cause epidemic hemorrhagic colitis but are negative for EAF. However, a plasmid-mediated antigenic fimbrial adherence factor has been identified on *E coli* O157:H7.

PATHOGENESIS

Escherichia coli strains belonging to the classic EPEC serogroups (Table 25-2) bind intimately to the epithelial surface of the intestine, usually the colon, via the adhesive EAF discussed above. The lesion caused by EPEC consists mainly of destruction of microvilli. There is no evidence of tissue invasion. Diarrhea is persistent, often chronic, and accompanied by fever. EPEC are negative for ST and LT, but most strains produce relatively small amounts of a potent Shiga-like toxin that has both enterotoxin and cytotoxin activity. Shiga-like toxin attacks the absorptive epithelial cells of the intestinal villi, blocking protein synthesis.

TABLE 25-2   Common Serologic Types of Non-ETEC *E coli* Grouped According to Their Mechanism of Pathogenesis[a]

Classic EPEC Serogroups	*Shigella*-Like (Enteroinvasive) Serogroups	Enterohemorrhagic Serogroups
O18, O26[b], O44, O55[b], O86[b], O111[b], O112, O114, O119[b], O125[b], O126[b], O127[b], O128ab[b], O142[b]	O28ac, O29, O124, O136, O143, O144, O152, O164	O26 : H11, O111, O157 : H7

[a] Occasional isolates fail to show the expected correlation between serogroup or serotype and disease type; this is due to the genetics of virulence factors (i.e., transmissibility of virulence-associated plasmids and phage between *E coli* strains in vivo as well as spontaneous loss of these factors in vitro).

[b] Usually EAF positive, other EPEC serogroups usually EAF negative.

The *E coli* strains associated with hemorrhagic colitis, most notably O157:H7, produce relatively large amounts of the phage-mediated Shiga-like toxin. This toxin was originally called Vero toxin after its cytotoxic effect on cultured Vero cells. Many strains of O157:H7 also produce a second cytotoxin (Shiga-like toxin 2, or Vero toxin 2), which is similar to Shiga toxin but is not neutralized by anti-Shiga toxin antibody.

The *Shigella*-like *E coli* strains are highly virulent; oral exposure to a very small number of these invasive bacteria causes severe illness. The site of the infection is the colon, where adherence is rapidly followed by invasion of the intestinal epithelial cells (Fig. 25-5). An acute inflammatory response and tissue destruction produce diarrhea with little fluid, much blood, and sheets of mucus containing polymorphonuclear cells. Invasive *E coli*, like *Shigella*, causes a rapid keratoconjunctivitis when placed on the conjunctiva of the guinea pig eye (Sereny test). Virulent Sereny test-positive isolates carry a large (usually 140-megadalton) plasmid responsible for this property.

HOST DEFENSES

Host defenses against EPEC are the same as those for ETEC. These defenses are frequently deficient or lacking in the infant and the elderly, which is consistent with the epidemiology of EPEC illness. An important example is the role of the immune system. Passive immune protection of infants by colostral antibody is important; breast-feeding is especially relevant where crowding and poor economic conditions prevail. Infection with these pathogens often excites an inflammatory cell response in the intestine, as is frequently reflected in the diarrheal symptoms.

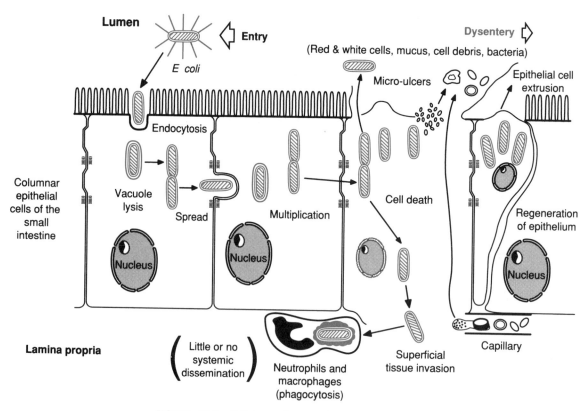

FIGURE 25-5 Cellular pathogenesis of invasive *E coli*.

EPIDEMIOLOGY

The geographic distribution of all EPEC is generally the same as for the ETEC, with a more severe disease in infants. Illness caused by the EPEC serogroups occurs most frequently in infants and young children, and so EPEC are much less important in traveler's diarrhea. Common-source community outbreaks are rare in geographic areas with satisfactory sanitation. However, sporadic cases are seen in the United States, Canada, and Europe, and outbreaks occur in these areas, most commonly in close-contact institutions such as hospital nurseries, day care centers, and nursing homes.

DIAGNOSIS

Diagnosis is usually based on the symptomatology described above. Enterohemorrhagic *E coli*, such as serotype O157:H7, is suspected in the setting of copious bloody diarrhea without fecal leukocytes or fever. *Escherichia coli* serotyping is useful in chronic cases and in outbreaks, because identification of the agent and its antibiotic sensitivity pattern are valuable in these situations. Testing for specific EPEC virulence factors is usually impractical because it can be done only in reference and specialized research laboratories.

CONTROL

Prevention and control are generally the same as for ETEC. Intervention of the fecal-oral transmission cycle is most effective in institutional situations. Broad-spectrum antibiotics are recommended in chronic and/or life-threatening cases.

REFERENCES

Evans DG, Evans DJ, Jr: New surface-associated heat-labile colonization factor antigen (CFA/II) produced by enterotoxigenic *Escherichia coli* of serogroups O6 and O8. Infect Immun 21:638, 1978

Evans DJ, Evans DG, DuPont HL: Hemagglutination patterns of enterotoxigenic and enteropathogenic *Escherichia coli* determined with human, bovine, chicken, and guinea pig erythrocytes in the presence and absence of mannose. Infect Immun 23:336, 1979

Gothefors L, Ahren C, Stoll B et al: Presence of colonization factor antigens on fresh isolates of fecal *Escherichia coli:* a prospective study. J Infect Dis 152:1128, 1985

Guerrant RL, Hughes JM: Nausea, vomiting, and noninflammatory diarrhea. In: Mandell GL, Douglas RG, Bennett JE (eds): Principles and Practice of Infectious Diseases. 3rd Ed. Churchill Livingstone, New York, 1989

Harris JR, Mariano J, Wells JG et al: Person-to-person transmission in an outbreak of enteroinvasive *Escherichia coli*. Am J Epidemiol 122:245, 1985

Harris JR, Wachsmuth IK, Davis BR et al: High-molecular-weight plasmid correlates with *Escherichia coli* invasiveness. Infect Immun 37:1295, 1982

Levine MM: *Escherichia coli* that cause diarrhea: enterotoxigenic, enteropathogenic, enteroinvasive, enterohemorrhagic, and enteroadherent. J Infect Dis 155:377, 1987

Nataro JP, Baldini MM, Kaper JB et al: Detection of an adherence factor of enteropathogenic *Escherichia coli* with a DNA probe. J Infect Dis 152:560, 1985

O'Brien AD, Newland JW, Miller SF et al: Shiga-like toxin-converting phages from *Escherichia coli* strains that cause hemorrhagic colitis or infantile diarrhea. Science 226:694, 1984

Robins-Browne RM: Traditional enteropathogenic *Escherichia coli* of infantile diarrhea. Rev Infect Dis 9:28, 1987

26
ESCHERICHIA, KLEBSIELLA, ENTEROBACTER, SERRATIA, CITROBACTER, AND PROTEUS

M. NEAL GUENTZEL

GENERAL CONCEPTS

Clinical Manifestations

The genera *Escherichia, Klebsiella, Enterobacter, Serratia,* and *Citrobacter* (collectively called the **coliform bacilli**) and *Proteus* include opportunistic pathogens responsible for a wide range of infections. Many species are members of the normal intestinal flora.

Nosocomial Infections: Coliform and *Proteus* bacilli cause about 45 percent of all nosocomial (hospital-acquired) infections in the United States. In order of decreasing frequency, the sites of primary infection are the urinary tract, lower respiratory tract, surgical wounds, bloodstream, and skin. *Escherichia coli* is the premier nosocomial pathogen.

Community-Acquired Infections: Escherichia coli is the major cause of urinary tract infections, including prostatitis and pyelonephritis; *Proteus, Klebsiella,* and *Enterobacter* species are also common urinary tract pathogens. *Proteus mirabilis* is the most frequent cause of infection-related kidney stones. *Klebsiella pneumoniae* causes a severe pneumonia; *K rhinoscleromatis* causes rhinoscleroma; and *K ozaenae* is associated with ozena, an atrophic disease of the nasal mucosa.

Structure, Classification, and Antigenic Types

The coliforms and *Proteus* are bacilli. All genera except *Klebsiella* are flagellated. Some strains produce capsules.

Virulence often depends on the presence of attachment pili (which can be characterized by specific hemagglutinating reactions). Sex pili also may be present. The major classes of antigens used in defining strains are H (flagellar), O (somatic), and K (capsular).

Pathogenesis

Specific serotypes with particular virulence factors often preferentially infect specific extraintestinal sites. *Escherichia coli* bacilli in extraintestinal infections have soluble and cell-bound hemolysins, siderophores, and adherence pili.

Host Defenses

Coliforms and *Proteus* species rarely cause disease unless host defenses are compromised. Destruction of the normal intestinal flora by antibiotic therapy may allow resistant nosocomial strains to colonize or overgrow. The skin and mucosae may be breached by disease, trauma, operation, venous catheterization, tracheal intubation, etc. Immunosuppressive therapy also increases the risk of infection.

Epidemiology

The epidemiology of coliform and *Proteus* infections involves many reservoirs and modes of transmission. The infecting organism may be endogenous or exogenous. Transmission may be direct or indirect; common vehicles include hospital food and equipment, intravenous solutions, and the hands of hospital personnel. Nosocomial strains progressively colonize the intestine with increasing length of hospital stay, resulting in an increased risk of infection.

Diagnosis

The clinical picture depends on the site of infection; diagnosis relies on culturing the organism and on biochemical and/or serologic identification.

Control

The most effective way to reduce transmission of nosocomial organisms is for hospital personnel to wash hands meticulously after attending to each patient. (This practice is ignored mainly by physicians.) Vaccines and hyperimmune sera are not currently available. Various antibiotics are the backbone of treatment; drug resistance (often multiple) due to conjugative plasmids is a major problem.

INTRODUCTION

The Gram-negative bacilli of the genera *Escherichia, Klebsiella, Enterobacter, Serratia, Citrobacter,* and *Proteus* (Table 26-1) are members of the normal intestinal flora of humans and animals and may be isolated from a variety of environmental sources. With the exception of *Proteus,* they are sometimes collectively referred to as the **coliform bacilli** because of shared properties, particularly the ability of most of these species to ferment the sugar lactose.

Many of these microorganisms used to be dismissed as harmless commensals. Today, they are known to be responsible for major health problems worldwide. A limited number of species, including *E coli, K pneumoniae, Enterobacter aerogenes, Enterobacter cloacae, S marcescens,* and *P mirabilis,* are responsible for most infections produced by this group of organisms. The increasing incidence of the coliforms, *Proteus,* and other Gram-negative organisms in disease reflects in part a better understanding of their pathogenic potential but more importantly the changing ecology of bacterial disease. The widespread and often indiscriminate use of antibiotics has created drug-resistant Gram-negative bacilli that readily acquire multiple resistance through transmission of drug resistance plasmids (R factors). Also, development of new surgical procedures, health support technology, and therapeutic regimens has provided new portals of entry and compromised many host defenses.

CLINICAL MANIFESTATIONS

As opportunistic pathogens, the coliforms and *Proteus* take advantage of weakened host defenses to colonize and elicit a variety of disease states. Together, the many disease syndromes produced by these organisms are among the most common infections in humans requiring medical intervention.

Nosocomial Infections

The coliforms and *Proteus* are responsible for approximately 45 percent of nosocomial (hospital-acquired) infections in the United States (Table 26-2). The mean nosocomial infection rate for 1984 was 3.3 percent of patients discharged from hospitals participating in the National Nosocomial Infections Survey (NNIS). Other recent estimates of nosocomial infections in mainstream U.S. hospitals suggest that about 5 percent of the estimated 40 million annual admissions, or 2 million patients, had at least one nosocomial infection. Thus, the coliforms and *Proteus* probably are responsible for hospital-acquired infections in approximately 900,000 patients each year. Aside from the enormous cost measured in human life, nosocomial infections prolong the duration of hospitalization by 3 to 13 days and increase the cost of medical care by more than $4 billion a year.

The highest rates of nosocomial infections in the NNIS occur in surgical and medicine services. In

TABLE 26-1 Taxonomy of the Coliform Bacilli
and *Proteus*

Organism	Other Designations
Escherichia	
E coli[a]	
Klebsiella	
K pneumoniae[a]	*Friedlander's bacillus*
K ozaenae	
K rhinoscleromatis	
K oxytoca	*K pneumoniae* (indole-positive, gelatin-positive)
K planticola[b]	
Enterobacter	
E aerogenes[a]	
E agglomerans	*Erwinia herbicola*
E cloacae[a]	
E sakazakii[b]	*E cloacae* (yellow pigmented)
E gergoviae[b]	
Serratia	
S marcescens[a]	
S rubidaea[b]	
S liquefaciens group[b]	*Enterobacter liquefaciens, S liquefaciens*
S fonticola[b]	
S odorifera[b]	
S plymuthica	
Citrobacter	
C freundii	
C diversus	*C intermedius* biotype[b]
C amalonaticus[b]	*C intermedius* biotype[a]
Proteus[c]	
P mirabilis[a]	
P penneri[b]	
P vulgaris	

[a] Major coliforms in nosocomial and/or community-acquired human diseases (prevalent in published reports).

[b] Relatively new species designations or organisms of questionable clinical significance.

[c] Organisms previously designated as *Proteus morganii* and *Proteus rettgeri* are now classified in the genera *Morganella* and *Providencia*, respectively.

order of decreasing frequency, the sites of infection are the urinary tract, lower respiratory tract, surgical wounds, bloodstream, and skin. *Escherichia coli*, the predominant nosocomial pathogen, is the major cause of infection in the urinary tract and is common in other sites. *Pseudomonas aeruginosa* is the most common pathogen in lower respiratory infections, followed by *Klebsiella*, whereas *Staphylococcus aureus* is predominant in cutaneous infections. Coagulase-negative staphylococci have replaced *E coli* as the predominant pathogen in primary bacteremias. The major causes of surgical wound infections are *S aureus*, enterococci, and *E coli*.

Other coliform bacilli and *Proteus* have been incriminated in various hospital-acquired infections. *Klebsiella*, *Enterobacter*, and *Serratia* species are frequent causes of bacteremia at some medical centers and are also frequently involved in infections associated with respiratory tract manipulations, such as tracheostomy and procedures using contaminated inhalation therapy equipment. *Klebsiella* and *Serratia* species commonly cause infections following intravenous and urinary catheterization and infections complicating burns. *Proteus* species frequently cause nosocomial infections of the urinary tract, surgical wounds, and lower respiratory tract. Less frequently, *Proteus* species cause bacteremia, most often in elderly patients. A series of nationwide outbreaks of bacteremia (1970 to 1971 and 1973) caused by contaminated commercial fluids for intravenous injections involved *Enterobacter cloacae*, *Enterobacter agglomerans*, and *C freundii*.

The role of *Citrobacter* species in human disease is not as great as that of the other coliforms and *Proteus*. *Citrobacter freundii* and *C diversus* have been isolated predominantly as superinfecting agents from urinary and respiratory tract infections. *Citrobacter* septicemia may occur in patients with multiple predisposing factors; Citrobacter species also cause meningitis, septicemia, and pulmonary infections in neonates and young children. Neonatal meningitis produced by *C diversus*, while uncommon, is associated with a very high frequency of brain abscesses, death, and mental retardation in survivors. Although *E coli* and group B

TABLE 26-2   Frequency of Selected Pathogens Causing Nosocomial Infections[a]

Organism	Percentage of Infections at Site						
	Bacteremia	Surgical Wound	Lower Respiratory	Urinary Tract	Cutaneous	Other	All Sites
E coli	10.1	11.5	6.4	30.7	7.0	7.4	17.8
Klebsiella	7.8	5.2	11.6	8.0	3.8	4.6	7.4
Enterobacter	6.3	7.0	9.4	4.8	4.5	3.9	5.9
Serratia	3.0	2.1	5.8	1.2	2.2	1.5	2.3
Citrobacter	0.7	8.2	1.5	3.4	11.5	11.6	6.3
Proteus	0.8	5.2	4.2	7.4	3.3	2.1	5.1
Pseudomonas aeruginosa	7.6	8.9	16.9	12.7	9.2	6.7	11.4
Staphylococcus aureus	12.3	18.6	12.9	1.6	28.9	14.6	10.3
Coagulase-negative staphylococci	14.9	8.2	1.5	3.4	11.5	11.6	6.3
Enterococci	7.1	12.1	1.5	14.7	8.8	7.0	10.4
Other pathogens	29.4	13.0	28.3	12.1	9.3	29.0	16.8
Cases/1,000 discharges	2.5	5.6	6.0	12.9	1.9	4.6	33.5

[a] Data from the Centers for Disease Control: Nosocomial infection surveillance, 1984. In CDC Surveillance Summaries 35:155, 1986. Centers for Disease Control, Atlanta, GA.

streptococci cause most cases of neonatal meningitis, the most common cause of brain abscesses in neonatal meningitis is *P mirabilis.*

Immunocompromised patients often develop non-hospital-acquired infections with coliforms. For example, group B streptococci and *E coli* are responsible for most cases of neonatal meningitis, with the latter accounting for about 40 percent of cases. Infections seen in cancer patients with solid tumors or malignant blood diseases frequently are caused by *E coli* and *Klebsiella, Serratia,* and *Enterobacter* species. Such infections often have a grave or lethal course. Individuals who are immunosuppressed by therapy (e.g., cancer patients or transplant recipients) or by congenital defects of the immune system may develop *Klebsiella, Enterobacter,* and *Serratia* infections. Many additional factors such as diabetes, trauma, and chronic lung disease may predispose to infection by coliforms and other microbes.

Community-Acquired Infections

The coliform organisms and *Proteus* species are major causes of diseases acquired outside the hospital; many of these diseases eventually require

hospitalization. *Escherichia coli* causes approximately 85 percent of cases of urethrocystitis (infection of the urethra and bladder), about 80 percent of cases of chronic bacterial prostatitis, and up to 90 percent of cases of acute pyelonephritis (inflammation of the renal pelvis and parenchyma). *Proteus, Klebsiella,* and *Enterobacter* species are among the other organisms most frequently involved in urinary tract infections. *Proteus,* particularly *P mirabilis,* is believed to be the most common cause of infection-related kidney stones, one of the most serious complications of unresolved or recurrent bacteriuria.

Klebsiella was first recognized clinically as an agent of pneumonia. *Klebsiella pneumoniae* accounts for approximately 3 percent of pneumonia cases; however, extensive damage produced by the organism results in high (up to 90 percent in untreated patients) case fatality rates. *Klebsiella rhinoscleromatis* is the agent of rhinoscleroma, a chronic destructive granulomatous disease of the respiratory tract that is endemic in Eastern Europe and Central America. *Klebsiella ozaenae,* a rare cause of serious infection, is classically associated only with ozena, an atrophy of nasal mucosal membranes with a mucopurulent discharge that tends to dry into crusts; however, recent studies indicate that the organism may cause various other diseases including infections of the urinary tract, soft tissue, middle ear, and blood.

DISTINCTIVE PROPERTIES

Structure and Antigens

The generalized structure and antigenic composition of coliform bacilli, as well as of *Proteus* and other members of the family Enterobacteriaceae, are depicted schematically in Figure 26-1. A more detailed figure of the structure is presented in Chapter 2. The major antigens of coliforms are referred to as H, K, and O antigens. The coliforms and *Proteus* are divided into serotypes on the basis of combinations of these antigens; different serotypes may have different virulence properties or may preferentially colonize and produce disease in particular body habitats. The H antigen determinants are flagellar proteins. *Escherichia coli, Enterobacter, Serratia, Citrobacter,* and *Proteus* organisms are peritrichous (i.e., they contain flagella that grow from many places on the cell surface). *Klebsiella* species are nonmotile and nonflagellated and thus have no H antigens.

Some strains of all coliform and *Proteus* species have pili (fimbriae). Pili are associated with adhesive properties and, in some cases, are correlated with virulence. Different pilial colonization factors generally are detectable as hemagglutinins that can be distinguished by the type of erythrocyte agglutinated and by the susceptibility of the hemagglutination to inhibition by the sugar mannose. Sex pili, which have receptors for specific bacterial viruses and are genetically determined by extrachromosomal plasmids, are important in coliform ecology and in the epidemiology of diseases produced by coliforms and *Proteus* species in that types F and I pili are involved in genetic transfer by conjugation (e.g., chromosome-mediated and plasmid-mediated drug resistances or virulence factors).

Major Surface Antigens

K antigens (capsule antigens) are components of the polysaccharide capsules. Certain K antigens (K88 and K99 of *E coli*) are piluslike proteins. The

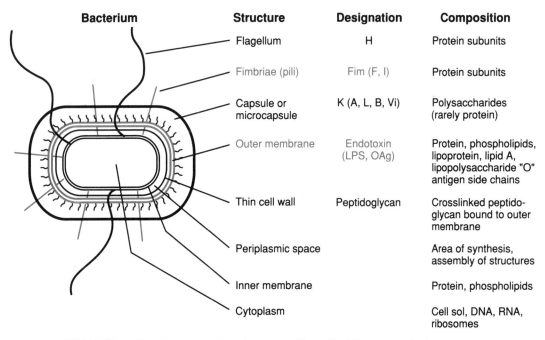

Bacterium	Structure	Designation	Composition
	Flagellum	H	Protein subunits
	Fimbriae (pili)	Fim (F, I)	Protein subunits
	Capsule or microcapsule	K (A, L, B, Vi)	Polysaccharides (rarely protein)
	Outer membrane	Endotoxin (LPS, OAg)	Protein, phospholipids, lipoprotein, lipid A, lipopolysaccharide "O" antigen side chains
	Thin cell wall	Peptidoglycan	Crosslinked peptidoglycan bound to outer membrane
	Periplasmic space		Area of synthesis, assembly of structures
	Inner membrane		Protein, phospholipids
	Cytoplasm		Cell sol, DNA, RNA, ribosomes

FIGURE 26-1 Structure and antigenic composition of coliforms and *Proteus* species.

K antigens often block agglutination by specific O antisera. In the past, K antigens routinely were differentiated into A, L, and B groups on the basis of differences in their lability to heat; however, these criteria are subject to difficulties that make the distinction tenuous. Some *Citrobacter* serotypes produce Vi (virulence) antigen, a K antigen also found in *Salmonella typhi*. Species of *Proteus, Enterobacter,* and *Serratia* apparently have no regular K antigens. However, the K antigens are important in the pathogenesis of some coliforms. A diffuse slime layer of variable thickness (the M antigen) also may be produced, but, unlike the K antigens, it is nonspecific and is serologically cross-reactive among different organisms.

The outer membrane of the bacterial cell wall of these species contains receptors for bacterial viruses and bacteriocins (plasmid-mediated, antibioticlike bactericidal proteins called **colicins** in *E coli* that are active against the same or closely related species). The outer membrane also contains lipopolysaccharide (LPS), of which the lipid A portion is endotoxic and the O (somatic) antigen is serotype specific. The serologic specificity of the O antigens is based on differences in sugar components, their linkages, and the presence or absence of substituted acetyl groups. Loss of the O antigen by mutation results in a **smooth-to-rough transformation,** which often involves changes in colony type and saline agglutination, as well as loss of virulence. Certain strains of *P vulgaris* (OX-19, OX-2, and OX-K) produce O antigens that are shared by some rickettsiae. These *Proteus* strains are used in an agglutination test (the Weil-Felix test) for serum antibodies produced against rickettsiae of the typhus and spotted fever groups (see Ch. 38).

Toxins

Enterotoxigenic strains of *Klebsiella, Enterobacter, Serratia, Citrobacter,* and *Proteus* also have been isolated from infants and children with acute gastroenteritis. The enterotoxins of at least some of these organisms are of the heat-labile and heat-stable types and have other properties in common with the *E coli* toxins (see Ch. 25).

PATHOGENESIS

The process of disease production by coliforms is, in many cases, poorly understood. Production of disease by coliforms or *Proteus* species in extraintestinal sites often involves specific serotypes of the organisms and special virulence factors (Table 26-1). For example, respiratory tract infections by *K pneumoniae* predominantly involve capsular types 1 and 2, whereas urinary tract infections often involve types 8, 9, 10, and 24. Similarly, only a few polysaccharide K antigens (types 1, 2, 3, 5, 12, and 13) of *E coli* are found with high frequency in urinary tract and other extraintestinal infections. These observations suggest that different serotypes may have specific pathogenicities. An alternative explanation is that such strains may simply be the most prevalent types in the normal gut flora.

There is good evidence for specific pathogenicity in *E coli* strains that cause extraintestinal infections (Table 26-3). Approximately 80 percent of *E coli* isolates involved in neonatal meningitis carry the K1 antigen, a fact attributable at least in part to the higher resistance to phagocytosis of K1-posi-

TABLE 26-3   Virulence Factors of *E coli* Isolates from Extraintestinal Infections

Virulence Factor	Proposed Role(s) in Pathogenesis
Col V plasmid	Codes for a siderophore (aerobactin) for Fe chelation
	Increases bacterial resistance to serum
Hemolysin	Damages host cells
	Releases Fe from red blood cells
Enterochelin	Chelates Fe for bacterial uptake
K1 antigen	Impedes phagocytosis
	Blocks binding of C3b opsonin
P-pili	Allow bacteria to bind to P blood group antigens on urinary tract cells (especially in kidneys)
Type 1 pili	Allow bacteria to bind to (1) bladder epithelium, (2) Tamm-Horsfall glycoprotein, and (3) polymorphonuclear neutrophils

tive strains. Certain O antigens (O7 and O18) are found in combination with K1, usually in strains that are isolated from cases of neonatal bacteremia and meningitis and that show increased resistance to the bactericidal effects of serum complement. Interestingly, the *E coli* K1 antigen, composed of neuraminic acid, shows immune cross-reactivity with the group B meningococcal polysaccharide capsule.

Escherichia coli strains isolated from extraintestinal infections often possess a number of properties not usually found in random fecal isolates. These include production of soluble and cell-bound hemolysins, the colicin V plasmid, enterochelin, and special pilial antigens for adherence to target cells. The hemolysin kills host cells and makes iron more available by releasing hemoglobin-bound iron from lysed red cells. To strip iron from the host iron-binding proteins, *Escherichia coli* produces siderophores of both the hydroxamate (aerobactin) and phenolate (enterochelin) types. Common or type 1 pili may mediate adherence to bladder cells; P-pili are virulence factors for strains causing pyelonephritis; S-pili, which recognize O-linked sialo-oligosaccharides of glycophorin A, are associated with meningitis; and X-pili form a heterogeneous group of mannose-resistant hemagglutinins with largely unknown receptor specificities.

The enzyme urease, produced by *Proteus* and to a lesser extent by *Klebsiella* species, is thought to play a major role in the production of infection-induced urinary stones. Urease hydrolyzes urea to ammonia and carbon dioxide. Alkalinization of the urine by ammonia can cause magnesium phosphate and calcium phosphate to become supersaturated and crystallize out of solution to form, respectively, struvite and apatite stones. Bacteria within the stones may be refractory to antimicrobial therapy. Large stones may interfere with renal function. The ammonia produced by urease activity may also damage the epithelium of the urinary tract.

Except in cases of bacteremia, there is little evidence that endotoxin plays a role in most coliform and *Proteus* diseases. Humans with coliform bacteremia show many of the typical effects of endotoxin, including fever, depletion of complement, release of inflammatory mediators, lactic acidosis, hypotension, vital organ hypoperfusion, irreversible shock, and death.

HOST DEFENSES

It cannot be overemphasized that coliforms and *Proteus* species are unlikely to cause disease unless the local or generalized host defenses fail in some way. The normal gastrointestinal flora, which includes *E coli* and frequently other coliforms and *Proteus* species in smaller numbers, is important in preventing disease through bacterial competition. Prolonged antibiotic therapy compromises this defense mechanism by reducing susceptible components of the normal flora, permitting nosocomial coliform strains or other bacteria to colonize or overgrow.

The organisms may breach anatomic barriers through third-degree burns, ulcers associated with solid tumors of the skin and mucous membranes, intravenous catheters, and surgical or instrumental procedures on the biliary, gastrointestinal, and genitourinary tracts. The lungs may be violated by instrumentation, as in tracheal intubation, or even by aerosols from contaminated nebulizers or humidifiers, which carry organisms to the terminal alveoli.

Corticosteroid administration, radiotherapy, and the increased steroid levels associated with pregnancy tend to decrease host control over infections (e.g., by depressing the immune response). Cytotoxic drugs also are immunosuppressive. Cancer- or drug-induced neutropenia is an important predisposing factor in bacteremia. Devitalized tissue or foreign bodies may be a source of organisms and may also shelter the organisms from phagocytes and antimicrobial factors.

The interaction of multiple predisposing factors often determines the clinical cause and outcome of coliform or *Proteus* infection. For example, the mortality of bacteremia increases progressively when the underlying disease (e.g., cancer or diabetes) is rated as nonfatal, ultimately fatal (death within 5 years), or rapidly fatal (death within 1 year). Similarly, coliform and *Proteus* infections commonly are more severe in the very old and very young.

EPIDEMIOLOGY

The epidemiology of coliform and *Proteus* infections is complex and involves multiple reservoirs and modes of transmission. *Klebsiella, Enterobacter, Serratia, Citrobacter,* and *Proteus* species live in water, soil, and occasionally food and, in some cases, form part of the intestinal flora of humans and animals. *Escherichia coli* is believed not to be free living, and its presence in environmental samples is taken as indicating recent fecal contamination.

Coliform and *Proteus* organisms causing infection may be exogenous or endogenous. Studies of hospitalized adults and infants have shown that the intestinal tract is progressively colonized by nosocomial coliforms with increasing length of hospitalization. Patients being treated with antibiotics, severely ill patients, and (probably) infants are more likely to be colonized, and other sites of colonization such as the nose and throat may be important in such patients. Colonized patients have a higher risk of nosocomial infection than patients who are not colonized.

The bacteria may be acquired indirectly via various vehicles or by direct contact. A variety of vehicles have been implicated in the spread of nosocomial pathogens. For example, *Klebsiella, Enterobacter,* and *Serratia* species have all been recovered in large numbers from hospital food, particularly salads, with the hospital kitchen being a primary source. An outbreak of urinary tract infections due to multiply drug-resistant *S marcescens* was associated with contaminated urine-measuring containers and urinometers. Serious outbreaks or individual cases of bacteremia due to coliforms have been associated with intrinsic contamination of intravenous fluids or caps during manufacture and with extrinsic contamination of intravenous fluids and administration sets in the hospital environment. Other medical devices and medications have served as vehicles for the spread of nosocomial pathogens. Occasionally, transmission may be via members of the hospital staff who are colonized with nosocomial pathogens in the rectum or vagina or on the hands; however, passive carriage on the hands of medical personnel constitutes the major mode of transmission.

Certain properties of the coliforms may be important in the epidemiology of hospital-acquired infections. Coliform bacteria other than *E coli* frequently are found in tap water or even distilled or deionized water. They may persist or actively multiply in water associated with respiratory therapy or hemodialysis equipment. *Klebsiella, Enterobacter,* and *Serratia* species, like *Pseudomonas* species, may exhibit increased resistance to antiseptics and disinfectants. The same group of coliforms has a selective ability over other common nosocomial pathogens (including *E coli, Proteus* species, *Pseudomonas aeruginosa,* and staphylococci) to proliferate rapidly at room temperature in commercial parenteral fluids containing glucose.

DIAGNOSIS

Because the coliforms and *Proteus* can cause almost any type of infection, the clinical symptoms rarely permit a diagnosis. Culturing and laboratory identification are usually used. The organisms have simple nutritional requirements and grow well on mildly selective media commonly used for members of the Enterobacteriaceae, but not on some moderately and highly selective enteric plating media (*Salmonella-Shigella,* bismuth sulfite, and brilliant green agar). Extraintestinal specimens such as urine, purulent material from wounds or abscesses, sputum, and sediment from cerebrospinal fluid should be plated for isolation on blood agar and a differential medium such as MacConkey or eosin-methylene blue agar. The finding of more than 10^5 organisms/ml in voided urine is often taken as "significant bacteriuria." However, in acutely symptomatic females and with other types of specimens (i.e., those obtained by catheterization or suprapubic aspiration) from either sex, a more appropriate threshold, particularly in the presence of pus cells and the absence of epithelial cells, might be more than 10^2 colonies of a known uropathogen/ml.

Isolation of selected coliforms or *Proteus* species from fecal specimens may be facilitated by adding a moderately selective medium such as xylose-lysine-desoxycholate (XLD) or Hektoen enteric agar. Use of tetrathionate or selenite broth for enrichment of enterotoxigenic strains from feces is not recommended because both media inhibit various genera of coliforms. The strong *(E coli, K pneumoniae, Enterobacter aerogenes)* and occasionally the slow or weak *(Serratia, Citrobacter)* lactose-fermenting coliforms produce characteristic pigmented colonies on the enteric plating media. A striking characteristic of *Proteus* species is their propensity to swarm over the surface of most plating media, making the isolation of other organisms in mixed cultures difficult. The swarming growth appears as a rapidly spreading thin film, sometimes with changing patterns of whirls and bands. Unless the physician specifically requests that the laboratory look for the possibility of *E coli* as an enteropathogen, tests for pathogenic strains, including toxin assays, serotyping, and serogrouping, will not be done.

In cases of suspected bacteremia, replicate bottles (one cultured aerobically, the other anaerobically) containing 50 to 100 ml of appropriate medium with anticoagulant (e.g., polyanetholesulfonate) are inoculated with 10-ml portions of blood. It is usually necessary to take multiple specimens, both before and after antibiotic therapy is started. It is important to take specimens after antibiotic treatment is started so that therapeutic failure can be recognized while the bacteremia may still be amenable to more aggressive medical or surgical treatment.

All the coliforms and *Proteus* species are Gram-negative, facultative anaerobic, non-spore-forming rods that are typically motile, except for *Klebsiella,* which is nonmotile. The oxidase test is negative, and nitrates are reduced to nitrites (except in certain *Enterobacter* species). *Proteus* species and all coliforms ferment glucose, but fermentation of other carbohydrates varies. Lactose usually is fermented rapidly by *Escherichia* and *Klebsiella*

species and more slowly by *Citrobacter* and some *Serratia* species. *Proteus,* unlike the coliforms, deaminates phenylalanine to phenylpyruvic acid, and it does not ferment lactose. Typically, *Proteus* is rapidly urease positive. Some species of *Klebsiella, Enterobacter,* and *Serratia* produce a positive urease reaction, but they do so more slowly. A battery of tests for biochemical properties is required to identify the coliforms and *Proteus* to the species level.

The coliforms are characterized by great antigenic diversity caused by various combinations of specific H, K, and O antigens. For example, approximately 50 H, 90 K, and 160 O antigens have been identified among various strains of *E coli.* In contrast, *Klebsiella,* with no H antigens, has 10 O antigens and approximately 80 K antigens. Serologic identification of the coliforms and *Proteus* species, commonly by reference laboratories and sometimes in combination with phage or bacteriocin typing, is an extremely important epidemiologic tool. Similarly, antibiograms (patterns of resistance to antimicrobial agents) and plasmid profiles (determined by agarose gel electrophoresis) are useful in epidemiologic studies, particularly of multiresistant isolates of coliforms and *Proteus.* In hospital-acquired infections, for example, the same or a small number of serologic or plasmid types suggests single sources of infection. The finding of multiple serotypes or plasmid profiles suggests multiple sources of infection or endogenous infections.

CONTROL

Prevention of coliform and *Proteus* infections, particularly those that are hospital acquired, is difficult and perhaps impossible. Sewage treatment, water purification, proper hygiene, and other control methods for enteric pathogens will reduce the incidence of *E coli* enteropathogens. However, these control measures are rarely available in less developed regions of the world. Breast-feeding is an effective means of limiting outbreaks of enteropathogens in infants. Aggressive infection control committees in hospitals can do much to reduce nosocomial infections through identification and control of predisposing factors, education and training of hospital personnel, and limited microbial surveillance. Except for investigations of potential outbreaks, routine culturing of personnel, patients, and the environment is not warranted. Meticulous hand washing after each patient contact—a highly effective means of reducing the transmission of nosocomial pathogens (Fig. 26-2)—is infrequently or poorly performed by some hospital personnel. Physicians often have the poorest hand-washing practices. In a recent study conducted in an intensive care unit following an educational campaign on the importance of hand washing, the compliance was 17 percent for physicians, 100 percent for nurses, 82 percent for respiratory technicians, and 88 percent for diagnostic services personnel.

Active or passive immunization against coliforms and *Proteus* species is not practiced; however, vaccines or hyperimmune sera for the six common pathogens (*E coli, Klebsiella, Enterobacter, Serratia, Pseudomonas aeruginosa,* and *Proteus*)

probably would have a major impact on morbidity and mortality from nosocomial infections. In one trial, the mortality was reduced markedly in a group of patients with Gram-negative bacteremia who had been given antiserum against a mutant *E coli* with an exposed lipopolysaccharide core.

Ampicillin, sulfonamides, cephalosporins, tetracycline, trimethoprim-sulfamethoxazole, nalidixic acid, and nitrofurantoin have been useful in treating urinary tract infections by coliforms and *Proteus* species. Gentamicin, amikacin, tobramycin, and a variety of third-generation cephalosporins may be effective for systemic infections; however, laboratory tests for drug susceptibility are essential. Antibiotic resistance is often a problem; some strains have multiple resistance due to the presence of R plasmids transmissible by conjugation. Conjugative resistance plasmids allow the transfer of resistance genes among species and genera that normally do not exchange chromosomal DNA (Ch. 5). In some cases, resolution of the infection may require drainage of abscesses or other surgical intervention.

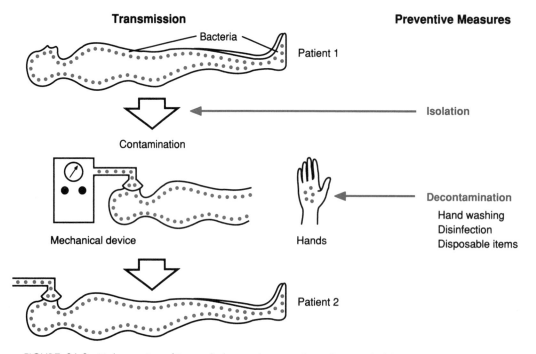

FIGURE 26-2 Major routes of transmission and prevention of spread of nosocomial pathogens.

REFERENCES

Bodey GP, Elting LS, Rodriguez S, Hernandez M: *Klebsiella* bacteremia: a 10-year review in a cancer institution. Cancer 64:2368, 1989

Boedeker EC: Enteroadherent (enteropathogenic) *Escherichia coli.* p. 123. In Farthing MJG, Keusch GT (eds): Enteric Infections: Mechanisms, Manifestations, and Management. Raven Press, New York, 1989

Brun-Buisson C, Legrand P, Philippon A et al: Transferable enzymatic resistance to third-generation cephalosporins during nosocomial outbreak of multiresistant *Klebsiella pneumoniae.* Lancet 2:302, 1987

Brun-Buisson C, Legrand P, Rauss A et al: Intestinal decontamination for control of nosocomial multiresistant gram-negative bacilli: study of an outbreak in an intensive care unit. Ann Intern Med 110:873, 1989

Conley JM, Hill S, Ross J et al: Handwashing practices in an intensive care unit: the effects of an educational program and its relationship to infection rates. Am J Infect Control 17:330, 1989

Evans DJ, Jr, Evans DG: Determinants of microbial attachment and their genetic control. p. 15. In Farthing MJG, Keusch GT (eds): Enteric Infections: Mechanisms, Manifestations, and Management. Raven Press, New York, 1989

Gordon MC, Hankins GDV: Urinary tract infections and pregnancy. Comp Ther 15:52, 1989

Griffith NC, Schell RE: Nosocomial infections. Am Fam Physician 35:179, 1987

Johnson JR, Stamm WE: Urinary tract infections in women: diagnosis and treatment. Ann Intern Med 111:906, 1989

Lipsky BA: Urinary tract infections in men: epidemiology, pathophysiology, diagnosis, and treatment. Ann Intern Med 110:138, 1989

Marshall JC, Christou NV, Horn R, Meakins JL: The microbiology of multiple organ failure: the proximal gastrointestinal tract as an occult reservoir of pathogens. Arch Surg 123:309, 1988

Mobley HLT, Chippendale GR: Hemagglutinin, urease, and hemolysin production by *Proteus mirabilis.* J Infect Dis 161:525, 1990

Morris JG, Lin FYC, Morrison CB et al: Molecular epidemiology of neonatal meningitis due to *Citrobacter diversus:* a study of isolates from hospitals in Maryland. J Infect Dis 154:409, 1986

Pai CH, Kelly JK: Shiga-like toxin-producing *Escherichia coli.* p. 141. In Farthing MJG, Keusch GT (eds): Enteric Infections: Mechanisms, Manifestations, and Management. Raven Press, New York, 1989

Saito H, Elting L, Bodey GP, Berky P: *Serratia* bacteremia: review of 118 cases. Rev Infect Dis 11:912, 1989

Sansonetti PJ: Enteroinvasive *Escherichia coli.* p. 283. *In* Farthing MJG, Keusch GT (eds): Enteric Infections: Mechanisms, Manifestations, and Management. Raven Press, New York, 1989

Segrati J: Nosocomial infections and secondary infections in sepsis. Crit Care Clin 5:177, 1989

Whimbey E, Kiehn TE, Brannon P et al: Bacteremia and fungemia in patients with neoplastic disease. Am J Med 82:723, 1987

27

PSEUDOMONAS

BARBARA H. IGLEWSKI

GENERAL CONCEPTS

Clinical Manifestations

Pseudomonas aeruginosa and *P maltophilia* account for 80 percent of opportunistic infections by pseudomonads. *Pseudomonas aeruginosa* infection is a serious problem in patients hospitalized with cancer, cystic fibrosis, and burns; the case fatality is 50 percent. Other infections caused by *Pseudomonas* species include endocarditis, pneumonia, and infections of the urinary tract, central nervous system, wounds, eyes, ears, skin, and musculoskeletal system.

Structure, Classification, and Antigenic Types

Pseudomonas species are Gram-negative, aerobic bacilli measuring 0.5 to 0.8 μm by 1.5 to 3.0 μm. Motility is by a single polar flagellum. Species are distinguished by biochemical and DNA hybridization tests. Antisera to lipopolysaccharide and outer membrane proteins show cross-reactivity among serovars.

Pathogenesis

Neutropenia in cancer patients and others receiving immunosuppressive drugs contributes to infection. *Pseudomonas aeruginosa* has several virulence factors, but their roles in pathogenesis are unclear. An alginate is antiphagocytic, and most strains isolated produce **toxin A,** a diphtheria-toxin-like exotoxin. All strains have **endotoxin,** which is a major virulence factor in bacteremia and septic shock.

Host Defenses

Phagocytosis by polymorphonuclear leukocytes is important in resistance to *Pseudomonas* infections. Antibodies to somatic antigens and exotoxins also contribute to recovery. Humoral immunity is normally the primary immune mechanism against *Pseudomonas* infection but does not seem to resolve infection in cystic fibrosis patients despite high levels of circulating antibodies.

Epidemiology

Pseudomonas species normally inhabit soil, water, and vegetation and can be isolated from the skin, throat, and stool of healthy persons. They often colonize hospital food, sinks, taps, mops, and respiratory equipment. Spread is from patient to patient via contact with fomites or by ingestion of contaminated food and water.

Diagnosis

Pseudomonas can be cultured on most general-purpose media and identified with biochemical media.

Control

The spread of *Pseudomonas* is best controlled by cleaning and disinfecting medical equipment. In burn patients, topical therapy of the burn with antimicrobial agents such as silver sulfadiazine, coupled with surgical debridement, has markedly reduced sepsis. Antibiotic susceptibility testing of clinical isolates is mandatory because of multiple antibiotic resistance; however, the combination of gentamicin and carbenicillin can be very effective in patients with acute *P aeruginosa* infections.

INTRODUCTION

The genus *Pseudomonas* contains more than 140 species, most of which are saprophytic. More than 25 species are associated with humans. Most pseudomonads known to cause disease in humans are associated with opportunistic infections. These include *P aeruginosa, P fluorescens, P putida, P cepacia, P stutzeri, P maltophilia,* and *P putrefaciens.* Only two species, *P mallei* and *P pseudomallei,* produce specific human diseases: glanders and melioidosis. *Pseudomonas aeruginosa* and *P maltophilia* account for approximately 80 percent of pseudomonads recovered from clinical specimens. Because of the frequency with which it is involved in human disease, *P aeruginosa* has received the most attention. It is a ubiquitous free-living bacterium and is found in most moist environments. Although it seldom causes disease in healthy individuals, it is a major threat to hospitalized patients, particularly those with serious underlying diseases such as cancer and burns. The high mortality associated with these infections is due to a combination of weakened host defenses, bacterial resistance to antibiotics, and the production of extracellular bacterial enzymes and toxins.

CLINICAL MANIFESTATIONS

Pseudomonas aeruginosa causes various diseases (Fig. 27–1). Localized infection following surgery or burns commonly results in a generalized and frequently fatal bacteremia. Urinary tract infections following introduction of *P aeruginosa* on catheters or in irrigating solutions are not uncommon. Furthermore, most cystic fibrosis patients are chronically colonized with *P aeruginosa.* Interestingly, cystic fibrosis patients rarely have *P aeruginosa* bacteremia, probably because of high levels of circulating *P aeruginosa* antibodies. However, most cystic fibrosis patients ultimately die of

localized *P aeruginosa* infections. Necrotizing *P aeruginosa* pneumonia may occur in other patients following the use of contaminated respirators. *Pseudomonas aeruginosa* can cause severe corneal infections following eye surgery or injury. It is found in pure culture, especially in children with middle ear infections. It occasionally causes meningitis following lumbar puncture and endocarditis following cardiac surgery. It has been associated with some diarrheal disease episodes. Since the first reported case of *P aeruginosa* infection in 1890, the organism has been increasingly associated with bacteremia and currently accounts for 15 percent of cases of Gram-negative bacteremia. The overall mortality associated with *P aeruginosa* bacteremia is about 50 percent. Some infections (e.g., eye and ear infections) remain localized; others, such as wound and burn infections and infections in leukemia and lymphoma patients, result in sepsis. The difference is most probably due to altered host defenses.

Pseudomonas maltophilia is the second most frequently isolated pseudomonad species in clinical laboratories. In nature, *P maltophilia* is found in water and in both raw and pasteurized milk. It has been associated with a variety of opportunistic infections in humans, including pneumonia, endocarditis, urinary tract infections, wound infections, septicemia, and meningitis. *Pseudomonas cepacia,* although primarily a plant pathogen (onion bulb rot), also is an opportunist. Most human infections caused by *P cepacia* are nosocomial and include endocarditis, necrotizing vasculitis, pneumonia, wound infections, and urinary tract infections. *Pseudomonas cepacia* causes chronic lung infections in cystic fibrosis patients. These infections differ from those caused by *P aeruginosa* in that *P cepacia* has become systemic in a number of cystic fibrosis patients, whereas *P aeruginosa* infections remain confined to the lungs. *Pseudomonas cepacia* is highly resistant to aminogly-

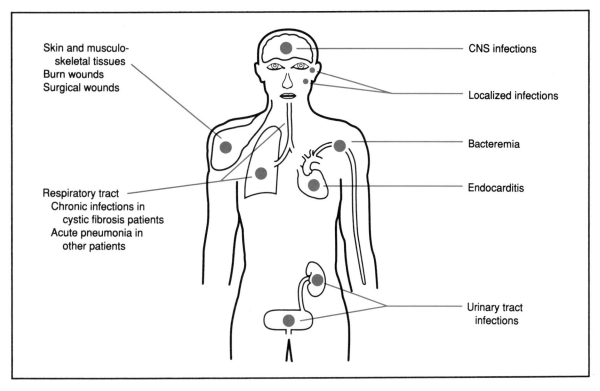

FIGURE 27-1   Diverse sites of infection by *P aeruginosa*. This opportunistic pathogen may infect virtually any tissue. Infection is facilitated by the presence of underlying disease (e.g., cancer, cystic fibrosis) or by a breakdown in nonspecific host defenses (as in burns).

cosides and other antibiotics, making it very difficult to control.

Unlike most pseudomonads, *P mallei* and *P pseudomallei* can cause disease in otherwise healthy individuals. *Pseudomonas mallei* is the agent of **glanders,** a disease primarily of equines. Humans generally become infected by inhalation or by direct contract through abraded skin. These infections are frequently fatal within 2 weeks of onset, although chronic infections also have been reported. Today, *P mallei* infections of equines are controlled and are rarely encountered in the western world. Similarly, **melioidosis,** an endemic glanderslike disease of animals and a human pulmonary infection caused by *P pseudomallei,* is rare in the western hemisphere. Melioidosis is still found in Southeast Asia, and travelers returning from that area are sometimes infected.

STRUCTURE, CLASSIFICATION, AND ANTIGENIC TYPES

Pseudomonas aeruginosa is a Gram-negative rod measuring 0.5 to 0.8 μm by 1.5 to 3.0 μm. Almost all strains are motile by means of a single polar flagellum, and some strains have two or three flagella (Fig. 27-2). The flagella yield heat-labile antigens (H antigen). The significance of antibody directed against these antigens, aside from its value in serologic classification, is unknown. Clinical isolates usually have pili, which may be antiphagocytic and probably aids in bacterial attachment, thereby promoting colonization.

The cell envelope of *P aeruginosa,* which is similar to that of other Gram-negative bacteria, consists of three layers: the inner or cytoplasmic membrane, the peptidoglycan layer, and the outer

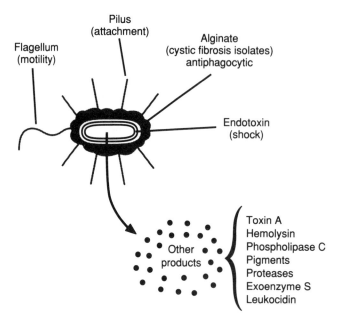

FIGURE 27-2 Structure and pathogenic mechanisms of *P aeruginosa*. The proposed role of other products is listed in Table 27-1.

membrane. The outer membrane is composed of phospholipid, protein, and lipopolysaccharide (LPS). The LPS of *P aeruginosa* is less toxic than that of other Gram-negative rods. The LPS of most strains of *P aeruginosa* contains heptose, 2-keto-3-deoxyoctonic acid, and hydroxy fatty acids, in addition to side-chain and core polysaccharides. Recent evidence suggests that the LPS of a large percentage of strains isolated from patients with cystic fibrosis may have little or no polysaccharide side chain (O antigen), and that this finding correlates with the polyagglutinability of these strains with typing sera.

Studies of isolated outer membranes suggest strong conservation of many of the outer membrane proteins of *P aeruginosa*. Although numerous serologic types exist (based on evaluations of O-specific antigens), many of the outer membrane proteins from these strains are antigenically cross-reactive.

Pseudomonas aeruginosa is a nonfermentative aerobe that derives its energy from oxidation rather than fermentation of carbohydrates. Although able to use more than 75 different organic compounds, it can grow on media supplying only acetate for carbon and ammonium sulfate for nitrogen. Furthermore, although an aerobe, it can grow anaerobically, using nitrate as an electron acceptor. This organism grows well at 25°C to 37°C, but can grow slowly or at least survive at higher and lower temperatures. Indeed, the ability to grow at 42°C distinguishes it from many other *Pseudomonas* species. In addition to its nutritional versatility, *P aeruginosa* resists high concentrations of salt, dyes, weak antiseptics, and many commonly used antibiotics. These properties help explain its ubiquitous nature and contribute to its preeminence as a cause of nosocomial infections.

PATHOGENESIS

Pseudomonas aeruginosa produces many factors that may contribute to its virulence. Table 27-1 lists some of them. Almost all strains of *P aeruginosa* are hemolytic on blood agar plates, and several different hemolysins have been described. A heat-stable hemolytic glycolipid consisting of two molecules each of L-rhamnose and 1-β-hydroxydecen-

TABLE 27-1   Products of *P aeruginosa* Strains

Product	Incidence of Production (%)	LD$_{50}$ in Mice	Proposed Role
Endotoxin	100	300 μg/IV	Terminal shock
Heat-stable hemolysin	95	5 mg/IP	Toxic to alveolar macrophages
Leukocidin	4	0.4 μg/IP	Depression of host defenses
Phospholipase C	70	?	Hydrolysis of lecithin
Pigments (pyocyanin and fluorescein)	90	?	Antibacterial agent
Proteases (elastase and alkaline protease)	90	200 μg/IP	Local tissue necrosis and spreading factor
Toxin A	90	0.2 μg/IP	Lethality and inhibition of host defenses
Exoenzyme S	90	?	Local and systemic toxicity

oic acid has been purified. Although this hemolytic glycolipid is not very toxic to animals (5 mg injected intraperitoneally is required to kill a mouse), it is toxic to alveolar macrophages. Furthermore, *P aeruginosa* strains isolated from respiratory tract infections produce more hemolysin than do environmental strains, suggesting that this glycolipid hemolysin may play a role in *P aeruginosa* pulmonary infections. Correlation of hemolysin production with infections of other sites has not been reported.

Several heat-labile protein hemolysins also have been described. One of these hemolysins may be identical to phospholipase C, which is produced by approximately 70 percent of all clinical strains of *P aeruginosa*. Phospholipase C, which hydrolyzes lecithin, is of unknown toxicity, and its role in *P aeruginosa* infections also remains unknown. Some strains of *P aeruginosa* produce a thermolabile protein (leukocidin), which lyses leukocytes from many species including humans but is nonhemolytic. This leukocidin (also called **cytotoxin**) damages lymphocytes and various tissue culture cells and is very toxic to mice (minimum lethal dose is 1 μg). Despite its toxicity, the role of leukocidin remains unknown.

Some strains of *P aeruginosa* produce large amounts of extracellular polysaccharide. These mucoid strains usually are isolated only from patients with cystic fibrosis. The role of these polysaccharides in the pathogenesis of *P aeruginosa*

chronic lung infections is unknown, but they may impede phagocytosis and impair diffusion of antibiotics and thus facilitate colonization and persistence. Interestingly, mucoid strains are frequently deficient in production of elastase, toxin A, and flagella, and their LPS lacks long polysaccharide side chains.

Most strains of *P aeruginosa* also produce one or more pigments, the most common being pyocyanin (a phenazine pigment) and fluorescein. These pigments are nontoxic in animals. Pyocyanin, however, retards the growth of some other bacteria and thus may facilitate colonization by *P aeruginosa*. One or more of these pigments appear to function in iron acquisition by *P aeruginosa*. Additional work is needed to clarify the role of these pigments in *P aeruginosa* infections.

Approximately 90 percent of *P aeruginosa* strains produce extracellular protease. Three separate proteases have been purified that differ in pH optimum, isoelectric point, and substrate specificity. Although all are capable of digesting casein, one of them, protease II, also digests elastin. When injected into the skin of animals, purified *P aeruginosa* proteases induce formation of hemorrhagic lesions, which become necrotic within 24 hours. These proteases also cause rapid tissue destruction when injected into the cornea of animal eyes or into rabbit lungs; they also probably contribute to the tissue destruction that accompanies *P aeruginosa* eye or lung infections and may aid bacteria in tissue invasion. Their effects, however, appear to be localized, and they are not highly toxic to animals (LD$_{50}$ = approximately 200 μg/mouse) (Table 27-1).

Toxin A

Toxin A, the most toxic known extracellular protein of *P aeruginosa,* is produced by 90 percent of all strains. The median lethal dose of pure toxin A is about 0.2 μg/mouse. Its toxicity has been attributed to its ability to inhibit protein synthesis in susceptible cells. It achieves this by catalyzing the transfer of the ADP-ribosyl moiety of nicotinamide adenine dinucleotide (NAD) onto elongation factor 2 (EF-2) according to the following reaction:

$$NAD + EF-2$$

$$\xrightleftharpoons{\text{toxin A}} ADP\text{-}ribosyl-EF\text{-}2 + nicotiamide + H^+$$

The resultant ADP-ribosyl–EF-2 complex is inactive in protein synthesis. This intracellular mechanism of action of toxin A is identical to that of diphtheria toxin fragment A (see Ch. 32). Also like diphtheria toxin, *Pseudomonas* toxin A is released by *P aeruginosa* as a proenzyme. Toxin A is toxic to animals and cultured cells, but the proenzyme has little or no enzymatic activity. Table 27-2 shows the relationship between the various forms of toxin A and their enzymatic activity and mouse toxicity. Evidence suggesting that toxin A may be a major virulence factor of *P aeruginosa* includes observations that toxin A-deficient mutants are less virulent in several animal models than their toxin

A-producing parental strains, as well as the observation that most patients surviving *P aeruginosa* sepsis have elevated levels of antitoxin A antibody or are infected with strains that produce little or no detectable toxin A in vitro. These studies need to be expanded before firm conclusions can be reached.

Exoenzyme S

A second ADP-ribosyltransferase, exoenzyme S, has been described. Exoenzyme S catalyzes the transfer of ADP-ribose onto a number of GTP-binding proteins, including the product of the proto-oncogene c-H-*ras* (p21$^{c\text{-}H\text{-}ras}$); however, it does not modify elongation factor 2. Exoenzyme S is produced by about 90 percent of clinical isolates of *P aeruginosa*. Transposon-induced S-deficient mutants are less virulent in several animal models than is their S-producing parental strain; thus, exoenzyme S may be involved in the pathogenesis of some *P aeruginosa* infections.

HOST DEFENSES

Although 85 percent of *P aeruginosa* isolates are resistant to serum alone, addition of polymorphonuclear leukocytes results in bacterial killing. Killing is most efficient in the presence of type-specific opsonizing antibodies, directed primarily at the antigenic determinants of LPS. This suggests that phagocytosis is an important defense and that opsonizing antibody is the principal functioning antibody in protecting from *P aeruginosa* infections; however, once a *P aeruginosa* infection is established, other antibodies, such as antitoxin, may be

TABLE 27-2 Comparison of the Structure and Function of Toxin A and Its Fragments

Toxin	Molecular Mass (Da)	Mouse LD$_{50}$	Maximum ADP-Ribosyltransferase Activity per μg of Protein (%)
Native toxin	70,000	0.2 μg	1–10
Reduced and denatured toxin[a]	70,000	>5.0 μg	35
Fragment A	27,000	>5.0 μg	100
Fragment B	43,000	Not tested	<1

[a] Toxin A was preincubated in 4 M urea plus 1 percent dithiothreitol for 15 minutes.

important in preventing death. Although evidence suggests interaction between *P aeruginosa* and the cellular immune system, patients with diseases characterized by impaired cellular immune responses (e.g., Hodgkin's disease) do not have an increased incidence of severe *P aeruginosa* infections; however, patients with diminished antibody responses caused by underlying disease or its associated therapy, have more serious *P aeruginosa* infections. This underscores the importance of the humoral response in controlling *P aeruginosa* infections. Cystic fibrosis is the exception; most cystic fibrosis patients have high levels of circulating antibodies to many bacterial antigens, but are unable to clear *P aeruginosa* efficiently from their lungs.

EPIDEMIOLOGY

Pseudomonas aeruginosa commonly inhabits soil, water, and vegetation. It is found in the skin of some healthy persons and has been isolated from the throat (5 percent) and stool (3 percent) of nonhospitalized patients. The gastrointestinal carriage rates increase in hospitalized patients to 20 percent within 72 hours of admission. Within the hospital, *P aeruginosa* finds numerous reservoirs: disinfectants, respiratory equipment, food, sinks, taps, and mops. Furthermore, it is constantly reintroduced into the hospital environment on fruits, plants, vegetables, and patients transferred from other facilities. Spread occurs from patient to patient on the hands of hospital personnel, by direct patient contact with contaminated reservoirs, and by the ingestion of contaminated foods and water.

Several different typing systems are available for epidemiologic studies: serologic, phage, pyocin, and DNA fingerprinting. In the pyocin system, pyocins (bacteriocins or aeruginocins) produced by the test strain are assayed for bactericidal activity against a series of indicator strains. A number of different serologic typing systems are used. Some employ combinations of heat-stable and heat-labile antigens, whereas others use only heat-stable antigens. No system is universally accepted. Recently, DNA fingerprinting has identified probes that are useful in typing *P aeruginosa* strains.

DIAGNOSIS

Diagnosis of *P aeruginosa* depends on its isolation and laboratory identification. It grows well on most laboratory media and commonly is isolated on blood agar plates or eosin-methylthionine blue agar. It is identified on the basis of its Gram morphology, inability to ferment lactose, a positive oxidase reaction, its fruity odor, and its ability to grow at 42°C. Fluorescence under ultraviolet radiation helps in early identification of *P aeruginosa* colonies and also is useful in suggesting its presence in wounds. Other pseudomonads are identified by specific laboratory tests.

CONTROL

The spread of *P aeruginosa* can best be controlled by observing proper isolation procedures, aseptic technique, and careful cleaning and monitoring of respirators, catheters, and other instruments. Topical therapy of burn wounds with antibacterial agents such as mafenide or silver sulfadiazine, coupled with surgical debridement, has dramatically reduced the incidence of *P aeruginosa* sepsis in burn patients.

Pseudomonas aeruginosa is frequently resistant to many commonly used antibiotics. Although many strains are susceptible to gentamicin, tobramycin, colistin, and amikacin, resistant forms have developed, making susceptibility testing essential. The combination of gentamicin and carbenicillin is frequently used to treat severe *Pseudomonas* infections, especially in patients with leukopenia. Several types of vaccines are being tested, but none is currently available for general use.

REFERENCES

Brown MRW (ed): Resistance of a *Pseudomonas aeruginosa.* John Wiley & Sons, New York, 1975

Clarke PH, Richman MN (eds): Genetics and Biochemistry of *Pseudomonas.* John Wiley & Sons, New York, 1975

Coburn J, Wyatt RT, Iglewski BH, Gill DM: Several GTP-binding proteins, including o24 C-H-ras, are preferred substrates of *Pseudomonas aeruginosa* exoenzyme S. J Biol Chem 264:9004, 1989

Cross AS, Sadoff JC, Iglewski BH, Sokol PA: Evidence

for the role of toxin A in the pathogenesis of infections with *Pseudomonas aeruginosa* in humans. J Infect Dis 142:538, 1980

Hancock REW, Mutharia LM, Chan L, et al: *Pseudomonas aeruginosa* isolates from patients with cystic fibrosis: a class of serum-sensitive, nontypable strains deficient in lipopolysaccharide O side chain. Infect Immun 42:170, 1983

Liu PV: Extracellular toxins of *Pseudomonas aeruginosa*. J Infect Dis, suppl. 130:S95, 1974

Mutharia LM, Nicas TI, Hancock REW: Outer membrane proteins of *Pseudomonas aeruginosa* serotyping strains. J Infect Dis 46:770, 1982

Pritchard AE, Vasal ML: Possible insertion sequences in a mosaic genome organization upstream of the exotoxin A gene in *Pseudomonas aeruginosa*. J Bacteriol 172:2020, 1990

Woods DE, Iglewski BH: Toxins of *Pseudomonas aeruginosa:* new perspectives. Rev Infect Dis, suppl. 5:S715, 1983

28
BRUCELLA

J. R. L. Forsyth
G. G. Alton

GENERAL CONCEPTS

Clinical Manifestations

Brucellosis is a severe acute febrile disease caused by bacteria of the genus *Brucella*. Relapses are not uncommon; focal lesions occur in bones, joints, the genitourinary tract, and other sites. Hypersensitivity reactions can follow occupational exposure. Infection may be subclinical. Chronic infections may occur.

Structure

Coccobacilli are Gram-negative, non-spore-forming, and nonmotile; they are aerobic, but may need added CO_2.

Classification and Antigenic Types

Three species (*B melitensis*, *B abortus*, and *B suis*) are important human pathogens; *B canis* is of lesser importance. Species are differentiated by production of urease and H_2S, dye sensitivity, cell wall antigens, and bacteriophage sensitivity. The major species are divided into multiple biovars.

Pathogenesis

Portals of entry are the mouth, conjunctivae, respiratory tract, and abraded skin. Organisms spread in mononuclear phagocytes to reticuloendothelial sites. Small granulomas reveal a mononuclear response; hypersensitivity is a major factor.

Host Defenses

Effective host defense depends primarily on cell-mediated immunity.

Epidemiology

Brucellosis is a **zoonosis** acquired from the handling of infected animals or by consuming contaminated milk or milk products. Exposure is frequently occupational. The disease is now uncommon in the United States and Britain, but common in the Mediterranean area, Arabian Gulf, Latin America, Africa, and parts of Asia.

Diagnosis

Diagnosis can be made clinically if there is a history of exposure. Blood cultures are positive in early disease, but serology is the mainstay of diagnosis. Interpretation is complicated by subclinical infections and persistent antibodies.

Control

Brucellosis is prevented by pasteurizing milk, eradicating infection from herds, and using safety precautions (protective clothing and laboratory safety). The disease is treated with doxycycline, streptomycin, and rifampin.

INTRODUCTION

Bacteria of the genus *Brucella* cause disease primarily in domestic and some wild animals, but most are also pathogenic for humans. In animals, brucellae typically affect the reproductive organs, and abortion is usually the only sign of the disorder. Human **brucellosis** is either an acute febrile disease or a chronic disease with a wide variety of symptoms. It is a true **zoonosis** in that virtually all human infections are acquired from animals. The disease is controlled by the routine practice of pasteurizing milk and milk products, as well as by widespread campaigns to eradicate the disease in domestic animals exhibiting positive serologic reactions to the organisms. Vaccines are available for protecting cattle, sheep, and goats.

CLINICAL MANIFESTATIONS

The presentation of brucellosis is characteristically variable. The incubation period is often difficult to determine but is usually 2 to 4 weeks. The onset may be insidious or abrupt. Subclinical infection is common.

In the simplest case, the onset is influenzalike, with fever reaching 38 to 40°C. Limb and back pains are unusually severe, however, and sweating and fatigue are marked. The leukocyte count tends to be normal or reduced, with a relative lymphocytosis. On examination, splenomegaly may be the only finding. If the disease is not treated, the symptoms may continue for 2 to 4 weeks. Many patients then recover spontaneously, but others may suffer a series of exacerbations. These may produce an **undulant fever,** in which the intensity of fever and symptoms recur and recede at about 10-day intervals. True relapses may occur months after the initial episode, even after apparently successful treatment.

Most patients recover entirely within 3 to 12 months, but some develop complications marked by involvement of various organs, and a few enter an ill-defined chronic syndrome. Complications include arthritis and spondylitis (in about 10 percent of cases), central nervous system effects including meningitis (in about 5 percent), uveitis,

and, occasionally, epididymo-orchitis. Although abortion is a common sign of brucellosis in domestic animals, it is not a feature of the disease in women. Hypersensitivity reactions, which may mimic the symptoms of an infection, may occur in individuals exposed to infective material after previous infection, even subclinical.

STRUCTURE

Brucellae are Gram-negative coccobacilli (short rods) measuring about 0.6 to 1.5 μm by 0.5 to 0.7 μm. They do not form spores, and they lack capsules or flagella and, therefore, are nonmotile. The outer cell membrane closely resembles that of other Gram-negative bacilli, with a dominant lipopolysaccharide (LPS) component and three main groups of proteins. The guanine-plus-cytosine content of the DNA is 55 to 58 moles/cm. Plasmids have not been found in any *Brucella* species.

The metabolism of the brucellae is mainly oxidative, and they show little action on carbohydrates in conventional media. They are aerobes, but some species require an atmosphere with added CO_2 (5 to 10 percent). Multiplication is slow at the optimum temperature of 37°C, and enriched medium is needed to support adequate growth.

Brucella colonies become visible on solid media in 2 to 3 days. Fresh strains from the principal species are smooth, but dissociation occurs readily to produce rough or mucoid colonies. Some species, which have relatively restricted host ranges, are normally rough or mucoid and lack the O chains.

CLASSIFICATION AND ANTIGENIC TYPES

The genus *Brucella* was originally classified according to the reservoir hosts. *Brucella melitensis* was described as early as 1886 as the cause of Malta fever in humans. Goats and some breeds of sheep were later shown to be the source. *Brucella melitensis, B abortus* (from cattle) and *B suis* (from pigs and reindeer) are the principal species that affect humans. *Brucella canis* (from dogs) causes only mild disease in humans, and *B ovis* (from sheep) and *B neotomae* (from the American desert wood rat) do not affect humans.

The species are differentiated in the laboratory by many criteria including colony morphology, a requirement for serum for growth, production of urease, the oxidase test, and the lytic action of controlled concentrations of certain bacteriophages (Table 28-1). Further differentiation into biovars may be useful: the criteria for this division include the requirement for added CO_2, the production of H_2S, reactions with monospecific sera, and the ability to grow on media containing low concentrations of certain dyes (Table 28-2). As a further refinement of differentiation, tests for the oxidative metabolism of certain amino acids and carbohydrates have been devised. Despite all this, modern DNA hybridization studies suggest that it would be more appropriate to reclassify the genus as consisting of a single species, as the currently named species show such a high degree of homology.

Two different O chains occur in the LPS of the brucellae with smooth colonies. These are called **A** and **M**, nominally indicating *abortus* and *melitensis* antigens; however, some *B abortus* biovars carry the M antigen and some common *B melitensis* biovars carry the A antigen. Both O chains are homopolymers of 4,6-dideoxy-4-formamido-D-mannopyranosyl; they differ only in that in the A chain the sugar molecules are always linked 2–1, whereas the M chain has a 3–1 linkage at every fifth junction. In routine serology, smooth species of brucellae cross-react almost completely with each other, but not with rough species, and vice versa. Monospecific sera reacting only to A or M antigens can be prepared by cross-absorption. Studies with monoclonal antibodies have shown that there is at least one unique epitope on each type of chain. (An epitope is the molecular site of an antigen that reacts with specific antibody.)

PATHOGENESIS

Brucellae are facultative intracellular parasites, multiplying mainly in cells of the reticuloendothelial system. This characteristic determines most aspects of the pathology, clinical manifestations, and therapy of the disease.

The organisms may gain entry into the body through a variety of portals (Fig. 28-1). Because the infection is systemic, it is often not possible to determine which portal was involved in a particular case. Oral entry, by ingestion of contaminated animal products (often raw milk or its derivatives) or by contact with contaminated fingers, probably represents the most common route of infection, even though this portal may not be the most vulnerable one. Inhalation of aerosols containing the bacteria, or aerosol contamination of the conjunctivae, is another route. Inhalation probably underlies some industrial outbreaks. Percutaneous infection through skin abrasions or by accidental inoculation has frequently been demonstrated.

Brucella species differ markedly in their capacity to cause invasive human disease. *Brucella melitensis* is the most pathogenic; *B abortus* is associated with less frequent infection and a greater proportion of subclinical cases. The virulence of *B suis* strains for humans varies but is generally intermediate.

Animal studies suggest that invading brucellae are rapidly phagocytosed by polymorphonuclear leukocytes. Brucellae are frequently able to survive and multiply in these cells because they inhibit the bactericidal myeloperoxidase-peroxide-halide system by releasing 5′-guanosine and adenine. Early in infection, macrophages are also relatively ineffectual in killing the intracellular brucellae (Fig. 28-2). It is not clear whether the bacteria are transported within polymorphonuclear leukocytes and macrophages or in the bloodstream outside cells. Organisms may disseminate widely from the regional lymphoid tissue appropriate to the portal of entry and may localize in certain target organs such as lymph nodes, spleen, liver, bone marrow, and (especially in animals) reproductive organs. The presence of *meso*-erythritol in the testicles and seminal vesicles of bulls, rams, goats, and boars and in the products of conception in pregnant ruminants and pigs stimulates enormous multiplication of brucellae. Erythritol represents a potent localizing factor in the relevant species, but is absent in humans.

In humans, the tissue lesions produced by *Brucella* species consist of minute granulomas that are composed of epithelioid cells, polymorphonuclear

TABLE 28-1 Differential Characteristics of *Brucella* Species

Species	Colony Morphology	Serum Requirement	Lysis by Phages Tb RTD[g]	Lysis by Phages Tb 10⁴ × RTD	Lysis by Phages R/C RTD	Oxidase	Urease	Preferred Host
B melitensis	Smooth	−	−	−	−	+	+[a]	Sheep, goats
B abortus	Smooth	−[b]	+	+	−	+[c]	+[d]	Cattle; Biovar 1; pigs; Biovar 2; hares and pigs
B suis	Smooth	−	−	+	−	+	+[e]	Biovar 3; pigs; Biovar 4; reindeer; Biovar 5; wild rodents
B neotomae	Smooth	−	−[f]	+	−	−	+[e]	Desert wood rats
B ovis	Rough	+	−	−	+	−	−	Rams
B canis	Rough	−	−	−	+	+	+[e]	Dogs

[a] Intermediate rate, some strains rapid.
[b] Except *B abortus* biovar 2, which generally requires serum for growth on primary isolation.
[c] Except *B abortus* biovar 3 strains isolated in Senegal and Guinea Bissau, which are negative.
[d] Intermediate rate except for reference strain 544 and occasional field strains, which are negative.
[e] High rate.
[f] Minute plaques.
[g] RTD, routine test dilution.

TABLE 28-2 Biovar Differentiation of *Brucella* Species

| Species | Biovar | CO_2 Requirement | H_2S Production | Growth on Dyes[a] | | Agglutination in Serum[b] | | |
				Thionine	Basic Fuchsine	A	M	R
B melitensis	1	−	−	+	+	−	+	−
	2	−	−	+	+	+	−	−
	3	−	−	+	+	+	+	−
B abortus	1	+[c]	+	−	+	+	−	−
	2	+[c]	+	−	−	+	−	−
	3	+[c]	+	+	+	+	−	−
	4	+[c]	+	−	+[d]	−	+	−
	5	−	−	+	+	−	+	−
	6	−	−	+	+	+	−	−
	9	±	+	+	+	−	+	−
B suis	1	−	+	+	−[e]	+	−	−
	2	−	−	+	−	+	−	−
	3	−	−	+	+	+	−	−
	4	−	−	+	−[f]	+	+	−
	5	−	−	+	−	−	+	−
B neotomae		−	+	−[g]	−	+	−	−
B ovis		+	−	+	−[f]	−	−	+
B canis		−	−	+	−[f]	−	−	+

[a] Dye concentration, 20μg/ml in serum dextrose medium (1 : 50,000).

[b] A, A monospecific antiserum; M, M monospecific antiserum; R, rough *Brucella* antiserum.

[c] Usually positive on primary isolation.

[d] Some strains isolated in Canada, Britain, and the United States do not grow on dyes.

[e] Some basic fuchsine resistant strains have been isolated in South America and South East Asia.

[f] Negative for most strains.

[g] Growth will occur at 10 μg of (1 : 100,000) thionine/ml.

leukocytes, lymphocytes, and some giant cells. In cases of infection with *B melitensis* these granulomas are particularly small, although the toxemia associated with this organism is great. Necrosis is not common, and abscesses do not form, except in *B suis* infection. The fact that humans rapidly develop hypersensitivity suggests that many of the symptoms of human brucellosis result from the reaction of the host defenses.

HOST DEFENSES

The specific host defenses against brucellae resemble those against other intracellular bacteria and are both humoral (antibody mediated) and cell mediated. Antibody, particularly that directed against the cell surface LPS, plays a part in protecting experimental animals against infection. Passively administered monoclonal antibody directed against LPS has reduced the number of brucellae surviving in the spleens and livers of experimental mice. However, the main effective defense against brucellae is cell mediated. Macrophages process brucellar antigen and present it to T lymphocytes, which produce lymphokines. These agents, of which interferon is the most active in this context, stimulate the formerly ineffective macrophages to greater bactericidal potency. T-cell-derived lymphokines also attract cells to the foci of infection, leading to granuloma formation. Although this contributes to the pathology, it also delivers the activated macrophages to the site

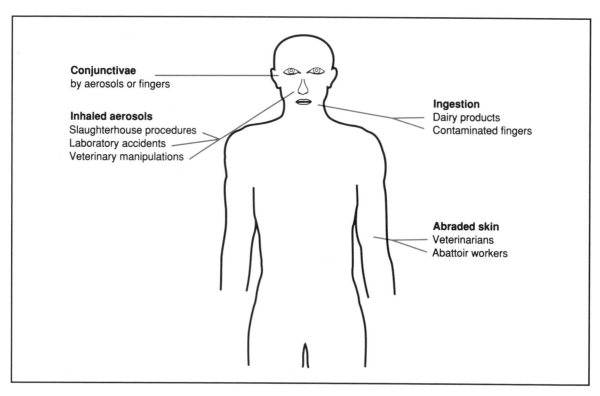

FIGURE 28–1 Portals of entry for *Brucella* species.

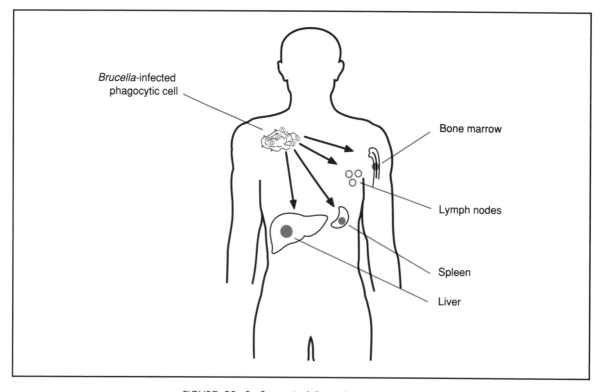

FIGURE 28–2 Spread of *Brucella* in the body.

where they are needed. The inflammatory response is enhanced by cytokines, such as the colony-stimulating factors, tumor necrosis factor, and interleukin-1, produced by a number of cell types.

Mice that survive brucellosis are protected against further challenge, and there is clinical evidence that complete recovery from a natural infection is associated with at least a degree of residual resistance in humans.

EPIDEMIOLOGY

The reservoirs of brucellosis are various wild and (particularly) domestic animals (Fig. 28-3). Humans are incidentally infected. The predilection of brucellae for the reproductive organs of ruminants is associated with abortion, often the only sign of disease. Huge numbers of brucellae are released during abortion, leading to massive contamination of the environment. Brucellae also often become established in the mammary glands for prolonged periods and are then shed in lesser,

but still significant, numbers in the milk. Such animals frequently show no sign of ill health. Brucellae are also released when infected animals, particularly pregnant females, are slaughtered. It is these circumstances that determine the epidemiology of brucellosis in humans.

Brucella melitensis is by far the most important species in human disease. It infects goats, some breeds of sheep, and camels and may also colonize the bovine udder. It is absent from North America and northern Europe as well as from Australasia and South East Asia. It is prevalent in the Mediterranean region, the Middle East, Central Asia, and some countries of Central and South America. Among the populations of the Arabian Gulf countries there is an extensive and continuing epidemic. Humans acquire *B melitensis* from handling animals, especially at parturition, and from ingesting unpasteurized milk and milk products. Fresh soft cheeses have been an important vehicle of spread. In many cases the route of infection is uncertain, and bacteria-laden dust has been suspected as the vehicle. Outbreaks of *B melitensis*

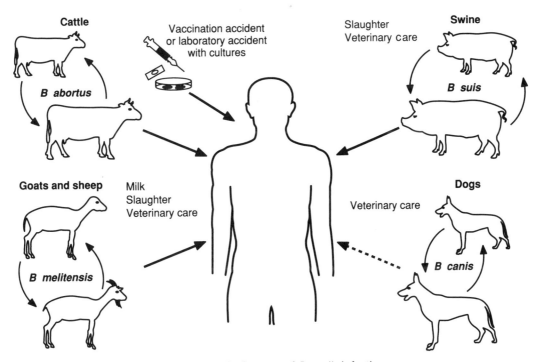

FIGURE 28-3 Sources of *Brucella* infection.

disease are important, and some have been extensive.

Brucella suis occurs sporadically in pig herds in many countries. It affects both sexes and causes chronic infertility and abortion. It can also colonize the bovine udder. Human infections, usually sporadic, occur among abattoir workers and pig keepers. However, the prevalence of disease has been markedly reduced in some countries, such as the United States, by an eradication campaign.

Bovine brucellosis (caused by *B abortus*) has been successfully eradicated in many areas, including Canada, Japan, northern Europe, Australia, and New Zealand. Human infections with *B abortus* are sporadic and occur as a result of occupational contact. Veterinarians are at substantial risk when removing retained products of conception, and they may also be infected by accidental inoculation of live vaccine. Slaughterhouse workers are also at risk. *Brucella abortus* has been transmitted by unpasteurized milk, but this is a relatively inefficient means of spread. Meat is not important.

Cases of *B canis* infection in humans occur largely in dog handlers. Close, frequent, contact usually seems to be necessary for transmission.

Although person-to-person spread is quite exceptional, the *Brucella* species of principal importance are all potent causes of laboratory infection. Aerosols are a very important medium of spread in this situation, and suitable precautions, with adequate equipment for containment, are essential when handling cultures.

DIAGNOSIS

The diagnosis of brucellosis is primarily clinical; it is made on the basis of the typical pattern of febrile disease combined with a history of possible exposure (Fig. 28-4). The history must include not only the patient's occupation and possible use of raw milk or milk products but also whether he or she has traveled to endemic areas. In some cases, however, the presentation of brucellosis is highly atypical. Unequivocal diagnosis depends on isolation of the organism. Blood culture is the method of

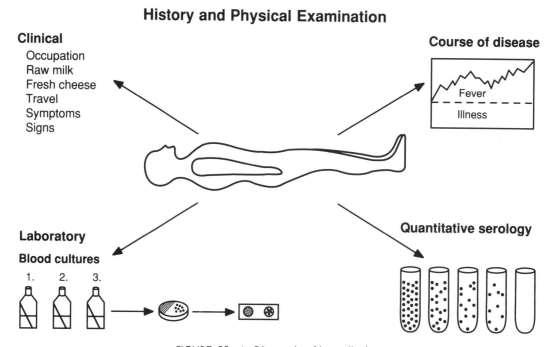

FIGURE 28–4 Diagnosis of brucellosis.

choice, but specimens must be obtained early in the disease and cultures may have to be incubated for up to 3 weeks. Even under these conditions, the organism often fails to grow, especially in cases of *B abortus* infection, and isolation rates of only 20 to 50 percent are reported even from experienced laboratories. Bone marrow culture has its advocates, but the improvement in the rate of diagnosis would not appear to justify the procedure. Cultured bacteria may be identified presumptively on the grounds of morphology, together with slide agglutination with specific antiserum. Further identification should be carried out at a reference facility.

Serology remains the mainstay of laboratory diagnosis, but the interpretation of results is fraught with difficulties. The standard serum agglutination test (SAT) has been augmented by the modified Coombs (antiglobulin) technique and supplemented by a complement fixation test. These classic methods may, in time, be replaced by enzyme-linked immunosorbent assay (ELISA), designed to differentiate between specific IgM and IgG antibodies. Although serum agglutination test titers commonly decline after recovery during infection and antiglobulin test levels are maintained much longer, the IgM antibody that is commonly measured by the serum agglutination test does not fall away as regularly as in some infections. Nevertheless, persisting levels of antibody may indicate a remaining focus of infection. Specific IgG levels rise again during a true relapse. Because cases often are investigated late in their course, rising titers are frequently missed; the variability of individual responses and the frequency of subclinical infections make the interpretation of single high titers difficult. All serologic tests must be interpreted with caution in the light of clinical data and in the context of the local prevalence of brucellosis.

Diagnosis of the chronic brucellosis syndrome, without specific localization, is often very unsatisfactory. Cultures are usually negative, and the results of serologic tests are equivocal. A confident diagnosis, which is needed when the question of compensation for an occupationally acquired disease arises, is often impossible. However, these cases do exist, and they represent a diagnostic dilemma.

CONTROL

Individuals who are occupationally exposed can protect themselves to some extent by wearing impermeable clothing, rubber boots, gloves, and face masks and by practising good personal hygiene. Pasteurization of milk for drinking and for incorporation into other dairy products is effective in protecting consumers. Vaccination of humans has not been used extensively outside the Soviet Union. If progress in the development of purified vaccines containing LPS, with or without outer membrane proteins, continues, this could change.

However, eradication of brucellosis from domestic animals eliminates the threat totally and has been successful in several countries. In eradication campaigns, the level of enzootic disease is first reduced by intensive use of live, attenuated vaccines (*B abortus* strain 19 in cattle, *B melitensis* strain Rev. 1 in sheep and goats), particularly in immature animals. Thereafter, the emphasis shifts to the detection of infected herds (by skin tests for sheep and by serologic tests on milk or blood samples taken at sale or slaughter for cattle) and individual animals (by serologic tests) and to the elimination of the latter by slaughter.

Human patients are treated with a combination of doxycycline and streptomycin; regimens of 2-week courses with intervals of 2 weeks between treatments have been successful. The addition of rifampin to reach intracellular organisms is indicated in complicated cases. Patients with chronic brucellosis frequently need symptomatic treatment in addition to antibiotics, and their response to antimicrobial chemotherapy may be disappointing.

REFERENCES

Alton GG, Jones LM, Angus RD et al: Techniques for the Brucellosis Laboratory. INRA, Paris, 1988

Joint FAO/WHO Expert Committee on Brucellosis: Sixth Report, Technical Report Series 740, World Health Organization, Geneva, 1986

Madkour MM (ed): Brucellosis. Butterworth, London, 1989

Spink WW: The Nature of Brucellosis. University of Minnesota Press, Minneapolis, 1956

World Health Organization: A Guide to the Diagnosis, Treatment and Prevention of Human Brucellosis. WHO, Geneva, 1983 (under revision)

Young EJ: Human brucellosis. Rev Infect Dis 5:821, 1983

Young EJ, Corbel MJ (eds): Brucellosis: Clinical and Laboratory Aspects, CRC Press, Boca Raton, FL, 1989

29 PASTEURELLA, YERSINIA, AND FRANCISELLA

FRANK M. COLLINS

GENERAL CONCEPTS

PASTEURELLA

Clinical Manifestations

In humans, *Pasteurella* causes chronic abscesses on the extremities or face after cat or dog bites.

Structure, Classification, and Antigenic Types

These bacteria are small, nonmotile, Gram-negative coccobacilli exhibiting bipolar staining. *Pasteurella multocida* is found in cattle, chickens, rabbits, and humans. There are four capsular types (A, B, D, and E), and 15 somatic antigens are recognized on cells stripped of capsular polysaccharides with acid or hyaluronidase. *Pasteurella haemolytica* affects cattle and horses.

Pathogenesis

Abscesses are characterized by extensive edema and fibrosis. Encapsulated organisms resist phagocytosis. Endotoxin contributes to tissue damage.

Host Defenses

Encapsulated bacteria are not phagocytosed unless specific opsonins are present. Acquired resistance is almost entirely humoral.

Epidemiology

Pasteurella species are primarily pathogens of cattle, sheep, fowl, and rabbits. Humans become infected while handling infected animals.

Diagnosis

Diagnosis depends on clinical appearance, history of animal contact, and results of culture on blood agar. Colonies are small, nonhemolytic, and iridescent. The organisms are identified by biochemical and serologic methods.

Control

No vaccines are available for human use. Treatment requires drainage of the lesion and prolonged multidrug therapy. *Pasteurella multocida* is susceptible to sulfadiazine, ampicillin, chloramphenicol, and tetracycline.

YERSINIA

Clinical Manifestations

Yersinia pestis causes **bubonic** and **pneumonic plague.** Bubonic plague is transmitted by the bite of infected fleas. Swollen, blackened lymph nodes (**buboes**) develop, followed by septicemia and hemorrhagic pneumonia. The pneumonic form spreads from human to human via respiratory droplets and is explosive and invariably lethal. *Yersinia enterocolitica* causes severe diarrhea and local abscesses, and *Y pseudotuberculosis* causes severe entercolitis.

Structure, Classification, and Antigenic Types

Yersinia organisms are small, Gram-negative coccobacilli showing bipolar staining. Three species are of medical importance; *Y pestis, Y enterocolitica,* and *Y pseudotuberculosis.* The capsular or envelope antigen is heat labile. Somatic antigens V and W are associated with virulence. Antigen 8 is a toxin.

Pathogenesis

In bubonic plague, the bacilli spread from a local abscess to draining lymph nodes; this is followed by septicemia and hemorrhagic pneumonia. *Yersinia enterocolitica* enters via Peyer's patches and causes severe liver and splenic abscesses. *Yersinia pseudotuberculosis* causes enlarged, caseous nodules in the Peyer's patches and mesenteric lymph nodes.

Host Defenses

Specific anti-envelope antibodies are opsonic and protective. Cell-mediated resistance is also involved.

Epidemiology

Yersinia pestis is primarily a rat pathogen. Human epidemics are initially transmitted by rat fleas, but may shift into the pneumonic form. *Yersinia enterocolitica,* a pathogen of deer and cattle, is spread to humans via water.

Diagnosis

Early clinical diagnosis of plague is essential. Blood culture is positive for *Y pestis,* and sputum may show small bacilli with fluorescent antibody staining. *Yersinia pestis* is extremely infectious and is a hazard for nursing and laboratory personnel.

Control

Control of rats and rat fleas is central. Laboratory personnel should be vaccinated with killed *Y pestis* vaccine. *Yersinia pestis* is susceptible to sulfadiazine, streptomycin, tetracycline, and chloramphenicol. *Yersinia enterocolitica* is controlled by purifying water and pasteurizing milk. *Yersinia pseudotuberculosis* disease requires aggressive treatment with ampicillin and tetracycline.

FRANCISCELLA

Clinical Manifestations

Francisella tularensis causes **tularemia,** with high fever and acute septicemia and toxemia. Oral infection causes typhoidlike disease.

Structure, Classification, and Antigenic Types

The organisms are small, nonmotile, Gram-negative coccobacilli. *Franciscella* is nutritionally demanding. It is biochemically similar to the brucellae, but antigenically distinct.

Pathogenesis

A local abscess at the site of infection is followed by septicemia with rapid spread to the liver and spleen; 30 percent of untreated patients die.

Host Defenses

Cell-mediated immunity is protective and long lasting.

Epidemiology

Franciscella is primarily a pathogen of squirrels and rabbits; humans are infected by the bite of an infected deerfly or tick or by handling or eating undercooked infected rabbit meat.

Diagnosis

Cultivation from blood or biopsy material is difficult and slow. Blood smears can be stained with specific fluorescent antibody. Hemagglutinins appear in 10 to 12 days; a rising titer is always diagnostic.

Control

A live attenuated vaccine is available for laboratory personnel. Goggles must be worn in the laboratory to prevent conjunctival infection. *Franciscella* is susceptible to streptomycin, tetracycline, and chloramphenicol.

INTRODUCTION

The genus *Pasteurella* was originally proposed and described by Trevisan in 1887. It consisted of a group of small (0.7 μm by 0.5 μm), nonmotile, Gram-negative coccobacilli often exhibiting a characteristic type of bipolar staining. (Fig. 29-1). The members of this genus are associated with severe, life-threatening systemic diseases involving both hemorrhagic pneumonia and septicemia. The

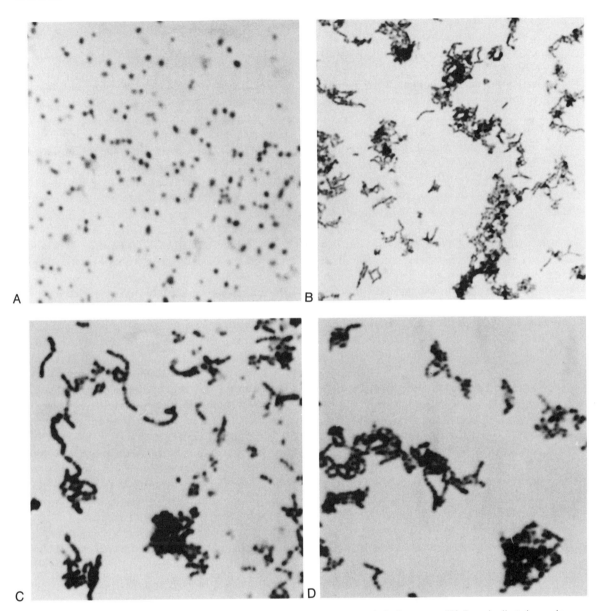

FIGURE 29-1 *(A) Pasteurella multocida* growth on brain-heart infusion agar. *(B) Francisella tularensis* growth on chocolate blood agar. *(C) Yersinia pestis* growth on tryptose soy agar. *(D) Yersinia entero-colitica* growth on tryptose soy agar. (Gram stain, ×1,200.)

first pathogen to be studied (then called *Pasteurella septica*) was responsible for hemorrhagic septicemia (shipping fever) in cattle and sheep and fowl cholera in chickens and was used by Pasteur for his milestone vaccination studies in 1880. This organism is now generally referred to as *Pasteurella*

multocida. Adult animals may carry this organism as part of their normal nasopharyngeal or gingival microflora and may infect young, susceptible animals, which develop a fulminating hemorrhagic pneumonia, especially following some form of stress (overcrowding or dehydration). The incubation period may be as short as 12 hours. The disease can spread explosively through an apparently normal herd or flock and has a very high mortality rate (80 to 100 percent).

Two other important pathogens were initially included in this genus. The first was *Pasteurella pestis* (the plague bacillus), which was isolated and described almost simultaneously by Kitasato and by Yersin in 1894. This organism is primarily a pathogen of the rat (one of a select group of acute bacterial pathogens for this host). For taxonomic reasons, it was decided in 1971 to place the plague bacillus in a new genus as *Yersinia pestis*, along with *Y pseudotuberculosis* and *Y enterocolitica*, both of which infect a variety of rodent species and can cause severe intestinal disease in humans. Finally, a third genus was created for an organism originally grouped with *P pestis*, but now separated as *Francisella tularensis*, the agent of tularemia in rodents and humans. The various diseases caused by these three genera, together with the vectors responsible for their spread to humans, are summarized in Table 29-1.

Metabolically, all of these organisms are facultative anaerobes which grow best on nutrient media enriched with blood, hematin, or catalase. Most members show a restricted fermentative capacity. Although they grow well when incubated at 37°C, they can also multiply at room temperature, some species produce putative virulence factors at room temperature that may help to establish them within the host tissues. Vaccines are of limited value. Aggressive treatment with broad-spectrum antibiotics is required for control.

◀ *PASTEURELLA* ▶

CLINICAL MANIFESTATIONS

Although *P multocida* is an awesome pathogen in young cattle, birds, and mice, it can also be a relatively benign member of the nasopharyngeal microflora of adult rabbits, cats, and dogs, often without the development of severe pulmonary involvement. There have been reports of pulmonary pasteurellosis in some cattle handlers, and it seems likely that this organism can colonize normal human nasopharyngeal membranes. These infections seldom progress to involve the lungs.

Most human infections with *Pasteurella* occur as localized abscesses of the extremities or the face as a result of cat or dog bites (Fig. 29-2). Historically, such infections were first associated with tiger bites in India. Domestic cats, as well as exotic felines, carry *P multocida* as part of the normal gingival microflora; the organism can thus be introduced into human tissues as a result of bites and scratches. *Pasteurella multocida* can be highly invasive, entering the subcutaneous tissues through apparently minor skin abrasions and quickly forming severe local abscesses, which eventually spread to the draining lymph nodes (Fig. 29-2). These abscesses may require surgical drainage because of the extensive associated edema and fibrosis (which also reduce the effectiveness of the chemotherapeutic intervention, even though this organism is susceptible to most antibiotics in vitro).

Adult cattle often carry virulent strains of *P multocida* as part of their normal nasopharyngeal flora

TABLE 29-1   Disease and Vector Comparisons for *Pasteurella, Yersinia,* and *Francisella*

Organism	Host Species	Vector	Disease
P multocida	Cattle, birds	Aerosols	Pneumonia and septicemia
	Humans	Cat and dog bites	Localized abscess
Y pestis	Rats, humans	Rat flea bite	Bubonic plague
		Aerosol	Pneumonic plague
Y enterocolitica	Cattle, birds, humans	Infected water and foods	Enterocolitis, systemic abscesses
Y pseudotuberculosis	Rodents, humans	Infected water	Enterocolitis
F tularensis	Rabbits, squirrels, humans	Ticks, deerflies, trauma, infected rabbit meat	Tularemia, septicemia, typhoidlike enteritis

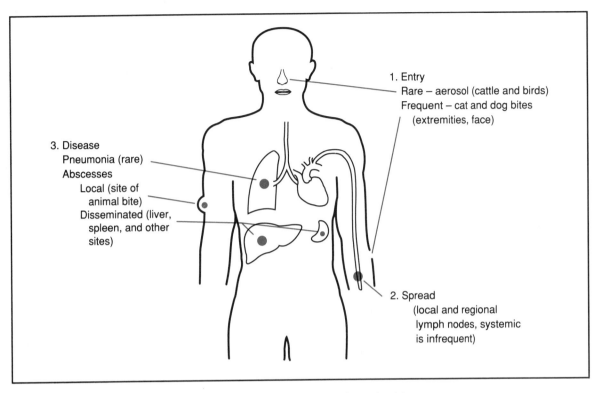

FIGURE 29-2 Pathogenesis of *P multocida*.

and show no obvious sign of infection unless they are stressed in some way (by dehydration, poor nutrition, overcrowding, or intercurrent viral infection). The dynamics of this pulmonary infection process are complex, and the controlling factors are still poorly understood. Animals are often infected by older carriers shortly after birth, when they are still immunologically immature, and may develop an acute pneumonia and septicemia when herded into crowded cattle transports or feedlots (hence the term **shipping fever**). Death can occur within 12 to 18 hours of onset of the symptoms. Similarly, chicken and turkey flocks can be decimated by an overwhelming pneumonia that sweeps through a previously healthy flock, apparently as a result of waterborne spread from a single infected carrier.

Rabbits are highly susceptible to chronic nasopharyngeal infections caused by *P multocida*, developing a characteristic "snuffles," often associated with a purulent otitis media. This infection may progress to a life-threatening hemorrhagic pneumonia if the animal is stressed (e.g., as a result of hyperimmunization procedures used during antibody production). Attempts to develop pasteurella-free rabbit breeding stocks have had only limited success.

Mice are extraordinarily susceptible to parenteral and aerogenic challenge with *P multocida*, especially with strains obtained from cattle and fowl sources. Introduction of fewer than 10 viable *P multocida* serotype A organisms into the lungs of a normal mouse is followed by logarithmic growth until the systemic disease overwhelms the host defenses, usually in a matter of hours. The virulent encapsulated organism readily resists phagocytosis and multiplies freely within the extracellular spaces and fluids of the lungs (Fig. 29-3). The host dies with no sign of any humoral or cellular immune response. In fact, the rate of growth by the

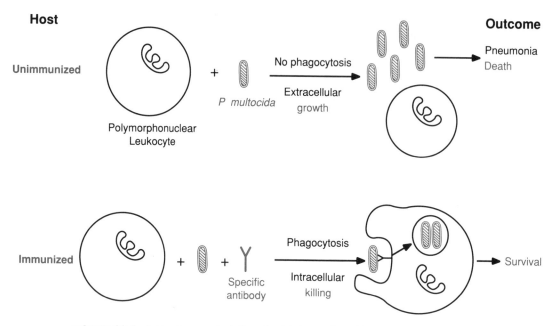

FIGURE 29-3 Protection against *P multocida* is mediated by opsonic antibodies.

pathogen in vivo seems little different from that observed in laboratory media. Large numbers of viable bacilli appear within the bloodstream in a matter of hours and can be recovered from virtually every organ of the moribund host. Curiously, the same organism shows little ability to cross the intact intestinal mucosa, and large numbers of viable bacilli can be introduced intragastrically with no harm to the host, provided that appropriate precautions are taken to prevent accidental infection of the lungs.

Pasteurella hemolytica causes a life-threatening hemorrhagic pneumonia in horses and cattle, but does not appear to infect humans.

STRUCTURE, CLASSIFICATION, AND ANTIGENIC TYPES

Pasteurella multocida is a small, nonmotile Gram-negative coccobacillus, which often exhibits **bipolar staining,** in which the ends of the bacilli stain more intensely than the middle. These bacteria possess both capsular and somatic antigens, and isolates can be divided into four distinct capsular types (A, B, D, and E) on the basis of an indirect

hemagglutination test. As many as 15 somatic antigens can be recognized once the capsular layer has been removed by acid or hyaluronidase treatment. Most fowl and human isolates are type A, whereas most cattle strains are type B. Type E strains are associated mostly with hemorrhagic septicemia cases in central Africa. Freshly isolated strains may produce large mucoid colonies rich in hyaluronic acid. However, after several transfers on solid media, most virulent strains produce smooth, translucent colonies that may become rough (untypable) following prolonged cultivation on laboratory media.

PATHOGENESIS

Abscesses are characterized by extensive edema and fibrosis. Encapsulated organisms resist phagocytosis. Endotoxin contributes to tissue damage.

HOST DEFENSES

Pasteurella multocida is an extracellular parasite that multiplies at the site of implantation despite the influx of polymorphonuclear leukocytes (PMNs) into the lesion. In the absence of specific opsonins (immune antibodies), the organisms within the lesion are not phagocytosed but continue to multiply freely within the tissue fluids. Acquired resistance to pasteurellosis is almost entirely humorally mediated. Protection can be passively transferred to naive recipients by means of hyperimmune serum but not by spleen cells harvested from the same donor. Once opsonized, the pasteurellae are rapidly phagocytosed and inactivated, so that the number of viable bacilli within the lesion declines sharply. More importantly, hematogenous spread (a feature of the normal infection pattern) is completely ablated by specific antibodies that prevent the establishment of a fatal pneumonia. This protective effect occurs long before any mononuclear cell response has time to develop. Killed whole-cell vaccines (**bacterins**) induce a substantial B-cell response, leading to copious plasma cell production and the release of specific anticapsular antibodies into the bloodstream (Fig. 29-3). These opsonins can passively transfer high levels of specific antibacterial immunity to naive recipients, at least in the laboratory. However, the situation seems more complicated in practice. Field trials with a number of multivalent *P multocida* vaccines containing adjuvants have yielded generally disappointing and inconsistent results, possibly owing to the large number of different serotypes in the environment of the test population under most field test conditions. Recently, several live attenuated vaccines (presented in drinking water) have been claimed to be effective against fowl cholera outbreaks in turkey flocks.

EPIDEMIOLOGY

Pasteurella species are primarily pathogens of cattle, sheep, fowl, and rabbits. Humans become infected while handling infected animals.

DIAGNOSIS

Pasteurella multocida grows readily on nutrient blood agar, giving rise to small, nonhemolytic, iridescent colonies. Highly mucoid colonies are occasionally seen on primary isolation. There is no growth on MacConkey agar, and most strains ferment only glucose and sucrose, with no gas production.

CONTROL

Pasteurella multocida is susceptible to sulfadiazine, ampicillin, chloramphenicol, and tetracycline in vitro. However, because of the acute nature of the animal infections, chemotherapy may be of limited use. In human cases, the localized abscesses resolve quite slowly and may require prolonged therapy with multiple antibiotics for effective results. The organism is susceptible to mild heat (55°C), as well as to exposure to most hospital disinfectants. Organisms in dried blood may remain viable at room temperature for several weeks. Vaccines are not available for human use.

◀ *YERSINIA* ▶

The genus *Yersinia* contains three species of medical importance: *Y pestis,* the agent of **bubonic** and **pneumonic plague,** and *Y pseudotuberculosis* and *Y enterocolitica,* both of which can induce severe gastroenteritis, with local abscess formation and peritonitis. The last two species will be presented after a complete discussion of *Y pestis.*

CLINICAL MANIFESTATIONS

Yersinia pestis is primarily a rodent pathogen, with humans being accidental hosts when bitten by an infected rat flea (Fig. 29-4). The flea draws viable *Y pestis* organisms into its intestinal tract with its blood meal. These organisms multiply in situ to block the proventriculus, so that some organisms are regurgitated into the next bite wound, transferring the infection to the new host. While growing in the invertebrate host, *Y pestis* loses its capsular layer, and most of the organisms are readily phagocytosed and killed by polymorphonuclear leukocytes, which enter the infection site in large numbers. A few bacilli are taken up by tissue macrophages, however, which are unable to kill them but provide a protected environment for them to resynthesize their capsular and other virulence antigens. The reencapsulated organisms kill the mac-

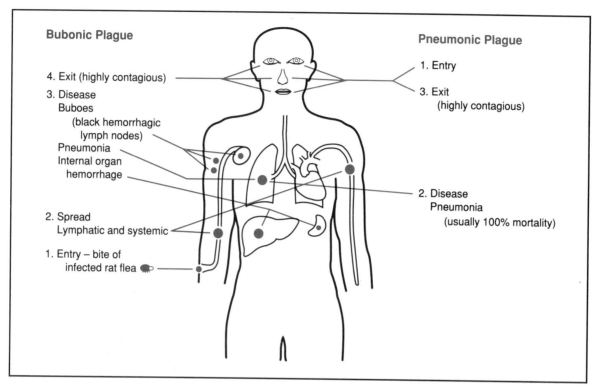

Bubonic Plague

4. Exit (highly contagious)
3. Disease
    Buboes
        (black hemorrhagic
        lymph nodes)
    Pneumonia
    Internal organ
        hemorrhage

2. Spread
    Lymphatic and systemic

1. Entry – bite of
    infected rat flea

Pneumonic Plague

1. Entry
3. Exit
    (highly contagious)

2. Disease
    Pneumonia
    (usually 100% mortality)

FIGURE 29-4 Pathogenesis of *Y pestis* in plague patients.

rophage and are released into the extracellular environment, where they resist phagocytosis. The resulting infection quickly spreads to the draining lymph nodes, which become hot, swollen, tender, and hemorrhagic, giving rise to the characteristic black **buboes** responsible for the name of this disease (Fig. 29-4). Within hours of the initial flea bite, the infection spills out into the bloodstream, leading to substantial involvement of the liver, spleen, and lungs. As a result, the patient develops a severe bacterial pneumonia, excreting large numbers of viable organisms into the air during coughing fits. Up to 90 percent of untreated patients die; patients represent a highly contagious health hazard to nursing staff. As an epidemic of bubonic plague develops (especially under conditions of severe overcrowding, malnutrition, and heavy ectoparasite infestation), it eventually shifts into a predominantly pneumonic form (Fig. 29-4), which is far more difficult to control and which has

100 percent mortality. Experimentally, a conjunctival infection route has been found in monkeys and guinea pigs, and it is likely that many laboratory-derived infections occur via this route.

STRUCTURE, CLASSIFICATION, AND ANTIGENIC TYPES

Yersinia pestis is a small, Gram-negative coccobacillus, which frequently shows strong bipolar staining. Pleomorphic and club-shaped forms are not unusual. Freshly isolated cultures often exhibit substantial slime production, with a so-called capsular or envelope antigen, which is heat labile and is readily lost when the organism is grown in vitro or in the insect vector (Table 29-2). Fully virulent strains possess V and W (virulence) antigens. Such strains are highly toxic for the mouse and, to a lesser extent, for the guinea pig (Table 29-2).

TABLE 29-2   Antigenic Makeup of *Y pestis*

Antigen	Composition	Function	Protection
Envelope (F1)			
A	Soluble polysaccharide-protein	Immunogen	+
B	Soluble polysaccharide	Species-specific antigen	−
C	Insoluble polysaccharide	Nonimmunogen	−
Somatic (O)			
1	Unknown	Virulence antigen	+
3	Corresponds to F1	Species-specific antigen	+
4	Heat-stable protein	Nonimmunogen	−
5	—	Shared with *Y pseudotuberculosis*	−
8	Heat-labile polypeptide	Toxin	−
V	Protein	Associated with virulence; inhibits phagocytosis	+
W	Protein	Shared with *Y pseudotuberculosis*	+
Rough	Heat-stable polysaccharide	Shared with *Y pseudotuberculosis*	−

PATHOGENESIS

The virulence of *Y pestis* strains can be equated to the rate of growth (or elimination) of the organism in the spleen following intravenous inoculation (Fig. 29-5). The most virulent strains multiply with no initial lag phase, increasing logarithmically to lethal numbers within 2 or 3 days. Infected animals exhibit progressive septicemia and usually die within 72 hours as a result of the hemorrhagic pneumonia. Less virulent strains begin to multiply in vivo only after an initial lag; this slowed growth allows the host defenses to mount an effective response (Fig. 29-5).

HOST DEFENSES

The major defense against *Y pestis* infections is the development of specific anti-envelope (F1) antibodies, which serve as opsonins for the virulent organisms, allowing their rapid phagocytosis and destruction while still within the initial infectious locus (Fig. 29-6). Although the V and W antigens are associated with virulence, a number of avirulent strains also possess them, and some individuals possessing high anti-VW antibody titers may nevertheless undergo second attacks of this disease. Therefore, the immune mechanism(s) against this disease is extremely complex and involves a combination of humoral and cellular factors. The convalescent host is solidly immune (at least for a time) to

virulent rechallenge, the inoculum being eliminated as though the organism were completely avirulent. Killed *Y pestis* vaccines (especially with suitable adjuvants) induce some measure of host protection, although this will be less effective than that afforded by the live infection.

EPIDEMIOLOGY

Bubonic plague—the Black Death—has been one of the great epidemic scourges of mankind, sweeping across Europe and Asia in a series of devastating pandemics throughout the Middle Ages. This disease may have been responsible for the death of one-third of the world's population during that time. Then, for largely unknown reasons, it suddenly ceased to be an important pandemic disease, and no major epidemics have occurred in Europe or North America for more than a century. Sporadic outbreaks of sylvatic plague still occur in wild rats, squirrels and prairie dogs in the western United States, and endemic plague has been reported in parts of Southeast Asia. Although no recent deaths due to plague have been reported in the United States, occasional isolates of *Y pestis* still appear to be fully virulent for experimental animals. The striking change in the epidemiology of this disease is probably due to such nonspecific factors as improved rodent control and the widespread use of insecticides against the

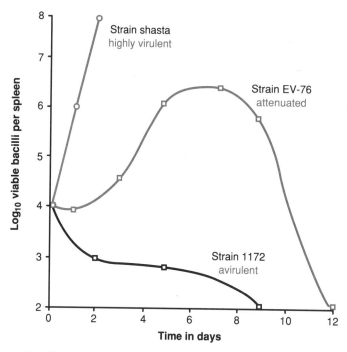

FIGURE 29-5 Growth of *Y pestis* in intravenously infected mice showing combined viable counts for spleen and liver homogenates. The virulence of *Y pestis* correlates with rate of growth in the mouse. The highly virulent Shasta strain killed 100 percent of infected animals within 3 days. The attenuated strain EV-76 gave rise to a self-limiting infection that induced an excellent immune response. The avirulent variant 1122 did not induce a protective immune response. (Data from Walker DL, Foster LE, Chen TH et al: Studies on immunization against plague. V. Multiplication and persistence of virulent and avirulent *P. pestis* in mice and guinea pigs. J Immunol 70:245, 1953.)

insect vector. Recent advances in our understanding of the molecular biology of microbial virulence factors associated with this pathogen offer the promise of improved immunogens capable of inducing a fully effective acquired resistance.

DIAGNOSIS

Yersinia infections must be diagnosed as quickly as possible owing to the extraordinary virulence of these organisms. Death from pneumonic plague may occur as soon as 24 hours after the first appearance of clinical symptoms. Sputum specimens from these patients contain large numbers of *Y pestis* organisms. Blood cultures are also positive, and lymph node biopsy material shows a massive inflammatory cell infiltrate, together with numerous cell-free coccobacilli. The organisms can be

identified rapidly by a fluorescent antibody staining technique, and the epidemiology of the outbreak may be traced by bacteriophage typing.

Yersinia pestis poses a serious infectious hazard for nursing and laboratory personnel. Protective goggles and a face mask must always be worn when working with this organism. Cultivation and virulence testing of this organism should be attempted only in P-3 containment facilities by staff who have been immunized recently with live attenuated vaccine. Animals should be checked to ensure that they are free of ectoparasites.

CONTROL

Yersinia can be killed by mild heat (55°C) and by treatment with 0.5 percent phenol for 15 minutes. It is susceptible to sulfadiazine, streptomycin, tet-

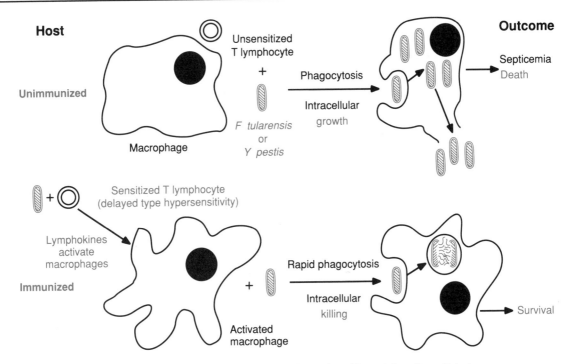

FIGURE 29-6   Protection against *F tularensis* or *Y pestis* is cell-mediated.

racycline, and chloramphenicol in vitro. Thus far, few drug-resistant strains have emerged. Control measures against plague center largely on rat flea eradication programs, which have been credited with preventing epidemics of plague in Europe in 1945 and in Southeast Asia during the Vietnam war. Attempts to eradicate the rodent reservoir have been unsuccessful, and it seems unlikely that plague will ever be completely eliminated worldwide.

YERSINIA PSEUDOTUBERCULOSIS

Yersinia pseudotuberculosis is a natural pathogen of rodents and birds but can infect humans, causing a severe enterocolitis with enlarged caseous nodules in the Peyer's patches and the mesenteric lymph nodes. These lesions often resemble those seen during intestinal tuberculosis. This organism is highly infectious for guinea pigs and can result in devastating outbreaks of pseudotuberculosis in breeding colonies, with very high mortality rates. The infection is virtually impossible to eliminate

once established. *Yersinia pseudotuberculosis* can be readily distinguished from other *Yersinia* species because of its motility when grown at 25°C.

In humans, *Y pseudotuberculosis* causes severe intestinal abscesses that require aggressive chemotherapy with ampicillin and tetracycline. No vaccine is available.

YERSINIA ENTEROCOLITICA

Yersinia enterocolitica is a natural pathogen of cattle, deer, pigs, and birds. Most infected animals recover from their primary disease, remaining healthy carriers indefinitely. The organism is excreted in large numbers in the feces of infected carriers and can contaminate drinking water and dairy products. Oral infection results in a severe diarrhea in humans, together with necrosis of the Peyer's patches, chronic lymphadenopathy, and liver and splenic abscesses (Fig. 29-7). An increasing number of human outbreaks have been reported in recent years, mostly in colder climates. This may reflect a greater awareness of this disease,

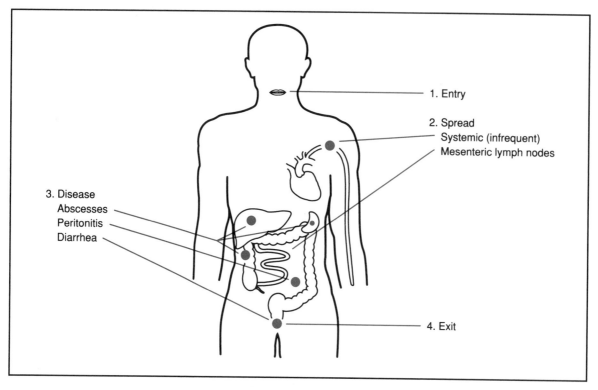

FIGURE 29-7 Pathogenesis of *Y enterocolitica.*

as well as improved isolation and diagnostic procedures, rather than an actual increase in its overall incidence.

Most human *Y enterocolitica* isolates have been avirulent for laboratory rodents. Recently, several strains virulent for mice have been isolated from human pathologic material. Orally infected mice develop progressive involvement of the ileal Peyer's patches, with abscess formation in the mesenteric lymph nodes, liver, and spleen. Eventually, most of the animals die from intestinal abscess perforation and peritonitis. The lesions typically contain large numbers of PMNs and a strong mononuclear cell response, which seems to be involved in any successful control of the infection.

The best prevention methods for *Y enterocolitica* infections are adequate water purification and milk pasteurization. Once the infection has become established in the gut-associated lymphoid tissues, it produces chronic abscesses, which re-

quire aggressive chemotherapy with a combination of ampicillin, chloramphenicol, and polymyxin. No vaccine is available for this infection.

◀ *FRANCISELLA* ▶

CLINICAL MANIFESTATIONS

Francisella tularensis causes **tularemia,** which is spread naturally to humans directly by ticks and deerflies (Fig. 29-8). Most strains that infect rabbits are highly infectious and virulent for humans. The subcutaneous infectious dose may be as low as 10 viable bacilli, with a mortality as high as 30 percent in untreated patients. Infections may result from local trauma incurred while skinning and dressing infected rabbit carcasses. Hence, protective gloves and goggles should always be worn while performing this chore in an endemic area.

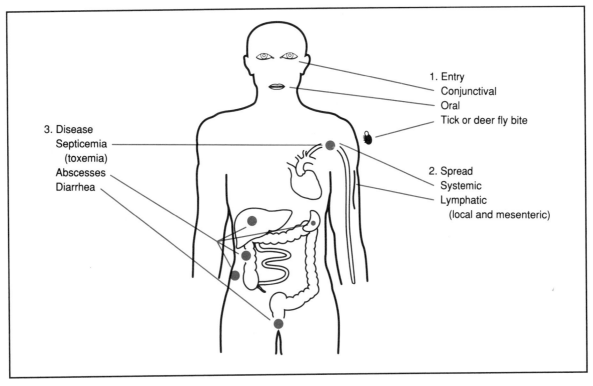

FIGURE 29-8 Pathogenesis of *F tularensis*.

Humans can also contract the disease by eating infected rabbit meat. Tularemia is a severe typhoidlike intestinal disease, resulting in local abscess formation in the Peyer's patches and the mesenteric lymph nodes (Fig. 29-7). It is associated with high fever and a severe toxemia (septicemia). *Francisella tularensis* is a facultative intracellular parasite, which induces a strong mononuclear cell immune response on the part of the host defenses (Fig. 29-3). A humoral response also develops, although the precise nature of the relationship between the specific antibodies and resistance to the naturally acquired disease is still not altogether clear. Actively infected mice develop a strong, delayed-type skin hypersensitivity to sensitins produced by this organism.

Laboratory infections may occur via the conjunctival membranes; this probably explains the high infection rate for this pathogen in laboratory personnel. Goggles and face mask should always be

worn when working with virulent strains of this organism, and staff should be immunized with the live attenuated vaccine. Animal infection studies must be performed under P-3 containment conditions, and, whenever possible, experimental studies should use the vaccine strain.

STRUCTURE, CLASSIFICATION, AND ANTIGENIC TYPES

Francisella tularensis is a nonmotile, Gram-negative coccobacillus, which forms small translucent colonies on glucose blood agar or on Dorset egg slants. The organism grows readily in developing chicken embryos. Nutritionally and biochemically it bears a close resemblance to the brucellae, but it has been differentiated from members of this genus on the basis of DNA homology tests. It is a natural pathogen of rodents (squirrels and rabbits mainly), but can be carried by birds, which usually develop latent infections.

PATHOGENESIS

Mice, rats, guinea pigs, and rabbits are readily infected with *F tularensis* by the subcutaneous, nasal, or conjunctival routes. Virulent strains multiply logarithmically within the liver and spleen (but not the lungs), and death usually occurs 5 to 8 days later. In sublethally challenged animals, the systemic infection peaks and declines rapidly; the response is associated with cell-mediated immunity, which can be transferred adoptively to naive recipients by splenic immune T cells, but not by hyperimmune serum. Most clinical isolates lose virulence when maintained for long periods on laboratory media and eventually cannot produce progressive disease in susceptible animals.

HOST DEFENSES

Acquired resistance following recovery from tularemia is long lasting and highly protective.

DIAGNOSIS

Isolation of *F tularensis* from pathologic material can be difficult and slow. Best growth occurs on cysteine-glucose-blood agar, but the plates should be incubated at 37°C for at least 3 weeks before being discarded as negative. Smears of pathologic material or blood cultures may be stained with fluorescent antibodies directed against specific surface antigens of the organism. Hemagglutinins appear in serum samples some 10 to 12 days after infection and slowly increase in titer for up to 8 weeks. A rising titer is always diagnostic of active disease.

CONTROL

Francisella tularensis is susceptible to inactivation by mild heat (55°C for 10 minutes) and disinfectants. It is susceptible to streptomycin, tetracycline, and chloramphenicol in vitro. Relapses are not uncommon if treatment is stopped before all the viable bacilli have been eliminated from the tissues. Infection control measures usually entail the elimination of the insect vectors.

Killed *F tularensis* vaccines are not very effective, even when presented in adjuvant. A live attenuated vaccine has been developed and should be used to immunize laboratory staff working with this organism.

REFERENCES

Bottone EJ: *Y. enterocolitica:* a panoramic view of a charismatic micro-organism. Crit Rev Microbiol 5:211, 1977

Collins FM: Mechanisms of resistance to *P. multocida* infection. A review. Cornell Vet 67:103, 1977

Falkow S: Molecular Koch's postulates applied to microbial pathogenicity. Rev Infect Dis 10:S274, 1988

Koskela P, Salminen A: Humoral immunity against *Francisella tularensis* after natural infection. J Clin Microbiol 22:973, 1985

Sanford JP: Landmark perspective: tularemia. J Am Med Assoc 250:3225, 1988

Tärnvik A, Löfgren ML, Löfgren S et al: Long-lasting cell-mediated immunity induced by live *Francisella tularensis* vaccine. J Clin Microbiol 22:527, 1985

Walker DL, Foster LE, Chen TH et al: Studies on immunization against plague. V. Multiplication and persistence of virulent and avirulent *P. pestis* in mice and guinea pigs. J Immunol 70:245, 1953

Weber DJ, Wolfson JS, Swartz MN, Hooper DC: *Pasteurella multocida* infections. Reports of 34 cases and a review of the literature. Medicine 63:133, 1984

30 HAEMOPHILUS SPECIES

DANIEL M. MUSHER

GENERAL CONCEPTS

Clinical Manifestations

Type b *Haemophilus influenzae* can cause meningitis, epiglottitis, bacteremia, and cellulitis. Nontypable *H influenzae* can cause otitis media, sinusitis, tracheobronchitis, and pneumonia. Other *Haemophilus* species and the syndromes they cause include *H parainfluenzae* (pneumonia and endocarditis), *H ducreyi* (genital chancre), and *H aegyptius* (conjunctivitis or Brazilian purpuric fever).

Structure, Classification, and Antigenic Types

Haemophilus species are Gram-negative coccobacilli similar in ultrastructural features to other pathogenic bacilli. *Haemophilus influenzae* requires hemin (factor X) and NAD^+ (factor V) for growth. Other *Haemophilus* species require only NAD^+ and therefore grow on blood agar. Typable *H influenzae* isolates are classified on the basis of seven antigenically distinct capsular polysaccharides; isolates lacking these polysaccharides are called **nontypable.**

Pathogenesis

Type b *H influenzae* colonizes the nasopharynx, and may penetrate the epithelium and capillary endothelium to cause bacteremia. Meningitis may result from direct spread via lymphatic drainage or from hematogenous spread. Nontypable *H influenzae* colonizes the pharynx and, to a lesser extent, the trachea and bronchi and may

infect mucosa damaged by viral disease or cigarette smoking. Lipooligosaccharide is largely responsible for inflammation; exotoxins do not play a role.

Host Defenses

Serum antibody to the capsule (in the case of typable *H influenzae*) or to somatic antigens is bactericidal and promotes phagocytosis.

Epidemiology

Haemophilus influenzae colonizes healthy children and adults (although the rate of colonization is far greater for nontypable than for type b *H influenzae*) and is spread by direct contact, secretions, and/or aerosol. *Haemophilus ducreyi* is spread by venereal contact. There is no animal reservoir for these organisms.

Diagnosis

Respiratory secretions and cerebrospinal fluid must be cultured on chocolate agar. Blood cultures are positive in meningitis. Capsular antigen may be detected in cerebrospinal fluid for early identification if Gram stain is unsuccessful. *Haemophilus ducreyi* grows on Mueller-Hinton agar with 5 percent sheep blood in a CO_2-enriched atmosphere.

Control

Recommended treatment includes ampicillin for strains of *H influenzae* that do not make β-lactamase and a third-generation cephalosporin or chloramphenicol for

421

strains that do. Ampicillin or amoxicillin together with a substance, such as clavulanic acid, that blocks the activity of β-lactamase is also effective, but does not reliably treat meningitis. Polyribosyl ribitol phosphate (PRP) vaccine and, more recently, protein-conjugated PRP have shown promise in stimulating antibody effective against type b *H influenzae*.

INTRODUCTION

The genus *Haemophilus* includes a number of species that cause a wide variety of infections but share a common morphology and a requirement for blood-derived factors during growth that has given the genus its name. *Haemophilus influenzae*, the major pathogen, can be separated into **encapsulated** or **typable** strains, of which there are seven types (a through f including e′) based on the antigenic structure of the capsular polysaccharide, and **unencapsulated** or **nontypable** strains. Type b *H influenzae* is by far the most virulent organism in this group, commonly causing bloodstream invasion and meningitis in children younger than 2 years. Nontypable strains are frequent causes of respiratory tract disease in infants, children, and adults.

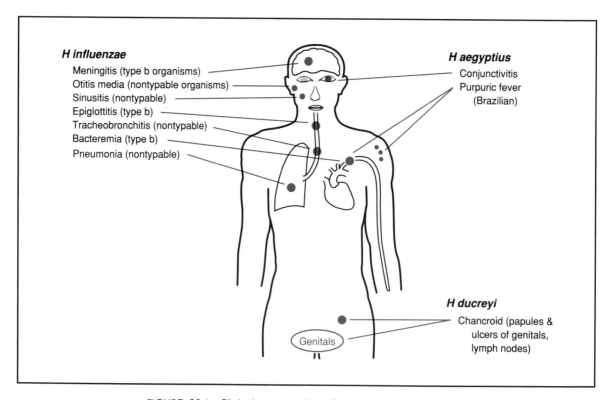

H influenzae
Meningitis (type b organisms)
Otitis media (nontypable organisms)
Sinusitis (nontypable)
Epiglottitis (type b)
Tracheobronchitis (nontypable)
Bacteremia (type b)
Pneumonia (nontypable)

H aegyptius
Conjunctivitis
Purpuric fever
(Brazilian)

H ducreyi
Chancroid (papules &
ulcers of genitals,
lymph nodes)

Genitals

FIGURE 30-1 Clinical presentation of *Haemophilus* infections.

Other *Haemophilus* species cause disease less frequently. *Haemophilus parainfluenzae* sometimes causes pneumonia or bacterial endocarditis. *Haemophilus ducreyi* causes chancroid. *Haemophilus aphrophilus* is a member of the normal flora of the mouth and occasionally causes bacterial endocarditis. *Haemophilus aegyptius,* which causes conjunctivitis and Brazilian purpuric fever, and *Haemophilus haemolyticus* used to be separated on the basis of their ability to agglutinate or lyse red blood cells, but both are now included among the nontypable *H influenzae* strains.

CLINICAL MANIFESTATIONS

Haemophilus species cause a variety of clinical syndromes (Fig. 30-1). Type b *H influenzae* is the most common cause of meningitis in children between the ages of 6 months and 2 years. In this situation, headache is followed rapidly by development of a stiff neck, with progression to coma and, in the absence of treatment, death. Emergent treatment reduces the incidence of, but does not eliminate, sequelae such as deafness and learning disabilities. Type b *H influenzae* also causes **cellulitis** and **epiglottitis,** a condition in which the epiglottitis becomes inflamed and swells, closing off the upper airway. Suffocation can be prevented in some cases only by performing a tracheostomy. Nontypable *H influenzae* strains commonly cause infection of the middle ear **(otitis media),** which manifests as an earache with fever in babies and young children. In adults, these organisms cause bronchitis and pneumonia, especially if some underlying disease of the bronchi and lungs is present. Nontypable *H influenzae* strains also commonly cause acute or chronic sinusitis in patients of all ages.

Chancroid is a venereal disease caused by *H ducreyi*. Lesions that resemble a syphilitic chancre result from sexual contact with an infected individual; they are usually found on the genitals. Unlike syphilitic chancres, the lesions are painful and are associated with a remarkable degree of swelling of lymph nodes in the inguinal area.

STRUCTURE, CLASSIFICATION, AND ANTIGENIC TYPES

Haemophilus species are Gram-negative coccobacilli that share common ultrastructural features with other Gram-negative bacilli. Their cell walls contain lipooligosaccharide, which resembles the lipopolysaccharide of Gram-negative bacilli but has shorter side chains (hence the designation **oligosaccharide** rather than polysaccharide). *Haemophilus* species have generally been thought not to make toxins or other extracellular products that account for their ability to produce infection. These organisms require hemin **(factor X)** and/or nicotinamide adenine dinucleotide (NAD^+) **(factor V)** for growth. Whereas NAD^+ is released into the medium by red blood cells and is available to the bacteria in blood agar, hemin is bound to red blood cells and is not released into the medium unless the cells are broken up, as in chocolate agar. *Haemophilus influenzae* requires both factors X and V; accordingly, it grows on chocolate agar but not on blood agar (Fig. 30-2), although it may appear on a blood agar plate as tiny satellite colonies around the colonies of other bacteria that have lysed red blood cells. *Haemophilus parainfluenzae* requires only factor V and therefore is able to grow on blood agar (however, recent reports suggest that many isolates identified as *H parainfluenzae* actually are *H paraphrophilus*). The long-prevailing notion that *H ducreyi* grows only in clotted rabbit blood has been dispelled by recent studies that show slow growth of this organism in Mueller-Hinton agar containing 5 percent sheep blood. All *Haemophilus* species grow more readily in an atmosphere enriched with CO_2; *H ducreyi* and some nontypable *H influenzae* strains will not form visible colonies on culture plates unless grown in a CO_2-enriched atmosphere.

Haemophilus influenzae strains are classified as either **serotypable** (if they display a capsular polysaccharide antigen) or **nontypable** (if they lack a capsule). The word "type" as applied to *H influenzae* refers to this serotyping scheme. There are six generally recognized types: a, b, c, d, e, and f. A seventh type has been designated e′ because its polysaccharide is closely related to that of type e.

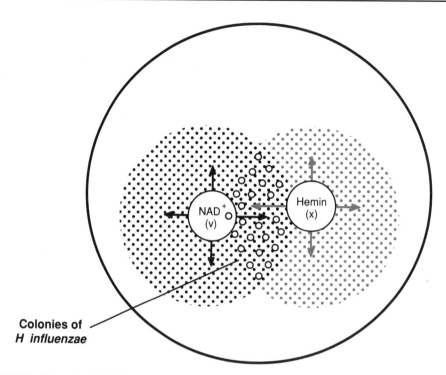

**Colonies of
H influenzae**

FIGURE 30-2   Growth of *H influenzae* requires both NAD⁺ (factor V) and hemin (factor X). Bacterial colonies occur only where both substances have diffused. (The hemin within intact erythrocytes is not accessible to the bacteria unless the erythrocytes are lysed by other bacteria or by heating the medium to make chocolate agar.)

Antiserum to type e′ *H influenzae* is not routinely available. These types may be identified by an agglutination reaction that uses antisera raised in rabbits; with this method, however, cross-reactions with somatic antigens may cause nontypable strains to be designated erroneously as typable. This kind of error is eliminated by using counterimmunoelectrophoresis, in which migration under an electric current removes somatic (protein) antigens from the reaction, leaving only capsular polysaccharides to react with antibody.

The presence of a polyribosyl ribitol phosphate (PRP) capsule is an important virulence factor: it renders type b *H influenzae* resistant to phagocytosis by polymorphonuclear leukocytes in the absence of specific anticapsular antibody. Susceptibility to the bactericidal effect of serum depends on the presence of antibodies to a number of antigenic sites, including the lipooligosaccharide or

outer membrane proteins designated as P1 and P2. Type b *H influenzae* is plainly the most virulent of the *Haemophilus* species; 95 percent of bloodstream and meningeal *Haemophilus* infections in children are due to this organisms. In contrast, in adults, nontypable strains of *H influenzae* are the most virulent, followed by type b isolates.

The relative place of *H influenzae* biogroup *aegyptius,* the cause of Brazilian purpuric fever, remains to be determined. Organisms that cause this syndrome differ from the other *H influenzae* biogroup *aegyptius* strains in having a plasmid that may mediate virulence. These organisms also have at least some of the genetic material that codes for encapsulation of type b *H influenzae*.

By using a series of biochemical reactions, *H influenzae* also may be classified into six biotypes designated I through VI. Most type b *H influenzae* strains fall into biotypes I or II, whereas most nontypable *H influenzae* strains fall into biotypes II through VI. Several interesting clinical correlations have recently emerged. Biotype I isolates appear to have a predilection for causing pneumonia. Nearly all genital isolates, as well as bloodstream isolates from infected neonates or from women with puerperal sepsis, are biotype IV. In addition, biotype III, which agglutinates red blood cells in vitro and includes *H influenzae* biogroup *aegyptius*, has been implicated as a common cause of conjunctivitis. There is no explanation for these clinically observed associations.

PATHOGENESIS

The pathogenesis of *H influenzae* infections is not completely understood, but the presence of the type b polysaccharide capsule is a major factor in virulence. Encapsulated organisms can penetrate the epithelium of the nasopharynx and invade blood capillaries directly. Nontypable strains are less invasive, but they, as well as typable strains, induce an inflammatory response that causes disease; production of exotoxins is not thought to play a role in pathogenicity. Nontypable *H influenzae* strains colonize the nasopharynx of most normal individuals, but type b *H influenzae* strains are found in only 1 to 2 percent of normal children. Outbreaks of type b infection occur, especially in nurseries and child care centers; prophylactic administration of antibiotics may be used. Vaccination with type b polysaccharide appears to be effective in preventing infection, and vaccines are now available for routine use.

Meningitis

The pathogenesis of meningitis due to type b *H influenzae* has been well studied. These organisms colonize the nasopharynx and spread from one human to another by direct contact or via secretions and/or aerosol. They penetrate epithelial layers and capillary endothelium by unknown mechanisms, reaching the meninges either directly via lymphatic drainage from the nasopharnyx or indirectly by causing bacteremia with subsequent seeding of the highly vascular choroid plexus. Type b *H influenzae* is the commonest cause of bacterial meningitis in children 6 months to 2 years old. In contrast, it is an uncommon cause of meningitis in adults. This difference is thought to be due to the much lower rate of colonization by type b *H influenzae* in later life, combined with the development of protective antibody over the first few years of childhood.

Most cases of *H influenzae* meningitis in adults are due to nontypable strains. The pathogenesis of these infections differs from that of type b *H influenzae*. Nontypable strains are unencapsulated and therefore less virulent, and they are unable to penetrate directly into capillaries. Rather, they gain entry to the central nervous system by direct extension, often associated with infection of the sinuses or middle ear and/or with trauma involving the sinuses or skull. Thus, about 50 percent of adults with *H influenzae* meningitis have a history of prior head trauma with or without a documented cerebrospinal fluid leak, and another 25 percent have chronic otitis media. Also, *H influenzae* is second only to *Streptococcus pneumoniae* as a cause of **recurring meningitis,** an unusual syndrome attributed to a connection between the sinuses and the subarachnoid space, usually via a tear in the dura. The clinical picture of meningitis caused by typable or nontypable *H influenzae* is similar to that caused by other bacteria, such as *S pneumoniae*. Since *Haemophilus* species do not produce substances that obviously damage mammalian tissues, bacterial replication is probably the usual pathway for disease production, with triggering of the complement cascade by classic and alternative pathways, followed by accumulation of inflammatory cells.

Cellulitis and Epiglottitis

Cellulitis and epiglottitis are discussed together because their pathogenesis is probably quite similar. Both are due to type b *H influenzae*, involve associated bacteremia, and occur more frequently in children than adults. Epiglottitis can be regarded as a cellulitis of the relatively loose submucosal connective tissues of the epiglottis. In this syndrome, a sore throat rapidly progresses to difficulty in breathing, stridor, obstruction of the airways, and respiratory arrest. Local extension from the colonized nasopharynx through soft tissues is probably responsible for epiglottitis. Cellulitis often involves the face or neck. It sometimes seems to start at the buccal mucosa and extend outward, supporting the idea that it also results from local extension. The often-repeated teaching that facial cellulitis due to *Haemophilus* causes a distinctive bluish tinge enabling it to be distinguished from cellulitis caused by other bacteria, defies reason and is best ignored.

Respiratory Disease

Nontypable *H influenzae* is a major pathogen that colonizes the human respiratory tract. Adherence of bacteria to mammalian tissues, which is mediated by pili (fimbriae), is thought to be an important precursor to colonization, and infection of the upper airways is associated with the presence of pili. Respiratory infections caused by these organisms include sinusitis, otitis media, acute tracheobronchitis, and pneumonia.

Purulent material aspirated from acutely infected paranasal sinuses in children or adults or from behind an infected tympanic membrane in babies and young children commonly contains nontypable *H influenzae*. Studies of outer membrane protein profiles have shown that middle ear and nasopharyngeal isolates are identical, supporting the notion that colonization of the eustachian tube, followed by obstruction and infection, is probably responsible. Repeated bouts of otitis media are thought to be due to different strains; each infection may be associated with emergence of antibody to distinctive surface proteins. The decreasing frequency of otitis media with age is due in part to anatomic changes and in part to immunity to *H influenzae*.

The situation is somewhat more complex for bronchopulmonary disease. Nontypable *H influenzae* is found in the nasopharynx and in sputum cultures of one-half to two-thirds of adults with chronic bronchitis. Not surprisingly, this organism is also recovered from the large airways via bronchoscopy, since upper-airway bacteria are carried along by the bronchoscope. On the basis of these observations, as well as of other observations on the presence of antibody in serum samples of patients with chronic bronchitis, some British investigators concluded that *H influenzae* actually plays a causative role in what they call chronic bronchitis—our chronic obstructive pulmonary disease. With the use of semiquantitative techniques, *H influenzae* have been shown to be very scarce in the sputum of patients with chronic bronchitis who are in a stable clinical state (and perhaps results from oropharyngeal contamination of the specimen), but that, at least in some patients, large numbers are present during an exacerbation. This observation fits with studies in which transtracheal aspiration has revealed the trachea to be free of *Haemophilus* isolates in stable patients with emphysema, but to contain these organisms in some patients who have purulent sputum.

In any case, nontypable *H influenzae* is certainly a prominent cause of acute tracheobronchitis or pneumonia in patients who have underlying chronic bronchitis, emphysema, or obstructive pulmonary disease. Other debilitating diseases such as malnutrition, lung cancer, and alcoholism are also often present. Symptoms of acute bronchitis include increased shortness of breath, cough, and production of purulent sputum; in more severe cases, fever and an increased white blood cell count may also be present. Pneumonia may result, with patchy or segmental pulmonary infiltrates detectable by radiography. Gram stain of sputum reveals a profusion of Gram-negative coccobacilli (Fig. 30-3), but no other pathogenic bacteria. A properly plated specimen yields a nearly pure growth of *Haemophilus*. When *S pneumoniae* organisms are present in small numbers (for example, 1 *S pneumoniae* colony to 100 *Haemophilus* colonies), it is less certain that *Haemophilus* is the sole pathogen. Blood cultures are positive in 10 to 15 percent of patients with *Haemophilus* pneumonia. Nontypable *H influenzae* is second only to *S pneumoniae* as the cause of bacterial pneumonia in middle-aged men. Although type b *H influenzae* is more virulent, pneumonia due to this organism is much less common, probably because of its vastly lower incidence of colonization. Compared with nontypable *H influenzae* pneumonia,

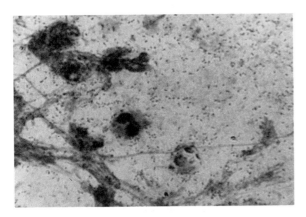

FIGURE 30-3 Gram-stained sputum showing profuse Gram-negative coccobacilli with no other bacterial forms present (original magnification × 440). Cultures showed nontypable *H influenzae* as the overwhelmingly predominant isolate. Quantitative culture showed 7×10^8 CFU/ml of sputum.

the underlying pulmonary disease may not be so prominent. In type b *H influenzae* disease, the onset is more acute and blood cultures are more likely to be positive. *Haemophilus influenzae* received its name because it was first isolated from the lungs of individuals who died during an epidemic of influenza virus infection in 1890. It is not possible to determine whether bacterial infection was due to typable or nontypable isolates.

Brazilian Purpuric Fever

In the past few years, a syndrome of fulminating illness with substantial mortality characterized by nausea, vomiting, hemorrhagic skin lesions, fever, prostration, and shock has been recognized under the name **Brazilian purpuric fever.** *Haemophilus influenzae* biogroup *aegyptius* can be cultured from the blood of affected patients. Many have had a history of conjunctivitis in the weeks preceding onset of the disease. As noted above, the responsible organisms differ from other *H influenzae* biogroup *aegyptius* strains that only cause conjunctivitis in having a unique plasmid, as well as containing genetic material that hybridizes with the capsular locus of *H influenzae.*

Miscellaneous

Type b *H influenzae* is a relatively common cause of septic arthritis in children and results from hematogenous dissemination. Interestingly, this organism only rarely causes osteomyelitis; the reasons for this discrepancy are unknown.

Nontypable *H influenzae* biotype IV tends to colonize the female genital tract and may cause puerperal fever and/or neonatal sepsis. Infection in the mother is relatively mild, but it may be fulminating in the newborn infant. It is unknown whether nontypable *H influenzae* biotype IV has any special virulence beyond the factors that promote adherence to vaginal epithelial cells.

Some patients have bacteremia due to type b *H influenzae* without an apparent focus of infection. There is good evidence that if this condition is left untreated in children, some source for the infection (e.g., meningitis) will become apparent within 24 to 48 hours. However, in this situation one cannot be certain that the meninges were not seeded secondarily to the bacteremia. In adults, there appears to be a syndrome of bacteremia due to nontypable *H influenzae* for which no focus ever becomes apparent.

HOST DEFENSES

For many years it was believed that bactericidal antibody directed against PRP capsule of type b *H influenzae* was entirely responsible for host resistance to infection. However, more recent studies have stressed a role for antibody to somatic antigens as well. For example, antibody to PRP can often be detected in the sera of children on admission to the hospital with sepsis due to type b *H influenzae*. In addition, adsorption of immune serum with PRP alone does not remove its protective capabilities, whereas adsorption with whole organisms does. Finally, immunization with ribosomes is protective in animal models of infection. Separation of the outer membrane of type b *H influenzae* into its many protein constituents by polyacrylamide gel electrophoresis (PAGE) combined with analysis of antibody responses during infection has suggested that antibody to any of a number of individual membrane proteins may be associated with immunity. Bactericidal antibodies that react with individual outer membrane proteins or with lipooligosaccharide constituents have been identified. These findings support, on a molecular basis, the potential importance of antibody to noncapsular antigens in immunity to type b *H influenzae* infection. Opsonizing antibody may also play a role in protection and may be directed against PRP or somatic constituents (Fig. 30-4).

Recent studies of nontypable *H influenzae* strains have shown that bactericidal antibody to outer membrane proteins develops in infants in response to otitis media caused by these organisms. Normal adults generally have both bactericidal and opsonizing antibodies directed against nontypable *H influenzae*. Although levels of opsonizing antibody may be low in adults who develop acute nontypable *H influenzae* infection, substantial levels of bactericidal activity are present in serum at the time infection is diagnosed. It is not clear why this should occur. In some instances a blocking effect by secretory IgA in bronchial secretions might be responsible. Alternatively, the extensive structural damage to the bronchi and lungs that predisposes to serious nontypable *H influenzae* infection may allow proliferation of the bacteria unchecked by normal serum defense mechanisms.

EPIDEMIOLOGY

Haemophilus organisms spread directly among individuals without a known contribution from environmental sources or animal reservoirs. Nontypable *H influenzae* strains are found in the nasopharynx of many healthy subjects, depending upon the frequency and intensity with which they are sought. By contrast, type b *H influenzae* is found only in 1 to 2 percent of healthy children, and its spread to previously uncolonized children in the early years is associated with a substantially increased risk of infection. Families and day care centers are important sources for dissemination of these organisms.

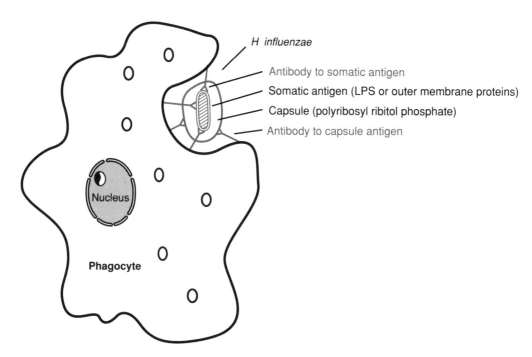

FIGURE 30-4 Macrophage or polymorphonuclear leukocyte phagocytosing *H influenzae* coated with antibodies specific for the capsule and somatic antigen.

DIAGNOSIS

Haemophilus influenzae meningitis cannot be distinguished on the basis of clinical presentation, physical examination, or cerebrospinal fluid abnormalities from meningitis due to other common bacterial pathogens. The cerebrospinal fluid in untreated patients contains an average of 2×10^7 bacteria/ml, so that microscopic examination, especially in the absence of prior antibiotic therapy, should reveal the infecting organisms. Detection of capsular material in the cerebrospinal fluid by counterimmunoelectrophoresis is helpful in cases in which the Gram stain is not conclusive; this technique is especially important in patients who have received enough antibiotic to suppress the growth of organisms in cultures of cerebrospinal fluid, but not enough to be curative.

The bacteriologic diagnosis of pneumonia or acute febrile purulent tracheobronchitis due to *H influenzae* is made by finding myriad small, somewhat pleomorphic, Gram-negative coccobacilli in Gram-stained sputum (Fig. 30-3) and by culturing *H influenzae* as the overwhelmingly predominant isolate; the mean number of viable organisms per milliliter of infected sputum is about 5×10^8. Blood cultures may be positive in 10 to 15 percent of patients with pneumonia and are negative in those with acute febrile tracheobronchitis.

Endocarditis due to *H parainfluenzae* tends to be associated with large vegetations that embolize to large arteries such as femoral or carotid, causing a limb to turn blue and cool, or producing a stroke. The etiologic diagnosis of endocarditis is, of course, established by blood culture. Recent studies have suggested that many isolates previously identified as *H parainfluenzae* are, in fact, *H paraphrophilus*. Chancres due to *H ducreyi* are tender, somewhat irregular, and slightly indurated; they may be confused with primary syphilitic chancres, traumatic lesions of the penis (especially with bacterial superinfection), fixed drug eruptions, or ulcerated herpetic lesions. The diagnosis is established by culturing the causative organism on Mueller-Hinton agar supplemented with 5 percent sheep blood and incubating it for 96 hours in a CO_2-enriched atmosphere.

CONTROL

Outbreaks of serious infection due to type b *H influenzae* can be prevented by vaccination or prophylactic therapy. Initial trials of vaccination with type b *H influenzae* PRP were disappointing, because this polysaccharide in its pure form is not immunogenic in infants, the group most at risk of infection. Later studies showed that injection of PRP conjugated to a protein, such as diphtheria toxoid, that serves as an adjuvant results in good antibody responses in infants. Clinical trials with these vaccines have been successful, and PRP-D (PRP-diphtheria toxoid) is now commercially available; other preparations in which PRP is linked to outer membrane proteins or ribosomes may be even more effective and are currently under study.

Once an outbreak of type b *H influenzae* infection has been documented, infants and toddlers who are in intimate contact with colonized or infected individuals have a greatly increased, albeit still small, likelihood of developing serious infection. The use of rifampin prophylaxis to prevent or eradicate naspharyngeal colonization has been recommended. This measure is controversial, however, because if widely applied it might encourage the emergence of rifampin-resistant organisms, and also because the cost to prevent each potential case of meningitis is high.

The mainstay of therapy for *H influenzae* infection used to be ampicillin, since isolates were uniformly susceptible to 0.5 µg/ml. In the last few years an increasing proportion of *H influenzae* isolates have produced β-lactamase. In most medical centers, 25 to 30 percent of type b isolates and a somewhat smaller percentage of nontypable isolates are now resistant to penicillin or ampicillin; in some centers, 50 to 60 percent of type b *H influenzae* isolates are ampicillin resistant. Very rarely, an isolate resists ampicillin but does not produce β-lactamase; decreased penetration into the bacterium is thought to be responsible. Treatment with a combination of amoxicillin and clavulanic acid (a substance that covalently binds β-lactamase) is effective against β-lactamase-producing strains, but has not been recommended for treating meningitis.Tetracycline and sulfa drugs are also effective. Erythromycin should not be used to treat *H influenzae* infections; many isolates are resistant, and documentation of susceptibility in routine clinical laboratories is subject to error.

Chloramphenicol was long considered the drug of choice for meningitis caused by a penicillin-resistant *H influenzae* strain, and it is still highly effective. Third-generation cephalosporins, such as ceftriaxone or cefotaxime, are effective against *H influenzae* and penetrate the meninges well; these drugs are useful in treating *H influenzae* meningitis. The addition of corticosteroids may reduce the incidence of complications such as deafness.

The spread of soft chancre due to *H ducreyi* is best prevented by use of a condom during sexual intercourse. Two-thirds of *H ducreyi* isolates produce β-lactamase. All isolates are susceptible in vitro to erythromycin, and excellent clinical results have been obtained.

REFERENCES

Doern GV, Jones RN: Antimicrobial susceptibility testing of *Haemophilus influenzae, Branhamella catarrhalis,* and *Neisseria gonorrhoeae.* Antimicrob Agents Chemother 32:1747, 1988

Eskola J, Peltola H, Takala AK et al: Efficacy of *Haemophilus influenzae* type b polysaccharide-diphtheria toxoid conjugate vaccine in infancy. N Engl J Med 317:717, 1987

Hammond GW, Slutchuk M, Scatliff J et al: Epidemiologic, clinical, laboratory, and therapeutic features of an urban outbreak of chancroid in North America. Rev Infect Dis 2:867, 1980

Harrison LH, de Silva GA, Pittman M et al: Epidemiology and clinical spectrum of Brazilian purpuric fever. J Clin Microbiol 27:599, 1989

Mason EO, Jr, Kaplan SL, Lamberth LB et al: Serotype and ampicillin susceptibility of *Haemophilus influenzae* causing systemic infections in children: 3 years of experience. J Clin Microbiol 15:543, 1982

Murphy TF, Apicella MA: Nontypable *Haemophilus influenzae:* a review of clinical aspects, surface antigens, and the human immune response to infection. Rev Infect Dis 9:1, 1987

Murphy TF, Berstein JM, Dryja DM et al: Outer membrane protein and lipooligosaccharide analysis of paired nasopharyngeal and middle ear isolates in otitis media due to nontypable *Haemophilus influenzae:* pathogenic and epidemiological observations. J Infect Dis 156:723, 1987

Musher D, Goree A, Murphy T et al: Immunity to *Haemophilus influenzae* type b in young adults: correlation of bactericidal and opsonizing activity of serum with antibody to polyribosylribitol phosphate and lipooligosaccharide before and after vaccination. J Infect Dis 154:935, 1986

Musher DM, Kubitschek KR, Crennan J et al: Pneumonia and acute febrile tracheobronchitis due to *Haemophilus influenzae.* Ann Intern Med 99:444, 1983

Osterholm MT, Pierson LM, White KE et al: The risk of subsequent transmission of *Haemophilus influenzae* type b disease among children in day care. N Engl J Med 316:1, 1987

Sell SH, Wright PF (eds): *Haemophilus influenzae:* Epidemiology, Immunology, and Prevention of Disease. Elsevier Biomedical, New York, 1982

Wallace RJ, Jr, Baker CJ, Quinones FJ et al: Nontypable *Haemophilus influenzae* (biotype 4) as a neonatal, maternal, and genital pathogen. Rev Infect Dis 5:123, 1983

31

BORDETELLA

HORST FINGER

GENERAL CONCEPTS

Clinical Manifestations

Bordetella pertussis causes **whooping cough (pertussis),** an acute respiratory infection marked by severe, spasmodic coughing episodes during the paroxysmal phase. Leukocytosis with lymphocytosis is also common during this phase of the illness. Dangerous complications are bronchopneumonia and acute encephalopathy. *Bordetella parapertussis* can cause a mild form of pertussis.

Structure

The bordetellae are small, Gram-negative, aerobic coccobacilli. *Bordetella pertussis* produces a number of virulence factors, including pertussis toxin, adenylate cyclase toxin, filamentous hemagglutinin, and hemolysin. Agglutinogens and other outer membrane proteins are important antigens.

Classification and Antigenic Types

The genus *Bordetella* contains the serologically related species *B pertussis*, *B parapertussis*, and *B bronchiseptica*, which cause pertussis and similar disorders in humans and animals. A fourth species, *B avium* (formerly *Alcaligenes faecalis*) may belong in this genus. Bordetellae are differentiated on the basis of biochemical and culture characteristics and by analysis of agglutinogen antigens. They show reversible antigenic modulation under certain culture conditions, and they mutate through several antigenically distinct phases when grown on agar.

Pathogenesis

Transmission is by droplets. The bacteria colonize only ciliated cells of the respiratory mucosa, and they multiply rapidly. Bacteremia does not occur. The roles of the various toxins in pathogenesis are unclear.

Host Defenses

Infection induces substantial immunity, although the protective antigens have not been identified conclusively. Both nonspecific and specific defenses participate in the response to disease.

Epidemiology

The human respiratory mucosa is the natural habitat for *B pertussis* and *B parapertussis*. Transmission is almost always directly from person to person. Patients are most infectous during the early, catarrhal phase of the disease and remain infectious for about 5 weeks. Pertussis is a common and dangerous childhood disease in unvaccinated populations.

Diagnosis

Pertussis is diagnosed rapidly by direct immunofluorescence of nasopharyngeal swabs. Modified Bordet-Gengou agar, charcoal agar, or supplemented Stainer-Scholte broth is used for culture. Circulating antibodies appear in week 3 of illness and peak in the eighth to tenth week. Antibodies can be demonstrated by an enzyme-linked immunosorbent assay. Detection of specific IgA provides evidence of natural infection.

431

Control

Treatment with erythromycin does not alter the course of disease, but reduces the infectious period to 5 to 10 days. Inactivated whole-cell vaccines are highly effective, but occasionally cause toxic side effects. Acellular vaccines are under development.

INTRODUCTION

The genus *Bordetella* contains three species (*B pertussis, B parapertussis,* and *B bronchiseptica*) of serologically related bacteria with similar morphology, size, and staining reactions. These bacteria cause **whooping cough (pertussis)** and similar respiratory syndromes in humans and animals.

Bordetella pertussis was first isolated in pure culture in 1906 and was for a long time believed to be the sole agent of whooping cough. Later, studies revealed that a mild form of this disease can be caused by *B parapertussis* and occasionally by *B bronchiseptica.*

CLINICAL MANIFESTATIONS

After an incubation period of 1 to 2 weeks, whooping cough begins with the **catarrhal phase** (Fig. 31-1). This phase lasts 1 to 2 weeks and is usually characterized by low-grade fever, rhinorrhea, and progressive cough; the patient is highly infectious. The subsequent **paroxysmal phase,** lasting 2 to 4 weeks, is characterized by severe and spasmodic cough episodes. At the end of the catarrhal phase, a leukocytosis with an absolute and relative lymphocytosis frequently begins, reaching its peak at the height of the paroxysmal stage. At this time, the total blood leukocyte levels may resemble those of leukemia ($\geq 100,000/mm^3$), with 60 to 80 percent being lymphocytes. The **convalescent phase,** lasting 1 to 3 weeks, is characterized by a continuous decline of the cough before the patient returns to normal. Serious complications, sometimes fatal, are bronchopneumonia and acute encephalopathy, the latter being characterized primarily by convulsions and frequently resulting in death or lifelong brain damage.

STRUCTURE

Bordetella pertussis is a small (approximately 0.8 μm by 0.4 μm), rod-shaped, coccoid, or ovoid Gram-negative bacterium that is encapsulated and does not produce spores. It is a strict aerobe. It is arranged singly or in small groups and is not easily distinguished from *Haemophilus* species. Whereas *B pertussis* and *B parapertussis* are nonmotile, *B bronchiseptica* are peritrichous and hence motile. Numerous antigens and biologically active structural components have been demonstrated in *B pertussis* (Fig. 31-2), although their exact chemical structure and location in the bacterial cell are known only in part.

Pertussis Toxin

Various immunologic, physiologic, and pharmacologic effects are induced by killed *B pertussis* cells in experimental animals (e.g., increased sensitivity to histamine and serotonin and active and passive anaphylaxis). Adjuvant activity, leukocytosis, splenomegaly, cell proliferation, hypoglycemia, and hypoproteinemia also occur. Many additional features have been described, including increased sensitivity to factors such as endotoxins, X irradiation, infection, cold stress, pollen extracts, peptone shock, and methacholine; increased resistance to infection; increased capillary permeability; and accelerated production of experimental "allergic" encephalomyelitis. These various biologic activities were assumed to be due to different products and structural components of the bacteria, which were accordingly designated the histamine-sensitizing factor, the lymphocytosis-promoting factor, islet-activating protein, and pertussis toxin or pertussigen. The latter toxin was prepared in crystalline form.

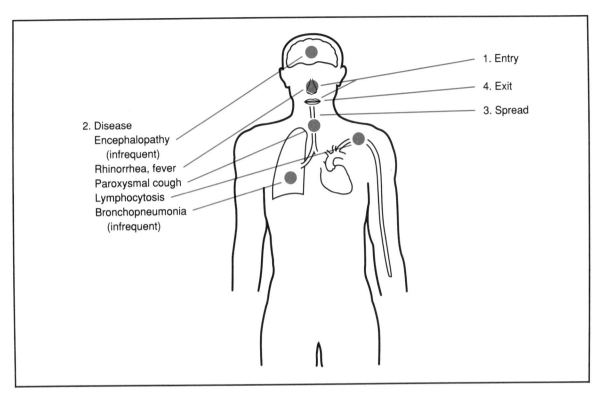

FIGURE 31-1 Pathogenesis of whooping cough.

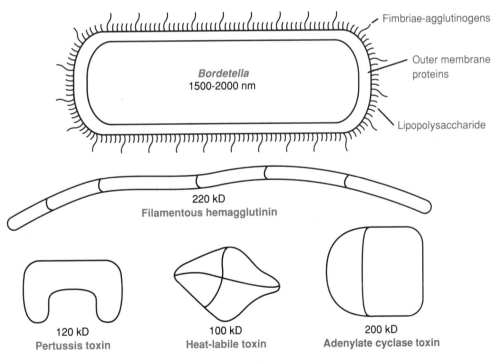

FIGURE 31-2 Virulence factors of *B pertussis*.

It is now generally accepted that all those biologic activities are caused by a single active protein produced by *B pertussis*. To avoid confusion caused by the many different names for this protein, the uniform term **pertussis toxin** was proposed by Pittman. Pertussis toxin is a protein exotoxin, secreted during in vivo and in vitro growth; it consists of five different subunits, designated S1, S2, S3, S4, and S5. Since the toxin molecule contains two S4 subunits, it is a hexamer. Like many other protein toxins, pertussis toxin consists of an A subunit that carries the biologic activity and a B subunit that binds the complex to the cell membrane. In pertussis toxin, the S1 subunit constitutes the A protomer and the B oligomer is formed by the remaining five subunits (Fig. 31-3). The toxin binds to cell receptors by two dimers, one consisting of S2 and S4 and the other of S3 and S4. Since glutaraldehyde-inactivated pertussis toxin is capable of adherence, this binding activity evidently has little to do with the various toxic activities of pertussis toxin. The toxin reacts with different cell types, including T lymphocytes, and acts on different cellular regulatory processes. Thus, it may interfere with the regulation of cyclic adenosine-5¹-monophosphate (cAMP)-mediated events (Fig.

31-4). Treatment of rat adipocytes with pertussis toxin increased the levels of cAMP 20-fold. Although pertussis toxin is synthesized solely by *B pertussis*, both *B parapertussis* and *B bronchiseptica* possess genes for pertussis toxin without expressing them. *Bordetella parapertussis* expresses pertussis toxin when the genes encoding the toxin in the *B pertussis* chromosome are introduced into *B parapertussis*.

Like many other bacteria, *B pertussis* possesses hemagglutinating activity, expressed as its capacity to agglutinate red cells from geese, chickens, and other animals. Pertussis toxin is one of the hemagglutinins, whereas another component with hemagglutinating activity is called **filamentous hemagglutinin.** This component appears as fine filaments, about 2 nm in diameter and 40 to 100 nm in length. Like pertussis toxin, it has hemagglutinating activity as well as the ability to effect the adherence of *B pertussis* to cilia.

Heat-Labile Toxin

The **heat-labile toxin** of *Bordetella* is a proteinaceous dermonecrotic toxin with a molecular weight of about 100,000, localized in the proto-

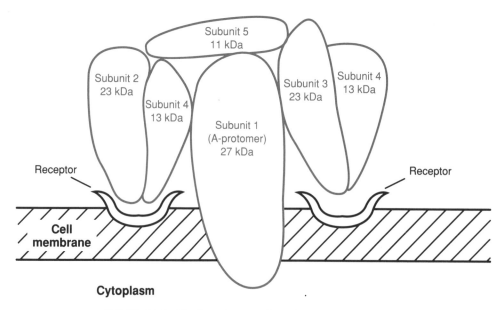

FIGURE 31-3 Binding of pertussis toxin to cell membranes.

Respiratory Tract Lumen

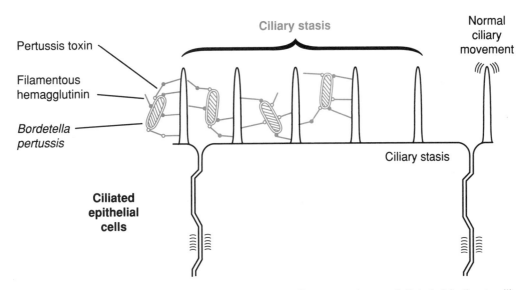

FIGURE 31-4 Synergy between pertussis toxin and the filamentous hemagglutinin in binding to ciliated respiratory epithelial cells.

plasm. This toxin produces strong vasoconstrictive effects, which are probably important during the initial phase of pertussis by their action on the respiratory tract. Thus, heat-labile toxin, in association with tracheal cytotoxin and lipopolysaccharide, possibly causes tissue damage in the respiratory tract.

Adenylate Cyclase Toxin

Like pertussis toxin, **adenylate cyclase toxin,** which is primarily extracytoplasmic, is a protein that interferes with cAMP regulation. The adenylate cyclase toxin-mediated increase in intracellular cAMP levels is associated with the inhibition of phagocytic cell oxidative reactions and natural killer (NK) cell activity. Thus, adenylate cyclase toxin appears to play a role in *B pertussis* virulence.

Tracheal Cytotoxin

Tracheal cytotoxin, which is chemically related to peptidoglycan, destroys the ciliated cell population of a hamster trachea in 60 to 96 hours.

Lipopolysaccharide

The heat-stable *Bordetella* **lipopolysaccharide** (LPS) endotoxin is similar in structure, chemical composition, and biologic activity to other endotoxins produced by Gram-negative bacteria. Endotoxin from *B pertussis* is serologically different from corresponding preparations from *B parapertussis* and *B bronchiseptica*. It is remarkable that heat-labile toxin, adenylate cyclase toxin, tracheal cytotoxin, and LPS are formed by the three *Bordetella* species, whereas pertussis toxin is produced solely by *B pertussis*.

Agglutinogens

The **agglutinogens** are surface antigens responsible for agglutination of the bacterial cells in the presence of their corresponding antibodies. To date, 14 different agglutinogens (AGG 1 through AGG 14) have been distinguished. AGG 1 is species specific for *B pertussis*, AGG 14 for *B parapertussis,* and AGG 12 for *B bronchiseptica*. In addition, the strain-specific AGGs 2, 3, 4, 5, 6, and 13 occur in *B pertussis,* AGGs 8, 9, and 10 in *B parapertussis,* and AGGs 8, 9, 10, 11, and 13 in *B bronchiseptica.* AGGs 2, 3, and 6 characterize three distinct types of pili (fimbriae).

Outer Membrane Proteins

At least four different outer membrane protein structures are distinguished on *B pertussis;* they are designated OMP 15, OMP 18, OMP 69, and OMP 91. They are believed to be protective antigens.

CLASSIFICATION AND ANTIGENIC TYPES

The genus *Bordetella* contains three species (*B pertussis, B parapertussis,* and *B bronchiseptica*) of serologically related bacteria with similar morphology, size, and staining reactions. Possibly, the genus should be amplified by a fourth species, *B avium,* a bird pathogen that was formerly designated *Alcaligenes faecalis.* DNA-DNA and DNA-rRNA hybridization analyses have shown a very close genetic relationship among *B pertussis, B parapertussis,* and *B bronchiseptica,* especially between the first two. *Bordetella avium* isolates are genetically more divergent.

Bordetella pertussis was first isolated in pure culture in 1906 and was long considered the sole agent of whooping cough. Later studies revealed that this disease also can be caused in a mild form by *B parapertussis* and occasionally by *B bronchiseptica.* A phenomenon of *B pertussis* organisms is their variation during growth on agar plates: the antigenically competent, smooth, virulent form (phase I) can mutate to the antigenically incomplete, nonvirulent, rough form (phase IV). This change is associated with a loss of capacity to synthesize pertussis toxin, filamentous hemagglutinin, heat-labile toxin, adenylate cyclase toxin, agglutinogens, and certain outer membrane proteins. There are also two intermediate forms, called phases II and III.

In addition to this spontaneous phase variation, *B pertussis* undergoes **antigenic modulation** in response to changes in environmental conditions, such as growth at low temperatures or on agar plates with high concentrations of $MgSO_4$ or nico-tinic acid. *Bordetella pertussis* organisms grown under such conditions are avirulent and are characterized by the loss of the capacity to synthesize the numerous toxic factors and other structural components. Both phase variation and antigenic modulation are reversible and also occur in *B parapertussis* and *B bronchiseptica.* Both phenomena are under the control of a single genetic locus. The virulent strains are therefore designated Vir^+, and the avirulent strains Vir^-. Phase variation has been observed in vivo. Another type of serotype variation in *B pertussis*—the loss of one or more agglutinogens—occurs independently of phase variation.

PATHOGENESIS

The agent of whooping cough is transmitted primarily via droplets. Infection results in colonization and rapid multiplication of the bacteria on the mucous membranes of the respiratory tract. Bacteremia does not occur. Electron microscopic studies have demonstrated that phase I strains of *B pertussis* adhere only to the tuft of ciliated cells in the mucosa of the human respiratory tract; no attachment to nonciliated cells was observed. Convincing experimental data indicate that the adherence of *B pertussis* to human cilia is effected by a synergistic action of pertussis toxin and filamentous hemagglutinin, each acting as a bivalent bridge between the bacterium and the ciliary receptor (Fig. 31-4).

Studies of numerous *B pertussis* toxins and their corresponding biologic activities have yielded plausible explanations for many of the symptoms of whooping cough. These include, for example, the frequent occurrence of absolute lymphocytosis (an unusual phenomenon in bacterial infections), hypoglycemia, and the adjuvant effect of pertussis toxin on the immune response to unrelated antigens. The finding that phase I isolates of *B bronchiseptica* produce almost complete ciliostasis within 3 hours in ciliated epithelial cell outgrowths from canine tracheal explants may be explained by the action of adenylate cyclase toxin and tracheal cytotoxin. The same toxins evidently inhibit the phagocytic activities of the host. In humans, an initial local peribronchial lymphoid hyperplasia occurs, accompanied or followed by necrotizing inflammation and leukocyte infiltration in parts of the larynx, trachea, and bronchi. Usually, peribronchiolitis and variable patterns of atelectasis and emphysema also develop.

To date, there is no plausible explanation for the development of the paroxysmal coughing syndrome characteristic of pertussis. According to Pittman, pertussis is mediated by pertussis toxin and is characterized by a two-stage process — infection (colonization) and disease — thus resembling other bacterial toxicoses such as diphtheria, tetanus, and cholera. This fascinating idea can be accepted only if it is clearly demonstrated that pertussis toxin causes paroxysmal coughing. Such a demonstration is lacking. Moreover, paroxysmal coughing occurs in infections with *B parapertussis*, which does not synthesize pertussis toxin. On the other hand, an additional infection with *B pertussis* cannot be excluded in such cases. There is no convincing explanation for the acute encephalopathy sometimes observed in pertussis. Research into the pathogenetic mechanisms of pertussis are hampered by the lack of an adequate animal model showing the characteristic paroxysmal coughing syndrome and by the limited opportunity to perform direct studies of the respiratory tract of babies and children.

HOST DEFENSES

A case of whooping cough confers substantial immunity, which usually lasts for many years. Second infections are rare. However, immunity acquired after infection with *B pertussis* does not protect against the other *Bordetella* species. Pertussis toxin is assumed to be the essential protective immunogen, but numerous findings indicate that other components, such as heat-labile toxin, agglutinogens, outer membrane proteins, and adenylate cyclase toxin, may also contribute to immunity after infection or vaccination. The immunogenicity of the substances is significantly increased by the presence of pertussis toxin. This synergism indicates that pertussis toxin could function as an ad-

juvant to a variety of protective antigens of *B pertussis*. Apart from reports of experimentally induced disease in monkeys, which could not be reproduced by other workers, animal diseases caused by *B pertussis* do not resemble whooping cough. There is evidence that the numerous active structural components of *B pertussis* cells are involved in the pathogenesis of whooping cough and in the defense mechanisms of the host. These defense mechanisms are both nonspecific (local inflammation, increase in macrophage activity, and production of interferon) and specific (proliferation of B and T cells). The basis of immunity in whooping cough is, however, incompletely understood. A role of circulating antibody in immunity is indicated by the correlation between protection of human vaccinees and their serum agglutinin titers. However, effective immunity does not necessarily depend on the presence of serum agglutinins, and immunity to whooping cough may therefore be mediated essentially by cellular mechanisms. This cell-mediated immunity may be considered the crucial carrier of long-term immunity, and titers of specific humoral antibodies may diminish over the years. This may be the reason why infants usually do not benefit significantly from maternal antibody.

EPIDEMIOLOGY

The mucous membranes of the human respiratory tract are the natural habitat for *B pertussis* and *B parapertussis*. Although *B pertussis* can survive outside the body for a few days and so may be transmitted by contaminated objects, most infections occur after direct contact with diseased persons — specifically, by inhalation of bacteria-bearing droplets expelled in cough spray. The patient is most infectious during the early catarrhal phase, when clinical symptoms are relatively mild and noncharacteristic (Fig. 31-5). Subclinical cases may have similar epidemiologic significance. Healthy carriers of *B pertussis* or *B parapertussis* are assumed to play no significant epidemiologic role. The natural habitat of *B bronchiseptica* is the respiratory tract of smaller animals such as rabbits, cats, and dogs. Therefore, human infections with *B*

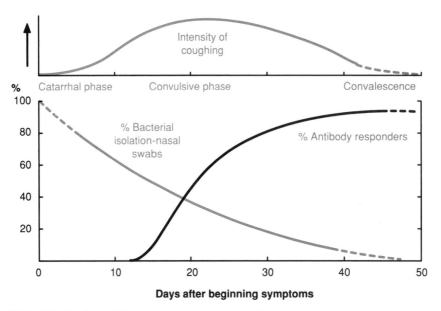

FIGURE 31-5   Relationship of *B pertussis* to the developing antibody response during whooping cough.

bronchiseptica are extremely rare and occur only after close contact with carrier animals.

Whooping cough, a highly communicable, worldwide infection, was once common and dangerous, killing many thousands of children per year. Widespread vaccination has caused a continuous decrease in incidence and mortality over the years, but large numbers of patients still die in countries where vaccination is inadequate. Therefore, in contrast to the situation in the United Kingdom and the United States, whooping cough continues to be a major cause of childhood disease in West Germany (about 100,000 cases per year), evidently because the rate of pertussis vaccination is as low as 7 percent in certain areas. Whooping cough is mainly an infection of infants, although susceptibility is general. The disease is especially dangerous in the first 6 months of life. Neither season nor climate seems to affect the morbidity rate.

DIAGNOSIS

Rapid diagnosis of pertussis is possibly by the fluorescent antibody procedure with nasopharyngeal swabs. However, findings should be evaluated with caution, as the quality of the results depends strongly on the experience of the investigator. The level of false-negative findings is reported to be between 10 and 50 percent, and false-positive findings are nearly as numerous. Therefore, the direct immunofluorescence test is recommended only when diagnosis by culture is also attempted. For culture isolation, Bordet-Gengou agar containing blood, potato extract, and glycerol remains one of the most effective means, although minor modifications regarding blood concentrations and addition of pencillin and nicotinamide have been recommended. Effective cultivation on charcoal agar is also possible. Considering that growth of *B pertussis* and production of pertussis toxin can be significantly increased by the presence of heptakis (2,6-*O*-dimethyl)-β-cyclodextrin, in the medium, it is not surprising that Stainer-Scholte broth, a synthetic medium intended primarily for mass culture of large inocula, is most sensitive for isolation of *B pertussis* and *B parapertussis* from clinical specimens, when supplemented with heptakis. The *Bordetella* species do not need factors X and V (NAD+ and hemin). For specimen collection, nasopharyngeal swabbing, in which the swab is introduced through one of the nostrils into the nasopharynx, is very effective. The material must be streaked immediately on growth medium or placed in a suitable transport medium, such as RL medium or Amies medium with charcoal.

Bordetella pertussis usually grows after 3 to 4 days of incubation at 37°C. The small, transparent colonies are indistinguishable from those of *B bronchiseptica*, but usually are smaller than those of *B parapertussis*. All three species produce hemolysis. Biochemically they are relatively inert and do not ferment carbohydrates or produce H_2S and indole. An important characteristic of *B parapertussis* is its capacity to produce brown pigmentation on blood-free peptone agar. The three *Bordetella* species may be differentiated on the basis of certain biochemical and culture characteristics (Table 31-1). In addition, slide agglutination tests are recommended. Whether the direct demonstration of adenylate cyclase toxin or the use of nucleic acid probes will prove suitable tools for routine diagnosis remains to be answered.

Circulating antibodies, appearing as late as week 3 of illness and reaching their maximum at weeks 8 to 10, have been demonstrated by agglutination and complement fixation tests. The agglutination test is applied mainly in epidemiologic studies. Although no direct relationship has been shown between the agglutinin concentration and the degree of protection, high agglutinin titers ($> 1:320$) are assumed to correlate with protection from disease. Modern serologic techniques, including radioimmunoassay and enzyme-linked immunosorbent assay (ELISA), have been used to detect IgG, IgM, IgA, and IgE antibodies to both whole *B pertussis* cells and certain isolated components. In accordance with other serologic methods, seroconversion could be observed only 2 to 4 weeks after the onset of the disease (Fig. 31-5). The detection of specific IgA and IgM antibodies, however, is indicative of recent infection and is useful for the differential diagnosis of pertussiform syndromes of longer duration. IgA antibodies to *B pertussis* and pertussis toxin are found mainly after natural infection; the same is true of secretory IgA in nasopharyngeal secretions, which usually appears during week 2 or 3 of illness and persists for at least 3 months. Unfortunately, infants do not produce IgA antibody before 6 months of age. Specific IgM antibodies may be used in infants as an indicator of acute infection.

CONTROL

Although *B pertussis* is susceptible in vitro to several antibiotics, such as tetracycline, erythromycin, and chloramphenicol, the efficacy of these drugs in patients during the paroxysmal phase is not convincing. Treatment with erythromycin, which is usually considered the antibiotic of choice, will eliminate viable *B pertussis* organisms from the respiratory tract within a few days. The treatment, however, has little influence on the course of the disease. Human hyperimmune pertussis globulin is still used occasionally, but no reliable data support its efficacy. Further treatment is symptomatic.

Susceptible children (unimmunized children without a history of whooping cough) should have no contact with pertussis patients during the first 4 weeks of illness, although such isolation is often difficult. A patient treated with erythromycin may

TABLE 31-1   Differential Characteristics of the Genus *Bordetella*

Characteristic	B pertussis	B parapertussis	B bronchiseptica
Motility	—[a]	—	+[a]
Growth on blood-free peptone agar	—	+	+
Pigment production	—	+	—
Nitrate reduction	—	—	+
Urea hydrolysis	—	+	+
Oxidase reaction	+	—	+

[a] +, Present; —, absent.

be contagious for only 5 to 10 days. Exposed immunized children younger than 4 years are given booster doses of pertussis vaccine. Exposed unimmunized children are given erythromycin for 10 days after contact is discontinued or after the patient ceases to be contagious.

Pertussis vaccine is produced from smooth forms (phase I) of the bacteria as a killed whole-cell vaccine. It is highly efficacious. In the United States, pertussis vaccination of infants and children is still recommended. Owing to a relatively mild course of disease and to occasional neurologic complications after vaccination, it has been argued by numerous pediatricians that general vaccination with the whole-cell vaccine is no longer justified.

Much progress has been made recently on the development of effective acellular vaccines of defined composition. Such endotoxin-free preparations have been used in Japan since 1981. Since then, several acellular vaccines have been produced in other countries; they consist of pure detoxified pertussis toxin, of mixed pertussis toxin and filamentous hemagglutinin, or of mixed pertussis toxin, filamentous hemagglutinin, and agglutinogens. However, no definite evaluation of vaccine efficacy can be made at this time.

REFERENCES

Arai H, Munoz J: Crystallization of pertussigen from *Bordetella pertussis*. Infect Immun 31:495, 1981

Bemis DA, Kennedy JR: An improved system for studying of *Bordetella bronchiseptica* on the ciliary activity of canine tracheal epithelial cells. J Infect Dis 144:349, 1981

Bordet J, Gengou U: Le microbe de la coqueluche. Ann Inst Pasteur 20:731, 1906

Finger H, Heymer B, Hof H et al: Ueber Struktur und biologische Aktivität von *Bordetella pertussis* Endotoxin. Zentralbl Bakteriol Mikrobiol Hyg 1 Abt Orig A 235:56, 1976

Finger H, Wirsing von Koenig CH: Enhancement and suppression of immune responsiveness by bacteria, bacterial products and extracts. p. 16. In Zschiesche W (ed): Immune Modulation by Infectious Agents. VEB Gustav Fischer Verlag, Jena, 1987

Finger H, Wirsing von Koenig CH: Serological diagnosis of whooping cough. Dev Biol Stand 61:331, 1985

Goldman WE, Klapper DG, Basemann JB: Detection, isolation and analysis of a released *Bordetella pertussis* product toxic to cultured tracheal cells. Infect Immun 36:782, 1982

Goodman YE, Wort AJ, Jackson FL: Enzyme-linked immunosorbent assay for detection of pertussis immunoglobulin A in nasopharyngeal secretions as an indicator of recent infection. J Clin Microbiol 13:286, 1981

Kersters K, Hinz K-H, Hertle A et al: *Bordetella avium* sp. nov., isolated from the respiratory tract of turkeys and other birds. Int J Syst Bacteriol 34:56, 1984

Monack D, Munoz JJ, Peacock MG et al: Expression of pertussis toxin correlates with pathogenesis in *Bordetella* species. J Infect Dis 159:205, 1989

Munoz JJ, Bergman RK: *Bordetella pertussis*. Vol. 4. Marcel Dekker, New York, 1977

Pittman M: Pertussis toxin: the cause of the harmful effects and prolonged immunity in whooping cough. A hypothesis. Rev Infect Dis 1:402, 1979

Pittman M: The concept of pertussis as a toxin-mediated disease. Pediatr Infect Dis J 3:467, 1984

Robinson A, Duggleby CJ, Gorringe AR et al: Antigenic variation in *Bordetella pertussis*. p. 147. In Birbeck TH, Penn CW (eds): Antigenic Variation and Infectious Diseases. Society for General Microbiology, IRL Press, Oxford, 1986

Tuomanen E: *Bordetella pertussis* adhesins. p. 75. In Wardlaw AC, Parton R (eds): Pathogenesis and Immunity in Pertussis. John Wiley & Sons, New York, 1988

Wardlaw AC, Parton R: Pathogenesis and Immunity in Pertussis. John Wiley & Sons, New York, 1988

Weiss AA, Falkow S: Genetic analysis of phase change in *Bordetella pertussis*. Infect Immun 43:263, 1984

Wirsing von Koenig CH, Tacken A, Finger H: Use of supplemented Stainer-Scholte broth for the isolation of *Bordetella pertussis* from clinical material. J Clin Microbiol 26:2558, 1988

32 CORYNEBACTERIUM DIPHTHERIAE

JOHN R. MURPHY

GENERAL CONCEPTS

Clinical Manifestations

Corynebacterium diphtheriae infects the nasopharynx or skin. Toxigenic strains may cause **diphtheria.** Symptoms are caused by diphtheria toxin and may include pharyngitis, fever, and swelling of the neck or area surrounding the skin lesion. Circulating toxin can cause paralysis and congestive heart failure.

Structure, Classification, and Antigenic Types

Corynebacterium diphtheriae is a nonmotile, noncapsulated, club-shaped, Gram-positive bacillus. Toxigenic strains are lysogenic for one of a family of corynebacteriophages that carry the structural gene for diphtheria toxin, *tox*. *Corynebacterium diphtheriae* is classified into biotypes (*mitis, intermedius,* and *gravis*), as well as into lysotypes. Most strains require nicotinic and pantothenic acids for growth; some also require thiamine, biotin, or pimelic acid. For optimal production of diphtheria toxin, the medium should be supplemented with amino acids and must be deferrated.

Pathogenesis

Asymptomatic nasopharyngeal carriage is common in some regions. In susceptible individuals, toxigenic strains cause disease by multiplying in either the nasopharynx or skin lesions and producing toxin. The diphtheritic lesion is often covered by a pseudomembrane composed of fibrin, bacteria, and inflammatory cells. Diphtheria toxin can be cleaved into two fragments. Fragment A catalyzes the NAD^+-dependent ADP-ribosylation of eukaryotic elongation factor 2. Fragment B binds to a cell surface receptor and facilitates the delivery of fragment A to the cytosol.

Host Defenses

Immunity involves an antibody response to diphtheria toxin or diphtheria toxoid (heat-denatured toxin).

Epidemiology

Unimmunized or immunocompromised individuals are at risk of infection. *Corynebacterium diphtheriae* is spread by droplets, secretions, or direct contact. In situ lysogenic conversion of nontoxigenic strains to a toxigenic phenotype has been documented. Infection is spread solely among humans. Isolated outbreaks of disease are often associated with a carrier who has recently visited a subtropical region where diphtheria immunization is not common.

Diagnosis

Clinical diagnosis depends on culture-proven toxigenic *C diphtheriae* infection of the skin, nose, or throat combined with clinical signs of nasopharyngeal diphtheria (e.g., sore throat, dysphagia, bloody nasal discharge,

441

pseudomembrane). Toxigenicity is identified by a variety of in vitro (e.g., gel immunodiffusion, tissue culture) or in vivo (e.g., rabbit skin test, guinea pig challenge) methods.

Control

Immunization with diphtheria toxoid is effective. Diphtheria patients must be treated with antitoxin to neutralize diphtheria toxin.

INTRODUCTION

Diphtheria is the paradigm of the toxigenic infectious diseases. In 1883, Klebs observed that *Corynebacterium diphtheriae* was the agent of diphtheria. One year later, Loeffler found that the organism could be cultured only from the nasopharyngeal cavity and not from damaged internal organs. These early observations led to the postulate that the systemic organ pathology in diphtheria was caused by the action of a soluble toxin. By 1888, Roux and Yersin showed that animals injected with sterile filtrates of *C diphtheriae* developed organ pathology indistinguishable from that of human diphtheria; this demonstrated that a potent exotoxin was the major virulence factor.

Diphtheria is most commonly an infection of the upper respiratory tract and causes fever, sore throat, and malaise. A thick, gray-green fibrin membrane, the **pseudomembrane,** often forms over the site(s) of infection as a result of the combined effects of bacterial growth, toxin production, necrosis of underlying tissue, and the host immune response. Recognition that the systemic organ damage was due to the action of soluble toxin led to the development of both an effective antitoxin-based therapy for acute infection and a highly successful toxoid vaccine.

Although toxoid immunization has made diphtheria a rare disease in countries where public health standards mandate vaccination, outbreaks of diphtheria still occur in immunocompromised and nonimmunized groups. Even though outbreaks of disease are rare, diphtheria has become one of the most successfully studied infectious diseases, and there is a detailed understanding of its pathogenesis at the molecular level.

CLINICAL MANIFESTATIONS

There are two types of clinical diphtheria: *nasopharyngeal* and *cutaneous*. Symptoms of nasopharyngeal diphtheria vary from mild pharyngitis to hypoxia due to airway obstruction by a gray-green pseudomembrane (Fig. 32-1). The involvement of cervical lymph nodes may cause swelling of the neck, and the patient may have a fever ($\geq 103°F$). The skin lesions in cutaneous diphtheria are usually covered by a gray-brown pseudomembrane. Life-threatening systemic complications, principally loss of motor function (e.g., difficulty in swallowing) and congestive heart failure, may develop; they are caused by the effects of absorbed toxin on the myocardium and peripheral motor neurons.

STRUCTURE, CLASSIFICATION, AND ANTIGENIC TYPES

Corynebacterium diphtheriae is a Gram-positive, nonmotile, club-shaped bacillus. Strains growing in tissue, or older cultures growing in vitro, contain thin spots in their cell walls that allow decolorization during the Gram stain and result in a Gram-variable reaction. Older cultures often contain metachromatic granules (polymetaphosphate) which stain bluish-purple with methylene blue. The cell wall sugars include arabinose, galactose, and mannose. In addition, a toxic 6,6'-diester of trehalose containing corynemycolic and corynemycolenic acids in equimolar concentrations may be isolated. Three distinct cultural types, *gravis, intermedius,* and *mitis,* have been recognized (Table 32-1).

Most strains require nicotinic and pantothenic acids for growth; some also require thiamine, bio-

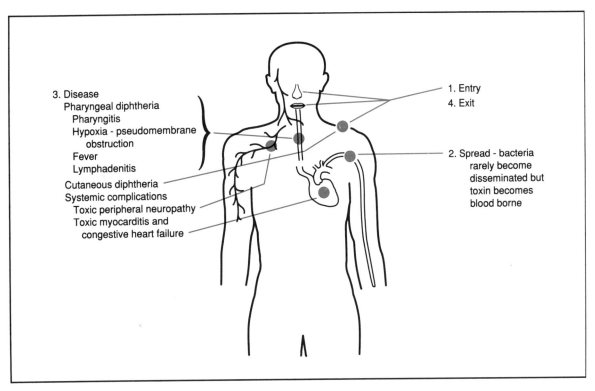

3. Disease
    Pharyngeal diphtheria
      Pharyngitis
      Hypoxia - pseudomembrane
        obstruction
      Fever
      Lymphadenitis
    Cutaneous diphtheria
    Systemic complications
      Toxic peripheral neuropathy
      Toxic myocarditis and
        congestive heart failure

1. Entry
4. Exit

2. Spread - bacteria
   rarely become
   disseminated but
   toxin becomes
   blood borne

FIGURE 32-1 Pathogenesis of diphtheria.

tin, or pimelic acid. For the optimal production of diphtheria toxin, the medium should be supplemented with amino acids and must be deferrated.

As early as 1887, Loeffler described the isolation from healthy individuals of avirulent (nontoxigenic) diphtheria bacilli that were indistinguishable from the virulent (toxigenic) strains isolated from patients. It is now recognized that avirulent strains of *C diphtheriae* may be converted to a toxigenic virulent phenotype following infection and lysogenization by one of a number of distinct corynebacteriophages that carry the structural gene for diphtheria toxin, *tox*. Moreover, it is now clear that lysogenic conversion of avirulent *C diphtheriae* may occur in situ, as well as in vitro. The nucleic acid sequences of the *tox* genes from a number of different strains of corynebacteriophage have now been determined. The *tox* gene is nonessential for either the corynebacteriophage or the bacterium. Despite this conclusion, genetic drift of diphtheria toxin has not been observed. Indeed, although

more than 50 years have passed between the isolation of the PW8 and C7 strains of *C diphtheriae*, the DNA sequences of their respective *tox* genes remain identical.

PATHOGENESIS

The pathogenesis of diphtheria is based upon two primary determinants: (1) the ability of a given strain of *C diphtheriae* to colonize the nasopharyngeal cavity and/or the skin, and (2) its ability to produce diphtheria toxin. Although the genetic determinants involving colonization are encoded by *C diphtheriae,* the diphtheria toxin structural gene is carried by toxigenic strains of corynebacteriophage. Therefore, the molecular basis for virulence in *C diphtheriae* results from the combined effects of determinants that are encoded on two genomes. Nontoxigenic strains of *C diphtheriae* are rarely associated with clinical disease; however, these strains may become highly virulent following lysogenic conversion to toxigenicity.

TABLE 32-1 Biochemical Properties Useful in Distinguishing *Corynebacterium* Species Isolated from the Human Oropharynx and Nasopharynx[a]

Strain	Production of					Fermentation of				
	Metachromatic Granules	Catalase	Pyrazinamidase	Gelatinase	Urease	Lactose	Maltose	Trehalose	Starch[b]	Glucose
C diphtheriae										
var *mitis*	+	+	−	−	−	−	+	−	−	+
var *gravis*	+	+	−	−	−	−	+	−	+	+
var *intermedius*	+	+	−	−	−	−	+	−	−	+
C ulcerans	+	+	−	⊕	⊕	−	+	⊕	+	+
C pseudotuberculosis[c]	+	+	−	−	+	−	+	−	+	+
C pseudodiphtheriticum	+	+	+	−	+	−	−	−	−	−
C xerosis	+	+	+	−	−	−	⊖	−	−	+

[a] +, All strains tested positive: ⊕, rare negative strains may be found; −, all strains tested negative: ⊖, rare positive strains may be found.
[b] Because soluble starch contains some glucose, laundry starch is used for starch fermentation tests.
[c] *C pseudotuberculosis* is found only rarely in the human throat.

(Data from Barksdale L et al: Phospholipase D activity of *Corynebacterium pseudotuberculosis* (*Corynebacterium ovis*) and *Corynebacterium ulcerans*, a distinctive marker within the genus *Corynebacterium*. *J Clin Microbiol* 13:335, 1981.)

Colonization

Little is known of the colonization factors of *C diphtheriae*. However, it is apparent that factors other than the production of diphtheria toxin contribute to virulence. Prolonged colonization with nontoxigenic lysotypes of *C diphtheriae* has been demonstrated in children. Indeed, epidemiologic studies have demonstrated that although a given lysotype may persist in the population for extended periods, it may also be supplanted by another lysotype. The emergence of new lysotypic strains in the population is presumably due to their ability to colonize and effectively compete in their segment of the nasopharyngeal ecologic niche. *Corynebacterium diphtheriae* may produce a neuraminidase that cleaves *N*-acetylneuraminic acid from the eukaryotic cell surface and further cleaves it into its pyruvate and *N*-acetylmannosamine components. Cord factor (6,6′-di-*O*-mycoloyl-α,α′-D-trehalose) is a surface component of the diphtheria bacilli, but its role in colonization of the host is unclear.

Diphtheria Toxin Production

The structural gene for diphtheria toxin, *tox*, is carried by a family of closely related corynebacteriophages. Corynebacteriophage *β* is the most extensively studied (Fig. 32-2). The expression of *tox* depends on the physiologic state of the corynebacterial host. Under conditions where iron becomes the growth rate-limiting substrate, the *tox* gene becomes derepressed and diphtheria toxin is synthesized and secreted into the culture medium at maximal rates. Diphtheria toxin is extraordinarily potent; in unimmunized sensitive species (e.g., humans, monkeys, rabbits, guinea pigs) as little as 100 to 150 ng of toxin/kg of body weight is lethal.

Diphtheria toxin is composed of a single polypeptide chain of 535 amino acids (Fig. 32-3). It contains at least three structural/functional domains that are essential for its action on sensitive intact eukaryotic cells: (1) an N-terminal ADP-ribosyltransferase, (2) a region that facilitates the delivery of the ribosyltransferase across the cell membrane and into the cytosol, and (3) the toxin receptor-binding domain. Following mild diges-

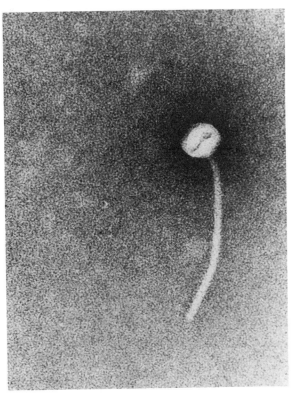

FIGURE 32-2 Electron micrograph of corynebacteriophage *β*, which carries *tox*. Following lysogenic conversion with corynebacteriophage *β*, or closely related corynebacteriophages, nontoxigenic strains of *C diphtheriae* become toxigenic.

tion with trypsin and reduction under denaturing conditions, diphtheria toxin may be separated into two polypeptide fragments. Fragment A is the N-terminal 21 kDa component of the toxin and contains the catalytic centers for the ADP-ribosylation of elongation factor 2 (EF-2) according to the following reaction:

$$NAD^+ + EF\text{-}2 \rightleftharpoons ADPR\text{-}EF\text{-}2 + \text{nicotinamide} + H^+$$

The C-terminal fragment, fragment B, carries the toxin receptor-binding domain and the hydrophobic membrane-associating region that facilitates the delivery of fragment A into the cytosol.

Diphtherial intoxication of a single cell involves at least four distinct steps (Fig. 32-4): (1) the bind-

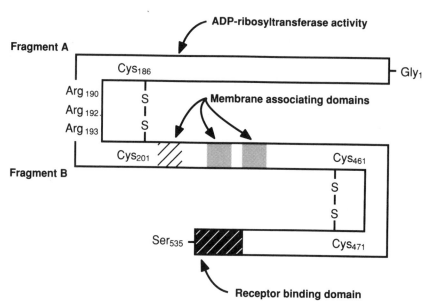

FIGURE 32-3 Schematic representation of diphtheria toxin. Intact toxin may be cleaved by trypsinlike proteases after Arg-190, Arg-192, and/or Arg-193. Following reduction of the disulfide bridge between Cys-186 and Cys-201, the toxin may be separated into fragments A and B.

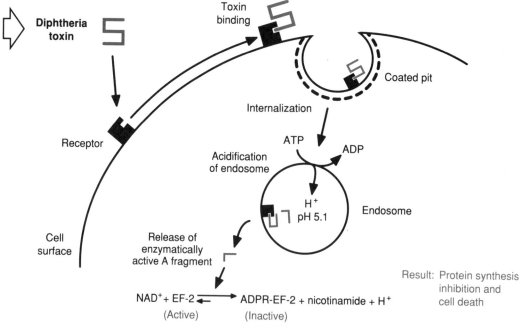

FIGURE 32-4 Schematic diagram of the diphtherial intoxication of a sensitive eukaryotic cell. The toxin binds to its cell surface receptor and is internalized by receptor-mediated endocytosis; upon acidification of the endosome, fragment A is delivered to the cytosol, resulting in inhibition of protein synthesis and death of the cell.

ing of diphtheria toxin to its receptor on the eukaryotic cell surface, (2) clustering of charged receptors into coated pits, (3) internalization of toxin by receptor-mediated endocytosis, and (following the acidification of the endosome by an ATP-driven proton pump) (4) the translocation of fragment A across the endocytic vesicle membrane and into the cytosol. Once in the cytosol, fragment A catalyzes the ADP-ribosylation of elongation factor 2. It has been shown that the introduction of a single molecule of fragment A into the cytosol is sufficient to be lethal for that cell.

HOST DEFENSES

Immunity to diphtheria involves an antibody response to diphtheria toxin or diphtheria toxoid vaccine.

EPIDEMIOLOGY

Before mass immunization of the U.S. population, diphtheria was typically a disease of children. However, with the almost complete disappearance of clinical diphtheria in the United States, a large percentage (20 to 70 percent) of adults have antitoxin titers below the protective level (0.01 IU/ml) and consequently are at risk. Both in Europe and in the United States, recent outbreaks of diphtheria have occurred largely among alcohol and/or drug abusers. Within this group, carriers of toxigenic *C diphtheriae* have moderately high levels of antitoxic immunity, whereas clinical disease is observed in those with less than 0.01 IU/ml. Fatal cases and cases with neurologic complications, however, occur almost exclusively in individuals without demonstrable antitoxin titers.

Focal outbreaks of diphtheria are almost always associated with an immune carrier who has recently returned from a region where mass immunization is not practised and disease is endemic. Toxigenic strains of *C diphtheriae* spread directly from person to person by droplet infection. It has been demonstrated recently that a given toxigenic strain may directly colonize the nasopharyngeal cavity. Alternatively, the *tox* gene may spread indirectly by the release of toxigenic corynebacteriophage and lysogenic conversion of autochthonous nontoxigenic *C diphtheriae* in situ.

In addition to the determination of biotype and lysotype of *C diphtheriae* isolates, it is now possible to use molecular epidemiologic techniques in the study of diphtheria outbreaks. Restriction endonuclease digestion patterns of chromosomal DNA, as well as the use of a cloned corynebacterial insertion sequence as a genetic probe, have been used effectively to study outbreaks of clinical diphtheria.

The Schick test has been used for many years to assess immunity to diphtheria toxin, although today it has been virtually replaced by serologic tests for specific antibodies to diphtheria toxin. In this test a small amount of diphtheria toxin (ca. 0.8 ng in 0.2 ml) is injected intradermally into the forearm (test site) and 0.0124 μg of diphtheria toxoid is injected at a control site. After 48 and 96 hours, readings are made. Nonspecific skin reactions generally peak by 48 hours. At 96 hours, an erythematous reaction with some possible necrosis at the test site indicates that there is insufficient antitoxic immunity to neutralize the test dose of toxin (less than 0.03 IU/ml). Inflammation at both the test and control sites at 48 hours indicates a hypersensitivity reaction to the antigen preparation. Since diphtheria toxin is only partially purified prior to inactivation with formaldehyde, preparations of diphtheria toxoid contain other corynebacterial products, which may elicit a hypersensitivity reaction in some individuals.

DIAGNOSIS

The clinical diagnosis of diphtheria requires bacteriologic laboratory confirmation of toxigenic *C diphtheriae* in throat or skin lesion cultures. For primary isolation, a variety of media may be used: Loeffler agar, Mueller-Miller tellurite agar, or Tinsdale tellurite agar. Sterile cotton-tipped applicators are used to swab the pharyngeal tonsils or their beds. Calcium alginate swabs may be inserted through both nares to collect nasopharyngeal samples for culture. Since diphtheritic lesions are often covered with a pseudomembrane, the surface of the lesion may have to be carefully exposed before swabbing with the applicator.

Following initial isolation, *C diphtheriae* may be identified as *gravis, intermedius,* or *mitis* biotype on

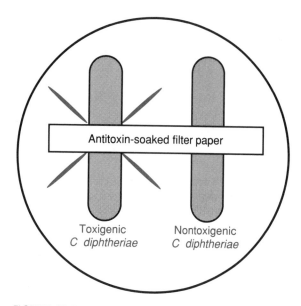

FIGURE 32-5 Elek immunodiffusion test. Filter paper impregnated with diphtheria antitoxin is imbedded in agar culture media. Then cultures of *C diphtheriae* are streaked across the plate at an angle of 90° to the antitoxin strip. Toxigenic *C diphtheriae* is detected because secreted toxin diffuses from the area of growth and reacts with antitoxin to form lines of precipitin.

the basis of carbohydrate fermentation patterns and hemolysis on sheep blood agar plates (Table 32-1). The toxigenicity of *C diphtheriae* strains is determined by a variety of in vitro and in vivo tests. The most common in vitro assay for toxigenicity is the Elek immunodiffusion test (Fig. 32-5). This test is based on the double diffusion of diphtheria toxin and antitoxin in an agar medium. A sterile, antitoxin-saturated filter paper strip is embedded in the culture medium, and *C diphtheriae* isolates are streak-inoculated at a 90° angle to the filter paper. The producton of diphtheria toxin can be detected within 18 to 48 hours by the formation of a toxin-antitoxin precipitin band in the agar. Many eukaryotic cell culture lines (e.g., African green monkey kidney, Chinese hamster ovary) are sensitive to diphtheria toxin, enabling in vitro tissue culture tests to be used for detection of toxin. Sev-

eral extremely sensitive in vivo tests for diphtheria toxin have also been described (e.g., guinea pig challenge test, rabbit skin test).

CONTROL

The control of diphtheria depends on adequate immunization with diphtheria toxoid, a denatured preparation of diphtheria toxin that is nontoxic but antigenically intact. The toxoid is prepared by incubating toxin with formaldehyde at 37°C under alkaline conditions. Immunization against diphtheria should begin in the second month of life with a series of three primary doses spaced 4 to 8 weeks apart followed by a fourth dose approximately 1 year after the last primary inoculation. The toxoid is widely used as a component in the DPT (diphtheria, pertussis, tetanus) vaccine. Epidemiologic surveys have shown that immunization against diphtheria is approximately 97 percent effective. Although mass vaccination against diphtheria is practiced in the United States and Europe and there is an adequate immunization rate in children, a large proportion of the adult population may have antibody titers that are below the protective level (0.01 IU/ml). This shows that the adult population should be reimmunized with diphtheria toxoid every 10 years. Indeed, booster immunization with tetanus-diphtheria toxoid should be administered to persons traveling to regions with high rates of endemic diphtheria (Central and South America, Africa, and Asia). In recent years, the use of highly purified toxoid preparations for immunization has minimized the occasional severe reaction.

Although antibiotics (e.g., penicillin and erythromycin) are used as part of the treatment of patients with diphtheria, *prompt* passive immunization with diphtherial antitoxin is most effective in reducing the fatality rate. The long half-life of specific antitoxin in the circulation is an important factor in ensuring effective neutralization of diphtheria toxin; however, to be effective, the antitoxin must react with the toxin before it becomes internalized in the target cells.

OTHER *CORYNEBACTERIUM* SPECIES

In addition to *C diphtheriae, C ulcerans* and *C pseudotuberculosis, C pseudodiphtheriticum* and *C xerosis* may occasionally cause infection of the nasopharynx and skin. The last two strains are recognized by their ability to produce pyrazinamidase. In veterinary medicine, *C renale* and *C kutscheri* are important pathogens and cause pyelonephritis in cattle and latent infections in mice, respectively.

REDESIGNING OF DIPHTHERIA TOXIN FOR THE DEVELOPMENT OF EUKARYOTIC CELL-RECEPTOR SPECIFIC CYTOTOXINS

Protein engineering is a new and rapidly developing area within the field of molecular biology; it brings together recombinant DNA methodology and protein chemistry. The study of diphtheria toxin structure-function relationships has clearly shown that the receptor-binding domain of the native toxin is positioned at the extreme C-terminal end of the protein (Fig. 32-3). In recent years it has been possible to genetically substitute the native toxin receptor-binding domain with a variety of polypeptide hormones, thus forming a new class of cell receptor-specific cytotoxic agents, the **fusion toxins.** Many of these fusion toxins may be important new biological agents for the treatment of specific tumors or other disorders in which cells with particular surface receptors play a major role in pathogenesis. Indeed, the first first of these new fusion toxins is currently being evaluated in human clinical trials, and the early results are most promising.

REFERENCES

Bishai WR, Murphy JR: Bacteriophage gene products that cause human disease. In Calendar R (ed): The Bacteriophages. Plenum, New York, 1988

Kiyokawa T, Shirono K, Hattori T, et al: Cytotoxicity of interleukin-2-toxin toward lymphocytes from patients with adult T-cell leukemia. Cancer Res 49:4042, 1989

Murphy JR, Strom TB: Diphtheria toxin-peptide hormone fusion proteins: protein engineering and selective action of a new class of biological response modifier. In Moss J, Vaughan M (eds): ADP-Ribosylating Toxin and G Proteins. American Society for Microbiology, Washington, DC, 1990

Pappenheimer AM, Jr: Diphtheria. Annu Rev Biochem 46:69, 1977

Pappenheimer AM, Jr: Diphtheria. In Germanier R (ed): Bacterial Vaccines. Academic Press, San Diego, 1984

Pappenheimer AM, Jr, Murphy JR: Studies on the molecular epidemiology of diphtheria. Lancet 2:923, 1983

Rappuoli R, Perugini M, Falsen E: Molecular epidemiology of the 1984–1986 outbreak of diphtheria in Sweden. N Engl J Med 318:12, 1988

33 MYCOBACTERIA AND *NOCARDIA*

DAVID N. MCMURRAY

GENERAL CONCEPTS

TYPICAL MYCOBACTERIA: *MYCOBACTERIUM TUBERCULOSIS, M BOVIS*

Clinical Manifestations

Tuberculosis primarily affects the lower respiratory system and is characterized by a chronic productive cough, low-grade fever, night sweats, and weight loss.

Structure

Mycobacteria are slender, curved *rods* that are acid fast and resistant to acids, alkalis, and dehydration. The cell wall contains complex waxes and glycolipids. Multiplication on enriched media is very slow, with doubling times of 18 to 24 hours; clinical isolates may require 4 to 6 weeks to grow.

Classification and Antigenic Types

On the basis of growth rate, catalase and niacin production, and pigmentation in light or dark, mycobacteria are classified into **typical** *(M tuberculosis, M bovis)* and **nontuberculous** species.

Pathogenesis

Mycobacteria enter the alveoli by airborne transmission. They resist destruction by alveolar macrophages and multiply, forming the primary lesion or tubercle; they then spread to regional lymph nodes, enter the circulation, and reseed the lungs. Tissue destruction results from cell-mediated hypersensitivity.

Host Defenses

Susceptibility is influenced by genetic and ethnic factors. Acquired resistance is mediated by T lymphocytes, which lyse infected macrophages directly or activate them via soluble mediators (e.g., gamma interferon) to destroy intracellular bacilli; antibodies play no protective role.

Epidemiology

Mycobacteria are highly contagious, but only 2 percent of infected normal individuals develop tuberculosis. Mycobacterial diseases are most common among the elderly, poor, malnourished, and immunocompromised. Persistent infection may reactivate after decades owing to deterioration of immune status; exogenous reinfection also occurs.

Diagnosis

The diagnosis depends on the clinical symptoms, conversion to a positive skin test (>10 mm induration) with purified protein derivative (PPD), an abnormal radiograph, and acid-fast bacilli in sputum or bronchoscopic specimens. A sputum culture is mandatory.

Control

Therapy consists of a 6-month course of isoniazid and rifampin; additional drugs (pyrazinamide or ethambutol) may be used if drug resistance is suspected (e.g., infection in Southeast Asian immigrants). PPD conversion without other signs or symptoms may warrant prophylactic isoniazid therapy, *M bovis* BCG vaccine is used in more than 120 countries and has been 80 percent effective in some trials.

NONTUBERCULOUS MYCOBACTERIA

Clinical Manifestations

Patients exhibit lower respiratory disease similar to tuberculosis *(M kansasii, M avium-intracellulare)*, cervical lymphadenitis *(M scrofulaceum)*, or skin and soft tissue infections *(M ulcerans, M marinum)*.

Structure

Nontuberculous mycobacteria resemble other mycobacteria. Multiplication is similar to that of other mycobacteria.

Classification and Antigenic Types

Nontuberculous mycobacteria are classified by pigmentation in the light or dark and by growth rate. Several species contain many serotypes, based upon lipooligosaccharides or peptidoglycolipids.

Pathogenesis

Pathogenesis is similar to that of other mycobacteria. There may be granuloma formation and delayed hypersensitivity.

Host Defenses

Host defenses are similar to those of other mycobacteria. Cell-mediated resistance is important.

Epidemiology

The infection is not transmissible between humans, but is acquired from natural sources (e.g., soil and water). Nontuberculous mycobacteria are important opportunistic pathogens in immunocompromised patients (e.g., AIDS patients).

Diagnosis

Diagnosis is as for other mycobacteria.

Control

These mycobacteria are resistant to multiple antimycobacterial drugs. Therefore, several drugs are often given simultaneously. Surgical resection is sometimes necessary. No vaccine is available.

MYCOBACTERIUM LEPRAE

Clinical Manifestations

Leprosy is an infection of the skin, peripheral nerves, and mucous membranes, leading to lesions, hypopigmentation, and loss of sensation (anesthesia), particularly in the cooler areas of the body.

Structure

Mycobacterium leprae is similar to other mycobacteria; the cell wall contains unique phenolic glycolipids. It cannot be cultivated in vitro; it multiplies very slowly in vivo (12-day doubling time).

Classification and Antigenic Types

All isolates of *M leprae*, both human and sylvatic, appear to be the same by DNA homology.

Pathogenesis

The spectrum of leprosy (Hansen's disease) ranges from **lepromatous** (disseminated, multibacillary, with loss of specific cell-mediated immunity) to **tuberculoid** (localized, paucibacillary, with strong cell-mediated immunity).

Host Defenses

Host defenses are similar to those against other mycobacteria.

Epidemiology

Transmission requires prolonged contact and occurs directly through intact skin, mucous membranes, or penetrating wounds. Armadillos in Louisiana and Texas are naturally infected.

Diagnosis

Diagnosis is based on acid-fast stain and cytologic examination of affected skin and response to the lepromin skin test; *M leprae* cannot be cultured.

Control

Treatment (including prophylaxis in close contacts) with dapsone, rifampin, and clofazimine is performed on an outpatient basis for 3 to 5 years; vaccination with *M bovis* BCG has been effective in some endemic areas.

NOCARDIA

Clinical Manifestations

Patients present with lower respiratory symptoms: fever, weight loss, cough, pleuritic chest pain, and dyspnea. In

20 percent of patients there are granulatomous skin lesions and/or central nervous system abnormalities.

Structure

The bacteria are Gram-positive, partially acid-fast rods, which grow slowly in branching chains resembling fungal hyphae.

Classification and Antigenic Types

Three species cause nearly all human infections: *N asteroides, N brasiliensis,* and *N caviae.* These are distinguished by proteolytic and fermentation patterns in culture.

Pathogenesis

Infection is by inhalation of airborne bacilli from an environmental source (soil or organic material); the disease is not contagious. *Nocardia* subverts antimicrobial mechanisms of phagocytes, causing abscess or granuloma formation with hematogenous or lymphatic dissemination to the skin or central nervous system. Mortality is up to 45 percent even with therapy.

Host Defenses

The natural resistance to infection is high in normal individuals, and the disease is usually associated with cellular immune dysfunction, immunoglobulin deficiencies, or leukocyte defects. Acquired resistance is complex and involves activated macrophages, cytotoxic T cells, and neutrophil inhibition.

Epidemiology

Nocardiosis is rare in normal persons but common in recipients of renal or cardiac transplants; in patients with leukemia, lymphoma, humoral, or leukocyte defects; or after prolonged steroid therapy.

Diagnosis

Diagnosis is by Gram stain, acid-fast stain, and culturing of organisms from sputum, bronchoscopic specimens (washing, brushing), or gastric washing, or by biopsy.

Control

Nocardiosis is treated by prolonged (up to 1 year) therapy with trimethoprim-sulfamethoxazole; these drugs may be used prophylactically in transplant patients.

INTRODUCTION

The genera *Mycobacterium* and *Nocardia* have been grouped into the family Mycobacteriaceae within the order Actinomycetales based upon similarities in staining and motility, lack of spore formation, and catalase production. These genera are characterized by the production of long-chain fatty acids, called **mycolic acids,** which have the following general structure:

$$R_1 - \overset{\beta}{C}H - \overset{\alpha}{C}H - COOH$$
$$\underset{OH}{|} \quad \underset{R_2}{|}$$

The side chains (R_1 and R_2) vary in length according to the genus: C_{60} to C_{90} in *Mycobacterium;* C_{40} to C_{56} in *Nocardia.* Several species produce disease in humans.

TYPICAL MYCOBACTERIA: *M TUBERCULOSIS, M BOVIS*

CLINICAL MANIFESTATIONS

The first sign of a new infection is often conversion of the intradermal skin test with **purified protein derivative (PPD)** to positive or detection of a lesion by chance on a chest x-ray in an otherwise asymptomatic individual (see Diagnosis below). Clinical signs and symptoms develop in only a small proportion (2 percent) of infected healthy people. These patients usually present with chest disease; prominent symptoms are chronic, productive cough, low-grade fever, night sweats, easy fatigability, and weight loss. Tuberculosis may present with or also exhibit extrapulmonary manifestations including lymphadenitis; kidney, bone, or joint involvement; meningitis; and disseminated (miliary) tuberculosis. The site of disease causing chronic, low-grade fever and weight loss may sometimes be difficult to identify. Lymphadenitis and meningitis are increased among otherwise normal infants with tuberculosis and all extrapulmonary manifestations are increased in frequency among immunocompromised individuals such as patients on chronic renal dialysis and elderly, malnourished, or human immunodeficiency virus (HIV)-infected individuals.

STRUCTURE

Mycobacteria are slender, curved rods in stained clinical specimens. The cell wall is composed of mycolic acids, complex waxes, and unique glycolipids. Figure 33-1 depicts the typical cell wall structure for *M tuberculosis* and other mycobacteria. The mycolic acids containing extremely long (C_{60} to C_{90}) side chains are joined to the muramic acid moiety of the peptidoglycan by phosphodiester bridges and to arabinogalactan by esterified glycolipid linkages. Species variations are characterized by variation in sugar substitutions in the glycolipids or peptidoglycolipids. The mycobacterial cell wall is **acid fast** (i.e., it retains carbolfuchsin dye when decolorized with acid-ethanol). This important property allows differential staining in contaminated clinical specimens such as sputum. Other important wall components are trehalose dimycolate (so-called **cord factor,** as it is thought to induce growth in serpentine cords on artificial medium) and mycobacterial sulfolipids, which may play a role in virulence.

This unusual cell wall structure endows mycobacteria with resistance to dehydration, acids, and alkalis. The resistance to acids and alkalis is useful in the isolation of mycobacteria from contaminated clinical specimens such as sputum. Treatment of sputum with dilute solutions of sulfuric acid or sodium hydroxide will allow mycobacteria to survive and grow on culture medium in the absence of other members of the respiratory flora.

Another important consequence of the unique

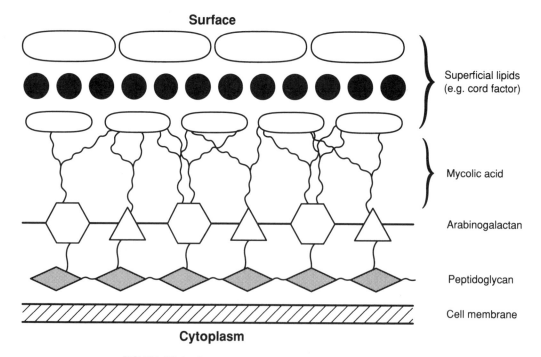

FIGURE 33-1 Complex cell wall structure of mycobacteria.

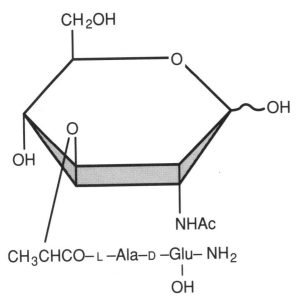

FIGURE 33-2   Structure of muramyl dipeptide from mycobacteria, which mediates adjuvanticity.

cell wall structure of mycobacteria is the adjuvant action of whole cells when mixed with a wetting agent (e.g., Tween) in an oil-water emulsion. Such a mixture is called **Freund's complete adjuvant.** Researchers have identified muramyl dipeptide as the peptidoglycan component that mediates adjuvanticity (Fig. 33-2).

Although mycobacteria are normally cultured from clinical material by inoculation onto enriched agar media containing bovine serum albumin, they can grow on a chemically defined medium containing asparagine, glycerol, and micronutrients. Even under ideal culture conditions *M tuberculosis* and *M bovis* grow very slowly, with doubling times on the order of 18 to 24 hours. This extremely slow growth, even in vivo, has two consequences of clinical significance: (1) the infection is an insidious, chronic process, which may take several weeks or months to become clinically patent, and (2) cultures inoculated with clinical material may take 4 to 6 weeks to exhibit identifiable mycobacterial colonies. When they do appear, the colonies are irregular, waxy, and white to cream, with bacteria piled up into clumps or ridges.

CLASSIFICATION AND ANTIGENIC TYPES

With the exception of *M leprae*, the mycobacteria are classified into two broad categories—typical *(M tuberculosis, M bovis, M africanum)* and atypical (virtually all other species)—based on their growth rate, pigmentation in the light **(photochromogenesis)** or dark **(scotochromogenesis),** catalase and niacin production, nitrate and tellurite reduction, and Tween 80 hydrolysis. Atypical mycobacteria are also referred to as **nontuberculous mycobacteria** and are discussed in some detail below. Although there are antigenic differences among species on the basis of serologic reactions to carbohydrate moieties in the glycolipids, such determinations are not clinically useful. Modern molecular biologic techniques have revealed a remarkable conservation of genes coding for the immunodominant antigens of all mycobacteria, including *M leprae*.

PATHOGENESIS

In this country, virtually all *M tuberculosis* infections occur by airborne transmission of droplets containing a few viable, virulent organisms produced by a sputum-positive individual (Fig. 33-3). The bacilli are deposited in the alveolar spaces of the lungs, where they are engulfed by alveolar macrophages. A portion of the infectious inoculum resists intracellular destruction and persists, eventually multiplying and killing the macrophage. The ability of virulent mycobacteria to survive within phagocytes justifies their designation as facultative intracellular pathogens. The mechanisms of intracellular survival are not clear and may vary from species to species. There is some evidence that *M tuberculosis* can prevent phagosome-lysosome fusion. In addition, some of the components of the mycobacterial cell wall (e.g., cord factor) may be directly cytotoxic to macrophages. Most of the tissue destruction associated with tuberculosis results from cell-mediated hypersensitivity, however, rather than direct microbial aggression.

Eventually, the accumulating mycobacteria stimulate an inflammatory focus, which matures into a granulomatous lesion characterized by a

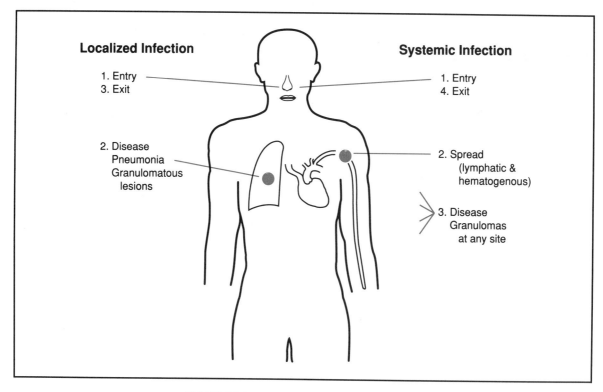

FIGURE 33-3 Pathogenesis of *M tuberculosis*.

mononuclear cell infiltrate surrounding a core of degenerating epithelioid and multinucleated giant cells. This lesion (called a **tubercle**) may become enveloped in fibrin, and its center often progresses to caseous necrosis. Erosion of the caseous tubercle into an adjacent airway may result in cavitation and the release of massive numbers of bacilli into the sputum. Often the tubercle becomes calcified and, along with calcified hilar lymph nodes, results in the classic radiologic picture associated with this disease.

Early in infection, mycobacteria may spread distally either indirectly through the lymphatics to the hilar or mediastinal lymph nodes and thence via the thoracic duct into the bloodstream or directly into the circulation by erosion of the developing tubercle into a pulmonary vessel. Extrapulmonary hematogenous dissemination results in the seeding of other organs (e.g., spleen, liver, and kidneys) and, eventually, reinoculation of the lungs. The

resulting secondary lung lesions (as opposed to the initial site of implantation) may serve as the origin of reactivation of clinical disease years or decades later owing to the persistence of viable tubercle bacilli. Figure 33-4 illustrates the radiologic differences between primary and postprimary tuberculosis. Primary disease is usually characterized by a single lesion in the middle or lower right lobe with enlargement of the draining lymph nodes. Endogenous reactivation is often accompanied by a single (cavitary) lesion in the apical region, with unremarkable lymph nodes and multiple secondary tubercles.

In parts of the world where bovine tuberculosis has not been eliminated and where dairy products are not properly treated, direct infection of the gastrointestinal tract may occur by ingestion of virulent *M bovis* organisms. The gut is also exposed occasionally in pulmonary tuberculosis when large numbers of viable *M tuberculosis* cells are coughed

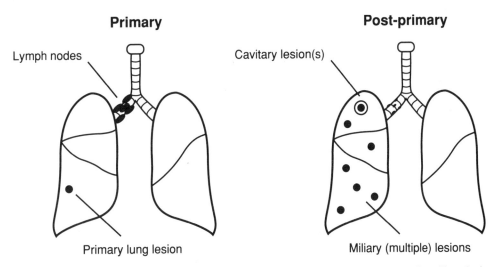

FIGURE 33-4 Radiologic differences between primary and post-primary tuberculosis. Miliary lesions, which are small granulomas, resemble millet seeds spread throughout the lung fields.

up and swallowed. In either case, the principal site of involvement is the mesenteric lymph nodes, with subsequent dissemination.

HOST DEFENSES

Innate susceptibility to pulmonary infection with *M tuberculosis* is clearly influenced by genetic and/or ethnic variables that have not been defined. Studies of mono- and dizygotic twins and siblings indicate a significant relationship between genotype and resistance to tuberculosis. Studies of inbred experimental animals point to genes both within and outside the major histocompatibility complex that apparently control resistance. The mechanism for this genetic effect may reflect the ability of macrophages to process and present mycobacterial antigens to the immune system.

Acquired immunity following mycobacterial infection usually develops within 4 to 6 weeks and is associated temporally with the onset of delayed hypersensitivity to mycobacterial antigens such as PPD. Successful acquired resistance is mediated by T lymphocytes. Antimycobacterial antibodies, although present in many patients, do not play a protective role in tuberculosis. Figure 33-5 depicts two of the principal mechanisms by which T lym-

phocytes activated by specific mycobacterial antigens can limit the replication of tubercle bacilli. Cells of the helper/inducer phenotype (CD4⁺) up regulate populations of antigen-specific effector T cells (CD4⁺) and cytotoxic T cells (CD8⁺). CD4 cells produce factors (e.g., gamma interferon) that activate macrophages and endow them with enhanced mycobacteriostatic or mycobactericidal capabilities. Unlike normal macrophages, these activated cells can limit the replication of intracellular *M tuberculosis* and may kill tubercle bacilli. CD8 cells attack infected macrophages expressing mycobacterial antigens and lyse the cells, releasing the mycobacteria from their protective niche and exposing them to activated macrophages.

Since the vast majority (98 percent) of otherwise healthy individuals who are infected with *M tuberculosis* never develop clinically apparent disease, acquired resistance must be quite effective. However, the immune response to mycobacteria is a double-edged sword: the intense cell-mediated hypersensitivity that usually accompanies infection is responsible for much of the pathology associated with clinical tuberculosis. Experimental evidence suggests that protection and hypersensitivity may be mediated by distinct subsets of T lymphocytes and may be directed against different mycobacter-

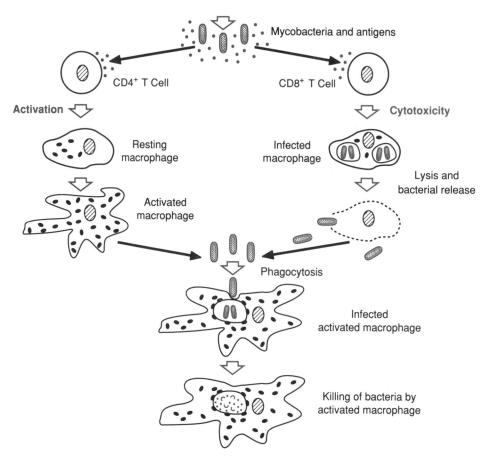

FIGURE 33-5 Principal mechanisms of T-lymphocyte activation or destruction of macrophages following stimulation by mycobacterial antigens. Activation of macrophages can result in bacterial killing while cytotoxicity may release bacteria from phagocytes and allow their engulfment and destruction by activated macrophages.

ial antigens. Much progress has been made in recent years in defining the important antigens of *M tuberculosis* and other mycobacteria by using gene cloning and monoclonal antibody technology. Table 33-1 lists the antigens identified to date from *M tuberculosis* and *M leprae*. Interestingly, some of these immunodominant mycobacterial antigens show remarkable homology with a family of stress (or heat shock) proteins that are widely conserved in both prokaryotes and eukaryotes, including humans. This observation may have relevance for the autoimmune phenomena (e.g., arthritis) associated with mycobacterial infection in some people.

EPIDEMIOLOGY

Numerous studies of tuberculosis epidemics in closed populations (e.g., on naval vessels and in nursing homes) document the highly contagious nature of this infection. Fortunately, overt clinical disease actually develops in only a small percentage of those infected (those who convert their PPD skin test). Identification of recently infected individuals is still important, however, because viable mycobacteria persisting in tissues may lead to endogenous reactivation tuberculosis later in life (see Control, below). Reactivation is usually associated with deterioration of the cell-mediated immune

TABLE 33-1 Mycobacterial Protein Antigens

| Protein Size (kDa) | | Sequence Known | Homology with Other Stress Proteins |
M tuberculosis	*M leprae*		
71	70	+	*E coli* DnaK, human
65	65	+	*E coli* GroEL, human
38	36	−	−
19	18	+	Plant
12	12	+	*E coli* GroES

response due to aging or to some associated clinical condition. Exogenous reinfection also has been documented, but most cases of so-called "post-primary" tuberculosis in this country are thought to be the result of endogenous reactivation.

Tuberculosis is particularly common in groups such as the elderly, the chronically malnourished, alcoholics, and the poor. The prevalence of clinical tuberculosis among the homeless in the United States may be up to 300 times higher than the national average rate. In recent years, the incidence of disease in nonwhite Americans has been more than five times that observed in whites or Hispanics. Of particular concern is the very high incidence of tuberculosis among recent immigrants from Southeast Asia.

Perhaps the most significant factor influencing the incidence of mycobacterial disease in the United States since 1984 has been the HIV epidemic. HIV-infected individuals have a high incidence of tuberculosis characterized by frequent extrapulmonary complications and treatment failure. Owing to the loss of T-cell function in these patients, the tuberculin skin test may not be reliable and the chest radiograph may not show the classic well-defined primary tubercle. Both of these observations make the diagnosis of tuberculosis in HIV-infected patients more challenging. *Mycobacterium tuberculosis* is the only microbe associated with HIV infection that can be transmitted easily to immunocompetent contacts.

DIAGNOSIS

Infection in an asymptomatic individual can be diagnosed with the help of the intradermal PPD skin test. Intracutaneous introduction of PPD into a previously infected, hypersensitive person results in the delayed appearance of an indurated (raised, hard) reaction with or without erythema. It is impossible to distinguish between present and past infection on the basis of a single positive tuberculin test. Recent conversion of reaction from negative to positive warrants clinical attention. Although multiple-puncture (or tine) tests have become popular for screening for tuberculin hypersensitivity, they are not as accurate or quantitative as the **Mantoux test.** The Mantoux test requires the intradermal injection of a measured volume (0.1 ml) containing a specified quantity (5 tuberculin units) of PPD. The diameter of induration is measured 48 to 72 hours later and interpreted as follows:

$$0 \text{ to } 4 \text{ mm} = \text{negative}$$

$$5 \text{ to } 10 \text{ mm} = \text{doubtful (retest)}$$

$$> 10 \text{ mm} = \text{positive}$$

In addition to the tuberculin skin test, clinical specimens from suspected patients (sputum, bronchial or gastric washings, pleural fluid, urine, or cerebrospinal fluid) should be stained for acid-fast bacilli. Culture and identification of mycobacteria in such specimens is mandatory for diagnosis. Although routine culture methods may take several weeks, newer techniques involving rapid identification of minute amounts of unique mycobacterial products by liquid or gas chromatography have shortened this period significantly.

CONTROL

In the United States, tuberculosis in the general population has been controlled by intensive case finding (by means of widespread PPD skin testing) and aggressive prophylactic chemotherapy in tuberculin converters. Short-term (6-month) ambulatory therapy with so-called first-line mycobactericidal drugs, such as isoniazid and rifampin, results in rapid disappearance of viable tubercle bacilli from the sputum, rendering the patient noninfectious. Prompt therapy, even in the absence of other signs or symptoms, is thought to sterilize the tissues and prevent endogenous reactivation of tuberculosis later in life. Patient compliance is probably the single most important varible affecting treatment outcome. If drug resistance is suspected, an additional drug (pyrazinamide or ethambutol) should be added to the antibiotic regimen. The emergence of primary drug resistance among clinical isolates of *M tuberculosis,* especially from Southeast Asian immigrants, suggests that establishment of drug sensitivity patterns may be necessary for all isolates in some parts of the country.

A viable, attenuated strain of *M bovis,* called **bacille Calmette-Guérin (BCG)** after the French microbiologists who developed the strain, has been used in more than 120 countries for many years as a vaccine to prevent clinical tuberculosis. Vaccination is the only feasible approach to controlling this disease in much of the developing world. The efficacy of BCG has varied in field trials from 0 to 85 percent, indicating an influence of unknown local environmental or host factors. BCG is not used in the United States because it results in PPD conversion, thereby interfering with the diagnostic value of the skin test.

NONTUBERCULOUS MYCOBACTERIA

CLINICAL MANIFESTATIONS

Nontuberculous mycobacteria, previously referred to as "atypical" mycobacteria, comprise several species, which may produce a wide range of clinical conditions involving several organ systems (Table 33-2). Clinically the pulmonary infection caused by these organisms is virtually indistinguishable from tuberculosis caused by *M tuberculosis.* Disseminated infection is usually limited to immunocompromised patients, particularly HIV-infected individuals, in whom the *M avium-intracellulare* complex is responsible for more than 90 percent of cases. Cervical lymphadenitis due to infection with *M scrofulaceum* is seen especially in children younger than 5 years. Granulomatous skin lesions and soft tissue infections are usually associated with *M marinum* (swimming pool granuloma) or *M ulcerans.*

CLASSIFICATION AND ANTIGENIC TYPES

Table 33-3 lists the nontuberculous mycobacteria associated with human disease and their classification within the **Runyon scheme,** in which the species in groups I to III are slow growers and those in group IV are rapid growers. The Runyon groups are further characterized by pigment production: **nonchromogens** (group III) are rarely pigmented;

TABLE 33-2 Clinical Presentation of Nontuberculous Mycobacterial Infections

Organ System	Involvement during Infection with					
	M avium complex	*M kansasii*	*M scrofulaceum*	*M fortuitum*	*M ulcerans*	*M marinum*
Pulmonary	+	+	−	+	−	−
Cutaneous	−	+	+	+	+	+
Gastrointestinal	+	−	−	−	−	−
Genitourinary	+	−	−	−	−	−
Ocular	−	−	−	+	−	−

TABLE 33-3   Classification of Nontuberculous Mycobacteria

Species	Runyon Group	Pigment Formation	Collective Designation of Complex
M kansasii *M marinum* *M simiae*	I I I	Photochromogens	–
M scrofulaceum *M szulgai*	II II	Scotochromogens	–
M avium *M intracellularae* *M ulcerans*	III III III	Nonchromogens	MAC[a]
M fortuitum *M chelonae*	IV IV	Rapid growers	*M fortuitum* complex

[a] MAC, *M avium* complex.

photochromogens (group I) are pigmented only when exposed to light; **scotochromogens** (group II) form pigment in the dark. Some of these species have been grouped into complexes based on similarities in the clinical condition which they cause. Other associations may be based upon biochemical similarities (e.g., the inclusion of *M scrofulaceum* with *M avium-intracellulare* to form the MAIS complex). Further distinction of multiple serotypes within some species (e.g., *M kansasii* and the MAIS complex) is based upon variations in the sugar residues on the lipooligosaccharides or the peptidoglycolipids.

EPIDEMIOLOGY

A crucial difference between *M tuberculosis* and nontuberculous mycobacteria is the lack of transmission of the latter from patient to patient (Fig. 33-3). There is no evidence that infections caused by nontuberculous mycobacteria are contagious. Rather, the organisms exist saprophytically in the soil or water, occasionally in association with some infected-animal reservoir (e.g., poultry infected with *M avium*). Inhalation of viable mycobacteria or introduction of bacilli through skin abrasions initiates the infection. Evidence for geographic concentrations of nontuberculous mycobacteria in the southeastern United States comes from skin test surveys with "tuberculins" made from specific nontuberculous mycobacteria (e.g., PPD-Y for *M kansasii;* PPD-A for *M avium*). In endemic areas many subclinical infections may occur. The ubiquity of nontuberculous mycobacteria makes them ideal opportunists for immunocompromised hosts. Up to 30 percent of patients with acquired immune deficiency syndrome (AIDS) may suffer disseminated infections, most of which are caused by members of the *M avium-intracellulare* complex. Such infections, which are associated with shortened survival, result from unpreventable environmental exposure.

CONTROL

Many nontuberculous mycobacteria are resistant to the drugs commonly used successfully in the treatment of tuberculosis (e.g., isoniazid, pyrazinamide, and streptomycin). Antibiotic regimens may require several (five or six) drugs including rifampin, which is quite effective against *M kansasii,* or clofazimine, which has marked activity against the *M avium-intracellulare* complex. Surgical resection is often recommended with or without chemotherapy. In treating disseminated infections in AIDS patients, a regimen of five or six drugs, including clofazamine and refabutin, should be considered.

MYCOBACTERIUM LEPRAE

CLINICAL MANIFESTATIONS

The clinical spectrum of **leprosy (Hansen's disease)** reflects variations in three aspects of the illness: bacterial proliferation and accumulation, immunologic responses to the bacillus, and the resulting peripheral neuritis. The disease affects peripheral nerves, skin, and mucous membranes. Skin lesions, areas of anesthesia, and enlarged nerves are the principal signs of leprosy. The disease manifestations fall on a continuum from **lepromatous leprosy** to **tuberculoid leprosy.** The polar lepromatous leprosy patient presents with diffuse or nodular lesions **(lepromas)** containing many acid-fast *M leprae* cells (multibacillary lesions). These lesions are found predominantly on the cooler surfaces of the body, such as the nasal mucosa and the peripheral nerve trunks at the elbow, wrist, knee, and ankle. Sensory loss results from damage to nerve fibers. On the other hand, polar tuberculoid leprosy consists of a few well-defined anesthetized lesions containing only a few acid-fast bacilli (paucibacillary lesions). Borderline forms of the disease are unstable conditions, presenting with intermediate signs and symptoms.

PATHOGENESIS

Since *M leprae* has never been cultured successfully in vitro, it appears to be an obligate intracellular pathogen that requires the environment of the host macrophage for survival and propagation. Estimates of the replication rate in vivo are on the order of 10 to 12 days. The bacilli resist intracellular degradation by macrophages, perhaps by escaping from the phagosome into the cytoplasm, and accumulate to high levels (10^{10} bacilli/g of tissue) in lepromatous leprosy. The peripheral nerve damage appears to be mediated principally by the host immune response to bacillary antigens. Tuberculoid leprosy is characterized by self-healing granulomas containing only a few, if any, acid-fast bacilli.

HOST DEFENSES

The successful host response in tuberculoid leprosy involves macrophage activation and recruitment by T lymphocytes that recognize *M leprae* antigens. Very little circulating antibody against the bacillus is present in tuberculoid leprosy. In contrast, lepromatous leprosy is associated with profound anergy (lack of T cell-mediated immunity against *M leprae* antigens) and high levels of circulating antibodies. These antibodies certainly play no protective role and may actually impair effective cell-mediated immunity. There is experimental evidence that components of the leprosy bacillus may induce suppressor T cells or interfere with macrophage function in the lesions. Figure 33-6 summarizes the immunologic and pathologic spectrum of leprosy. Much of the pathology is caused by the host immune response.

EPIDEMIOLOGY

More than 10 million cases of leprosy are estimated to exist worldwide, predominantly in Asia (two-thirds) and Africa (one-third). Human-to-human transmission requires prolonged contact and is thought to occur via intact skin, penetrating wounds, or insect bites or by inhalation of *M leprae* and deposition on respiratory mucosa (Fig. 33-7). The source of the organism in nature is unknown. Natural infections have been documented in mangabey monkeys and wild armadillos in Texas and Louisiana. Several human infections have been reported following contact with armadillos, but their role in the epidemiology of this disease is controversial. Armadillos experimentally infected with *M leprae* serve as an important source of bacilli for researchers.

DIAGNOSIS

The diagnosis of leprosy is based on the clinical signs discussed above, along with cytologic examination of biopsy specimens taken from lepromas or other skin lesions. The presence of acid-fast bacilli, which retain the carbolfuchsin dye when extracted with pyridine, is presumptive evidence

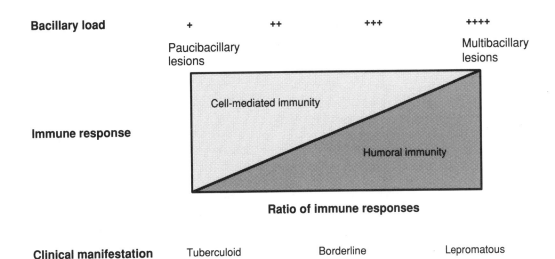

FIGURE 33-6 Pathologic (bacillary load), immunologic, and clinical spectrum of leprosy.

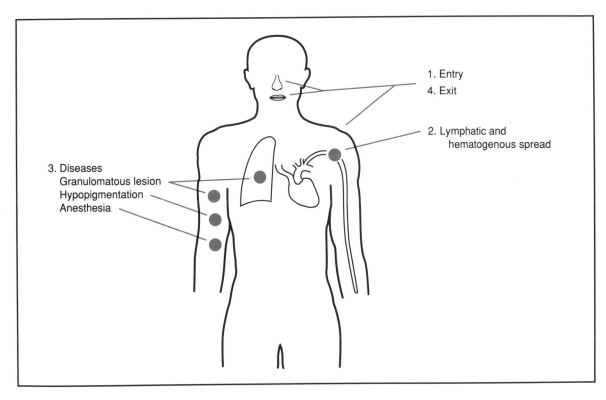

FIGURE 33-7 Pathogenesis of leprosy.

of infection with *M leprae*. Although *M leprae* cannot be grown in vitro, bacteriologic cultures of clinical material may rule out the presence of other mycobacteria. The **lepromin skin test,** in which a heat-killed suspension of armadillo-derived *M leprae* is injected into the skin of the patient, has little diagnostic value but will provide information of prognostic importance about the immune status of the individual.

CONTROL

A variety of combinations of the following drugs are used to treat leprosy: dapsone, rifampin, clofazimine, and either ethionamide or prothionamide. Paucibacillary cases (tuberculoid and borderline tuberculoid) can be treated in 6 months, although dapsone alone is usually given for up to 3 years after disease inactivity. Therapy for patients with lepromatous or borderline lepromatous leprosy may require primary treatment for 3 years, with dapsone alone continued for the rest of the patient's life. In many cases patient management must include anti-inflammatory therapy to alleviate the immunologic sequelae. Irreversible nerve damage leading to loss of sensation may result in paralysis or occult wounds and deformities. Wound prevention techniques and proper wound care are important.

◁ *NOCARDIA* ▷

CLINICAL MANIFESTATIONS

Nocardia rarely causes clinical disease except in immunocompromised individuals, especially organ transplant recipients, in whom it is the agent of **nocardiosis.** Ninety percent of such patients present with pulmonary involvement, including cough, pleuritic chest pain, dyspnea, and radiologic abnormalities such as nodules and nodular infiltrates. Other clinical findings include weight loss, malaise, fever, and night sweats. About 20 per cent of patients with nocardiosis present with cutaneous lesions, both localized and disseminated, and/or central nervous system abnormalities. About 50 percent of patients have an associated

disease process (another infection or a tumor). Cutaneous infection with *N brasiliensis* results in localized development of granulomata and abscesses with soft tissue and bone involvement (Fig. 33-8).

STRUCTURE

Nocardia organisms are Gram-positive rods, which in old cultures or clinical specimens may appear as branching chains resembling fungal hyphae. Figure 33-9 illustrates a typical colony of *N asteroides* and shows these organisms infecting rabbit alveolar macrophages. The filamentous morphology is evident. Nocardia are weakly acid-fast following staining with the modified Ziehl-Neelsen or Kinyoun stain. Cultures may grow in a few days, but typically require 2 to 3 weeks of incubation. The colony in Figure 33-9 is 3 weeks old.

CLASSIFICATION AND ANTIGENIC TYPES

Three species of *Nocardia* are associated with human disease. *Nocardia asteroides* causes most nocardial pulmonary infections in this country (80 to 90 percent), with *N brasiliensis* (5 to 6 percent) and *N caviae* (3 percent) being recovered from only a few patients with nocardiosis. In the southern United States and in the tropics, *N brasiliensis* is an important agent of cutaneous nocardiosis. The three species can be distinguished by their patterns of proteolytic hydrolysis or of acid fermentation of several substrates.

PATHOGENESIS

Nocardia cells have been isolated from soil and organic material throughout the world. Natural infections occur in domestic animals. Human infection usually results from the inhalation of airborne bacilli or the traumatic inoculation of organisms into the skin. The infection is not transmissible between individuals. Natural resistance, mediated by intact mucous membranes and alveolar and tissue phagocytes, is quite strong.

In immunocompromised hosts, pulmonary infection results in the formation of abscesses and

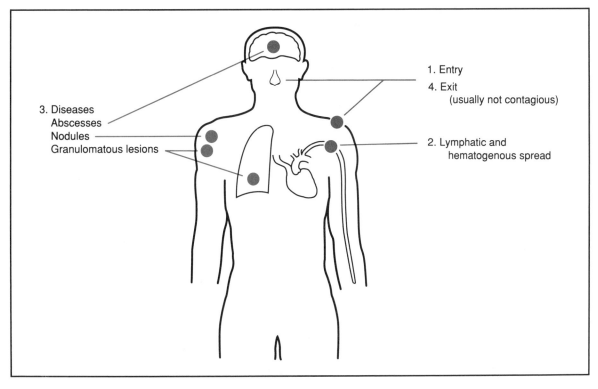

FIGURE 33-8 Pathogenesis of nocardiosis.

occasional granulomas, with hematogenous or lymphatic dissemination to the skin or central nervous system. *Nocardia* can subvert the antimicrobial mechanisms of phagocytes by inhibiting phagosome-lyosome fusion. Owing to the debilitated nature of the infected patients, morality is quite high (up to 45 percent), even with appropriate therapy.

HOST DEFENSES

Nocardiosis is usually associated with T-cell dysfunctions, immunoglobulin deficiencies, and leukocyte abnormalities. Acquired resistance to *Nocardia* is complex, involving antibody-dependent phagocytosis by neutrophils, macrophage activation by the products of immune T cells, and the development of cytotoxic T lymphocytes. Neutrophils ingest opsonized bacteria but may not kill them. Macrophage activation is associated with containment and clearance of *Nocardia* organisms

from the lungs. In a murine model, resistance to nocardiosis can be transferred with whole spleen cells or splenic T cells from immune mice.

EPIDEMIOLOGY

Although nocardiosis has been diagnosed in individuals with no detectable deficiency of humoral or cell-mediated immunity, it usually occurs in patients whose immune status has been compromised by posttransplant immunosuppressive therapy, leukemia, lymphoma, dysgammaglobulinemia, pancytopenia, humoral defects, chronic granulomatous disease, or steroid therapy. The male/female ratio in nocardiosis is approximately 2 : 1, and infections occur from infancy to old age. There is no apparent geographic clustering of cases in the United States, except for cutaneous infection with *N brasiliensis*, which is more common in the south.

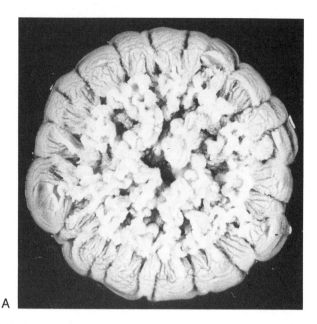

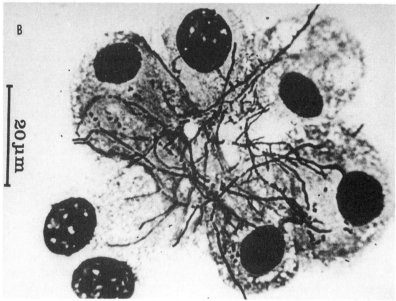

FIGURE 33-9 (*A*) Colony of *N asteroides* after 3 weeks of growth at 37°C on brain heart infusion agar (×11). (*B*) Interaction of *N asteroides,* virulent strain 14795, with seven (rabbit) alveolar macrophages (some in the process of fusing) 24 hours postinfection. At 3 hours postinfection, only rod-shaped, intracellular forms were apparent. At 6 hours postinfection, elongation into filaments was evident. Some bacterionemata shown here are intact, and others are fragmenting. Gram-stained cover slip preparation. (Fig. A courtesy of Cynthis Vistica and Blaine L. Beaman. Fig. B from Beaman BL: In vitro response of rabbit alveolar macrophages to infection with *Nocardia asteroides.* Infect Immun 15:934, 1977, with permission.)

DIAGNOSIS

Nocardia can be identified presumptively by Gram and acid-fast stains and definitively by culture from appropriate clinical specimens. Sputum culture is useful for patients with a productive cough. The presence of branching, weakly acid-fast organisms in histologic sections, pus, or sputum usually establishes the clinical diagnosis. In one series, nearly 40 percent of cases required more invasive procedures (e.g., thoracentesis, transtracheal aspiration, bronchial washing, or biopsy) to obtain useful material for stain or culture of *Nocardia*.

CONTROL

Antimicrobial therapy with sulfa drugs (e.g., trimethoprim-sulfamethoxazole) is the treatment of choice. The duration of therapy ranges from 2–3 months for minor infections to 1 year for major infections. In immunocompromised patients, lifelong maintenance therapy is recommended. Trimethoprim-sulfamethoxazole can also be used prophylactically in candidates for renal or cardiac transplants. Owing to the ubiquitous nature of these bacteria and the possibility that some infections are nosocomial, some authorities recommend respiratory isolation for transplant recipients.

REFERENCES

Bendinelli M, Friedman H (eds): *Mycobacterium tuberculosis.* Interactions with the Immune System. Plenum, New York, 1988

Chapman JS: The Atypical Mycobacteria and Human Mycobacterioses. Plenum, New York, 1977

Gangadharam PRJ: Pathophysiology and clinical presentation of infections caused by nontuberculous mycobacteria. In: Revillard J-P, Wierzbicki N (eds): Immune Disorders and Opportunistic Infections. Vol. 5. Fondation Franco-Allemande, Suresnes, France, 1989

Grange JM: Mycobacteria and Human Disease. Edward Arnold, London, 1988

Hastings RC (ed): Leprosy. Churchill Livingstone, Ltd., Edinburgh, 1985

Hastings RC, Gillis TP, Krahenbuhl JL et al: Leprosy. Clin Microbiol Rev 1:330, 1988

Horsburgh CR, Selik RM: The epidemiology of disseminated nontuberculous mycobacterial infection in the acquired immunodeficiency syndrome (AIDS). Am Rev Respir Dis 139:4, 1989

Ratledge C, Stanford J, Grange JM (eds): Biology of the Mycobacteria. Vol. 3. Clinical Aspects of Mycobacterial Disease. Academic Press, San Diego, 1989

Wilson JP, Turner HR, Kirchner KA et al: Nocardial infections in renal transplant recipients. Medicine 68:38, 1989

Woods GL, Washington WA: Mycobacteria other than *Mycobacterium tuberculosis:* review of microbiologic and clinical aspects. Rev Infect Dis 9:275, 1987

34 ACTINOMYCES, ARACHNIA, AND STREPTOMYCES

MARY ANN GERENCSER

GENERAL CONCEPTS

ACTINOMYCES AND ARACHNIA

Clinical Manifestations

Actinomycosis is a chronic disease characterized by persisting swelling, suppuration, and formation of abscesses with draining sinuses. Major types are cervicofacial, thoracic, and abdominal.

Structure

Gram-positive rods grow as filaments, branching rods, and diphtheroidal rods.

Classification and Antigenic Types

There are 11 species of *Actinomyces* and 1 of *Arachnia*. Each species represents a serologic group with subtypes. Classification is based on cell wall structure, metabolic end products, biochemical reactions, and serology.

Pathogenesis

Endogenous oral bacteria are introduced into tissue. Abscesses with fibrous walls and pus with sulfur granules develop. Lesions spread by direct extension.

Host Defenses

An intact mucosa is the first line of defense. Another possible defense is cell-mediated immunity.

Epidemiology

Actinomycosis is endogenous; sporadic cases occur worldwide. Disease outbreak is unrelated to age, sex, season, or occupation.

Diagnosis

The disease is suggested by a suppurative lesion with Gram-positive filaments in the exudate. Sulfur granules may be present. The diagnosis is confirmed by isolation and identification of the bacteria.

Control

Good oral hygiene may help in prevention. Actinomycosis is treated with antibiotics and surgical drainage of lesions. Penicillin is the drug of choice.

STREPTOMYCES

Clinical Manifestations

Symptoms of **mycetoma** include actinomycotic mycetoma. Lesions are swollen and localized at the site of the trauma. There are multiple abscesses, draining sinuses, and pus with granules.

Structure

Gram-positive bacteria form filaments and branching filaments, nonfragmenting substrate mycelium, and aerial mycelium with spores.

Classification and Antigenic Types

More than 400 species are defined on the basis of pigmentation, cell wall type, lipid composition, and numerical taxonomy.

Pathogenesis

Most species are not pathogenic. *Streptomyces somaliensis* causes mycetoma. Some species cause plant diseases.

Host Defenses

Resistance depends on a well-developed cell-mediated immune system.

Epidemiology

Streptomyces species are found worldwide in soil. They are important in soil ecology and as antibiotic pro-ducers. Mycetoma occurs mainly in tropical and sub-tropical areas.

Diagnosis

The diagnosis is suggested by clinical features of myce-toma and characteristic pus granules; it is confirmed by isolation and identification of microorganisms.

Control

Treatment is with long-term antibiotics and surgery.

INTRODUCTION

Actinomyces and *Arachnia* are members of a large group of Gram-positive bacteria, all of which have some tendency toward mycelial growth. Both gen-era are common members of the oral flora of humans or animals. *Actinomyces* species, in particu-lar, are major components of dental plaque. *Acti-nomyces* and *Arachnia* cause actinomycosis in humans and animals.

ACTINOMYCES AND ARACHNIA

CLINICAL MANIFESTATIONS

Actinomycosis is a chronic disease characterized by the production of suppurative abscesses or granulomas that eventually develop draining si-nuses (Fig. 34-1). These lesions discharge pus con-taining the organisms (Fig. 34-2). In long-standing cases, the organisms are found in firm, yellowish granules called **sulfur granules** (Fig 34-3). The disease is usually divided into three major clinical types, cervicofacial, thoracic, and abdominal, but primary infections may involve almost any organ. Secondary spread of the disease is by direct exten-sion of an existing lesion without regard to ana-tomic barriers. Hematogenous spread of the orga-nisms is not common.

Actinomycosis is almost always a mixed infec-tion; a variety of other oral bacteria can be found in the lesion with *Actinomyces* or *Arachnia*. The role of these associated bacteria is not clear, but *Eiken-ella corrodens* and *Actinobacillus actinomycetemcomi-tans* enhance actinomycosis in experimental infec-tions in mice. The presence of the associated bacteria may add to the difficulty of treating the disease.

Cervicofacial infections involve the face, neck, jaw, or tongue and usually occur following an in-jury to the mouth or jaw or a dental manipulation such as extraction. The disease begins with pain and firm swelling along the jaw and slowly pro-gresses until draining sinuses are produced.

Thoracic actinomycosis results from aspiration of bits of infectious material from the teeth and may involve the chest wall, the lungs, or both. The symptoms are similar to those of other chronic pulmonary diseases, and the disease is often diffi-cult to diagnose. Thoracic disease may spread ex-tensively to adjacent tissues or organs and often disseminates through the bloodstream, resulting in abscesses in distant sites such as the brain.

Abdominal actinomycosis is often associated with abdominal surgery, accidental trauma, or acute perforative gastrointestinal disease. Persist-ent purulent drainage after surgery or abdominal masses resembling tumors may be the first sign of infection.

Actinomycosis may affect almost any organ. For example, *Actinomyces* and *Arachnia* cause a lacrimal

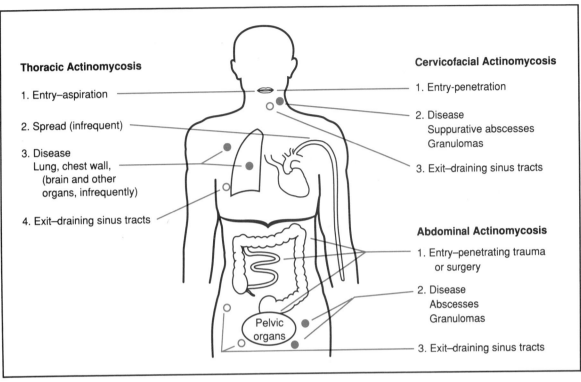

Thoracic Actinomycosis

1. Entry–aspiration

2. Spread (infrequent)

3. Disease
   Lung, chest wall,
   (brain and other
   organs, infrequently)

4. Exit–draining sinus tracts

Cervicofacial Actinomycosis

1. Entry–penetration

2. Disease
   Suppurative abscesses
   Granulomas

3. Exit–draining sinus tracts

Abdominal Actinomycosis

1. Entry–penetrating trauma
   or surgery

2. Disease
   Abscesses
   Granulomas

3. Exit–draining sinus tracts

Pelvic
organs

FIGURE 34-1 Pathogenesis and disease sites of three major forms of actinomycosis.

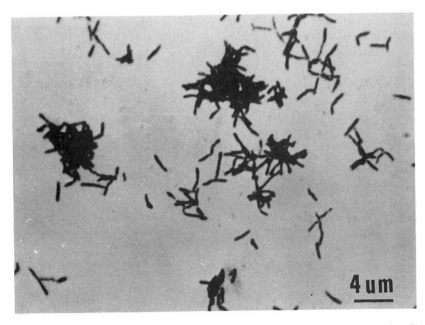

4 um

FIGURE 34-2 Gram stain of *A israelii* showing diphtheroidal rods and short branching filaments.

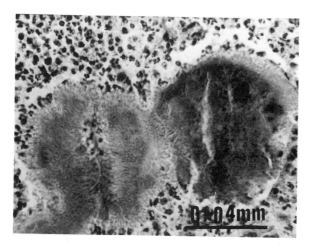

FIGURE 34-3 Sulfur granule from human actinomycosis tissue section (hematoxylin and eosin stain). (From Slack JM, Gerencser MA: *Actinomyces,* Filamentous Bacteria: Biology and Pathogenicity. p. 95. Burgess, Minneapolis, 1975, with permission.)

canaliculitis with concretions in the canaliculi and persistent drainage. In recent years, female pelvic infections associated with wearing an intrauterine contraceptive device have been reported with increasing frequency. There has been considerable interest in the possible role of *Actinomyces* in human periodontal disease. Evidence suggests that these bacteria are not involved in the more destructive forms of periodontal disease. *Actinomyces viscosus* and possibly other species may be involved in gingivitis and mild forms of periodontitis. *Achinomyces viscosus* has also been associated with root surface caries.

STRUCTURE

Despite their name, which means "ray fungus," *Actinomyces* species are typical bacteria. Both *Actinomyces* and *Arachnia* are Gram-positive filamentous rods that are not acid fast and are nonmotile (Fig. 34-4A). As in other Gram-positive bacteria, the cell wall peptidoglycan contains muramic acid, *N*-acetylglucosamine, glutamic acid, and one or two additional amino acids. *Actinomyces* species have lysine or lysine plus ornithine in the peptidoglycan, whereas *Arachnia propionica* contains L-diaminopimelic acid and glycine.

Most strains of *A viscosus* and *A naeslundii* bear well-developed long, thin surface fibrils. Pili (fimbriae) on *A viscosus* and *A naeslundii* are of two types. Type 1 pili are involved in attachment of the bacteria to hard surfaces in the mouth, whereas type 2 pili are involved in coaggregation reactions with other bacteria.

CLASSIFICATION AND ANTIGENIC TYPES

Actinomyces and *Arachnia* are irregular, non-spore-forming, Gram-positive rods. *Actinomyces* contains 11 species (Table 34-1), of which *A israelii* is the most common human pathogen. There is only one species of *Arachnia, Arachnia propionica.*

Actinomyces and *Arachnia* species grow well on most rich culture media. They are best described as aerotolerant anaerobes. The species vary in oxygen requirements: *A viscosus,* for example, grows best in an aerobic environment with carbon dioxide, whereas *A israelii* requires anaerobic conditions for growth. Both genera obtain energy from the fermentation of carbohydrates. The major end products of glucose fermentation by *Actinomyces* are acetic, lactic, formic, and succinic acids, whereas *Arachnia* produces propionic, acetic, and formic acids with a trace of succinic acid.

All the *Actinomyces* species that have been studied can be separated serologically from the other species and from *Arachnia. Actinomyces israelii, A*

TABLE 34-1   Species of *Actinomyces*[a]

Human Pathogens[b]	Animal Pathogens
A israelii	*A bovis*
A naeslundii	*A denticolens*
A viscosus	*A howellii*
A odontolyticus	*A hordeovulneris*
A meyeri	*A slackii*
A pyognes	

[a] Data from Schaal KP: Genus *Actinomyces.* p. 1383. In Sneath PH, Mair NS, Sharpe ME, Holt JG (eds): Bergey's Manual of Systematic Bacteriology. Vol. 2. Williams & Wilkins, Baltimore; and Dent VE, Williams RAD: *Actinomyces slackii* sp. nov. from dental plaque of dairy cattle. Int J Syst Bacteriol 36:392, 1986.
[b] All of these species except *A odontolyticus* and *A meyeri* have also been isolated from animals.

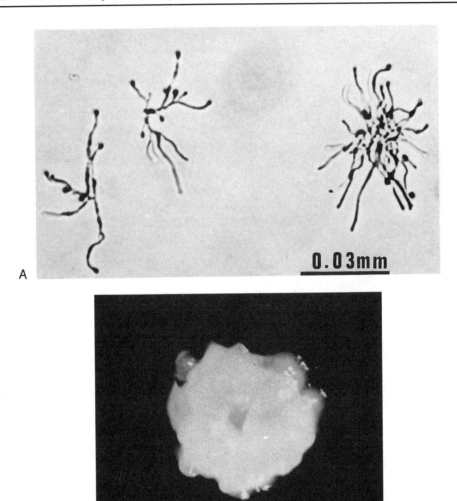

FIGURE 34-4   Characteristic colonies of *A israelii.* (*A*) Microcolony at 24 hours. Brain heart infusion agar shows branching filaments with no distinct center: a spider colony. (*B*) Mature colony at 14 days. Brain heart infusion agar shows rough, heaped colony with central depression. (From Slack JM, Landfried S, Gerencser MA: Morphological, biochemical, and serological studies on 64 strains of *Actinomyces israeli.* J Bacteriol 97:873, 1969, with permission.)

naeslundii, A viscosus, A odontolyticus, and *A bovis* each have at least two serovars. *Arachnia propionica* strains can also be separated into two serovars.

The chemical composition and cellular location of some *Actinomyces* antigens are known. One group of carbohydrate antigens is cell wall associated, protease resistant, and heat stable. *Actinomyces viscosus* has an amphipathic antigen that is a fatty-acid-substituted heteropolysaccharide and is different from the teichoic and lipoteichoic acids found in most Gram-positive bacteria. The pili of *A viscosus* and *A naeslundii* are of two antigenic types, which correlate with the different functions of type 1 and 2 pili (see above).

PATHOGENESIS

Actinomycosis results when bacteria resident in the mouth are introduced into the tissues. The mechanism by which *Actinomyces* and *Arachnia* produce disease is not clear. Pathogenesis may involve the ability of these organisms to suppress some of the immune functions of the host. Studies of oral disease have shown that *Actinomyces* organisms are chemotactic, activate lymphocyte blastogenesis, and stimulate the release of lysosomal enzymes from polymorphonuclear leukocytes and macrophages.

With the exception of *A pyogenes*, which produces a soluble toxin and a hemolysin that can be neutralized by antiserum, *Actinomyces* and *Arachnia* do not produce exotoxins or significant amounts of other toxic substances. Factors that would aid in tissue invasion and abscess formation have not been demonstrated.

HOST DEFENSES

Antibodies to *Actinomyces* circulate in some healthy individuals and in individuals with gingivitis and periodontitis, as well as in those with clinical actinomycosis. This humoral response probably does not play a major role in defense against actinomycosis. An intact mucosa is the first line of defense, because *Actinomyces* and *Arachnia*, like other anaerobes in the normal flora, must gain access to tissue with an impaired blood supply to establish an infection. Once the organisms have gained access to tissues, the cell-mediated immune response of the host may limit the extent of the infection, but may also contribute to tissue damage.

EPIDEMIOLOGY

Actinomyces israelii, A naeslundii, A viscosus, A odontolyticus, A pyogenes, A meyeri, and *Arachnia propionica* are normal inhibitants of the human mouth and are found in saliva, on the tongue, in gingival crevice debris, and frequently in tonsils in the absence of clinical disease. *Actinomyces bovis* is not found in humans and, to date, the four newly described species, *A denticolens, A slackii, A howellii,* and *A hordeovulneris,* have not been found in human speci-

mens. *Actinomyces bovis, A denticolens, A howellii* and *A slackii* are found in cattle, *A viscosus* in rodents and dogs, and *A naeslundii* and *A viscosus* in zoo animals, including primates and herbivores. *Actinomyces pyogenes* is found in cattle, sheep, goats, and other domesticated animals; *A hordeovuneris* was isolated from dogs. *Actinomyces* and *Arachnia* are not found in the soil or on vegetation.

Actinomycosis occurs worldwide. No relationship to race, age, or occupation has been noted, but the disease appears more often in men than in women. Except for human bite wounds, no evidence exists to support person-to-person or animal-to-human transmission.

DIAGNOSIS

A search for *Actinomyces* and *Arachnia* usually is based on a tentative clinical diagnosis of actinomycosis, but these bacteria should be considered whenever a direct Gram stain of pus or suppurative exudate shows Gram-positive, non-acid-fast rods in diphtheroidal arrangements with or without branching. Specimens are first examined for the presence of granules. If present, the granules are crushed, Gram stained, and examined for Gram-positive rods or branching filaments. Washed, crushed granules or well-mixed pus in the absence of granules is cultured on a rich medium, such as brain heart infusion blood agar and incubated anaerobically and aerobically with added carbon dioxide. Plates are examined after 24 hours and after 5 to 7 days for the characteristic colonies of *Actinomyes* (Fig. 34-4B). *Arachnia propionica* colonies are identical to those of *A israelii*. Isolates morphologically resembling *Actinomyces* and *Arachnia* are identified by determining the metabolic end products by gas-liquid chromatography and by performing a series of biochemical tests. Immunofluorescence tests are useful for serologic identification if antiserum is available.

CONTROL

Successful treatment of actinomycosis requires long-term antibiotic therapy combined with surgical drainage of the lesions and excision of damaged tissue. *Actinomyes* is susceptible to penicillins, the cephalosporins, tetracycline, chloramphenicol, and a variety of other antibiotics. Penicillin is the drug of choice.

STREPTOMYCES

Like *Actinomyces* and *Arachnia*, *Streptomyces* belongs to the large group of filamentous bacteria known as actinomycetes, but *Streptomyces* species have a well-developed substrate mycelium, produce an aerial mycelium with chains of spores, and are strict aerobes. *Streptomyces* bacteria are common in soil and give it its characteristic earthy odor. They seldom produce human infections, but are important as producers of antibiotics.

CLINICAL MANIFESTATIONS

Some *Streptomyces* species, principally *S somaliensis*, cause **actinomycotic mycetoma**, which is indistinguishable from that caused by *Nocardia* species (see Ch. 33), other actinomycetes, and some fungi. Lesions usually occur on the extremities, most often on the feet (Fig. 34-5). They appear as localized swollen nodules that slowly enlarge. Multiple ab-

scesses form, and draining sinuses open to the surface and discharge pus and granules.

STRUCTURE

Streptomyces species are Gram-positive, aerobic, filamentous bacteria with an extensive substrate mycelium that does not fragment and aerial hyphae with chains of spores produced by hyphal segmentation. Colonies are initially smooth but become powdery or cottony as the aerial mycelium and spores develop. The colonies grow slowly, requiring 7 to 10 days to develop aerial hyphae.

CLASSIFICATION AND ANTIGENIC TYPES

Species identification within the genus *Steptomyces* is complicated. More than 400 species have been described on the basis of morphology, pigmentation, cell wall structure, chemical composition, some biochemical tests, and serologic relationships.

Streptomyces species have been divided into seven groups on the basis of the color of the mature aerial mycelium. Further subdivision is based on the morphology of the spore chains. In addition,

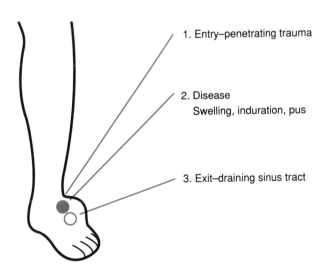

1. Entry–penetrating trauma

2. Disease
   Swelling, induration, pus

3. Exit–draining sinus tract

FIGURE 34-5 Pathogenesis of actinomycotic mycetoma.

cell wall peptidoglycan structure and the types of sugars in whole-cell hydrolysates are used extensively to characterize aerobic actinomycetes. *Streptomyces* organisms have a type 1 cell wall containing L-diaminopimelic acid and glycine and do not have a characteristic cell wall sugar.

PATHOGENESIS

Soil organisms are introduced into the tissue by trauma, most often minor trauma caused by thorns, splinters, or an abrasion (Fig. 34-5). The initial lesions spread to subcutaneous tissue and then into bone. Radiographs show multiple small granulomas with pus in the center and cavities in the bone. Continued spread of the cutaneous lesions leads to the formation of draining sinuses. The discharged pus contains granules, whose size and color provide a clue to the etiologic agent. For example, *S somaliensis* granules are large and yellow to brown.

HOST DEFENSES

Mycetoma develops in only some of the many individuals exposed to the organisms. Development of disease seems to be dependent on a deficiency in cell-mediated immunity. A relationship between susceptibility to mycetoma and deficiency in cell-mediated immunity has been shown in animal studies.

EPIDEMIOLOGY

Streptomyces organisms occur worldwide in the soil, in water, and on organic debris. They play an important role in soil ecology by decomposing organic matter and contributing to soil fertility. The major medical significance of this genus is as a producer of antibiotics. About 85 percent of the known antibiotics, including streptomycin, chloramphenicol, and tetracycline, are produced by streptomycetes.

Mycetoma occurs mainly in tropical and subtropical areas. The dominant agent in a particular area depends on the prevalence of these agents in the soil.

DIAGNOSIS

Diagnosis is usually based on clinical grounds when there is a well-established lesion. Determination of antibodies in serum, usually by counterimmunoelectrophoresis, is useful. Pus should be examined for the color, size, consistency, and microscopic appearance of granules, which will usually identify the agent of mycetoma. Definitive diagnosis depends on isolation and identification of the bacteria.

CONTROL

Long-term antibiotic treatment and surgical management are necessary. For *S somaliensis* infection, treatment with streptomycin and either co-trimoxazole or dapsone is recommended. The average duration of treatment is about 10 months.

REFERENCES

Brown DA, Fischlschweiger S, Birdsell DC: Morphological, chemical and antigenic characterization of cell walls of the oral pathogenic strains *Actinomyces viscosus* T14V and T14AV. Arch Oral Biol 25:451, 1980

Brown JR: Human actinomycosis: a study of 181 subjects. Hum Pathol 4:319, 1973

Causey WA: Actinomycosis. p. 383. In Vinken PV, Bruyn GW (eds): Handbook of Clinical Neurology. Vol. 35. North Holland, Amsterdam, 1978

Gerencser MA: Actinomycosis. p. 551. In Balows A, Hausler WJ, Jr, Ohashi M, Turano A (eds): Laboratory Diagnosis of Infectious Diseases: Principles and Practice. Vol. 1. Bacterial, Mycotic and Parasitic Diseases. Springer-Verlag, New York, 1988

Goodfellow M, Mordarski M, William ST (eds): The Biology of the Actinomycetes. Academic Press (London), London, 1984

Jordan HV, Kelley DM, Heeley JD: Enhancement of experimental actinomycosis in mice by *Eikenella corrodens*. Infect Immun 46:367, 1984

Lerner PI: Pneumonia due to *Actinomyces, Arachnia,* and *Nocardia.* p. 514. In Pennington JE (ed): Respiratory Infections: Diagnosis and Management. 2nd ed. Raven Press, New York, 1988

Lopatin DE, Peebles FL, Woods RW, Syed SS: In-vitro evaluation in man of immuno-stimulation by subfractions of *Actinomyces viscosus.* Arch Oral Biol 25:23, 1980

Mahgoub ES: Mycetoma. p. 633. In Balows A, Hausler WJ, Jr, Ohashi M, Turano A, (eds): Laboratory Diagnosis of Infectious Diseases: Principles and Practice. Vol. 1. Bacterial, Mycotic and Parasitic Diseases. Springer-Verlag, New York, 1988

Schaal KP: Genus *Arachnia,* p. 1332, and Genus *Actinomyces,* p. 1383: In Sneath PH, Mair NS, Sharpe ME, Holt JG (eds): Bergey's Manual of Systematic Bacteriology. Vol. 2. Williams & Wilkins, Baltimore, 1986

Slack JM, Gerencser MA: *Actinomyces.* Filamentous Bacteria: Biology and Pathogenicity. Burgess, Minneapolis, 1975

35 LEPTOSPIRA, BORRELIA (INCLUDING LYME DISEASE), AND *SPIRILLUM*

RUSSELL C. JOHNSON

GENERAL CONCEPTS

LEPTOSPIRA

Clinical Manifestations

Leptospira interrogans causes **leptospirosis,** a usually mild febrile illness that may result in liver or kidney failure.

Structure, Classification, and Antigenic Types

Leptospira is a flexible, spiral-shaped, Gram-negative spirochete with internal flagella. *Leptospira interrogans* has many serovars based on cell surface antigens.

Pathogenesis

Leptospira enters the host through mucosa and broken skin, resulting in bacteremia. The spirochetes multiply in organs, most commonly the central nervous system, kidneys, and liver. They are cleared by the immune response from the blood and most tissues but persist and multiply for some time in the kidney tubules. Infective bacteria are shed in the urine. The mechanism of tissue damage is not known.

Host Defenses

Serum antibodies are responsible for host resistance.

Epidemiology

Leptospirosis is a worldwide zoonosis affecting many wild and domestic animals. Humans acquire the infection from the urine of infected animals. Human-to-human transmission is extremely rare.

Diagnosis

Clinical diagnosis is confirmed by serology. Isolation of spirochetes is time-consuming and difficult.

Control

Animal vaccination and eradication of rodents are important. Treatment with tetracycline and penicillin G is effective. No human vaccine is available.

BORRELIA

Clinical Manifestations

Borrelia recurrentis (louse borne) and *B hermsii* and *B turicatae* (tick borne) cause **relapsing fevers:** influenza-like febrile diseases that follow a relapsing and remitting course. Myocarditis is a rare sequela. *Borrelia burgdorferi* causes **Lyme disease,** a multisystem, relapsing febrile disease with a rash and manifestations such as arthritis, carditis, and neuritis.

Structure, Classification, and Antigenic Types

Like *Leptospira, Borrelia* is a flexible, spiral-shaped, Gram-negative spirochete with internal flagella. *Borrelia* species are differentiated primarily on the basis of vectors and DNA homology.

Pathogenesis

Borrelia is transmitted by tick or louse bites. The relapsing-fever borreliae cause recurrent febrile bacteremias

479

separated by remissions during which the borreliae are sequestered in tissues; each resurgence involves a change in cell surface antigens. Lyme disease also follows a relapsing course, with different manifestations at different times; recurrences and late sequelae may appear for many years. The pathogenesis of borrelial diseases is not understood.

Host Defenses

Serum antibodies are responsible for host resistance.

Epidemiology

The tick-borne relapsing fevers and Lyme disease are zoonoses with rodents as the major reservoir; incidence and distribution depend mainly on the biology of the tick vectors. Louse-borne relapsing fever has no animal reservoir and causes epidemics in crowded, unsanitary populations.

Diagnosis

The clinical diagnosis is confirmed by serology.

Control

Areas known to harbor infected ticks and lice should be avoided. Tetracycline is an effective treatment. No vaccines are available.

SPIRILLUM

Clinical Manifestations

Spirillum causes **rate bite fever,** with ulceration at the site of the bite, lymphadenopathy, rash, and a relapsing fever.

Structure, Classification, and Antigenic Types

Spirillum is Gram negative but, unlike *Leptospira* and *Borrelia*, has a rigid cell wall and external flagela. *Spirillum* species are differentiated on the basis of cell morphology.

Pathogenesis

Spirillum is transmitted by the bite of an infected rat. The mechanism of pathogenesis is not understood.

Host Defenses

Serum antibodies are responsible for host resistance.

Epidemiology

Rat bite fever occurs worldwide but is most common in Asia.

Diagnosis

Clinical diagnosis is confirmed by serology.

Control

Eradication of rodents is the main means of control. Treatment with penicillin is effective. No vaccine is available.

INTRODUCTION

Leptospira, Borrelia, and *Spirillum* cause disease characterized by clinical stages with remissions and exacerbations. *Leptospira* organisms are very thin, tightly coiled, obligate aerobic spirochetes characterized by a unique flexuous type of motility. The genus is divided into two species: the pathogenic leptospires *L interrogans* and the free-living leptospire *L biflexa*. Serotypes of *L interrogans* are the agents of **leptospirosis,** a zoonotic disease. The primary hosts for this disease are wild and domes-

tic mammals, and the disease is a major cause of economic loss in the meat and dairy industry. Humans are accidental hosts in whom this disseminated disease varies in severity from subclinical to fatal. The first human case of leptospirosis was described in 1886 as a severe icteric illness and was referred to as **Weil's disease;** however, most human cases of leptospirosis are nonicteric and are not life-threatening. Recovery usually follows the appearance of a specific antibody.

In contrast to the pathogenic leptospires, serotypes of *L biflexa* exist in water and soil as free-living organisms. Although *L biflexa* has been isolated from mammalian hosts on occasion, no pathology has been found, and it does not infect experimental animals. Because of the widespread distribution of *L biflexa* in fresh water and the capability of leptospires to pass through 0.45 to 0.22-μm-pore-size sterilizing filters, they have been found as contaminants of filter-sterilized media.

Borrelia species are responsible for the **relapsing fevers** and **Lyme disease.** The organisms are transmitted to humans primarily by lice or ticks. Relapsing fevers are acute recurrent illnesses characterized by febrile episodes that recede spontaneously but generally reappear with decreasing intensity and duration. *Borrelia recurrentis* is responsible for the louse-borne or epidemic type of relapsing fever with humans serving as the reservoir host. The disease does not occur in the United States. In the western United States and Canada *B hermsii* and *B turicatae* are the most frequent causes of tick-borne or endemic relapsing fever, with *B hermsii* responsible for most human cases. Rodents are the primary reservoir for these borreliae. Lyme disease is another tick-borne illness and is caused by *B burgdorferi.* The disease occurs worldwide. It is found in most areas of the United States, with the majority of cases occurring in the north central and northeastern states. Rodents are the major reservoir for this spirochete. Antibodies play an important role in immunity to borrelial infections.

A single member of the genus *Spirillum, S minum,* is pathogenic for humans *Spirillum minum* causes one type of rat bite fever, which is characterized by recurrent fever. The pathogenesis of the organism is obscure, but the host can produce a spirillicidal antibody.

◄ *LEPTOSPIRA* ►

CLINICAL MANIFESTATIONS

Clinical manifestations of leptospirosis are associated with a general febrile disease and are not sufficiently characteristic for diagnosis. As a result, leptospirosis often is initially misdiagnosed as men-

ingitis or hepatitis. Typically, the disease is biphasic, with an acute **leptospiremic phase** followed by the immune **leptospiruric phase.** The three organ systems most frequently involved are the central nervous system, kidneys, and liver (Fig. 35-1). After an average incubation period of 7 to 14 days, the leptospiremic acute phase is evidenced by abrupt onset of fever, severe headache, muscle pain, and nausea; these symptoms persist for approximately 7 days. Jaundice occurs during this phase in more severe infections. With the appearance of antileptospiral antibodies, the acute phase of the disease subsides and leptospires can no longer be isolated from the blood. The immune leptospiruric phase occurs after an asymptomatic period of several days. It is manifested by a fever of shorter duration and central nervous system involvement (meningitis). Leptospires appear in the urine during this phase and are shed for various periods depending on the host. The more severe form of leptospirosis is frequently associated with infections having the serotype *icterohaemorrhagiae* and is often referred to as Weil's disease.

STRUCTURE, CLASSIFICATION, AND ANTIGENIC TYPES

Leptospira has the general structural characteristics that distinguish spirochetes from other bacteria (Fig. 35-2). The cell is encased in a three- to five-layer outer membrane or envelope. Beneath this outer membrane are the flexible, helical peptidoglycan layer and the cytoplasmic membrane; these encompass the cytoplasmic contents of the cell. The structures surrounded by the outer membrane are collectively called the *protoplasmic cylinder.* An unusual feature of the spirochetes is the location of the flagella, which lie between the outer membrane and the peptidoglycan layer. They are referred to as **periplasmic flagella.** The periplasmic flagella are attached to the protoplasmic cylinder subterminally at each end and extend toward the center of the cell. The number of periplasmic flagella per cell varies among the spirochetes. The motility of bacteria with external flagella is impeded in viscous environments, but that of spirochetes is enhanced. The slender (0.1 μm by 8 to

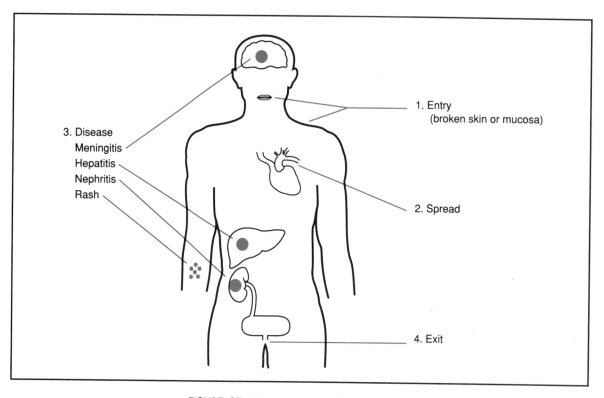

FIGURE 35-1   Pathogenesis of leptospirosis.

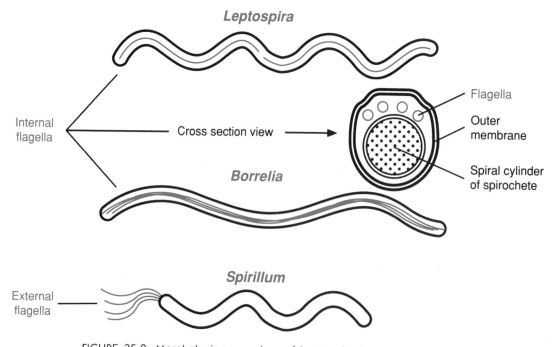

FIGURE 35-2   Morphologic comparison of *Leptospira, Borrelia,* and *Spirillum.*

20 μm) leptospires are tightly coiled, flexible cells (Fig. 35-3). In liquid media, one or both ends are usually hooked. Leptospires are too slender to be visualized with the bright-field microscope but are clearly seen by dark-field or phase microscopy. They do not stain well with aniline dyes.

The leptospires have two periplasmic flagella, one originating at each end of the cell. The free ends of the periplasmic flagella extend toward the center of the cell, but do not overlap as they do in other spirochetes. The basal bodies of *Leptospira* periplasmic flagella resemble those of Gram-negative bacteria, whereas those of other spirochetes are similar to the basal bodies of Gram-positive bacteria. *Leptospira* differs from other spirochetes in lacking glycolipids and having diaminopimelic acid rather than ornithine in its peptidoglycan.

The leptospires are the most readily cultivated of the pathogenic spirochetes. They have relatively simple nutritional requirements; long-chain fatty acids and vitamins B_1 and B_{12} are the only organic compounds known to be necessary for growth. When cultivated in media of pH 7.4 at 30°C, their average generation time is about 12 hours. Aeration is required for maximal growth. They can be cultivated in plates containing soft (1 percent) agar medium, in which they form primarily subsurface colonies.

The two species, *L interrogans* and *L biflexa*, are further divided into serotypes based on their antigenic composition. More than 200 serotypes have been identified in *L interrogans*. The most prevalent serotypes in the United States are *canicola, grippotyphosa, hardjo, icterohaemorrhagiae,* and *pomona.* Genetic studies have demonstrated that serologically diverse serotypes may be present in the same genetic group. At least seven genetic groups are known to exist in this genus.

PATHOGENESIS

The musosa and broken skin are the most likely sites of entry for the pathogenic leptospires (Fig. 35-1). A generalized infection ensues, but no lesion develops at the site of entry. Bacteremia occurs during the acute, leptospiremic phase of the disease. The host responds by producing antibodies that, in combination with complement, are

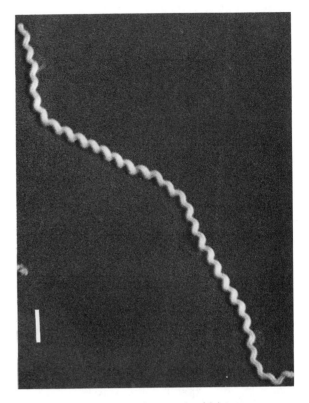

FIGURE 35-3 Electron micrograph of *L interrogans* serovar *icterohaemorrhagiae.* Bar, 0.5 μm.

leptospiricidal. The leptospires are rapidly eliminated from all host tissues except the brain, eyes, and kidneys. Leptospires surviving in the brain and eyes multiply slowly if at all; however, in the kidneys they multiply in the convoluted tubules and are shed in the urine (the leptospiruric phase). The leptospires may persist in the host for weeks to months; in rodents they may be shed in the urine for the lifetime of the animal. Leptospiruric urine is the vehicle of transmission of this disease.

The mechanism by which leptospires cause disease remains unresolved, as neither endotoxin nor exotoxins have been associated with them. The marked contrast between the extent of functional impairment in leptospirosis and the scarcity of histologic lesions suggests that most damage occurs at the subcellular level. Damage to the endothelial lining of the capillaries and subsequent interference with blood flow appear responsible for the lesions associated with leptospirosis. The most notable feature of severe leptospirosis is the progressive impairment of hepatic and renal function. Renal failure is the most common cause of death. The lack of substantial cell destruction in leptospirosis is reflected in the complete recovery of hepatic and renal function in survivors. Although spontaneous abortion is common in infected cattle and swine, only recently has a human case of fatal congenital leptospirosis been documented.

The host immunologic response to leptospirosis is thought to be responsible for lesions associated with the late phase of this disease; this helps to explain the ineffectiveness of antibiotics once symptoms of the disease have been present for 4 days or more.

HOST DEFENSES

Nonspecific host defenses appear ineffective against the virulent leptospires, which are rapidly killed in vitro by the antibody-complement system; virulent strains are more resistant to this leptospiricidal activity than are avirulent strains. Immunity to leptospirosis is primarily humoral; cell-mediated immunity does not appear to be important in immunity, but may be responsible for some of the late manifestations of the disease. Immunity to leptospirosis is serotype specific and may persist for years. Immune serum has been used to treat human leptospirosis and passively protects experimental animals from the disease. The survival of leptospires within the convoluted tubules of the kidneys may be related to the ineffectiveness of the antibody-complement system at this site. Previously infected animals can become seronegative and continue to shed leptospires in their urine, possibly because of the lack of antigenic stimulation by leptospires in the kidneys.

EPIDEMIOLOGY

Leptospirosis is a worldwide zoonosis with a broad spectrum of animal hosts. The primary reservoir hosts are wild mammals such as rodents, which can shed leptospires throughout their lifetimes. Domestic animals are also an important source of human infections. Leptospires have been isolated from approximately 160 mammalian species in the temperate zone. The disease is more widespread in tropical countries, where the infectious agent may be one of many serotypes carried by a large variety of hosts.

Direct or indirect contact with urine containing virulent leptospires is the major means by which leptospirosis is transmitted. As mentioned above, leptospires from urine-contaminated environments, such as water and soil, enter the host through the mucous membranes and through small breaks in the skin. Moist environments with a neutral pH provide suitable conditions for survival of leptospires outside the host. Urine-contaminated soil can remain infective far as long as 14 days. In humans, leptospirosis has occurred in an infant being breast-fed by a mother with the disease. The cellular structure of leptospires causes them to be susceptible to killing by adverse conditions such as dehydration, exposure to detergents, and temperatures above 50°C. Most cases of leptospiroses occur during summer and fall.

DIAGNOSIS

Because clinical manifestations of leptospirosis are too variable and nonspecific to be diagnostically useful, microscopic demonstration of the organisms, serologic tests, or both are used in diagnosis. The microscopic agglutination test is most frequently used for serodiagnosis. The organisms can be isolated from blood or urine on commercially available media. Isolation of the organisms confirms the diagnosis.

CONTROL

Human leptospirosis can be controlled by reducing its prevalence in wild and domestic animals. Although little can be done about controlling the disease in wild animals, leptospirosis in domestic animals can be controlled through vaccination with inactivated whole cells or an outer membrane preparation. If vaccines do not contain a sufficient immunogenic mass, the resulting immune response protects the host against clinical disease but not against development of the renal shedder state. Because a multiplicity of serotypes may exist in a given geographic region and the protection afforded by the inactivated vaccines is serotype specific, the use of polyvalent vaccines is recommended. Vaccines for human use are not available in the United States.

Although the leptopsires are susceptible to antibodies such as penicillin and tetracycline in vitro, use of these drugs in the treatment of leptospirosis is somewhat controversial. Treatment is most effective if initiated within a week of disease onset. At later times, immunologic damage may already have begun, rendering antimicrobial therapy less effective. Doxycycline has been used successfully as a chemoprophylactic agent for military personnel training in tropical areas.

◀ *BORRELIA* ▶

CLINICAL MANIFESTATIONS

Once the relapsing-fever borreliae have entered the host, they cause a generalized infection, apparent after an incubation period of approximately 1 week (Fig. 35-4). The onset of the disease, which is associated with numerous spirochetes in the blood is abrupt, with fever, headache, and muscle pain that persists for 4 to 10 days, followed by an afebrile period of 5 to 6 days correlated with the absence of spirochetemia. Usually, a single relapse occurs in louse-borne relapsing fever. The clinical features of relapsing fever, other than its recurrent pattern, are not diagnostic. The mortality in untreated epidemic relapsing fever can be higher than 40 percent, and myocarditis probably is the most common cause of death. The tick-borne relapsing fever is similar to the louse-borne disease, but is less severe (mortality, 0 to 8 percent), and several relapses of decreasing intensity are commonly experienced.

STRUCTURE, CLASSIFICATION, AND ANTIGENIC TYPES

Borrelia has morphologic characteristics similar to those of *Leptospira,* except that cells average 0.2 to 0.5 μm by 4 to 18 μm and have fewer coils (Fig.

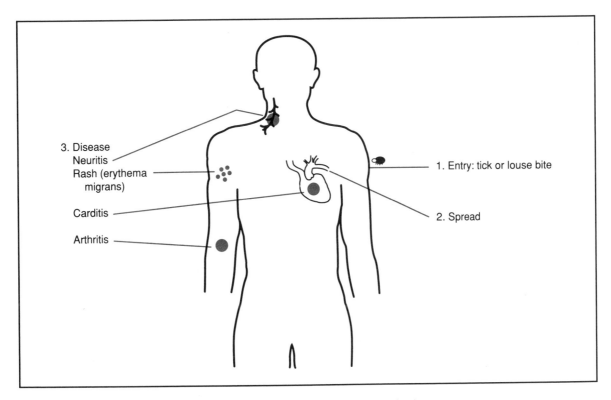

3. Disease
   Neuritis
   Rash (erythema migrans)

   Carditis

   Arthritis

1. Entry: tick or louse bite

2. Spread

FIGURE 35-4 Pathogenesis of *Borrelia* infection.

35-5). Seven to twenty periplasmic flagella originate at each end and overlap at the center of the cell. In contrast to the *Leptospira* peptidoglycan, that of *Borrelia* contains ornithine rather than diaminopimelic acid. Basal bodies of periplasmic flagella of borreliae resemble those in Gram-positive bacteria. Because of their larger diameter, borreliae are more readily stained with aniline dyes than are other spirochetes. Their lipid components are unusual in that they include cholesterol; this substance has been found in only one other bacterial genus, *Mycoplasma*.

The nutritional requirements of the borreliae are more complex than those of leptospires. Glucose, amino acids, long-chain fatty acids, *N*-acetylglucosamine, and several vitamins are some of their required organic nutrients. The borreliae are microaerophilic organisms. *Borrelia hermsii* has a generation time of 12 hours when cultivated in artificial media at 35°C compared with only 6 to 10 hours in the mouse.

PATHOGENESIS

In most cases, borreliae must rely on an insect vector to transmit the organisms through the epidermis (Fig. 35-4). The site of entry is usually not prominent as the organisms are not clinically recognized until they enter the blood. The mechanisms by which they reach the bloodstream are unknown. The relapses are due to the ability of borreliae to undergo multiple cyclic antigenic variations (Fig. 35-6). As antibodies for the predominant antigenic type multiplying within the host appear, these organisms "disappear" from the peripheral blood and are replaced by a different antigenic variant within a few days. This process may occur several times in an untreated host, depending on the infecting *Borrelia* strain.

The mechanism by which borreliae cause Lyme disease has not been elucidated. Early Lyme disease is characterized by an expanding annular red rash, erythema migrans, in approximately 70 percent of patients, which is frequently accompanied by fever, fatigue, headache, and muscle and joint pain. Arthritis, neuritis, and carditis may also be present during early Lyme disease. Persistent neurologic and arthritic infections (lasting for months to years) may occur in some patients. In contrast to the relapsing fevers, there are very few spirochetes in Lyme disease, but viable *B burgdorferi* organisms are necessary for the disease to manifest itself. Although the disease has the same general features in the United States and Europe, arthritis occurs more frequently in the former and neurologic disease in the latter.

HOST DEFENSES

Borrelia appears to be resistant to nonspecific host defense mechanisms and elicits only a minimal inflammatory response consisting of mononuclear cells. These spirochetes are rapidly killed in vitro by the antibody-complement system. Immunity to the borrelioses is primarily humoral, and immune serum passively protects experimental animals

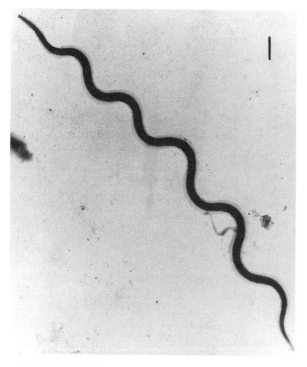

FIGURE 35-5   Electron micrograph of *B hispanica*. Bar, 1 μm.

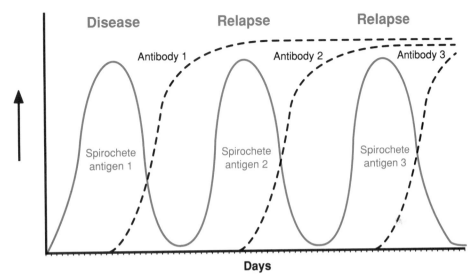

FIGURE 35-6 Immunoavoidance mechanism of *Borrelia,* illustrating the emergence of antigenic variants during infection.

from infection. Several immunotypes of *B burgdorferi* have been reported.

EPIDEMIOLOGY

Borrelia is transmitted to humans by the body louse or ticks. *Borrelia recurrentis,* the cause of louse-born (epidemic) relapsing fever, is carried by the human louse *Pediculus humanus.* The louse ingests the bacterium while feeding on a borrelemic host. The organisms multiply in the hemolymph and central ganglion of the louse. Because other organs are not invaded, transovarial transmission does not occur in the louse. In addition, *Borrelia* organisms are released when the louse is injured by host activities such as scratching. Accordingly, one louse can infect only a single host and is infective only for its lifespan of around 1 month. Therefore, humans rather than the louse are the reservoir of this disease. The louse-borne disease is called **epidemic relapsing fever** because it can be rapidly disseminated under conditions of overcrowding and poor personal hygiene, such as during wars and natural disasters. Relapsing fever, which depends on the aforementioned conditions favoring the multiplication and transfer of the human

louse, has disappeared from the United States except for imported cases. Ethiopia appears to have the highest incidence of this disease.

The tick-borne relapsing fever is called endemic relapsing fever because it occurs whenever humans are exposed to infected ticks. The soft ticks *Ornithodoros hermsi* and *O turicata* most frequently transmit the disease in the United States. These ticks often obtain their blood meal at night, and because the tick bite is usually painless and feedings are short (5 to 20 minutes), people may not be aware of having been bitten. The designation of species of these borreliae is based on their vector (e.g., *B hermsii* is associated with *O hermsi*). Genetic studies have shown that this basis is incorrect. The three North American species, *B hermsii, B parkeri,* and *B turicatae,* actually represent a single species. The ticks usually become infected by feeding on borrelemic rodents. In contrast to the louse, all tissues of the tick are invaded, resulting in transovarial transmission and the presence of borreliae in salivary and coxal (basal segment of appendage) secretions. These spirochetes in the salivary and coxal secretions enter the host through the bite wound while the tick is feeding (less than 1 minute may be required for transmission). The largest outbreak of tick-borne relapsing fever in the western hemisphere occurred in 1973 on the north rim of the Grand Canyon, where 62 persons staying in log cabins developed the disease.

Borrelia burgdorferi, the agent of Lyme disease, is transmitted by members of the *Ixodes ricinus* complex (hard ticks). In the northeastern and midwestern United States the spirochete is transmitted by the deer tick, *I dammini,* whereas the western black-legged tick, *I pacificus,* is the primary vector in the western United States. However, only one *Borrelia* species, *B burgdorferi,* appears responsible for the disease in the various geographic areas, and it does not undergo the major antigenic changes of the relapsing-fever borreliae. Transovarial transmission of the spirochete is infrequent, with fever than 1 percent of the larvae infected. The pinhead-sized nymph form of the tick is the primary source of human infections, but the disease can also be transmitted by the large adult female tick. Feedings are lengthy and require several days. The spirochetes are present in the midgut of the tick, and 12 to 24 hours is required before the spirochetes are transmitted. Within endemic areas of Lyme disease, 20 to 60 percent of *I dammini* may be carriers of *B burgdorferi* and a similar percentage of white-footed mice, a major reservoir host, are infected. The white-tailed deer, although not a reservoir host for the spirochete, plays a critical role in the life cycle of the tick, and Lyme disease occurs in areas in which deer are present. Dogs and birds are important in the dispersal of infected ticks to new locations. The number of cases of Lyme disease is increasing rapidly, and it occurs worldwide.

DIAGNOSIS

Clinical features of the relapsing fevers other than their recurring pattern are not diagnostic. Diagnosis is based primarily on demonstration of the spirochetes in blood during febrile episodes by dark-field examination, use of stained blood smears, or mouse inoculation. Antibody detection by indirect immunofluorescence assay is available. There is strong cross-reactivity with antibodies to *B*

burgdorferi and weaker reactivity with those to *Treponema pallidum.*

The characteristic expanding red skin lesion, erythema migrans, is diagnostic for Lyme disease. However, 30 percent of patients do not develop this rash. The usual symptoms of early disease (fever, fatigue, headache, and muscle and joint pain) are too nonspecific to be diagnostic. Although *B burgdorferi* has been isolated from blood, skin, and cerebrospinal fluid, this is a low-yield procedure and is not recommended. Determination of antibody titers is presently the most useful laboratory test. The serologic tests used to detect total immunoglobulins or class-specific IgM and IgG are the indirect immunofluorescence assay and the enzyme-linked immunosorbent assay (ELISA). These serologic tests will not discriminate between Lyme disease and relapsing fevers. As with the relapsing-fever borreliae, cross-reactivity occurs between *B burgdorferi* and the pathogenic *Treponema* species. The rapid plasma reagin and Venereal Disease Research Laboratory (VDRL) tests can be used to differentiate borreloses from treponemal infections.

Lyme disease usually begins with a characteristic red skin lesion called **erythema migrans;** 50 percent of patients have multiple annular secondary lesions. Lesions are not found in all cases. The patient usually experiences malaise and fatigue, headache, fever and chills, generalized aches, and enlargement of regional lymph nodes. Lyme disease can be diagnosed serologically by the indirect immunofluorescence assay and the ELISA. Cross-reactions have been found in sera of patients with syphilis, but the diseases can be distinguished by the nontreponemal test for syphilis.

CONTROL

Relapsing fevers and Lyme disease are prevented by avoiding the vectors. It is important to be aware of endemic areas and to take proper precautions. When in potential tick habitats, one should wear clothing that covers as much of the skin as possible and use tick repellants. Periodic skin inspection and tick removal may prevent Lyme disease. A

Lyme disease vaccine may be available in the near future. The relapsing-fever and Lyme disease borreliae have similar antibiotic susceptibilities.

Early Lyme disease can be effectively treated with oral tetracyclines and semisynthetic penicillins. Arthritic and neurologic disorders are treated with high-dose intravenous penicillin G or ceftriaxone. Patients who have failed to respond to penicillin or tetracycline therapy have been effectively treated with ceftriaxone.

◀ SPIRILLUM ▶

Spirillum causes one form of **rat bite fever.** Spirillar rat bite fever is characterized by ulceration at the site of the bite, lymphadenopathy, rash, and a relapsing fever. The spirilla differ from the spirochetes in that the former possess the rigid cell wall and external flagella typical of Gram-negative bacterial morphology. A single species, *S minus,* is pathogenic for humans and is the agent of one type of rat bite fever, referred to as **spirillar fever** to distinguish it from that caused by *Streptobacillus moniliformis* (streptobacillary fever). *Spirillum minus* is an aerobic, short, spiral-shaped, Gram-negative rod (0.2 to 0.5 μm by 3 to 5 μm) with two to three coils and bipolar tufts of flagella. It has not been cultivated successfully on an artificial medium.

Rat bite fever is primarily a disease of wild rodents. Human infection follows the bite of a rodent or rodent-ingesting animal (Fig. 35-7). After an incubation period of about 2 weeks, the site of the bite becomes inflamed and painful, and a chancrelike ulceration may occur. Associated with this eruption are inflammation and enlargement of the adjacent lymphatics and lymph nodes, fever,

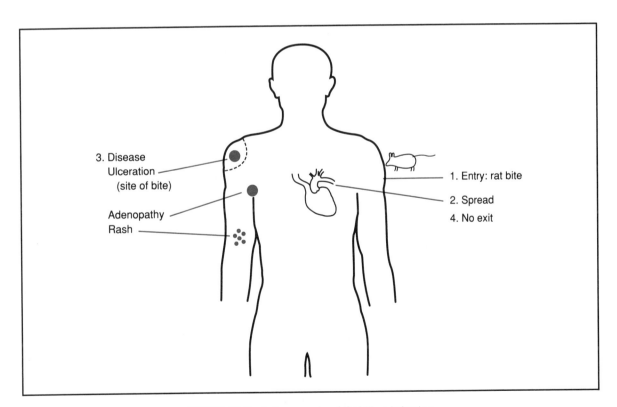

FIGURE 35-7 Pathogenesis of *Spirillum* infection.

headache, and a rash radiating from the wound site and lasting about 48 hours. In untreated patients the symptoms subside, only to reappear in 3 to 9 days. This relapsing fever may last for weeks to months. Because of the low incidence of this disease, little is known of its pathogenesis. Diagnosis is established by demonstrating *S minus* in darkfield preparations of lesions and adjacent lymph node exudates or blood. If this fails, laboratory animals free of spirilla are inoculated and examined for the development of a spirillemia. The disease has been successfully treated with streptomycin and penicillin. Improvement of sanitary conditions to minimize rodent contact with humans is the best preventive measure for rat bite fever.

REFERENCES

Alexander AD: *Leptospira.* p. 473. In Lennette E, Balows A, Hausler WJ, Jr, Shadomy HJ (eds): Manual of Clinical Microbiology. 4th Ed. American Society for Microbiology, Washington DC, 1985

Benach JL, Bosler EM: Lyme disease and related disorders. Ann NY Acad Sci 539:1, 1988

Burgdorfer W, Barbour AG, Hayes SF et al: Lyme disease: a tick-borne spirochetosis. Science 216:1317, 1982

Canale-Parola E: Physiology and evolution of spirochetes. Bacteriol Rev 41:181, 1977

Felsenfeld O: *Borrelia:* Strains, Vectors, Human and Animal Borreliosis. Warren Green, St. Louis, 1971

Holt SC: Anatomy and chemistry of spirochetes. Microbiol Rev 42:114, 1978

Hyde FW, Johnson RC: Genetic relationship of Lyme disease spirochetes to *Borrelia, Treponema,* and *Leptospira.* J Clin Microbiol 20:151, 1984

Johnson RC (ed): The Biology of Parasitic Spirochetes. Academic Press, San Diego, 1976

Johnson RC: The spirochetes. Annu Rev Microbiol 31:89, 1977

Johnson RC (ed): Lyme disease. Rheum Dis Clin North Am 15:627, 1989

Smibert RM: Spirochaetales: a review. Crit Rev Microbiol 2:491, 1973

Steere AC, Grodzicki RL, Kornblatt AN et al: The spirochetal etiology of Lyme disease. N Engl J Med 308:733, 1983

36

TREPONEMA

THOMAS J. FITZGERALD

GENERAL CONCEPTS

Clinical Manifestations

Treponemes cause diverse clinical manifestations in almost all tissues. In patients with **syphilis** there is an initial genital tract lesion (primary stage), followed by disseminated lesions (secondary stage) and cardiovascular and neurologic problems (tertiary stage). Infection during pregnancy **(congenital syphilis)** results in fetal death or numerous birth defects. Infections are chronic. **Yaws, pinta,** and **endemic syphilis** are usually present as skin or mucous membrane lesions. Soft tissue and bone lesions also can occur.

Structure

Treponemes are helically coiled, corkscrew-shaped cells, 6 to 15 μm long 0.1 to 0.2 μm wide. They have an outer membrane, axial filaments (membrane-covered flagella), cytoplasmic tubules, an inner cytoplasmic membrane, and a high content of lipids. Multiplication is by binary transverse fission. Treponemes have not yet been cultured in vitro.

Classification and Antigenic Types

Classification is based on clinical manifestations. *Treponema pallidum* subsp *pallidum* causes syphilis; *T pallidum* subsp *pertenue* causes yaws; *T pallidum* subsp *carateum* causes pinta; and *T pallidum* subsp *endemicum* causes endemic syphilis. Syphilis is transmitted by sexual contact; the other diseases are transmitted by casual contact.

Pathogenesis

Pathogenesis depends on cellular attachment of pathogens. The cell coating of glycosaminoglycans and sialic acid is anticomplementary. *Treponema*-induced prostaglandin E_2 is immunosuppressive.

Host Defenses

The body defends itself by a combination of antibodies, macrophages, and T lymphocytes that kill and lyse treponemes. Macrophage suppressor activity may prematurely down regulate immune responses, leading to the next clinical stage.

Epidemiology

Worldwide epidemics are due to the extreme contagiousness of the disease. The highest incidence of syphilis occurs in the most sexually active age group (ages 20 to 24 years).

Diagnosis

Diagnosis relies heavily on clinical manifestations. In addition, the finding of treponemes within exudative lesions and positive serology aid the diagnosis.

Control

Condom use minimizes the spread of syphilis. Penicillin treatment eradicates all stages, including congenital infection in pregnancy.

INTRODUCTION

The genus *Treponema* contains both pathogenic and nonpathogenic species. Human pathogens cause four treponematoses: **syphilis** (*T pallidum* subsp *pallidum*), **yaws** (*T pallidum* subsp *pertenue*), **pinta** (*T pallidum* subsp *carateum*), and **endemic syphilis** (*T pallidum* subsp *endemicum*). Nonpathogenic treponemes may be part of the normal flora of the intestinal tract, the oral cavity, or the genital tract; at least six such species have been identified. Some of the oral nonpathogens have been associated, along with other anaerobic species, in gingivitis and periodontal disease.

CLINICAL MANIFESTATIONS

Syphilis exhibits diverse clinical manifestations that mimic many other bacterial or viral infections (Fig. 36-1). Yaws, pinta, and endemic syphilis also have highly variable manifestations. Infections by these four treponemes are unique in that they are characterized by distinct clinical stages. Multiplication of the organisms at the initial site of entry produces the **primary stage** (localized infection). The dissemination of treponemes to other tissues results in the **secondary stage.** After a relatively prolonged period, in some cases 20 to 30 years, the **tertiary** or **late stage** evolves. *Treponema pallidum* subsp *pallidum* is the most invasive organism; it produces highly destructive lesions in almost any tissue of the body. *Treponema pallidum* subsp *carateum* is the least invasive and remains within the dermal and epidermal regions. *Treponema pallidum* subspp *pertenue* and *endemicum* are intermediate in invasiveness and cause destructive lesions only in bones and soft tissues.

Syphilis is the prototype treponemal disease; it is the most common treponematosis in developed countries. It is the subject of most of this chapter. *Treponema pallidum* subsp *pallidum* infects almost every tissue of the body, resulting in a wide variety of clinical manifestations. For this reason, it is called the great imitator. The spirochete that causes Lyme disease, *Borrelia burgdorferi,* also causes diverse clinical manifestations and has received the same epithet.

Clinical manifestations of syphilis are complex and widely diffuse, and the periods associated with each stage vary greatly; Figure 36-2 depicts averages. As the number of treponemes increases, clinical manifestations result; as the number decreases as a result of effective host responses, asymptomatic periods occur.

After an incubation period of 10 to 90 days, extensive multiplication of treponemes at the site of entry produces erythema and induration. A papule forms that eventually progresses to a superficial ulcer with a firm base, which is the **hard chancre** of the primary stage. (*Haemophilus ducreyi* causes *soft chancre,* which differs in that it is flat, centrally umbilicate, tender, and painful.) Numerous treponemes are present in this highly contagious, open lesion. Regional lymph nodes enlarge, causing regional lymphademopathy. After 2 to 6 weeks of symptoms, this primary lesion heals, leaving only remnants of scar tissue.

After an asymptomatic period to 2 to 24 weeks, the secondary stage begins. Organisms multiply in many different tissues. Clinical manifestations include slight fever, generalized lymphadenopathy, malaise, and a mucocutaneous rash. The rash initially appears on the palms and soles and eventually spreads to other areas; this is highly diagnostic. The rash may be macular, papular, follicular, papulosquamous, or pustular. On mucous membranes of the mouth, vagina, or anus, either white mucoid patches of moist papules or condylomata occur. These patches and draining skin lesions teem with treponemes and are highly contagious. If the kidneys are involved, immune complexes of treponemal antigens and host antibodies may be deposited on the glomerular basement membrane, resulting in a nephrotic syndrome. After 2 to 6 weeks of secondary syphilis, host defenses bring about healing. About 25 percent of patients experience up to three relapses of this secondary stage.

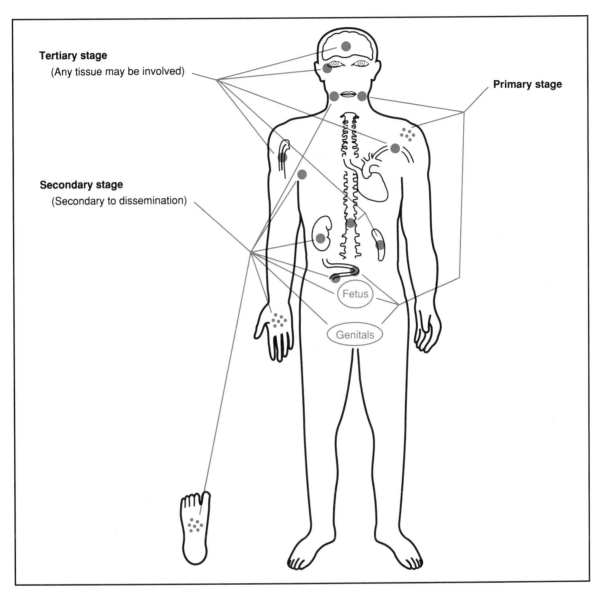

Tertiary stage
(Any tissue may be involved)

Secondary stage
(Secondary to dissemination)

Primary stage

Fetus

Genitals

FIGURE 36-1 Clinical manifestations of syphilis.

The period between secondary and tertiary syphilis, termed **latency,** lasts 3 to 30 years. **Early latency** refers to the first 4 years; **late latency** is the period beyond 4 years. No clinical manifestations are apparent, but the patient harbors infectious organisms, especially in the spleen and lymph nodes. Blood serology remains positive throughout this period.

Tertiary syphilis can affect almost any tissue. Ap-

proximately 80 percent of fatalities are caused by cardiovascular involvement; most of the remaining 20 percent are from neurologic involvement. Cardiovascular problems are attributed to multiplication of treponemes within the aorta. The subsequent aortitis produces complications such as stenosis, angina, myocardial insufficiency, and aneurysms. Neurologic syphilis is meningovascular or parenchymatous. If the parenchymatous form

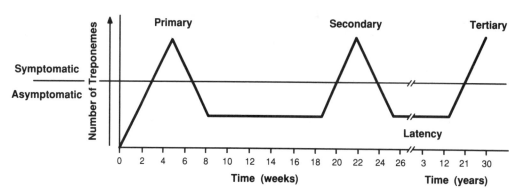

FIGURE 36-2 Development of the clinical stages of syphilis over time.

involves the brain, it is called **general paresis;** if it involves the spinal column, it is called **tabes dorsalis.** Complications of neurosyphilis are paralytic dementia, amyotropic lateral sclerosis, seizures, or blindness from optic atrophy.

Gummas are highly destructive tertiary syphilitic lesions that usually occur in skin and bones but may also occur in other tissues. They are large granulomas with extensive caseation necrosis and contain numerous lymphocytes, giant cells, epithelioid cells, and few treponemes. Delayed hypersensitivity similar to that found in tuberculosis may be responsible.

Besides the three stages of disease in adults, *T pallidum* subsp *pallidum* also damages fetuses. If a woman is pregnant and has symptomatic or asymptomatic syphilis, the organism passes through the placenta and infects most organs and tissues of the fetus. Approximately 50 percent of fetuses are aborted or stillborn; the rest exhibit diverse syphilitic stigmata. In **early congenital syphilis,** symptoms are apparent before age 2 years. They include cutaneous lesions, mucous membrane lesions, osteochondritis (especially within the long bones), anemia, and hepatosplenomegaly. In **late congenital syphilis,** an infected child appears normal past age 2 years and then exhibits syphilitic manifestations, such as interstitital keratitis and blindness, tooth deformation (notched incisors and moon molars), eighth-nerve deafness, neurosyphilis, rhagades (fissures at mucocutaneous junctions), cardiovascular lesions, Clutton's joints (fluid accumulation on knee), and bone deformation of the

legs, nasal septum, and hard palate. Combinations of these stigmata usually occur. In late congenital syphilis, three commonly observed manifestations, called **Hutchinson's triad,** are interstitial keratitis, notched incisors, and eighth-nerve deafness.

STRUCTURE

Treponemes are helically coiled, corkscrew-shaped, Gram-negative organisms 6 to 15 μm long and 0.1 to 0.2 μm wide (Figs. 36-3 and 36-4). The organisms stain readily but are almost too slender to be seen by light microscopy. They can be visualized by using the silver impregnation method of Krajian, in which silver precipitates are deposited on the surface of the organism. Alternatively, live treponemes can be visualized by using dark-field microscopy. *Treponema pallidum* subsp *pallidum* exhibits characteristic motility that consists of rapid rotation about its longitudinal axis and bending, flexing, and snapping about its full length.

Treponemes differ in structure from other bacteria. Figure 36-5 is a diagrammatic cross-section of *T pallidum* subsp *pallidum.* The organism has a coating of glycosaminoglycans that contains *N*-acetyl-*D*-glucosamine and *N*-acetyl-*D*-galactosamine. It is not clear whether this coating is host-derived material adhering to the treponemal surface or capsular material synthesized by the treponemes. Just below this coating is an outer membrane (outer envelope) that is responsible for structural integrity; the susceptibility of trepon-

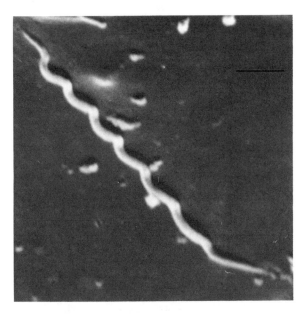

FIGURE 36-3 Scanning electron micrograph of *T palli-dum*. (From Fitzgerald TJ, Cleveland P, Johnson RC et al: Scanning electron microscopy of *Treponema pallidum* (Nichols strain) attached to cultured mammalian cells. J Bacteriol 130:1333, 1977, with permission.)

emes to penicillin indicates a peptidoglycan cell wall structure. This membrane covers three flagella (axial filaments) that wind around the surface of the organism. These flagella arise at each end of the treponeme and extend halfway down the organism, overlapping at the midpoint. A cytoplasmic membrane (wall membrane) that acts as an osmotic barrier covers the protoplasmic cylinder; six to eight cytoplasmic tubules (body fibrils) are located on the inner surface of this membrane. These tubules also arise at each end and wind around the organism to the midpoint.

Treponema pallidum subsp *pallidum* is a fastidious organism that exhibits narrow optimal ranges of pH (7.2 to 7.4), E_h (-230 to -240 mV), and temperature (30 to 37°C). It is rapidly inactivated by mild heat, cold, desiccation, and most disinfectants. Traditionally this organism has been considered a strict anaerobe, but recent evidence indicates that it is microaerophilic and requires low concentrations of oxygen (1 to 4 percent).

The composition of *T pallidum* subsp *pallidum* (dry weight) is approximately 70 percent proteins, 20 percent lipids, and 5 percent carbohydrates. This lipid content is relatively high for bacteria. Of the total lipids, 68 percent are phospholipids (primary phosphatidylcholine, sphingomyelin, and cardiolipin) and 32 percent are neutral lipids (primarily cholesterol).

Antigenic analysis of *T pallidum* subsp *pallidum* is hampered by the inability to grow this organism in vitro. The appearance of many different antibodies during infection indicates that the antigenic makeup of the organism is complex. A genus-specific antigen is shared with nonpathogenic treponemes. A species-specific antigen exclusive for *T*

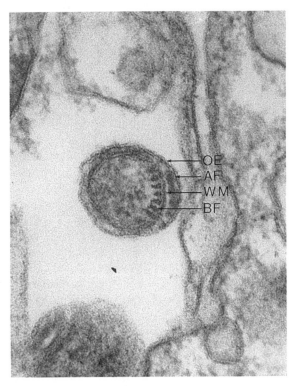

FIGURE 36-4 Transmission electron micrograph of cross-section of *T pallidum*. Abbreviations: OE, outer envelope (membrane); AF, axial filament; WM, cell wall membrane; BF, body fibrils. (From Johnson RC, Ritzi DM, Levermore BP et al: Outer envelope of virulent *Treponema pallidum*. Infect Immun 8:294, 1973, with permission.)

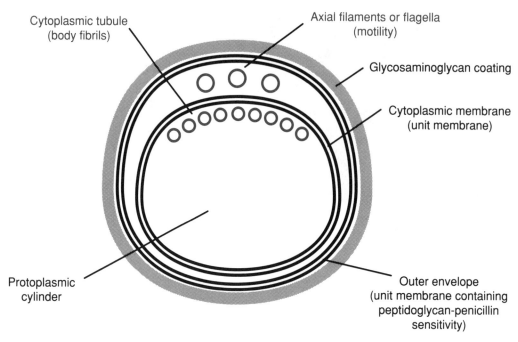

FIGURE 36-5 Treponemal structure (cross-section).

pallidum subsp *pallidum* has not yet been found. Many antigens are shared with the other pathogenic treponemes; in fact, *T pallidum* subspp *pallidum, pertenue, carateum,* and *endemicum* are antigenically indistinguishable.

Cardiolipin is part of the treponemal structure. This antigen elicits Wassermann antibodies, which form the basis for a group of serologic tests. It is also found in human and animal tissues as part of the mitochondrial membrane. In addition, newer methods involving gel electrophoresis and immunoblotting have revealed more than 100 separate protein antigens.

Multiplication occurs through binary transverse fission. The in vivo generation time is relatively long (30 hours). Despite intense efforts over the past 75 years, *T pallidum* subsp *pallidum* has not been successfully cultured in vitro. Viable organisms can be maintained for 18 to 21 days in complex media. The other three pathogenic treponemes have also not been successfully grown.

CLASSIFICATION AND ANTIGENIC TYPES

The pathogenic treponemes cannot be distinguished by morphology, biochemical capabilities, physiologic criteria, or DNA homology. Specific antigenic differences have not yet been identified, and serologic reactions positive for one disease are also positive for the other three. Differentiation of the treponematoses is based on geographic location, modes of transmission, and clinical manifestations (Table 36-1). Similarities in treponemal infections include their generalized nature, regional and general lymphadenopathy, chronicity, spontaneous healing, asymptomatic periods, and relatively painless symptoms.

Although specific strain differentiation is not available, different human isolates have been characterized. These isolates exhibit various degrees of virulence; the more virulent isolates cause more intense manifestations and slower healing.

TABLE 36-1   Characteristics of the Four Treponematoses

Characteristic	Syphilis (subsp *pallidum*)	Yaws (subsp *pertenue*)	Pinta (subsp *carateum*)	Endemic Syphilis (subsp *endemicum*)
Epidemiology				
Other names	Venereal syphilis	Frambesia, pian	Carate, cute	Bjel, dichuchwa
Prevalence	Worldwide	Hot, humid areas	Hot, humid areas	Hot, dry areas
Locations	Worldwide	Tropics	Central and South America	Deserts
Age group	Adults	Children	Children, adolescents	Children, adults
Spread	Venereal	Skin	Skin	Mucous membranes
Congenital infection	Yes	No	No	Rarely
Disease charac-teristics				
Incubation period	10–90 days	14–28 days	2–6 months	?
Invasiveness	High	Intermediate	Low	Intermediate
Perivascular (cuffing)	Yes	No	Yes	Yes
Tissues	All	Skin, bones, soft tissues	Skin	Mucous membranes, skin, muscles, bones
Predominant cellular infiltrate	Lymphocytes, plasma cells	Mostly plasma cells	Mostly lympho-cytes	Lymphocytes, plasma cells
Destructive lesions	Yes	Yes	No	Yes
Granulomas	Yes	Yes	No	Yes
Gummas	Yes	Yes	No	Yes
Condylomata lata	Yes	Yes	No	Yes

PATHOGENESIS

Syphilis is a painless, slowly evolving chronic granulomatous disease that fluctuates between short symptomatic stages and rather prolonged asymptomatic stages. The host-parasite relationship is constantly changing; multiplication of organisms results in disease (primary, secondary, and tertiary stages); host responses, in turn, produce healing.

Humans are the only natural host for *T pallidum* subsp *pallidum*, and infection occurs through sexual contact. The organisms penetrate mucous membranes or enter minuscule breaks in the skin. Once inside the host, organisms localize at the site of entry and begin to multiply. *Treponema pallidum* subsp *pallidum* immediately gains access to the blood and lymphatics and disseminates to other tissues. Thus, from the outset, syphilis is a disseminated disease. Target tissues include lymph nodes, skin, mucous membranes, liver, spleen, kidneys, heart, bones, joints, larynx, eyes, meninges, brain, and central nervous system. In women the initial lesion is usually on the labia, the walls of the vagina, or the cervix; in men it is on the shaft or glans of the penis. A primary lesion may also occur on lips, tongue, tonsils, anus, or other skin areas.

The most prominent feature of syphilitic infection is perivascular involvement of arterioles and capillaries. Periarteritis (proliferation of adventitial cells and cuffing), endarteritis (swelling and proliferation of endothelial cells that reduce the vessel lumen), and infiltration of lymphocytes and plasma cells are characteristic of syphilitic histopathology. *Treponema pallidum* subsp *pallidum* appears to lack potent toxins, and it has been suggested that at least some of the histopathology results from activation of host defenses. Treponemes readily attach to tissues. Antibodies, in association with complement or macrophages and T lymphocytes that interact with organisms, may indirectly damage the host tissues.

In recent years new concepts of treponemal pathogenesis have emerged (Fig. 36-6). In vitro studies have shown that *T pallidum* subspp *pallidum* and *pertenue* specifically attach to numerous and different types of tissues. This probably reflects their in vivo ability to infect most tissues and organs of the body. Importantly, nonpathogenic treponemes do not attach; this directly relates attachment to pathogenesis. To disseminate away from the site of initial entry, organisms must traverse the viscous ground substance between tissue cells. *Treponema pallidum* subsp *pallidum* has a hyaluronidase that degrades the hyaluronic acid within the ground substance to facilitate the spread of the organisms. To gain access to the blood and lymphatic channels, treponemes must degrade the intact basement membrane surrounding these vessels, and then pass between endothelial cells to enter the lumen (Fig. 36-6). At distant sites, the process is reversed and organisms eventually localize perivascularly. *Treponema pallidum* subsp *pallidum* specifically attaches to laminin and collagen type IV, which are integral components of the

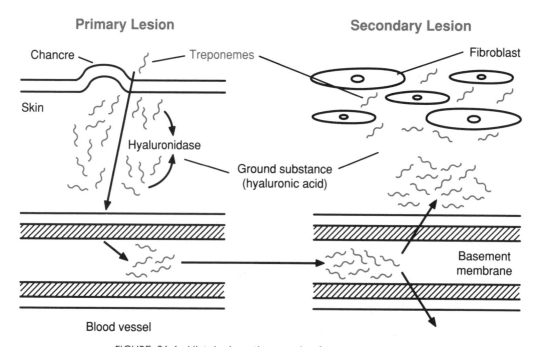

FIGURE 36-6 Histologic pathogenesis of treponemal disease.

basement membrane. It also attaches to fibronectin, collagen type I, and hyaluronic acid, which are integral components of the intercellular ground substance.

In addition to attachment, *T pallidum* subsp *pallidum* possesses at least three virulence factors that partially neutralize elements of the immune response (Table 36-2). Glycosaminoglycans similar to hyaluronic acid act as anticomplement factors. These long, straight-chain polysaccharides coat the outer surface of the organisms. They may represent a capsulelike material synthesized by the organism or may merely reflect passive coating by host-derived glycosaminoglycans. Whatever their origin, they interfere with treponemal killing by the classic (antibody-dependent) complement pathway. In addition, *T pallidum* subsp *pallidum* carries surface-associated sialic acid. This component retards the activation and killing by the alternative (non-antibody-dependent) complement pathway. Glycosaminoglycans and sialic acid conceivably allow the organisms to disseminate in the bloodstream, despite the detrimental effect of the complement.

Treponema pallidum subsp *pallidum* appears to contain an intact cyclooxygenase pathway and can synthesize its own prostaglandin E_2. These autocoids are potent immunomodulators. It has been proposed that prostaglandin E_2 down regulates early immune processing by stimulating macrophage suppressor activity. This suppression could be an important factor in the exacerbation of infection that leads to the next clinical stage.

HOST DEFENSES

Immunity develops in untreated syphilis. In the 19th century, experiments involving reinoculation of syphilitic patients demonstrated that an infected individual was somewhat resistant. The Oslo study, begun in the early 1900s, involved 1,000 untreated patients observed for 30 to 50 years. Approximately 25 percent of these patients developed secondary syphilis and 13 percent developed tertiary syphilis; the fact that 75 percent of the patients did not progress beyond primary syphilis indicates a certain degree of immunity. The Sing-Sing and

TABLE 36-2   Immune System Evasion by Treponemal Factors

Treponemal Surface-Activated Factor	Immune System Evasion Mechanism
Glycosaminoglycans	Inhibit complement activation of the classic (antibody dependent) pathway
Sialic acid	Inhibits complement activation of the alternative (antibody-independent) pathway
Treponemal secretion of prostaglandin E_2	Inhibits many different immune functions and enhances development of macrophage suppressor activity

Tuskegee studies, involving humans and experimental syphilitic rabbits, confirm these observations. (The ethics of performing such studies, in which some syphilis victims were used as controls and were not treated, is now a highly controversial issue.) Immunity develops very gradually during the infection.

Syphilis generates a wide variety of antibodies that are the basis for numerous diagnostic tests. The precise contribution of humoral antibodies to host defenses in syphilitic infection is not clear. Within lesions, *T pallidum* subsp *pallidum* exhibits a predilection for perivascular areas. A lymphocyte and plasma cell infiltration occurs early in infection and is especially prominent in perivascular areas. The presence of both organisms and antibody-synthesizing host cells in the same tissue areas suggests some role for antibodies. Passive transfer of immune serum does not protect experimental syphilitic rabbits against challenge inoculation, although some modification of treponemal lesions occurs. However, injection of immune serum before *T pallidum* subsp *pallidum* challenge lengthens the incubation period, reduces the severity of lesions, and speeds healing. Thus, antibodies appear to be partially but not solely responsible for healing and immunity.

Within syphilitic lesions, macrophages and T lymphocytes predominate. The role of these two cell types is now being clarified. Macrophages readily phagocytose and process treponemal organisms. Activated macrophages, in turn, amplify T-cell stimulation. Both cell types secrete soluble substances that kill and lyse *T pallidum* subsp *pallidum*. The paradox is that most but not all treponemes are cleared from the infected tissues and that macrophages play a key role in prematurely down regulating the activated immune responses. The treponemal prostaglandin E_2 appears to enhance macrophage synthesis of prostaglandin E_2, which elicits a macrophage-suppressive activity that prematurely accelerates immunologic turn-off. The end result is that the immune system is down regulated before all organisms are cleared. The residual treponemes then multiply and induce the next clinical stage.

EPIDEMIOLOGY

Treponema pallidum subsp *pallidum* is distributed worldwide and occurs in epidemic proportions in virtually every country. Humans are the only source of this highly contagious infection. In almost all cases, syphilis is transmitted through sexual contact. Infectivity rates correspond to the most sexually active age groups, being highest in the 20 to 24 year age group; slightly lower in the 15 to 19 year age group, and lower in the 25 to 29-year age group.

In the late 1940s, penicillin was found to be effective in eradicating syphilis in each of its three clinical stages, in latent infections, and in congenital infections. The peak incidence of syphilis was observed in 1946 to 1947 (Fig. 36-7). The number of cases progressively decreased until 1958, after which the trend reversed and a steady increase has occurred. Fortunately, the incidence of late manifestations has greatly declined, probably because of the widespread use of penicillin and related antibiotics to treat many other nonsyphilitic diseases. Better surveillance methods have also helped. In addition, approximately 1 to 10 percent of persons with gonorrhea may have concurrent syphilitic infection. Because gonorrhea has a shorter incubation period (2 to 8 days) and has painful symptoms,

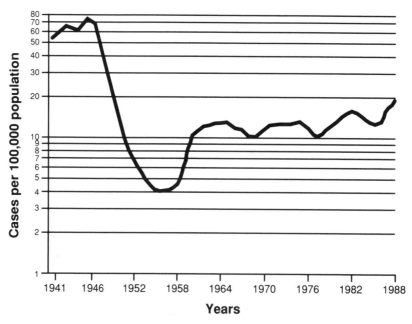

FIGURE 36-7   Incidence of syphilis (primary and secondary) by year in the United States between 1941 and 1988.

the patient seeks treatment before syphilitic lesions develop. Penicillin therapy of gonorrhea eradicates syphilis before it becomes clinically apparent.

The treponemes have many cross-reacting antigens, and untreated infection confers partial protection against the other treponemal diseases. In areas in which yaws is endemic, the incidence of syphilis is low. After effective campaigns to eradicate yaws, the incidence of syphilis eventually increases. Similar epidemiologic observations have been made after local eradication of pinta and endemic syphilis. The treponematoses are highly contagious: syphilis is distributed throughout the world, yaws is widespread in the tropics, pinta is highly endemic in Central and South America, and endemic syphilis is present in certain desert regions.

DIAGNOSIS

Definitive diagnosis of syphilis is complicated by the inability to cultivate *T pallidum* subsp *pallidum* in vitro. Clinical manifestations, demonstration of treponemes in lesion material, and serologic reactions are used for diagnosis. In most cases, clinical manifestations are sufficiently characteristic. If manifestations include exudative lesion, treponemes should be detectable within lesion material. Dark-field microscopy is used to visualize motile and nonmotile organisms.

Serologic tests are important in diagnosis, especially in cases in which clinical manifestations are confusing or exduative material is not present. More than 200 serologic tests have been developed over the years; they fall into two general categories. (1) **Nontreponemal tests** measure levels of Wassermann antibody, which is elicited in response to cardiolipin antigens, presumably from host tissue; many variants of these tests are used. (2) **Treponemal tests** measure levels of antibodies elicited in response to antigenic components of *T pallidum* subsp *pallidum;* these include the fluorescence of treponemes (FTA-ABS), *T pallidum* immobilization (TPI), agglutinin, and hemagglutinin tests.

Serologic reactions vary with the stage of the disease. The results of nontreponemal tests usually parallel the severity of infection: titers are high during clinical infection and subside during subclinical infection (latency) or following antibiotic therapy. The treponemal tests may not become positive until well after the initial clinical manifestations; titers remain high in latency.

The World Health Organization recommends that sera be screened by the Venereal Disease Research Laboratory (VDRL) test, rapid plasma reagin (RPR) test, or automated reagin test (ARTR) and that positive sera be confirmed by the FTA-ABS test. Recently, a group of hemagglutination tests have been developed that are easier to perform than the FTA-ABS test and appear to be as good.

Two terms relevant to serologic testing are sensitivity and specificity. The perfect test, not yet developed, would detect 100 percent of the treponemal infections and would be nonreactive in all other diseases. **Sensitivity** refers to the ability to detect the tested variable, in this case syphilis. A biologic false-negative occurs when serum from a syphilitic patient fails to react; for example, the FTA-ABS test is nonreactive early in the primary stage. **Specificity** refers to the ability to recognize when the variable is not present (i.e., to exclude syphilis in nonsyphilitic patients). A biologic false-positive occurs when serum from a nonsyphilitic patient reacts positively; for example, serum samples from patients with leprosy, tuberculosis, malaria, infectious mononucleosis, collagen disorders, systemic lupus erythemotosus, rheumatoid arthritis, and thyroiditis frequently show positive reactions in the VDRL test. Pregnancy, old age, and drug abuse are also associated with false-positive results.

Congenital syphilis of the newborn is somewhat difficult to diagnose. Maternal antibodies (IgG) pass through the placenta and enter the fetal circulation. Therefore, at birth the baby is serolopositive, although these maternal antibodies disappear after 3 months. Because of the presence of maternal antibodies in the newborn, quantitative VDRL or RPR tests should be performed monthly over the first 6 months. If the titer increases or stabilizes and does not decrease, congenital syphilis is indicated and the baby should be treated accordingly.

CONTROL

The current worldwide epidemic of syphilis emphasizes the need for developing preventive measures. Unfortunately, effective measures are limited (Table 36-3). The condom remains the method of choice. Topical application of antibiotics, chemicals, creams, or lotions and thorough washing with soap and water after sexual contact are highly ineffective. A vaccine appears to be the only hope for future control of syphilis. Despite intense research in this area, only limited progress has been made. Two other control measures are important. The first is to educate people about the early clinical manifestations of primary syphilis, so that they can seek treatment before infecting others. The second, for which epidemiology programs have been established, is to trace contacts of syphilitic patients; these contacts are then treated prophylactically before onset of clinical manifestations.

Penicillin remains the drug of choice for treating syphilis. Penicillin resistance has not yet emerged, unlike the situation for gonorrhea. Long-acting penicillin is used to maintain high levels in serum for 7 to 10 days. Infection may be treated with any one of the following: procaine penicillin G, clemizole penicillin, procaine penicillin G with 2 percent aluminum monostearate, or benzathine penicillin G. If allergy to penicillin exists, tetracycline, erythromycin, and cephaloridine are alternatives. The dosage depends on the stage of infection. However, antibiotics are effective during each clinical stage, latency, and congenital syphilis in utero and after birth.

A Jarisch-Herxheimer reaction occasionally follows treatment of secondary or tertiary syphilis.

TABLE 36-3 Effective and Ineffective Preventive
Measures against Syphilis

Very Effective	Totally Ineffective
Condoms	Topical antibiotics
	Topical chemicals
	Topical creams, including spermicides
	Thorough washing with soap and water

This focal and systemic reaction is associated with the rapid death of treponemes. Between 2 and 12 hours after antibiotic therapy, headache, malaise, slight fever, chills, muscle aches, and intensification of syphilitic lesions occur. These manifestations resolve in fewer than 12 hours. This benign reaction requires no prophylactic measures and, importantly, indicates effective therapy.

Both Wassermann and treponemal antibodies remain detectable for long periods, even after effective treatment. The recommended procedure for verifying a cure involves tracking the number of Wasermann antibodies, which disappear more rapidly than treponemal antibodies. Patients with primary syphilis should be Wassermann seronegative 6 to 12 months after treatment; patients with secondary syphilis should be Wassermann seronegative 12 to 18 months after treatment. A cure is difficult to verify if infection has endured beyond 2 years; in these patients, Wassermann and treponemal antibodies may be detected 12 to 25 years after treatment.

OTHER TREPONEMATOSES

Yaws

Yaws, caused by *T pallidum* subsp *pertenue*, predominates in the tropical areas of Africa, South America, India, Indonesia, and the Pacific Islands. Its highly contagious nature is indicated by an estimated 50 million cases worldwide. Transmission occurs through human-to-human nonsexual contact. Most cases are in children and adolescents. In endemic areas, 75 percent of the population contract yaws before reaching 20 years of age.

The primary lesion, or mother yaw, develops within 2 to 4 weeks at the site of skin entry as a painless erythematous papule or group of papules. Lesions enlarge and ulcerate, exuding a serous fluid with a bloody tinge that is swarming with organisms. These lesions heal within 1 to several months, leaving an atrophic, depressed scar. The treponemes disseminate, and, within 1 to 12 months, secondary lesions evolve that are quite similar to the mother yaw. Crops of these lesions develop initially on the face and moist areas of the body and then spread to the trunk and arms. Infection of the soles and palms is characteristic, as it is in syphilis. Elevated granulomatous papules may enlarge to a diameter of 5 cm and then heal, leaving areas of depigmentation. Successive crops of these lesions occur for many months. Histopathology is similar to that observed in syphilis, with minimal vascular changes and no endothelial cell proliferation. The late destructive stage, sometimes called tertiary yaws, involves treponemal infection of the bones and periosteum, especially the long bones of legs and forearms, and the bones of the feet and hands. Pathologic findings are similar to those seen in the tertiary stage of syphilis. Highly destructive gummas also may occur within the bones and soft tissues.

Diagnosis depends on geographic location, clinical manifestations, demonstration of treponemes within exudates, and positive serology. In areas in which syphilis and yaws coexist, definitive diagnosis is unnecessary since both can be readily eradicated by penicillin.

Pinta

Pinta, caused by *T pallidum* subsp *carateum*, is endemic in the tropical areas of Central and South America. Recently, the total number of cases has been estimated at 500,000. Transmission occurs through human-to-human nonsexual contact. Most cases initially occur in children and adolescents.

The primary lesion develops within 2 to 6 months at the site of skin entry as a flat, erythematous papule or group of papules. These lesions and occasional satellite lesions enlarge over several months and produce plaques with scaly surfaces. Secondary lesions occur after 2 to 18 months or longer and involve ulceration and hyperchromic patches. Typically the hands, feet, and scalp are infected. Late stages of pinta involve patches of hyperchromia and achromia, irregular acanthosis, and epidermal atrophy. Lesions heal initially with hyperpigmentation. Then, with scarring, the lesions become depigmented and hyperkeratotic. The treponemes disturb normal melanin pigmentation and produce the characteristic skin manifestations within 2 to 5 years.

The different stages of this disease are not clearly separated, and overlap of manifestations is common. Diagnosis relies on geographic location, clinical manifestations, demonstration of organisms in exudates, and positive serology. Penicillin is the antibiotic of choice. Contrary to syphilis and yaws, in which the lesions heal rapidly following antibiotic treatment, pinta lesions may require 1 year to fully resolve. After primary or early secondary manifestations, skin pigmentation returns to normal. In later manifestations, however, pigmentation remains altered permanently.

Endemic Syphilis

Endemic syphilis, caused by *T pallidum* subsp *endemicum*, is found in the desert areas of the Middle East and Central and South Africa. Transmission is through human-to-human nonsexual contact. Most cases are contracted by children past the age of 2 years. Transmission of endemic syphilis, like that of yaws and pinta, is associated with poor hygiene.

Clinical manifestations can be quite similar to those of syphilis and yaws. The site of entry is usually the mucous membranes of the eyes and mouth. The primary lesion, a small papule, is detectable in only 1 percent of cases. After 2 to 3 months, secondary lesions or plaques develop in mucous membranes, skin, muscles, and bone. These oozing papules erode, harden, become condylomatous, and eventually heal. Clinical manifestations are then not apparent for 5 to 15 years (latency). Late endemic syphilis develops in the skin and skeletal system. Skin lesions may be superficial, nodular, or tuberous, or they may be highly destructive, deep gummas. Destructive bone lesions frequently localize in the tibia.

Diagnosis depends on geographic location, clinical manifestations, treponemes in the exudate, and positive serology. Penicillin eradicates endemic syphilis.

REFERENCES

Crissey JT, Denenholz DA: Syphilis. Clin Dermatol 2:1, 1984

Hovind-Haugen K: Determination by means of electron microscopy of morphological criteria of value for classication of some spirochetes, in particular treponemes. Acta Pathol Microbiol Scand Suppl 255:1, 1976

Johnson RC (ed.): The Biology of Parasitic Spirochetes. Academic Press, San Diego, 1976

Lomholt G: Textbook of Dermatology. Vol. 1. Blackwell Scientific Publications, Oxford, 1972

Miller JN: Value and limitations of non-treponemal and treponemal tests in the laboratory diagnosis of syphilis. Clin Obstet Gynecol 18:191, 1975

Schell RG, Musher DM, (eds): Pathogenesis and Immunology of Treponemal Infection. Marcel Dekker, New York, 1983

US Department of Health, Education, and Welfare: Syphilis: A Synopsis. Public Health Service Publication no. 1660, 1968

Vegas FK: Clinical, Tropical Dermatology. Blackwell Scientific Publications, Oxford, 1985

Wicher K, Wicher V: Experimental syphilis in guinea pig. Crit Rev Microbiol 16:181, 1989

37 MYCOPLASMAS

SHMUEL RAZIN

GENERAL CONCEPTS

Clinical Manifestations

Mycoplasma pneumoniae infection is a disease of the upper and lower respiratory tracts. Cough, fever, and headache may persist for several weeks. Convalescence is slow. *Ureaplasma urealyticum* infection causes nongonococcal urethritis in *men,* resulting in dysuria, urgency, and frequency of urination with urethral discharge.

Structure, Classification, and Antigenic Types

Mycoplasmas are spherical to filamentous cells with no cell walls. There is an attachment organelle at the tip of filamentous *M pneumoniae, M genitalium,* and several other pathogenic mycoplasmas. Fried-egg-shaped colonies are seen on agar. The mycoplasmas presumably evolved by degenerative evolution from Gram-positive bacteria and are most closely related to some clostridia. Mycoplasmas are the smallest self-replicating organisms with the smallest genomes (a total of about 500 to 1,000 genes); they are low in guanine and cytosine. Mycoplasmas are nutritionally very exacting. Many require cholesterol, a unique property among prokaryotes. Ureaplasmas require urea for growth, another unusual property. Mycoplasmas have surface antigens such as membrane proteins, glycolipids, and lipoglycans. Antibodies to these antigens inhibit growth; various serologic tests have been developed and are useful in classification.

Pathogenesis

Mycoplasmas are surface parasites of the human respiratory and urogenital tracts. *Mycoplasma pneumoniae* attaches to sialoglycoprotein or sialoglycolipid receptors on the tracheal epithelium via protein adhesins on the attachment organelle. The major adhesin is a 170-kilodalton (kDa) protein, named P1. Hydrogen peroxide and superoxide radicals (O_2^-) excreted by the attached organisms cause oxidative tissue damage. Pneumonia is induced largely by local immunocyte and phagocytic responses to the parasite. Sequalae of *M Sequalae pneumoniae* infection (mainly hematologic and neurologic) apparently have an autoimmune etiology.

Host Defenses

IgM antibodies, followed by IgG and secretory IgA, are important in *host resistance.* The importance of cell-mediated immunity is unclear.

Epidemiology

Mycoplasma pneumoniae infection is worldwide and more prevalent in colder months. It affects mainly children ages 5 to 9 years. It is spread by close personal contact and has a long incubation period. *Ureaplasma urealyticum* is spread primarily through sexual contact. Women may be asymptomatic reservoirs.

Diagnosis

Culture of *M pneumoniae* from sputum is possible, but very slow. Diagnosis is based on serologic tests of relatively low specificity. Specific diagnostic DNA probes are being developed.

Control

There is no certified vaccine for *M pneumoniae*. Treatment with erythromycin and tetracyclines is effective in reducing symptoms in both *M pneumoniae* and *U urealyticum* infections.

INTRODUCTION

Mycoplasmas are the smallest and simplest self-replicating bacteria. The mycoplasma cell contains a set of organelles minimally essential for growth and replication: a plasma membrane, ribosomes, and a double-stranded DNA molecule (Fig. 37-1). Unlike all other prokaryotes, the mycoplasmas have no cell walls, and they are consequently placed in the separate class Mollicutes (*mollis,* soft; *cutis,* skin).

Mycoplasmas have been nicknamed the "crabgrass" of cell cultures because their infections are persistent, frequently difficult to detect and diagnose, and difficult to cure. Contamination of cell cultures by mycoplasmas presents serious problems in research laboratories and in biotechnological industries using cell cultures. The origin of contaminating mycoplasmas is in components of the cell culture medium, particularly serum, or in the flora of the technician's mouth, spread by droplet infection.

CLINICAL MANIFESTATIONS

Mycoplasmal Pneumonia

The term **primary atypical pneumonia** was coined in the early 1940s to describe pneumonias different from the typical lobar pneumonia caused by pneumococci. Several common respiratory viruses, including influenza virus and adenovirus, were shown to be responsible for a significant number of these pneumonias. From other cases, many of which developed antibodies agglutinating red blood cells in the cold (**cold agglutinins**), an unidentified filterable agent was isolated by Eaton and associates and was called **Eaton agent.** This agent was identified as a new *Mycoplasma* species after its successful cultivation on cell-free media in 1962. Named *Mycoplasma pneumoniae,* it was the first clearly documented mycoplasma pathogenic for humans.

The effects of *M pneumoniae* on humans include subclinical infection, upper respiratory disease, and bronchopneumonia. Most human infections

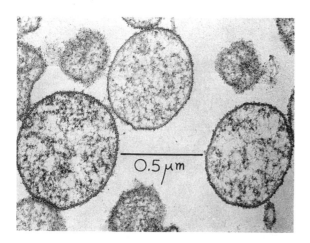

FIGURE 37-1 Electron micrograph of thin-sectioned mycoplasma cells. Cells are bounded by a single membrane showing in section the characteristic trilaminar shape. The cytoplasm contains thin threads representing sectioned chromosome and dark granules representing ribosomes. (Courtesy of RM Cole, Bethesda, MD.)

do not progress to a clinically evident pneumonia. When pneumonia occurs, the onset generally is gradual and the clinical picture is one of a mild to moderately severe illness, with early complaints referable to the lower respiratory passages. Radiography frequently reveals evidence of pneumonia before physical signs are apparent. Involvement is usually limited to one of the lower lobes of the lungs, and the pneumonia is interstitial or bronchopneumonic. The course of the disease varies; remittent fever, cough, and headache persist for several weeks. One of the most consistent clinical features is a long convalescence, which may extend from 4 to 6 weeks. Few fatal cases have been reported. Several unusual complications have been noted, including hemolytic anemia, polyradiculitis, encephalitis, aseptic meningitis, and central nervous system illness such as Guillain-Barré syndrome. In addition, pericarditis and pancreatitis have been observed. These sequelae may be related to the suspected immunopathology of *M pneumoniae* disease (see below).

Nongonococcal Urethritis and Salpingitis

Growing evidence suggests that *Ureaplasma urealyticum* causes **nongonococcal urethritis** in men free of *Chlamydia trachomatis*, an established agent of nongonococcal urethritis. The wide occurrence of *U urealyticum* in sexually active, symptom-free adults hampers research in this field. Evidence is based primarily on the production of nongonococcal urethritis symptoms in ureaplasma-free and chlamydia-free volunteers by intraurethral inoculation of *U urealyticum* and on a report that this disease could be cured in a chlamydia-free man only when he and his partner were treated simultaneously with tetracycline, which eliminated *U urealyticum* from both. Ureaplasmas have also been associated with chorioamnionitis, habitual spontaneous abortion, and low-birth-weight infants. *Mycoplasma hominis*, a common inhabitant of the vagina of healthy women, becomes pathogenic once it invades the internal genital organs, where it may cause pelvic inflammatory diseases such as tuboovarian abscess or salpingitis.

It has been suggested that *Mycoplasma genitalium*, isolated in 1981 from the urethral discharge of two homosexual men, may account for the tetracycline-responsive, nongonococcal urethritis cases in which chlamydias and ureaplasmas cannot be isolated (about 20 percent of all cases). However, the failure to isolate additional *M genitalium* strains from the genital tract and the recent isolation of *M genitalium* from throat specimens of *M pneumoniae* pneumonia patients raise serious doubts about the possible role of *M genitalium* in urogenital disease.

STRUCTURE, CLASSIFICATION, AND ANTIGENIC TYPES
Distinguishing Properties

The coccus is the basic form of all mycoplasma cultures. The diameter of the smallest coccus capable of reproduction is about 300 nm. In most mycoplasma cultures, elongated or filamentous forms (up to 100 μm long and about 0.4 μm thick) also occur. The filaments tend to produce truly branched mycelioid structures, hence the name mycoplasma (*myces*, a fungus; *plasma*, a form). Mycoplasmas reproduce by binary fission, but cytoplasmic division frequently may lag behind genome replication, resulting in formation of multinuclear filaments (Fig. 37-2).

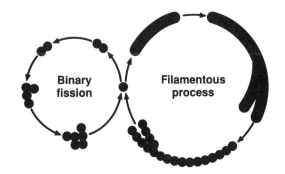

FIGURE 37-2 Schematic presentation of the mode of mycoplasma reproduction. Cells may either divide by binary fission or first elongate to multinucleate filaments, which subsequently break up to coccoid bodies. (From Razin S (ed): Special Issue on *Mycoplasma* Infections. Isr J Med Sci 17:510, 1981, with permission.)

Some mycoplasmas possess unique attachment organelles, which are shaped as a tapered tip in *M pneumoniae* and *M genitalium*. *Mycoplasma pneumoniae* is a pathogen of the respiratory tract, adhering to the respiratory epithelium, primarily through the attachment structure. Interestingly, these two human mycoplasmas exhibit gliding motility on liquid-covered surfaces. The tip structure always leads, again indicating its importance in attachment.

One of the most useful distinguishing features of mycoplasmas is their peculiar fried-egg colony shape, consisting of a central zone of growth embedded in the agar and a peripheral one on the agar surface (Fig. 37-3).

The lack of cell walls and intracytoplasmic membranes facilitates isolation of the mycoplasma membrane in a relatively pure form. The isolated mycoplasma membrane resembles that of other prokaryotes in being composed of approximately two-thirds protein and one-third lipid. The mycoplasma lipids resemble those of other bacteria,

apart from the large quantities of cholesterol in the sterol-requiring mycoplasmas.

Membrane proteins, glycolipids, and lipoglycans exposed on the cell surface are the major antigenic determinants in mycoplasmas. Antisera containing antibodies to these components inhibit growth and metabolism of the mycoplasmas and, in the presence of complement, cause lysis of the organisms. These properties are used in various serologic tests that differentiate between mycoplasma species and serotypes and detect antibodies to mycoplasmas in sera of patients (see below).

Molecular Biology

The mycoplasma genome is typically prokaryotic, consisting of a circular, double-stranded DNA molecule. The *Mycoplasma* and *Ureaplasma* genomes are the smallest recorded for any self-reproducing prokaryote (Table 37-1). Therefore, there are very few genes; the number is estimated at fewer than 500, about one-fifth the number of

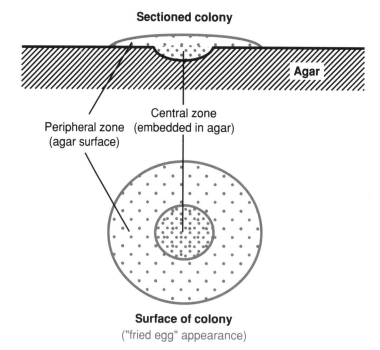

FIGURE 37-3 Morphology of a typical "fried-egg" mycoplasma colony.

TABLE 37-1   Taxonomy and Properties of
Mycoplasmas Capable of Infecting Humans[a]

Genus	Number of Established Species	Genome		Cholesterol Requirement	Distinctive Properties	Hosts
		Size (×10⁸ Da)	G + C Content (mol%)			
Mycoplasma	87	5–10	23–41	+	None	Humans, other animals
Ureaplasma	5	5–8	27–30	+	Urease positive	Humans, other animals

[a] The table includes only *Mycoplasma* and *Ureaplasma*, the mycoplasma genera that contain species capable of infecting humans. The genera *Acholeplasma*, *Anaeroplasma*, *Asteroleplasma*, and *Spiroplasma* contain species infecting only animals, plants, and arthropods.

genes in *Escherichia coli.* Mycoplasmas accordingly express a small number of cell proteins and lack many enzymatic activities and metabolic pathways. Their nutritional requirements are correspondingly complex, and they are dependent on a parasitic mode of life.

The dependence of mycoplasmas on their host for many nutrients explains the great difficulty of cultivation in the laboratory. The complex media for mycoplasma culture contain serum, which provides fatty acids and cholesterol for mycoplasma membrane synthesis. The requirement of most mycoplasmas for cholesterol is unique among prokaryotes. The consensus is that only a small fraction of mycoplasmas existing in nature have been cultivated so far. Despite many efforts, none of the mycoplasma like organisms causing a variety of diseases in plants has been cultivated. Some of the cultivable mycoplasmas, including the human pathogen *M pneumoniae,* grow very slowly, particularly on primary isolation. *Ureaplasma urealyticum,* a pathogen of the human urogenital tract, grows very poorly in vitro, reaching maximal titers of 10^7 organisms/ml of culture. *Mycoplasma genitalium,* apparently another human pathogen, grows so poorly that only a few successful isolations have been achieved.

Glucose and other metabolizable carbohydrates can be used as energy sources by the fermentative mycoplasmas possessing the Embden-Meyerhof-Parnas glycolytic pathway. All mycoplasmas examined thus far possess a truncated, flavin-termi-nated respiratory system, which rules out oxidative phosphorylation as an ATP-generating mechanism. Breakdown of arginine by the arginine dihydrolase pathway has been proposed as the major source of ATP in nonfermentative mycoplasmas. Ureaplasmas have a requirement, unique among living organisms, for urea. Because they are nonglycolytic and lack the arginine dihydrolase pathway, it has been suggested that ATP is generated through an electrochemical gradient produced by ammonia liberated during the intracellular hydrolysis of urea by the organism's urease.

The mycoplasma genome is characterized by a low guanine-plus-cytosine content and by a corresponding preferential utilization of codons containing adenine and uracil. Most interesting is the use of the universal stop codon UGA as a tryptophan codon in mycoplasmas, a rare property found so far only in mycoplasmas and in the mitochondrial DNA. Resistance of mycoplasmal RNA polymerase to rifampin is another property distinguishing mycoplasmas from the conventional eubacteria. However, apart from this resistance to rifampin, the mycoplasmas are susceptible to antibiotics, such as tetracyclines and chloramphenicol, that inhibit protein synthesis on prokaryotic ribosomes.

Phylogeny

As the smallest and simplest self-replicating prokaryotes, the mycoplasmas pose an intriguing question: do they represent the descendants of exceedingly primitive bacteria that existed before the development of a peptidoglycan-based cell wall, or do they represent evolutionary degenerate eubacterial forms that have lost their cell walls? The balance of the molecular evidence, based largely on comparison of base sequences of highly conserved 5S and 16S rRNA molecules, favors the hypothesis of **degenerative evolution.** According to Woese and his colleagues, the mycoplasmas evolved as a branch of the low-guanine-plus-cytosine Grampositive bacteria and are most closely related to two clostridia, *Clostridium innocuum* and *C ramosum.* However, the marked phenotypic and genotypic variability among mycoplasmas has led some workers to conclude that mycoplasmas evolved from a variety of walled bacteria and accordingly have a polyphyletic origin. Woese maintains that the origin of mycoplasmas is monophyletic and explains the great variety of mycoplasmas by a process of rapid evolution characteristic of the group.

PATHOGENESIS

All mycoplasmas cultivated and identified thus far are parasites of humans, animals, plants, or arthropods. The primary habitats of human and animal mycoplasmas are the mucous surfaces of the respiratory and urogenital tracts and the joints in some animals. Although some mycoplasmas belong to the normal flora, most species are pathogens, causing various diseases that tend to run a chronic course (Fig. 37-4).

Most mycoplasmas that infect humans and other animals are surface parasites, adhering to the epithelial linings of the respiratory and urogenital tracts. Adherence is firm enough to prevent the elimination of parasites by mucous secretions or urine. The intimate association between the adhering mycoplasmas and their host cells provides an environment in which local concentrations of toxic metabolites excreted by the parasite build up and cause tissue damage (Fig. 37-5). Moreover, be-

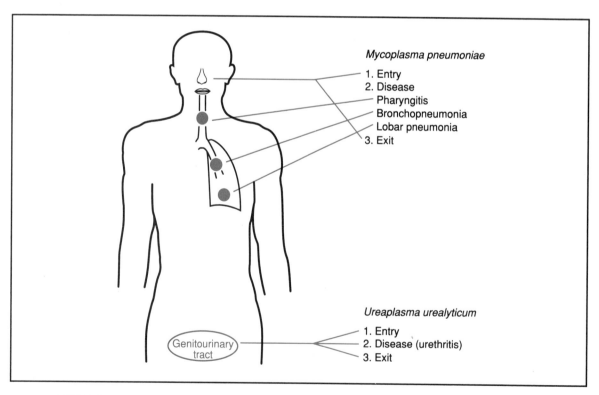

FIGURE 37-4 Pathogenesis and disease sites of infection by *M pneumoniae* and *U urealyticum.*

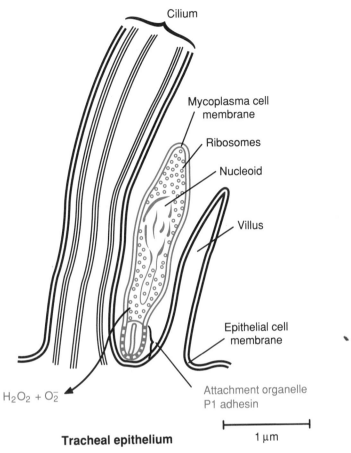

Cilium

Mycoplasma cell membrane

Ribosomes

Nucleoid

Villus

Epithelial cell membrane

Attachment organelle P1 adhesin

$H_2O_2 + O_2^-$

Tracheal epithelium

1 μm

FIGURE 37-5   Schematic presentation of a *M pneumoniae* organism attaching to the surface of the ciliary tracheal epithelium, as seen by electron microscopy of a thin section. The clustering of the P1 adhesin on the surface of the attachment organelle at the tip of the mycoplasma is depicted. The H_2O_2 and O_2^- excreted by the mycoplasma penetrate into the host cell and cause oxidative damage.

cause mycoplasmas lack cell walls, fusion between the membranes of the parasite and host has been suggested, but experimental evidence is insufficient. Several studies suggest that the parasite and host membranes exchange antigenic components, an event that may help the parasite to evade the host immunologic response and perhaps also trigger autoimmune reactions. Because attachment of *M pneumoniae* and *M genitalium* is affected by pretreatment of the host cells with neuraminidase, sialoglycoproteins and/or sialoglycolipids of the host cell membrane appear to be receptor sites for these mycoplasmas. There is evidence that several *M pneumoniae* membrane proteins act as adhesins

and that they have high affinity for the specific receptors for *M pneumoniae* on host cells. Monoclonal antibodies to one of these proteins, protein P1 (molecular weight, 170,000), inhibit attachment of the parasite. Ferritin labeling of the antibodies has shown that P1 concentrates on the tip structure of the mycoplasma, a finding that further supports the theory that the tip serves as an attachment organelle.

The results obtained with *M pneumoniae* were essentially duplicated recently with *M genitalium* and showed that in this organism, which closely resembles *M pneumoniae* morphologically and physiologically, a major adhesin protein, named

MgPa, is clustered at the tip organelle. The genes of the major adhesins of *M pneumoniae* (P1) and of *M genitalium* (MgPa) were recently cloned and sequenced, allowing the characterization of these proteins. The two adhesins are alike in many respects and in fact contain extensive areas of homology, as expressed also by shared epitopes. These two proteins may be the product of an ancestral gene that underwent a horizontal gene transfer event.

The nature of the toxic factors that damage the mucosal surfaces infected by mycoplasmas is still unclear. Toxins are rarely found in mycoplasmas. Consequently, researchers considered whether the end products of mycoplasma metabolism were responsible for tissue damage. Hydrogen peroxide, the end product of respiration in mycoplasmas, has been implicated as a major pathogenic factor ever since it was shown to be responsible for the lysis of erythrocytes by myco-

plasmas in vitro; however, the production of H_2O_2 alone does not determine pathogenicity, as the loss of virulence in *M pneumoniae* is not accompanied by a decrease in H_2O_2 production. For the H_2O_2 to exert its toxic effect, the mycloplasmas must adhere closely enough to the host cells surface to maintain a toxic, steady-state concentration of H_2O_2 sufficient to cause direct damage, such as lipid peroxidation, to the cell membrane. The accumulation of malonyldialdehyde, an oxidation product of membrane lipids, in cells exposed to *M pneumoniae* supports this notion. Moreover, *M pneumoniae* inhibits host cell catalase by excreting superoxide radicals (O_2^-). This would be expected to further increase the accumulation of H_2O_2 at the site of parasite-host cell contact (Fig. 37-6).

There is evidence that both organism-related and host-related factors are involved in the pathogenesis of *M pneumoniae* pneumonia. The host may be largely responsible for the appearance of pneu-

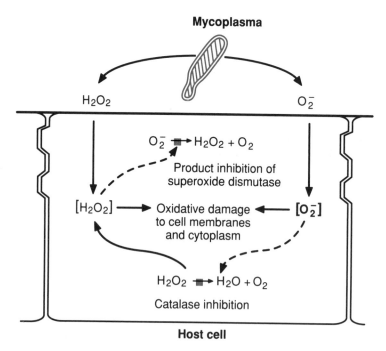

FIGURE 37-6 Proposed mechanism of oxidative damage to host cells by adhering *M pneumoniae* by increasing concentrations of H_2O_2 and O_2^-. (Modified from Almagor M, Kahane I, Yatziv S: Role of superoxide anion in host cell injury induced by *Mycoplasma pneumoniae* infection. J Clin Invest 73:842, 1984, with permission.)

monia by mounting a local immunocytic and phagocytic response to the parasite. Syrian hamsters inoculated intranasally with *M pneumoniae* show patchy bronchopneumonic lesions consisting of infiltration of mononuclear cells. The ablation of thymic function before the experimental infection prevents development of the characteristic pulmonary infiltration, but lengthens the period during which the organisms can be isolated from the lungs. When thymic animals are allowed to recover and then reinfected, an exaggerated and accelerated pneumonic process occurs. Epidemiologic data also suggest that repeated infections in humans are required before symptomatic disease occurs: serum antibodies to *M pneumoniae* can be found in most children 2 to 5 years of age, although the illness occurs with greatest frequency in individuals 5 to 15 years of age.

An immunopathologic mechanism also may explain the complications affecting organs distant from the respiratory tract in some *M pneumoniae* patients. Various autoantibodies have been detected in the sera of many of these patients, including cold agglutinins reacting on the erythrocyte I antigen, antibodies reacting with lymphocytes, smooth muscle antibodies, and antibodies reacting with brain and lung antigens. Serologic cross-reactions between *M pneumoniae* and brain and lung antigens have been demonstrated, and these antigens probably are related to the glycolipids of *M pneumoniae* membranes, which are also found in most plants and in many bacteria. Clearly, host reaction varies markedly, as only about half the patients develop cold agglutinins and complications are rare, even among individuals with antitissue globulins.

HOST DEFENSES

Infection with *M pneumoniae* induces the development of serum antibodies that fix complement, inhibit growth of the organism, and lyse the organism in the presence of complement. Generally, the first antibodies produced are of the IgM class, whereas later in convalescence the predominant antibody is IgG. Secretory IgA antibodies also develop and appear to be important in host resist-

ance. The first infection in infancy usually is asymptomatic and generates a brief serum antibody response. Recurrent infections, which occur at approximately 2- to 4-year intervals, generate a more prolonged systemic antibody response and increasing numbers of circulating antigen-responsive lymphocytes. By late childhood, clinically apparent lower respiratory disease, including pneumonia, becomes more common. Therefore, mycoplasma respiratory disease manifestations appear to vary, depending on the state of local and systemic immunity at the time of reinfection. One hypothesis holds that local immunity mediates resistance to infection and that systemic immunity contributes substantially to the pulmonary and systemic reactions characteristic of *M pneumoniae* pneumonia.

The relative importance of humoral and cell-mediated immunity in resistance to respiratory mycoplasma infections is still unclear. For many mycoplasma infections, such as bovine pleuropneumonia, resistance can be transferred with convalescent-phase serum. Although these results indicate that antibody can mediate resistance to mycoplasma infections of the respiratory tract, this may not be true for all mycoplasma respiratory diseases. For example, resistance of rats to pulmonary disease induced by *M pulmonis* can be transferred only with spleen cells obtained from previously infected animals. Although IgA antibody may be important in upper respiratory tract resistance to mycoplasmas, other factors seem to be involved in resistance to pulmonary disease, and these factors may not be the same for all mycoplasma infections.

EPIDEMIOLOGY

One of the most puzzling features of *M pneumoniae* pneumonia is the age distribution of patients. In a survey conducted between 1964 and 1975 of more than 100,000 individuals in the Seattle area, the age-specific attack rate was highest among 5- to 9-year-old children. Rates of *M pneumoniae* pneumonia in the youngest age group, 0 to 4 years old, were about one-half those in school-age children, but considerably higher than in adults. *Mycoplasma pneumoniae* pneumonia was rarely observed in infants younger than 6 months, suggesting maternally conferred immunity (Fig. 37-7). *Mycoplasma pneumoniae* accounts for 8 to 15 percent of all pneumonias in young school-age children. In older children and young adults, the organism is responsible for approximately 15 to 50 percent of all pneumonias. Infection with *M pneumoniae* is worldwide and endemic; it occurs all year round but shows a predilection for the colder months, apparently because of greater opportunity for transmission by droplet infection. *Mycoplasma pneumoniae* appears to require close personal contact to spread; successful spreading usually occurs in families, schools, and institutions. The incubation period is relatively long, ranging from 2 to 3 weeks.

Ureaplasma urealyticum is spread primarily through sexual contact. Colonization has been linked to the frequency of sexual intercourse and the number of sexual partners. Women may be asymptomatic reservoirs of infection.

DIAGNOSIS

Diagnosis on the basis of microscopy alone is equivocal; therefore, culture is essential for definitive diagnosis.

Culture

A routine mycoplasma medium consists of heart infusion, peptone, yeast extract, salts, glucose or arginine, and horse serum (5 to 20 percent). Fetal or newborn calf serum is preferable to horse serum. To prevent the overgrowth of the fast-growing bacteria that usually accompany mycoplasmas in clinical materials, penicillin, thallium acetate or both are added as selective agents. For *Ureaplasma* culture, the medium is supplemented with urea and its pH is brought to 6.0. *Ureaplasma* and *M genitalium* are relatively sensitive to thallium, which, therefore, is omitted from their culture media. For *M pneumoniae* isolation, nasopharyngeal secretions are inoculated into a selective diphasic medium (pH 7.8) made of mycoplasma broth and agar and supplemented with glucose and phenol red. When *M pneumoniae* grows in this medium, it produces acid, causing the color of the medium to change from purple to yellow. Broth from the diphasic medium is subcultured to mycoplasma agar when a color change occurs, or at weekly intervals for a minimum of 8 weeks.

Identification

Colonies appearing on the plates can be identified as *M pneumoniae* by staining directly on agar with

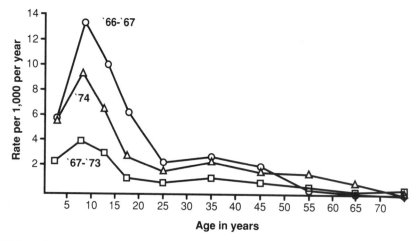

FIGURE 37-7   Incidence of *M pneumoniae* pneumonia in Seattle by age, for two epidemics (1966–67 and 1974) and the endemic periods (1967–73). (From Foy HM, Kenny GE, Cooney MK, Allan ID: Long-term epidemiology of infections with *Mycoplasma* pneumonia. J Infect Dis 139:681, 1979, with permission.)

homologous fluorescein-conjugated antibody or by demonstrating that a specific antiserum to *M pneumoniae* inhibits their growth on agar. Colonies of ureaplasmas are usually minute (less than 100 μm in diameter); because of urea hydrolysis and ammonia liberation, the medium becomes alkaline. When manganous sulfate is added to the medium, the *Ureaplasma* colonies stain dark brown. Isolates can be characterized in more detail by a variety of routine biochemical and serologic tests, supplemented when required by more sophisticated tests, including electrophoretic analysis of cell proteins, crossed immunoelectrophoresis of cell proteins, DNA hybridization tests, and DNA cleavage pattern evaluations by use of restriction endonucleases.

Serodiagnosis

Serodiagnosis consists of examining serum samples for antibodies that inhibit the growth and metabolism of the organism or fix complement with mycoplasmal antigens. Antibody response in mycoplasmal pneumonia is most easily demonstrated by complement fixation, reacting acute- and convalescent-phase sera with intact organisms or their lipid extract as antigen. A fourfold or greater antibody rise is considered indicative of recent infection, whereas a sustained high antibody titer may not be significant, because a relatively high level of antibody may persist for at least 1 year after infection. The cold agglutinin test is less useful because only about one-half of patients develop cold agglutinins and because these antibodies also are induced by a great many other conditions. Serologic tests employing as antigens the purified adhesin P1 or synthetic oligopeptides representing the N terminus of this molecule are much more specific, but these antigens are not commercially available and, in addition, have epitopes in common with the *M genitalium* adhesin MgPa.

Present techniques for laboratory diagnosis of *M pneumoniae* infections are of little use to the clinician because recovery and identification of the mycoplasmas take at least 1 to 2 weeks. Methods for rapid laboratory diagnosis, such as direct demonstration of organisms in the sputum by immunofluorescence, electron microscopy, or enzyme-linked immunosorbent assay (ELISA) are at various stages of development. Most promising is the new approach based on the use of specific DNA probes. The probes consist of species-specific DNA fragments selected from genomic libraries of the organisms. Dot-blot hybridization with the probes can detect as few as 10^4 organisms. Diagnostic kits containing specific DNA probes for *M pneumoniae* and *M genitalium* are now at the stage of clinical evaluation. Once introduced commercially, the DNA probes are expected to overcome the difficulties encountered in cultivation and serodiagnosis of infections by the two mycoplasmas.

CONTROL

Prevention

Chemoprophylaxis of mycoplasma infections is not recommended because it does not cure the infection, although it may modify the secondary cases to subclinical disease. Attempts at control by immunoprophylaxis fail in most cases. Prior natural infection appears to provide the most effective resistance; however, evidence shows that *M pneumoniae* infections recur at intervals of several years. These observations suggest that immunity to a single natural infection is relatively short-term, particularly in children, and it may be unrealistic to expect more, or even as much, from artificially induced immunity.

Attenuation of mycoplasma strains tends to reduce virulence and immunogenicity. In most cases, attenuated viable vaccines do not reach the level of protective efficiency required from a commercial vaccine. Killed *M pneumoniae* vaccines administered intranasally to hamsters are relatively ineffective unless boosted by parenteral inoculation of vaccine. Intranasal immunization may be ineffective because the antigenic mass is not retained for a sufficient period in the lungs. On the other hand, parenteral killed vaccines, particularly if combined with adjuvant, do produce adequate protection in terms of reducing pneumonia, although there is only a minimal effect on the number of organisms growing in the lungs. A similar protective effect can be achieved briefly by inoculation with hyperimmune serum. In summary, a single dose of vaccine in a form suitable for clinical use is unlikely to produce lasting immunity to mycoplasma infection. Stimulation of systemic antibodies may prevent the clinical manifestations of pneumonia, but additional local stimulation with live or killed organisms may be necessary to evoke resistance to colonization.

An approach worth pursuing is the preparation of vaccines made of antigenic components specifically related to the mycoplasma-host cell interaction, such as components of the mycoplasma membrane responsible for attachment of the parasites to the epithelial cell surface. Guinea pigs preimmunized with purified P1 adhesin protein and subsequently infected with *M pneumoniae* showed increased *M pneumoniae*-specific IgG, IgA, and adherence-inhibiting antibodies. However, these animals developed severe lung lesions on challenge, suggesting that it may well be harmful to vaccinate the host with the P1 protein, as it may sensitize the host so that subsequent infection will potentiate host response and lead to a more severe disease.

Treatment

The mycoplasmas are sensitive to most broad-spectrum antibiotics, such as tetracyclines and chloramphenicol, but are resistant to antibiotics that specifically inhibit bacterial cell wall synthesis. Tetracycline combined with erythromycin therapy reduces the duration of fever and pulmonary infiltration in *M pneumoniae* patients. Effective treatment of the symptoms, however, usually is not accompanied by eradication of the organism from the infected host. To prevent recurrence of non-gonococcal urethritis caused by *U urealyticum,* sexual partners should be treated simultaneously with tetracycline. Tetracycline-resistant strains of *U urealyticum* and *M hominis* were recently shown to harbor the tetracycline resistance element *tetM* integrated into their chromosome. The resistance factor could be transferred from other tetracycline-resistant bacteria by a process resembling conjugation.

REFERENCES

Baseman JB, Dallo SF, Tully JG, Rose DL: Isolation and characterization of *Mycoplasma genitalium* strains from the human respiratory tract. J Clin Microbiol 26:2266, 1988

Bernet C, Garret M, De Barbeyrac B et al: Detection of *Mycoplasma pneumoniae* by using the polymerase chain reaction. J Clin Microbiol 27:2492, 1989

Dallo SF, Chavoya A, Su CJ, Baseman JB: DNA and protein sequence homologies between the adhesins of *Mycoplasma genitalium* and *Mycoplasma pneumoniae.* Infect Immun 57:1059, 1989

Hyman HC, Yogev D, Razin S: DNA probes for detection and identification of *Mycoplasma pneumoniae* and *Mycoplasma genitalium.* J Clin Microbiol 25:726, 1987

Razin S: Molecular biology and genetics of mycoplasmas *(Mollicutes).* Microbiol Rev 49:419, 1985

Razin S, Barile MF (eds): Mycoplasma Pathogenicity. In: The Mycoplasmas. Vol. 4. Academic Press, San Diego, 1985

Razin S, Yogev D: Molecular approaches to characterization of mycoplasmal adhesins. p. 52. In Switalski L, Hook M, Beachy E (eds): Molecular Mechanisms of Microbial Adhesion. Springer-Verlag, New York, 1989

Woese C: Bacterial evolution. Microbiol Rev 51:221, 1987

38

RICKETTSIAE

DAVID H. WALKER

GENERAL CONCEPTS

Rickettsiae

The rickettsiae are a diverse collection of obligate intracellular Gram-negative bacteria found in ticks, lice, fleas, mites, chiggers, and mammals. They include the genera *Rickettsia, Ehrlichia, Coxiella,* and *Rochalimaea.* These zoonotic pathogens cause infections that disseminate in the blood to many organs.

RICKETTSIA

Clinical Manifestations

Rickettsia species cause Rocky Mountain spotted fever, rickettsialpox, other spotted fevers, epidemic typhus, murine typhus, and scrub typhus. Patients present with febrile exanthems and visceral involvement; symptoms may include nausea, vomiting, abdominal pain, encephalitis, hypotension, acute renal failure, and respiratory distress.

Structure, Classification, and Antigenic Types

Rickettsia species are small, Gram-negative bacilli that are obligate intracellular parasites of eukaryotic cells. This genus consists of three antigenically defined groups: spotted fever group, typhus group, and scrub typhus group. The first two groups are related; scrub typhus rickettsiae differ in lacking lipopolysaccharide, peptidoglycan, and a slime layer.

Pathogenesis

Rickettsia species are transmitted by the bite of infected ticks, mites, or chiggers or by the feces of infected lice or fleas. From the portal of entry in the skin, *Rickettsia* species spread via the bloodstream to infect the endothelium and sometimes the vascular smooth muscle cells. *Rickettsia* species enter their target cells, multiply by binary fission in the cytosol, and damage heavily parasitized cells directly.

Host Defenses

T-lymphocyte-mediated immune mechanisms and lymphokines, including gamma interferon, play a more important role than antibodies.

Epidemiology

The geographic distribution of these zoonoses is determined by that of the infected arthropod, which for most rickettsial species is the reservoir host.

Diagnosis

Rickettsioses are difficult to diagnose both clinically and in the laboratory. Cultivation requires viable eukaryotic host cells, such as antibiotic-free cell cultures, embryonated eggs, and susceptible animals. Confirmation of the diagnosis requires comparison of acute- and convalescent-phase serum antibody titers.

517

Control

Rickettsia species are susceptible to the broad-spectrum antibiotics, doxycycline, tetracycline, and chloramphenicol. Prevention of exposure to infected arthropods offers some protection. A vaccine exists for epidemic typhus but is not readily available.

EHRLICHIA

Clinical Manifestations

Ehrlichia species cause ehrlichioses that vary in severity from a life-threatening febrile disease that resembles Rocky Mountain spotted fever, except for less frequent rash, to an infectious mononucleosis-like syndrome.

Classification and Antigenic Types

Ehrlichia sennetsu, E canis, and other ehrlichiae of veterinary importance share some antigens.

Pathogenesis

Although the reservoir of ehrilichiae is unknown, it is presumed that ticks or other arthropods bite human skin and inoculate organisms, which then spread by the bloodstream. Lymphocytes, macrophages, and other leukocytes have cytoplasmic vacuoles that contain ehrlichiae dividing by binary fission.

Host Defenses

Host defenses are unknown.

Epidemiology

Sennetsu ehrlichiosis has been documented in Japan. Human infections with *E canis*-like organisms have been found recently; these originate in most of the Atlantic, southeastern, and south central states from New Jersey to Texas.

Diagnosis

Clinical and laboratory clues must be confirmed serologically.

COXIELLA

Clinical Manifestations

Coxiella burnetii causes Q fever, which may present as an acute febrile illness with pneumonia or as a chronic infection with endocarditis.

Structure, Classification, and Antigenic Types

Coxiella burnetii varies in size and may have an endospor-elike form. This species has lipopolysaccharide types and phage types that correlate with pathogenicity.

Pathogenesis

Coxiella burnetii organisms are transmitted to the human lungs by aerosol from heavily infected placentas of sheep an other mammals and disseminate in the bloodstream to the liver and bone marrow, where they are phagocytosed by macrophages. Growth within phagolysosomes is followed by formation of T-lymphocyte-mediated granulomas. In the few patients who develop serious chronic Q-fever, heart valves contain organisms within macrophages.

Host Defenses

Host defense depends on T lymphocytes and gamma interferon.

Epidemiology

Q fever is found worldwide. It is associated mainly with exposure to infected placentas and birth fluids of sheep and other mammals.

Diagnosis

The disease is difficult to diagnose clinically, and cultivation poses a biohazard. Therefore, serology is the mainstay of laboratory diagnosis.

Control

Antibiotics are effective against acute Q fever. A vaccine containing killed phase I organism shows promise in protecting against infection.

ROCHALIMAEA

Rochalimaea quintana, the agent of trench fever, is the only rickettsial agent that can be cultured outside of eukaryotic cells. It is transmitted to humans via lice. Trench fever was a significant medical problem during World War I.

INTRODUCTION

Rickettsiae are small, Gram-negative bacilli that have evolved in such close association with arthropod hosts that they are adapted to survive within the host cells. They represent a rather diverse collection of bacteria, and so listing characters that apply to the entire group is difficult. The common threads that hold the rickettsiae into a group are their epidemiology, their obligate intracellular lifestyle, and the laboratory technology required to work with them. In the laboratory, rickettsiae cannot be cultivated on agar plates or in broth, but only in viable eukaryotic host cells (e.g., in cell culture, embryonated eggs, or susceptible animals). The exception, which shows the artificial nature of using obligate intracellular parasitism as a defining phenotypic characteristic, is *Rochalimaea quintana*, which is cultivable axenically, yet remains classified in the family Rickettsiaceae. The diversity of rickettsiae is demonstrated in the variety of specific intracellular locations where they live and the remarkable differences in their major outer membrane proteins and guanine-plus-cytosine content (Table 38-1). An example of extreme adaptation is that the metabolic activity of *Coxiella burnetii* is greatly increased in the acidic environment of the phagolysosome, which is a harsh location for survival for most other organisms. Obligate intracellular parasitism among bacteria is not unique to rickettsiae. Chlamydiae also have evolved to occupy an intracellular niche, and numerous bacteria (e.g., *Legionella*, *Salmonella*, *Shigella*, and *Brucella*) are facultative intracellular parasites. In contrast with chlamydiae, all rickettsiae can synthesize ATP. *Coxiella burnetii* is the only rickettsia that has a developmental cycle.

Some organisms in the family *Rickettsiaceae* are closely related genetically (e.g., *Rickettsia rickettsii*, *R prowazekii*, *R typhi*, and *Rochalimaea quintana*); others are related remotely (e.g., *Rickettsia* and *Ehrlichia*); and others not related (e.g., *C burnetii* and *Rickettsia* species). The phenotypic traits of the medically important organism *Rickettsia tsutsugamushi* suggest that the species may be an example of convergent evolution in a similar ecologic niche by organisms possibly unrelated to other *Rickettsia* species.

Rickettsioses are zoonoses. Except for Q fever, most are usually transmitted to humans by arthropods (tick, mite, flea, louse, or chigger) (Table 38-2). Therefore, their geographic distribution is determined by that of the infected arthropod, which for most rickettsial species is the reservoir host. Rickettsiae are important causes of human diseases in the United States (Rocky Mountain spotted fever, Q fever, murine typhus, sylvatic typhus, ehrlichiosis, and rickettsialpox) and around the world (Q fever, murine typhus, scrub typhus, epidemic typhus, boutonneuse fever, and other spotted fevers) (Table 38-2).

RICKETTSIAE OF THE SPOTTED FEVER AND TYPHUS GROUPS

The rickettsial diseases are arranged into several major categories (Table 38-2), the first two of which are the spotted fever and typhus fever groups.

CLINICAL MANIFESTATIONS

Rocky Mountain Spotted Fever

Rocky Mountain spotted fever is among the most severe of human infectious diseases, with a mortality of 20 to 25 percent unless treated with appropriate antibiotics. The severity and mortality are greater for men, elderly persons, and black men with glucose-6-phosphate dehydrogenase deficiency. Although, in theory, the disease is always curable by early, appropriate treatment, the case fatality rate is still 4 percent. The incidence of disease parallels the geographic distribution of infected *Dermacentor variabilis* ticks in the eastern United States and *D andersoni* in the Rocky Mountain states, where the infection was first recognized. Rocky Mountain spotted fever was subsequently recognized in the eastern United States. The incidence has declined in the Rocky Mountain

TABLE 38-1 Properties of Selected
Rickettsial Organisms

Species	Cellular Location	Developmental Cycle	Axenic Cultivation	Lipopolysaccharide	Major Outer Membrane Proteins (kDa)	Percent G + C Content
Rickettsia rickettsii	Endothelial and smooth muscle cytosol and nucleus	No	No	Yes	155, 120	33
Rickettsia prowazekii	Endothelial cytosol	No	No	Yes	120	29
Rickettsia tsutsugamushi	Cytosol, rarely nucleus	No	No	No	70, 54–56, 46–47	Unknown
Ehrlichia sennetsu	Leukocytic cytoplasmic membrane-bound vacuole	No	No	Unknown	58, 30	Unknown
Coxiella burnetii	Macrophage phagolysosome	Yes	No	Yes	60, 28	39
Rochalimaea quintana	Extracellular, attached to louse gut epithelium	No	Yes	Yes	Unknown	43

TABLE 38-2 Distinguishing Characteristics of Rickettsial Diseases

Disease	Organism	Geographic Distribution	Ecologic Niche	Transmission to Humans	Pathologic Basis (Injury)	Rash	Eschar	Serologic Diagnosis
Rickettsia								
Spotted fever group								
Rocky Mountain spotted fever	*R rickettsii*	North, Central, and South America	Ticks	Tick bite	Microvascular	90%	Rare	IFA, LA, IHA, EIA, CF
Boutonneuse fever	*R conorii*	Mediterranean Basin, Africa, Indian subcontinent	Ticks	Tick bite	Microvascular	97%	50%	IFA, LA, CF
Rickettsialpox	*R akari*	North America, USSR, Korea	Mites	Mite bite	Microvascular	100%	92%	IFA, CF
North Asian tick typhus	*R sibirica*	USSR, China, Mongolia, Pakistan	Ticks	Tick bite	Microvascular	100%	77%	IFA, CF
Queensland tick typhus	*R australis*	Australia	Ticks	Tick bite	Microvascular	92%	75%	CF
Oriental spotted fever	*R japonica*	Japan	Unknown	Arthropod bite	Microvascular	100%	48%	IFA, CF
Typhus group								
Epidemic typhus	*R prowazekii*	Africa, South America, Mexico, Asia, eastern United States	Louse	Louse feces	Microvascular	100%	None	IFA, IHA, EIA, CF
Murine typhus	*R typhi*	Worldwide	Fleas	Flea feces	Microvascular	80%	None	IFA, IHA, EIA, LA, CF
Scrub typhus group								
Scrub typhus	*R tsutsugamushi*	Asia, south Pacific, Australia	Chiggers	Chigger bite	Microvascular	50%	35%	IFA, EIA
Ehrlichia								
Sennetsu rickettsiosis	*E sennetsu*	Japan	Unknown	Unknown	Lymphoid hyperplasia	Very rare	None	IFA, CF
Human ehrlichiosis	*E canis*-like	North America	Unknown	Tick bite	Perivasculitis, granulomas	40%	None	IFA
Coxiella								
Q fever	*C burnetii*	Worldwide	Ticks, ungulates	Aerosol from infected placenta of sheep, goats, cattle	Pneumonia, granulomas of liver and bone marrow, chronic endocarditis	Rare	None	IFA, EIA, CF
Rochalimaea								
Trench fever	*R quintana*	North America, Europe, Africa	Humans	Louse bite and feces	Perivasculitis	Yes	None	IHA, EIA, CF

a IFA, Indirect fluorescent antibody test; IHA, indirect hemagglutination test; CF, complement fixation test; LA, latex agglutination test; EIA, enzyme immunoassay.

states and increased dramatically in the southeastern United States and Oklahoma. Currently most cases actually occur in the Atlantic states from Maryland to Georgia, as well as in Oklahoma, Missouri, Kansas, Ohio, Tennessee, Arkansas, and Texas, although cases are reported in nearly every state. In the southeastern states, the disease occurs during the seasonal activity of *D variabilis* ticks (April through September) and affects children more frequently than adults. Significant changes in incidence do occur. From a low of 199 cases reported in 1959, the annual number of cases rose steadily to a peak of 1,192 cases in 1981, with a subsequent decline to 700 cases in 1985. The reasons for these fluctuations are unclear.

The rickettsiae are maintained in nature principally by transovarial transmission from infected female ticks to infected ova that hatch into infected larval offspring (Fig. 38-1). A low rate of acquisition

of rickettsiae by uninfected ticks occurs when the ticks feed upon small mammals with enough rickettsiae in their blood to establish tick infection. This effect replenishes lines of infected ticks that are occasionally killed by massive rickettsial overgrowth. A recently observed factor of potential importance in this balance of nature is the interference phenomenon, by which infection of ticks with nonpathogenic spotted fever group rickettsiae prevents the establishment of infection by *R rickettsii*.

The clinical gravity of Rocky Mountain spotted fever is due to severe damage to blood vessels by *R rickettsii*. This organism is unusual among rickettsiae in its ability to spread and invade vascular smooth muscle cells as well as endothelium. Damage to the blood vessels in the skin in locations of the rash leads to visible hemorrhages in half the infected persons (Fig. 38-2). Attempted plugging of vascular wall destruction consumes platelets,

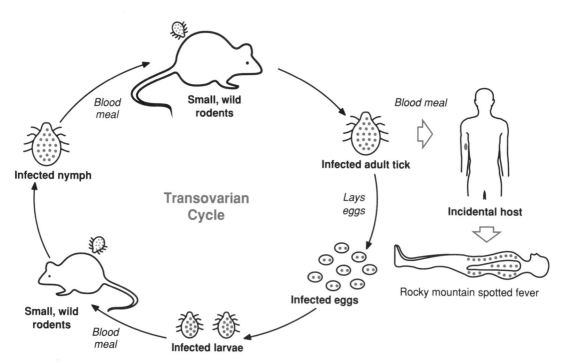

FIGURE 38-1 Transovarian passage of *R rickettsii* in the tick vector is an important cycle in maintaining the infection in nature from one generation of tick to another. Horizontal transmission (i.e., acquisition of the bacteria by uninfected ticks feeding on infected animals) occurs less often and is not shown. Humans become incidental hosts after being bitten by an infected adult tick.

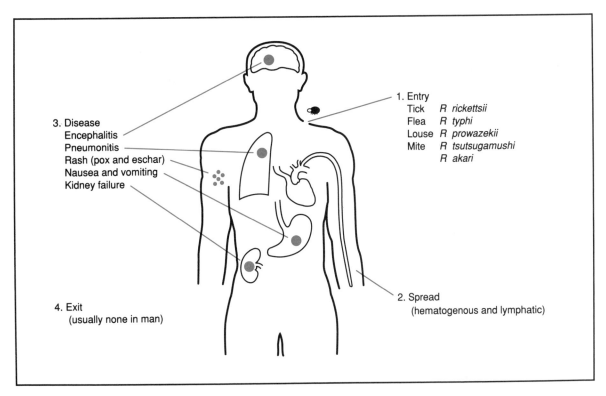

FIGURE 38-2   Common clinical manifestations of the rickettsial diseases.

with consequent thrombocytopenia also affecting approximately half of the patients.

Rickettsialpox and Other Spotted Fevers

In the late 1940s an epidemic of disease characterized by fever, rash, and cutaneous necrosis appeared in one area of New York City. The etiology was traced to *R akari* transmitted by the bite of mites *(Liponyssus sanguineus)* that infested the numerous mice in an apartment house in this area. The disease was named **rickettsialpox** because many patients had blisterlike rashes resembling those of chickenpox. Epidemics were diagnosed in other cities, and *R akari* has been isolated in other countries (e.g., the USSR). Perhaps because this nonfatal disease is seldom considered by physicians, or its incidence is truly low, the diagnosis is rarely made. Transovarial transmission in the mite and periodic documentation of cases assure us that the etiologic agent is still with us.

Boutonneuse fever, so called because of the buttonlike appearance of the papular rash in some cases, has many synonyms, reflecting different geographic regions of occurrence (e.g., Mediterranean spotted fever, Kenya tick typhus, and South African tick bite fever). Cases are observed in the United States in travelers returning from endemic areas. The agent, *R conorii,* is closely related to *R rickettsii.* Severe disease resembling Rocky Mountain spotted fever can cause death in high-risk groups (e.g., elderly, alcoholic, and glucose-6-phosphate dehydrogenase-deficient patients). Cutaneous necrosis caused by rickettsial vascular infection at the tick bite site of inoculation, known as an **eschar** or **tache noire,** is observed in only half the patients with boutonneuse fever. The curiously high prevalence of antibodies reactive with *R conorii* in healthy populations in endemic regions might be explained by missed diagnosis of prior illness, subclinical infection, infection with an antigenically related but less pathogenic rickettsia, or nonspecificity of the laboratory test.

Other spotted fevers occur in geographic distributions of little concern to many physicians in the United States. North Asian tick typhus caused by *R sibirica,* Queensland tick typhus caused by *R australis,* and the recently discovered oriental spotted fever caused by *R japonica* demonstrate that spotted fever group rickettsiae occur worldwide.

Epidemic Typhus and Brill-Zinsser Disease

Epidemics of louse-borne **typhus fever** have had important effects on the course of history; for example, typhus in one army but not in the opposing force has determined the outcome of wars. Populations have been decimated by epidemic typhus. During and immediately after World War I, 30 million cases occurred, with 3 million deaths. Unsanitary, crowded conditions in the wake of war, famine, flood, and other disasters and in poor countries today encourage human louse infestation and transmission of *R prowazekii.* Epidemics usually occur in cold months in poor highland areas, such as the Andes, Himalayas, Mexico, Central America, and Africa. Lice live in clothing, attach to the human host several times daily to take a blood meal, and become infected with *R prowazekii* if the host has rickettsiae circulating in the blood. If the infected louse infests another person, rickettsiae are deposited on the skin via the louse feces or in the crushed body of a louse. Scratching inoculates rickettsiae into the skin.

Between epidemics *R prowazekii* persists as a latent human infection. Years later, when immunity is diminished, some persons suffer recrudescent typhus fever **(Brill-Zinsser disease).** These milder sporadic cases can ignite further epidemics in a susceptible louse-infested population. In the United States Brill-Zinsser disease is seen in immigrants who suffered typhus fever before entering the country. In the eastern United States, sporadic human cases of *R prowazekii* infection have been traced to a zoonotic cycle involving flying squirrels and their own species of lice and fleas.

Murine Typhus

Murine typhus is prevalent throughout the world, particularly in ports, countries with warm climates, and other locations where rat populations are high. *Rickettsia typhi* is associated with rats and fleas, particularly the oriental rat flea, although other ecologic cycles (e.g., opossums and cat fleas) have been implicated. Fleas are infected by transovarian transmission or by feeding on an animal with rickettsiae circulating in the blood. Rickettsiae are shed from fleas in the feces, from which humans acquire the infection through the skin, respiratory tract, or conjunctiva. During the 1940s more than 4,000 cases of murine typhus occurred annually in the United States. The incidence declined coincident with increased utilization of the insecticide DDT. Although the infection and clinical involvement affects the brain, lungs, and other visceral organs in addition to the skin, mortality in humans is less than 1 percent.

STRUCTURE, CLASSIFICATION, AND ANTIGENIC TYPES

Rickettsia species include two antigenically defined groups that are closely related genetically but differ in their surface-exposed protein and lipopolysaccharide antigens. These are the spotted fever and typhus groups. The organisms in these groups are smaller (0.3 μm by 1.0 μm) than most Gram-negative bacilli that live in the extracellular environment (Fig. 38-3). They are surrounded by a poorly characterized structure that is observed as an electron-lucent zone by transmission electron microscopy and is considered to represent a polysaccharide-rich slime layer or capsule. The cell wall contains lipopolysaccharides, a major component that differ antigenically between the typhus group and the spotted fever group. These rickettsiae also contain major outer membrane proteins with both cross-reactive antigens and surface-exposed epitopes that are species specific and easily denatured by temperatures above 54°C. The major outer membrane protein of typhus group rickettsiae has an apparent molecular mass of 120,000 Da. Spotted fever group rickettsiae generally have a pair of analogous proteins with apparent molecular masses characteristic of each species. *Rickettsia prowazekii* has a transport mechanism that exchanges ATP for ADP in its environment, thus providing a means to usurp host cell energy sources under favorable circumstances. Rickett-

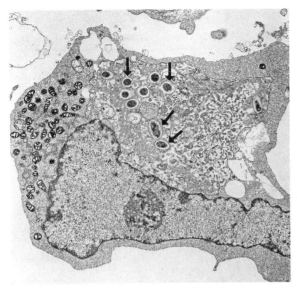

FIGURE 38-3 Electron micrograph showing *R rickettsii* (arrows) localized in the cytoplasm of a human vascular endothelial cell. (Courtesy of David J. Silverman, Ph.D., University of Maryland School of Medicine, College Park, MD.)

siae also are able to synthesize ATP via metabolism of glutamate. Adaptation to the intracellular environment is further evidenced in a variety of transport mechanisms to obtain crucial substances such as particular amino acids from cytoplasmic pools in the host cell. These adaptations and the presence of numerous independent metabolic activities demonstrate that rickettsiae are not degenerate forms of bacteria, but, rather, have evolved successfully for survival with an intracellular lifestyle.

PATHOGENESIS

Rickettsiae are transmitted to humans by the bite of infected ticks and mites and by the feces of infected lice and fleas. They enter via the skin and spread through the bloodstream to infect vascular endothelium in the skin, brain, lungs, heart, kidneys, liver, gastrointestinal tract, and other organs (Fig. 38-1). Rickettsial attachment to the endothelial cell membrane induces phagocytosis, soon followed by escape from the phagosome into the cytosol (Fig. 38-4). Rickettsiae divide inside the cell. *Rickettsia prowazekii* remains inside the apparently

healthy host cell until massive quantities of intracellular rickettsiae accumulate and the host cell bursts, releasing the organisms. In contrast, *R rickettsii* leaves the host cell via long, thin cell projections (**filopodia**) after a few cycles of binary fission. Hence, relatively few *R rickettsii* organisms accumulate inside any particular cell, and rickettsial infection spreads rapidly to involve many other cells. Perhaps because of the numerous times the host cell membrane is traversed, there is an influx of water that is initially sequestered in cisternae of cytopathically dilated rough endoplasmic reticulum in the cells more heavily infected with *R rickettsii*.

The bursting of endothelial cells infected with *R prowazekii* is a dramatic pathologic event. The mechanism is unclear, although phospholipase activity, possibly of rickettsial origin, has been suggested. Injury to endothelium and vascular smooth muscle cells infected by *R rickettsii* seems to be caused directly by the rickettsiae, possibly through the activity of a rickettsial phospholipase or rickettsial protease or through free-radical peroxidation of host cell membranes. Host immune, inflammatory, and coagulation systems are activated and appear to benefit the patient. Rickettsial lipopolysaccharide is biologically relatively nontoxic and does not appear to cause the pathogenic effects of these rickettsial diseases.

The pathologic effects of these rickettsial diseases originate from the multifocal areas of endothelial injury with loss of intravascular fluid into tissue spaces (**edema**), resultant low blood volume, reduced perfusion of the organs, and disordered function of the tissues with damaged blood vessels (e.g., encephalitis, pneumonitis, and hemorrhagic rash).

DIAGNOSIS

Diagnosis of rickettsial infections is often difficult. The clinical signs and symptoms (e.g., fever, headache, nausea, vomiting, and muscle aches) resemble many other diseases during the early stages when antibiotic treatment is most effective. A history of exposure to the appropriate vector tick, louse, flea, or mite is helpful but cannot be relied upon. Observation of a rash, which usually appears

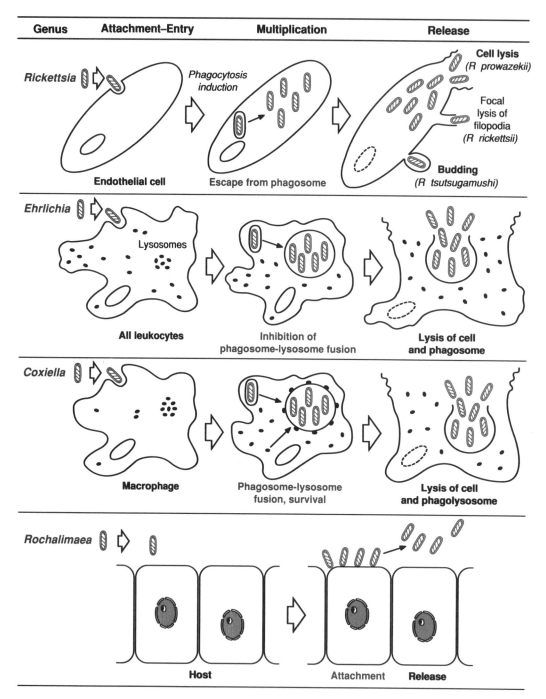

FIGURE 38-4   Pathogenesis of the rickettsial agents illustrating unique aspects of their interactions with eukaryotic cells.

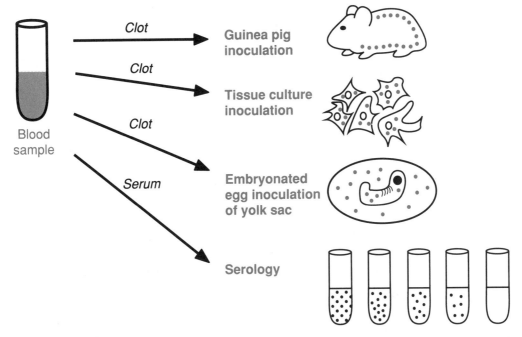

FIGURE 38-5 Laboratory methods used in confirming a diagnosis of rickettsial infection. These bacteria can be cultivated as indicated, but use of serology is more common.

on or after day 3 of illness, should suggest the possibility of a rickettsial infection but, of course, may occur in many other diseases also. Knowledge of the seasonal and geographic epidemiology of rickettsioses is useful, but is inconclusive for the individual patient. Except for epidemic louse-borne typhus, rickettsial diseases strike mostly as isolated single cases in any particular neighborhood. Therefore, clinico-epidemiologic diagnosis is ultimately a matter of suspicion, empirical treatment, and later laboratory confirmation of the specific diagnosis.

Because rickettsiae are both fastidious and hazardous, few laboratories undertake their isolation and diagnostic identification (Fig. 38-5). Some laboratories are able to identify rickettsiae by immunohistology in skin biopsies as a timely, acute diagnostic procedure, but to establish the diagnosis physicians usually rely on serologic demonstration of the development of antibodies to rickettsial antigens in serum collected after the patient has recovered. Currently, assays that demonstrate antibodies to rickettsial antigens themselves (e.g., the

indirect fluorescence antibody test or latex agglutination) are preferable to the nonspecific, insensitive Weil-Felix test that is based on the cross-reactive antigens of OX-19 and OX-2 strains of *Proteus vulgaris*.

CONTROL

Although early treatment with doxycycline, tetracycline, or chloramphenicol is effective in controlling the infection in the individual patient, this action has no effect on rickettsiae in their natural ecologic niches (e.g., ticks). Human infections are prevented by control of the vector and reservoir hosts. Massive delousing with insecticide can abort an epidemic of typhus fever. Prevention of attachment of ticks and their removal before they have injected rickettsiae into the skin reduces the likelihood of a tick-borne spotted fever. Control of rodent populations and of the access of rats and mice to homes and other buildings may reduce human exposure to *R typhi* and *R akari*.

Vaccines against spotted fever and typhus group

rickettsiae have been developed empirically by propagation of rickettsiae in ticks, lice, embryonated hen eggs, and cell culture. Vaccines containing killed organisms have provided incomplete protection. A live attenuated vaccine against epidemic typhus has proved successful, but is accompanied by a substantial incidence of side effects, including a mild form of typhus fever in some persons. The presence of strong immunity in convalescent subjects indicates that vaccine development is feasible, but it requires further study of rickettsial antigens and the effective antirickettsial immune response. T-lymphocyte-mediated immune mechanisms, including effects of the lymphokine gamma interferon, seem most important.

◁ SCRUB TYPHUS ▷
RICKETTSIA GROUP

Although the agents of **scrub typhus** bear a single taxonomic name, *Rickettsia tsutsugamushi*, these interrelated organisms are quite heterogeneous and differ strikingly from other *Rickettsia* species.

CLINICAL MANIFESTATIONS

Patients with scrub typhus often have only fever, headache, and swollen lymph nodes and in some cases myalgia, gastrointestinal complaints, or cough beginning 6 to 21 days following exposure to the vector. Fewer than half of patients have an eschar at the site where the larval mite fed and the classic rash. The mortality varies but averages 7 percent without antirickettsial treatment.

STRUCTURE, CLASSIFICATION, AND ANTIGENIC TYPES

Rickettsia tsutsugamushi is very labile rickettsia that is particularly difficult to propagate and separate from the host cells in which it grows. In contrast with spotted fever group and typhus group ticketts-siae, *R tsutsugamushi* does not seem to possess lipopolysaccharides, peptidoglycan, a slime layer, or other T-independent antigens. The rickettsial cell wall consists of proteins linked by disulfide bonds. The three well-recognized, antigenically distin-

guishable prototype strains (Karp, Gilliam, and Kato) represent only part of what seems to be a great antigenic mosaic. Immunity to infection with the homologous strain wanes within a few years; cross-protective immunity to heterologous strains disappears within a few months. The reasons for this lack of long-term immunity are unclear.

PATHOGENESIS

Rickettsia tsutsugamushi is injected into the skin during feeding by a larval trombiculid mite (chigger). An eschar often forms at this location. Rickettsiae spread via the bloodstream and damage the microcirculation of the skin (rash), lungs (pneumonitis), brain (encephalitis), and other organs. The generalized enlargement of lymph nodes is unique among rickettsial diseases. *Rickettsia tsutsugamushi* is phagocytosed by the host cell, escapes from the phagosome into the cytosol, divides by binary fission, and is released from projections of the cell membrane (Fig. 38-4). The pathogenic mechanism of *R tsutsugamushi* is not known.

EPIDEMIOLOGY

Scrub typhus occurs where chiggers infected with virulent rickettsial strains feed upon humans. *Leptotrombidium deliense* and other mites are found particularly in areas where regrowth of scrub vegetation harbors the *Rattus* species that are hosts for the mites. Some of these foci are quite small and have been referred to as mite islands. Because *R tsutsugamushi* is transmitted transovarially from one generation of mites to the next, these dangerous areas tend to persist for as long as the ecologic conditions, including scrub vegetation, persist. Truly one of the neglected diseases, scrub typhus occurs over a vast area, including Japan, China, the Philippines, New Guinea, Indonesia, other islands of the southwest Pacific Ocean, southeastern Asia, northern Australia, India, Sri Lanka, Pakistan, USSR, and Korea. Recognized in western countries mainly because of large numbers of infections of military personnel during World War II and the Vietnam War, scrub typhus perennially affects native populations. Reinfection and undiagnosed infections are highly prevalent. Mortality ranges from 0 to 35 percent and has not been correlated with any specific factor.

DIAGNOSIS

Classic textbook cases with fever, headache, eschar, and rash are far outnumbered by cases that lack rash or eschar. Such cases are usually misdiagnosed. Laboratory diagnosis is unavailable in many areas where scrub typhus occurs. Isolation of rickettsiae requires inoculation of mice or cell culture. Serologic diagnosis is made by specific methods (indirect fluorescence antibody test or enzyme immunoassay) or by the older method of demonstrating cross-reactive antibodies that agglutinate the OXK strain of *P mirabilis*.

CONTROL

Scrub typhus can be treated with doxycycline, tetracycline, or chloramphenicol. Chigger repellents may prevent exposure. Prophylaxis with weekly doses of doxycycline during and for 6 weeks after exposure protects against scrub typhus. Attempts to develop a safe, effective vaccine have failed.

◁ EHRLICHIA ▷

According to the evolutionary scheme suggested by 16S rRNA sequence homology, ehrlichiae are genetically related to typhus group rickettsiae. The genus *Ehrlichia* contains Gram-negative bacteria that reside in a cluster (**morula**) within membrane-bound cytoplasmic vacuoles of lymphocytes, monocytes, and polymorphonuclear leukocytes. Ehrlichiae have been implicated as the agents of diseases of horses (*E risticii* and *E equi*), dogs (*E canis* and *E platys*, a platelet pathogen), and other animals. *Ehrlichia sennetsu* causes a human disease in Japan resembling infectious mononucleosis.

In 1987 the first case of human **ehrlichiosis** was reported in the United States. A severely ill man with multiorgan system involvement had morula inclusions demonstrated in peripheral blood leukocytes. He developed antibodies reactive with *E canis* antigens. Subsequently, cases of human ehrlichiosis have been documented mainly in eastern and southern states between New Jersey and Texas. The infection has varied from severe and sometimes fatal, mimicking Rocky Mountain spotted fever, to oligosymptomatic and asymptomatic forms. A history of tick bite and the seasonal and geographic occurrence favor a tick vector. Illness is often accompanied by leukopenia, thrombocytopenia, and damage to the liver. Lesions differ little from rickettsial vasculitis in the central nervous system, kidney, heart, and lungs, as is observed in canine ehrlichiosis. Clinical diagnosis is difficult. Laboratory diagnosis by indirect fluorescence antibody assay with antigens of *E canis* is not widely available. Ehrlichial morulae are difficult to detect in peripheral blood leukocytes.

◁ COXIELLA BURNETII ▷ AND Q FEVER

Coxiella burnetii is sufficiently different genetically from the other rickettsial agents that it is placed in a separate group. Unlike the other agents, it is very resistant to chemicals and dehydration. Additionally, its transmission to humans is by the aerosol route, although a tick vector is involved in spread of the bacteria among the reservoir animal hosts.

CLINICAL MANIFESTATIONS

Q fever is a highly variable disease, ranging from asymptomatic infection to fatal chronic infective endocarditis (Fig. 38-6). Some patients develop an acute febrile disease that is a nonspecific influenza-like illness or an atypical pneumonia. Other patients are diagnosed after identification of granulomas in their liver or bone marrow. The most serious clinical conditions are chronic *C burnetii* infections, which may involve cardiac valves, the central nervous system, and bone.

STRUCTURE, CLASSIFICATION, AND ANTIGENIC TYPE

Coxiella burnetii is an obligate intracellular bacterium with some peculiar characteristics. It is small, generally 0.25 μm by 0.5 to 1.25 μm. However, there is considerable ultrastructural pleomor-

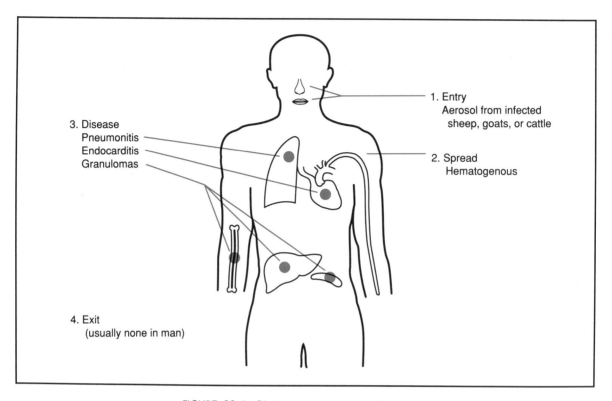

FIGURE 38-6 Clinical manifestations of Q fever.

phism, including small- and large-cell variants and possible endosporelike forms, suggesting a hypothetical developmental cycle. Among rickettsiae, *C burnetii* is the most resistant to environmental conditions, is the only species that resides in the phagolysosome, is activated metabolically by low pH, and has a plasmid. The extensive metabolic capacity of *C burnetii* suggests that its obligate intracellular parasitism is a highly evolved state rather than a degenerate condition. The cell wall is typical of Gram-negative bacteria and contains peptidoglycan, proteins, and lipopolysaccharide. When propagated under laboratory conditions in embryonated eggs or cell culture, *C burnetii* undergoes phase variation analogous to the smooth to rough lipopolysaccharide variation of members of the Enterobacteriaceae. Phase I is the form found in nature and in human infections. The phase II variant contains truncated lipopolysaccharide, is avirulent, and is a poor vaccine.

PATHOGENESIS

Human Q fever follows inhalation of aerosol particles derived from heavily infected placentas of sheep, goats, cattle, and other mammals. *Coxiella burnetii* proliferates in the lungs, causing atypical pneumonia in some patients. Hematogenous spread occurs, particularly to the liver, bone marrow, and spleen. The disease varies widely in severity, including asymptomatic, acute, subacute, or chronic febrile disease, granulomatous liver disease, and chronic infection of the heart valves. The target cells are macrophages in the lungs, liver, bone marrow, spleen, heart valves, and other organs. *Coxiella burnetii* is phagocytosed by Kupffer cells and other macrophages and divides by binary fission within phagolysosomes (Fig. 38-3). Apparently it is minimally harmful to the infected macrophages. Some strains have genetic and phenotypic characteristics that correlate with establishment of the most serious infection caused by *C burnetii*, chronic endocarditis. Other strains are associated with acute, self-limited infection or with natural environmental sources. The lipopolysaccharides are relatively nonendotoxic. Host-mediated pathogenic mechanisms appear to be important, especially immune and inflammatory reactions, such as T-lymphocyte-mediated granuloma formation.

EPIDEMIOLOGY

Coxiella burnetii infects a wide variety of ticks, domestic livestock, and other wild and domestic mammals and birds throughout the world. Most human infections follow exposure to heavily infected birth products of sheep, goats, and cattle, as occurs on farms, in research laboratories, and in abattoirs. *Coxiella burnetii* is also shed in milk, urine, and feces of infected animals. Animals probably become infected by aerosol and by the bite of any of the 40 species of ticks that carry the organisms.

DIAGNOSIS

Clinical diagnosis depends upon a high index of suspicion, careful evaluation of epidemiologic factors, and, ultimately, confirmation by serologic testing. Although *C burnetii* can be isolated by inoculation of animals, embryonated hen eggs, and cell culture, very few laboratories undertake this biohazardous approach. Likewise, the diagnosis is seldom made by visualization of the organisms in infected tissues. Acute Q fever is diagnosed by demonstration of the development of antibodies to protein antigens of *C burnetii* phase II organisms. Chronic Q fever endocarditis is diagnosed by demonstration of a high titer of antibodies, particularly IgG and IgA, against the lipopolysaccharide antigens of *C burnetii* phase I organisms in patients with signs of endocarditis whose routine blood cultures contain no organisms.

CONTROL

Antibiotic treatment is more successful in ameliorating acute, self-limited Q fever than in curing life-threatening chronic endocarditis. Reduction in exposure to these widespread organisms is difficult because some serologically screened animals that have no detectable antibodies to *C burnetii* still shed organisms at parturition. Persons with known occupational hazards (e.g., Australian abattoir workers) have benefited from a vaccine composed of killed phase I organisms. This vaccine is not readily available, but offers promise for development of safe, effective immunization.

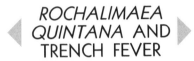

ROCHALIMAEA QUINTANA AND TRENCH FEVER

Rochalimaea quintana is the agent of trench fever, a widespread disease in soldiers during World War I. This Gram-negative bacillus has been cultivated extracellularly and hence does not fit the criterion of definition of rickettsiae as obligate intracellular bacteria. *Rochalimaea quintana* is an extracellular pathogen that infects the gut of human body lice, where it attaches to the surface of epithelial cells (Fig. 38-3). Individuals who have recovered from trench fever continue to have *R quintana* circulating in their blood for months. Therefore, persons in this stage of infection may serve as sources of infection for lice, which can transmit the infection to others.

REFERENCES

Audy JR (ed): Red Mites and Typhus. University Press, New York, 1968

Baca OG, Paretsky D: Q fever and *Coxiella burnetii*: a model for host-parasite interactions. Microbiol Rev 47:127, 1983

Brettman LR, Lewin S, Holzman RS et al: Rickettsialpox: report of an outbreak and a contemporary review. Medicine (Baltimore) 60:363, 1981

Burdorfer W, Anacker RL (eds): Rickettsiae and Rickettsial Diseases. Academic Press, San Diego, 1981

Fishbein DB, Kemp A, Dawson JE, et al: Human ehrlichiosis: prospective active surveillance in febrile hospitalized patients. J Infect Dis 160:803, 1989

Helmick CG, Bernard KW, D'Angelo LJ: Rocky Mountain spotted fever: clinical, laboratory and epidemiological features of 262 cases. J Infect Dis 150:480, 1984

Kaplowitz LG, Fischer JJ, Sparling PF: Rocky Mountain spotted fever: a clinical dilemma. Curr Clin Top Infect Dis 2:89, 1981

McDade JE, Newhouse VF: Natural history of *Rickettsia rickettsii*. Annu Rev Microbiol 40:287, 1986

McDade JE, Shepard CC, Redus MA et al: Evidence of *Rickettsia prowazekii* infections in the United States. Am J Trop Med Hyg 29:277, 1980

Moulder JW (ed): Intracellular Parasitism. CRC Press, Boca Raton, Fla, 1989

Sawyer LA, Fishbein DB, McDade JE: Q fever: current concepts. Rev Infect Dis 9:935, 1987

Walker DH (ed): Biology of Rickettsial Disease. Vols I and II. CRC Press, Boca Raton, FL, 1988

Walker DH: Rocky Mountain spotted fever: a disease in need of microbiological concern. Clin Microbiol Rev 2:227, 1989

Wolbach SB, Todd JL, Palfrey FW: Pathology of typhus in man. p. 152. In: Etiology and Pathology of Typhus. The League of Red Cross Societies Harvard Press, Cambridge, Mass, 1922

Zinsser H (ed): Rats, Lice, and History. Little, Brown, New York, 1935

39

CHLAMYDIA

YECHIEL BECKER

GENERAL CONCEPTS

Clinical Manifestations

Ocular Infections: Chlamydia trachomatis causes **trachoma** and **inclusion conjunctivitis.** Trachoma is characterized by the development of follicles and inflamed conjunctivae. The cornea may become cloudy and vascularized; repeated infections are a common cause of blindness. Inclusion conjunctivits is a milder inflammatory conjunctival infection with purulent discharge.

Genital Infections: Some *C trachomatis* strains cause genital infections, including nongonococcal urethritis in men and acute salpingitis and cervicitis in women. Other strains cause lymphogranuloma venereum, a venereal disease with genital lesions and regional lymph node involvement (buboes).

Respiratory Infections: Chlamydia psittaci usually causes an influenzalike illness called **psittacosis.** *Chlamydia pneumoniae* (TWAR organism) causes atypical pneumonitis in humans.

Structure, Classification, and Antigenic Types

Chlamydiae are obligate intracellular bacteria. They lack several metabolic and biosynthetic pathways and depend on the host cell for intermediates, including ATP. Chlamydiae exist as two stages: (1) infectious particles called **elementary bodies** and (2) intracytoplasmic, reproductive forms called **reticulate bodies.** The chlamy-

diae consist of three species, *C trachomatis, C psittaci,* and *C pneumoniae.* The first two contain many serovars based on differences in cell wall and outer membrane proteins. *Chlamydia pneumoniae* contains one serovar—the TWAR organism.

Pathogenesis

Chlamydiae have a hemagglutinin that may facilitate attachment to cells. The cell-mediated immune response is largely responsible for tissue damage during inflammation, although an endotoxinlike toxin has been described.

Host Defenses

Antibodies develop during infection, but they do not prevent reinfection. The precise role of cell-mediated immunity is not known.

Epidemiology

Trachoma occurs worldwide and is prevalent in Africa and Asia. *Chlamydia trachomatis* usually is inoculated into the eye by contaminated fingers or fomites or, in neonates, by passage through an infected birth canal. Genital infections are spread venereally, and respiratory infections usually by inhalation. Psittacosis is acquired from infected birds.

Diagnosis

The clinical presentation is often diagnostic; the diagnosis may be confirmed by serology (complement fixation or microimmunofluorescence tests) on sera and/or tears.

Control

Tetracycline and erythromycin are the drugs of choice. Penicillin is not effective.

INTRODUCTION

The chlamydiae are a small group of nonmotile coccoid bacteria that are obligate intracellular parasites of eukaryotic cells. Chlamydial cells are unable to carry out energy metabolism and lack many biosynthetic pathways; therefore they are entirely dependent on the host cell to supply them with ATP and other intermediates. Because of their dependence on host biosynthetic machinery, the chlamydiae were originally thought to be viruses; however, they have a cell wall and contain DNA, RNA, and ribosomes and therefore are now classified as bacteria. The group consists of a single genus, *Chlamydia* (order Chlamydiales, class Chlamydiaceae). This genus contains the species *C trachomatis* and *C psittaci,* as well as a new organism, the TWAR organism, which has recently been proposed as a third species *(C pneumoniae)*. All three species cause disease in humans. *Chlamydia psittaci* infects a wide variety of birds and a number of mammals, whereas *C trachomatis* is limited largely to humans. *Chlamydia pneumoniae* (TWAR organism) has been found only in humans.

CLINICAL MANIFESTATIONS

Chlamydia tracomatis Infections

The diseases caused by chlamydiae are summarized in Table 39-1 and Figure 39-1.

Trachoma, a *C trachomatis* infection of the conjunctival epithelial cells, results in subepithelial infiltration of lymphocytes, leading to the development of follicles. The infected epithelial cells contain cytoplasmic inclusion bodies. As a result of damage to the epithelial cells, fibroblasts and blood vessels invade the infected area, a pannus forms, and the cornea becomes vascularized and clouded. The eyelids become scarred and malformed, causing **trichiasis,** an abnormal inward growth of the eyelashes. Continual scraping of the cornea by the eyelashes leads to corneal opacification and blindness.

Chlamydia trachomatis also causes **inclusion conjunctivitis,** an eye disease of children and adults that is milder than trachoma. It consists of purulent conjunctivitis that heals spontaneously without scarring.

TABLE 39-1   Human Diseases Caused by Chlamydia

Species	Serotypes	Disease(s)
C trachomatis	A, B, Ba, C	Trachoma (hyperendemic, a leading cause of blindness in humans); sexually transmitted infections of the genitals
	D, E, F, G, H, I, J, K	Inclusion conjunctivitis (adult and newborn); cervicitis; salpingitis; proctitis, epididymitis, and pneumonia of newborns; lymphogranuloma venereum
C psittaci	L-1, L-2, L-3, many unidentified	Pneumonia (psittacosis)
C pneumoniae	TWAR[a]	Pneumonia

[a] The name is derived from the isolates TW-183 and AR-39.
(Modified from Schachter J: Chlamydial infections. N Engl J Med 298:428, 1978, with permission.)

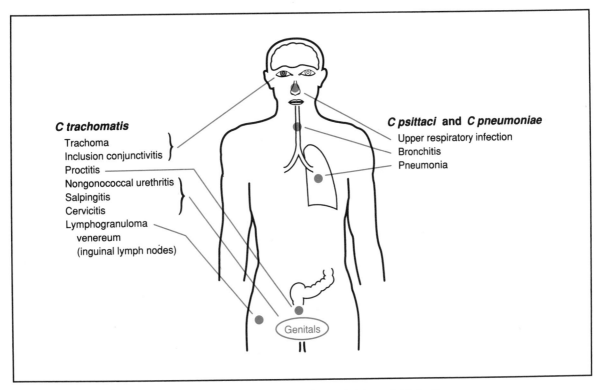

C trachomatis
Trachoma
Inclusion conjunctivitis
Proctitis
Nongonococcal urethritis
Salpingitis
Cervicitis
Lymphogranuloma
    venereum
    (inguinal lymph nodes)

C psittaci and C pneumoniae
Upper respiratory infection
Bronchitis
Pneumonia

Genitals

FIGURE 39-1 Clinical manifestations of chlamydial infections.

Chlamydia trachomatis also causes sexually transmitted genital and rectal infections. The frequency of *C trachomatis* infections in men may equal or exceed the frequency of gonorrhea. Nongonoccocal urethritis, epididymitis, and proctitis in men can result from infection with *C trachomatis*. Superinfection of gonorrhea patients with *C trachomatis* also occurs. Acute salpingitis and cervicitis in young women can be caused by a *C trachomatis* infection ascending from the cervix. A high rate genital tract coinfection by *C trachomatis* in women with gonorrhea has been reported. *Chlamydia trachomatis* was isolated from the fallopian tubes of infected women. In one report *C trachomatis* elementary bodies attached to spermatozoa were recovered from the peritoneal cavity of patients with salpingitis.

Neonates exposed to *C trachomatis* in an infected birth canal may develop acute conjunctivitis within 5 to 14 days. The disease is characterized by marked conjunctival erythema, lymphoreticular proliferation, and purulent discharge. Untreated infections can develop into pneumonitis; this type of pneumonitis occurs only during the first 4 to 6 months of life.

Recently, *C trachomatis* has been suspected of causing lower respiratory tract infections in adults, and several cases of *C trachomatis* pneumonia have been reported in immunocompromised patients from whom the pathogen was isolated. Evidence also indicates that *C trachomatis* may cause pneumonia or bronchopulmonary infections in immunocompetent persons.

Polyarthritis in lambs, calves, and possibly humans also may be caused by *C trachomatis*.

Lymphogranuloma venereum is a human venereal disease caused by *C trachomatis* strains different from the strains that cause trachoma (Table 39-1). The disease usually occurs in men and involves inguinal lymphadenopathy. Signs of lymphogranuloma venereum appear a few days after venereal exposure. The initial lesions, or vesicles, appear in the urogenital tract in men and women. If the disease does not heal spontaneously, regional lymph nodes become involved.

Chlamydia psittaci Infections

Chlamydia psittaci infects birds through the respiratory tract. Humans exposed to dead or living infected birds may develop fever, a mild influenzalike disease, or toxic fulminating pneumonitis after an incubation period of 2 to 4 weeks. *Chlamydia psittaci* can cause pneumonia in cats and sheep as well as in humans. Other strains of *C psittaci* can cause abortions in animals.

TWAR Organism Infections

Recently, a new *Chlamydia* strain (designated *C pneumoniae* serovar TWAR organism) that spreads from person to person in human populations was reported to cause outbreaks of respiratory tract infections in immunocompetent persons.

Latent Chlamydia Infections

Latent and inapparent infections of humans, other mammals, and birds are sometimes caused by chlamydiae. The agents of lymphogranuloma venereum, for example, may persist in infected humans for years before the disease becomes apparent. Individuals may develop acute trachoma years after leaving areas endemic for trachoma.

STRUCTURE

The chlamydiae exist in nature in two forms: (1) a nonreplicating, infectious particle called the **elementary body (EB)**, 0.25 to 0.3 μm in diameter, that is released from ruptured infected cells and can be transmitted from one individual to another *(C trachomatis, C pneumoniae)* or from infected birds to humans *(C psittaci)*, and (2) an intracytoplasmic form called the **reticulate body** (RB), 0.5 to 0.6 μm in diameter, that engages in replication and growth (Fig. 39-2 and 39-3). The elementary body, which is covered by a rigid cell wall, contains a DNA genome with a molecular weight of 66×10^7 (about 600 genes, one-quarter of the genetic information present in the DNA of *Escherichia*

coli). A cryptic DNA plasmid (7,498 base pairs) is also found. It contains an open reading frame for a gene involved in DNA replication. In addition, the elementary body contains an RNA polymerase responsible for the transcription of the DNA genome after entry into the host cell cytoplasm and the initiation of the growth cycle. Ribosomes and ribosomal subunits are present in the elementary bodies. Throughout the developmental cycle, the DNA genome, proteins, and ribosomes are retained in the membrane-bound prokaryotic cell (reticulate body).

A complex series of events occurs during the developmental cycle of chlamydiae. These and the effects on the host cell are summarized in Figure 39-4 and Table 39-2. Studies on the growth cycle of *C trachomatis* and *C psittaci* in cell cultures in vitro revealed that the infectious elementary body develops into a noninfectious **reticulate body (RB)** within a cytoplasmic vacuole in the infected cell. There is an eclipse phase of about 20 hours after entry of the elementary body into the infected cell, during which the infectious particle develops into a reticulate body. In these structures the chlamydial genome is transcribed into RNA, proteins are synthesized, and the DNA is replicated. The reticulate body divides by binary fission to form particles which, after synthesis of the outer cell wall, develop into new infectious elementary body progeny. The yield of chlamydial elementary bodies is maximal 36 to 50 hours after infection.

CLASSIFICATION AND ANTIGENIC TYPES

Several distinct antigenic components have been recognized in *C trachomatis* and *C psittaci,* some group specific and others species specific. Detergents have been used to extract antigens from elementary bodies and reticulate bodies. *Chlamydia pneumoniae* (TWAR organism) is serologically unique and differs from *C trachomatis* species and all *C psittaci* strains tested.

The outer chlamydial cell wall contains several antigenic proteins, including a 40-kilodalton (kDa) major outer membrane protein (MOMP), a 60- to 62-kDa and 15-kDa, cysteine-rich proteins, a 74-

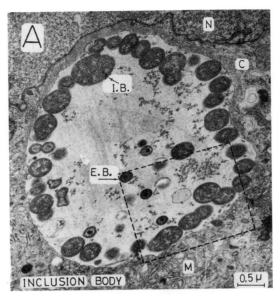

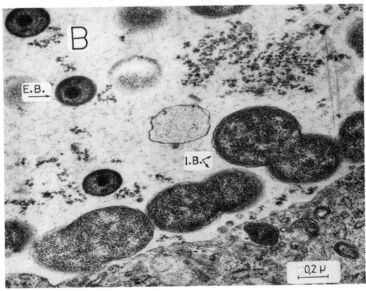

FIGURE 39-2 (*A*) Electron micrograph of *C trachomatis* inclusion body in cytoplasm (C) of infected cell. Part of the nucleus (N) and mitochondria (M) can also be seen. (*B*) Enlarged view of inclusion body showing elementary bodies (E.B.) and reticulate (initial) bodies (I.B.). (Courtesy of Y. Becker, Jerusalem, Israel.)

kDa species-specific protein, and 31- and 18-kDa eukaryotic cell-binding proteins, which share the same primary sequence.

Hyperimmune mouse antiserum against the 40-kDa MOMP protein from serotype L2 reacted with elementary bodies of *C trachomatis* serotypes Ba, E, D, K, L1, L2, and L3 during indirect immunofluorescence but failed to react with serotypes A, B, C, F, G, H, I, and J or with *C psittaci*. Indeed, cloning and sequencing of the *C trachomatis* MOMP gene

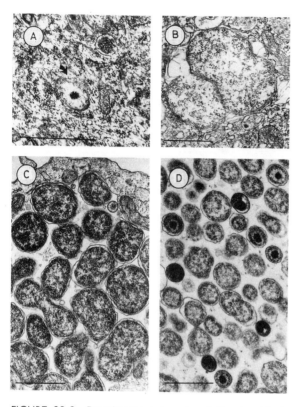

FIGURE 39-3   Developmental cycle of *C psittaci* in L cells (mouse fibroblasts). (*A*) Bar, 1 μm. At 2.5 hours after infection, the figure shows an elementary body (arrow) that has just begun to differentiate into a reticulate body (× 36,000). (*B*) Twelve hours after infection (× 23,000). (*C*) Twenty hours after infection (× 23,000). (*D*) Thirty hours after infection (× 23,000). (From Tribby IIE, Friis RR, Moulder JW: Effect of chloramphenicol, rifampicin, and nalidixic acid on *Chlamydia psittaci* growing in L cells. J Infect Dis 127:158, 1973, with permission.)

distantly related serovars. When MOMP is inserted into the outer elementary body envelope, exposed domains of MOMP serve as both serotyping and protective antigenic determinants. Predominantly conserved regions of C and B serotypes are interspersed with short variable domains.

Three monoclonal antibodies that recognize epitopes on cysteine-rich membrane proteins interact with all 15 human *C trachomatis* serotypes, establishing the species specificity of this antigen. Monoclonal antibodies to the 15-kDa cysteine-rich protein showed biovar specificity and species specificity. The 60- to 62-kDa and 15-kDa cysteine-rich proteins are highly immunogenic in the natural infection, but the antibodies do not neutralize the infectivity of *C trachomatis* elementary bodies.

PATHOGENESIS

Spread of Agents

Human diseases caused by chlamydiae can be divided into two types: (1) chlamydial agents transmitted by direct contact (*C trachomatis* genital and ocular infections, *C pneumoniae* ocular infection) and (2) chlamydial agents that are transmitted by the respiratory route (*C psittaci* and *C pneumoniae*.)

The spread of *C trachomatis* from person to person may cause trachoma, inclusion conjunctivitis, or lymphogranuloma venereum. Transmission of *C trachomatis* from the urogenital tract to the eyes and vice versa occurs via contaminated fingers, towels, or other fomites and, in neonates, by passage through an infected birth canal. These diseases appear in an epidemic form in populations with low standards of hygiene. *Chlamydia trachomatis* genital infections are sexually transmitted. *Chlamydia psittaci* is transmitted from infected birds or animals to humans through the respiratory tract. *Chlamydia pneumoniae* spreads from infected individuals by respiratory tract infections but is not sexually transmitted.

Chlamydial Diseases

Chlamydial agents are intracytoplasmic obligate parasites of mammalian cells and can damage infected cells in tissues. The elementary bodies are

revealed the same number of amino acids for serovars L2 and B, while the MOMP gene of serovar C contained codons for three additional amino acids. The antigenic diversity of the chlamydial MOMP was reflected in four sequence-variable domains, two of which are candidates for the putative type-specific antigenic determinants. The basis for MOMP differences among *C trachomatis* serovars were clustered nucleotide substitutions for closely related serovars and insertions and deletions for

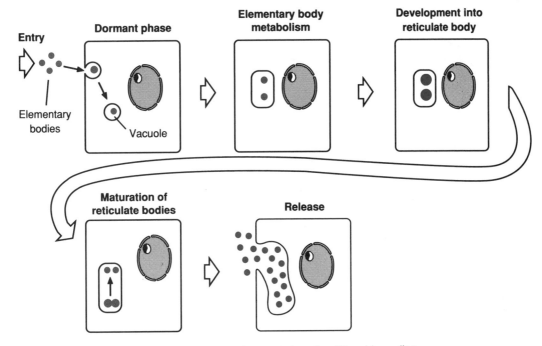

FIGURE 39-4 Developmental cycle of the chlamydiae.

TABLE 39-2 Stages in the Developmental Cycle
of Chlamydiae

Agent	Host Cell
Stage 1. Dormant phase. Elementary bodies (EBs) have no or little metabolic activity, contain a DNA genome (ca. 600 genes), plasmid DNA (ca. 8 kbp), ribosomal subunits, cytoplasm, cell membrane, and cell wall containing a major outer membrane protein (MOMP), three cysteine-rich outer membrane proteins (60 to 62, 15 and 74 kDa), and two cell-binding proteins (31 and 18 kDa).	Host cell can be in any phase of its growth cycle at infection.
Stage 2. Initiation of EB metabolism. EBs adsorb to host cell membrane. The organization of the EB cell wall changes (deficiency of the cysteine-rich proteins; no change in MOMP). EBs adsorb to host cells and utilize glucose-6-phosphate as substrate. EBs utilize mitochondrial functions. DNA in EBs changes conformation from compact organization to loose arrangement, possibly for transcriptional processes.	Duration: 0–12 h after infection. Cell phagocytizes EBs. Cell forms vacuole around EBs. Mitochondria support EB development. Cellular enzyme in glucose metabolic pathway is utilized by EB. Host cell nucleic acid metabolism continues. Nucleotides in host cell pool are available for the prokaryotic parasite.

Continued

TABLE 39-2 *(continued)*

Agent	Host Cell
DNA-dependent RNA polymerase molecules attached to DNA genome, are activated, and transcribe the genome. At this stage, EB development becomes sensitive to rifampin. Protein synthesis with existing ribosomes begins in EBs. Low level of DNA synthesis in EB is detected since development is sensitive to 5×10^{-4} M hydroxyurea. EB mass increases because of macromolecule synthesis.	

Stage 3. Development of EB into reticulate body.

Agent	Host Cell
Rate of DNA biosynthesis increases. DNA is replicated by a DNA-dependent DNA polymerase encoded by chlamydial and plasmid DNAs. Replication of DNA is semiconservative, with synthesis of short Okazaki-like fragments on the DNA template.	Duration: 12–35 h after infection. Cell responds to enlargement of EB by increasing the size of vacuole in which the agent develops.
DNA synthesis is accompanied by endogenous synthesis of thymidine, probably from deoxycytidine precursor. DNA synthesis is inhibited by folic acid analogs and hydroxyurea.	Host cell can supply some of the nucleotide precursors.
DNA-dependent RNA polymerase transcribes ribosomal genes in chlamydial DNA. Precursors of rRNA are synthesized and processed to yield two RNA species, of 1.1 and 0.55 MDa. rRNA species assemble into 50S and 30S ribosomal subunits by combining with ribosomal proteins synthesized according to genetic information in the chlamydial DNA.	
Glucose 6-phosphate is catabolized by enzymes in the agent. In *C trachomatis* only, glycogen is synthesized and deposited in vacuole, where RBs develop.	
Synthesis of DNA, ribosomes, and proteins is coupled with formation of new RBs by a binary fission-like process. At this stage the cytoplasmic vacuoles are filled with RBs.	Duration: 20–48 h after infection. Inhibition of protein synthesis of cytoplasmic polyribosomes by chloramphenicol does not affect chlamydial life cycle. The cytoplasmic vacuole containing the RBs is markedly enlarged. In *C psittaci* the vacuole fills most of the cell cytoplasm. In *C trachomatis* the vacuole is more rigid and defined.
Chlamydial enzymes are involved in the biosynthesis of the RB-limiting membranes.	DNA synthesis in the nucleus is affected.
Chlamydial enzymes synthesize RB cell walls.	

Stage 4. Maturation of RBs, formation of EBs.

Agent	Host Cell
DNA synthesis in RBs is coupled with division of particles into two smaller daughter cells (pre-EBs).	
Internal organization in pre-EB particles: the DNA genome is condensed in the center of the particle, with cell wall loosely arranged around the particle.	
RBs start the synthesis of cysteine-rich proteins.	Vacuole is disrupted, and host cell death is inevitable.
Cell wall synthesis leads to rigid EB particles. At this stage, EBs are formed and the life cycle is completed. EBs are released from the ruptured cells.	

(Modified from Becker Y: *Chlamydia*: Molecular biology of procaryotic obligate parasites of eucaryocytes. Microbiol Rev 42:299, 1978, with permission.)

infectious particles that can be transmitted from the infected tissues to uninfected tissues in the same person (transfer of *C trachomatis* elementary bodies from an infected genital tract to the eyes and vice versa) or from a person with atypical pneumonia (caused by *C psittaci* or *C pneumoniae*) to healthy individuals (respiratory release of elementary bodies). In the infected individuals the chlamydial agent causes tissue damage and induction of interleukin-1α, interleukin-1β, and tumor necrosis factor alpha, which are cytokines involved in the inflammation process. Ocular infections by *C trachomatis* and sometimes *C pneumoniae* strains cause acute purulent conjunctivitis either due to infection of the neonate during passage through the birth canal or due to subsequent infections leading to scarring of the conjunctiva and to blindness subsequent to mucopurulent follicular conjunctivitis. *Chlamydia trachomatis* infection also spreads through sexual contact when urethritis or cervicitis is present. The genital tract infection serves as a source of infectious elementary bodies for the eyes.

The recently recognized *C pneumoniae* isolates cause mild to severe pneumonia, prolonged bronchitis, pharyngitis, sinusitis, and a febrile illness in humans. The agent does not cause death in patients without complications.

HOST DEFENSES
Nonspecific Responses

Infections with chlamydial agents evoke responses from the blood vessels (ocular trachoma), connective tissue (scars in *C trachomatis* infections), and lymphocyte infiltration (pannus). Chlamydial infections are characterized by chronic inflammation. The mechanisms that trigger migration of lymphocytes or connective tissue to the site of *C trachomatis* infection in the eyes are not known. However, coculture of *C trachomatis* (serovar L2) with human blood monocytes induced the production of interleukin-1, an important mediator of inflammation and scarring. Interleukin-1α and interleukin-1β can be induced in human monocytes by *C trachomatis* lipopolysaccharide. Release of angiogenesis factors from infected cells may cause

proliferation of blood vessels in the infected eye. Fever accompanies *C psittaci* pneumonitis. It was reported that tumor necrosis factor is induced by *C trachomatis* infection in athymic nude mice.

Cultured chlamydiae are sensitive to interferon, which is produced by cultured cells infected with chlamydiae.

Immune Response in Humans

All chlamydial infections induce IgM, IgG, IgA, and IgE antibodies, but these antibodies do not prevent reinfection. Although secretions from trachomatous eyes contain specific antitrachoma IgG and IgA antibodies, these antibodies do not impede the infection. Moreover, antibodies that bind to *C trachomatis* elementary bodies do not impair their infectivity in cell cultures. However, the addition of anti-gamma globulin to antibody-treated elementary bodies neutralizes their infectivity. Monoclonal antibodies to proteins in the outer elementary body envelope were reported to neutralize elementary body infectivity. Most patients with *C trachomatis* infections have antibodies that react with the *C trachomatis* cell wall proteins. Sera from individuals with genital infections caused by *C trachomatis* also reacted with the 60- to 62-kDa cysteine-rich proteins of all the *C trachomatis* serotypes. The precise role of cell-mediated immunity is not known.

EPIDEMIOLOGY

Trachoma is still prevalent in Africa and Asia (more than 500 million people are estimated to have the disease), and sporadic cases occur all over the world. The disease flourishes in hot, dry areas where there is a shortage of water and where standards of hygiene are low. The agent is spread to the eyes by flies, dirty towels, fingers, or cosmetic eye pencils. The initial infection usually occurs in childhood, and the active disease eventually appears (mostly by 10 to 15 years of age). Trachoma may leave a residuum of permanent lesions that can lead to blindness. *Chlamydia trachomatis* also resides in the genital tract, cervix, and urethra of adults, and genital infection is spread sexually. Lymphogranuloma venereum persists in the genital tract of infected persons. Because *C trachomatis* is able to infect both the eyes and the urogenital tract, antitrachoma campaigns involving only ocular treatments are futile.

Chlamydia psittaci, the cause of psittacosis in birds and occasionally in humans, is carried by wild and domestic birds, including poultry. The severity of psittacosis in humans has been considerably reduced by the susceptibility of *C psittaci* to antibiotics.

Chlamydia pneumoniae spreads in human populations by respiratory tract infections. It is the agent of atypical pneumonia in hospitalized patients as well as in young individuals with an acute respiratory disease. It has caused epidemics in Scandinavia. Studies of the prevalence of antibodies to *C pneumoniae* in humans around the world showed that it also prevails in Japan, Panama, and North America.

DIAGNOSIS

Most diseases caused by the chlamydiae are diagnosed on the basis of their clinical manifestations. Eye damage caused by *C trachomatis* is typical, as are the vesicles in the infected urogenital tract. Diagnosis of penumonitis requires laboratory testing.

Chlamydia trachomatis can be identified microscopically in scrapings from the eyes or the urogenital tract. Inclusion bodies in scraped tissue cells are identified by iodine staining of glycogen present in the cytoplasmic vacuoles in infected cells. To isolate the agent, cell homogenates that contain the chlamydial elementary bodies are centrifuged onto the cultured cells (e.g., irradiated McCoy cells). After incubation, typical cytoplasmic inclusions are seen in the cells stained with Giemsa stain or iodine. Staining with iodine can distinguish between inclusion bodies of *C trachomatis* and *C psittaci,* as only the former contain glycogen. Each chlamydial agent can also be identified by using specific immunofluorescent antibodies prepared against either *C trachomatis* or *C psittaci.* Homogenates or exudates of infected tissues also have been used to isolate the agent in the yolk sac of embryonated eggs.

Sera and tears from infected humans are used to detect anti-*Chlamydia* antibodies by the complement fixation or microimmunofluorescence tests. The latter is useful for identifying specific serotypes of *C trachomatis;* however, even detection of anti-*C trachomatis* antibodies of the IgM class cannot be used diagnostically for genital infections, because similar antibodies are found in *Chlamydia*-negative patients. Fluorescent monoclonal antibodies are used to stain *C trachomatis* elementary bodies in urethral and cervical exudates.

It is possible to diagnose *C trachomatis* in tissue biopsy specimens by in situ DNA hybridization with cloned *C trachomatis* DNA probes.

DNA from *C trachomatis* isolates can be examined by restriction endonuclease analysis. The DNA cleavage pattern of *C trachomatis* isolates differs greatly from that of DNA from *C psittaci* isolates. DNAs of the agents of trachoma and lymphogranuloma venereum differ in their cleavage patterns, and this allows identification of the biovars.

Chlamydia pneumoniae DNA has 10 percent homology with *C trachomatis* or *C psittaci; C pneumoniae* isolates have 100 percent homology. *Chlamydia pneumoniae* isolates can be diagnosed by hybridization with a specific DNA probe that does not hybridize to other chlamydiae. Two additional serologic tests are in use: the microimmunofluorescence test with *C pneumoniae*-specific elementary body antigen, and the complement fixation test, which measures *Chlamydia* antibodies.

CONTROL

Attempts to use *C trachomatis* vaccines for prophylaxis and treatment of trachoma have failed. The course of trachoma is more severe in immunized than in nonimmunized individuals. Specific anti-*Chlamydia* antibodies fail to neutralize chlamydial elementary bodies in vivo.

Tetracycline and erythromycin are the antiobiotics commonly used to treat chlamydial infections in humans. Penicillin is not effective. Patients with trachoma have been treated effectively with erythromycin, rifampin, sulfonamides, chloramphenicol, and tetracyclines. Repeated treatment cycles of long-acting sulfonamides also have been used in local or systemic treatment of trachoma infections. In trachoma patients with trichiasis, corrective surgery is necessary. Patients with inclusion conjunctivitis usually are not treated, because the infection is self-limiting and relatively mild.

Tetracyclines or sulfonamides sometimes are effective in patients with lymphogranuloma venereum, but treatment does not always improve the condition. Tetracycline treatment of gonorrhea in patients infected with gonococci or *Chlamydia* is more effective against postgonococcal urethritis than is treatment with penicillin.

REFERENCES

Baehr W, Zhang YX, Joseph T, et al: Mapping antigenic domains expressed by *Chlamydia trachomatis* major outer membrane protein genes. Proc Natl Acad Sci USA 85:4000, 1988

Becker Y: The agent of trachoma. Monogr Virol 7, 1974

Becker Y: *Chlamydia:* molecular biology of procaryotic obligate parasites of eucaryotes. Microbiol Rev 42:274, 1978

Grayston JT: *Chlamydia pneumoniae,* strain TWAR. Chest 95:664, 1989

Hatch TP, Miceli M, Sublett JE: Synthesis of disulfide-bonded outer membrane proteins during the developmental cycle of *Chlamydia psittaci* and *Chlamydia trachomatis.* J Bacteriol 165:379, 1986

Hatt C, Ward ME, Clarke IN: Analysis of the entire nucleotide sequence of the cryptic plasmid of *Chlamydia trachomatis* serovar L1. Evidence for involvement in DNA replication. Nucleic Acids Res 16:4053, 1988

Moulder JW: Order II Chlamydiales Storz and Page 1971, 334[AL]. p. 729. In Krieg NR, Holt JG (eds), Bergey's Manual of Systematic Bacteriology. Vol 1. Williams & Wilkins, Baltimore, 1984

Peterson EM, de la Maza LM: Restriction endonuclease analysis of DNA from *Chlamydia trachomatis* biovars. J Clin Microbiol 26:635, 1988

Rothermel CD, Schachter J, Lavrich P, et al: *Chlamydia trachomatis*-induced production of interleukin-1 by human monocytes. Infect Immun 57:2705, 1989

Schachter J: Chlamydiae: exotic and ubiquitous. West J Med 132:238, 1980

Schachter J, Grossman M: Chlamydial infections. Annu Rev Med 32:45, 1981

Stephens RS, Tam MR, Kuo CC, Nowinski RC: Monoclonal antibodies to *C. trachomatis:* antibody specificity and antigen characterizations. J Immunol 128:1083, 1982

Tribby IIE, Friis RR, Moulder JW: Effect of chloramphenicol, rifampicin and nalidixic acid on *Chlamydia psittaci* growing in L cells. J Infect Dis 127:155, 1973

Wenman WM, Lovett MA: Expression in *E coli* of *C trachomatis* antigen recognized during human infection. Nature (London) 296:68, 1982

Williams DM, Bonewald LF, Roodman GD, et al: Tumor necrosis factor alpha is a cytotoxin induced by murine *Chlamydia trachomatis* infection. Infect Immun 57:1351, 1989

Yong EC, Chinn GS, Caldwell HD, Kuo CC: Reticulate bodies as single antigen in *Chlamydia trachomatis* serology with microimmunofluorescence. J Clin Microbiol 10:351, 1979

Zhang YX, Morrison SG, Caldwell HD, Baehr W: Cloning and sequence analysis of the major outer membrane protein genes of two *Chlamydia psittaci* strains. Infect Immun 57:1621, 1989

40 LEGIONELLA

WASHINGTON C. WINN, JR.

GENERAL CONCEPTS

Clinical Manifestations

The most common presentation of *Legionella pneumophila* is acute pneumonia (**legionellosis**); potentially any species of *Legionella* may cause the disease. Extrapulmonary disease (e.g., pericarditis and endocarditis) is rare. Less often, disease presents as a nonpneumonic epidemic influenzalike illness called **Pontiac fever.**

Structure, Classification, and Antigenic Types

Legionella species are Gram-negative bacilli. There are currently 27 species and 43 distinct antigenic types of *Legionella*.

Pathogenesis

Legionella bacilli reside in surface and drinking water and are usually transmitted to humans in aerosols. The bacteria multiply intracellularly in alveolar macrophages. Recruited neutrophils and monocytes as well as bacterial enzymes produce destructive alveolar inflammation. Direct inoculation of surgical wounds by contaminated tap water has been described.

Host Defenses

Nonspecific physical and inflammatory pulmonary defenses are important, but cell-mediated immunity is critical. Immunologically activated monocytes and macrophages restrict intracellular bacterial growth. The role of humoral immunity is unclear.

Epidemiology

Legionella species are widespread in nature. Interactions with other environmental organisms may facilitate growth. Disease may be sporadic or epidemic and may occur in the community or in hospitals. People with compromised host defenses are at increased risk.

Diagnosis

Legionellosis can be suspected clinically, but diagnosis can be confirmed only by laboratory testing. The preferred method is culturing on special charcoal-containing agar.

Control

Decontamination of identified environmental sources is of primary importance for prevention. The drug of choice is erythromycin. Immunization works in experimental animals but has not been attempted in humans.

INTRODUCTION

Legionella was first recovered from the blood of a soldier almost 50 years ago, but its importance as a human pathogen was not recognized until 1976, when a mysterious epidemic of pneumonia struck members of the Pennsylvania American Legion. The disease was dubbed **legionnaire's disease** by the press. Within 6 months a bacterium, subsequently named *Legionella pneumophila,* had been isolated and definitively established as the agent, thanks to the efforts of many investigators from Pennsylvania and the Centers for Disease Control in Atlanta. A general term for disease produced by *Legionella* species is **legionellosis.**

CLINICAL MANIFESTATIONS

The clinical manifestations of *Legionella* infections are primarily respiratory (Fig. 40-1). Two very different kinds of respiratory illness may result from infection; the reasons for this dichotomy are not understood (Table 40-1). The most common presentation is acute pneumonia, which varies in severity from mild illness that does not require hospitalization (**walking pneumonia**) to fatal multilobar pneumonia. Typically, patients have high, unremitting fever and cough but do not produce much sputum. Extrapulmonary symptoms, such as headache, confusion, muscle aches, and gastrointestinal disturbances, are common. Most patients respond promptly to appropriate antimicrobial therapy, but convalescence is often prolonged (lasting many weeks or even months).

The second form of respiratory illness is called **Pontiac fever** after the city in Michigan where the first epidemic was recognized. This uncommon manifestation of infection resembles acute influenza, including fever, headache, and severe muscle aches. It is self-limited, and convalescence is uneventful.

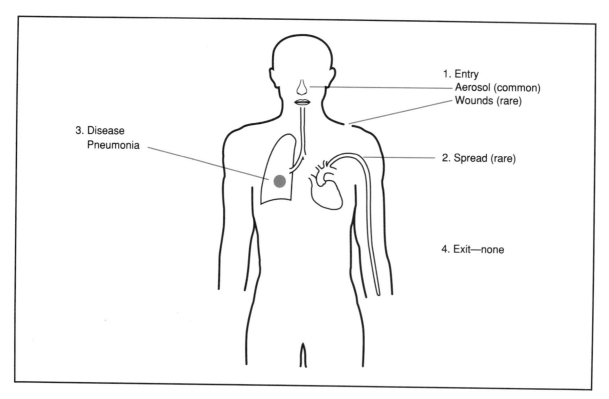

FIGURE 40-1   Pathogenesis of legionellosis.

TABLE 40-1 Clinical Manifestations of *Legionella* Infections

Disease	Pneumonia	Occurrence	Attack Rate	Incubation Period	Species Implicated
Legionnaire's disease	Almost always	Epidemic, sporadic, nosocomial, community	Low	Long (days)	All, especially *L pneumophila* and *L micdadei*
Pontiac fever	Never	Epidemic, community	High	Short (hours)	*L pneumophila, L micdadei, L feelei*
Disseminated infection	Usually		Rare		*L pneumophila*
Primary wound infection	Rarely	Sporadic, nosocomial	Rare		*L pneumophila, L dumoffii*

Bacteremia occurs during *Legionella* pneumonia, and symptomatic infection outside the lungs occasionally develops. Under special conditions, bacteria introduced through portals other than the lungs, such as surgical wounds, may cause disease.

STRUCTURE

Legionella cells are thin, somewhat pleomorphic Gram-negative bacilli that measure 2 to 20 μm by approximately 0.5 to 1.0 μm (Fig. 40-2). Long, filamentous forms may develop, particularly after growth on the surface of agar. Ultrastructurally, *Legionella* has the inner and outer membranes typical of Gram-negative bacteria. It possesses pili (fimbriae), and most species are motile by means of a single polar flagellum.

It is ironic that *Legionella* species are sometimes referred to as fastidious bacteria, because they grow luxuriantly in tap water and can multiply in the usually hostile environment of phagocytic cells. They are fastidious only in the media commonly used in laboratories. The primary growth factor required is L-cysteine, a nutrient that is also essential for *Francisella tularensis*. Ferric iron is also essential, and other compounds are necessary for optimal growth. Energy is derived from amino acids rather than carbohydrates.

CLASSIFICATION AND ANTIGENIC TYPES

Molecular characterization of strains isolated from patients in Pennsylvania led to the creation of a new family of bacteria, Legionellaceae, as well as a new genus, *Legionella*. The genus now has 27 species, defined by studies of DNA homology. Only one genus within the family has been recognized. Immunologic diversity within species is reflected in the creation of serogroups (Table 40-2). *Legionella pneumophila* holds the record, with 14 distinct serologic types. Important antigens include outer membrane proteins, some of which are species-specific antigens, and the lipopolysaccharide that is the major serogroup-specific antigen. Strains may be divided into subtypes by antigenic analysis,

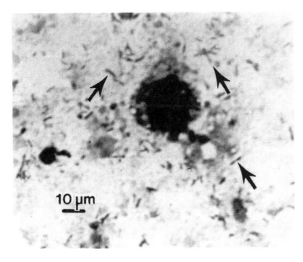

FIGURE 40-2 Impression smear from the lung of a patient fatally infected with *L pneumophila* serogroup 1, demonstrating many thin, Gram-negative bacilli (arrows). These bacteria stain less intensely with safranin than do enteric bacilli.

TABLE 40-2   Pathogenic *Legionella* Species
Isolated from Humans[a]

Species	Number of Serogroups
L pneumophila	14
L micdadei	1
L dumoffii	1
L bozemanii	2
L gormanii	1
L longbeachae	2
L jordanis	1
L wadsworthii	1
L feelei	2
L maceachernii	1
L cincinnatiensis	1
L birminghamensis	1
L tucsonensis	1
L anisa	1

[a] *Legionella oakridgensis, L sainthelensi, L jamestowniensis, L rubrilucens, L erythra, L spiritensis, L parisiensis, L cherrii, L steigerwaltii, L santicrucis, L israelensis, L moravica,* and *L brunensis* have been isolated only from the environment.

using panels of monoclonal antibodies, or by characterization of bacterial enzyme systems. These increasingly fine distinctions can be very valuable for epidemiologic study but do not affect clinical decisions.

PATHOGENESIS

The pathogenesis of *Legionella* infections begins with a supply of water containing virulent bacteria and with a means for their dissemination to humans (Fig. 40-1). Person-to-person transmission has never been demonstrated, and *Legionella* is not a member of the bacterial flora of humans.

Infection begins in the lower respiratory tract. Alveolar macrophages, which are the primary defense against bacterial infection of the lungs, engulf the bacteria; however, *Legionella* is a facultative intracellular parasite and multiplies freely in macrophages (Fig. 40-3). The bacteria bind to alveolar macrophages via the complement receptors and are engulfed into a phagosomal vacuole. However, by an unknown mechanism, the bacteria **block the fusion of lysosomes with the phagosome,** preventing the normal acidification of the phagolysosome and keeping the toxic myeloperoxidase system segregated from the susceptible bacteria. The bacilli multiply within the phagsosome. Thus, a cellular compartment that should be a death trap instead becomes a nursery. Eventually, the cell is destroyed, releasing a new generation of microbes to infect other cells.

Bacterial growth, activation of the complement system, and/or the death of alveolar macrophages produces powerful chemotactic factors that elicit an influx of monocytes and polymorphonuclear neutrophils (Fig. 40-4). Leaky capillaries allow the transudation of serum and deposition of fibrin in the alveoli. The result is a destructive pneumonia that obliterates the air spaces and compromises respiratory function (Fig. 40-5). Dissemination of bacteria to sites outside the lung occurs at least partially via macrophages, but only rarely does an inflammatory response develop.

The symptoms of *Legionella* infection undoubtedly result from a combination of physical interference with oxygenation of blood, ventilation-perfusion imbalance in the remaining lung tissue, and release of toxic products from bacteria and inflammatory cells. Bacterial factors include a protease that may be responsible for tissue damage. Cellular factors include interleukin-1, which produces fever after it is released from monocytes, and tumor necrosis factor, which may be responsible for some of the systemic symptoms.

HOST DEFENSES

Risk factors for legionnaire's disease include conditions that compromise both the specific and nonspecific defenses. The fact that patients with chronic heart and lung diseases are at increased risk of developing serious *Legionella* pneumonia suggests that the integrity of physical clearance mechanisms, such as the mucociliary escalator of the tracheobronchial tree, is an important element of the defenses. Nonimmunologic antibacterial factors normally found in respiratory secretions, such as lactoferrin or lysozyme, may also play a role.

Inflammatory cell defenses play both positive

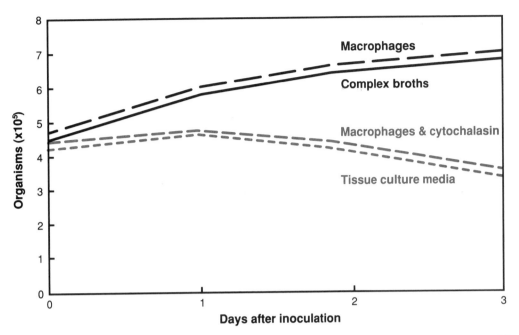

FIGURE 40-3 Growth of *Legionella* cells in vitro. This facultative intracellular pathogen grows well in complex broths that provide all necessary nutrients. The usual tissue culture media, which are adequate to support the growth of human and animal cells, cannot support the growth of *Legionella* cells. The bacteria also grow well within alveolar macrophages that have been maintained in cell culture. If phagocytosis is prevented by treatment with cytochalasin, however, the bacteria are denied access to the intracellular environment and growth does not occur.

and negative roles. The human alveolar macrophage and its relation, the recruited blood monocyte, abdicate their normal roles as primary antibacterial defenses in *Legionella* infections. The major reason why mice are very resistant to experimental *Legionella* pneumonia is probably that their alveolar macrophages do not support intracellular bacterial growth.

The role of polymorphonuclear leukocytes is less clear. These cells do not support bacterial growth in vitro and are only minimally bactericidal. Treatment with cytokines such as gamma interferon marginally increases their bactericidal activity. Neutropenia is not an important risk factor.

The most impressive risk factors for human disease are various types of immunosuppression. In a small outbreak of disease caused by contaminated nebulizers, pneumonia developed most often in patients being treated with corticosteroids.

The critical component of the immune system in resistance to legionellosis has not yet been pinpointed. Attention has focused on cell-mediated immunity because *Legionella* is a facultative intracellular pathogen. Infected patients produce a cell-mediated immune response that can be detected by measuring lymphocyte blastogenesis after exposure to *Legionella* antigen. Lymphocytes appear in the air spaces of experimentally infected animals about 5 days after an acute infection (Fig. 40-4). In contrast to naive alveolar macrophages, which are permissive for intracellular bacterial growth, activated alveolar macrophages or peripheral blood monocytes restrict bacterial multiplication in vitro (Fig. 40-6). The macrophages can be activated by treatment with lymphokines produced by specifically stimulated lymphocytes. Gamma interferon, which can substitute for the lymphokines, is an important mediator. It has been sug-

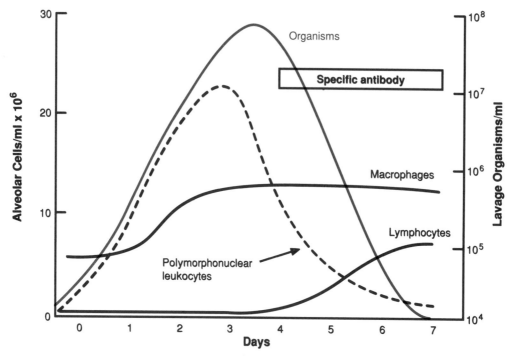

FIGURE 40-4 Inflammatory response in experimental *Legionella* pneumonia. Alveolar macrophages are the only resident cells in the air spaces of the lungs. Exponential bacterial growth begins soon after infection at a time when only macrophages are present; bacteria are most numerous 3 to 4 days later, but have virtually disappeared by the end of the first week. Infection elicits a large influx of polymorphonuclear leukocytes, followed by monocytes from the peripheral blood. Fluid exudation into the alveoli follows the pattern of the polymorphonuclear leukocytes. Specific immunologic responses (i.e., antibody and lymphocyte influx) are detectable 4 to 5 days after infection.

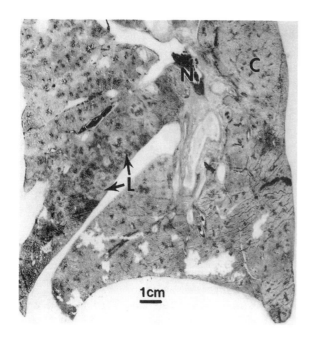

FIGURE 40-5 Acute *L pneumophila* pneumonia. Paper-mounted whole-lung section, unstained. The air spaces are filled with fibrin and inflammatory cells. The consistency of the completely consolidated lower lobe (C) resembles that of an adjacent hilar lymph node (N). The lobular nature of the process is accentuated by gray carbon accumulation around the terminal bronchioles in the centers of the lobules (L).

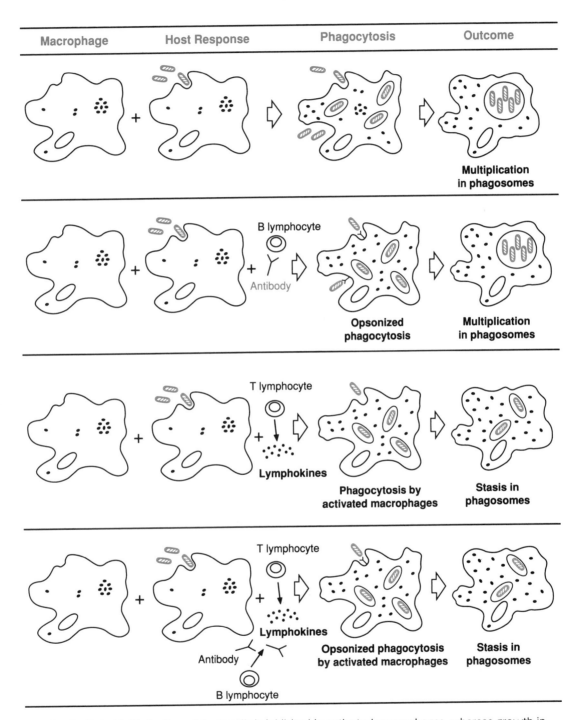

FIGURE 40-6 Multiplication of *Legionella* is inhibited in activated macrophages, whereas growth in normal macrophages provides a preferred environment, enhancing bacterial growth.

gested that restriction of entry of iron (an important growth factor for *Legionella*) into the phagosome inhibits intracellular growth.

The role of humoral immunity is less clear. Antibody in all immunoglobulin classes is made after human or experimental infection. This antibody serves an opsonizing function in vitro, facilitating the phagocytosis of bacteria by polymorphonuclear leukocytes, macrophages, and monocytes. Antibody does not kill most strains of *Legionella*, however, so that the outcome of the interaction depends on the capabilities of the phagocytic cell (Fig. 40-6). The classic pathway of the complement system is activated by *L pneumophila*, enhancing phagocytosis still further. *Legionella micdadei* activates the alternative complement pathway as well, so that opsonization of this species can occur even before an immunologically specific antibody response is mounted. One can construct scenarios from in vitro data in which antibody is deleterious as well as helpful. Experimental studies with animals support a protective role for antibody.

EPIDEMIOLOGY

The epidemiology of *Legionella* infections is a complex equation that is composed of the aquatic environment (including representatives of multiple microbial phyla, humans, mechanical devices, and medical facilities), dissemination from the environment to the host, and host susceptibility. The complexity of the environmental interactions rivals those of viral and parasitic infections.

The only documented source of *Legionella* species is water, particularly the surface waters of rivers and lakes and drinking water. *Legionella* does not multiply in sterile tap water, but the addition of other bacteria, certain types of algae, or free-living amoebae results in growth of *Legionella* in vitro. The relationship with a variety of amoebae is particularly interesting. These single-cell animals, which can be viewed as nature's macrophages, occur in the same aquatic environment as do *Legionella* organisms (Fig. 40-7) and support the intracellular growth of *Legionella* in much the same way. Another factor that favors the survival of *Legionella* in natural or treated waters is its rela-

tive resistance to the effects of chlorine and heat; *Legionella* can find refuge in relatively inhospitable environments such as hot-water tanks.

The second factor in the epidemiology equation is dissemination of bacteria from the environment to the host. In most cases the link is an aerosol of water contaminated with the organisms. Evaporative condensers and cooling towers are proven sources of outdoor infection. Indoors, nebulizers and humidifiers filled with contaminated drinking water have disseminated *Legionella* to susceptible patients. The automatic misting devices that keep supermarket produce fresh have even been fingered as culprits in outbreaks of pneumonia. Aerosols are produced in numerous ways in our environment, from taking a shower to flushing the toilet. In most cases we do not know the source of the infection. Direct infection of surgical wounds has been linked to washing of patients with tap water that harbored pathogenic *Legionella* organisms.

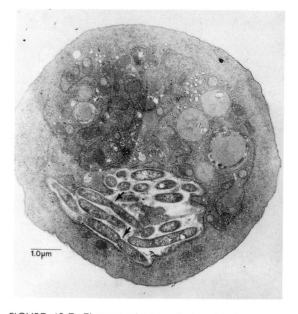

FIGURE 40-7   Electron micrograph showing *L pneumophila* serogroup 1 in the process of dividing (arrows) within a vesicle of an amoeba (*Hartmanella vermiformis*) cell. (× 18,500.) (Courtesy of Barry S. Fields, Centers for Disease Control.)

The final factor in the equation is the susceptibility of patients. The diseases and conditions that serve as risk factors are concentrated in health care facilities, so it should be no surprise that many of the epidemics of disease have been nosocomial.

Legionella infections may be sporadic or epidemic, community acquired or nosocomial. There is great geographic variation in the frequency of infection, even within communities, presumably reflecting the presence of suitable aquatic environments and susceptible subjects. Both sporadic and epidemic cases are more common during summer than winter months, perhaps because of increased use of air-cooling equipment that generates aerosols.

DIAGNOSIS

There are no reliable distinguishing clinical features of *Legionella* pneumonia, so the diagnosis must come from the laboratory. Some clinical features suggest legionnaire's disease, however, and should prompt the selection of appropriate laboratory tests (Table 40-3). The diagnosis is confirmed in the laboratory by culture, demonstration of bacterial antigen in body fluids, or detection of a serologic response.

The preferred diagnostic method is culturing, because it is both sensitive and specific; however, appropriate specimens are not always available. The laboratory must be alerted to the possibility of legionellosis, because specially designed media must be used. The medium of choice is buffered charcoal–yeast extract–α-ketoglutarate medium. This medium contains yeast extract, iron, L-cysteine, and α-ketoglutarate for bacterial growth; activated charcoal to inactivate toxic peroxides that develop in the media; and a buffer with a pK at pH 6.9, the optimum for growth of *Legionella* organisms. For contaminated specimens such as sputum, antibiotics should be added and/or the specimen should be decontaminated with acid. Morphologically distinctive bacterial colonies can usually be detected within 3 to 5 days and identified presumptively as *Legionella* species if the isolated bacteria depend on cysteine for growth. The identification can be confirmed by specific immunologic typing of the isolated bacteria or, in problematic cases, by molecular analysis.

Direct detection of bacterial antigen in clinical specimens is potentially much faster than culturing. Unfortunately, direct immunofluorescence detection of *Legionella* antigen in respiratory specimens is neither sensitive nor specific enough to warrant general use. A commercially available radioimmunoassay for bacterial antigen in urine is satisfactory, but is available only for serogroup 1 of *L pneumophila* and requires the use and disposal of radiochemicals.

Serologic diagnosis is sensitive and reasonably specific. Indirect immunofluorescence has been used most frequently, but enzyme immunoassays

TABLE 40-3 Clinical Clues to *Legionella* Pneumonia

Clue	Example
Patient's history and physical examination	
Presence of an epidemic or documented source of infection	Family, friends, or associates with similar infection and similar exposure
Prominent neurologic or gastrointestinal symptoms	Pneumonia with confusion, nausea, and vomiting
Nonresponse to aminoglycoside or β-lactam antibiotics	Worsening condition after 5 days on antibiotics
Patient's laboratory data	
Gram stain of sputum with many neutrophils but no bacteria	Laboratory report showing many neutrophils and few normal flora or no bacteria
Nodular peripheral infiltrates in chest radiograph	Progression of unilateral opacities to bilateral nodular infiltrates over several days

also are available. It is important to use an assay that detects IgM and IgG. The advantages of serologic diagnosis are that it is performed on easily obtained blood specimens and can detect mild or even asymptomatic infection. The major disadvantage of the technique is that paired acute- and convalescent-phase sera are essential. The convalescent-phase specimen must be obtained at least 6 weeks after onset of the infection, by which time the physician and patient have often lost interest in the enterprise.

CONTROL

Because the interactions between *Legionella* organisms, the environment, and the host are so complex, the incidence of disease may be controlled in several ways. If an aquatic source of infection can be found, elimination of *Legionella* from the source is an effective control mechanism. This genus is so common in water systems that molecular analysis of environmental and clinical strains is often helpful in pinpointing the source. Unfortunately, decontamination can be expensive. The two most common means of eradicating *Legionella* are periodic superheating of water, with attendant dangers of scalding, and continuous chlorination, which accelerates deterioration of plumbing systems unless carefully monitored. Even "chlorinated" drinking water must be treated because the levels of chlorine decrease with increasing distance from the distribution center, particularly in hot water. Constant vigilance must be maintained to prevent return of the unwanted pathogens.

Immunization has been proposed as a means of preventing *Legionella* infection in susceptible populations. This approach works in experimental animals but has not been attempted in humans.

Pontiac fever does not require antimicrobial therapy. The preferred drug for symptomatic *Legionella* infections is erythromycin. If the patient is seriously ill, it is important to deliver the antibiotic intravenously at first; subsequently, oral therapy may be used. Rifampin is sometimes added as a second antibiotic in seriously ill patients. Retrospective analysis of the antibiotics used to treat the Pennsylvania Legionnaires suggests that erythro-

mycin was the most effective agent. If these patients had been hospitalized in major medical centers, they would undoubtedly have received the latest antimicrobial agents and it might have taken us years to determine that erythromycin is the drug of choice. Experimentally, both erythromycin and rifampin inhibit the growth of *Legionella* organisms in infected macrophages, but do not kill the bacteria.

It may appear that we are defenseless against *Legionella* infection, because the most effective type of host defense shows only very modest bactericidal abilities in vitro. In fact most infections are subclinical, and mortality is low in patients who are not immunocompromised. Similarly, even susceptible experimental animals survive infection unless moderately large doses of bacteria are given. The defense mechanisms probably function better in vivo than in vitro. The action of host defenses may also be additive in vivo. One can construct a scenario by which bacteria are increasingly phagocytosed by cells that do not permit bacterial growth. The net result is a decreasing number of extracellular bacteria and hence a decreased source of infection for a decreasing population of permissive cells. Obsolescent inflammatory cells in the lungs are removed by the mucociliary escalator and expectorated as sputum. Therefore, the infection may begin with a bang, but it ends in most cases with a whimper.

REFERENCES

Balows A, Fraser DW (eds): International Symposium on Legionnaires' Disease. Ann Intern Med 90:491, 1978

Byrd TF, Horwitz MA: Interferon gamma-activated human monocytes downregulate transferrin receptors and inhibit the intracellular multiplication of *Legionella pneumophila* by inhibiting the availability of iron. J Clin Invest 83:1457, 1989

Horwitz MA: Cell-mediated immunity in Legionnaires' disease. J Clin Invest 71:1686, 1983

Thornsberry C, Balows A, Feeley JC, Jakubowski W (eds): *Legionella*. Proceedings of the 2nd International Symposium. American Society for Microbiology, Washington, DC, 1984

Winn WC, Jr: Legionnaires disease: historical perspective. Clin Microbiol Rev 1:60, 1988

II

VIROLOGY

Recent epidemiologic reports show that viral infections in developed countries are the most common cause of acute disease that does not require hospitalization. In developing countries, viral diseases also exact a heavy toll in mortality and permanent disability, especially among infants and children. Now that antibiotics effectively control most bacterial infections, viral infections pose a relatively greater and less controlled threat to human health. Some data suggest that the already broad gamut of established viral diseases soon may be expanded to include other serious human ailments such as juvenile diabetes, rheumatoid arthritis, various neurologic and immunologic disorders, and some tumors.

Viruses can infect all forms of life (bacteria, plants, protozoa, fungi, insects, fish, reptiles, birds, and mammals); however, this section covers only viruses capable of causing human infections. Like other microorganisms, viruses may have played a role in the natural selection of animal species. A documented example is the natural selection of rabbits resistant to virulent myxoma virus during several epidemics deliberately induced to control the rabbit population in Australia. Indirect evidence suggests that the same selective role was played by smallpox virus in humans. Another possible, though unproved, mechanism by which viruses may affect evolution is by introducing viral genetic material into animal cells by mechanisms similar to those that govern gene transfer by bacteriophages. For example, genes from avirulent retrovirus integrated into genomes of chickens or mice produce resistance to reinfection by related, virulent retroviruses. The same relationship may exist for human retroviruses, since human leukemia-causing retroviruses have been reported.

Viruses are small, subcellular agents that are unable to multiply outside a host cell (intracellular obligate parasitism). The assembled virus (virion) is formed by only one type of nucleic acid (RNA or DNA) and, in the simplest viruses, a protective protein coat. The nucleic acid contains the genetic information necessary to program the synthetic machinery of the host cell for viral replication. The protein coat serves two main functions: first, it protects the nucleic acid from extracellular environmental insults such as nucleases; second, it permits attachment of the virion to the membrane of the host cell, the negative charge of which would repel a naked nucleic acid. Once the viral genome has penetrated and thereby infected the host cell, virus replication mainly depends on host cell machinery for energy and synthetic requirements.

The various virion components are synthesized separately within the cell and then assembled to form progeny particles. This assembly type of replication is unique to viruses and distinguishes them from all other small, obligate, intracellular parasites. The basic structure of viruses can cause them to be simultaneously adaptable and selective. Many viral genomes are so adaptable that once they have penetrated the cell membrane under experimental conditions, viral replication can occur in almost any cell. On the other hand, intact viruses are so selective that most virions can infect only a limited range of cell types. This selectivity exists largely because penetration of the nucleic acid usually requires a specific reaction for the coat to attach to the host cell membrane.

Another important feature of viral infections is that most viruses, unlike most other microorganisms, cannot establish a mutual relationship with the host. In fact, although some viruses may establish some forms of silent infection, their multiplication usually causes cell damage or death; however, since viruses must depend on host survival for their own survival, they tend to establish mild infections in which death of the host is more an aberration than a regular outcome.

Viruses are distinct among microorganisms in their extreme dependence on the host cell. Since a virus must grow within a host cell, the virus must be viewed together with its host in any consideration of pathogenesis, epidemiology, host defenses, or therapy. The bilateral association between the virus and its host imposes specific conditions for pathogenesis. For example, rhinoviruses require a temperature not exceeding 34°C; this requirement restricts their growth to only those cells in the cool outer layer of the nasal mucosa, thereby preventing spread to deeper cells where temperatures are higher.

The intracellular location of the virus often protects the virus against some of the host's immune mechanisms; at the same time, this location makes the virus vulnerable because of its dependence on the host cell's synthetic machinery, which may be altered by even subtle physical and chemical changes produced by the viral infection (inflammation, fever, circulatory alterations, and interferon).

Epidemiologic properties depend greatly on the characteristics of the virus-host association. For example, some arthropod-borne viruses require a narrow range of temperature to multiply in insects; as a result, these viruses are found only under certain seasonal and geographic conditions. Other environmental conditions determine the transmissibility of viruses in aerosols and in food.

Viruses are difficult targets for chemotherapy because they replicate only within host cells, mainly utilizing many of the host cell's biosynthetic processes. The similarity of host-directed and virus-directed processes makes it difficult to find antiviral agents specific enough to exert a greater effect on viral replication in infected cells than on functions in uninfected host cells. It is becoming increasingly apparent, however, that each virus may have a few specific steps of replication that may be used as targets for highly selective, carefully aimed chemotherapeutic agents. Therefore, proper use of such drugs requires a thorough knowledge of the suitable targets, based on a correct diagnosis and a precise understanding of the replicative mechanisms for the offending virus.

Knowledge of the pathogenetic mechanisms by which virus enters, spreads within, and exits from the body also is critical for correct diagnosis and treatment of disease and for prevention of spread in the environment. Effective treatment with antibody-containing immunoglobulin requires knowing when virus is susceptible to antibody (for example, during viremic spread) and when virus reaches target organs where antibody is less effective. Many successful vaccines have been based on knowledge of pathogenesis and immune defenses. Comparable considerations govern treatment with interferon.

Clearly, viral infections are among the most difficult and demanding problems a physician must face. Unfortunately, some of these problems still lack satisfactory solutions, although tremendous progress has been made during the last several decades. Many aspects of medical virology are now understood, others are being clarified gradually, and many more are still completely obscure. Knowledge of the properties of viruses and the relationships they establish with their hosts is crucial to successful investigation and clinical management of their pathologic processes.

Our plan for conveying this knowledge is to present, first, concepts of viral structure, and then relate them to principles of viral multiplication. Together these concepts form the basis for understanding how viruses are classified, how they affect cells, and how their genetic system functions. These molecular and cellular mechanisms are combined with the concepts of immunology to explain viral pathogenesis, nonspecific defenses, persistent infections, epidemiology, evolution, and control. The important virus families are then discussed. Having studied the virology section, the reader should be able to use most principles of virology to explain individual manifestations of virus infection and the processes that bring them about.

Thomas Albrecht
Ferdinando Dianzani
Samuel Baron

41 STRUCTURE AND CLASSIFICATION OF VIRUSES*

CARL F. T. MATTERN

GENERAL CONCEPTS

Structure and Function

Because viruses are obligate intracellular parasites, they do not need to contain the complex metabolic and biosynthetic machinery of eukaryotic and prokaryotic cells. A complete infectious virus particle is called a **virion.** The main function of the virion is to deliver its DNA or RNA genome into the host cell so that the genome can be expressed (transcribed and translated) by the host cell's synthetic machinery. The genomic DNA or RNA, sometimes with associated basic proteins, is packaged inside a symmetric protein **capsid.** The capsid plus nucleic acid or nucleoprotein is called the **nucleocapsid.** In **enveloped** viruses, the nucleocapsid is surrounded by an envelope that usually has a lipid bilayer component derived from a modified host cell membrane plus a projecting outer layer of glycosylated proteins.

Classification of Viruses

Morphology: Viruses are classified on the basis of morphology, chemical composition of the genome, and mode of replication. **Helical morphology** is seen in nucleocapsids of many filamentous and pleomorphic vi-

ruses. Helical nucleocapsids consist of a helical array of capsid proteins **(protomers)** wrapped around a helical filament of nucleic acid. **Icosahedral morphology** is characteristic of the nucleocapsids of many "spherical" viruses. The number and arrangement of the **capsomeres** (morphologic subunits of the icosahedron) is useful in identification and classification.

Chemical Composition and Mode of Replication: The genome of a virus may consist of DNA or RNA, which may be single stranded or double stranded, linear or circular. The entire genome may occupy either one nucleic acid molecule **(monopartite genome)** or several nucleic acid segments **(multipartite genome).** The different types of genome necessitate different replication strategies.

Nomenclature

Several factors pertaining to the mode of replication play a role in the classification and nomenclature of viruses, including the configuration of the nucleic acid, whether the genome is monopartite or multipartite. The genomic RNA strand of single-stranded RNA viruses is called **sense** *(positive sense, plus sense)* in orientation if it can serve as mRNA, and **antisense** *(negative sense, minus sense)* if a complementary strand synthesized by a viral RNA transcriptase serves as mRNA. Also considered in viral classification is the site of capsid assembly and, in enveloped viruses, the site of envelopment.

---

* Included herein, with updating, is most of the chapter of the late Natalie J. Schmidt on virus classification and nomenclature appearing in the second edition of *Medical Microbiology.*

559

STRUCTURE AND FUNCTION

Because viruses are obligate intracellular parasites, they do not require the complicated structure needed to carry out the multiple functions of eukaryotic and prokaryotic cells. The main action of a virus is to deliver its **genome** (nucleic acid) into the host cell so that the genome can be expressed (transcribed and translated) by the synthetic machinery of the host cell.

A fully assembled infectious virus is called a **virion.** The simplest virions consist of two basic components: **nucleic acid** (single- or double-stranded RNA or DNA) and a protein coat, the **capsid,** which protects the viral genome from nucleases and attaches the virion to the host cell membrane. Capsid proteins are specified by the virus genome. The limited amount of genomic nucleic acid can code for only a few structural proteins. Viral coats that consist of only one or a few structural proteins must therefore **self-assemble** to form the continuous capsid structure. Such self-assembly arrangements follow two basic patterns: **helical symmetry,** in which the protein subunits and the nucleic acid are arranged in a helix, and **icosahedral symmetry,** in which the protein subunits assemble into a symmetric shell covering the viral core of nucleic acid or nucleoprotein. Some of the larger viruses have more complex structures.

Some virions with these symmetries have an additional covering, called the **envelope,** which is usually derived in part from modified host cell membranes. Viral envelopes usually contain a lipid bilayer in contact with virus-encoded proteins internally and with glycosylated proteins externally. Under the electron microscope, viral envelopes often appear to be studded with glycoprotein spikes called **peplomers.** In viruses that pick up their envelope by budding through the plasma or another cell membrane, the lipid composition of the viral envelope frequently reflects that of the host cell membrane. The envelope glycoproteins of viruses are important in determining the **viral host range.**

CLASSIFICATION OF VIRUSES

Viruses currently are classified on the basis of morphology, chemical composition, and mode of replication. The viruses that cause human disease reflect only a small part of the morphologic spectrum of the multitude of different viruses whose host ranges extend from vertebrates to protozoa and from plants and fungi to bacteria.

Morphology

Helical Symmetry

In the replication of viruses with helical symmetry, identical protein subunits **(protomers)** self-assemble into a helical array surrounding the nucleic acid, which follows a similar spiral path. The entire structure (nucleic acid within capsid) is referred to as a **nucleocapsid.** Such structures appear as rigid, highly elongated rods or as flexible filaments; in either case, details of the capsid structure are often discernible by electron microscopy. In addition to classification as flexible or rigid and as naked or enveloped (by a membrane), helical nucleocapsids are characterized by length, width, pitch of the helix, and number of protomers per helical turn. The most extensively studied helical virus is tobacco mosaic virus (Fig. 41-1). Many important structural features of this plant virus have been detected by x-ray diffraction studies. Figure 41-2 shows Sendai virus, another virus with helical symmetry. (This virus was originally considered a paramyxovirus, but now is thought not to be a human pathogen.)

Icosahedral Symmetry

An **icosahedron** is a polyhedron having 20 equilateral triangular faces and 12 vertices (Fig. 41-3).

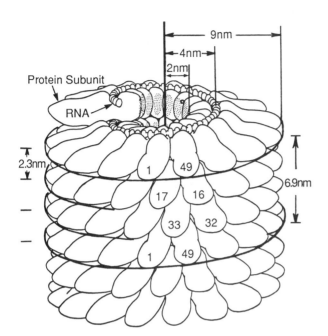

FIGURE 41-1   The helical structure of the rigid, filamentous tobacco mosaic virus. About 5 percent of the length of the virion is depicted. Individual 17,400-Da protein subunits assemble in a helix with an axial repeat of 6.9 nm (49 subunits per three turns). Each turn contains a nonintegral number of subunits (16-⅓), producing a pitch of 2.3 nm. The RNA (2×10^6 Da) is sandwiched internally between adjacent turns of capsid protein, forming an RNA helix of the same pitch, 8 nm in diameter, that extends the length of virus, with three nucleotide bases in contact with each subunit. Some 2,130 subunits per virion cover and protect the RNA. The complete virus is 300 nm long and 18 nm in diameter with a hollow cylindrical core 4 nm in diameter. (From Mattern CFT: Symmetry in virus architecture. In Nayak DP (ed): Molecular Biology of Animal Viruses. Marcel Dekker, New York, 1977, as modified from Caspar DLD: Adv Protein Chem, 18:37, 1963, with permission.)

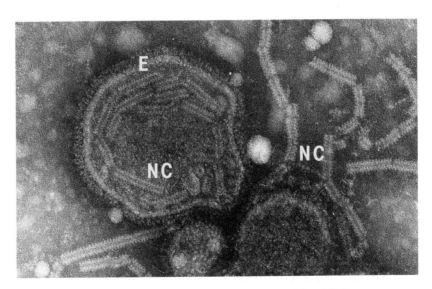

FIGURE 41-2   Fragments of flexible helical nucleocapsids (NC) of Sendai virus, a paramyxovirus, are seen either within the protective envelope (E) or free, after rupture of the envelope. The intact nucleocapsid is about 1,000 nm long and 17 nm in diameter; its pitch (helical period) is about 5 nm. (×200,000.) (Courtesy of A. Kalica, National Institutes of Health.)

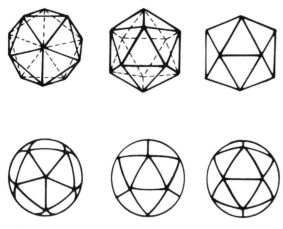

FIGURE 41-3   Icosahedral models seen, left to right, on fivefold, threefold, and twofold axes of rotational symmetry. These axes are perpendicular to the plane of the page and pass through the centers of each figure. Both polyhedral (upper) and spherical (lower) forms are represented by different virus families.

Lines through opposite vertices form axes of fivefold rotational symmetry: all structural features of the polyhedron repeat five times within each 360° of rotation about any of the fivefold axes. Lines through the centers of opposite triangular faces form **axes** of threefold rotational symmetry; twofold rotational symmetry axes are formed by lines through midpoints of opposite edges. Icosahedra (polyhedral or spherical) with fivefold, threefold, and twofold axes of rotational symmetry (Fig. 41-3) are defined as having 532 symmetry (read as 5,3,2). Because 32 symmetry is also exhibited by the **cubic** or **isometric** crystal systems, these terms also have been used to describe the 532 symmetry of viruses.

Viruses were first found to have 532 symmetry by x-ray diffraction studies and subsequently by electron microscopy with negative-staining techniques. In several icosahedral viruses, the protomers (protein subunits) are conveniently arranged in relatively large clusters called **capsomeres,** which are readily delineated by electron-dense stains (Fig. 41-4). The arrangement of capsomeres into icosahedral symmetry (compare Fig. 41-4 with the upper right model in Fig. 41-3)

permits the classification of such viruses by capsomere number. This requires the identification of a closest pair of vertex capsomeres (those through which the fivefold symmetry axes pass) and the distribution of capsomeres between them.

In the adenovirus model in Figure 41-4, one of the capsomeres on a fivefold axis is arbitrarily assigned the indices $h = 0$, $k = 0$ (origin), where h and k are the indicated axes of the inclined (60°) net of capsomeres. The net axes are formed by lines of the closest-packed neighboring capsomeres. In adenoviruses, the h and k axes also coincide with the edges of the triangular faces. Any second neighboring vertex capsomere has indices $h = 5$, $k = 0$ (or $h = 0$, $k = 5$). The capsomere number (C) can be determined to be 252 from the h and k indices and the equation: $C = 10(h^2 +$

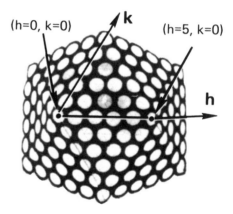

FIGURE 41-4   Adenovirus model. Capsomeres are depicted as circles delineated by an electron dense stain. The inclined axes, h and k, are indicated. The second vertex has indices $h = 5$, $k = 0$. The total number of capsomeres $C = 10(h^2 + hk + k^2) + 2 = 252$. Capsomere organization is also expressed by the triangulation number, T, the number of unit triangles on each of the 20 faces of the icosahedron. A unit triangle is formed by lines joining the centers of three adjacent capsomeres. $T = (h^2 + hk + k^2) = 25$ for adenoviruses, and $C = 10T + 2$. Adenoviruses also have 12 antennalike protein structures (pentons), one projecting from each of the 12 vertices (not shown; see Ch. 67). Protomers are the smallest protein units assembled into capsomeres and are usually not delineated by negative staining.

$hk + k^2) + 2$. This number of capsomeres is found in all members of the adenovirus group.

Virus Core Structure

Except in helical nucleocapsids, little is known about the packaging or organization of viral nucleic acid (RNA or DNA) within the virion core. It is known, however, that some virions are simple nucleocapsids and that others have a core containing nucleic acid and basic protein(s) surrounded by capsid protein.

Chemical Composition and Mode of Replication

RNA Virus Genomes

RNA viral genomes of different viruses vary remarkably in structure (Fig. 41-5). The RNA may be single stranded or double stranded, and the genome may occupy a single RNA segment or be distributed on two or more separate segments **(segmented genomes).** In addition, the RNA strand of a single-stranded genome may be either a sense strand (plus strand), which can function as messenger RNA (mRNA), or an antisense strand (minus strand), which is complementary to the sense strand and cannot function as mRNA in protein translation (see Ch. 42). Sense viral RNA alone can replicate if injected into cells, since it can function as mRNA and initiate translation of virus-encoded proteins. Antisense RNA, on the other hand, has no translational function and cannot per se produce viral components.

Double-stranded RNA viruses such as the reoviruses contain 10 to 12 separate genome segments, each consisting of complementary sense and antisense strands that are hydrogen bonded into linear double-stranded molecules. The replication of these viruses is complex; only the sense RNA strands are released from the infecting virion to initiate replication.

Retroviruses represent a unique RNA virus group. Their genome consists of two identical, single-stranded, sense RNA molecules that are noncovalently linked over a short terminal region. These viruses contain **reverse transcriptase** (RNA-dependent DNA polymerase), which transcribes the viral RNA to produce a double-stranded, circular proviral DNA. This DNA becomes covalently bonded into the DNA of the host cell to make possible the subsequent transcription of the sense strands that form the progeny retrovirus virions.

DNA Virus Genomes

Most DNA viruses (Fig. 41-5) contain a single genome of double-stranded linear DNA. The papovaviruses, however, have a circular DNA genome. Double-stranded DNA serves as a template both for mRNA and for self-transcription. Because the sense (plus) RNA strand is complementary to only one of the DNA strands, that strand is called the minus DNA strand.

Single-stranded linear DNA is found only in the small viruses of the parvovirus group (see Ch. 64). Both the adeno-associated virus (AAV) parvovirus and parvovirus B19 have very small genomes incapable of producing progeny virions except in the presence of **helper viruses** (adenovirus or herpesvirus) for AAV strains or in the presence of rapidly dividing cells for serum parvovirus-like strains. In both cases progeny virions in about equal number contain a single strand of either sense or antisense RNA. Adeno-associated virus is said to be **replication defective** because it is unable to manage its own replication; serum parvovirus-like strains, in contrast, are **autonomous.** As with all viruses, these two viruses depend on the host cell environment to provide some replicative functions that they lack.

NOMENCLATURE

Viral morphology is determined by the combined expression of the viral genes, and it provides a basis for grouping viruses into families. A virus family may consist of members that replicate only in vertebrates, only in invertebrates, only in plants, or only in bacteria. Certain families contain viruses that replicate in more than one of these hosts. This section concerns only families and genera of medical importance.

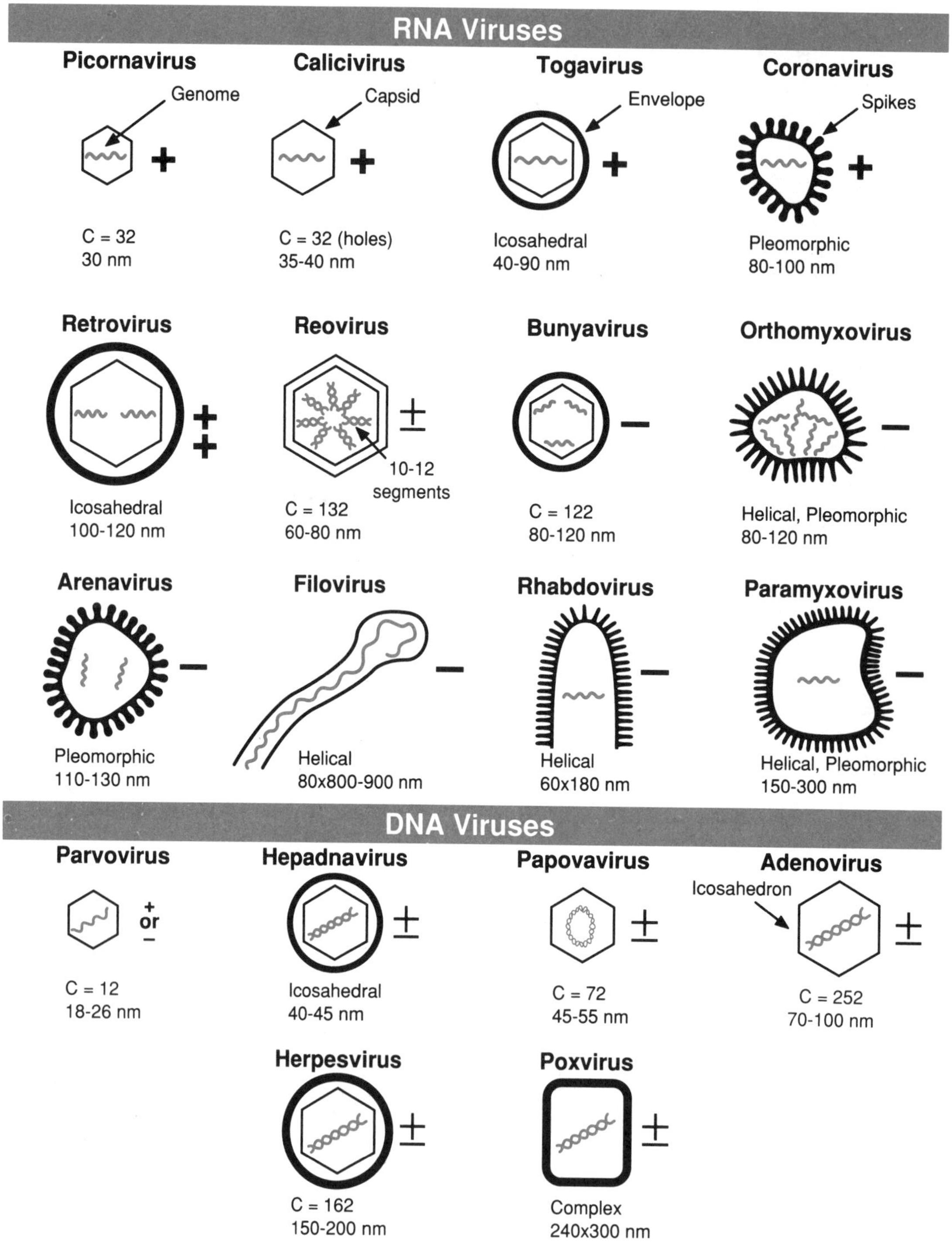

RNA Viruses

Picornavirus

Genome

C = 32
30 nm

Calicivirus

Capsid

C = 32 (holes)
35-40 nm

Togavirus

Envelope

Icosahedral
40-90 nm

Coronavirus

Spikes

Pleomorphic
80-100 nm

Retrovirus

Icosahedral
100-120 nm

Reovirus

10-12 segments

C = 132
60-80 nm

Bunyavirus

C = 122
80-120 nm

Orthomyxovirus

Helical, Pleomorphic
80-120 nm

Arenavirus

Pleomorphic
110-130 nm

Filovirus

Helical
80x800-900 nm

Rhabdovirus

Helical
60x180 nm

Paramyxovirus

Helical, Pleomorphic
150-300 nm

DNA Viruses

Parvovirus

+ or −

C = 12
18-26 nm

Hepadnavirus

Icosahedral
40-45 nm

Papovavirus

C = 72
45-55 nm

Adenovirus

Icosahedron

C = 252
70-100 nm

Herpesvirus

C = 162
150-200 nm

Poxvirus

Complex
240x300 nm

FIGURE 41-5 Distinctive structures of 18 virus families showing outer envelope, capsid and internal nucleic acid genome. +, Sense strand; −, antisense strand; ±, double-stranded RNA or DNA; 0, circular DNA; C, number of capsomeres or holes, where known; nm, dimensions of capsid, or envelope when present; the hexagon designates an icosahedral structural feature (capsid).

Several factors pertaining to the mode of replication play a role in classification and nomenclature: the configuration of the nucleic acid (single or double stranded, linear or circular), whether the genome consists of one molecule of nucleic acid or is segmented, and whether the strand of single-stranded RNA is sense or antisense. Also considered in viral classification is the site of viral capsid assembly and, in enveloped viruses, the site of nucleocapsid envelopment. Table 41-1 lists the major chemical and morphologic properties of the families of viruses that cause disease in humans.

The use of Latinized names ending in -viridae for virus families and ending in -virus for viral genera has gained wide acceptance. The names of subfamilies end in -virinae. There is less support for a Latinized binomial nomenclature for viruses, and vernacular names continue to be used to describe the viruses within a genus. In this text, Latinized endings for families and subfamilies usually are not used. Table 41-2 shows the current classification of medically significant viruses.

From the early 1950s until the mid-1960s, when many new viruses were being discovered, it was popular to compose virus names by using *sigla* (abbreviations derived from a few or initial letters). Thus the name Picornaviridae is derived from pico (small) and RNA; the name Reoviridae is derived from *r*espiratory, *e*nteric, and *o*rphan viruses because the agents were found in both respiratory and enteric specimens and were not related to other classified viruses; Papovaviridae is from *pa*pilloma, *po*lyoma, and *va*cuolating agent (simian virus 40 [SV40]); retrovirus is from *re*verse *tra*nscriptase; Hepadnaviridae is from the replication of the virus in *hepa*tocytes and their *DNA* genomes, as seen in hepatitis B virus. Hepatitis A virus is classified in the family Picornaviridae, genus *Heparnavirus* (from *hepa*tocytes and their *RNA* genome). Although the current rules for nomenclature do not prohibit the introduction of new sigla, they require that the siglum be meaningful to workers in the field and be recognized by international study groups.

The names of the other families that contain viruses pathogenic for humans are derived as follows: Parvoviridae (*parvo* means small); Adenoviridae (*adeno*, "gland"; refers to the adenoid tissue from which the viruses were first isolated); Herpesviridae (*herpes*, "creeping," describes the nature of the lesions); Poxviridae (*pock* means pustule); Togaviridae (*toga*, "cloak" refers to the viral envelope); Orthomyxoviridae (*ortho*, "true," plus *myxo* "mucus," a substance for which the viruses have an affinity); Paramyxoviridae (*para*, "closely resembling" and *myxo*); Rhabdoviridae (*rhabdo*, "rod" describes the shape of the viruses); Arenaviridae (*arena* "sand" describes the sandy appearance of the virion); Coronaviridae (*corona*, "crown" describes the appearance of the peplomers protruding from the viral surface); Bunyaviridae (from Bunyamwera, the place in Africa where the type strain was isolated); *Calicivirus* (*calici*, "cup" or "goblet" from the cup-shaped depressions on the viral surfaces); and Filoviridae (from the Latin *filo*, "thread" or "filament" which describes the morphology of these viruses). In the early days of virology, it was also popular to name viruses after their discoverers; however, by the current rules persons' names may no longer be used in viral nomenclature.

Several viruses of medical importance remain unclassified. Some are difficult or impossible to propagate in standard laboratory host systems and thus cannot be obtained in sufficient quantity to permit more precise characterization. The hepatitis A virus is now classified as a picornavirus, and a new family, Hepadnaviridae, has been proposed to include human hepatitis B virus and related viruses from other species (see Ch. 70). The family Filoviridae has been accepted for the pleomorphic Marburg and Ebola viruses, the agents of African hemorrhagic fever, which do not appear to fit into any of the currently classified groups of animal viruses. The Norwalk virus and similar agents (Chapter 65) that cause nonbacterial gastroenteritis in humans are now recognized to be more similar to caliciviruses than to parvoviruses. The viruses that cause degenerative diseases in humans and other animals (scrapie in sheep; kuru and Kreutzfeldt-Jakob disease in humans) (see Ch. 71) have been likened to viroids because of their resistance to certain chemical and physical agents, particularly ultraviolet radiation. They are also similar to "prions," a name

TABLE 41-1 Chemical and Morphologic Properties of
Animal Virus Families

Family	Nucleic Acid Genome		Virion						
	Type and Configuration[a]	MW × 10^6	Shape[b]	Diameter (nm)	Enveloped[c]	Capsid Symmetry	No. of Capsomeres[d]	Site of Capsid Assembly	Transcriptase Present in Virion
Parvoviridae	ssDNA; sense or antisense	1.5–2.0	S	18–26	0	Icosahedral	32	Nucleus	None
Papovaviridae	dsDNA; circular	3–5	S	45–55	0	Icosahedral	72	Nucleus	None
Adenoviridae	dsDNA	20–25	S	70–90	0	Icosahedral	252	Nucleus	None
Herpesviridae	dsDNA	80–150	S	120–200	+	Icosahedral	162	Nucleus	None
Iridoviridae	dsDNA	100–250	S	125–300	+	Icosahedral	ca. 1,500	Cytoplasm	DNA-dependent RNA polymerase[e]
Poxviridae	dsDNA	85–240	X	240 × 300	+	Complex	—	Cytoplasm	DNA-dependent RNA polymerase
Hepadnaviridae	dsDNA; circular; one ss region	1.6–2.3	S	40–50	0	?	—	?	DNA-dependent DNA polymerase
Picornaviridae	ssRNA; sense	2.5	S	22–30	0	Icosahedral	32	Cytoplasm	None
Caliciviridae	ssRNA; sense	2.6–2.8	S	35–39	0	Icosahedral	32	Cytoplasm	None
Togaviridae	ssRNA; sense	4	S	40–70	+	Icosahedral	?	Cytoplasm	None
Reoviridae	dsRNA; 10–12 pieces	12–20	S	60–80	0	Icosahedral	32 or 92	Cytoplasm	RNA-dependent RNA polymerase

Orthomyxoviridae	ssRNA; 8 molecules, anti-sense	5	S^f	80–120	+	Helical	—	Cytoplasm	RNA-dependent RNA polymerase
Paramyxoviridae	ssRNA; mostly antisense	5–7	S^f	150–300	+	Helical	—	Cytoplasm	RNA-dependent RNA polymerase
Rhabdoviridae	ssRNA; antisense	3.5–4.6	U	60 × 180	+	Helical	—	Cytoplasm	RNA-dependent RNA polymerase
Bunyaviridae	ssRNA; 3 molecules, antisense	6–7	S	90–100	+	Helical	—	Cytoplasm	RNA-dependent RNA polymerase
Coronaviridae	ssRNA; sense	5.5–6.1	S	75–160	+	Helical	—	Cytoplasm	None
Arenaviridae	ssRNA; 5 molecules, 2 virus-specific	3–5	S	50–300	+	?	—	Cytoplasm	RNA-dependent RNA polymerase
Retroviridae	ssRNA; inverted dimer of sense strand	6–7	S	80–100	+	?	—	Cytoplasm	RNA-dependent DNA polymerase
Filoviridae	ssRNA; antisense	4.2	Pleomorphic	80 × 800–900	+	Complex	—	Cytoplasm	?

^{a} ss, Single stranded; ds, double-stranded.

^{b} S, spherical; X, brickshaped or ovoid; U, elongated with parallel sides and a round end.

^{c} Most enveloped viruses are sensitive to lipid solvents; however, some members of the Poxviridae are resistant to ether, and conversely, some members of Reoviridae (orbiviruses) are only partially resistant to lipid solvents.

^{d} Applicable to viruses with icosahedral symmetry.

^{e} Some members, including African swine fever virus.

^{f} Filamentous forms also occur.

TABLE 41-2   Current Classification of Major Groups of Viruses of Medical Significance

Family	Genera (or Subfamilies)	Vernacular Name of Type Species or Typical Member	Viruses Shown to Produce Infection in Humans
DNA Viruses			
Parvoviridae	*Parvovirus*	Latent rat virus	B19 virus associated with erythema infectiosum and aplastic crisis of sickle cell anemia
	Dependovirus	Adeno-associated virus (AAV) type 1	Defective viruses (infect humans in presence of a helper adenovirus)
Papovaviridae	*Papillomavirus*	Rabbit papilloma virus	Human papilloma (wart) viruses
	Polyomavirus	Polyomavirus (mouse)	JC and BK viruses, simian virus 40 (SV40)
Adenoviridae	*Mastadenovirus*	Human adenovirus type 2	≥40 human adenovirus serotypes (species)
Herpesviridae	Alphaherpesvirinae	Human herpesvirus 1	Herpes simplex virus type 1
		Human herpesvirus 2	Herpes simplex virus type 2
	Varicellovirus	Human herpesvirus 3	Varicella-zoster virus
	Gammaherpesvirinae	Human herpesvirus 4	Epstein-Barr virus
	Bethaherpesvirinae	Human herpesvirus 5	Human cytomegalovirus
		Human herpesvirus 6	Human B-lymphotropic virus
Poxviridae	Orthopoxvirus	*Vaccinia virus*	*Vaccinia, variola, cowpox, monkeypox viruses*
	Parapoxvirus	Orf virus	Orf, bovine pustular stomatitis, milker's node, molluscum contagiosum viruses
Hepadnaviridae	*Hepadna virus*	Hepatitis B virus	Hepatitis B virus
RNA Viruses			
Picornaviridae	*Enterovirus*	Poliovirus type 1	67 enterovirus serotypes
	Heparnavirus	Hepatitis A virus	Hepatitis A virus
	Rhinovirus	Human rhinovirus type 1	Over 100 rhinovirus serotypes
	Aphthovirus	Foot-and-mouth disease virus	Foot-and-mouth disease virus (rarely)

Continued

TABLE 41-2   *(continued)*

Family	Genera (or Subfamilies)	Vernacular Name of Type Species or Typical Member	Viruses Shown to Produce Infection in Humans
Caliciviridae	*Calicivirus*	Vesicular exanthem virus (swine)	Human gastroenteritis viruses (e.g., Norwalk virus)
Togaviridae	*Alphavirus*	Sindbis virus	Various group A arboviruses
	Rubivirus	Rubella virus	Rubella virus
Flaviviridae	*Flavivirus*	Yellow fever virus	Various group B arboviruses with segmented genomes
Reoviridae	*Reovirus*	Reovirus type 1	Reovirus types 1, 2, and 3
	Orbivirus	Bluetongue virus	Colorado tick fever virus
	Rotavirus	Human rotavirus	Human rotavirus
Orthomyxoviridae	*Influenzavirus*	Influenza virus type A, strain A/WS/33(H0N1)	Influenza virus types A and B
	Probable separate genus	Influenza virus type C	Influenza virus type C
Paramyxoviridae	*Paramyxovirus*	Newcastle disease virus (NDV)	Parainfluenza virus types 1 to 4, mumps virus, NDV
	Morbillivirus	Measles virus	Measles virus
	Pneumovirus	Respiratory syncytial virus	Respiratory syncytial virus
Rhabdoviridae	*Vesiculovirus*	Vesicular stomatitis virus (VSV)	VSV and Chandipura virus
	Lyssavirus	Rabies virus	Rabies, Mokola, Duvenhage viruses
Bunyaviridae	*Bunyavirus*	Bunyamwera virus	Various arthropod-transmitted viruses
	Phlebovirus	Sandfly fever Sicilian virus	Sandfly fever virus, Rift Valley fever virus
	Nairovirus	Crimean-Congo hemorrhagic fever virus	Crimean-Congo hemorrhagic fever virus, Nairobi sheep disease virus
	Hantavirus	Hantaan virus	Hemorrhagic fever with renal syndrome
Coronaviridae	*Coronavirus*	Avian infectious bronchitis virus	Human coronaviruses, several types
Arenaviridae	*Arenavirus*	Lymphocytic choriomeningitis virus	Lymphocytic choriomeningitis virus, Lassa viruses, viruses of the Tacaribe complex

Continued

TABLE 41-2   *(continued)*

Family	Genera (or Subfamilies)	Vernacular Name of Type Species or Typical Member	Viruses Shown to Produce Infection in Humans
Retroviridae	Oncovirinae	Type B or C oncovirus	Human T cell leukemia viruses
	Spumavirinae	Foamy virus group	Human foamy virus
	Lentivirinae	Maedi/visna virus group	Probably virus(es) associated with acquired immuno-deficiency syndrome
Filoviridae	*Filovirus*	Marburg virus	Marburg virus, Ebola virus

coined for replicating agents that have no demonstrable nucleic acid. Their properties do not fit completely into either of these categories, however, and they are still considered to be unconventional viruses within the group of agents that cause the subacute spongiform viral encephalopathies.

REFERENCES

Brown F: The classification and nomenclature of viruses: summary of results of meetings of the International Committee on Taxonomy of Viruses in Edmonton, Canada 1987. Intervirology 30:181, 1989

Caspar DLD: Design principles in virus particle construction. In Horsfall FL, Tamm I (eds): Viral and Rickettsial Infections in Man. 4th Ed. JB Lippincott, Philadelphia, 1975

Compans RW, Klenk H-D: Virus Membranes. In Fraenkel-Conrat H, Wagner RR (eds): Comprehensive Virology. Vol. 13. Plenum, New York, 1979

Fischer HW: Use of electron microscopy in virology. In Fraenkel-Conrat H, Wagner RR (eds): Comprehensive Virology. Vol. 17. Plenum, New York, 1981

Gajdusek DC: Unconventional viruses and the origin and disappearance of kuru. Science 197:943, 1977

Holmes IA: Rotaviruses. In Joklik WK (ed): Reoviridae. Plenum, New York, 1983

Jacrot B: Structural studies of viruses with x-rays and neutrons. In Fraenkel-Conrat H, Wagner RR (eds): Comprehensive Virology. Vol. 17. Plenum, New York, 1981

Kiley MP, Bowen ET, Eddy GA et al: Filoviridae: a taxonomic home for Marburg and Ebola viruses? Intervirology 18:24, 1982

Mattern CFT: Symmetry in virus architecture. In Nayak DP (ed): Molecular Biology of Animal Viruses. Marcel Dekker, New York, 1977

Matthews REF: Classification and nomenclature of viruses. Fourth report of the International Committee on Taxonomy of Viruses. Intervirology 17:1, 1982

Melnick JL: Taxonomy and nomenclature of viruses. Prog Med Virol 28:208, 1982

Palmer EL, Martin ML: Electron Microscopy in Viral Diagnosis. CRC Press, Boca Raton, FL, 1988

Siegl G: The human parvovirus. In Berns KI (ed): The Parvoviruses. Plenum, New York, 1984

42 MULTIPLICATION

BERNARD ROIZMAN

GENERAL CONCEPTS

Introductory Principles

Virus-induced pathology results from (1) a toxic effect of virus gene products, (2) host reactions to cells expressing virus genes, and (3) virus-induced modifications of host gene expression. Host **susceptibility** is the capacity of a cell or animal to become infected; the **host range** is the range of tissue cells and animal species in which a virus can multiply; the **portal of entry** is the host site where cells first become infected; and **target cells** are the cells in which infection leads to disease. The virus reproductive cycle is divided into the **eclipse** phase, just after the virus genome has been exposed to the host and viral synthetic machinery, and the **maturation** phase, in which progeny virions accumulate. Infection of a cell may be **productive** (yielding infectious viruses), **restrictive,** or **abortive** (not yielding infectious virus). Abortive infection may result either from infection of susceptible but nonpermissive cells, or from infection by defective or incomplete virus. Persistence of the viral genome is a more common consequence of restrictive and abortive than of productive infections.

Initiation of Infection

Initiation of viral infection has three phases: (1) **attachment** (specific binding of a virion protein to a constituent of the cell surface); (2) **penetration** (an energy-dependent step that may occur by translocation of the virion across the plasma membrane, by endocytosis, or by fusion of virion envelope with the cell membrane);

and (3) **uncoating** (exposure of the viral genome to host or viral synthetic machinery).

Strategies of Viral Multiplication

Requirements: The synthesis of viral proteins from viral mRNA by the protein-synthesizing machinery is a key event. Constraints: For some viruses, the host cell lacks enzymes to synthesize mRNA on the viral RNA genoma or enzymes capable of transcribing viral DNA in the cytoplasm. Eukaryotic cells rarely recognize internal initiation sites within viral mRNAs.

Encoding and Organization of Viral Genomes

Viral genes are encoded on either RNA or DNA; viral DNA may be either single stranded or double stranded. Some viruses have a single chromosome **(monopartite);** in others the genome consists of several chromosomes **(multipartite).**

Assembly, Maturation, and Egress

Nonenveloped viruses are assembled within the cell and released by cell lysis (e.g., picornaviruses, reoviruses, papovavirus, parvovirus, and adenoviruses). In enveloped viruses, the last step of virion assembly is combined with egress by budding through a cell membrane (e.g., antisense ((−)-strand) RNA viruses, togaviruses, and retroviruses). The herpesvirus nucleocapsid is assembled in the nucleus, and envelopment and maturation occur at the nuclear membrane.

Variability in Viral Genomes and Multiplication

A major focus of research is the role of genetic variation within the various species of viruses, on defective viruses, and on the viral genes expressed during restrictive and abortive infections as they influence the broad spectrum of clinical disease.

INTRODUCTION

The pathologic effects of virus diseases result from (1) a toxic effect of virus gene products on the metabolism of infected cells, (2) reactions of the host to infected cells expressing virus genes, and (3) modifications of host gene expression by structural or functional interactions with viral genetic material. In many instances, the symptoms and signs of acute viral diseases are directly related to destruction of cells by the infecting virus.

To multiply, a virus must first infect a cell. The **susceptibility** of a cell or animal is its capacity to become infected. The **host range** of a virus defines both the kinds of tissue cells and the animal species that it can infect and in which it can multiply. Viruses differ considerably in their host range. Some viruses (e.g., St. Louis encephalitis virus) have a wide host range, whereas the host range of others may be a specific set of differentiated cells of one species (e.g., human papillomaviruses multiply only in human keratinocytes). Determinants of the host range and susceptibility are discussed in the next section.

When an individual becomes exposed to a virus with a human host range, the cells that become immediately infected are the susceptible cells at the **portal of entry** (the host site where cells first become infected). Infection of these cells, however, may not be sufficient to cause clinically demonstrable disease. Disease is often the consequence of infection of target cells (e.g., in the central nervous system), by virus introduced into the body directly (e.g., via the bite of a mosquito), or made in the susceptible cells at the portal or entry. The target cells are often at the portal of entry (e.g., respiratory infections, genital herpes simplex infections).

In the course of infection, the virus introduces its genetic material—RNA or DNA—and often its essential proteins into the cell. The size, composition, and gene organization of viral genomes vary enormously. Viruses appear to have evolved by different routes, and although no single pattern of replication has prevailed, two concepts are vital to the understanding of how viruses multiply. First, the ability of a virus to multiply and the fate of an infected cell hinge on the synthesis and function of virus gene products—the proteins. Nowhere is the correlation between structure and function—between the sequence and arrangement of genetic material and the mechanism of expression—more apparent than in viruses. The diversity of mechanisms by which viruses ensure that their proteins are made is reflected in (but unfortunately not always deduced from) their genomic structure. Second, although viruses differ considerably in the number of genes they contain, all viruses encode a minimum of three sets of functions, which are expressed by the proteins they specify. Viral proteins (1) ensure the replication of the viral genomes, (2) package the genome into virus particles (the **virions**), and (3) alter the structure and/or function of the infected cell. The capacity to remain latent, a feature essential for the survival of some viruses in the human population, is an additional function expressed by the proteins of some viruses.

The strategy used by viruses to ensure the execution of these functions varies. In a few instances (papovaviruses), viral proteins merely assist host enzymes to replicate the viral genome. In most instances (e.g., picornaviruses, reoviruses, herpesviruses), the viral proteins replicate the virus genome; however, even the most self-reliant virus uses at least some host proteins in this process. In all instances, the viral proteins package the genome into virions, even though host proteins or polyamines may complex with viral genomes (e.g., papovaviruses) before or during the biogenesis of the virus particle. The effects of viral multiplication may range from cell death to subtle but potentially very significant changes in cell function and in the spectrum of antigens expressed on the cell surface.

A few years ago, our knowledge of viral reproductive cycles stemmed mainly from analyses of the events in synchronously infected cells in culture; we knew little concerning viruses that had not yet been grown in cultured cells. Recently, molecular cloning and expression of viral genes has enriched enormously our knowledge of viruses that grow poorly if at all in cells in culture (e.g., human hepadnaviruses, human papillomaviruses).

The reproductive cycles of all viruses have several common features (Fig. 42-1). First, shortly after infection and for up to several hours thereafter, only small amounts of parental infectious virus can be detected. This interval is known as the **eclipse phase;** it signals the fact that the viral genomes are exposed to host or viral machinery necessary for their expression, but that progeny virus production has not yet reached a detectable level. There follows the **maturation phase,** an interval in which viral components continue to be synthesized and progeny virions accumulate at exponential rates in the cell or in the extracellular environment. After several hours (e.g., in picornaviruses) or days (e.g., in cytomegalovirus), cells infected with lytic viruses cease all metabolic activity and lose their structural integrity. Cells infected with nonlytic viruses may continue to synthesize viruses indefinitely. The reproductive cycle of viruses ranges from 8 hours (picornaviruses) to more than 72 hours (some herpesviruses). The virus yields per cell range from several thousand poxvirus particles to more than 100,000 poliovirus particles.

Infection of a susceptible cell does not automatically ensure that viral multiplication will follow and that viral progeny will emerge. This is among the most important conceptual developments in virology and should be stressed in some detail. Infection of susceptible cells may be **productive, restrictive,** or **abortive.** Productive infection occurs in **permissive** cells and is characterized by produc-

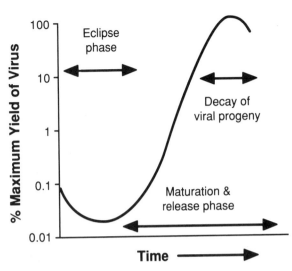

FIGURE 42-1   Reproductive cycle of viruses that infect eukaryotic cells. The time scale varies for different viruses; it may range from 8 hours (e.g., poliovirus) to more than 72 hours (e.g., cytomegalovirus).

tion of infectious progeny. Abortive infection can occur for two reasons. Although a cell may be susceptible to infection, it may be **nonpermissive,** allowing a few (but not all) viral genes to be expressed, for reasons that are rarely known. Abortive infection may also result from infection of either permissive or nonpermissive cells with defective viruses, which lack a full complement of viral genes. Lastly, cells may be only transiently permissive, with the consequence either that the virus persists in the cell until the cell becomes permissive or that only a few of the cells in a population produce viral progeny at any time. This type of infection has been called **restrictive** by some and **restringent** by others. This classification is neither trivial nor gratuitous; its significance stems from the observation that cytolytic viruses, which normally destroy permissive cells during productive infection, may merely injure abortively infected, permissive, or nonpermissive cells. The consequences of this injury may be the expression of host functions that transform the cell from normal to malignant. Persistence of the viral genomes is a more common consequence of restrictive and abortive infections.

INITIATION OF INFECTION

To infect a cell, the virus must attach to the cell surface, penetrate the cell, and become sufficiently uncoated to make its genome accessible to viral or host machinery for transcription or translation.

Attachment

Attachment constitutes specific binding of a virion protein (the antireceptor) to a constituent of the cell surface (the receptor). The classic example of an antireceptor is the hemagglutinin of influenza virus (an orthomyxovirus). The antireceptors are distributed throughout the surfaces of viruses that infect human and animal cells. Complex viruses, such as herpes simplex virus (a herpesvirus), may carry more than one species of antireceptor molecule. Mutations in the genes specifying antireceptors may result in a loss of the capacity to interact with certain receptors. The cellular receptors identified thus far are largely glycoproteins.

Attachment requires ions in concentrations sufficient to reduce electrostatic repulsion, but it is largely temperature and energy independent. The susceptibility of a cell is limited by the availability of appropriate receptors, and not all cells in an otherwise susceptible organism express receptors. Human kidney cells lack receptors for poliovirus in situ, but receptors appear when the cells are propagated in cell culture. Susceptibility should not be confused with permissiveness. Although chicken cells are not susceptible to poliovirions because they lack receptors for attachment of the virus, they are fully permissive: they produce infectious virus following transfection with intact viral RNA extracted from poliovirus particles. Attachment of viruses to cells in some instances (e.g., picornaviruses) leads to irreversible changes in the structure of the virion. In other instances (e.g., orthomyxoviruses and paramyxoviruses, which carry a neuraminidase on their surface), if penetration does not ensue, the virus can detach and readsorb to a different cell. These viruses can elute from their receptors by cleaving neuraminic acid from the polysaccharide chains of the receptors.

Penetration

Penetration is an energy-dependent step that occurs almost instantaneously after attachment and involves one of three mechanisms: (1) translocation of the virion across the plasma membrane; (2) endocytosis of the virus particle, resulting in accumulation of virions inside cytoplasmic vacuoles; and (3) fusion of the cellular membrane with the virion envelope. Nonenveloped viruses penetrate by one of the first two mechanisms. For example, during adsorption of poliovirus, the capsid becomes modified and loses its integrity as it is translocated into the cytoplasm. For viruses that penetrate as a consequence of fusion of their envelopes with the plasma membrane (e.g., herpesviruses), the envelope remains in the plasma membrane but the internal constituents spill into the cytoplasm. Fusion of viral envelopes with the plasma membrane requires the interaction of specific viral proteins in the viral envelope with proteins in the cellular membrane.

Uncoating

Uncoating is a general term applied to the events that occur after penetration and set the stage for the viral genome to express its functions. For most viruses, the virion disaggregates, alone or with the aid of cellular components (enzymes), and only the nucleic acid or a nucleic acid-protein complex remains before expression of viral functions. In the exceptional case of reoviruses, only portions of the capsid are removed and the viral genome expresses all of its functions, even though it is never fully released from the capsid. The poxvirus genome is uncoated in two stages: although in the first stage the outer covering is removed by host enzymes, the release of viral DNA from the core appears to require the participation of viral gene products made after infection.

STRATEGIES OF VIRAL MULTIPLICATION
Requirements and Constraints

In the course of their evolution, viruses have developed several different strategies to deal with encoding and organization of viral genes, gene expression, genome replication, and assembly and maturation of viral progeny. Before these strategies are considered in detail, it should be reiterated that the synthesis of viral proteins by the host protein-synthesizing machinery is the key event in viral replication. Irrespective of the size, composition, and organization of its genome, the virus must present to the protein-synthesizing machinery of the eukaryotic cell a messenger RNA (mRNA) that the cell can recognize as such and translate. The cell does impose two constraints on viruses. First, the cell synthesizes its own mRNA in the nucleus by transcription of its DNA, followed by posttranscriptional processing of the transcript. The cell therefore lacks (1) the enzymes necessary to synthesize mRNA on a viral RNA genome, either in the nucleus or in the cytoplasm; and (2) enzymes capable of transcribing viral DNAs in the cytoplasm. The consequence of this constraint is that only viruses whose genomes consist of DNA that reaches the nucleus can take advantage of cell transcriptases to synthesize their mRNAs. All other viruses have had to develop their own transcriptases to generate mRNA. The second constraint is that the protein-synthesizing machinery of eukaryotic cells is equipped to translate monocistronic mRNAs, inasmuch as it does not usually recognize internal initiation sites within mRNAs. The consequences of this constraint are that viruses direct the synthesis of a separate mRNA for each polypeptide (functionally monocistronic mRNAs) or of one or more mRNAs encoding a large precursor "polyprotein," which is subsequently cleaved into individual proteins. In rare instances (e.g., retroviruses), by using a specific frameshift determined by its structure, the same mRNA directs the synthesis of two distinct sets of proteins.

Encoding and Organization of Viral Genomes

Viral genes are encoded in either RNA or DNA genomes, which may be either single stranded or double stranded. In addition, the genome can be **monopartite** (carried on a single chromosome) or **multipartite** (distributed on several chromosomes and, together, constituting the viral genome). To avoid confusion, we shall designate as "genomic" only the nucleic acid found in virions. Among the RNA viruses, the reoviruses represent the best-known family that contains a double-stranded genome, and this genome is multipartite, consisting of 10 segments or chromosomes. The genomes of single-stranded RNA viruses are either monopartite (picornaviruses, togaviruses, paramyxoviruses, rhabdoviruses, coronaviruses, and retroviruses) or multipartite (orthomyxoviruses, arenaviruses, and bunyaviruses). All RNA genomes are linear. Some (e.g., picornaviruses) contain a covalently linked polypeptide or an amino acid at the 5' end of the RNA.

All known DNA viruses that infect vertebrate hosts contain a monopartite genome. Except for the parvovirus genomes, all are at least partially double stranded. Individual parvovirus virions contain linear single-stranded DNA; in some genera (e.g., adeno-associated virus), both complementary strands of the DNA are packaged, but in different virus particles. The genomes of papovaviruses and papillomaviruses are closed-circular DNA molecules. While the genomes of adenoviruses and herpesviruses are linear double-stranded molecules, one strand at each end of the adenovirus genome is covalently linked to a protein, whereas the herpesvirus DNAs exhibit a 3' single nucleotide extension at each terminus. The DNAs of poxviruses are also linear, but in this instance the 3' terminus of each strand is covalently linked to the 5' terminus of the complementary strand, forming a continuous loop. The DNA of hepatitis B virus is a circular, double-stranded molecule, in which each strand has a gap.

Expression and Replication of Viral Genomes

It is convenient to discuss the RNA viruses first and to focus primarily on the function of the genomic RNA.

Single-Stranded RNA Viruses

The linear single-stranded RNA viruses form three groups. Picornaviruses and togaviruses are examples of the first group. These genomes have two functions (Figs. 42-2 and 42-3). The first of these functions is to serve as an mRNA. By convention, viruses whose genomes can and do serve as mRNAs are known as **sense-strand** (or **(+)-strand**) **viruses.** After entering the cell, the picornavirus RNA binds to ribosomes and is translated in its entirety (Fig. 42-2). The product of this translation—the polyprotein—is then cleaved by proteolytic enzymes. While secondary cleavages clearly involve virus-specified proteases, there is good evidence that the polyprotein itself is enzymatically active in that each molecule cleaves other polyproteins *(trans)* but not itself. The second function of the genomic RNA is to serve as a template for the synthesis of a complementary **antisense ((−)- strand)** RNA strand by a polymerase derived from cleavage of the polyprotein. The antisense (−) strand then serves in turn as a template to make additional sense (+) strands. The progeny sense strands can then serve as (1) mRNA, (2) templates to make more antisense strands, and (3) constituents of progeny virus particles.

Togaviruses and some of the other sense (+)- strand RNA viruses differ in one respect from picornaviruses (Fig. 42-3). Specifically, only a portion of the genomic RNA is available for translation in the first round of protein synthesis (Fig. 42-3). The probable function of the resulting products is to transcribe the genomic RNA to yield a full-length antisense (−) RNA strand. This antisense (−) strand serves as a template for two size classes of sense RNA molecules. The first class is a small mRNA encompassing the region of the genomic RNA not translated in the first round; the resulting polyprotein is cleaved into proteins whose main function is to serve as structural components of the virions. The second class is the full-sized genomic RNA, which is packaged into virions. Several mRNA species (nested RNAs) are made in cells infected with coronaviruses.

Central to the replication of sense-strand viruses is the capability of the genomic RNA to serve as mRNA after infection. There are two consequences. First, enzymes responsible for the replication of the genomes are made after infection and

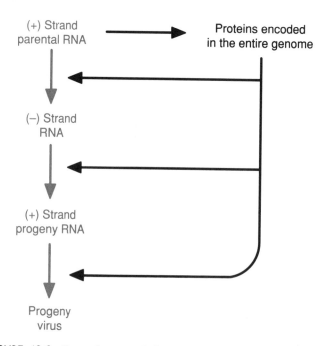

FIGURE 42-2 Flow of events during the replication of picornaviruses.

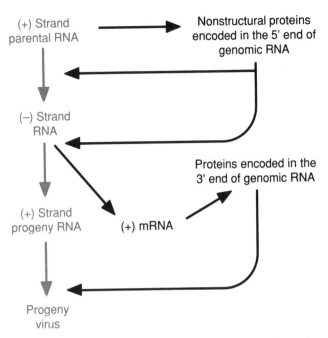

FIGURE 42-3 Flow of events during the replication of togaviruses.

need not be brought into the infected cell by the virion. This is why naked RNA extracted from virions is infectious. Second, because all sense-strand genomes are monopartite, having all their genes linked in a single chromosome, the initial products of translation of both genomic RNA and of mRNA species are necessarily a single protein. The translation products of picornaviruses and togaviruses must then be cleaved to yield the individual proteins found in the virion or in the infected cell.

The multipartite orthomyxoviruses, bunyaviruses, and arenaviruses, paramyxoviruses, and the monopartite and rhabdoviruses (Fig. 42-4) make up the second set of single-stranded RNA viruses, defined as the *antisense-strand viruses.* Characteristically, their genomic RNAs must serve two template functions, first for transcription and then for replication. Because the genome must be transcribed to make mRNA and the cell lacks the appropriate enzymes, all antisense viruses package a transcriptase along with the viral genome in the virion. The transcription of the viral genome is the first event after entry of the virus into cells; the

process yields functionally monocistronic sense mRNAs, each specifying a single protein. Replication begins under the direction of newly synthesized viral proteins; a full-length sense strand is made and serves as a template for the synthesis of antisense-strand genomic RNAs (Fig. 42-4).

To reiterate, in contrast to the sense-strand viruses, the antisense virus genome serves as a template for transcription only, first for the synthesis of mRNA and then for the transcription of a sense strand which in turn serves as the template for an antisense strand. There are three consequences. First, the virus must bring into the infected cell the transcriptase to make its mRNAs. Second, it follows that naked RNA extracted from virions is not infectious. Third, the mRNAs produced are gene unit length (e.g., they specify a single polypeptide). However, selective (but not arbitrary) observance of RNA synthesis initiation and termination signals or splicing signals may result in multiple mRNAs, each specifying a different protein transcribed from the same region of genomic RNA. Consequently the sense transcript that functions as mRNA is different from the sense-strand RNA

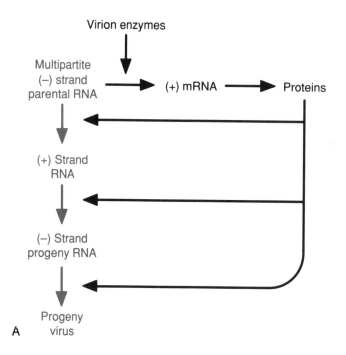

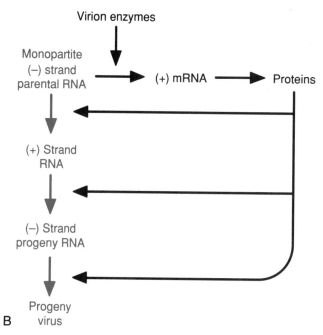

FIGURE 42-4 Flow of events during the replication of multipartite orthomyxoviruses, bunyaviruses, and arenaviruses (A) and monopartite paramyxoviruses and rhabdoviruses (B).

that serves as the template for progeny virus, even though both are synthesized on the genomic RNA! The advantages of the transcription of multiple mRNAs from the same region through splicing of the RNA are obvious. Monocistronic mRNA is advantageous because the virus can control the abundance of the individual proteins; they need not be made in equimolar amounts.

Retroviruses comprise the third group of RNA viruses (Fig. 42-5). Characteristically, retrovirus genomes are monopartite but diploid, and the two strands are either partially hydrogen bonded to another macromolecule or base paired in an unknown fashion. Following infection, the sole known function of the genomic RNA is to serve as a template for the synthesis of viral DNA. Inasmuch as eukaryotic cells lack enzymes competent to perform this function, the virion contains, in addition to the genome, an RNA-dependent DNA polymerase **(reverse transcriptase),** as well as a mixture of host transfer RNAs (tRNAs), one of which serves as the primer for transcription. The key steps in the genome transcription are (1) binding of the tRNA-reverse transcriptase complex to the genomic RNA; (2) synthesis of a DNA molecule complementary to the genomic RNA, coupled with the digestion of the RNA by a viral ribonuclease (RNase H, also packaged in the virion) specific for RNA in RNA-DNA hybrids; and (3) synthesis of the complementary DNA strand and completion of a linear DNA molecule containing in its entirety the sequences contained in the genomic RNA, but with the duplication of two small sequences, one from the 3′ terminus of the RNA duplicated at the 5′ terminus of the DNA, and one from the 5′ terminus of the RNA duplicated at the 3′ terminus of the DNA. The double-stranded DNA is then translocated into the nucleus, where it is integrated into the host genome by viral proteins (see Ch. 47 and Fig. 47-1). Virus gene expression may or may not ensue. When it does occur, the integrated viral DNA is transcribed by the host RNA polymerase II. The products of transcription are genome-length RNA molecules and shorter, gene-cluster-length mRNAs, which are translated to yield polyproteins. The polyproteins are then cleaved to yield the individual viral proteins. Only genome-length transcripts are packaged into virions.

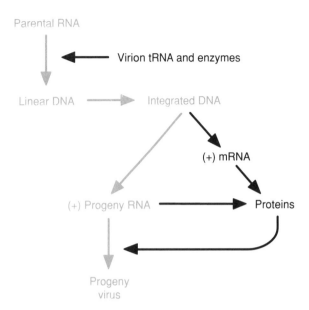

FIGURE 42-5 Flow of events during the replication of retroviruses.

Double-Stranded RNA Viruses

The double-stranded, multipartite reovirus genome is transcribed within the partially opened capsid by a polymerase packaged into the virion, and the 10 different mRNA (sense) species are extruded through the exposed vertices of the capsid (Fig. 42-6). The mRNA molecules have two functions. First, they are translated as monocistronic mRNAs to yield the viral proteins. Second, one of each of the 10 RNA species assembles within a precursor particle, in which they serve as a template for the synthesis of the complementary strand, yielding double-stranded genome segments.

DNA Virus Genomes

The DNA viruses can be split into four groups. The papovavirus, adenovirus, and herpesvirus genomes are transcribed and replicated in the nucleus and therefore can utilize the transcriptional enzymes of the host for generation of mRNA. As expected, the DNAs of these viruses are infectious. The transcriptional program consists of at least

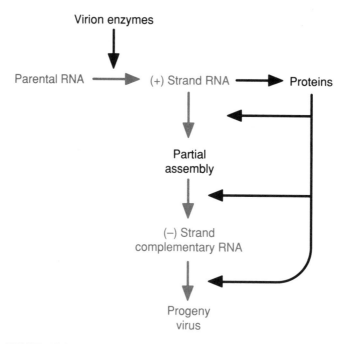

FIGURE 42-6   Flow of events during the replication of reoviruses.

two cycles of transcription for papovaviruses and at least three for herpesviruses (Fig. 42-7) and adenoviruses. In each instance, the structural or virion polypeptides are made from mRNA generated from the last cycle of transcription.

The poxviruses constitute the second group. Although poxvirus DNAs have been detected in the nucleus, the transcription and most of the other events in the reproductive cycle appear to take place in the cytoplasm. The genome is transcribed by a viral enzyme. The initial transcription occurs in the core of the virion. Many questions concerning the reproductive cycle of poxviruses remain unresolved.

Parvoviruses constitute the third group. One human parvovirus, the adeno-associated virus, requires adenoviruses or herpes simplex viruses as helper viruses for its multiplication. In the absence of a helper virus, the genome appears to integrate into a specific locus of a human chromosome. Other human parvoviruses are capable of multiplying without the assistance of a helper virus. Viral replication involves the synthesis of a DNA

strand complementary to the single-stranded genomic DNA in the nucleus and the transcription of the genome.

The hepatitis B virus exemplifies the fourth group (Fig. 42-8). The gaps in the DNA of this virus are first repaired by a DNA polymerase packaged in the virion, converting the DNA into a closed-circular molecule, and the genome is then transcribed into two classes of RNA molecules: an mRNA specifying proteins and a genomic RNA that is transcribed by a reverse transcriptase to make the genomic DNA.

ASSEMBLY, MATURATION, AND EGRESS OF VIRUSES FROM INFECTED CELLS

Viruses have evolved two fundamental strategies to achieve assembly, maturation, and egress from the infected cell. The first, exemplified by the nonenveloped viruses (e.g., picornaviruses, reoviruses, papovaviruses, parvoviruses, and adenoviruses) involves intracellular assembly and

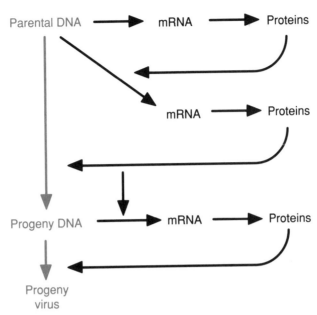

FIGURE 42-7 Flow of events during the replication of herpesviruses (e.g., herpes simplex virus).

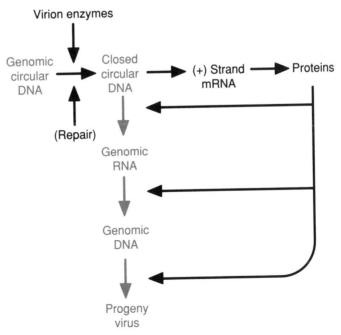

FIGURE 42-8 Flow of events during the replication of hepadna viruses (e.g., hepatitis B virus).

maturation. For picornaviruses, 60 copies each of virion proteins, designated as VP0, VP1, and VP3, assembly in the cytoplasm into a **procapsid.** Viral RNA is then packaged into the procapsid and, in the process, VP0 is cleaved to yield two polypeptides, VP2 and VP4. The cleavage causes a rearrangement of the capsid into a thermodynamically stable structure in which the RNA is shielded from access by nucleases. Reoviruses also assemble in the cytoplasm. In contrast, adenoviruses, papovaviruses, and parvoviruses assemble in the nucleus. As a rule, all viruses that assemble and acquire infectivity inside the nucleus depend largely but not entirely on the disintegration of the infected cell for their egress. The disintegration of the cell and the shutoff of host macromolecular metabolism, however, are frequently the functions of viral structural proteins.

The second strategy is used by enveloped viruses, including all antisense RNA viruses, togaviruses, and retroviruses. In this strategy the last step of virion assembly is combined with its egress from the infected cell. In these enveloped viruses, the viral proteins carrying appropriate signal sequences or other recognition markers become inserted into both the inner and outer surface of the plasma membrane or of other cytoplasmic membranes. The proteins projecting from the outer surface usually become glycosylated by host enzymes and aggregate into patches, displacing host membrane proteins. Viral nucleocapsids bind to special virus-specified proteins lining the cytoplasmic side of these patches or to cytoplasmic domains of viral glycoproteins (e.g., in togaviruses) and become wrapped up by the patch. In the process, the nascent virion is "extruded" or "buds" into the extracellular environment. In some instances (e.g., in orthomyxoviruses and paramyxoviruses), cleavage and rearrangement of one species of surface protein occurs during or after extrusion and imparts to the newly formed virion the capability of infecting cells. Virus assembly and maturation by extrusion from the cell surface provide a more efficient mechanism of egress, in that they do not depend on the disintegration of the infected cell. Indeed, viruses that mature and exit in this fashion vary considerably in their effects on

host cell metabolism and integrity. They range from highly cytolytic (e.g., togaviruses, paramyxoviruses, and rhabdoviruses) to frequently noncytolytic (e.g., retroviruses). By virtue of the insertion of the viral glycoproteins into the cell surface, however, these viruses impart to the cell a new antigenic specificity, and the infected cell becomes a target for the immune mechanisms of the host.

The herpesvirus nucleocapsid is assembled in the nucleus. Unlike other enveloped viruses, envelopment and maturation of herpesviruses occur at the inner lamella of the nuclear membrane. The enveloped virus accumulates in the space between the inner and outer lamellae of the nuclear membrane, in the cisternae of the cytoplasmic reticulum, and in vesicles carrying the virus to the cell surface. The enveloped virus is uniquely shielded from contact with the cytoplasm. Herpesviruses are cytolytic and invaraibly destroy the cells in which they multiply. Like other enveloped viruses, herpesviruses impart new antigenic specificities to the infected cell.

VARIABILITY IN VIRAL GENOMES AND VIRAL MULTIPLICATION

A major focus of research in virology is on the role of genetic variation within the various species of viruses, on defective viruses, and on restrictive and abortive infections in human disease. Interest in these phenomena stems from several observations, including the observations that the spectrum of clinical disease caused by many of the viruses that infect humans varies considerably in severity and symptomatology; that some viruses (e.g., human lentiviruses, a subfamily of retroviruses) vary considerably in nucleotide sequence; and that many years after a primary infection, individuals may exhibit symptoms of recurrent infection, of chronic debilitating diseases of the central nervous system, and of cancer apparently related to that infection. Our understanding of the relationship of these phenomena to the various manifestations and sequelae of virus infection is summarized in the following discussion.

Viruses belonging to the same species and family may differ enormously. For example, no two epidemiologically unrelated strains of herpes simplex virus are identical with respect to the nucleotide sequence of their genomes. Human immunodeficienty viruses (HIV) vary considerably in nucleotide sequence. The notion that some naturally occurring strains are more likely to cause severe illness than others is more anecdotal than proven, but it is not farfetched.

It is convenient to classify defective viruses into two groups. Viruses in the first group lack one or more essential genes and therefore are incapable of independent replication without a helper virus. Interest in this group stems from the suspicion that specific types of defective viruses (e.g., papillomaviruses) can transform infected cells from normal to malignant or (e.g., herpesviruses) can transactivate oncogenic viruses, causing the cell to become malignant. The second group comprises viruses that contain mutations and deletions and therefore cannot replicate in an efficient fashion. Interest in this group stems largely from the suspicion that chronic debilitating infections of the central nervous system might be related to viruses that are sluggish in their replication, in their ability to destroy the infected cells, or in their ability to alter the infected cell sufficiently to make it a target for the host immune system.

Restrictive and abortive infections are of interest chiefly because the cell may survive and perpetuate the viral genome indefinitely for the life of the host. A cell restrictively infected with a competent virus may be a latent reservoir of virus, which can replicate and disseminate when the cell is triggered to become permissive. A cell abortively infected with a defective virus may also survive and, given the appropriate stimulus, may become malignant. In some instances, restrictive infections are related to the requirement that the virus be maintained in a specific cell to be perpetuated with its natural host. To reiterate, the role of these phenomena in human disease is strongly suspected, but not proven. Undoubtedly they will be the focus of investigation for many years.

REFERENCES

Baltimore D: Expression of animal virus genomes. Bacteriol Rev 35:235, 1971

Fields BN, Knipe DM, Chanock RM et al (eds): Virology. 2nd Ed. Raven Press, New York, 1990

Narayan O, Clements JE: Biology and pathogenesis of lentiviruses. J Gen Virol 70:1617, 1989

Palese P, Roizman B (eds): Genetic variation of viruses. Ann NY Acad Sci 354:1, 1980

43

VIRAL GENETICS

W. ROBERT FLEISCHMANN, JR.

GENERAL CONCEPTS

Genetic Change in Viruses

Viruses are continuously changing as a result of genetic selection. They undergo subtle genetic changes through **mutation** and major genetic changes through **recombination.** Mutation occurs when an error is incorporated in the viral genome. Recombination occurs when coinfecting viruses exchange genetic information, creating a novel virus.

Mutations

Mutation Rates and Outcomes: The mutation rates of DNA viruses approximate those of eukaryotic cells, yielding in theory one mutant virus in several hundred to many thousand genome copies. RNA viruses have much higher mutation rates, perhaps one mutation per virus genome copy. Mutations can be deleterious, neutral, or occasionally favorable. Only mutations that do not interfere with essential virus functions can persist in a virus population.

Phenotypic Variation by Mutations: Mutations can produce viruses with new antigenic determinants. The appearance of an antigenically novel virus through mutation is called **antigenic drift.** Antigenically altered viruses may be able to cause disease in previously resistant or immune hosts.

Vaccine Strains from Mutation: Mutations can produce viruses with a reduced pathogenicity, altered host range, or altered target cell specificity but with intact antigenicity. Such viruses can sometimes be used as vaccine strains.

Recombination

Recombination involves the exchange of genetic material between two related viruses during coinfection of a host cell.

Recombination by Independent Assortment: Recombination by independent assortment can occur among viruses with segmented genomes. Genes that reside on different pieces of nucleic acid are randomly assorted. This can result in the generation of viruses with new antigenic determinants and new host ranges. Development of viruses with new antigenic determinants through independent assortment is called **antigenic shift.**

Recombination of Incompletely Linked Genes: Genes that reside on the same piece of nucleic acid may undergo recombination. The closer two genes are together, the rarer is recombination between them (partial linkage).

Phenotypic Variation from Recombination: Development of viruses with new antigenic determinants by either type of recombination may allow viruses to infect and cause disease in previously immune hosts.

Vaccines through Recombination: Vaccine strains of viruses can be used to create recombinant viruses that carry extra genes coding for a specific immunogen. During viral vaccination, the replicating virus will express the specific immunogen. Specific antibody production will be stimulated, and the host will be protected from the immunogen as well as from the vaccine virus.

INTRODUCTION

Viruses are simple entities, lacking an energy-generating system and having very limited biosynthetic capabilities. The smallest viruses have only a few genes; the largest viruses have as many as 200. Genetically, however, viruses have many features in common with cells. Viruses are subject to mutations, the genomes of different viruses can recombine to form novel progeny, the expression of the viral genome can be regulated, and viral gene products can interact. By studying viruses, we can learn more about the mechanisms by which viruses and their host cells function.

GENETIC CHANGE IN VIRUSES

This chapter covers the mechanisms by which genetic changes occur in viruses. Two principal mechanisms are involved: **mutation** and **recombination.** Alterations in the genetic material of a virus may lead to changes in the function of viral proteins. Such changes may result in the creation of new viral serotypes or viruses of altered virulence.

MUTATIONS

Mutations arise by one of three mechanisms: (1) by the effects of physical mutagens (UV light, x-rays) on nucleic acids; (2) by the natural behavior of the bases that make up nucleic acids (resonance from keto to enol and from amino to imino forms), and (3) through the fallibility of the enzymes that replicate the nucleic acids. The first two mechanisms act similarly in all viruses; hence, the effects of physical mutagens and the natural behavior of nucleotides are relatively constant. However, viruses differ markedly in their mutation rates, which is due primarily to differences in the fidelity with which their enzymes replicate their nucleic acids. Viruses with high-fidelity transcriptases have relatively low mutation rates and vice versa.

Mutation Rates and Outcomes

DNA viruses have mutation rates similar to those of eukaryotic cells because, like eukaryotic DNA polymerases, their replicatory enzymes have proofreading functions. The error rate for DNA viruses has been calculated to be 10^{-8} to 10^{-11} errors per incorporated nucleotide. With this low mutation rate, replication of even the most complex DNA viruses, which have 2×10^5 to 3×10^5 nucleotide pairs per genome, will generate mutants rather rarely, perhaps once in several hundred to many thousand genome copies. The RNA viruses, however, lack a proofreading function in their replicatory enzymes, and some have mutation rates that are many orders of magnitude higher — 10^{-3} to 10^{-4} errors per incorporated nucleotide. Even the simplest RNA viruses, which have about 7,400 nucleotides per genome, will generate mutants frequently, perhaps as often as once per genome copy.

Not all mutations that occur persist in the virus population. Mutations that interfere with the essential functions of attachment, penetration, uncoating, replication, assembly, and release are rapidly lost from the population. However, because of the redundancy of the genetic code, many mutations are neutral, resulting either in no change in the viral protein or in replacement of an amino acid by a functionally similar amino acid. Only mutations that do not cripple essential viral functions can persist or become fixed in a virus population.

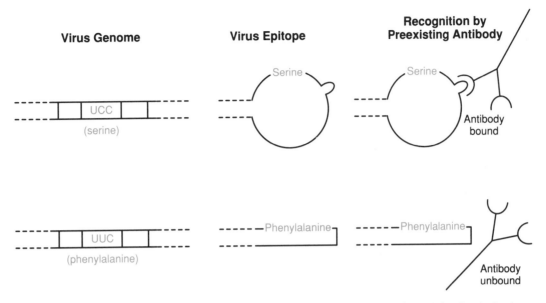

FIGURE 43-1 Mutation causing phenotypic (antigenic) variation. Mutation of the codon for the hydrophilic amino acid serine to the codon for the hydrophobic amino acid phenylalanine can change an epitope on the viral hemagglutinin protein and thereby alter its recognition by specific antibody. The mutant virus may then be able to infect a previously immune host.

Phenotypic Variation by Mutations

Mutations that alter the viral phenotype but are not deleterious may be important. For example, mutation can create novel antigenic determinants. A mutation in the hemagglutinin gene of influenza A virus can give rise to a hemagglutinin molecule with an altered antigenic site (epitope) (Fig. 43-1). Provided the attachment function of the new hemagglutinin is intact, the mutant virus may be able to initiate an infection in an individual immune to viruses expressing the previous hemagglutinin. For example, from 1968 to 1979, mutations altered 10 percent of the amino acids in the influenza virus hemagglutinin serotype H_3 molecule. This relatively modest mechanism of antigenic change through mutation, called **antigenic drift,** may allow a virus to outflank host defenses and cause disease in previously immune individuals.

Vaccine Strains from Mutation

Mutation has been a principal tool of virologists in developing attenuated live virus vaccines (Table 43-1). For example, the Sabin vaccine strains of poliovirus were developed by growing polioviruses in monkey kidney cells. Mutation and selection produced variant polioviruses that were adapted for efficient replication in these cells. Some of the mutations in these variants affected the genes coding for the poliovirus coat proteins in such a way as to produce mutants unable to attach to human neural cells but still able to infect human intestinal cells. Infection of human intestinal cells does not produce paralytic disease but does induce immunity. Poliovirus vaccine strains 1 and 2 have multiple mutations in the coat proteins and are very stable. The type 3 vaccine strain is less stable and is subject to back-mutations (reversions) that restore neural virulence. This vaccine strain therefore causes paralytic disease in one out of every several million vaccinated individuals. Despite the possibility of back-mutations, the generation and selection of attenuated viral mutants remains an important mechanism for producing viral vaccines.

TABLE 43-1   Live Attenuated Virus Vaccines

Viral Vaccine	Cell Used for Production of Attenuated Virus
Measles virus (rubeola virus)	Chick embryo cells
German measles virus (rubella virus)	Monkey kidney cells
Mumps virus	Embryonated chicken egg
Poliovirus	Monkey kidney cells
Yellow fever virus	Chick embryo cells

RECOMBINATION

Viral recombination occurs when viruses of two different parent strains coinfect the same host cell and interact during replication to generate virus progeny that have some genes from both parents. Recombination generally occurs between members of the same virus type (e.g., between two influenza viruses or between two herpes simplex viruses. Two mechanisms of recombination have been observed for viruses: **independent assortment** and **incomplete linkage.** Either mechanism can produce new viral serotypes or viruses with altered virulence.

Recombination by Independent Assortment

Independent assortment occurs when viruses that have multipartite (segmented) genomes trade segments during replication (Fig. 43-2). These genes are unlinked and assort at random. Recombination by independent assortment has been reported, for example, for the influenza viruses and

Steps

1. Dual infection (coinfection)

2. Uncoating of segmented virus genomes

3. Replication of genome segments

4. Assortment of genome segments

5. Progeny virus with independently assorted genome segments

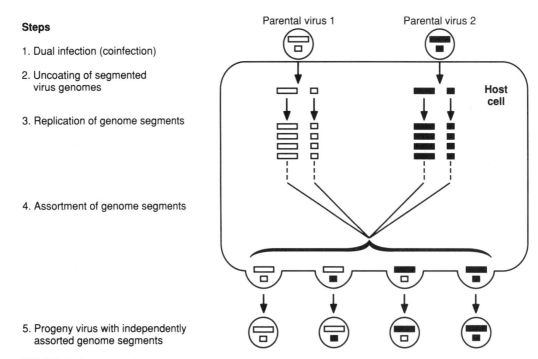

FIGURE 43-2 Recombination by independent assortment during dual infection. After infection of a cell with two viruses with two or more genetic segments ("chromosomes"), reassortment of the replicated segments can occur. Independent assortment results in the generation of progeny viruses whose genomes contain segments of genome from both types of parental virus.

TABLE 43-2 Antigenic Shifts
Resulting from Reassortment of
Genome Segments

Year	Strain
1890	H2N8
1900	H3N8
1918	H1N1
1957	H2N2 (Asian flu)
1968	H3N2 (Hong Kong flu)
1977	H1N1

other orthomyxoviruses (8 segments of single-stranded RNA) and for the reoviruses (10 segments of double-stranded RNA). The frequency of recombination by independent assortment is 6 to 20 percent for orthomyxoviruses. Independent assortment between an animal and a human strain of influenza virus (see Ch. 58) during a mixed infection can yield an antigenically novel influenza virus strain capable of infecting humans but carrying animal-strain hemagglutinin and/or neuraminidase surface molecules. This recombinant can infect individuals immune to the parent human virus. This mechanism results in an immediate, major antigenic change and is called **antigenic shift.** Antigenic shifts in influenza virus antigens can give rise to pandemics (worldwide epidemics) of influenza. Such antigenic shifts have occurred relatively frequently during recent history (Table 43-2). Because the number of different serotypes of hemagglutinin and neuraminidase are limited, a given strain reappears from time to time. For example, the H1N1 influenza virus strain was responsible for the 1918 to 1919 influenza pandemic that caused 20 million deaths. The same virus also caused pandemics in 1934 and in 1947, then disappeared after 1958 and reappeared in 1977. The reappearance of virus strains after an absence is believed to be the result of recombinational events involving the independent assortment of genes from two variant viruses.

Recombination of Incompletely Linked Genes

Recombination also occurs between genes residing on the same piece of nucleic acid (Fig. 43-3).

Genes that generally segregate together are called **linked genes.** If recombination occurs between them, the linkage is said to be **incomplete.** Recombination of incompletely linked genes occurs in all DNA viruses that have been studied and in several RNA viruses.

In DNA viruses, as in prokaryotic and eukaryotic cells, recombination between incompletely linked genes occurs by means of a break-rejoin mechanism. This mechanism involves the actual severing of the covalent bonds linking the bases of each of the two DNA strands in a DNA molecule (Fig. 43-3). The severed DNA strands are then rejoined to the DNA strands of a different DNA molecule that has been broken in a similar site. Recombination rates for herpesviruses, which are DNA viruses that replicate in the nucleus of infected cells, approximate those expected for a eukaryotic genome of the size of the herpesvirus genome. Herpesviruses have an average recombination frequency of 10 to 20 percent for any two loci. However, the rate of recombination between a specific pair of genetic loci depends on the distance between them and varies from less than 1 percent to approximately 50 percent. Measurement of the recombination frequencies for different loci can be used to map the virus genome. In this type of genetic map, loci with high recombination frequencies are far apart and loci with low recombination frequencies are close together.

Recombination has been shown to occur in several positive-sense single-stranded RNA virus groups: retroviruses, picornaviruses, and coronaviruses. That is initially surprising, as recombination between RNA molecules has not been observed in prokaryotic or eukaryotic cells. In retroviruses, recombination actually occurs at the point in replication when the retrovirus genome is in a DNA form and takes place by the same break-rejoin mechanism as in cells and DNA viruses. Recombination can occur both between two related retroviruses and between the retrovirus DNA and the host cell DNA. Recombination between two retroviruses gives rise to novel viral progeny with reassorted genes. Recombination between retroviruses and the host cell can give rise to novel viral progeny that carry nonviral genes. If these host

Steps

1. Dual infection

2. Uncoating of virus genomes

3. Interaction of some replicating genomes

4. Break in some replicating genomes

5. Crossover between broken genomes

6. Progeny virus with recombined (break-rejoin) or parental genomes

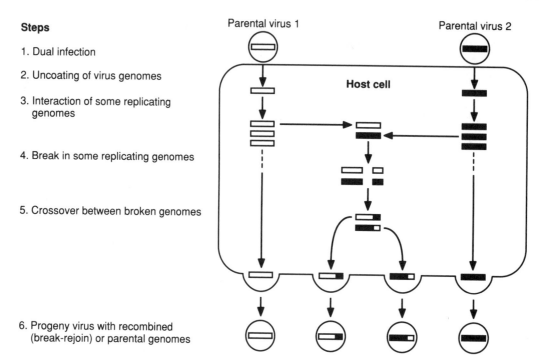

FIGURE 43-3 Recombination by break-rejoin of incompletely linked genes. The genetic interaction of DNA viruses can result in break-rejoin recombination, in which the two DNA molecules of different viruses break and then cross over. Break-rejoin recombination results in novel progeny viruses with some DNA sequences of both types of parental viruses.

genes code for growth factors, growth factor receptors, or a number of other specific cellular proteins, the recombinant retroviruses may be oncogenic (see Ch. 47).

In picornaviruses and coronaviruses, recombination takes place at the level of the interaction of the viral RNA genomes and is not believed to occur by a break-rejoin mechanism. The mechanism is currently believed to be a **copy-choice** mechanism (Fig. 43-4). Copy choice may occur in these RNA viruses because the viral RNA polymerase binds to only a few bases of the template RNA at any one time. Such a weak interaction of the polymerase with the template RNA would permit the polymerase, carrying its RNA strand, to disassociate from the original template nucleic acid strand and then associate with a new template RNA strand. Recombination frequencies in the range of 0.2 to 0.4 percent have been reported. Therefore, the efficiency of this mechanism of recombination is low.

Phenotypic Variation from Recombination

As mentioned above, viral recombination is important because it can generate novel progeny viruses that express new antigenic and/or virulence characteristics. For example, the novel progeny viruses may have new surface proteins that permit them to infect previously resistant individuals; they may have altered virulence characteristics; they may have novel combinations of proteins that make them infective to new cells in the original host or to new hosts; or they may carry material of cellular origin that gives them oncogenic potential.

Vaccines through Recombination

Recombination is being used experimentally by virologists to create new vaccines. Vaccinia virus, a DNA virus of the poxvirus group, was used as a live vaccine in the eradication of smallpox. Recombi-

Steps

1. Dual infection

2. Uncoating of virus genomes

3. Initiation of genome replication

4. Dissociation of polymerase with nascent genome

5. Association of polymerase and nascent genome with another parental genome

6. Completion of replication of genomes

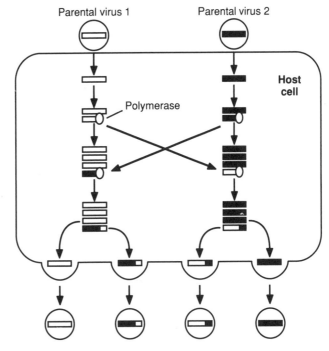

7. Progeny virus with recombined (copy-choice) or parental genomes

FIGURE 43-4 Recombination by copy choice of incompletely linked genes. The genetic interaction of certain RNA viruses can result in copy-choice recombination. In this mechanism, the polymerase begins replicating RNA from one viral RNA template. By an unknown mechanism, which may involve a high degree of secondary structure in the viral RNA template, the polymerase complex (with its nascent viral RNA molecule) dissociates from the initial viral RNA template. The polymerase complex (with its nascent viral RNA molecule) may then reassociate with the original or a second viral RNA template. If the polymerase complex (with its nascent viral RNA molecule) reassociates with the template viral RNA of a different parental virus, the nascent RNA molecule will be synthesized as a novel recombinant virus whose RNA genome contains genes from each parental virus type.

FIGURE 43-5 Development of recombinant vaccinia virus for immunization against cholera toxin. Vaccinia virus genomic DNA is cut with an endonuclease. A specific sequence of DNA (with appropriate regulatory sequences) coding for a protein (e.g., cholera toxin) to be used as an immunogen is ligated into the vaccinia virus genome, making a recombinant vaccinia virus. The DNA will be transcribed and the immunogen will be produced along with vaccinia virus proteins in infected cells following vaccination. The immunogen will then elicit antibody production by the host, providing protective immunity.

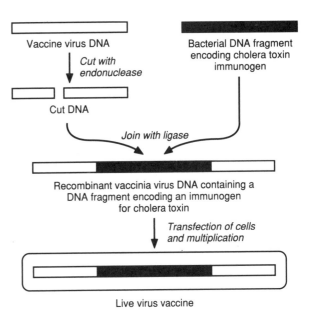

nant vaccinia viruses are being developed that carry vaccinia virus DNA recombined with DNA from other sources (exogenous DNA) (Fig. 43-5). For example, vaccinia virus strains carrying DNA coding for bacterial and viral antigens have been produced. It is expected that after vaccination with the recombinant vaccinia virus, the bacterial or viral antigen **(immunogen)** will be produced. The presence of this immunogen will then stimulate specific antibody production by the host, resulting in protection of the host from the immunogen. Studies with these live, recombinant vaccinia viruses are currently under way to determine whether inoculation of the skin with the recombinant virus can induce a protective host antibody response to the bacterial or viral antigens. Other studies are investigating the use of live, recombinant adenoviruses containing bacterial or viral genes to infect the gastrointestinal tract and induce both mucosal and systemic immunity. If these studies give positive results, such directed generation of recombinant viruses may become an important tool in the development of vaccines.

REFERENCES

Holland J, Spindler K, Horodyski F et al: Rapid evolution of RNA genomes. Science 215:1577, 1982

Honess RW, Buchan A, Halliburton IW, Watson DH: Recombination and linkage between structural and regulatory genes of herpes simplex virus type I: study of the functional organization of the genome. J Virol 34:716, 1980

Palese P, Young JF: Variation of influenza A, B, and C viruses. Science 215:1468, 1982

Paoletti E, Perkus ME, Piccini A: Live recombinant vaccines using genetically engineered vaccinia virus. Antiviral Res, suppl 1:301, 1985

Radding CM: Homologous pairing and strand exchange in genetic recombination. Annu Rev Genet 16:405, 1982

Romanova LI, Blinov VM, Tolskaya EA et al: The primary structure of crossover regions of intertypic poliovirus recombinants: a model of recombination between RNA genomes. Virology 155:202, 1986

Schaffer PA, Tevethia MJ, Benyesh-Melnick M: Recombination between temperature sensitive mutants of herpes simplex virus type 1. Virology 58:219, 1974

Smith FI, Palese P: Variation in influenza virus genes: epidemiological, pathogenic, and evolutionary consequences. p. 319. In Krug RM (ed): The Influenza Viruses. Plenum, New York, 1989

44 EFFECTS ON CELLS

THOMAS ALBRECHT
MICHAEL FONS
ALAN S. RABSON

GENERAL CONCEPTS

Definitions

Cells that support viral replication are called **permissive.** Infections of permissive cells are called **productive** because infectious progeny virus is produced. Most productive infections are called **cytocidal (cytolytic)** because they kill the host cell. Infections of nonpermissive cells yield no infectious progeny virus and are called **abortive.** In **persistent infections,** viral nucleic acid remains in specific host cells indefinitely; progeny virus may or may not be produced.

Cytocidal Infections

The effects of cytocidal infections on host cells may be classified as follows.

Morphologic Effects: The changes in cell morphology caused by infecting virus are called **cytopathic effects.** Common examples are rounding of the infected cell, fusion with adjacent cells to form a syncytium, and the appearance of nuclear or cytoplasmic inclusion bodies. Inclusion bodies may represent either altered host cell structures or accumulations of viral components. Noncytocidal infections may change the pattern of cell growth.

Effects on Cell Physiology: The interaction of virus and cell may result in rapid changes in the cell membranes, including movement of ions and the metabolism of secondary messengers such as cyclic nucleotides.

Effects on Cell Biochemistry: Viruses often inhibit the synthesis of host cell macromolecules, including DNA, RNA, and protein.

Biologic Effects: Expression of viral genes may alter the biologic functioning of infected cells. For example, virus-specified proteins inserted in the membrane may alter the cell's antigenic or immune properties, and changes in cytoskeletal elements may alter the cell's shape and behavior.

Genotoxic Effects: Alterations of cellular genetic material occur following some viral infections including chromosome damage.

Persistent Infections

Persistent infections can produce virus continuously (chronic infection) or intermittently (latent infection).

Chronic Infection: The cellular effects of chronic infection are usually the same as those of acute cytocidal infections, except that their progression may be slower. The long-term cellular changes may result in the shedding of products that may injure cells or tissues or in immune damage to cells or tissues.

Latent Infection: These intermittently productive infections are characterized by the maintenance of the virus genome as an episome or integrated into cellular DNA. Although some virus genes may be expressed, there are usually few, if any, changes in the infected cell.

Transforming Infections

Some persistent infections in which part or all of the viral genome is retained in the host cell (either as episomes or integrated into the host DNA) can cause the host cell to undergo **oncogenic transformation.**

Stages of Transformation: Transformation generally takes place in more than one step. For example, a first **(initiating)** event that immortalizes a cell (makes it capable of dividing indefinitely) will not result in a tumor unless a second **(promoting)** event releases the cell from contact inhibition. Viruses may either initiate or promote transformation.

Restriction of Virus Expression in Transforming Infections: Because DNA viruses are often cytocidal, transformation by DNA viruses takes place usually in abortive infections; few or no viral genes are expressed. Transforming RNA viruses, in contrast, may produce infectious progeny.

Mechanisms of Oncogenic Transformation: Viruses transform cells either via the expression of viral oncogenes or by altering the expression of cellular oncogenes. In the former case, the relevant segments of the viral genome must be retained intact in the host cell.

INTRODUCTION

In most cases, the disturbances of bodily function that are manifested as the signs and symptoms of viral disease result from the direct effects of viruses on cells. Knowledge of the morphologic, biologic, biochemical, and physiologic effects of viruses on cells is essential in understanding the pathophysiology of viral disease and developing accurate diagnostic procedures and effective treatment.

Virus-host cell interactions (Table 44-1) may produce either **cytocidal (cytolytic) infections,** in which production of new infectious virus kills the cell, **persistent infections,** in which the virus or its genome resides in some or all of the cells without killing most of them, or **transformation,** in which the virus does not kill the cell but produces morphologic, biochemical, physiologic, and biologic changes that may result in the acquisition of malignant properties by the cell (malignant transformation) (see also Ch. 47). The type of virus infection and the virus-induced effects on cells are dependent on the virus, the cell type and species, and often the physiologic state of the cell.

TABLE 44-1   Virus-Cell Interactions and Representative Effects on Cells

Type of Infection	Fate of Infected Cell	Release of Infectious Virus	Effects on Cells				
			Morphologic	Physiologic	Biochemical	Biologic	Genotoxic
Cytocidal	Death	+	+	+	+	+	+
Persistent							
Chronic	Variable	±	Variable	+	+	+	+
Latent	Survival	0[a]	0	0	0	0	0
Transforming	Survival	0 or + (retroviruses); 0 (DNA viruses)	0 or +	0 or +	0 or +	0 or +	0 or +

[a] None or minimal

CYTOCIDAL INFECTION

Morphologic Effects

Infection of permissive cells with virus leads to **productive (cytocidal, cytolytic) infection,** which often results in cell death. The first effects of the replication of cytocidal viruses to be described were the morphologic changes known as **cytopathic effect.** Cultured cells that are infected by viruses undergo morphologic changes, which can be observed easily in unfixed, unstained cells by a light microscope. Some viruses cause characteristic cytopathic effects; thus, observation of the cytopathic effect is an important tool for virologists concerned with isolating and identifying viruses from infected animals or humans (Fig. 44-1).

Many types of cytopathic effect occur. Often the first sign of viral infections is a rounding of the cells. In some diseased tissues, intracellular structures called **inclusion bodies** appear in the nucleus and/or cytoplasm of infected cells. Inclusion bodies were first identified by light microscopy in smears and stained sections of infected tissues, but their composition has been clarified by electron microscopy. In an adenovirus infection, for example, crystalline arrays of adenovirus capsids accumulate in the nucleus to form an inclusion body. Inclusions may alternatively be host cell structures altered by the virus. For example, in reovirus-infected cells, virions associate with the microtubules, giving rise to a crescent-shaped perinuclear inclusion. Some characteristics of inclusion bodies produced by various viruses are listed in Table 44-2.

A particularly striking cytopathic effect of some viral infections is the formation of **syncytia,** or **polykaryocytes,** which are large cytoplasmic masses that contain many nuclei (*poly,* many; *karyon,* nucleus) and are usually produced by fusion of infected cells (Fig. 44-2). The mechanism of cell fusion during viral infection probably results from the interaction between viral gene products and host cell membranes. Cell fusion may be a mechanism by which virus spreads from infected to uninfected cells.

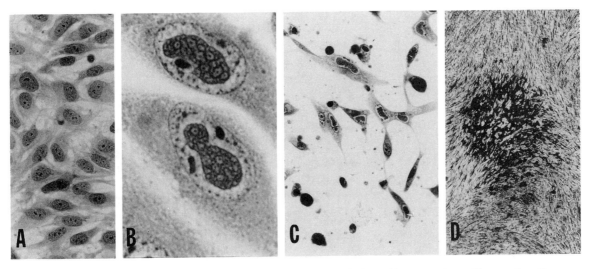

FIGURE 44-1 Development and progression of viral cytopathology. Human embryo skin muscle cells were infected with human cytomegalovirus and stained at selected times to demonstrate *(A)* uninfected cells, *(B)* late virus cytopathic effects (nuclear inclusions, cell enlargement), *(C)* cell degeneration, and *(D)* foci of infected cells in a cell monolayer (i.e., a plaque). Bouins fixative; hematoxylin and eosin stain. (A, × 255; B, × 900; C, × 225; D, × 20.)

TABLE 44-2   Viral Inclusion Bodies in Some
Human Diseases

Virus	Location in Cell	
	Nucleus	Cytoplasm
Papovaviruses	+ (Cowdry type A)	
Adenovirus	+ (Cowdry type A)	
Herpes simplex virus	+ (Cowdry type A)	
Varicella-zoster virus	+ (Cowdry type A)	
Cytomegalovirus	+ (Cowdry type A)	+
Measles virus	+ (Cowdry type A)	+
Vaccinia virus		+ (Guarnieri bodies)
Rabies virus		+ (Negri bodies)
Reovirus		+

Effects on Cell Physiology

Many morphologic alterations have physiologic and/or biochemical correlates. A number of viruses bind to receptors that have important physiologic functions (Table 44-3). Although research into the cellular physiologic effects of virus infections has been limited, there may be a close correlation between cellular physiologic responses and the replication of some viruses (Fig. 44-3). For example, human cytomegalovirus infection induces a cascade of cellular physiologic responses

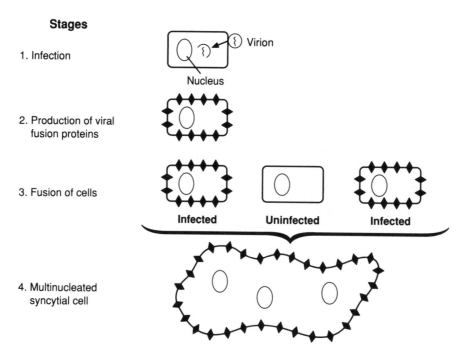

Stages

1. Infection

Virion

Nucleus

2. Production of viral fusion proteins

3. Fusion of cells

Infected   Uninfected   Infected

4. Multinucleated syncytial cell

FIGURE 44-2   Formation of fused multinucleated cells. The figure represents the cytopathology of measles virus-induced syncytia.

TABLE 44-3   Proposed Virus Receptors on
Cell Membranes

Virus	Proposed Receptor Molecule	Representative Cell Types with Receptor
Influenza virus type A	Glycophorin A Sialyloligosaccharides	Respiratory epithelium
Rabies virus	Acetylcholine receptor	Neurons
Epstein-Barr virus	Complement component 3D (CR2) receptor	B lymphocytes
Vaccinia virus	Epidermal growth factor (EGF) receptor	Skin cells
Human immunodeficiency virus	CD4	T lymphocytes
Reovirus T3	β-Adrenergic receptor	Neurons, lymphocytes
Semliki Forest virus	HLA-A and B	Many
Sindbis virus	Catecholamine receptor	Skeletal muscle
Hepatitis B virus	IgA	Liver
Poliovirus	Immunoglobulin superfamily molecules	Orthopharyngeal cells, motor neurons
Rhinovirus	Intracellular adhesion molecule 1 (ICAM-1)	Nasal epithelium

that resemble those associated with cell activation, including membrane-associated responses and specific increases in secondary messengers (e.g., Ca^{2+}, cAMP, cGMP). In the virus-infected cells, however, perturbed regulation of the cellular responses associated with the cell activation cascade results in protraction of some of the responses. These protracted responses appear to have two consequences. First, synthesis of some macromolecules, particularly cellular DNA, is inhibited. Second, the infected cells enlarge, developing the cytomegaly that is characteristic of cytomegalovirus infection. Under these conditions, the virus is able to replicate its DNA without competition from replicating cellular DNA for a limited supply of substrates. The virus thus takes advantage of cellular pathways to modify the cell so that viral replication is favored. There is a close correlation between virus-induced cellular physiologic responses, biochemical and morphologic cellular responses, virus-specific macromolecule synthesis, and replication of the virus (Fig. 44-3).

Alterations in cell physiology, including increased arachidonic acid metabolism and an increase in cytosolic Ca^{2+}, have been demonstrated in cells following infection with human immunodeficiency virus (HIV). These physiologic alter-

ations may be related to cell activation signals triggered, at least in part, by the HIV receptor molecule, CD4.

Other virus-associated alterations in cell physiology are related to insertion of viral proteins or other changes in the cell membrane. One example is the leaky cell membrane that appears after infection with picornaviruses or Sindbis virus; the change in intracellular ion concentrations that results from the leaky membrane may favor translation of the more salt-stable viral mRNA over cellular mRNA.

Effects on Cell Biochemistry

As indicated above, biochemical activity is often affected by the virus. Cellular protein synthesis frequently is inhibited during the replicative cycle of cytocidal viruses. This inhibition occurs in characteristic ways. In poliovirus or herpes simplex infections, for example, selective inhibition of host protein synthesis ("host shutdown") occurs prior to the maximal synthesis of viral proteins. In some cases, viral products inhibit both protein and nucleic acid synthesis ("total shutdown"). Purified adenovirus penton fibers can shut down the synthesis of host protein, RNA, and DNA (Fig. 44-4).

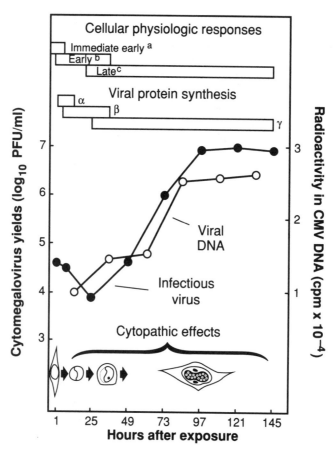

FIGURE 44-3 Relationship of morphologic, physiologic, and biochemical cellular effects to the replication of human cytomegalovirus.

Total shutdown also may occur when excess viral products accumulate in the cell late in the viral replicative cycle. Some picornaviruses specify a protein that causes cell damage independent of the viral proteins that inhibit cell macromolecular synthesis.

The mechanisms underlying virus-induced inhibition of host cell protein synthesis vary, but appear to depend on viral structural proteins. Cellular mRNA may be degraded. For example, in influenza virus and herpes simplex virus infections, cellular mRNA stops binding with ribosomes to form polyribosomes; only virus-specific mRNA is bound. In addition, specific virus gene products degrade host mRNAs, giving viral mRNAs a selec-

tive advantage. Cell DNA synthesis is inhibited in most cytolytic virus infections, but in most cases the inhibition of DNA synthesis seems to be a passive result of the decrease in cellular protein synthesis. Reoviruses and some herpesviruses may be exceptions in that they cause a decrease in cell DNA synthesis before a substantial decline in protein synthesis occurs. Direct degradation of host DNA is seen in vaccinia virus infections due to a virion-associated DNAse.

Biologic Effects

The biologic effects observed in cells following cytocidal virus infections are primarily those asso-

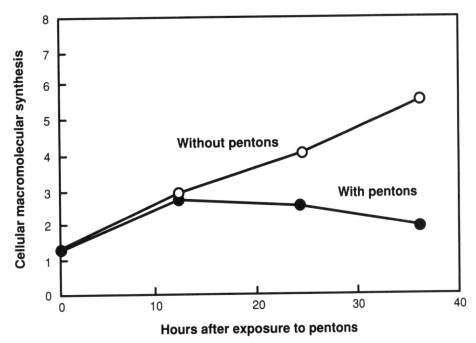

FIGURE 44-4 Effect of purified adenovirus pentons on cellular macromolecular synthesis. DNA, RNA, and protein synthesis are all decreased after treatment with adenovirus pentons. Symbols: O, cellular DNA, RNA, or protein synthesis in the absence of pentons; ●, cellular DNA, RNA, or protein synthesis in the presence of 250 μg of adenovirus penton fiber antigen/ml. (Adapted from Levine AJ, Ginsberg HS: Mechanism by which fiber antigen inhibits multiplication of type 5 adenovirus. J Virol 1:747, 1967, with permission.)

ciated with high yields of progeny virus. Some of these effects result from viral proteins that appear in the host cell membrane. Virus-specific attachment proteins usually appear in the cell membrane during the replication of enveloped viruses. Virus-specific proteins inserted into the plasma membrane are thought to be involved in syncytium formation. These effects are important in the diagnosis of some virus infections. Some viruses (for example, herpes simplex virus), insert proteins into the plasma membrane that bind the Fc fragment of antibody. It has been proposed that binding antibody through the Fc portion to infected cells may compromise the ability of the immune system to recognize the cell as infected.

Infection of cells by other viruses causes specific alterations in the cytoskeleton of cells. Reoviruses bind to cellular microtubules, which become associated with the virus-induced perinuclear inclusion bodies. In addition, reoviruses and cytomegalovirus disrupt cellular intermediate filaments (Fig. 44-5).

Genotoxic Effects

Replication of viruses may alter the morphologic characteristics of the cellular chromosomes. Chromosome breaks, fragments, and pulverization are often observed (Fig. 44-6). The chromosomal breaks are apparently nonrandom, since they most often affect the same chromosomes that are preferentially damaged by radiation or radiomimetic drugs.

Relation of Cellular Effects to Viral Pathogenesis

Although most of the events that damage or modify the host cell during lytic infection are difficult

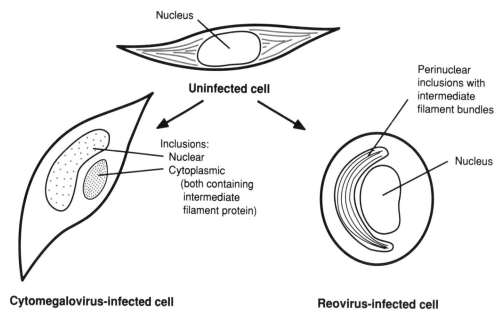

FIGURE 44-5 Alteration of cytoskeleton organization by virus infection. Normal cells have a network of intermediate filaments (IFs) throughout the cytoplasm. Infection with reovirus causes a perinuclear aggregation of IFs, and infection with cytomegalovirus causes a modification of IF proteins, including their relocation into the nuclear and cytoplasmic inclusion bodies.

to separate from viral replication, the effects are not always linked directly to the production of progeny virions. For example, changes in cell size, shape, and physiologic parameters may occur before progeny virions or even many virus proteins are produced. These alterations in cell structure and function may be important aspects of the pathogenesis of some viral infections. A particularly devastating result of this interaction with cells is evident in the virus-induced birth defects associated with rubella virus and cytomegalovirus infections. The long-term structural and functional effects of persistent virus infections (see below) may also be related to such progressive diseases as atherosclerosis and demyelination in multiple sclerosis, although viral involvement in these diseases has not been proven.

PERSISTENT INFECTIONS

Types of Persistent Infection

In a **persistent infection** the virus is not eliminated from all of the host tissues after the acute phase of

disease. The several types of persistent infection (chronic, latent, and transformation (Table 44-1; see Chs. 46 and 47) differ in the mechanisms controlling pathogenesis. In **chronic persistent infections,** a limited number of cells (often in a few target organs) are infected. These infected cells may demonstrate a cytopathic effect, synthesize virus macromolecules, and release infectious virus. The spread of infection is limited by host factors such as interferons and other nonspecific inhibitors and by humoral and cell-mediated immune responses. Thus, although infectious virus is often detected, only a few cells are usually involved at any given time. In **latent persistent infections,** infectious virus is seldom detected. Few cells are infected, and virus expression and replication are usually completely restricted. Common features of latent persistent infection are their ability to reactivate in response to various environmental stimuli (e.g., heat, ultraviolet irradiation) and alterations in the immune system brought on by disease, hormones, or chemicals. In **transforming persistent infections,** infectious virus may or may not be re-

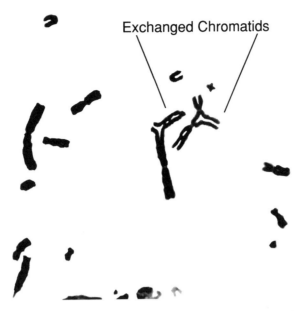

FIGURE 44-6 Chromosomal aberrations resulting from cytomegalovirus infection of hamster fibroblasts. Note chromatid exchange. (From Deng CZ, unpublished results.)

leased, but cells undergo transformation that may lead to malignancy (the ability to keep dividing when normal cells would stop).

Cellular Effects

Autoimmune injury and other forms of cell damage may occur during persistent infections. Budding virions and viral peptides associated with the cell membrane change the antigenic characteristics of the cell so that the immune system may recognize it as foreign (see Chs. 1 and 50). The cell then may be attacked by the humoral and cellular immune system of the host and will die even though it was infected by a noncytocidal virus.

The immune response also may cause formation of circulating antigen-antibody complexes involving viral antigens. These complexes may deposit in the kidneys and lead to renal disease (e.g., lymphocytic choriomeningitis virus infection in mice). The long-term association of the virus with specific target cells may lead to altered function or responses;

this type of mechanism is responsible for the progressive neurologic disease associated with slow virus-type persistent infections such as kuru, Creutzfeldt-Jakob disease, or subacute sclerosing panencephalitis (see Ch. 71).

TRANSFORMING INFECTIONS

In the context of persistent virus-cell interactions, the term **transformation** (oncogenic transformation) refers to the process by which the control of cell proliferation is modified so that the cell becomes cancerous (see Ch. 47). Transformation of a cell involves at least two components: first, the cell gains the capacity for unlimited cell division in culture (**immortalization**), and second, the transformed cells acquire the ability to produce a tumor in an appropriate host. The second process is associated with cell multiplication. Immortalization is necessary but not sufficient for oncogenic transformation. Cells can also undergo various types of nononcogenic transformation, involving biochemical, antigenic, morphologic, and physiologic alterations that are not themselves oncogenic (Table 44-4).

Stages of Cellular Transformation

Current data indicate that oncogenic transformation occurs in cumulative steps resulting in modification of the control of cell proliferation. For example, in the first step, the cell may undergo changes that result in immortalization; in the second step, one of these cells may become able to produce tumors; and in a third step, a tumor cell may acquire the ability to invade and metastasize. Different steps are usually caused by different agents (chemical, physical, or viral) acting at different loci in the cell. For example, mouse polyomavirus middle T protein alone can transform immortalized cells to malignant cells, whereas both the large T and middle T proteins are required to transform nonimmortalized cells. Since transformation is most often a multistep process, the first exposure of an animal or cells to a tumor virus or chemical carcinogen (initiator) usually does not induce a tumor, but does produce heritable

TABLE 44-4 Cellular Effects of Transformation

Cell proliferation
    In vivo: tumor formation
    In vitro: fewer restrictions for proliferation (e.g., lower requirement for serum and attachment surface; higher requirement for cell density inhibition [contact inhibition]; decreased orientation of cells)
Metabolic and molecular changes
    Increased proliferation (e.g., increased expression of cell oncogenes; cytoskeletal changes; increased metabolism)
    Increased invasiveness and surface changes (e.g., decreased fibronectin; increased proteolysis; fetal antigens; agglutinability; altered membrane components)
Virus products
    Surface antigens
    Intracellular antigens, nucleic acids, and sometimes virus

changes in some cells. Exposure to a second agent (promoter) then results in tumor formation, even though the promoter would not induce tumors if used alone. Tumor viruses, chemicals, and radiation may all serve as either initiators or promoters. Some agents are referred to as complete carcinogens because they are capable of both initiation and promotion. The term progression is often used for the multiple steps of promotion that cause the transformed cells and the tumors derived from these cells to manifest increased malignancy.

Restriction of DNA Virus Expression in Transforming Infections

Since DNA viruses are usually lytic in natural hosts, DNA viruses induce transformation only under conditions that restrict virus replication and permit survival of infected cells (e.g., in nonlytic infections of selected cell types or animal hosts or in infection with incomplete virions). Under such conditions, infectious progeny virions are seldom produced. In contrast, because RNA virus replication is usually noncytocidal, they can cause oncogenic transformation in their natural hosts, and viral products may be produced whether or not virus is released.

Mechanisms of Viral Transformation

Basically, oncogenic transformation requires an altered expression of oncogenes of virus or cell origin that modify control of the cell proliferation. Transforming viruses often integrate all or part of their genome into the cell DNA. (For RNA tumor viruses, a DNA copy of the RNA genome is integrated.) Herpesvirus and papillomavirus DNA may be maintained in transformed cells as episomes or be randomly integrated into cell DNA. Expression of virus oncogenes can result in the generation of tumor cells (see Ch. 47), although it is not clear whether all integration sites permit sufficient expression of these genes. For example, expression of viral regulatory genes such as the simian virus 40 T antigen (Fig. 44-7) can cause transformation of cells. Some viral oncogenes represent mutated versions of cellular growth-regu-

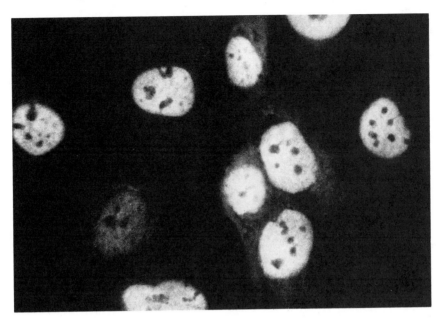

FIGURE 44-7   Intranuclear transforming T antigen specified by simian virus 40 in transformed human cells.

lating genes. Alternatively, integration of a defective retrovirus adjacent to a cellular oncogene may activate or deregulate it to transform the cell. Thus, genetic rearrangements after integration may be an important aspect of the expression of the oncogene. One of the major unanswered questions of modern oncology and molecular biology is how the expressed oncogenes modify the affected cell and cause it to exhibit a transformed phenotype.

REFERENCES

Albrecht T, Boldogh I, Fons M et al: Cell-activation responses to cytomegalovirus infection: relationship to the phasing of CMV replication and to the induction of cellular damage. Subcell Biochem 15:157, 1989

Butel JS: SV40 large T-antigen: dual oncogene. Cancer Surv 5:343, 1986

Fenner FJ, White DO: Medical Virology. 2nd Ed. Academic Press, San Diego, CA, 1976

Nigg EA: Mechanisms of signal transduction to the cell nucleus. Adv Cancer Res 55:271, 1990

Schneider RJ, Shenk T: Impact of virus infection on host cell protein synthesis. Annu Rev Biochem 56:317, 1987

45

VIRAL PATHOGENESIS

SAMUEL BARON
MICHAEL FONS
THOMAS ALBRECHT

GENERAL CONCEPTS

Pathogenesis

Pathogenesis is the process by which an infection leads to disease. Pathogenic mechanisms of viral disease include (1) implantation of virus at the portal of entry, (2) local replication, (3) spread to target organs (disease sites), and (4) spread to sites of shedding of virus into the environment. Factors that affect pathogenic mechanisms are (1) accessibility of virus to tissue, (2) cell susceptibility to virus multiplication, and (3) virus susceptibility to host defenses. Natural selection favors the dominance of low-virulence virus strains.

Cellular Pathogenesis

Direct cell damage and death from viral infection may result from (1) diversion of the cell's energy, (2) shutoff of cell macromolecular synthesis, (3) competition of viral mRNA for cellular ribosomes, (4) competition of viral transcriptional enhancers for cellular transcriptional factors such as RNA polymerases, and inhibition of the interferon defense mechanisms. Indirect cell damage can result from integration of the viral genome into the cell genome, inflammation, and the host immune response.

Tissue Tropism

Viral affinity for specific body tissues (**tropism**) is determined by (1) cell receptors for virus, (2) cell transcription factors that recognize viral enhancer sequences, (3) ability of the cell to support virus replication, (4) physi-

cal barriers, (5) local temperature, pH, and oxygen tension, and (6) digestive enzymes and bile in the gastrointestinal tract that may inactivate some viruses.

Implantation at the Portal of Entry

Virions implant onto living cells mainly via the respiratory, gastrointestinal, and skin-penetrating routes, although other routes can be used. The final outcome of infection may be determined by the dose and location of the virus as well as its infectivity and virulence.

Local Replication and Local Spread

Most virus types spread among cells extracellularly, but some may also spread intracellularly. Establishment of local infection may lead to localized disease and localized shedding of virus.

Dissemination from the Portal of Entry

Viremic: The most common route of systemic spread from the portal of entry is the circulation, which the virus reaches via the lymphatics. Virus may enter the target organs from the capillaries by (1) multiplying in endothelial cells or fixed macrophages, (2) diffusing through gaps, and (3) being carried in a migrating leukocyte.

Neural: Dissemination via nerves usually occurs with rabies virus and sometimes with herpesvirus and poliovirus infections.

Incubation Period

The incubation period is the time between exposure to virus and onset of disease. During this usually asymptomatic period, implantation, local multiplication, and spread (for disseminated infections) occur.

Multiplication in Target Organs

Depending on the balance between virus and host defenses, virus multiplication in the target organ may be sufficient to cause disease and death.

Shedding of Virus

Although the respiratory tract, alimentary tract, and blood are the most frequent sites of shedding, diverse viruses may be shed at virtually every site.

Congenital Infections

Infection of the fetus as a target "organ" is special because the virus must traverse additional physical barriers, the early fetal immune and interferon defense systems may be immature, transfer of the maternal defenses are partially blocked by the placenta, the developing first-trimester fetal organs are vulnerable to infection, and hormonal changes are taking place.

INTRODUCTION

Pathogenesis is the process by which virus infection leads to disease. Pathogenic mechanisms include implantation of the virus at a body site (the portal of entry), replication at that site, and then spread to and multiplication within sites (target organs) where disease or shedding of virus into the environment occurs. Most viral infections are subclinical, suggesting that body defenses against viruses arrest most infections before disease symptoms become manifest. Knowledge of subclinical infections comes from serologic studies showing that sizeable portions of the population have specific antibodies to viruses even though the individuals have no history of disease. These inapparent infections have great epidemiologic importance: they constitute major sources for dissemination of virus through the population, and they confer immunity (see Ch. 48).

Many factors affect pathogenic mechanisms. An early determinant is the extent to which body tissues and organs are accessible to the virus. Accessibility is influenced by physical barriers (such as mucus and tissue barriers), by the distance to be traversed within the body, and by natural defense mechanisms. If the virus reaches an organ, infection occurs only if cells capable of supporting virus replication are present. Cellular susceptibility requires a cell surface attachment site (receptor) for the virions and also an intracellular environment that permits virus replication and release. Even if virus initiates infection in a susceptible organ, replication of sufficient virus to cause disease may be prevented by host defenses (see Chs. 49 and 50).

Other factors that determine whether infection and disease occur are the many virulence characteristics of the infecting virus. To cause disease, the infecting virus must be able to overcome the inhibitory effects of physical barriers, distance, host defenses, and differing cellular susceptibilities to infection. The inhibitory effects are genetically controlled and therefore may vary among individuals and races. Virulence characteristics enable the virus to initiate infection, spread in the body, and replicate to large enough numbers to impair the target organ. These factors include the ability to replicate under certain circumstances during inflammation, during the febrile response, in migratory cells, and in the presence of natural body inhibitors and interferon. Extremely virulent strains often occur within virus populations. Occasionally, these strains become dominant as a result of unusual selective pressures (see Ch. 48). The viral proteins and genes responsible for specific virulence functions are only just beginning to be identified.

Fortunately for the survival of humans and animals (and hence for the infecting virus), most natural selective pressures favor the dominance of less virulent strains. Because these strains do not cause severe disease or death, their replication and transmission are not impaired by an incapacitated host. Mild or inapparent infections can result from absence of one or more virulence factors. For example, a virus that has all the virulence characteristics except the inability to multiply at elevated temperatures is arrested at the febrile stage of infection and causes a milder disease than its totally virulent counterpart. Live virus vaccines are composed of viruses deficient in one or more virulence factors; they cause only inapparent infections and yet are able to replicate sufficiently to induce immunity.

Disease does not always follow successful virus replication in the target organ. Disease occurs only if the virus replicates sufficiently to damage essential cells directly, to cause the release of toxic substances from infected tissues, or to damage organ function indirectly as a result of the host immune response to the presence of virus antigens.

As a group, viruses use all conceivable portals of entry, mechanisms of spread, target organs, and sites of excretion. This abundance of possibilities is not surprising considering the astronomic numbers of viruses and their variants (see Ch. 43).

CELLULAR PATHOGENESIS

Direct cell damage and death may result from disruption of cellular macromolecular synthesis by the infecting virus. Also, viruses cannot synthesize their genetic and structural components, and so they rely almost exclusively on the host cell for these functions. Their parasitic replication therefore robs the host cell of energy and macromolecular components, severely impairing the host's ability to function and often resulting in cell death and disease. Damage of cells by replicating virus and damage by the immune response are considered further in Chapters 44 and 50, respectively.

Pathogenesis at the cellular level can be viewed as a process that occurs in progressive stages leading to cellular disease. As noted above, an essential aspect of viral pathogenesis at the cellular level is the competition between the synthetic needs of the virus and those of the host cell. Since viruses must use the cell's machinery to synthesize their own nucleic acids and proteins, they have evolved various mechanisms to subvert the cell's normal functions to those required for production of viral macromolecules and eventually viral progeny. The function of some of the viral genetic elements associated with virulence may be related to providing conditions in which the synthetic needs of the virus compete effectively for a limited supply of cellular macromolecule components and synthetic machinery, such as ribosomes.

Tables 45-1 and 45-2 give examples of mechanisms that have evolved to facilitate the preferen-

TABLE 45-1 Selected Mechanisms of Molecular Pathogenesis of DNA Viruses

Virus	Inhibition of Host Macromolecule Synthesis	Inhibition of Interferon Action	Transcriptional Enhancer Element
Polyomavirus	+	−	+
Adenovirus	+	+	+
Herpes simplex virus	+	−	−
Epstein-Barr virus	±	+	+
Cytomegalovirus	±	?	+
Vaccinia virus	+	+	−

TABLE 45-2   Selected Mechanisms of Molecular
Pathogenesis of RNA Viruses

Virus	Inhibition of Host Cell Macromolecule Synthesis	Stealing of 5' from Cellular mRNA	Mimicry of Cellular 5'
Influenza virus	+	+	−
Picornavirus	+	−	+
Reovirus	+	−	−
Togavirus	+	−	−
Bunyavirus	+	+	−

tial expression of viral gene products, often at the expense of the synthetic needs of the host cell. These mechanisms include the following:

1. Viruses can shut off host cell macromolecular synthesis; this may occur in adenovirus, picornavirus, togavirus, polyomavirus, and herpes simplex virus infections. Inhibition of cellular macromolecular synthesis can preclude cell product formation and can permit the almost exclusive production of virally encoded gene products.

2. Both the picornaviruses and the orthomyxoviruses have evolved viral mRNA that is more efficient than cellular mRNA for translation by the host ribosomes. Picornaviruses encode a protein, VPg, which mimics the cellular cap at the 5′ end of mRNA. This cap analog increases the chance that viral messages will be translated. On the other hand, in cells infected with orthomyxoviruses such as influenza virus, the 5′ cap is stripped from cellular mRNA and attached to virus-specific mRNA, thereby ensuring efficient and preferential translation of the virus-specific messages.

3. Strong transcriptional enhancers that effectively compete for cellular RNA polymerases and other transcriptional factors are used by polyomaviruses, adenoviruses, and cytomegaloviruses to ensure efficient transcription of viral genes.

4. Epstein-Barr virus, adenovirus, and possibly cytomegalovirus have virus-associated RNA molecules that inhibit activation of an interferon-induced protein kinase that phosphorylates protein synthesis initiation factor eIF-2α. Phosphorylation of eIF-2α by interferon is associated with inhibition of translation. The presence of virus-associated RNAs may therefore allow for translation of viral messages, even in the presence of interferon.

Additional details pertaining to the specific mechanisms used by different viruses for preferential synthesis of viral gene products are discussed in Chapter 44, Chapter 45, and specific chapters pertaining to each virus group.

TISSUE TROPISM

Most viruses have an affinity for specific tissues; that is, they display **tissue specificity** or **tropism.** This specificity is determined by selective susceptibility of cells, physical barriers, local temperature and pH, and host defenses. Many examples of viral tissue tropism are known. Polioviruses selectively infect and destroy certain nerve cells, which have a higher concentration of surface receptors for polioviruses than do virus-resistant cells. Rhinoviruses multiply exclusively in the upper respiratory tract because they are adapted to multiply best at low temperature and pH and high oxygen tension. Enteroviruses can multiply in the intestine, partly because they resist inactivation by digestive enzymes, bile, and acid.

The cell receptors for some viruses have been identified. Rabies virus uses the acetylcholine receptor present on neurons as a receptor, and hepatitis B virus binds to polymerized albumin receptors found on liver cells. Similarly, Epstein-Barr virus uses complement C3d receptors on B lymphocytes, and human immunodeficiency virus uses the CD4 molecules present on T lymphocytes as specific receptors.

Viral tropism is also dictated in part by the presence of specific cell transcription factors that require enhancer sequences within the viral genome. Recently, enhancer sequences have been shown to participate in the pathogenesis of certain viral infections. Enhancer sequences within the long terminal repeat (LTR) regions of Moloney murine leukemia retrovirus are active in certain host tissues. In addition, JV papovavirus appears to have an enhancer sequence that is active specifically in oligodendroglia cells, and hepatitis B virus enhancer activity is most active in hepatocytes.

SEQUENCE OF VIRUS SPREAD IN THE HOST

Implantation at Portal of Entry

Viruses may be carried to the body by all possible routes (air, food, bites, and any contaminated ob-

ject). Similarly, all possible sites of implantation (all body surfaces and internal sites reached by mechanical penetration) may be used. The frequency of implantation is greatest where virus contacts living cells directly (in the respiratory tract, in the alimentary tract, and subcutaneously). With some viruses, implantation in the fetus may occur at the time of fertilization through infected germ cells, as well as later in gestation via the placenta, or at birth.

Even at the earliest stage of pathogenesis (implantation), certain variables may influence the final outcome of the infection. For example, the dose, infectivity, and virulence of virus implanted and the location of implantation may determine whether the infection will be inapparent (subclinical) or will cause mild, severe, or lethal disease.

Local Replication and Local Spread

Successful implantation may be followed by local replication and local spread of virus (Fig. 45-1). Virus that replicates within the initially infected cell may spread to adjacent cells extracellularly or

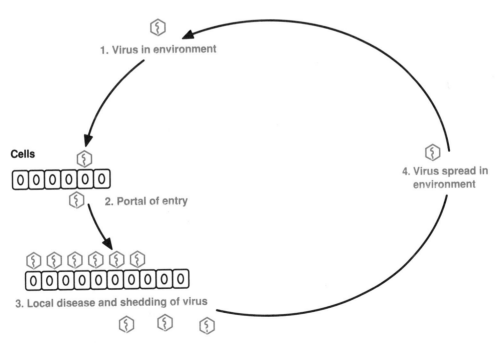

1. Virus in environment

Cells

2. Portal of entry

4. Virus spread in environment

3. Local disease and shedding of virus

FIGURE 45-1 Virus spread during localized infection. Numbers indicate sequence of events.

intracellularly. Extracellular spread occurs by release of virus into the extracellular fluid and subsequent infection of the adjacent cell. Intracellular
spread occurs by fusion of infected cells with adjacent, uninfected cells or by way of cytoplasmic
bridges between cells. Most viruses spread extracellularly, but herpesviruses, paramyxoviruses,
and poxviruses may spread through both intracellular and extracellular routes. Intracellular spread
provides virus with a partially protected environment because the antibody defense does not penetrate cell membranes.

Spread to cells beyond adjacent cells may occur
through the liquid spaces within the local site (e.g.,
lymphatics) or by diffusion through surface fluids
such as the mucous layer of the respiratory tract.
Also, infected migratory cells such as lymphocytes
and macrophages may spread the virus within local
tissue.

Establishment of infection at the portal of entry
may be followed by continued local virus multiplication, leading to localized virus shedding and localized disease. In this way, local sites of implantation also are target organs and sites of shedding in
many infections (Table 45-3). Respiratory tract infections that fall into this category include influenza, the common cold, and parainfluenza virus
infections. Alimentary tract infections caused by
several gastroenteritis viruses (e.g., rotaviruses
and picornaviruses) also may fall into this category.
Localized skin infections of this type include warts,
cowpox, and molluscum contagiosum. Localized
infections may spread over body surfaces to infect
distant surfaces. An example of this is the picornavirus epidemic conjunctivitis shown in Figure
45-2; in the absence of viremia, virus spreads directly from the eye (site of implantation) to the

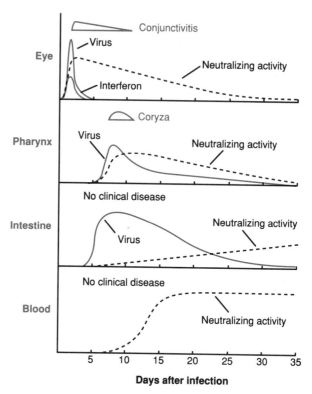

FIGURE 45-2 Spread of picornavirus over body surfaces
from eye to pharynx and intestine during natural infection. Local neutralizing antibody activity is shown.
(Adapted from Langford MP, Stanton GJ, Barber JC: Early
appearing antiviral activity in human tears during a case of
picornavirus epidemic conjunctivitis. J Infect Dis 139:653,
1979, with permission.)

pharynx and intestine. Other viruses may spread
internally to distant target organs and sites of excretion (disseminated infection). A third category
of viruses may cause both local and disseminated
disease, as in herpes simplex and measles.

TABLE 45-3   Pathogenesis of Selected Virus Infection:
Localized Infections

Disease	Site of Implantation	Route of Spread	Target Organ	Site of Shedding
Influenza	Respiratory tract	Local	Respiratory tract	Respiratory tract
Coryza	Respiratory tract	Local	Respiratory tract	Respiratory tract
Gastroenteritis	Alimentary tract	Local	Alimentary tract	Alimentary tract
Warts	Skin and mucosa	Local	Skin and mucosa	Skin and mucosa

Dissemination from the Portal of Entry

Dissemination in the Bloodstream

At the portal of entry, multiplying virus contacts pathways to the blood and peripheral nerves, the principal routes of widespread dissemination through the body. The most common route of systemic spread of virus involves the circulation (Fig. 45-3 and Table 45-4). Viruses such as those causing poliomyelitis, smallpox, and measles disseminate through the blood after an initial period of replication at the portal of entry (the alimentary and respiratory tracts), where the infection often causes no significant symptoms or signs of illness because the virus kills cells that are expendable and easily replaced. Virus progeny diffuse through the afferent lymphatics to the lymphoid tissue and then through the efferent lymphatics to infect cells in close contact with the bloodstream (e.g., endothelial cells, especially those of the lymphoreticular

organs). This initial spread may result in a brief primary viremia. Subsequent release of virus directly into the bloodstream induces a secondary viremia, which usually lasts several days and puts the virus in contact with the capillary system of all body tissues. Virus may enter the target organ from the capillaries by replicating within a capillary endothelial cell or fixed macrophage and then being released on the target organ side of the capillary. Virus may also diffuse through small gaps in the capillary endothelium or penetrate the capillary wall through an infected, migrating leukocyte. The virus may then replicate and spread within the target organ or site of excretion by the same mechanisms as for local dissemination at the portal of entry. Disease occurs if the virus replicates in a sufficient number of essential cells and destroys them. For example, in poliomyelitis the central nervous system is the target organ, whereas the alimentary tract is both the portal of entry and the site of shedding. In some situations, the target

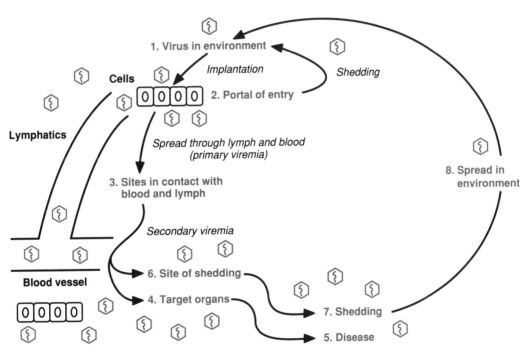

FIGURE 45-3 Virus spread through bloodstream during a generalized infection. Numbers indicate sequence of events.

TABLE 45-4   Pathogenesis of Selected Virus Infections:
Disseminated Infections

Disease	Common Site of Implantation	Route of Spread	Target Organ(s)	Site of Shedding
Poliomyelitis	Alimentary tract	Blood (nerves)	Central nervous system	Alimentary tract
Hepatitis A	Alimentary tract	Blood	Liver	Alimentary tract
AIDS	Injection, trauma, intestine	Blood	Immune system, brain	Blood, semen
Kuru	Alimentary tract	Blood	Brain	Brain (transmitted by ingestion)
Rubella	Respiratory tract	Blood	Skin, lymph nodes, fetus	Respiratory tract, excreta in newborn
Measles	Respiratory tract	Blood	Skin, lungs, brain	Respiratory tract
Chickenpox	Respiratory tract	Blood, nerves (to site of latency)	Skin, lungs	Respiratory tract, skin
Herpes simplex type 1				
Acute	Respiratory tract	Nerves, leukocytes	Many (e.g., brain, liver, skin)	Respiratory tract, epithelial surfaces
Recurrent	Ganglion	Nerves (to site of latency)	Skin, eye	Skin, eyes
Rabies	Subcutaneously (bite)	Nerves	Brain	Salivary glands
Arbovirus infection	Subcutaneously (bite)	Blood	Brain and others	Lymph and blood (via insect bite)
Hepatitis B	Penetration of skin	Blood	Liver	Blood
Herpes simplex type 2	Genital tract	Nerves (to site of latency)	Genital tract	Genital tract

organ and site of shedding may be the same. Table 45-4 presents other examples.

Dissemination in Nerves

Dissemination through the nerves is less common than bloodstream dissemination, but is the means of spread in a number of important diseases (Fig. 45-4). This mechanism occurs in rabies virus, herpesvirus, and, occasionally, poliomyelitis virus in-

fections. For example, rabies virus implanted by a bite from a rabid animal replicates subcutaneously and within muscular tissue to reach nerve endings. Evidence indicates that the virus spreads centrally in the neurites (axons and dendrites) and perineural cells, where virus is shielded from antibody. This nerve route leads rabies virus to the central nervous system, where disease originates. Rabies virus then spreads centrifugally through the nerves to reach the salivary glands, the site of shed-

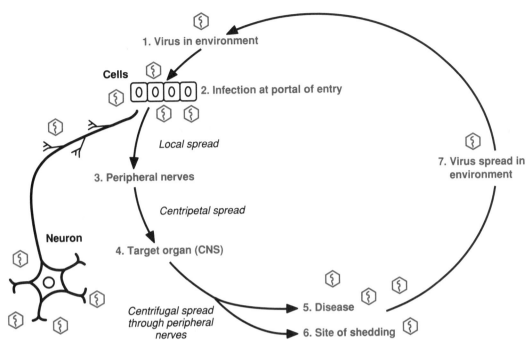

FIGURE 45-4   Virus spread through nerves during a generalized infection. Numbers indicate sequence of events.

ding. Table 45-4 shows other examples of nerve spread.

INCUBATION PERIOD

During most virus infections, no signs or symptoms of disease occur through the stage of virus dissemination. Thus, the incubation period (the time between exposure to virus and onset of disease) extends from the time of implantation through the phase of dissemination, ending when virus replication in the target organs causes disease. Occasionally, mild fever and malaise occur during viremia, but they often are transient and have little diagnostic value.

The incubation period tends to be brief (1 to 3 days) in infections in which virus travels only a short distance to reach the target organ (i.e., in infections in which disease is due to virus replication at the portal of entry). Conversely, incubation periods in generalized infections are longer because of the stepwise fashion by which the virus

moves through the body before reaching the target organs. Other factors also may influence the incubation period. Generalized infections produced by togaviruses may have an unexpectedly short incubation period because of direct intravascular injection (insect bite) of a rapidly multiplying virus. The mechanisms governing the long incubation period (months to years) of persistent infections are poorly understood. The persistently infected cell is often not lysed, or lysis is delayed. In addition, disease may result from a late immune reaction to viral antigen (e.g., arenaviruses in rodents) or from unknown mechanisms in slow viral infections during which no immune response has been detected (as in the scrapie-kuru group).

MULTIPLICATION IN TARGET ORGANS

Virus replication in the target organ resembles replication at other body sites except that (1) the target organ in systemic infections is reached late during the stepwise progression of virus through the body, and (2) clinical disease originates there. At each step of virus progression through the body, the local recovery mechanisms (local body defenses, including interferon, local inflammation, and local immunity) are activated. Thus, when the target organ is infected, the previously infected sites may have reached various stages of recovery. Figure 45-2 illustrates this staging of infection and recovery in different tissues during a spreading surface infection. Circulating interferon and immune responses probably account for the termination of viremia, but these responses may be too late to prevent seeding of virus into the target organ and into sites of shedding. Nevertheless, these systemic defenses can diffuse in various degrees into target organs and thereby help retard virus replication and disease.

Depending on the balance between virus and host defenses (see Chs. 49 and 50), virus multiplication in the target organ may be sufficient to produce dysfunction manifested by disease or death. Additional constitutional disease such as fever and malaise may result from diffusion of toxic products of virus replication and cell necrosis, as well as from release of lymphokines and other inflammatory mediators. Release of leukotriene C4 during respiratory infection may cause bronchospasm. Viral antigens also may participate in immune reactions, leading to disease manifestations. In addition, impairment of leukocytes and immunosuppression by some viruses may cause secondary bacterial infection.

SHEDDING OF VIRUS

Because of the diversity of viruses, virtually every possible site of shedding is utilized (Table 45-4); however, the most frequent sites are the respiratory and alimentary tracts. Blood and lymph are sites of shedding for the arboviruses, since biting insects become infected by this route. HIV is shed in blood and semen. Milk is a site of shedding for viruses such as some RNA tumor viruses (retroviruses) and cytomegalovirus (a herpesvirus). Several viruses (e.g., cytomegaloviruses) are shed simultaneously from the urinary tract and other sites more commonly associated with shedding. The genital tract is a common site of shedding for herpesvirus type 2 and may be the route through which the virus is transmitted to sexual partners or the fetus. Saliva is the primary source of shedding for rabies virus. Cytomegalovirus is also shed from these last two sites. Finally, viruses such as tumor viruses that are integrated into the DNA of host cells can be shed through germ cells.

CONGENITAL INFECTIONS

Infection of the fetus is a special case of infection in a target organ. The factors that determine whether a target organ is infected also apply to the fetus, but the fetus presents additional variables. The immune and interferon systems of the very young fetus are immature. This immaturity, coupled with the partial placental barrier to transfer of maternal immunity and interferon, deprive the very young fetus of important defense mechanisms. Another variable is the high vulnerability to disruption of the rapidly developing fetal organs, especially during the first trimester of pregnancy. Furthermore, susceptibility to virus replication may be modulated by the undifferentiated state of the fetal cells and by hormonal changes during pregnancy. Interestingly, although virus multiplication in the fetus may lead to congenital anomalies or fetal death, the mother may have only a mild or inapparent infection.

To cause congenital anomalies, virus must reach the fetus and multiply in it, thereby causing maldeveloped organs. Generally, virus reaches the fetus during maternal viremia by infecting or passing through the placenta to the fetal circulation and then to fetal target organs. Sufficient virus multiplication may disrupt development of fetal organs, especially during their rapid development (the first trimester of pregnancy). Although many viruses occasionally cause congenital anomalies, cytomegalovirus and rubella virus are the most common offenders. Virus shedding by the congenitally infected newborn infant may occur as a result of persistence of the virus infection at sites of shedding.

REFERENCES

Albrecht T, Boldogh I, Fons M et al: Cell activation signals and the pathogenesis of human cytomegalovirus. Intervirology 31:68, 1990

Buller RML, Chakrabarti S, Cooper JA et al: Deletion of the vaccinia virus growth factor gene reduces virus virulence. J Virol 62:866, 1988

Fenner F, White DO: Medical Virology. 2nd Ed. Academic Press, San Diego, 1976

Fields BN: How do viruses cause different diseases? J Am Med Assoc 250:1754, 1983

Galasso GJ, Merigan TC, Buchanan RA (eds): Antiviral Agents and Viral Diseases of Man. Raven Press, New York, 1984

Kauffman RS, Wolf JL, Finberg R et al: The sigma 1 protein determines the extent of spread of reovirus from the gastrointestinal tract of mice. Virology 124:403, 1983

Strayer DS, Laybourne KA, Heard HK: Determinants of the ability of malignant fibroma virus to induce immune dysfunction and tumor dissemination in vivo. Microb Pathog 9:173, 1990

46 PERSISTENT VIRAL INFECTIONS

ISTVAN BOLDOGH
THOMAS ALBRECHT
DAVID D. PORTER

GENERAL CONCEPTS

Definitions

There are three types of persistent viral infection. In **latent infections,** no infectious virus is detectable between episodes of recurrent disease. In **chronic infection,** the acute primary infection is followed by chronic, low-level production of virus; disease may be chronic or recurring. **Slow infections** have a long incubation period followed by progressive disease.

Models of Persistence in Vitro

Three kinds of persistent infection can be maintained in cell cultures: chronic focal, chronic diffuse, and latent. These infections may model key aspects of persistent infections in living hosts.

Pathogenesis

The mechanisms by which persistent infections are maintained involve both modulation of virus gene expression and modification of the host immune response. Reactivation of a latent or chronic infection may be triggered by various stimuli, including superinfection by another virus, physical stress or trauma, and changes in cell physiology. Immunosuppression is particularly associated with reactivation of a number of persistent virus infections.

Persistent Infections by Organ System

Immune System: The viruses that establish persistent infections in cells of the immune system include human immunodeficiency virus, human T-cell leukemia viruses (HTLV-1 and HTLV-2), Epstein-Barr virus, human cytomegalovirus, and human herpesviruses 6 and 7.

Nervous System: Viruses that can establish latent infections of the nervous system include herpes simplex virus types 1 and 2, varicella-zoster virus, measles virus, and human papovaviruses. Unconventional agents cause the slow infections known as subacute spongiform virus encephalopathies.

Digestive System: Hepatitis B virus can establish a chronic infection of hepatocytes (which may exacerbate to acute hepatitis upon superinfection with the defective virus known as delta agent). Hepatitis B virus can also latently infect some cell types. Adenoviruses can establish latent infections, most often in the adenoids and tonsils.

Skin and Mucous Membranes: The human papillomaviruses persistently infect epithelial cells. In some cases the infection is latent and may be tumorigenic.

Control

No measures to eradicate persistent viruses have been developed. Vaccination can sometimes prevent infection and may reduce the frequency of clinical recurrences.

INTRODUCTION

Medical science has begun to control a number of acute virus infections, many by immunization, but persistent virus infections are largely uncontrolled. Diseases caused by persistent virus infections include acquired immune deficiency syndrome (AIDS), chronic hepatitis B, subacute sclerosing panencephalitis (chronic measles encephalitis), chronic papovavirus encephalitis (progressive multifocal leukoencephalopathy, PML), spongiform encephalopathies (caused by unconventional viruses), several herpesvirus-induced diseases, and some neoplasias. The pathogenic mechanisms by which these viruses cause disease include disorders of biochemical, cellular, immune, and physiologic processes. Ongoing studies are rapidly advancing our understanding of many persistent infections. Viruses have evolved a wide variety of strategies by which they maintain long-term infection of populations (see Ch. 48), individuals, and tissue cultures. This chapter primarily describes persistent infections in vivo and focuses on viruses that persist in humans.

DEFINITIONS

Persistent infections are those in which the virus is not cleared from the host following primary infection, but remains associated with specific cells. Figure 46-1 presents a classification scheme of the principal types of persistent infections in vivo. **Latent infection** is characterized by the lack of demonstrable infectious virus between episodes of recurrent disease. **Chronic infection** is characterized by the continued presence of virus following the primary infection and may include chronic or

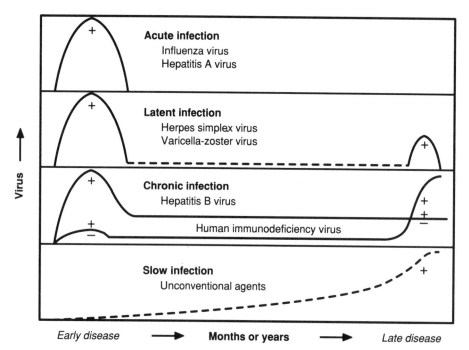

FIGURE 46-1 Natural history of acute and persistent human infections. Solid line, shedding of infectious virus; dashed line, virus not readily demonstrable; +, disease episode.

recurrent disease. **Slow infection** is characterized by a prolonged incubation period followed by progressive disease. Unlike latent and chronic infections, slow infection may not begin with an acute period of viral multiplication. During persistent infections, the viral genome may be either stably integrated into the cellular DNA or maintained episomally.

Some viruses can maintain more than one type of persistent infection at the same time, but in different cells. The type of persistent infection may or may not be dependent on the cell type and the physiologic state of the cell. For example, Epstein-Barr virus (EBV) latently infects B cells, but in the same individual it is released for long periods from productively infected pharyngeal epithelial cells (chronic infection). Therefore, in one individual persistent infection with a single virus may involve multiple types of persistence, each of which may become more or less important as the individual responds to the disease.

MODELS OF VIRUS PERSISTENCE IN VITRO

Three types of persistent infection can be distinguished in cultured cells (Table 46-1). In the first, known as **chronic focal infection** (carrier culture), only a small portion of the cell population is infected. These cells release virus and are killed. Low concentrations of antiviral substances (e.g., interferon) reduce extracellular virus to a low level so that only a small number of susceptible cells are infected at any time, maintaining the infection. Such chronic focal persistent infections can be "cured" by increasing the concentration of antiviral antibody, interferon, or nonspecific inhibitor. In **chronic diffuse infections** (steady-state infections), all the cells are infected and both virus and cell multiplication proceed without the cells being killed. Virus is continually released from the cells, and the infection cannot be eliminated by antiviral antibodies. The third type is the so-called **true latent infection,** in which the viral genome is replicated and segregated to the daughter cells either within the chromosomes or extrachromosomally. In some persistent infections, the viral genome may be integrated into the cellular DNA.

PATHOGENESIS OF PERSISTENT VIRUS INFECTIONS

Persistent infections are caused by a wide variety of viruses through diverse pathogenetic mechanisms that may cause strikingly different diseases (see Chs. 57, 59, 62, 66, 67, 68, 70, and 71 for thorough discussions of the viruses that cause persistent infections). Although the mechanisms by which any of these viruses produce persistent infection are not completely understood, some common factors have been identified.

The first is immune modulation. Many viruses that cause persistent infection avoid the nonspecific and specific immune defenses in several ways. Examples include

1. Limitation of recognition molecules on infected cells:
    a. Restricted expression of viral antigens (e.g., measles virus in subacute sclerosing panencephalitis).
    b. Antiviral antibody-induced internalization and modulation of viral antigens (e.g., measles virus).
    c. Viral antigenic variation (e.g., human immunodeficiency virus [HIV]).
    d. Blocking antibody that prevents the binding of neutralizing antibody (e.g., measles virus).
    e. Decreased expression of cell major histocompatibility complex recognition molecules (e.g., adenovirus).
    f. Restricted expression of the cell adhesion molecules LFA-3 and ICAM-1 (e.g., Epstein-Barr virus).
2. Altered lymphocyte and macrophage functions, including modified production of cytokines and immunosuppression (e.g., human immunodeficiency virus).
3. Infection in immunologically privileged anatomic sites (e.g., herpesviruses in the central nervous system).
4. Compromised nonspecific defenses (e.g., interferon).
5. Immune tolerance (?).

The second factor is modulation of viral expression. Examples include down regulation of some

TABLE 46-1   Virus-Cell Interactions In Vivo

Types of Infection	Fraction of Cells Infected	Cell Death	Infectious Virus	Schematized Mechanism	Disease Examples	Controlling Mechanism
Acute Cytocidal	All	+	+		Influenza Poliomyelitis Togavirus encephalitis	None
Persistent Chronic diffuse	All	0	+		Rubella Lymphocytic choriomeningitis	Noncytocidal viruses
Chronic focal	Few	+	+		Adenovirus infections	Antiviral substances (e.g., antibody, interferon)
Latent	Few	0 (during latency)	+ (with reactivation)		Herpes simplex	Not known

viral genes by viral or cellular regulatory gene products and possibly by synthesis of latency-associated transcripts and viral variants.

Further work is being directed toward defining the relative importance of various mechanisms in the initiation and maintenance of persistent viral infections.

REACTIVATION OF PERSISTENT VIRUSES

For disease to recur in a latent infection, the virus must be reactivated and begin replicating. Some factors associated with reactivation are infection with other viruses (as in HIV), nerve trauma (e.g., herpes facialis following surgery of the trigeminal ganglion), physiologic and physical changes (e.g., fever, menstruation, and sunlight), and immunosuppression (as in cytomegalovirus disease). Papovavirus encephalitis in immunosuppressed patients may represent exacerbation and spread of a chronic infection.

PERSISTENT INFECTIONS BY ORGAN SYSTEM

Immune System

A number of viruses can infect cells of the lymphoid system during acute infection, and some of these viruses persist (Table 46-2). Thus, the lymphoid system also may serve as a reservoir for seeding other organs with the persisting virus. Persistent infection of the immune system may lead to evasion of immunologic surveillance.

Human Immunodeficiency Virus

HIV infection is often followed by a clinical latent period of many years before AIDS develops. A variety of immune cells (e.g., CD4$^+$ lymphocytes, B cells, monocyte-macrophages, promyelocytes, dentritic cells) can be infected by the virus. The long lag time between infection and development of AIDS is called clinical latency. During the lag phase, about 0.01 percent of lymphocytes or macrophages are infected and only 1 percent of these produce virus. Because of the long-term produc-

tion of low levels of virus, the monocyte-macrophages are important reservoirs for persistent HIV in vivo, and these cells may seed other tissues and organs with the virus.

The restricted production of virus during the lag period may be due to three HIV regulatory proteins (Tat, Rev, and Nef) that appear to be involved in the development and maintenance of chronic persistent infection (Fig. 46-2). Tat is a transactivator of all HIV sequences, augmenting increased RNA levels. The *rev* gene encodes a protein (Rev) that causes the viral DNA to produce selectively either regulatory proteins or viral structural components. The interaction between Tat and Rev and HIV DNA results in a controlled, often noncytocidal infection. The *nef* gene is a negative regulator whose product (Nef) slows the replication of the virus. The effects of these three regulatory proteins result in a well-controlled, persistent HIV infection.

The transition from a latent to a productive infection may occur in response to mitogens that activate T cells to proliferate. Gene products from other viral infections, including cytomegalovirus, human herpesvirus 6, Epstein-Barr virus, and human T-cell leukemia virus, can enhance and/or activate HIV transcription and may be important in HIV pathogenesis. How do HIV-infected cells escape immune surveillance? Several mechanisms have been proposed.

1. Expression of HIV and HIV-induced cellular proteins may be down regulated.
2. HIV may escape neutralizing antibodies by spreading directly from cell to cell.
3. Budding of virus particles into cytoplasmic vacuoles instead of budding from the cell surface may occur, resulting in masked virus production.
4. Extracellular Tat protein may inhibit antigen-induced lymphocyte proliferation.
5. There may be genetic (antigenic) variation among HIV isolates.
6. Multiplication in immunologically privileged sites may occur.
7. Immune and nonspecific defenses may be inhibited.

TABLE 46-2   Persistent Virus Infections Primarily
Associated with the Immune System

Virus	Cells Harboring Virus	Physical State of Virus Genome	Mechanism of Persistence	Reactivation Syndromes
HIV	CD4+ T cells, monocytes, macrophages	Integrated into cell DNA; episomal	Immune avoidance	AIDS
EBV	B lymphocytes	Episomal	Decreased synthesis (?) of cell adhesion molecules (ICAM-1, LFA-3)	Neoplasias and AIDS-related conditions
CMV	CD4+, CD8+ T cells, interstitial mononuclear inflammatory cells	Episomal	Limited viral gene expression	Birth defects, multiple diseases associated with immunosuppression
HHV-6	B and T cells	Episomal?	Limited viral genome expression	AIDS-related conditions
HTLV-1 and 2	T lymphocytes	Integrated	Down regulation of viral gene expression	Leukemia, neurologic disorders

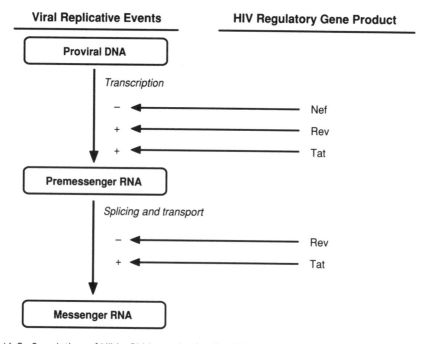

FIGURE 46-2   Regulation of HIV mRNA production by HIV gene products during persistent infection. Host regulatory mechanisms also are important in modulating HIV expression and replication.

Human T-Cell Leukemia Viruses

Infection by these viruses is followed by a 10- to 30-year clinically latent period before development of leukemias or neurologic disorders. As with HIV, the long lag period may be due to the HTLV regulatory proteins (Rex and Tax) encoded by the integrated proviral DNA. The virus may persist in the form of an integrated genome in cells not expressing viral antigens.

Epstein-Barr Virus

EBV persistently infects hematopoietic cells, both the large light B blasts and the small heavy B cells, presumably in the G_0 phase of the cell cycle. The estimated frequency of EBV-carrying cells in the blood is in the range of 10^{-6} to 10^{-7}, with limited expression of viral genes in latently infected cells.

The EBNA-1 EBV gene and a *cis*-acting sequence, *oriP*, together constitute a plasmid replicon that ensures replication of the EBV genome in latently infected cells. Also, the viral latent membrane proteins down regulate viral and cellular genes to avoid immune responses. In addition, latent membrane proteins and EBNA-2 appear to

function in the immortalization of latently infected cells in vitro (Fig. 46-3). Production of infectious virus requires the activation of the BZLF-1 gene, which encodes a regulatory protein that transactivates additional EBV genes, leading to a replication cycle.

After the initial infection, humoral and cellular immunity to EBV develops. Since virus-specific antigen(s) is present in the membrane of latently infected B cells, it is appropriate to examine how these cells escape immune surveillance. This phenomenon has been studied in EBV-positive Burkitt lymphoma (BL) cells. These cells were not killed by major histocompatibility complex (MHC)-matched, virus-specific cytotoxic lymphocytes (CTL) in assays in which EBV-transformed B lymphoblastoid cells derived from the normal B cells of the patients were readily lysed. Resistance of EBV-transformed cells to cytotoxic T lymphocytes is correlated with a reduced level of the cellular adhesion molecules LFA-3 and ICAM-1 on the cell surface (Fig. 46-3). Therefore, the initial interaction that normally occurs between cytotoxic T lymphocytes and target cells does not take place, and the infected cells may survive even though they

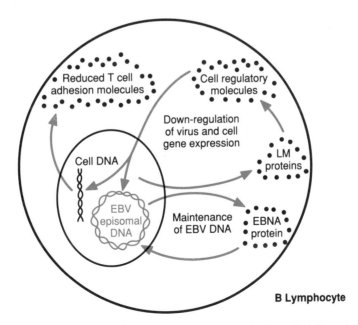

FIGURE 46-3 Maintenance of EBV DNA and immune avoidance by latently infected cells. LM, EBV-latent membrane protein; EBNA, EBV nuclear antigen.

express class 1 major histocompatibility complex molecules and the EBV-encoded latent membrane proteins.

Human Cytomegalovirus

The strongest evidence for the existence of latent CMV infection comes from the increased incidence of reactivated infection in seronegative individuals who undergo transplants of organs from seropositive donors. Endogenous sources of cytomegalovirus are also found in immunosuppressed AIDS patients. The best candidate cells for latent infection are thought to be leukocytes, particularly mononuclear cells, bearing either CD4 or CD8 markers.

The physical state of viral DNA and the extent of its expression during the latent state are not yet characterized. Gene expression of latent virus is very limited.

Human Herpesviruses 6 and 7

These viruses are latent in resting T cells, but may replicate in T cells stimulated to proliferate, including those in lymphoproliferative disorders. Also, both viruses are activated in immunosuppressive disorders such as AIDS.

Nervous System

Many chronic, degenerative nervous system diseases are related to viral persistence (Table 46-3).

Persistence in the nervous system probably involves some unique mechanisms that take advantage of the many types of specialized cells and the immunologically privileged status of the central nervous system.

Herpes Simplex Virus Types 1 and 2

During acute herpes simplex virus (HSV) infection (see Ch. 68), virus and/or viral components (e.g., nucleocapsids) containing viral genetic material ascend in nerve axons from the initial site of infection to the sensory ganglia—mainly the trigeminal ganglia in the case of HSV-1; mainly the lumbar and sacral ganglia in the case of HSV-2 (Fig. 46-4A). In the sensory ganglia, the virus may cause a cytolytic infection or establish a latent, noncytolytic infection. Sympathetic ganglia and other cell types of the central nervous system may also serve as sites of virus latency. In the neuron, viral DNA is maintained as an extrachromosomal plasmid (episome) with 1 to 20 copies per cell. Reactivation with recurrent productive infection and disease is induced by various factors, such as heat, cold, ultraviolet light, unrelated immune hypersensitivity reactions, pituitary or adrenal hormones, immunosuppression, and emotional disturbance. Current studies are examining the possibility that latent virus is restricted by virus DNA-encoded antisense RNA molecules known as latency-associated transcripts (LATs). When the latent virus is reactivated, its genome passes anterograde in

TABLE 46-3   Persistent Infections Primarily
Associated with the Nervous System

Virus	Cells Harboring Virus	Virus Genome	Mechanism of Persistence	Reactivation Syndromes
HSV-1 and 2	Neurons	Episomal?	Restricted viral and cell MHC gene expression	Surface lesions and CNS
VZV	Neurons and satellite cells	Episomal?	Restricted viral genome expression	Herpes zoster
JC	Oligodendrocytes, and other cells of the CNS	Integrated/episomal	?	Progressive multifocal leukoencephalopathy
Measles	Neurons and supporting cells	?	Restricted viral multiplication	Subacute sclerosing panencephalitis

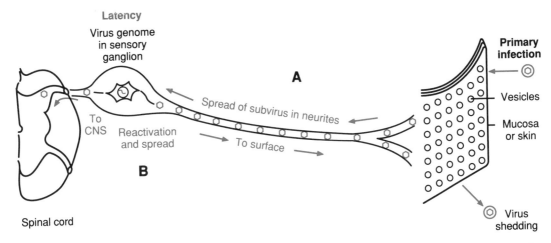

FIGURE 46-4 Establishment and reactivation of latent herpesvirus infections. *(A)* Establishment of herpes simplex virus or varicella-zoster virus latency in ganglia after primary infection of skin or mucosa. *(B)* Reactivation of virus in ganglion and spread through nerves to skin or mucosa to cause surface lesions or retrograde spread through nerves to central nervous system to cause encephalitis (infrequent).

axons to the epithelium, where productive replication takes place (Fig. 46-4B).

Varicella-Zoster Virus

After recovery from acute varicella, virus remains within the sensory ganglia (Fig. 46-4A). Years later, virus may reactivate, possibly owing to suppression of cell-mediated immunity or local trauma. In most patients, virus spreads unilaterally down the peripheral nerve to productively infect the corresponding dermatome (Fig. 46-4B). However, in immunocompromised patients, life-threatening disseminated infections can occur. Studies suggest that the virus is harbored in sensory ganglia (trigeminal and/or dorsal) and satellite cells. In these cells, limited transcription of the latent viral genome has been reported. Expression of latent varicella-zoster virus genes seems to be more extensive than in the case of herpes simplex virus: only one HSV DNA region is transcribed whereas at least five diverse regions of the varicella-zoster virus genome produce latency-associated transcripts. No virus-specific protein synthesis is detectable. The virus genome appears to be episomal during latency. The molecular basis for reactivation of latent virus is not known.

Measles Virus

Measles is normally an acute self-limited disease in which the virus appears to be eliminated. In rare individuals, however, virus persists in the brain. Possible mechanisms of persistence include the immunologically privileged status of the brain, antiviral antibody-induced internalization of viral antigens, and restricted virus expression and replication.

A late (5 to 15 years) sequela of acute measles virus infection is subacute sclerosing panencephalitis (SSPE), which occurs in about 1/100,000 individuals who have had measles. This slow virus infection is manifested by progressive mental deterioration, involuntary movements, muscular rigidity, and coma. Mature virions, containing antisense RNA, are rarely produced. The affected neurons contain the sense strand of measles RNA, inclusion bodies containing nucleocapsids, cell surface proteins (hemagglutinin, fusion protein) and the matrix (M) protein, which is important for viral assembly. Virus-infected cells may avoid immune surveillance by a defect in virus M protein production in subacute sclerosing panencephalitis. This defect could contribute to the lack of virus budding, which favors persistence. Subacute sclerosing panencephalitis patients have high titers of anti-measles antibody in both serum and cerebrospinal fluid; however, antibody to M protein is often lacking.

Human Papovaviruses

The JC papovavirus is widely distributed in the human population. The virus is thought to persist in the kidney, perhaps via an integrated or episomal form, and is reactivated when the host immune system is impaired (e.g., HIV infection, immunosuppressive therapy, pregnancy). JC virus is regularly isolated from brain cells of patients with progressive multifocal leukoencephalopathy (PML), a fatal demyelinating disease.

The mechanism of persistence may be related to an integrated infection, as with other papovaviruses (simian virus 40, BK virus). The latent JC virus genome can randomly integrate into cellular DNA and encode T antigen(s). When excision of viral DNA is induced by certain conditions, the latent genome becomes activated, infectious virus is produced, and disease may develop.

Persistent Infections Caused by Unconventional Agents

The subacute spongiform virus encephalopathies are a unique type of slow virus infection caused by agents called unconventional viruses. The infective component of these agents is a protein related to a normal cell protein, and the agents lack detectable amounts of nucleic acid. A long incubation period (often years to decades) with slowly rising and spreading infection precedes the onset of clinical illness and is followed by a chronic progressive disease (months to years). The mechanisms responsible for slow multiplication are unknown. The host shows no inflammatory response, no humoral or cellular immune response, and no interferon production. Immunosuppression of the host has no effect on pathogenesis or progression of disease. The human subacute spongiform virus encephalopathies include kuru, Creutzfeldt-Jakob disease, and Gerstmann-Straussler-Schenker syndrome.

Digestive System

Of the numerous viruses that infect the digestive system, most (the enteroviruses and reoviruses) are considered to be acute viruses that cause infections even though some may continue for months or even years. Persistent infections may be caused by hepatitis B virus (HBV), adenoviruses, and the dependovirus group of parvoviruses (Table 46-4).

Hepatitis B Virus

Among the hepatitis viruses only HBV is able to develop a persistent infection. Persistent HBV infection may be either chronic or latent, depending

TABLE 46-4   Persistent Infections Primarily Associated with the Digestive System and Skin

Virus	Cells Harboring Virus	Physical State of Virus Genome	Mechanism of Persistence	Reactivation Syndromes
Digestive system				
Hepatitis B virus	Hepatic, pancreatic	Integrated/episomal	Restricted viral gene expression	Chronic hepatitis, hepatocellular carcinoma (?)
Adenovirus	Epithelial, adenoidal, lymphocytes (?)	Integrated/episomal	Restricted cell MHC gene expression	None known
Skin and mucous membranes				
Human papilloma virus	Germinal epithelial cells	Episomal	Restricted viral gene expression	Warts and carcinomas

on the host cell type. Chronic hepatitis develops in about 10 percent of hepatitis B patients. The presence of viral surface antigen (HBsAg) in serum serves as a marker of persistent infection. In chronic infections, HBV productively infects hepatocytes and maintains a low level of virus production over a long period. It is not known whether the destruction of hepatocytes in these infections is due to cytotoxic effects of the virus or to specific cells of the immune system. In addition, HBV is capable of causing latent infections (e.g., of peripheral blood lymphocytes or bone marrow cells) in which viral gene expression is very limited.

The mechanism of viral latency is mostly unknown, but may involve random incorporation of viral DNA into the cellular chromosomes. Integrated HBV DNA is also present in hepatocytes during active disease. Integration is not required for virus replication, but it may be a crucial event for long-term perpetuation of the virus genome. It is a common finding in hepatocellular carcinomas and cell lines derived from hepatocellular carcinomas. There is either limited or no detectable expression of viral genes in these cells.

Other Hepatitis Viruses (Hepatitis C, Delta Agent and Non-A, Non-B Viruses)

At present there is no evidence available regarding long-term persistence of hepatitis C and non-A, non-B viruses. However, delta agent, a defective virus that requires active replication of coinfecting HBV for its own reproduction, may exacerbate hepatitis B (see Ch. 70). The mechanism of this interaction is being studied.

Adenoviruses

The high incidence of adenovirus infections in organ transplant (kidney, bone marrow) recipients and AIDS patients suggests that these infections most probably represent reactivation of a latent adenovirus infection. For example, adenoviruses can persist latently for years in adenoids and tonsils and often are shed in the feces for many months after the initial infection.

The mechanism and the cell type harboring the latent virus in vivo is presently unknown. In vitro studies suggest that the mechanism used to avoid immune surveillance is the suppression of major histocompatibility complex expression. For example, the adenovirus type 2 early protein can bind to major histocompatibility complex antigens and prevent them from being correctly glycosylated. Adenovirus type 12 early protein (E1a) inhibits class 1 major histocompatibility complex expression at the transcriptional level and blocks the transport of major histocompatibility complex mRNA molecules into the cytoplasm. It is possible that down regulation of class 1 major histocompatibility complex antigen operates in the host during natural persistent infection.

Dependovirus Group of Parvoviruses

The dependovirus group of parvoviruses (the adeno-associated viruses) can be isolated from fecal, ocular, or respiratory specimens and from penile and condylomatous lesions during simultaneous adenovirus infections. The adeno-associated viruses integrate into host cell DNA and replicate with it, only to be excised and induced to replicate when the latently infected cells are superinfected with adenoviruses. The dependoviruses are not known to be pathogenic.

Skin

Of the viruses that cause acute infections of the skin and mucous membranes, the papillomaviruses (Table 46-4) and herpesviruses (see above) are capable of establishing persistent infections.

Human Papillomaviruses

The ubiquity of latent papillomavirus infections is emphasized by the frequent, often acute outbreak of warts in immunosuppressed patients and pregnant women. Human papillomaviruses specifically infect cells of the basal layer of the epidermis. When the basal cells divide, one cell remains as a basal cell and the other enters the suprabasal level. The latent virus genome, possibly in episomal form, replicates along with the host cells. This persistent infection is associated with some skin cancers and cervical cancer. Productive viral replication occurs only in terminally differentiated skin cells (see Fig. 66-4). At present, little is known about the mechanisms regulating papillomavirus latency and replication.

CONTROL OF PERSISTENT INFECTIONS

Studies of treatment of persistent infections are beginning. Promising findings are that persistent lymphocytic choriomeningitis virus infection of mice can be cured by immune T cells and some persistent hepatitis B infections of humans can be cured with alpha interferon. Health education is an important component in preventing the spread of infections that tend to persist.

REFERENCES

Ahmed R, Jamieson BD, Porter BD: Immune therapy of a persistent and disseminated viral infection. J Virol 61:3920, 1987

Arthur RR, Shah KV: Occurrence and significance of papovaviruses BK and JC in the urine. Prog Med Virol 36:42, 1989

Berns KL, Bohenzky RA: Adeno-associated viruses: an update. Adv Virus Res 32:243, 1987

Black FL: Measles active and passive immunity in a worldwide perspective. Prog Med Virol 36:1, 1989

Evans LA, Levy JA: Characteristics of HIV infection and pathogenesis. Biochim Biophys Acta 989:237, 1989

Galloway DA, McDougall JK: Human papillomaviruses and carcinomas. Adv Virus Res 37:125, 1989

Hammarskjold ML, Rekosh D: The molecular biology of the human immunodeficiency virus. Biochim Biophys Acta 989:269, 1989

Howard CR: The biology of hepadenaviruses. J Gen Virol 67:1215, 1986

Hull R, McGeoch DJ: Some highlights of virus research in 1988. J Gen Virol 70:2815, 1989

Hwang LY, Beasley RP: Hepatitis B virus as the major cause of hepatocellular carcinoma. Cancer Bull 40:258, 1988

Klein G: Viral latency and transformation: the strategy of Epstein Barr virus. Cell 58:5, 1989

Narayan O, Clements JE: Biology and pathogenesis of lentiviruses. J Gen Virol 70:1617, 1989

Oldstone MBA: Viral persistence. Cell 56:5, 1989

Spalholz BA, Howley PM: Papillomavirus-host cell interactions. Adv Viral Oncol 8:27, 1989

Stevens JG: Human herpesviruses: a consideration of the latent state. Microbiol Rev 53:318, 1989

Sugden B: An intricate route to immortality. Cell 57:5, 1989

Valerie LN, McGrath MS: Human t-cell leukemia virus involvement in adult leukemia. Cancer Bull 40:276, 1988

47 TUMOR VIRUSES

JOAN C. M. MACNAB
DAVID ONIONS

GENERAL CONCEPTS

CAUSATION OF TUMORS

Biologic criteria for causal association of viruses with tumors include the presence of virus in tumor tissues, the presence of virus before disease onset, viral persistence, the location of virus at appropriate sites, and prevention of disease by prevention of viral infection.

HUMAN ONCOGENIC RNA VIRUSES

Classification of Retroviruses

Retroviruses are divided into oncoviruses, lentiviruses, and spumaviruses. These in turn can be divided into three broad groups.

1. Feline, murine, and avian leukemogenic retroviruses replicate efficiently in their hosts, produce a broad range of diseases, and interact with cellular proto-oncogenes to produce leukemia.
2. Human leukemogenic retroviruses are exemplified by the human viruses HTLV-1 and HTLV-2 and the related bovine and simian viruses; they often establish a latent infection in their host cells, have a narrow disease spectrum, and carry a transactivating gene, *tax,* associated with transformation.
3. Simian type-D retroviruses and mouse mammary tumor virus make up the final group.

Replication

Retroviruses generally replicate by binding to a cellular receptor and causing transcription of genomic RNA into proviral DNA and integration of proviral DNA into chromosomal DNA. Latency may be established at this point, or transcription may occur to produce new genomes and mRNA. Virus is released by budding, usually without cytopathology. HTLV-1 has a specific pattern of replication involving transactivation by *tax,* followed by a switch to viral structural proteins as the level of *rex* protein builds up, by means similar to those of HIV replication.

Oncogenic Transformation

The mechanisms of oncogenic transformation by HTLV-1 are areas of active research. Studies of other oncogenic retroviruses have identified viral genes (v-*onc*) that have been acquired by recombination from cellular genes (c-*onc*). The c-*onc* genes mainly regulate cellular growth and differentiation, but like their viral counterparts, they can be disregulated or mutated, a process associated with their oncogenic capacity. The general classes of oncogenes encode growth factors, cellular receptors, signaling proteins, DNA binding proteins, and other regulatory proteins.

HTLV-1 appears to have a distinct transforming mechanism. It carries a viral gene *tax* that is required for replication but that can transactive cellular genes. Among these are the interleukin-2 and interleukin-3 receptor genes, whose expression could lead to transformation by an autocrine mechanism. Ongoing studies of secondary events in the development of HTLV-induced leukemia in vivo illustrate that multiple genetic events are necessary for transformation.

629

ONCOGENIC DNA VIRUSES

Oncogenic human DNA viruses include hepatitis B virus, herpesviruses, and papillomaviruses. Their mechanisms of replication and epidemiology are considered in each of the specific chapters describing these viruses.

Human Hepatitis B Virus

Clinical Manifestations: Patients develop cirrhosis caused by persistent infection, which progresses to primary hepatocellular carcinoma.

Epidemiology and Geographic Distribution: Hepatitis B virus is prevalent in Southeast Asia and Africa. Tumors are associated with an early age at first infection and with viral persistence.

Molecular Mechanisms of Transformation: One possible mechanism to account for the oncogenicity of hepatitis B virus could be integration within or near a cellular gene responsible for growth control or regulation (e.g., an oncogene). Other possible mechanisms of viral involvement in oncogenesis are (1) repression of the cell interferon beta promoter by a *trans* mechanism; (2) integration within a cell cycle control gene, cyclin; and (3) integration near a hormone response gene, thus altering control.

Diagnosis: Viral DNA is detected commonly by Southern blotting with a radiolabeled probe.

Control: Control by vaccination is possible.

Herpesviruses: Epstein-Barr Virus and Burkitt's Lymphoma

Clinical Manifestations: Epstein-Barr virus may cause a B-cell lymphoma of childhood.

Epidemiology and Geographic Distribution: Epstein-Barr virus is present in regions of equatorial Africa where vector-borne disease is common. Primary infection occurs at a very early age.

Host Response to the Tumor: Epstein-Barr virus-encoded proteins are produced, especially Epstein-Barr virus nuclear antigen 1, whose expression has been correlated with tumor expression.

Molecular Mechanism of Transformation: The most important molecular mechanism associated with Burkitt's lymphoma is the increased transcription of the proto-oncogene c-*myc*, which is transferred from its location in chromosome 8 to chromosome 14, where it is much more actively transcribed under control of the heavy chain of the immunoglobulin gene.

Cofactors: Immune suppression at an early age by infection with malaria may influence the pathogenesis of Epstein-Barr virus infection.

Other B-Cell Lymphomas: Other lymphomas are seen in immunocompromised patients in whom the tumors do not behave like Burkitt's lymphoma because they arise quickly and often in immune-privileged sites, such as the central nervous system.

Diagnosis: Episomal Epstein-Barr virus DNA is detected in the tumor by Southern blotting with a radiolabeled probe.

Control: The tumor responds at least primarily to drug therapy.

Herpesviruses: Epstein-Barr Virus and Nasopharyngeal Carcinoma

Clinical Manifestations: The presentation is squamous carcinoma of the nasopharynx.

Epidemiology and Geographic Distribution: Nasopharyngeal carcinoma is prevalent in China and Southeast Asia. The tumor most often is present in the fifth and sixth decades of life.

Persistence of the Virus: The virus is mainly latent in a monoclonal tumor, and the Epstein-Barr virus genome persists as multiple copies of episomes in the tumor cells.

Molecular Mechanisms of Transformation: Only Epstein-Barr virus nuclear antigen 1 has been detected in nasopharyngeal carcinoma.

Cofactors: Genetic factors and dietary carcinogens may be cofactors.

Diagnosis: Epstein-Barr virus DNA is detected by Southern blotting with a radiolabeled probe.

Control: The tumor may respond to chemotherapy.

Herpesviruses: Herpes Simplex Virus Type 2

Clinical Manifestations: Herpes simplex virus type 2 is associated with cervical intraepithelial neoplasia or cervical uterine tumors.

Diagnosis: Virus DNA is present in only about 10 percent of tumors detected by Southern blotting with a radiolabeled probe.

Persistence of the Virus: Herpes simplex virus type 2 infections generally are persistent and latent.

Host Response to the Tumor: Studies have detected higher antibody titers and a greater incidence of herpes simplex virus antibody-positive individuals in patients with cervical cancer of the uterus.

Molecular Mechanisms of Transformation: Cloned fragments, corresponding to the large and small subunits of the ribonucleotide reductase and to stem-loop structure downstream of the small subunit, initiate transformation; the transformed cells are oncogenic. Herpes simplex virus type 2 may act as a cocarcinogen in the evolution of cervical cancer of the uterus, and herpes simplex virus DNA is not required to retain the transformed phenotype. Important mechanisms for this "hit-and-run" type of transformation include mutagenesis, gene amplification, induction of endogenous retroviruses, and increased or altered expression of cellular genes (oncogenes). Herpes simplex virus type 2 DNA from the transforming *BglII* N fragment can convert keratinocytes, immortalized by human papillomavirus to oncogenicity in the nude mouse by regulating growth or differentiation or by induction of cellular oncogenes.

Control: Control measures include the use of condoms and avoidance of first intercourse at an early age and of multiple sexual partners.

Herpesviruses: Human Cytomegalovirus

Epidemiology: The total genome of human cytomegalovirus is reported to be present in a high percentage of cervical tumors, and the virus has been linked with Kaposi's sarcoma.

Diagnosis: The virus is detected in tumors by Southern blotting.

Host Response: It has not been conclusively shown that antibody titers to human cytomegalovirus are raised in patients with cervical carcinoma of the uterus.

Persistence of the Virus: The virus persists in its host and frequently causes no illness.

Molecular Mechanisms of Transformation: Two separate regions of human cytomegalovirus DNA can transform rodent cells in vitro, but the viral DNA may not be retained. Induction of cell genes involved in growth control has been demonstrated for human cytomegalovirus.

Human Papillomaviruses

Clinical Manifestations: Genital strains are closely associated with cervical intraepithelial neoplasia or cervical or vulval cancer. Macular skin lesions of epidermodysplasia verruciformis precede squamous skin carcinomas.

Epidemiology: The virus is ubiquitous. Genital strains are sexually transmitted.

Classification: The different strains (now 60 by DNA homology) show host cell and tissue tropism.

Cofactors: In cervical carcinoma of the uterus, other viruses (e.g., herpes simplex virus type 2 or human cytomegalovirus) or other infectious agents (e.g., chlamydiae) have been implicated as cofactors with human papillomavirus 16. For decades, multiple sexual partners and early age of first intercourse have been recognized as cofactors. In epidermodysplasia verruciformis, impaired cell-mediated immune responses and exposure to sunlight are characteristic.

Host Response to the Tumor: In epidermodysplasia verruciformis, host-mediated immunity is significantly impaired. This disease is associated with several human papillomavirus strains that correlate with impaired immunity. The exact role of the host immune response in patients with cervical intraepithelial neoplasia and cervical carcinoma of the uterus is not clear.

Molecular Mechanisms of Transformation: Human papillomavirus can immortalize cells, but does not code for a virus-encoded oncogene.

State of the HPV genome in tumors: In cervical carcinoma of the uterus the human papillomavirus genome is detected as an integrated 8-kb DNA fragment.

Control: Recommendations for prevention include the use of condoms and avoidance of early age of first intercourse and of multiple sexual partners.

VACCINES IN THE PREVENTION OF CANCERS ASSOCIATED WITH VIRUSES

Experimentally, live vaccinia virus recombinant vaccine which contains a gP340 Epstein-Barr virus glycoprotein prevents the cotton top tamarin from developing lymphomas when challenged with Epstein-Barr virus. Other vaccines also are potentially possible, but problems of safety, efficacy, implementation, and cost must be overcome.

CAUSATION OF TUMORS

Viruses whose association with human oncogenic disease is considered to be causative should ideally fulfill certain criteria:

1. The virus or part of its genome should be closely associated with the oncogenic disease (e.g., should be present in tumor tissues).
2. The virus should persist throughout the disease.
3. A prospective study should show that infection with the virus precedes disease.
4. Prevention of virus infection (e.g., by vaccine) should prevent disease.
5. The location of the virus should be appropriate to account for disease.

In the absence of the ability to test whether the infected virus will induce the tumor, several of these criteria are good evidence for some causative role for the virus in the development of the tumor. Almost always, further cofactors are essential. Viruses from three DNA and one RNA genera fulfill at least some of these criteria, and their association with human tumors deserves further study.

HUMAN ONCOGENIC RNA VIRUSES (RETROVIRUSES)

CLASSIFICATION OF RETROVIRUSES

Although several groups of DNA viruses are oncogenic in their natural hosts, only one group of RNA viruses, the **retroviruses,** have this property. The retroviruses are classified into three major subfamilies.

1. The **oncoviruses** contain the oncogenic retroviruses and are divided into type B, type C, and type D viruses on the basis of their morphology and genome structure.

2. The **lentiviruses** contain viruses (e.g., human immunodeficiency virus [HIV]) associated with slowly progressive, usually fatal conditions (see Ch. 62).
3. The **spumaviruses** are believed to be apathogenic.

ONCOVIRUS GROUPS

Type B Oncoviruses

Only one member of the type B oncoviruses— mouse mammary tumor virus (MMTV)—has been clearly identified. This virus has a distinctive morphology and is produced when a preformed core buds through a cytoplasmic membrane (Fig. 47-1).

Type C Oncoviruses

The type C oncoviruses include the human and animal leukemogenic retroviruses. Neoplastic transformation is induced by these viruses through direct interaction with cellular genes called proto-oncogenes.

One group of type C oncoviruses includes human T-cell leukemia viruses types 1 and 2 (HTLV-1 and HTLV-2) as well as bovine (BLV) and simian (STLV-1) leukemogenic viruses. These viruses establish predominantly latent infections, often with the concurrent production of antiviral antibody. They produce a narrower disease spectrum than the other type C oncoviruses (such as avian leukemia virus); for HTLV-1, the disease spectrum includes adult T-cell leukemia and lymphoma and tropical spastic paraparesis. The HTLV group of viruses carry a viral gene, *tax,* which is probably involved in neoplastic transformation.

Type D Oncoviruses

Type D oncoviruses have been isolated only from nonhuman primates, in which they induce both immunosuppression and proliferative syndromes.

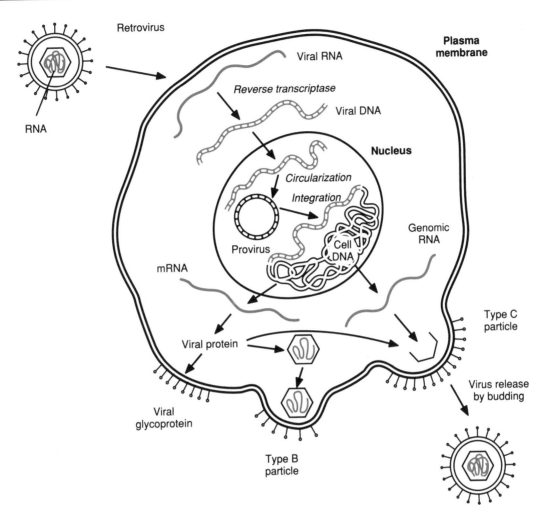

FIGURE 47-1 Replication of retroviruses. Type B and D particles develop from the budding of pre-formed cores known as type A particles.

REPLICATION

General Features

Although there are important differences in the replication strategies among the oncogenic retroviruses, there is a strong common theme. Retroviruses are enveloped RNA viruses, and two copies of the viral genome are enclosed within a core, together with the virion-associated enzyme reverse transcriptase. Surrounding the core is an envelope containing the viral glycoproteins, which serves as the antireceptor for the virus to bind to its target cell (Fig. 47-1). Once bound, the core is released into the cytoplasm and the RNA genome of the virus is transcribed into double-stranded DNA by reverse transcriptase. The double-stranded DNA copy of the viral genome—called the **provirus**—migrates in a nucleoprotein complex to the nucleus, where it becomes covalently integrated into the chromosomal DNA. Integration of the provirus is dependent on an integrase function of reverse transcriptase.

At the gross level, integration appears to be a random process occurring anywhere within open chromatin, although fine-structural features of the chromosomal target may influence the exact integration point. In HTLV infection, the proviral copy number usually ranges from one to three proviruses per cell. The HTLV replication cycle may be halted at this point, and then a latent infection is established within the cell.

Once transcription is initiated, new genomic RNA and mRNA encoding viral proteins are transcribed from the provirus. Viral glycoproteins become substituted into the plasma membrane, and in the type C viruses internal core proteins assem-

ble beneath this region, forming a nascent virion, which is released by a budding process (Fig. 47-1). In contrast to infection with HIV, release of the type C oncoviruses is not usually a cytopathic process; hence, a cell can continue to divide and function normally while releasing virions. These features, coupled with the integration of the provirus into chromosomal DNA, lead to persistent, usually lifelong infections with these viruses.

Genomic Organization

The genomic organization of the oncoviruses is discussed in Chapter 62 and illustrated in Figure 47-2.

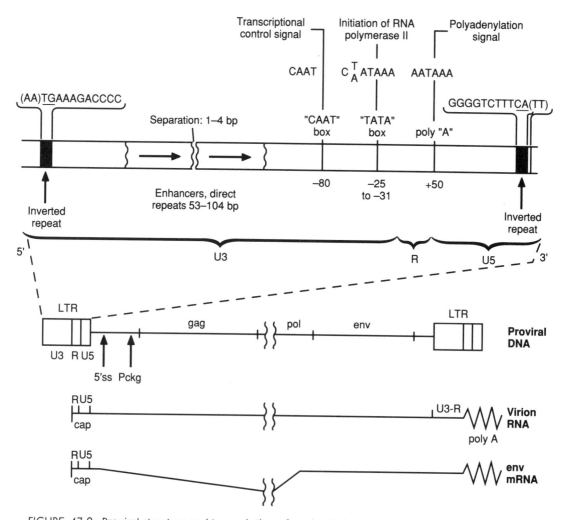

FIGURE 47-2   Proviral structure and transcription of murine leukemia virus.

ONCOGENIC TRANSFORMATION

Oncogenes

Oncogenes are cellular and viral genes that influence cell growth and differentiation and may lead to oncogenic disease. The discovery of the human oncogenic and immunosuppressive retroviruses has been of major importance in human medicine; however, study of animal retroviruses has led to the discovery of the cellular oncogenes, whose mutation or dysregulation leads to oncogenic disease.

When avian leukemia virus infects a chicken, many months may pass before tumors occur, if they occur at all. However, when viruses are isolated from tumor tissue, they may contain acutely transforming viruses (e.g., Rous sarcoma virus [RSV]) that are capable of rapidly reproducing the same type of tumor. Rous sarcoma virus was found

to contain an additional gene, *src,* which is responsible for the transforming activity of the virus. This gene is of cellular origin and becomes incorporated into the virus by recombination (Fig. 47-3).

Subsequently, other acutely transforming retroviruses were characterized, and the generic term **viral oncogene (v-onc)** became used to describe the transduced cellular gene within the viral genome. The cellular homologs of the viral oncogenes are referred to as **c-oncs** or **proto-oncogenes,** to indicate that the cellular genes fulfill normal functions governing replication and differentiation in healthy cells. Rous sarcoma virus is unique in that it is replication competent. Other viral oncogene-containing retroviruses have lost viral sequences and require the presence of a conventional leukemia virus to complement their defectiveness and permit their replication and dis-

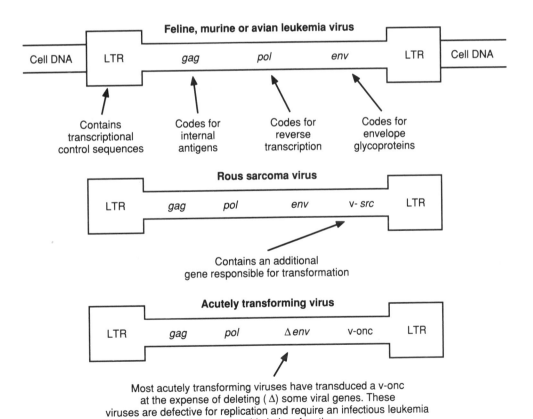

FIGURE 47-3 Proviral structure of rapidly transforming oncogene-containing viruses.

semination throughout the body. Most of the evidence suggests that viral oncogene-containing viruses are generated de novo in each individual and are not transmitted from animal to animal.

Viral Oncogenes Are Derived from Processed Cellular RNA

Examination of viral oncogenes indicates that they differ from their normal cellular counterparts. The most obvious difference is that viral oncogenes lack introns, indicating that they were derived by reverse transcription of spliced mRNA from which the introns have been removed.

Often, there are other important differences, ranging from point mutations to deletions of large domains of the gene, that affect its transforming capacity. Viral oncogenes may also be expressed as a fusion protein with part of the viral *gag* sequences, a factor that can also influence their transforming activity.

Features that influence the transforming properties of an oncogene have been described for the oncogene v-*myc*, which encodes a phosphoprotein that localizes in the nucleus. A major factor governing the target cell that can be transformed resides in the properties of the enhancers within the viral long terminal repeat sequences (LTRs), although other factors, including mutations within *myc*, may play a part.

In one form of insertional mutagenesis, a defective retrovirus integrates upstream of exon 2 and a hybrid mRNA is produced from the promoter within the viral long terminal repeat. This process disrupts the normal feedback regulation of c-*myc* expression, leading to uncoordinated production of the *myc* gene product. Hybrid virus-*myc* RNAs of this form are probably precursors of v-*myc*-containing viruses.

A more complex situation is also shown in Figure 47-4. In this case, the virus integrates some distance from the *myc* gene, but the enhancers within the viral long terminal repeat influence the transcription from the normal c-*myc* promoters. Again, this process disrupts the normal feedback control of *myc* expression.

Nature of Oncogenes

A wide range of genes are activated or transduced by retroviruses, and where their gene products have been identified, it has been possible to assign them to putative functional groups (Fig. 47-5).

A clearly defined group in Figure 47-5 consists of the growth factors interleukin-2 (IL-2) and interleukin-3, which are expressed in response to insertional activation. Since receptors for these factors were present in the cells in which these genes were activated, an autocrine mechanism governing cellular proliferation appears likely in these cases.

Growth factor receptors have been identified as viral oncogenes, and genes for other cell surface structures, like the beta chain of the T-cell antigen receptor, have also been found in retroviruses. For instance, the oncogene v-*erb*-B is the homolog of the epidermal growth factor (EGF) receptor. In this case, there has been extensive modification of the protein, including deletion of the extracellular domain, forming the putative epidermal growth factor-binding site. Other changes in the cytoplasmic domain include the loss of a site for autophosphorylation. Phosphorylation of proteins is an important method of regulating protein activity and of communicating signals intracellularly. Consequently, the net effect of these changes is to produce a receptor that is constitutively active in the absence of its natural ligand.

Another large group of oncogenes, which includes the *src* gene of Rous sarcoma virus (Fig. 47-5, III), also have a tyrosine-protein kinase activity (i.e., they phosphorylate proteins on tyrosine residues). The products of this group of oncogenes appear to be associated with the plasma membrane and may act as second messengers, transducing signals from cell surface receptors.

A distinct group of oncogenes, the *ras* oncogenes, appears to be related to the signal-transducing G proteins, which are regulated by binding to GTP and GDP, the GTP-bound forms being active and the GDP-bound forms inactive. The active form of *ras* bound to GTP is regulated by another protein, GAP, which has a GTPase activity, converting GTP to GDP. However, both v-*ras*

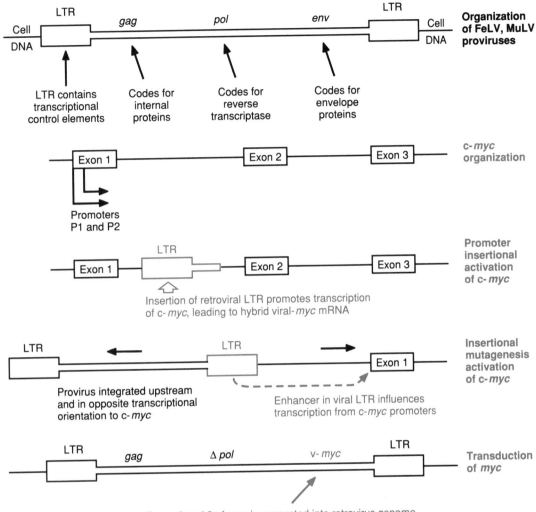

Organization of FeLV, MuLV proviruses

LTR contains transcriptional control elements

Codes for internal proteins

Codes for reverse transcriptase

Codes for envelope proteins

c-*myc* organization

Promoters P1 and P2

Promoter insertional activation of c-*myc*

Insertion of retroviral LTR promotes transcription of c-*myc*, leading to hybrid viral-*myc* mRNA

Insertional mutagenesis activation of c-*myc*

Provirus integrated upstream and in opposite transcriptional orientation to c-*myc*

Enhancer in viral LTR influences transcription from c-*myc* promoters

Transduction of *myc*

Exons 2 and 3 of *myc* incorporated into retrovirus genome. Viruses of this type are rapidly oncogenic and defective for replication.

FIGURE 47-4   Examples of insertional mutagenesis of c-*myc* by a retroviral provirus. The c-*myc* gene consists of three exons: exons 2 and 3 code for the protein, and exon 1 contains promoters.

genes within retroviruses and *ras* genes activated in nonviral cancers possess point mutations that prevent GAP-mediated GTPase activity. Consequently, these *ras* gene products remain in their GTP-bound activated state.

Other oncogene products, such as those of *myc, myb, fos, ski,* and *erb*-A genes, are located within the nucleus. The c-*erb*-A gene is the thyroid hormone receptor gene. Like other receptors of this class, the normal thyroid hormone receptor activates

transcription through the binding of a hormone-receptor complex to enhancer elements of their target genes. The v-*erb*-A gene is unable to bind thyroid hormone and is likely to be constitutively active.

Role of Multiple Genetic Events in Transformation

A common theme in viral oncogenesis is the concept that viruses act as initiators of transformation,

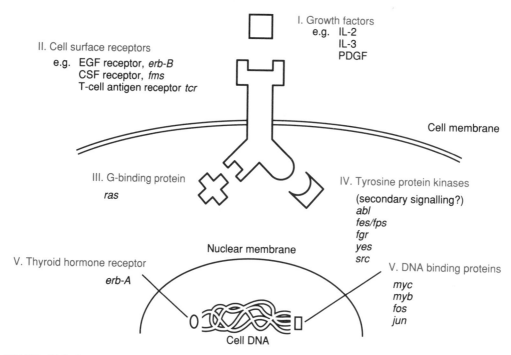

FIGURE 47-5 Representative types of substances derived from oncogene groups.

with secondary genetic events being required for progression to the full neoplastic phenotype. Many of the oncogenes identified as retrovirus-activated genes are also activated in nonviral cancers. Moreover, different groups of oncogenes appear to complement one another in transformation. For example, genes such as *myc* exert an immortalizing function on primary embryo fibroblasts, which are normally capable of only a restricted number of divisions in vitro. Such immortalized cells are not tumorigenic, but become so when other genes such as *ras* are activated.

Recently, attention has been directed to a new, important class of repressor genes that exert an anti-oncogenic effect. The best-characterized example is the p53 protein, which suppresses the function of intranuclear transforming gene products such as the large T antigen of simian virus 40. Mutation of the p53 gene or insertional inactivation by retroviruses can ablate the anti-oncogenic effects of this gene, thus contributing to tumor progression.

HTLV Replication

HTLV-1 and HTLV-2, as well as the bovine and simian leukemia viruses, have a genomic organization and replication pattern that distinguish them from other animal leukemia viruses (Fig. 47-6). In addition to the *gag*, *pol*, and *env* genes, these viruses contain a px region encoding two genes, *tax* and *rex*, which are generated from a double-spliced message.

HTLV-1 appears to remain as a latent infection in most infected cells in vivo. However, when the virus is activated, *tax* and *rex* transcripts are produced. The *tax* gene product acts as a transactivator, up-regulating the transcription of the provirus and thus creating a positive feedback loop. The effects of the *tax* protein are not direct and require interaction with cellular proteins, which, in turn, bind to target regions within the viral long terminal repeat.

The Rex protein has a different regulatory function. It favors the accumulation of unspliced and

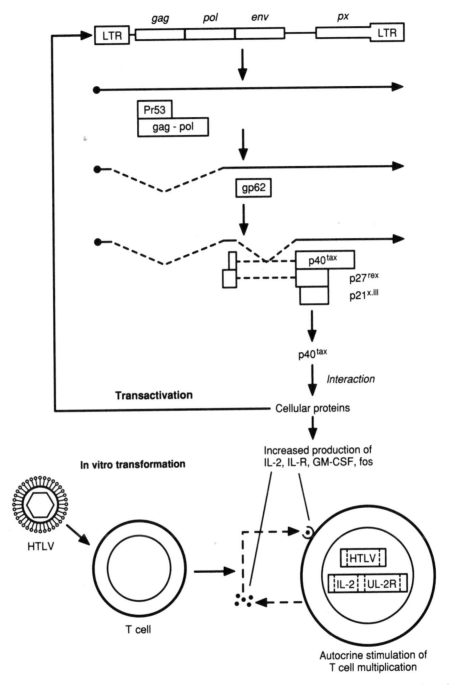

FIGURE 47-6 Genomic structure and transcription of the HTLV-1 provirus leading to autocrine stimulation of T cell multiplication.

single-spliced mRNA encoding structural proteins over the double-spliced mRNAs encoding the regulatory proteins. The mode of action of Rex is not fully resolved, but the protein may be involved in the nuclear export of the structural mRNAs. The balance between Rex and Tax production leads to an early/late switch in replication. When the provirus is first activated, all of the mRNA will be double spliced because of the low level of Rex. As Tax increases the level of transcription, Rex also increases, switching the balance toward the production of structural proteins.

Mode of Action of Tax

When HTLV-1 infects cord blood lymphocytes, a polyclonal proliferation of T cells occurs, and these events are associated with the expression of interleukin-2 and the interleukin-2 receptor by these cells. The genes for both interleukin-2 and the interleukin-2 receptor are among the cellular genes transactivated by Tax, indicating that HTLV-1 can initiate this autocrine stimulatory pathway.

However, the pathogenesis of HTLV-1-associated T-cell leukemia and lymphoma remains an enigma. Although clonal HTLV-1 proviruses can be detected in the neoplastic cells, viral RNA transcripts are not usually detected. This situation is analogous to the role of Epstein-Barr virus (EBV) (a herpesvirus) in Burkitt's lymphoma and suggests that secondary genetic events are important in the development of HTLV-1-associated T-cell leukemia and lymphoma. These events remain to be elucidated, but the possibility that Tax is also modulating signals from cell surface receptors such as CD4 and the T-cell antigen receptor remains an interesting speculation.

◀ ONCOGENIC DNA ▶ VIRUSES

HUMAN HEPATITIS B VIRUS
Clinical Manifestations and Epidemiology
One DNA virus with a strong association with a human tumor is the hepatitis B virus (HBV) (see Ch. 70), which

is implicated as an agent of primary hepatocellular carcinoma in about 80 percent of patients with this disease. In common with many other tumors, primary hepatocellular carcinoma is prevalent in certain geographic areas, principally in Africa and Asia. Its study has produced a convincing association of HBV with primary hepatocellular carcinoma. The prevalence of primary hepatocellular carcinoma in these countries correlates with a high level of infection by HBV.

Prospective Studies

Infection with HBV prior to the onset of primary hepatocellular carcinoma has been demonstrated in a study of 22,707 patients in Taiwan. The study showed a very strong association between infection with HBV and the subsequent development of primary hepatocellular carcinoma. The 10 percent of individuals in this series who were HBV carriers had a 223-fold higher risk of developing primary hepatocellular carcinoma than did the individuals not carrying the virus. That this is a very high risk is shown by the fact that moderate cigarette smoking increases the risk of developing lung cancer only 10-fold.

Cofactors

As previously noted, impaired immunity is a risk factor in the development of HBV-associated primary hepatocellular carcinoma. Another risk factor is alcohol-associated hepatic cirrhosis. A potent fungal carcinogen, aflatoxin, is frequently found in the areas in which primary hepatocellular carcinoma is prevalent. It has been pointed out that it would be difficult to distinguish between the contributions of aflatoxin and HBV to primary hepatocellular carcinoma. Both factors may act synergistically to increase the risk of carcinogenesis.

Host Response and Viral Persistence

Because HBV cannot yet be cultured in vitro, another method is necessary to diagnose the continuing presence of the virus in patients. Therefore, the presence of HBV antigen in serum is monitored; in particular, the presence of HBV surface antigen (HBsAg) is used to indicate persistent infection. Patients with a poor antibody response (HBsAb) to HBsAg are those who frequently progress to develop primary hepatocellular carcinoma. Low levels of HBsAb indicate an impaired immune response. Another factor implicated in primary hepatocellular carcinoma is early age of infection of the patient. The virus is often spread from mother to infant, and close family members also spread the virus. Low standards of living are also a contributing factor; in more developed Western countries, where primary hepatocellular carcinoma is not common, the initial infection takes place later in life (i.e., in the teens). Early infection may occur before maturation of the immune system.

Diagnosis and Persistence of Hepatitis B Virus DNA in Primary Hepatocellular Carcinoma Cells

Biopsy material from patients with primary hepatocellular carcinoma has been tested for the presence of HBV DNA. HBV DNA is integrated into the host genome, and isolation of restriction fragments larger than the HBV genome confirms HBV integration within the cell genome, as do DNA-sequencing studies, which show that integration is usually random. The total genome is frequently not retained, and deletions, rearrangements, and insertions are observed in the HBV insert, indicating that this integrated HBV genome is probably not the source of the persistent infection. This finding also suggests that the primary role of HBV in carcinogenesis does not require the continuing expression of the integrated HBV genome (i.e., a hit-and-run mechanism).

Molecular Mechanisms of Transformation

Despite numerous studies, no viral oncogene has been detected in HBV. One possible mechanism for the oncogenicity of HBV is integration of the HBV genome in or near a proto-oncogene. Such an integration event has been observed: in this case integration took place near a gene with homology to v-*erb*-A, the putative DNA-binding domain of

the human glucocorticoid and estrogen receptors. This gene might subsequently be inappropriately transcribed. In addition, integration of HBV DNA within the DNA sequences coding for human cyclin A has been recorded. Cyclin, which exists in A and B forms, is an important protein in the control of the cell cycle. Integration of HBV at such a site could alter the growth control of the normal cell.

The fact that HBV encodes a reverse transcriptase and replicates via an RNA intermediate similar to that of the retroviruses suggests that the mechanism of oncogenicity may be similar in the two virus groups. The X open reading frame of HBV DNA (Fig. 47-7) corresponds in position to the HTLV *tax* gene discussed above. Experimental evidence has shown that the X gene can transactivate promoters and enhancers and stimulate itself and other genes in the presence of cellular factors. Integrated HBV retains the X gene, in contrast to other HBV genes, which are frequently lost.

Another possible mechanism of HBV oncogenesis is repression of the cellular interferon beta promoter by a *trans* mechanism. This event could promote persistent infection by HBV, leading to cirrhosis and ultimately to cancer. Infection with HBV correlates with a deletion in chromosome 4, suggesting that one mechanism by which the virus achieves oncogenicity is deletion of an anti-oncogene.

Animal Models

Receptors for HBV are present only in human and chimpanzee cells. Other viruses of this genus have been clearly demonstrated to be tumorigenic (e.g., woodchuck hepatitis virus, which induces tumors in 90 percent of infected woodchucks within 1 to 2 years, and duck hepatitis virus, which is oncogenic in ducks).

Conclusions

HBV is strongly associated with primary hepatocellular carcinoma by its presence in the tumor cell and by the striking role of persistent HBV infection as a risk factor for the development of primary hepatocellular carcinoma. If it is shown that vaccination significantly decreases the incidence of pri-

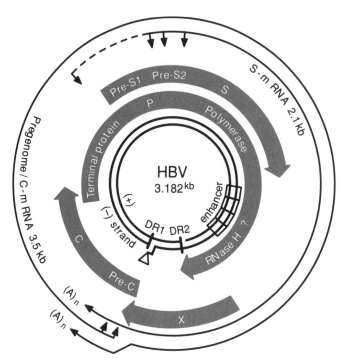

FIGURE 47-7 Genome map of HBV. (From Schlicht H-J, Schaller H: Analysis of hepatitis B virus gene functions in tissue culture and in vivo. Curr Top Microbiol Immunol 144:253, 1989, with permission.)

mary hepatocellular carcinoma in individuals with persistent infection, that will be a clear indication that HBV is involved in the development of primary hepatocellular carcinoma.

HERPESVIRUSES

Epstein-Barr Virus: Association with Burkitt's Lymphoma

Epidemiology and Geographic Distribution

Burkitt's lymphoma is the most frequent childhood tumor in Africa, and a high incidence is also found in New Guinea. It is present in regions where malaria is endemic and could be associated with a vector-borne disease. The most common age of onset is 6 to 8 years. Boys are two to five times more often affected than girls. The tumor, a poorly differentiated lymphocytic lymphoma, is of monoclonal origin, indicating that it is derived from a single viral transforming event.

Diagnosis and State of the Viral Genome

The presence of EBV genes in Burkitt's lymphoma is shown by Southern blot hybridization or by in situ hybridization with a radiolabeled DNA probe. Transformation-specific EBV nuclear antigens (EBNAs) are detected in tumor cells by anti-complementary immunofluorescence. The viral genome is maintained mostly as multiple episomal copies, although some EBV DNA is also integrated into the cell genome.

Host Response to the Tumor

The EBV genome codes for many proteins, including five EBNAs, of which EBNA 1 is essential for maintenance of viral DNA in episomal form. Antibody to this protein can be found together with antibody to other EBV-encoded proteins whose expression has been correlated with tumor expression. The amount of antibody to viral capsid antigen is proportional to the tumor mass. Successful therapy and remission are correlated with a decrease in the viral capsid antigen titer. A subsequent increase in viral capsid antigen titer indicates tumor recurrence. Burkitt's lymphoma is also associated with a high titer of antibodies to the *restricted* (i.e., restricted to the cytoplasm) and *diffuse* (i.e., diffused throughout the cell) components of the early antigen complex. Rising titers to the restricted complex indicate relapse and tumor recurrence. High titers of anti-membrane antigen and antibody-dependent cellular cytotoxic antibodies are associated with good prognosis in therapeutically induced remission.

Persistence of the Virus

Burkitt's lymphoma tumors may contain cells that shed no virus or a very low percentage of cells (called **producer cells**) that shed infectious virus. Producer cells can be identified by staining with antibody to viral capsid antigens. In addition, Burkitt's lymphoma is a monoclonal tumor, and the presence of multiple EBV genome copies indicates persistence of the virus from the time of the initial transformation event.

Molecular Mechanism of Transformation

The most important mechanism of transformation associated with Burkitt's lymphoma is the increased transcription of the cellular oncogene c-*myc*. This event, which can be observed cytogenetically, is brought about by a translocation in which c-*myc* is transferred from its location on chromosome 8 to chromosome 14, where it is much more actively transcribed under control of the gene for the immunoglobulin heavy chain. Translocation to chromosomes 2 and 22 is also seen, in this case into the light immunoglobulin chain gene. The translocation event leads directly to transcriptional activation of the c-*myc* oncogene.

The virus itself can infect lymphocytes and immortalize them, thus displaying the ability to code for immortalizing functions. No single oncogene has been identified. Translocations of c-*myc* are not seen in lymphocytes immortalized in vitro. Recently, the virus BNLF-1 gene product, also known

as latent membrane protein 1, has been shown to transform Rat-1 or murine BALB/c 3T3 cells to multiplication without attachment to a substrate (anchorage independence). A similar tumor function for the latent membrane protein has not yet been shown in human B cells or epithelial cells, the target cells for EBV-induced human proliferative diseases.

Cofactors

Cofactors thought to be involved in EBV-associated carcinogenesis are the early age at which the initial infection with EBV occurs in endemic areas (i.e., at a time when the immune system is not fully developed). Malaria is considered to be a cofactor because it impairs the host cell-mediated immunity at an early age. Cytotoxic T cells from patients with malaria cannot suppress EBV-induced lymphoproliferation.

Animal Models

EBV is capable of infecting cotton-top tamarins as well as humans. EBV-induced tumors in cotton-top tamarins have been used as an animal model for disease and to test the efficacy of possible EBV vaccines. Several animal herpesviruses are associated with tumors. The most convincing of these associations is that involving Marek's disease herpesvirus, a virus that causes fatal lymphomas in chickens. The disease is efficiently prevented by a vaccine, indicating a true cause-and-effect relationship between infection with this virus and tumor development.

Other B-Cell Lymphomas

Some patients with persistent EBV infection develop lymphomas that apparently are associated with EBV but do not behave like Burkitt's lymphoma. These patients are immunocompromised as a result either of another infection (with HIV, for example) or of therapeutic immunosuppression after transplant surgery. These lymphomas arise quickly (e.g., within 4 months after transplant surgery) and often in immune-privileged sites such as the central nervous system. Cytogenetic translocations are not always seen, but have been reported in such lymphomas as develop in patients with acquired immune deficiency syndrome (AIDS). In addition, patients with genetic immunodeficiencies are prone to B-cell lymphomas.

Epstein-Barr Virus: Association with Nasopharyngeal Carcinoma

Epidemiology and Geographic Distribution

Nasopharyngeal carcinoma is prevalent in distinct geographic regions, namely South China, other parts of Southeast Asia, and Alaska. The incidence may be as high as 98 cases per 100,000 population per year among Cantonese Chinese. The disease affects men twice as often as women. Incidence peaks between ages 50 and 70. The tumor is an undifferentiated or poorly differentiated monoclonal carcinoma of the nasopharynx.

Diagnosis and State of the Viral Genome

Viral DNA is detected by Southern blotting or in situ hybridization with a radiolabeled DNA probe. The viral DNA is present in tumor cells as multiple episomal copies. In addition, EBNA can be detected by anticomplement immunofluorescence.

Persistence of the Virus

As mentioned above, the tumor is monoclonal and the EBV genome persists as multiple episomal copies. Few cells in a tumor give rise to infectious virus, and latency is the most common state of the viral genome.

Host Response to the Tumor

The host response to nasopharyngeal carcinoma differs from that of Burkitt's lymphoma. Patients with nasospharyngeal carcinoma develop high IgG anti-viral capsid antigen titers and high titers to the diffuse component of the early antigen complex. IgA antibodies to viral capsid antigen and diffuse early antigens and antibodies to membrane proteins reach high levels in patients with nasopharyn-

geal carcinomas. High titers of antibodies to EBV-specific DNase are also found in these patients. Antibodies are used in diagnosis, and when anti-diffuse early antigen IgG, anti-viral capsid antigen IgA, and anti-diffuse early antigen IgA are all found, nasopharyngeal carcinoma is extremely likely to be present. The characteristic pattern may not be detectable if the tumor is very small and is limited to the postnasal space, however, or if the tumor has spread through the bones but has a small mass. Patients who respond well to therapy show declining antibody titers, and an increase in these titers may signal relapse. High titers of antibody-dependent cellular cytotoxic antibodies correlate with a good prognosis.

Molecular Mechanisms of Transformation

An analysis of EBV transcription in nasopharyngeal carcinoma has been made by screening a cDNA library from these tumor cells to identify transcriptionally active EBV genes. The pattern of transcription of the EBV genome in nasopharyngeal carcinoma was found to be quite different from that in Burkitt's lymphoma, and the splicing was also different. Only EBNA-1 was detected (not EBNA-2 through EBNA-5); EBNA-1 may be an RNA-binding protein. In nasopharyngeal carcinoma, transcripts are detected that could be related to transcripts thought to be important to latency for herpes simplex virus (i.e., transcripts of the lat [latency-related] gene). The alkaline exonuclease is transcribed in nasopharyngeal carcinoma, as usually is latent membrane protein, but the significance of this finding is not known. The transcription patterns of the EBV genome in Burkitt's lymphoma and nasopharyngeal carcinoma suggest that the type of cell that is infected or harbors the EBV genome exerts control over the ultimate viral gene expression.

In an attempt to understand the role of EBV in nasopharyngeal carcinoma, epithelial cells of human and primate origin were transfected with restriction fragments representing different EBV genes. A region of the EBV genome was found that could immortalize these cells, but the maintenance of this function did not depend on retaining the EBV genome sequences. The EBV fragments transcribed in nasopharyngeal carcinoma are similar to the fragments that confer immortalization to epithelial cells in vitro. Transfection of latent membrane protein into immortalized keratinocytes inhibits terminal differentiation, a process possibly involved in multistage carcinogenesis.

Cofactors

In contrast to the case in Burkitt's lymphoma, no translocations of c-*myc* are detected in nasopharyngeal carcinoma. In addition, the age of onset of the tumor does not suggest that infection at a very early age leads to an immunocompromised state. South Chinese who emigrate to the United States still show a high incidence of EBV-associated nasopharyngeal carcinoma, suggesting that genetic factors are involved in the etiology of this tumor. Dietary factors may also be involved. Sprouting fern shoots, which are consumed in Asia, are thought to have high levels of carcinogens similar to those that have been found in bracken and shown to act as cofactors in the development of alimentary tumors in cows infected with bovine papillomavirus.

Herpes Simplex Virus Type 2

Epidemiology

Numerous studies have demonstrated that patients with cancer of the cervix have both a greater incidence and a higher titer of antibodies to herpes simplex virus type 2 (HSV-2) than do controls. Although some studies have not supported this conclusion, it has always been difficult to decide which test is important and which HSV-2-encoded antigen should be monitored for antibody response. This dilemma has not been resolved. Certainly, the virus infects the cervix, can be isolated from cervical cancer patients and from normal individuals, and causes painful lesions in the male penis as well as in female genitalia. The infection is sexually transmitted.

Persistence of the Virus

HSV-2 infections generally are persistent and latent; virus can even be recovered from normal persons in whom there is no sign of disease.

Diagnosis and the State of the Viral Genome

Evidence that the total HSV-2 genome is present in tumor cells is lacking, but fragments of the HSV-2 genome have been detected in cervical cancer cells by Southern hybridization to radiolabeled probes and by the polymerase chain reaction. Gene coding regions predominantly represented are the large and small subunits of the ribonucleotide reductase, the DNA polymerase, and the major DNA-binding protein. However, the exact function of these fragments in tumorigenicity, if any, is not understood. Numerous studies have shown the presence of potentially virus-encoded antigens in cervical cancer cells and cervical intraepithelial neoplasia (the precursor to cervical cancer) cells. The data are difficult to interpret, but may represent the detection of cells in which fragments of the HSV-2 genome are retained and expressed. It is of interest that HSV-2 fragments are rarely, if ever, found integrated into normal cervical cells.

Host Response to the Tumor

Antibodies to HSV are present in at least 90 percent of all individuals, even when no HSV lesions are present. The significance of these antibodies with respect to cervical carcinogenesis is unclear. However, as stated above, tests have distinguished higher antibody titers and a greater incidence of HSV-2 antibody-positive individuals among patients with cervical cancer than in the rest of the population.

Molecular Mechanisms of Transformation

Cloned fragments of HSV-2 DNA have been used to transform rodent fibroblasts in vitro. Fragments corresponding to the large and small subunits of the ribonucleotide reductase initiate transformation, and the transformed cells are oncogenic. In addition, fragments of the HSV-2 genome cloned from regions outside these known reading frames initiate oncogenic transformation, suggesting that the system is complex. Recently, a *BglII* N fragment encoding the small subunit of ribonucleotide reductase and the host shut off gene was used to convert to tumorigenicity human keratinocytes that had been immortalized by human papillomavirus type 16.

HSV-2 may act as a cocarcinogen in the evolution of cervical cancer. If that is the case, the HSV genome need not necessarily be retained in the cell. Several important mechanisms of this type have been reported (Fig. 47-8): mutagenesis, gene amplification, the induction of endogenous retroviruses, decreased methylation of DNA, and increased or altered expression of cellular genes. In the last case, oncogenes or proteins involved in altering the immune response of the host cell could be important. An analogous system is the putative involvement of bovine papillomavirus

type 4 in bovine alimentary carcinoma, in which the DNA is not retained in the tumor cell.

Animal Models

The mouse has been used as a model system; typical tumors of the cervix can be induced in mice by both HSV-2 and its DNA. Moreover, a vaccine against HSV-2 protects mice against cervical carcinoma.

Human Cytomegalovirus

Epidemiology

The total genome of human cytomegalovirus (HCMV) is reported to be present in a high percentage of cervical tumors from patients in Taiwan, Africa, Finland, and the United States. In western Scotland, HCMV DNA fragments have been identified in cervical intraepithelial neoplasia tissue. The virus has been most strongly linked with

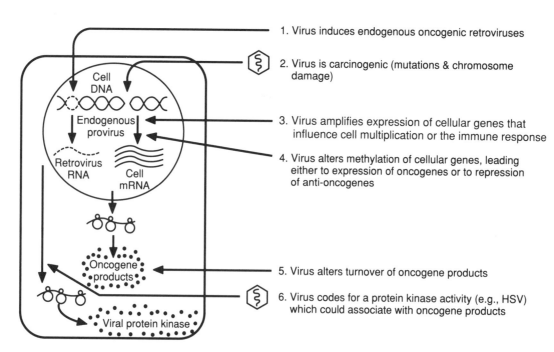

FIGURE 47-8   Possible mechanisms by which HSV and HCMV may induce one stage of multistage carcinogenesis.

Kaposi's sarcoma, a fibrosarcoma that previously was found mostly in Africa but now is common in AIDS patients.

Diagnosis and State of the Viral Genome

The virus is detected in tumors by Southern blotting with a radiolabeled probe. The total genome has been found in tumors. In studies of cervical intraepithelial neoplasias, fragments of the genome were found in 5 percent of the specimens investigated. The DNA fragments in these cases were integrated. The function of the HCMV genome in tumorigenesis is not understood, but HCMV does induce cell macromolecular synthesis, which in turn can induce cell proliferation.

Host Response

The host response to HCMV has not been studied in depth, but no data clearly suggest that antibody titers to HCMV are unusually elevated in patients with cervical cancer.

Persistence of the Virus

The virus persists in its host, frequently causing no illness. It can, however, be detected in the throat and in urine; it becomes a problem only in immunosuppressed patients.

Molecular Mechanisms of Transformation

Experiments show that two separate regions near the major immediate-early HCMV gene can transform rodent cells in vitro; however, in one of these regions, the viral DNA is not retained. The mechanism of transformation is not fully understood. It may involve transcriptional activation by the HCMV fragment that appears to be retained in the transformed cells.

Studies investigating the association of HCMV infection with tumorigenicity have shown that the virion itself is involved in the rapid induction of RNA of the cellular oncogenes *fos, jun,* and *myc.* The induction of endogenous retroviruses has also been described by virus and by subgenomic fragments of viral DNA. The induction of protooncogenes (Fig. 47-8) or alterations in the host cell response to immune mechanisms could also be important.

HUMAN PAPILLOMAVIRUSES
Epidemiology and Association with Disease

The papillomaviruses are specifically associated with proliferative lesions. The virus can multiply only in differentiating keratinocytes. The proliferative lesions are mainly benign, giving rise to warts of the skin and mucosa. However, certain types of human papillomavirus are strongly associated with the development of carcinoma. This association is supported by the presence of papillomavirus DNA in the tumor cells.

The papillomaviruses have a close association with cancer of the uterine cervix; they are associated with at least 70 percent of cervical tumors. Cancer of the uterine cervix is associated with sexual transmission of the infecting papillomaviruses. The virus is also found in vulval tumors. Epidermodysplasia verruciformis, a tumor of the skin, is strongly associated with several different human papillomaviruses.

Some 60 different types of human papillomaviruses have been described. The viruses are ubiquitous but highly tropic. The cancers with which they are associated are monoclonal, moderately to poorly differentiated carcinomas.

Diagnosis and State of the Viral Genome

Viral DNA is detected in tumor cells usually by Southern blotting with radiolabeled probes, although in situ hybridization and, more recently, the polymerase chain reaction (which uses a polymerase to amplify regions of the viral DNA within selected synthetic oligonucleotides) have also been used. Integration does not occur frequently in normal tissue, and the transcription of the episomal viral DNA in normal tissues has not been investigated. In benign lesions, the virus usually persists as multiple episomes. However, in cervical cancers the viral genome is integrated. The viral genome is often integrated in cells from cervical intraepithelial neoplasias as well.

In cervical cancer cells, the genome can be detected as an integrated 8-kb DNA fragment by Southern blotting. However, careful investigation of the integration sites of human papillomavirus types 16 and 18 has revealed that the viral E1, E6, and E7 open reading frames are integrated, whereas the genome is frequently cut through the viral E2 open reading frame and integrated into the cellular DNA at that point (Fig. 47-9). Thus, viral open reading frames E2 through E5 are lost and are not transcribed in tumors.

Classification

The 60 different strains of human papillomavirus show host cell tropism. The criteria for deciding that an isolate is a new strain is based on the DNA homology to existing known strains. If a strain shows less than 50 percent DNA homology to other strains under stringent conditions of hybridization, it is considered to be a new strain. Cervical intraepithelial neoplasia, some cervical cancers, and some vulval intraepithelial neoplasias have been associated with human papillomavirus types 11, 16, 18, 30, 31, 33, 34, 35, 39, 40, 41, 42, 43, 44, 45, 51, 52, 56, and 57. Types 5 and 8 in particular, and to a lesser extent types 14, 17, and 20, are found in patients with epidermodysplasia verruciformis, a condition that progresses to carcinoma in 30 to 50 percent of patients.

Early studies of human papillomavirus implied that the presence of certain virus types (e.g., type 16) is prognostically significant and is associated with more advanced stages of cervical intraepithelial neoplasia or other tumors. Human papillomavirus types 6 and 11 are associated with lower grades of cervical intraepithelial neoplasia. Studies from West of Scotland on patients attending a colposcopy clinic as a follow-up measure after an abnormal result on a cytology smear test showed human papillomavirus type 16 to be the prevalent strain in that area. Human papillomavirus types 6 and 11 were rarely detected in specimens from cervical intraepithelial neoplasias. Moreover, human papillomavirus type 16 was found fre-

quently in histologically normal tissue adjacent to the tumor and was present in histologically normal women without either cervical intraepithelial neoplasia or cancer. In some of these specimens of normal tissue, the genome was integrated; thus, factors other than the presence of human papillomavirus type 16 may contribute to the formation of cancer. Women in other areas of the United Kingdom also have a high incidence of human papillomavirus type 16 in both normal tissue and cervical intraepithelial neoplasia.

Host Response to the Tumor

It has been clearly shown for epidermodysplasia verruciformis that host cell-mediated immunity is significantly impaired. The fact that the disease is associated with several strains of human papillomavirus strengthens the correlation with impaired immunity.

The exact role of the host immune response in patients with cervical intraepithelial neoplasia and cervical cancer is not clear, but the immune system could be involved in the disease process. Humoral antibody to type-common human papillomavirus antigen is abundant and ubiquitous, and the use of genetically engineered constructs expressing different open reading frames has shown that antibody to different open reading frames is present at different times of life. Antibody to the viral E4 antigen is associated with replicating virus and increases in the mid-teens. Its appearance is thought to coincide with first intercourse. Antibody to the viral E7 antigen is present in patients with cervical intraepithelial neoplasia and cervical cancer.

Molecular Mechanisms of Transformation

Human papillomavirus type 16 transforms rodent cells in vitro by using the E6 and E7 open reading frames (Fig. 47-10). Rat embryo fibroblasts can be transformed by the viral E7 open reading frame of human papillomavirus type 16, in the presence of dexamethasone, to cell multiplication not requiring attachment. Moreover, the viral E7 open reading frame can immortalize human keratinocytes. It is clear that human papillomavirus can immortal-

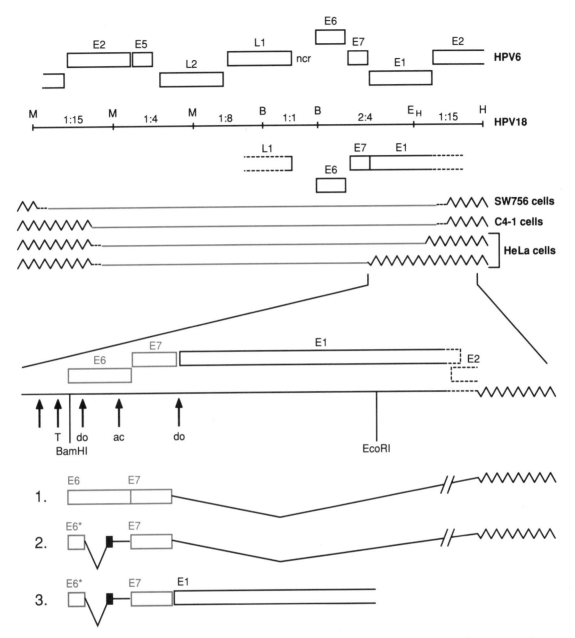

FIGURE 47-9 Integration and transcription patterns of human papillomavirus type 18 sequences in human cervical carcinoma cell lines HeLa, C4-1, and SW756. (Top) Solid lines indicate integrated viral DNA sequences, and zigzag lines indicate host cell sequences. A restriction map of the linearized prototype human papillomavirus type 18 DNA is shown above, indicating the cleavage sites for *Bam*HI (B), *Eco*RI (E), and *Hind*II (H). Open reading frames and the noncoding region (ncr) of human papillomavirus types 18 and 6 DNAs are also given. (Bottom) E6-E7-E1 are part of integrated human papillomavirus DNA and cDNA structures. Open boxes indicate the open reading frames, and "do" and "ac" denote splice donor and acceptor sites, respectively. Open arrows indicate TATA box sequences. (Adapted from Schwartz E, Schneider-Gädicke A, Zur Hausen H: Human papillomavirus type 18 transcription in cervical carcinoma cell lines. Cancer Cells 5:48, 1987, with permission.)

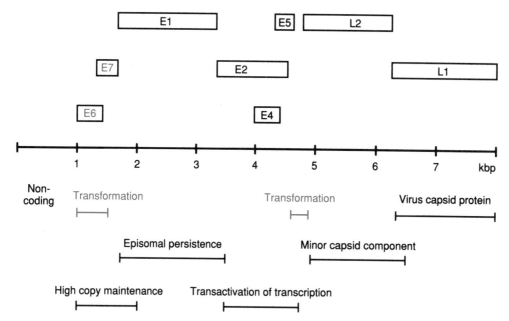

FIGURE 47-10 Genome organization of papillomaviruses. Open bars represent open reading frames, which are labeled E or L depending on their position in the early or late region of the genome. The position of reading frame E5 is rather variable. This prototype example is derived for bovine papillomavirus type 1. Gene functions that have been mapped for bovine papillomavirus type 1 are listed below the genome. This organization formed a model with which other virus types were compared. (Adapted from Pfister H, Krubke J, Dietrich W et al: Classification of the papillomaviruses—mapping of the genome. CIBA Found Symp 120:10, 1986, with permission.)

ize cells; however, it does not code for a viral oncogene. Human papillomavirus type 8, which is associated with epidermodysplasia verruciformis, has two different genome regions involved with transformation—E7 and parts of E2, E4, and L2. Human papillomavirus type 16 will cooperate with activated oncogenes such as v-*fos* and EJ *ras* to produce oncogenic cells.

Cofactors

In cervical cancer, other viruses (e.g., HSV-2 and HCMV) and other infectious agents (e.g., *Chlamydia* species) have been implicated as cofactors acting in concert with human papillomavirus type 16. For decades, it has been realized that multiple

sexual partners and an early age at first intercourse contribute to the development of the disease.

In cases of epidermodysplasia verruciformis, an impaired cell-mediated immune response is characteristically present, and numerous human papillomavirus strains are often detected in the same patient. Exposure to sunlight is another cofactor: the cancers typically develop on skin sites exposed to the sun.

Animal Models

Bovine papillomavirus is strongly associated with alimentary carcinoma in cattle. The viral genome is not retained in the cancer cells in this disease, indicating that the virus plays a role in initiation but that further cofactors are needed for progression. The disease progresses to cancer in regions where bracken is eaten by the cattle (e.g., West of Scotland). The carcinogen quercetin, found in bracken, is thought to be a cofactor. However, bracken also contains immunosuppressive agents, and these may act synergistically with the virus.

Cottontail rabbits can be infected by the cottontail rabbit papillomavirus. These animals develop warts in which the DNA is episomal. In a high percentage of laboratory animals, the benign infection progresses to carcinomas in which the papillomavirus genome is integrated. This is an excellent animal model for the situation in which integration of the viral genome is strongly associated with progression to malignancy.

VACCINES IN THE PREVENTION OF VIRUS-ASSOCIATED CANCERS

It has been popular to respond to the problem of virus-associated carcinogenesis by vaccination. Live attenuated virus vaccines have been used, but a more popular approach recently has been to construct live recombinant virus vaccines that are specifically engineered to express a viral protein known to be immunogenic and to confer immunity to the virus. Such a vaccine is the vaccinia virus recombinant that contains a gP340 EBV glycoprotein. This vaccine prevents the cotton-top tamarin from developing lymphomas when challenged with EBV. However, there are two problems. First, primary hepatocellular carcinoma, Burkitt's lymphoma, and nasopharyngeal carcinoma occur with high incidence in geographic areas where the standard of living is low; however, the vaccine is expensive. Second, the high incidence of HIV causing AIDS, which is so specifically immunosuppressive, has altered the approach to live vaccines, since such vaccines could be more deadly than the disease in an HIV-positive recipient who is unable to raise antibodies.

REFERENCES
RNA Viruses

Alt FW, Harlow E, Ziff EB: Nuclear Oncogenes: Current Communications in Molecular Biology. Cold Spring Harbor Laboratory, Cold Spring Harbor, NY, 1987

Bishop JM, Varmus H: Functions and origins of retroviral transforming genes. p. 999. In Weiss R, Teich N, Varmus H, Coffin J (eds): RNA Tumor Viruses. Cold Spring Harbor Laboratory, Cold Spring Harbor, NY, 1984

Greene WC, Bohnlein E, Ballard DW: HIV-1, HTLV-1 and normal T-cell growth: transcriptional strategies and surprises. Immunol Today 10:272, 1989

Land H, Parada LF, Weinberg RA: Tumorogenic conversion of primary embryo fibroblasts requires at least two cooperating oncogenes. Nature 304:596, 1983

Neil JC, Forrest D, Loggett DL, Mullins JC: The role of feline leukemia virus in naturally occurring leukaemias. Cancer Surv 6:117, 1987

Onions D, Lees G, Forrest D, Neil JC: Feline leukaemia virus carrying the *myc* gene rapidly produce clonal tumours expressing T-cell antigen receptor genes. Int. J. Cancer 40:40, 1987

Poiesz BJ, Ruscetti FN, Gazadar AF et al: Detection and isolation of type C retrovirus particles from fresh and cultured lymphocytes of a patient with cutaneous T-cell lymphoma. Proc. Natl. Acad. Sci. USA 77:7415, 1980

Stehelin D, Varmus HE, Bishop JM, Vogt PK: DNA related to the transforming gene(s) of avian sarcoma viruses is present in normal avian DNA. Nature 260:170, 1976

Varmus H, Swantstrom R: Replication of retroviruses. p. 369. In: Weiss R, Teich N, Varmus H, Coffin J (eds): RNA Tumor Viruses. Cold Spring Harbor Laboratory, Cold Spring Harbor, NY, 1984

Yoshida M, Inoue J-I, Fujisawa J-I, Seiki M: Trans-Regulation of HTLV-1 expression. p. 251. In: Franza B, Jr, Cullen BR, Wong-Staal F (eds): The Control of Human Retrovirus Gene Expression. Cold Spring Harbor Laboratory, Cold Spring Harbor, NY, 1988

DNA Viruses

Baichwal VR, Hammerschmidt W, Sugden B: Characterization of the BNLF-1 oncogene of Epstein-Barr virus. Curr Top Microbiol Immunol 144:233, 1989

Boldogh I, Abubakar S, Albrecht T: Activation of proto-oncogenes: an immediate early event in human cyto-megalovirus infection. Science 247:561, 1990

Hitt MM, Allday MJ, Hara T et al: EBV gene expression in an NPC-related tumour. EMBO J 8:2639, 1989

Koshy R, Hofschneider PH: Transactivation by hepatitis B may contribute to hepatocarcinogenesis. Curr Top Microbiol Immunol 144:265, 1989

Levine AJ: The cellular and molecular biology of Epstein-Barr virus. Curr Top Microbiol Immunol 144:217, 1989

Macnab JCM: Herpes simplex virus and human cyto-megalovirus: their role in morphological transformation and genital cancers. J Gen Virol 68:2525, 1987

Macnab JCM, Walkinshaw SA, Cordiner JW, Clements JB: Human papillomavirus in clinically and histologically normal tissue of patients with genital cancer. N Engl J Med 315:1052, 1986

Schlicht H-J, Schaller H: Analysis of hepatitis B virus gene functions in tissue culture and in vivo. Curr Top Microbiol Immunol 144:253, 1989

Schwartz E, Schneider-Gädicke A, Zur Hausen H: Human papillomavirus type 18 transcription in cervical carcinoma cell lines and in human cell hybrids. Cancer Cells 5:47, 1987

48

EPIDEMIOLOGY AND EVOLUTION

FRANK FENNER

GENERAL CONCEPTS

Aspects of Viral Epidemiology

Viruses must enter cells to multiply. Transmission may be **horizontal** (between different individuals) or **vertical** (from mother to offspring either before, during, or immediately after birth).

Portals of Entry and Exit

Portals of entry and exit in horizontal transmission include all body surfaces. Vertical transmissions may occur in the ovum, via the placenta, during birth, or in the colostrum or milk. The mode of exit is not necessarily the same as the portal of entry.

Viral Zoonoses

Some human viral infections are acquired from an animal source, which may be an arthropod, in which the virus may multiply.

Epidemiologic Features of Viral Infections

Each kind of viral infection is characterized by a particular mode(s) of transmission, a reasonably defined incubation period, a typical period of communicability, and a proportion of subclinical cases. Many infections have a seasonal incidence.

Evolution of Viruses

Viruses, especially those with RNA genomes, have a very high rate of mutation. Many viruses undergo recombination, and those with segmented genomes may undergo reassortment. Evolutionary changes are due to the interplay of genetic variability and natural selection, often during the transmission phase.

INTRODUCTION

Within the field of medical virology, **pathogenesis** (see Ch. 45) concerns the processes by which viruses infect individuals, whereas **epidemiology** examines the transfer and persistence of viruses in human populations. Epidemiology and evolution are linked because epidemiologic mechanisms of transfer largely determine the natural selection component of viral evolution. Since viruses multiply only within cells, the epidemiology of viral diseases does not involve multiplication in food, water, or soil. Transmission may be **horizontal** (between different individuals) or **vertical** (from mother to offspring, either antenatally or perinatally). Some viruses that affect humans may multiply and persist in other animals, such as arthropods, rodents, and bats.

PORTALS OF ENTRY AND EXIT

The human body presents three large epithelial surfaces to the environment—the skin, the respiratory mucosa, and the alimentary tract—and two lesser surfaces—the genital tract and the conjunctiva—(Fig. 48-1). To gain entry to the body, viruses must (1) infect cells in one of these surfaces, (2) otherwise breach the surface (by trauma, the bite of an arthropod or mammal, or injection, transfusion, or transplantation), or (3) be transmitted congenitally. Viruses escape from the body via the same surfaces, but not necessarily by the route used as the portal of entry.

Infection via the Skin

Intact skin has a tough outer layer of cornified cells; this barrier protects the body from infection but is frequently breached by trauma or by inoculation (e.g., by a needle or an insect bite) (Table 48-1). Virus inoculation by injection or transfusion is now common as a result both of medical procedures and of social practices such as sharing of needles by intravenous drug users. In Western society, hepatitis B virus is usually transmitted in this way; less often, cytomegalovirus, Epstein-Barr virus (EBV), and human immunodeficiency virus (HIV) are transferred in this manner. Hepatitis B is transferred in some parts of the world by minor "surgical" procedures such as tattooing, dentistry, ear piercing, and even arm-to-arm vaccination.

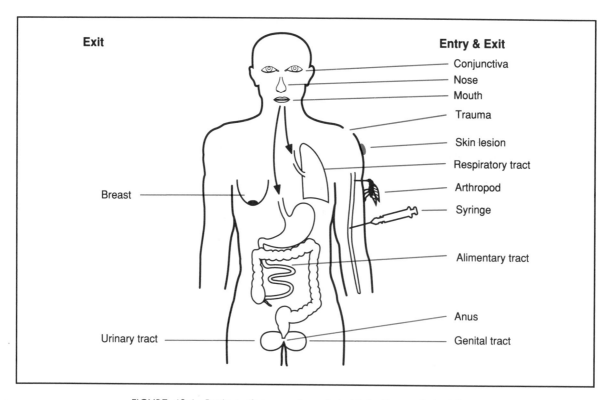

FIGURE 48-1 Body surfaces as sites of viral infection and shedding.

TABLE 48-1   Viruses That Initiate Infection by Penetration of Skin or
That Cause Direct Infection of Genital and Conjunctival Mucosa

Route	Family or Genus	Specific Viruses
Penetration		
Minor trauma	Hepadnaviridae	Hepatitis B virus
	Papillomavirus	All types
	Herpesviridae	HSV-1, HSV-2
	Poxviridae	Molluscum contagiosum virus, milker's node parapoxvirus, vaccinia virus, cowpox virus, orf parapoxvirus
	Retroviridae	HIV-1, HIV-2
Arthropod bite		
Mechanical	Poxviridae	Tanapox virus
Biologic	*Alphavirus*	All species
	Flaviviridae	All species
	Reoviridae	Colorado tick fever virus
	Bunyaviridae	La Crosse virus, sandfly fever virus, Rift Valley fever virus
Bite of vertebrate	Rhabdoviridae	Rabies virus
	Herpesviridae	B herpes virus
Injection	Hepadnaviridae	Hepatitis B virus
	Herpesviridae	Cytomegalovirus, EBV
	Filoviridae	Ebola virus, Marburg virus
	Retroviridae	HIV-1, HIV-2, HTLV-1
	Unclassified	Hepatitis C virus
Direct infection		
Genital tract	Hepadnaviridae	Hepatitis B virus
	Papillomavirus	Genital types
	Herpesviridae	HSV-2
	Retroviridae	HIV-1, HIV-2, HTLV-1
Conjunctiva	Adenoviridae	Some types
	Picornaviridae	Enterovirus 70

This mode of transfer used to occur in Western society also.

Infection by arthropod bite is improtant for the large number of viruses that multiply in both arthropods and vertebrates (the arboviruses, which include most togaviruses and flaviviruses, the *Orbivirus* genus of the reoviruses, and all bunyaviruses except Hantaan virus).

In contrast to the many viruses that enter the body through the skin, only a few are shed from it in an infectious form. Herpes zoster lesions in the skin usually shed few viruses, but they are epidemiologically important in that adults shedding virus may transmit chickenpox to susceptible children. Some viruses that infect humans via the respiratory tract may be shed from superficial lesions of the oral mucosa (e.g., measles and, in the past, smallpox viruses) or from infected salivary glands (e.g., mumps virus).

Infection via the Respiratory Tract

In modern Western society the respiratory tract is by far the most common route of viral infection. The average human adult breathes in about 600 L of air every hour; small suspended particles (<2 μm diameter) pass down the pharynx, and a few reach the alveoli. Viruses in such droplets may initiate infection if they attach to cells of the respiratory tract. Many respiratory viruses are also transferred by contact with contaminated fingers or fomites (inanimate carriers). The viruses commonly referred to as the respiratory viruses multiply only in the respiratory tract and cause influenza, colds, pharyngitis, bronchiolitis, and pneumonia; other viruses that initiate infection via the respiratory tract can produce generalized infections (Table 48-2).

The respiratory tract sheds many different viruses and is the main route of excretion for all viruses that initiate infection by respiratory means.

Infection via the Alimentary Tract

Although the surface of the alimentary tract is potentially exposed to a great number and variety of viruses, the harsh conditions in the stomach and duodenum protect it from many viruses. For instance, viruses that have a lipid-containing envelope are usually inactivated by the acid, bile salts, and enzymes in the stomach and duodenum. Infection via the gut, therefore, is due to viruses that resist these chemicals. These viruses multiply in the cells of the small intestine and are excreted in the feces (Table 48-3). Such viruses usually resist environmental conditions and may cause water- and food-borne epidemics.

Recently, the significance of trauma to the mucosa of the lower rectum as a result of anal intercourse has been highlighted by the frequency of sexually transmitted viruses, notably HIV in homosexual men.

Infection via the Genital Tract

The list of sexually transmitted viruses (Table 48-4) of the female genital tract has been enlarged recently by the discovery of heterosexual transmission of acquired immune deficiency syndrome (AIDS), especially in Africa, and transmission of the leukomogenic virus human T-cell lymphotrophic virus type 1 (HTLV-1). The importance of genital transmission of particular papillomaviruses in the development of cervical carcinoma is receiving more attention (see Ch. 66). Genital ulcers due to herpes simplex virus type 2 (HSV-2), a sexually transmitted virus, are important in themselves and may increase the likelihood of heterosexual transmission of HIV.

A few viruses are shed in the urine of humans or, in the case of arenavirus infections, of rodents. The arenaviruses in rodent urine may then cause human infection (e.g., hemorrhagic fever) as a re-

TABLE 48-2   Viruses That Initiate Infection via the Respiratory Tract

Type of Infection	Family	Specific Viruses
Local respiratory infection		
	Orthomyxoviridae	Influenza A and B viruses
	Paramyxoviridae	Parainfluenza virus, respiratory syncytial virus
	Picornaviridae	Rhinoviruses, a few enteroviruses
	Coronaviridae	Many serotypes
	Adenoviridae	Many serotypes
Generalized disease, usually without initial respiratory symptoms		
	Herpesviridae	Varicella virus, EBV, cytomegalovirus
	Papovaviridae	BK and JC viruses
	Parvoviridae	Erythema infectiosum virus
	Paramyxoviridae	Mumps, measles viruses
	Togaviridae	Rubella virus
	Picornaviridae	Some enteroviruses
	Bunyaviridae	Hantaan virus
	Arenaviridae	Lymphocytic choriomeningitis virus, Lassa fever virus
	Poxviridae	Smallpox virus (in the past)

TABLE 48-3   Viruses That Initiate Infection via the
Alimentary Tract

Site of Infection	Family	Specific Viruses
Mouth or oropharynx		
	Poxviridae	Monkeypox virus
	Herpesviridae	HSV, EBV, cytomegalovirus
Intestinal tract		
Producing enteritis		
	Reoviridae	Rotaviruses
	Caliciviridae	Norwalk agent and related viruses
	Adenoviridae	Several types
Producing generalized disease, usually without local symptoms		
	Picornaviridae	Many enteroviruses including polioviruses and hepatitis A virus
Usually symptomless		
	Picornaviridae	Some enteroviruses
	Adenoviridae	Some adenoviruses
	Reoviridae	Reoviruses
	Coronaviridae	Coronaviruses (rarely)

TABLE 48-4   Viruses That Initiate Infection of the Eyes
or Genitourinary Tract or Are Excreted in Urine

Site	Family	Specific Viruses	Disease
Eyes	Adenoviridae	Human type 8 viruses and others	
	Herpesviridae	HSV-1	
	Poxviridae	Accidental vaccinia virus	Conjunctivitis
	Picornaviridae	Enterovirus 70, coxsackievirus A24	
	Paramyxoviridae	Newcastle disease virus	
Genital tract	Poxviridae	Molluscum contagiosum virus	Molluscum contagiosum
	Herpesviridae	HSV-2	Genital herpes
		Cytomegalovirus	Congenital disease
	Papoviridae	Human papillomaviruses 16, 18; others	Genital warts
	Hepadnaviridae	Hepatitis B virus	Hepatitis
	Retroviridae	HIV-1, HIV-2	AIDS
		HTLV-1	Adult T-cell leukemia
Excretion in urine	Herpesviridae	Cytomegalovirus	Generalized disease
	Togaviridae	Rubella virus	Rubella
	Paramyxoviridae	Measles virus	Measles
		Mumps virus	Mumps
	Hepadnaviridae	Hepatitis B virus	Hepatitis

sult of inhalation of dust containing virus particles in dried urine.

Infection of the Conjunctiva

Viruses of several families occasionally infect the conjunctiva directly (Table 48-4), but conjunctivitis in generalized diseases such as measles is caused by virus that reaches the conjunctiva through the bloodstream.

Vertical Transmission

Vertical transmission refers to the transfer of virus from parent to offspring and may occur via the ovum, across the placenta, during birth, or via the mother's milk. Viruses that cross the placenta include rubella virus and cytomegalovirus, which may cause congenital defects or severe neonatal disease, and HIV.

The classic examples of vertical transmission of viruses in animals are lymphocytic choriomeningitis virus in mice, transmitted via the cytoplasm of the egg or the placenta, and the retroviruses that cause avian leukosis and sarcoma and murine leukemia. The retroviruses are transferred either as an integrated DNA copy of the viral RNA genome or, more rarely, in birds, as infectious virions via the egg. HTLV-1, the retrovirus that causes human adult T-cell leukemia/lymphoma (see Ch. 62), appears to be transmitted horizontally, although integrated provirus is found in the lymphocytes of affected individuals.

Vertical transmission of cytomegalovirus may occur through the mother's milk, and both cytomegalovirus and herpes simplex virus type 1 can be transmitted from parents to infants by salivary contamination. Then, because of its long latency and the periodic recurrence of lesions, the same virus may be transferred to the next generation. In small, isolated human populations, infections with zoster-chickenpox may be maintained by a similar cycle, although, strictly speaking, infection transmitted perinatally is horizontal transmission. Perinatal transmission of hepatitis B virus is important in much of Africa and Asia because it is common and often produces a persistent infection that may lead to cirrhosis of the liver or primary hepatocellular carcinoma.

VIRAL ZOONOSES

A wide range of viruses that can cause human diseases survive in nature as reservoir infections of other animals; humans are only occasionally infected, and infection of humans is usually unimportant for viral survival. These infections are called **zoonoses** (Table 48-5); many are caused by arboviruses (viruses that are transmitted by arthropod vectors), and some are due to direct infection. Important exceptions to arbovirus transmission of animal infections to humans are dengue and yellow fever viruses, which can be maintained indefinitely by human-to-human infection, although both have animal reservoir hosts also.

EPIDEMIOLOGIC FEATURES OF VIRAL INFECTIONS

Some epidemiologically important features of human viral diseases are presented in Table 48-6. The control of these infections requires knowledge not only the mode of transmission but also of the incubation period, period of communicability, and seasonal incidence. Not all infections cause disease; inapparent infection (which may nevertheless be responsible for new cases) is the rule with many viruses, especially enteroviruses and some of the herpesviruses. Only in a few diseases, such as measles, does virtually every infection of a susceptible individual cause obvious clinical disease.

Humoral immunity affects the behavior of viral infections as much in human populations as in individuals. The frequency of immunity in a population is sometimes called the **herd immunity.** Generalized virus diseases are associated with lifelong immunity; therefore, in the absence of an animal reservoir or of recurrent infectivity, these diseases survive only in large populations and die out in small, isolated communities. For example, measles and poliomyelitis do not occur as endemic infections in Eskimos and the populations of small islands.

In superficial infections of the respiratory and alimentary tracts, humoral antibodies are less important than secretory antibodies (IgA). However, IgA is produced for a much shorter period, so that

TABLE 48-5   Viruses Responsible for Viral Zoonoses

Family and Genus	Specific Viruses	Reservoir Host	Mode of Transmission	Disease
Direct Transmission				
Poxviridae	Cowpox virus	Cattle, cats, rodents	Contact, skin abrasions	Skin pustule
	Milker's node virus	Cattle	Contact, skin abrasions	Skin nodule
	Orf virus	Sheep, goats	Contact, skin abrasions	Skin ulcer
	Monkeypox virus	Squirrels, primates	Contact, including oral	Generalized rash
	Tanapox virus	? Rodents, monkeys	Insect bite (mechanical)	Skin nodule
Bunyaviridae	Hantaan virus	Rodents	Contact	Hemorrhagic fever
Rhabdoviridae	Rabies virus	Carnivores, bats	Animal bite, respiratory	Central nervous system disease
Filoviridae	Ebola, Marburg viruses	? Monkeys	Contact, injection	Hemorrhagic fever
Orthomyxoviridae	Influenza A virus	Pigs, horses, birds	Respiratory[a]	Fever and cough
Arenaviridae	Lymphocytic choriomeningitis virus, Lassa virus, Junin virus, Machupo virus	Rodents	Respiratory, contact	Hemorrhagic fever
Arthropod-Borne (with Replication in Arthropod)				
Togaviridae *Alphavirus*	Chikungunya virus	Birds	Mosquitoes	Fever, polyarthritis
	Eastern equine encephalitis virus	Mammals		Fever, encephalitis
	Venezuelan equine encephalitis virus	Mammals		Fever, encephalitis
	Western equine encephalitis virus	Birds		Fever, encephalitis
	O'Nyong-nyong virus	Mammals		Fever, polyarthritis
	Ross River virus	Mammals		Fever, polyarthritis
Flaviviridae	Dengue virus	Primates	Mosquitoes	Fever (shock syndrome)
	Japanese encephalitis virus	Birds and pigs		Fever, encephalitis
	Murray Valley encephalitis virus	Birds		Fever, encephalitis
	Yellow fever virus	Primates		Hemorrhagic fever
	Kyasanur Forest disease virus	Primates	Ticks	Hemorrhagic fever
	Louping ill virus	Mammals		Fever, encephalitis
	Omsk hemorrhagic fever virus	Mammals		Hemorrhagic fever
	Powassan virus	Mammals		Fever, encephalitis
	Tick-borne encephalitis virus	Mammals and birds		Fever, encephalitis

Continued

TABLE 48-5   Viruses Responsible for Viral Zoonoses (continued)

Family and Genus	Specific Viruses	Reservoir Host	Mode of Transmission	Disease
Bunyaviridae				
Bunyavirus	California encephalitis virus	Mammals		Fever, encephalitis
	La Crosse virus	Mammals	Mosquitoes	Fever, encephalitis
	Tahyna virus	Mammals		Fever, encephalitis
Phlebovirus	Sandfly fever virus	Gerbils	Sand flies	Fever, myalgia
	Rift Valley fever virus	Mammals	Mosquitoes	Fever (encephalitis)
Nairovirus	Crimean-Congo hemorrhagic fever virus	Mammals	Ticks	Hemorrhagic fever
Reoviridae	Colorado tick fever virus	Mammals	Ticks	Fever, myalgia

a Reassortment involved

TABLE 48-6   Epidemiologic Features of Some Common Human Viral Diseases

Disease	Mode of Transmission	Incubation Period[a] (days)	Period of Communicability[b]	Incidence of Subclinical Infections[c]	Season of Maximum Incidence
Influenza	Respiratory	1–2	Short	Moderate	Winter
Common cold	Respiratory	1–3	Short	Moderate	Spring, autumn
Bronchiolitis, croup	Respiratory	3–5	Short	Moderate	Winter
ARD (adenovirus)	Respiratory	5–7	Short	Moderate	Winter
Dengue	Mosquito bite	5–8	Short	Moderate	Summer
Herpes simplex	Salivary	5–8	Long	Moderate	Nil
Enterovirus diarrhea	Alimentary	6–12	Long	High	Summer
Rotavirus diarrhea	Alimentary	2–4	Moderate	Moderate	Winter
Norwalk diarrhea	Alimentary	2–4	Moderate	Moderate	Nil
Poliomyelitis	Enteric	5–20	Long	High	Summer
Measles	Respiratory	9–12	Moderate	Low	Spring
Chickenpox	Respiratory	13–17	Moderate	Moderate	Spring
Mumps	Respiratory	16–20	Moderate	Moderate	Spring
Rubella	Respiratory, congenital	17–20	Moderate	Moderate	Spring
Mononucleosis	Contact	30–50	Long	High	Nil
Hepatitis A	Alimentary	15–40	Long	High	Summer
Hepatitis B	Inoculation	50–150	Very long	High	Nil
Rabies	Animal bite	30–100	Nil	Nil	Nil
Warts	Contact	50–150	Long	Low	Nil
AIDS	Sexual contact, inoculation, congenital	1–8 years	Very long	Low	Nil

a Until first appearance of symptoms. Diagnostic signs (e.g., rash or paralysis) may not appear until a few days later.

b Many viral diseases are transmissible beginning a few days before symptoms occur. Long, >10 days; short, <4 days.

c High, >90 percent; low, <10 percent.

d ARD, Acute respiratory disease.

reinfections with viruses such as respiratory syncytial virus are relatively common. Futhermore, the effect of antibody in preventing respiratory and enteric infections is often circumvented by the great number of non-cross-reacting antigenic types of most viruses that cause superficial infections of these surfaces.

In conclusion, the main variables that determine the transmissibility of viruses are excretion (manner, duration, quantity of virus, and infectivity), environment (stability of the virus and the chance of contact with a new host), and immunity (the level of herd immunity among possible hosts). Many viral diseases have been brought under control by manipulating certain of these variables, for example, by immunization and by improving sanitation to reduce the possibility of contact (see Ch. 51).

EVOLUTION OF VIRUSES

Viral genomes undergo genetic change by mutation and by recombination. Recombination may be either intramolecular or, among viruses with divided genomes, by reassortment. Mutation in RNA viruses may be extremely rapid because there is no proofreading mechanism for RNA polymerases, such as there is for DNA polymerases. This situation is compounded in the retroviruses, for there is no proofreading mechanism for the reverse transcriptase either. Most of these mutations result in nonviable phenotypes. Whether the genetic changes lead to an altered phenotype depends on natural selection, which may occur within the infected cell, during spread of virus in the body, or during transmission of the virus from one host to the next.

For the practicing physician, virus evolution may appear to be an academic matter, because evolutionary changes usually occur over a time scale that is long compared with human life. However, sometimes genetic changes in viruses occur rapidly as a result of evolutionary pressure. For instance, the highly virulent myxoma virus introduced into Australia to control the wild rabbit population evolved in a few years to a much more attenuated strain, enabling infected rabbits to survive for weeks instead of days, thereby increasing chances for transmission. Among influenza viruses, antigenic variation evolves toward decreased affinity for preexisting neutralizing antibodies during the course of an outbreak. Periodically, pandemics of influenza occur (most recently in 1957 and 1968) as a result of the spread of reassortant viruses with a novel hemagglutinin antigen. Because the survival of a virus depends largely on its ability to circulate among its natural hosts, natural selection tends to favor viruses that are better transmitted (usually less virulent), have a lower susceptibility to antibody, and have a greater ability to persist. Also, the ability of the virus to produce reactions that promote excretion, such as coughing and sneezing in respiratory infections and diarrhea in many enteric infections, is likely to be retained.

Contemporary society seems to be experiencing an increased development of new serotypes of several kinds of respiratory and enteric viruses because of the evolutionary potential afforded by the human population explosion and the great increase in international travel. Evolution allows influenza to remain potentially the most important of all human viral diseases (see Ch. 58). Genetic reassortment and exchange of influenza viruses between humans and animals, producing antigenic shift, periodically introduce new viruses to the human population; mutation and selection, producing antigenic drift, accounts for year-to-year variations in influenza A virus subtypes.

REFERENCES

Evans AS (ed): Viral Infections of Humans: Epidemiology and Control. 3rd Ed. Plenum, New York, 1989

Mims CA: The Pathogenesis of Infectious Disease. 3rd Ed. Academic Press, Ltd., London, 1987

Nathanson N: Epidemiology, p. 267. In Fields BN, Knipe DM, Chanock RM et al (eds): Virology. 2nd Ed. Raven Press, New York, 1990

Strauss EG, Strauss JH, Levine AJ: Virus Evolution. p. 167. In Fields BN, Knipe DM, Chanock RM et al (eds): Virology. 2nd Ed. Raven Press, New York, 1990

White DO, Fenner F: Medical Virology. 3rd Ed. Academic Press, San Diego, 1986

49 NONSPECIFIC DEFENSES

FERDINANDO DIANZANI
SAMUEL BARON

GENERAL CONCEPTS

Most viral infections are limited by nonspecific and/or specific host defenses. Nonspecific defenses act sooner than specific defenses. Some are always in place (anatomic barriers, nonspecific inhibitors, and phagocytic cells); others are evoked by the infection (fever, inflammation, and interferon).

Anatomic Barriers

Anatomic barriers are located at body surfaces (skin and mucosa) or within the body (endothelial cells and basement membranes). They are partly effective in preventing virus spread but may be breached by large numbers of virus, by trauma, by increased permeability, by replication of virus in endothelial cells, or by transportation of virus in leukocytes.

Nonspecific Inhibitors

Body fluids and tissues normally contain soluble viral inhibitors. Most prevent viral attachment, some directly inactivate viruses, and others act intracellularly. These inhibitors may be overwhelmed by sufficient virus.

Phagocytosis

Viruses may be phagocytosed to different degrees by polymorphonuclear leukocytes and macrophages. The effect of phagocytosis may be virus inactivation, persistence, or multiplication; consequently, the result may be clearance of virus, transportation to distant sites, or enhanced infection.

Fever

Replication of most viruses is reduced by even a modest rise in temperature. During viral infection, fever can be induced by at least three endogenous pyrogens: (1) interleukin-1, (2) interferon, and (3) tumor necrosis factor.

Inflammation

Inflammation inhibits viral replication through (1) elevated local temperature, (2) reduced oxygen tension, (3) metabolic alterations, and (4) acid production. The effects of these mechanisms are often additive.

Viral Interference and Interferon

Viral interference occurs when infection by one virus renders cells resistant to the same or other superinfecting viruses. Interference is usually mediated by the host cell protein **interferon.** Secreted interferon binds to cells and causes them to block various stages of viral replication. Interferon also (1) inhibits growth of some normal and tumor cells and of many intracellular parasites, such as rickettsiae and protozoa; (2) modulates the immune response; and (3) promotes cell differentiation. There are three main types of interferon, alpha, beta, and gamma interferons. Alpha interferon is produced mainly by leukocytes other than T lymphocytes, beta interferon by epithelial cells and fibroblasts, and gamma interferon by T lymphocytes.

INTRODUCTION

Most viral infections are limited by **nonspecific defenses,** which (1) restrict initial virus multiplication to manageable levels, (2) initiate recovery that is completed by a combination of these early nonspecific and subsequent specific immune defenses, and (3) enable the host to cope with the peak numbers of virus that, if presented as the infecting dose, could be lethal. Although immune and nonimmune (nonspecific) defenses operate together to control viral infections, this chapter considers only nonspecific defenses. Some nonspecific defenses exist independently of infection (e.g., genetic factors, anatomic barriers, nonspecific inhibitors in body fluids, and phagocytosis). Others (e.g., fever, inflammation, and interferon) are produced by the host in response to infection. All nonspecific defenses begin to act before the specific defense responses develop.

The fact that viruses replicate intracellularly and the ability of some viruses to spread by inducing cell fusion partly protect viruses against such extracellular defenses as neutralizing antibody, phagocytosis, and nonspecific inhibitors. However, because they replicate within the cell, viruses are vulnerable to intracellular alterations caused by host responses to infection. Nonspecific responses that alter the intracellular environment include fever, inflammation, and interferon.

These multiple defenses function with great complexity because of their interactions with one another. This complexity is compounded by the varying effectiveness of the defenses that results from the diversity of viruses, hosts, and sites and stages of infection.

DEFENSE MECHANISMS THAT PRECEDE INFECTION

Anatomic Barriers

Anatomic barriers to viruses exist at the body surfaces and within the body. At the body surfaces, the dead cells of the epidermis and any live cells that may lack viral receptors resist virus penetration and do not permit virus replication. However, this barrier is easily breached, for example, by animal bites (rabies virus), insect bites (togaviruses), and minor traumas (wart virus). At mucosal surfaces, only the mucus layer stands between invading virus and live cells. The mucus layer forms a physical barrier that entraps foreign particles and carries them out of the body; it also contains nonspecific inhibitors (see following section). The mucus barrier is not absolute, however, since sufficient quantities of many viruses can overwhelm it and infect by this route. In fact, most viruses use mucous surfaces as the portal of entry and initial replication site.

Within the body, anatomic barriers to virus spread are formed by the layer of endothelial cells that separates blood from tissues (e.g., the blood-brain barrier). Under normal conditions, these barriers have a low permeability for viruses unless the virus can penetrate them by replicating in the capillary endothelial cells or in circulating leukocytes. These internal barriers may explain, in part, the high level of viremia required to infect organs such as the brain, placenta, and lungs.

Nonspecific Inhibitors

A number of viral inhibitors occur naturally in most body fluids and tissues. They vary chemically (lipids, polysaccharides, proteins, lipoproteins, and glycoproteins) and in the degree of viral inhibition and types of viruses affected. Some inhibitors are related to the viral receptors of the cell surface, but most are of unknown origin. Many inhibitors act by preventing virus from attaching to cells, others by directly inactivating virus, and a few by inhibiting virus replication. In the gastointestinal tract, some susceptible viruses are inactivated by acid, bile salts, and enzymes. Whereas most inhibitors block only one or a few viruses, some have a broad antiviral spectrum. Although the effectiveness of the inhibitors has not been fully established in vivo, their importance as host defenses is suggested by their antiviral activity in tissue culture and in vivo and by the direct correlation between the degree of virulence of some viruses and their degree of resistance to certain inhibitors. Examples are the serum and mucus inhibitors of influenza viruses during experimental infections. However, even sensitive viruses may overwhelm these inhibitors when the infecting dose of virus is sufficiently high. Therefore, the presence of these inhibitors may explain the relatively high dose of virus required to initiate infection in vivo, compared with the dose needed in cell cultures.

Phagocytosis

The limited information available suggests that phagocytosis is less effective against viral infections than against bacterial infections. However, few of the factors that control uptake of virions or infected cells by phagocytes and their digestion by lysosomal enzymes have been studied systemically. Different viruses are affected differently by the various phagocytic cells. Some viruses are not engulfed, whereas others are engulfed but may not

be inactivated. In fact, some viruses, such as human immunodeficiency virus (HIV), may even multiply in the phagocytes (e.g., macrophages), which may serve as a persistent reservoir of virus (Fig. 49-1). Recently, cytomegalovirus has been reported to replicate in granulocytes. Macrophages seem to be more effective against viruses than are granulocytes, and some viruses seem to be more susceptible to phagocytosis than others. Macrophages and polymorphonuclear leukocytes can afford important protection by markedly reducing the viremia caused by virus strains susceptible to phagocytosis. The virulence of several strains of herpes simplex virus correlates with their ability to survive or multiply in macrophages. Infected macrophages may carry virus across the blood-brain barrier.

Viruses may stimulate macrophages to produce **monokines,** which can reduce viral multiplication. For example, macrophage-produced **alpha interferon (IFN-α)** inhibits viral multiplication both directly and also indirectly by activating natural killer cells. **Interleukin 1 (IL-1),** produced by macrophages, can interfere with viral multiplication in a

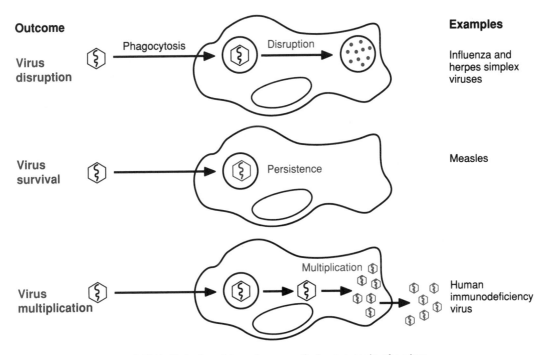

FIGURE 49-1 Possible outcomes of phagocytosis of a virus.

number of ways: (1) by inducing T lymphocytes to produce interleukin-2, which in turn induces gamma interferon (IFN-γ), which then induces alpha and beta interferons; (2) by inducing the production of beta interferon (IFN-β) by fibroblasts and epithelial cells; (3) by inducing fever, which inhibits viral replication; (4) by performing macrophage-mediated cytolysis of infected cells; and (5) by inducing production of **tumor necrosis factor** (TNF), which inhibits virus multiplication both directly and also indirectly by inducing interferon and augmenting inflammation. Therefore, depending on the situation, macrophages acting as phagocytes may reduce the number of viruses, help spread the infection, augment or depress immune defenses, or have little effect.

DEFENSE MECHANISMS EVOKED BY INFECTION

Fever

Viral replication is influenced strongly by temperature. Fever can be induced during viral infection by at least three independent **endogenous pyro-gens:** interleukin-1, interferon, and tumor necrosis factor. Even a modest increase can cause strong inhibition: a temperature rise from 37°C to 38°C drastically decreases the yield of many viruses. This phenomenon has been observed in tissue culture as well as in many experimental (including primate) and natural infections. Artificial induction of fever reduces mortality in mice infected with viruses (Fig. 49-2). Artificial lowering of the temperature during infection may increase mortality, as in suckling mice infected with coxsackieviruses and taken away from the warmth of their mother's nest. Fever also augments the generation of cytotoxic T lymphocytes.

Several observations suggest strongly that fever reduces virus multiplication during human viral infections. Retrospective studies have shown that the incidence and severity of paralysis among children infected with polioviruses were significantly greater in patients treated with antipyretic drugs (e.g., aspirin) than in untreated children. Also consistent with these findings is the observation that virus strains that replicate best at fever temperature are usually virulent, whereas virus strains that replicate poorly at fever temperature are usually

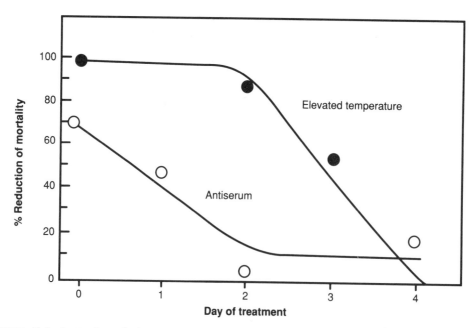

FIGURE 49-2   Protection of mice by elevated temperature or antibody administered before or after intracerebral infection with the picornavirus EMC strain.

low in virulence and therefore often are used as live virus vaccines.

Temperatures as low as 33°C are normal at body surfaces exposed to air; viruses that infect these sites and replicate optimally at these temperatures establish only local infections that do not spread to deeper tissues, where the body temperature is higher. For example, rhinoviruses that cause common colds replicate optimally at 33°C to 34°C (found in normally ventilated nasal passages); however, they are inhibited at 37°C (found when swelling of the edematous mucosa and secretions interrupt air flow). An interesting question is whether this temperature increase is important for recovery from coryza. The same general considerations of temperature probably apply to other human viral infections such as measles, rubella, and mumps, although, unfortunately, suitable and controlled studies have not been conducted. Nevertheless, available information suggests that antipyretic drugs be used conservatively.

Inflammation

Several antiviral mechanisms are generated by the local inflammatory response to virus-induced cell damage or to virus-stimulated mediators such as activated complement. The major components of the inflammatory process are circulatory alterations, edema, and leukocyte accumulation. The resulting phenomena are elevated local temperature, reduced oxygen tension in the involved tissues, altered cell metabolism, and increased levels of CO_2 and organic acids. All of these alterations, which occur in a cascading and interrelated fashion, drastically reduce the replication of many viruses. For instance, the altered energy metabolism of the infected and surrounding cells, as well as the accumulating lymphocytes, can generate local hyperthermia. At superficial sites where the temperature is normally lower, hyperthermia can also be generated by hyperemia during the early stages of inflammation. As inflammation progresses, hyperemia becomes passive, thereby greatly reducing blood flow and decreasing oxygen tension. Two factors account for this decrease in oxygen tension: limited influx of erythrocytes, and lower diffusion of oxygen through edema fluid. In turn, the decreased oxygen tension causes less ATP produc-

tion, thus reducing the energy available for viral synthesis and increasing anaerobic glycolysis, which increases the accumulation of CO_2 and organic acids in the tissues. These acid catabolites may decrease the local pH to levels that inhibit the replication of many viruses. Local acidity also may increase by accumulation and subsequent degradation of the leukocytes in the affected area. It is possible that other less well defined factors are also significant.

Therefore, the local inflammation resulting from viral infection clearly activates several metabolic, physicochemical, and psysiologic changes; acting individually or together, these changes interfere with virus multiplication. Although further animal and human studies are required, this interpretation is supported by the finding that anti-inflammatory drugs (corticosteroids) often increase the severity of infection in animals. Therefore, these drugs should be used with caution in treating viral diseases.

VIRAL INTERFERENCE AND INTERFERON
Viral Interference

Generally, infection by one virus renders host cells resistant to other, superinfecting viruses. This intriguing phenomenon, called **viral interference,** occurs frequently in cell cultures and in animals (including humans). Although interference occurs between most viruses, it may be limited to homologous viruses under certain conditions. Some types of interference are caused by competition among different viruses for critical replicative pathways (extracellular competition for cell surface receptors, intracellular competition for biosynthetic machinery and genetic control). Similar interference may result from competition between **defective** (nonmultiplying) and **infective** viruses that may be produced concurrently. Another type of interference—the most important type in natural infections—is directed by the host cells themselves. These infected cells may respond to viral infection by producing interferon (a protein), which can react with uninfected cells to render them resistant to infection by a wide variety of viruses.

Interferon

The important role played by interferon as a defense mechanism is clearly documented by three types of experimental and clinical observations: (1) for many viral infections, a strong correlation has been established between interferon production and natural recovery; (2) inhibition of interferon production or action enhances the severity of infection; and (3) treatment with interferon protects against infection. In addition, the interferon system is one of the earliest appearing of known host defenses, becoming operative within hours of infection. Figure 49-3 compares the early production of interferon with the level of antibody during experimental infection of humans with influenza virus. Clinical studies of interferon and its inducers have shown protection against certain viruses, including hepatitis B and C viruses, papovaviruses, rhinoviruses, and herpes simplex virus.

Although interferon was first recognized as an extraordinarily potent antiviral agent, it was found subsequently to affect other vital cell and body functions. For example, it may enhance killing by granulocytes, macrophages, natural killer (NK) cells, and cytotoxic lymphocytes and affect the humoral immune response and the expression of cell membrane antigens and receptors. It may also lyse or inhibit the division of certain cells, influence the body's response to ionizing radiation, and cross-activate hormone functions such as those of epinephrine and adrenocorticotropin (ACTH). The effect of these modulations on viral infections is under study.

Interferon Production and Types

Interferon is produced de novo by cellular protein synthesis. The three types (alpha, beta, and

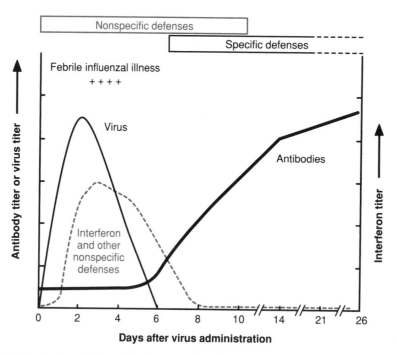

FIGURE 49-3 Production of virus, interferon, and antibody during experimental infection of humans with influenza wild-type virus. Nonspecific defenses include anatomic barriers, inhibitors, phagocytosis, fever, inflammation, and IFN. Specific defenses include antibody and cell-mediated immunity. Data from a study by B. Murphy et al, National Institutes of Health (personal communication).

gamma) differ both structurally and antigenically and have molecular weights ranging from 16,000 to 45,000. Interferons are secreted by the cell into the extracellular fluids (Fig. 49-4). Usually, virus-induced interferon is produced at about the same time as the viral progeny are released by the infected cell, thus protecting neighboring cells from the spreading virus.

The three known types of interferon are induced by different stimuli. Beta interferon is induced by viral and other foreign nucleic acids in most body cells (fibroblasts, epithelial cells, and macrophages). This induction mechanism is illustrated in Figure 49-4 and the top portion of Figure 49-5.

Alpha interferon can be induced by foreign cells, virus-infected cells, tumor cells, bacterial cells, and viral envelopes that stimulate B lymphocytes, null lymphocytes, and macrophages to produce it (Fig. 49-4, middle). Mitogens for B cells may mimic this induction. An unusual, acid-labile alpha interferon may occur during some retrovirus infections and is found in patients with immune perturbations such as lupus erythematosus, rheumatoid arthritis, pemphigus, and acquired immune deficiency syndrome (AIDS).

Gamma interferon is produced (along with other lymphokines) by T lymphocytes induced by foreign antigens to which the T lymphocytes have been presensitized (Fig. 49-4). Mitogens for T cells may mimic this induction. Gamma interferon has several unusual properties: (1) it exerts greater immunomodulatory activity, including activation of macrophages, than the other interferons; (2) it exerts greater lytic effects than the other interferons; (3) it potentiates the actions of other interferon; (4) it activates cells by a mechanism different from that of the other interferons; and (5) it inhibits intracellular microorganisms other than viruses (e.g., rickettsia).

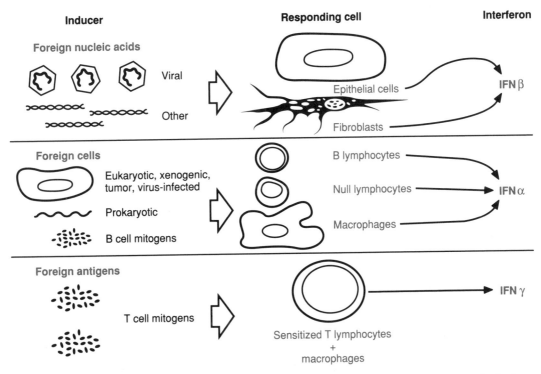

FIGURE 49-4 Induction of beta interferon, alpha interferon, and gamma interferon, respectively, by foreign nucleic acids, foreign cells, and foreign antigens.

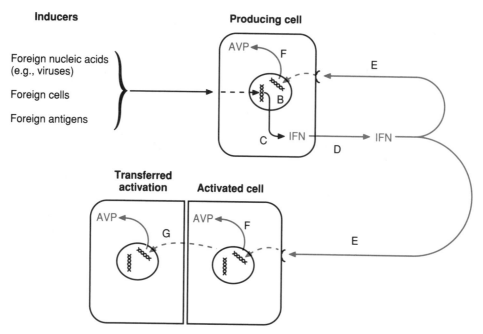

FIGURE 49-5 Cellular events of the induction, production, and action of interferon. Inducers of interferon react with cells to depress the interferon gene(s) (A). This leads to the production of mRNA for interferon (B). The mRNA is translated into the interferon protein (C), which is secreted into the extracellular fluid (D), where it reacts with the membrane receptors of cells (E). The interferon-stimulated cells derepress genes (F) for effector proteins (AVP) that establish antiviral resistance and other cell changes. The activated cells also stimulate contacted cells (G) to produce AVP by a still unknown mechanism.

Mechanism of Action

Interferon does not inactivate viruses directly. Instead, it prevents viral replication in surrounding cells by reacting with specific receptors on the cell membranes to derepress cellular genes that encode intracellular effector antiviral proteins, which must be synthesized before virus replication can be inhibited (Figs. 49-5 and 49-6). Alpha and beta interferons both bind to the same type of membrane receptor; gamma interferon binds to a different receptor. The antiviral proteins probably inhibit viral multiplication by inhibiting the synthesis of essential viral proteins, but alternative or additional inhibitory mechanisms (i.e., inhibition of transcription and viral release) also occur. Viral protein synthesis may be inhibited by several biochemical alterations of cells, which may, in theory,

inhibit viral replication at the different steps shown in Figure 49-6.

It has been shown that the antiviral state may be transferred from interferon-treated cells to adjacent untreated cells without the continued presence of interferon (Fig. 49-4); this transfer mechanism may further amplify and spread the activity of the interferon system.

The interferon system is nonspecific in two ways: (1) various viral stimuli induce the same type of interferon, and (2) the same type of interferon inhibits various viruses. On the other hand, the interferon molecule is mostly specific in its action for the animal species in which it was induced: interferon produced by animals or humans generally stimulates antiviral activity only in cells of the same or closely related families (e.g., human inter-

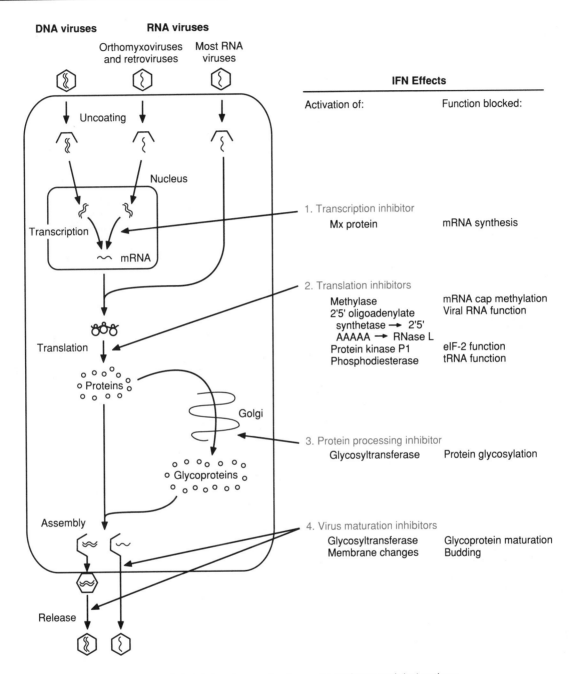

FIGURE 49-6 Molecular mechanisms of interferon antiviral actions.

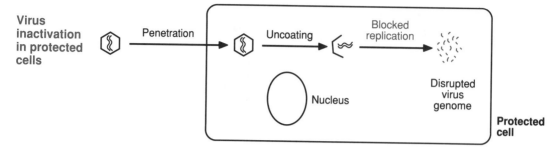

FIGURE 49-7 Nonspecific elimination of viruses by cells.

feron protects human and monkey cells, but not chicken or mouse cells).

Interferon during Natural Infection

The importance of interferon in the response to certain natural virus infections varies. Much depends on the effectiveness of the virus in stimulating interferon production and on its susceptibility to the antiviral action of interferon. Interferon protects solid tissues during virus infection; it is also disseminated through the bloodstream during viremia, thereby protecting distant organs against the spreading infection. Cells protected against viral replication may eliminate virus by degrading the virus genome (Fig. 49-7).

Medical Applications

Interferons have been approved in several nations for treatment of viral infections (papillomas and condylomata, herpes simplex, and hepatitis B and C) and cancers (hairy cell leukemia, chronic myelogenous leukemia, non-Hodgkin's lymphomas, and Kaposi sarcoma in AIDS patients). Clinical trials also have shown effectiveness against cryoglobulinemia and thrombocytosis and maintenance of remission in multiple myeloma. Studies of effectiveness in other viral infections and cancers are continuing, as are studies with substances capable of inducing endogenous interferon.

CONCLUSION

In conclusion, individual defense mechanisms assume roles of varying importance during different viral infections; in most cases, the recovery process is probably carried out by the simultaneous or sequential action of several mechanisms. The presence of multiple defenses helps explain why suppression of one or several mechanisms does not entirely abrogate host resistance to viral infections; however, impairment of host defenses by medications used for symptomatic relief of viral infections may lead to more severe illness. For example, aspirin and corticosteroids reduce the nonspecific defenses. Therefore, the well-established principle of the ancient physician—"primum non nocere" (primarily do not harm)—is still valid.

REFERENCES

Baron JL, Li JL, McKerlie ML et al: A new subtype of a natural viral inhibitor (CVI) that is stable in the gastrointestinal tract. Microb Pathog 1:241, 1986

Baron S, Dianzani F, Stanton GJ: The interferon system. Texas Rep Biol Med (I and II):1, 1982

Baron S, Niesel D, Singh IP et al: Recently described innate broad spectrum virus. Microb Pathog 7:237, 1989

Fleischmann WR Jr, Ramamurthy V, Stanton GJ et al: Interferon: mode of action and clinical applications. p. 1. In Smith RA (ed): Interferon Treatment of Neurologic Disorders. Marcel Dekker, New York, 1988

Isaacs A: Interferon. Adv Virus Res 10:1, 1963

Kumar S, Baron S: Non-interferon cellular products capable of virus inhibition. Texas Rep Biol Med 41:395, 1981

Wasserman FE: Methods for the study of viral inhibitors. In Marmarosh K, Koprowski H (eds): Methods in Virology. Academic Press, San Diego, 1988

Yilma T, Owens S, Adams DS: Preliminary characterization of a serum viral inhibitor. Am J Vet Res 46:2360, 1985

50

IMMUNE DEFENSES

GARY R. KLIMPEL

GENERAL CONCEPTS

Viral Activation of Immunity

Immunity to viral infection is caused by a variety of specific and nonspecific mechanisms. The activation of different immune functions and the duration and magnitude of the immune response depend on how the virus interacts with host cells (on whether it is a cytolytic, steady-state, latent, and/or integrated infection) and on how the virus spreads (by local, primary hematogenous, secondary hematogenous, and/or nervous system spread).

Humoral Immunity: Virus and/or virus-infected cells can stimulate B lymphocytes to produce antibody (specific for viral antigens) that neutralizes virus either by direct binding with the virus or by antibody-directed lysis of infected cells by complement or killer leukocytes. Antibody neutralization is most effective when virus is present in large fluid spaces (e.g., serum) or on moist surfaces (e.g., the gastrointestinal and respiratory tracts).

Cell-Mediated Immunity: The term **cell-mediated immunity** refers to (1) the recognition and/or killing of virus and virus-infected cells by leukocytes (T lymphocytes, natural killer (NK) cells, and/or macrophages) and (2) the production of different soluble factors **(cytokines)** by these cells when stimulated by virus or virus-infected cells.

Virus-Induced Immunopathology

Immune mediated disease may develop in certain virus infections in which viral antigens and uncontrolled immune hypersensitivity to them persist for a long period.

Roles of Immune Functions during Viral Infections

The early, nonspecific responses (nonspecific inhibition, natural killer cell activity, and interferon) limit virus multiplication during the acute phase of virus infections. The later specific immune (humoral and cell-mediated) responses function to help eliminate virus at the end of the acute phase, and subsequently to maintain specific resistance to reinfection.

TABLE 50-1 Host Effector Functions Important
against Primary Viral Infections

Host defense	Time of First Appearance	Effector	Target of Effector
Early nonspecific responses	Hours	Fever	Virus replication
		Phagocytosis	Virus
		Inflammation	Virus replication
		NK cell activity	Virus-infected cells
		Interferon	Virus replication, immunomodulation
Cell-mediated immune responses	Days	Cytotoxic T lymphocytes	Virus-infected cells
		Activated macrophages	Virus, virus-infected cells
		Lymphokines	Virus-infected cells, immunomodulation
		ADCC	Virus-infected cells
Humoral immune responses	Days	Antibody	Virus, virus-infected cells
		Antibody plus complement	Virus, virus-infected cells

INTRODUCTION

The general principles of immunology are presented in Chapter 1. The present chapter discusses viral activation of immunity, humoral and cell-mediated immunity, virus-induced immunopathology, and roles of immune functions during viral infections.

VIRAL ACTIVATION OF IMMUNITY

The term **immunity** as used in this chapter covers the mechanisms by which a host may specifically recognize and react to viruses. The nonspecific defenses are considered in Chapter 49. The host immune response may be beneficial, detrimental, or both. An immune response to a virus appears first during the primary infection of a susceptible, nonimmune host (Table 50-1) and increases during reinfection of an immune host. The specific immune responses that are effective against viruses are (1) cell-mediated immunity involving T lymphocytes and cytotoxic effector T lymphocytes, (2) antibody, with and without its interaction with complement and antibody-dependent cell-mediated cytotoxicity (ADCC), (3) natural killer (NK) cells and macrophages, and (4) lymphokines and monokines (Fig. 50-1). Some of these immune

FIGURE 50-1 The immune system response to a virus. (1) Virus bearing an antigenic epitope. (2) Processing of antigen to fragments. (3) Presentation of antigen (Ag) to T cells (on the infected cell surface) and B cells (free antigenic pieces or viruses). (4 and 5) Regulator T cells help (4) or suppress (5) both B and T effector responses. (6) Antigen-specific cytotoxic (killer) T cells. (7) T cells (helper as well as cytotoxic) produce lymphokines. (8) Some lymphocytes (both T and B) activated by antigen differentiate into a long-lived pool of memory cells responsible for rapid, secondary response to the same antigen. (9) Antibody combines with antigen (neutralization, elimination). (10 and 11) Products of T cells activate macrophages for killing of ingested virus (10) and natural killer cells (11) for nonspecific cytotoxicity against virus-infected cells. (12) Interferons are produced for protection of surrounding cells against virus infection. (13) Complexing of antibody with virus (opsonization) increases the engulfment of the virus by phagocytes and can neutralize virus. (14) Binding of antibody to infected target cells activates the antibody-dependent cytotoxic cell (ADCC). (15) Complement enzymatic cascade is activated by antigen-antibody complex (in this case, the antigen is on the cell surface). (16) Antibody binds to immunoglobulin receptors on basophils and mast cells.

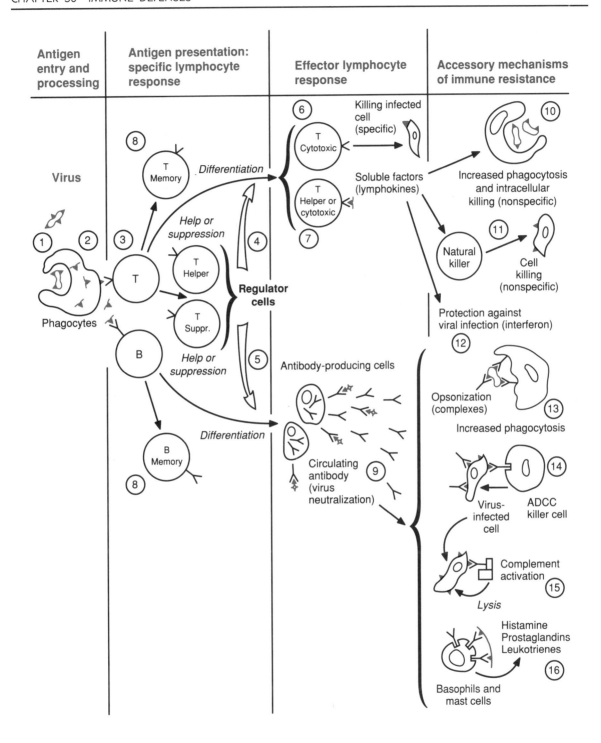

functions may interact, often synergistically, with nonimmune defense mechanisms (see Ch. 49).

Viral Antigens

The degree to which viral antigens are exposed to the host immune defenses is governed by the intracellular replication of viruses and by the several possible types of virus-host cell interaction (Fig. 50-2; see also Ch. 1).

Acute Cytolytic Infection

Acute cytolytic infection, the most common form of virus-host cell interaction (Fig. 50-2a–c), results in destruction of the infected cell. There are three ways in which the immune system can encounter the virus or virus-specific antigens of cytolytic viruses. In some cases, the immune system encounters viral antigen only when cell lysis releases the virions (Fig. 50-2a). Many viruses (e.g., reoviruses and coxsackieviruses), however, also induce virus-specific antigens on the cell surface before cell death occurs and sometimes before viral multiplication is complete (Fig. 50-2b). In the third type of cytolytic infection (Fig. 50-2c), common among enveloped viruses (e.g., herpesviruses, poxviruses, paramyxoviruses), virus-specific antigens are present on the cell surface and the cells release the infectious virions by budding for a short period before cell death. These viruses (e.g., herpesviruses, poxviruses, and paramyxoviruses) sometimes are disseminated by contiguous spread from cell to cell without exposure to extracellular antibody. Cell-mediated immune responses are believed to be important in controlling the local spread of this type of infection.

Persistent Infections

Some viruses produce a chronic (steady-state) infection rather than an acute infection of the host cell: progeny virions are released continuously, with little adverse effect on cellular metabolism. These cells express virus-specific antigens on their surface and produce abundant virus progeny, but are not killed by the infectious process. In some steady-state infections the progeny virus is released by budding through the cell membrane, and

virus can spread from cell to cell without being exposed to the extracellular environment. DNA viruses do not produce steady-state infections, but some RNA viruses (paramyxoviruses and retroviruses) do.

Latent Infections

Latent infections result when an infecting virus (e.g., a herpesvirus) is maintained within a cell for a long time (sometimes years) without giving rise to progeny virus or damaging the cell. Cells infected in this way may express virus-specific antigens on their cell surface. Months to years after infection, the virus in these cells can be reactivated, replicate, and cause disease. The mechanisms by which viruses are maintained intracellularly for long periods and then reactivated are only incompletely understood. Many latent infections occur in sequestered areas of the body (such as the nervous system), where recognition of infected cells by the immune system is believed to be difficult. In addition, any cell that harbors a virus but does not express viral antigens is not recognized by the immune system.

Integrated Virus Infection

There is another type of persistent virus-host cell interaction, **integrated virus infection,** in which all or part of the viral nucleic acid becomes integrated into the genome of the host cell. Progeny virions may never be assembled or released from the host cell. New virus-specific antigens, however, can be detected within the cell or on the cell surface. Infection with retroviruses is a classic example of this mechanism.

In most cases, the immune system is activated because the virus and its antigens appear in the extracellular fluid or on the cell membrane.

Virus Spread

Another important consideration in how viral infections trigger an immune response is the way in which a particular virus spreads in the host. In animal hosts, four types of viral spread are recognized: (1) **local spread,** in which the infection is confined largely to a mucosal surface or organ (as

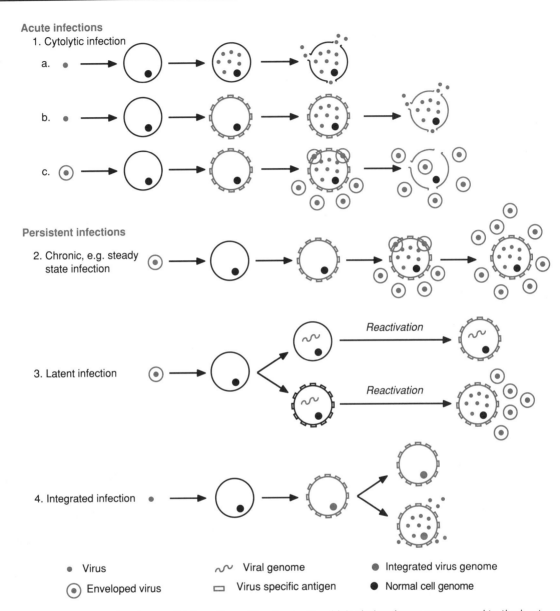

FIGURE 50-2 Virus-host cell interactions. The degree to which viral antigens are exposed to the host immune defenses is governed by the obligate intracellular replication of viruses. This exposure varies according to the virus-host cell interactions shown here; i.e., acute (cytolytic infections); persistent (steady-state infections, latent infections, and integrated infections).

in infection of the respiratory epithelium by rhinoviruses or of the gastrointestinal epithelium by rotaviruses); (2) **primary hematogenous spread,** in which the virus is inoculated directly into the bloodstream (e.g., insect-transmitted viruses) and then disseminates to target organs; (3) **secondary hematogenous spread,** in which the initial virus infection and replication (often relatively asymptomatic) occur on a mucosal surface with subsequent dissemination to target organs via the bloodstream (e.g., common viral exanthems, poliomyelitis, and mumps); and (4) **nervous system spread,** in which viruses (such as herpesviruses and rabiesviruses) disseminate via the nervous system. Therefore, viral antigens may be present in different parts of the body depending on the route of spread and phase of infection. Different immune mechanisms may operate at the various sites of virus spread and infection.

Virus Location

The location of the virus in the host is important not only for understanding the immune response, but also for developing and administering a vaccine. For example, local infections on surfaces such as the mucosa of the respiratory or gastrointestinal tract may elicit cell-mediated and humoral (IgA) immune responses, but not systemic immunity. The reverse is also true: systemic immunity does not always lead to local mucosal immunity. For example, the Salk polio vaccine, which consists of killed virus administered systemically, elicits serum IgG as the major antibody and induces little or no secretory response. As a result, the immunized individual resists systemic infection, but may become a temporary carrier, with virus persisting at the intestinal portal of entry because of the lack of secretory antibody. The orally administered, live Sabin polio vaccine, on the other hand, induces secretory antibody in the intestine and is effective in preventing replication and subsequent mucosal penetration by the virus.

Multiplicity of Immune Defenses

Recent studies have revealed a great complexity of host immune defenses against viral infections. This complexity arises from the many components of the host immune defenses and their interactions with one another. The existence of a variety of defenses is not surprising in view of the diversity of viruses, hosts, routes of infection, body compartments, cells, and mechanisms of virus multiplication and spread. The situation is further complicated by the varying effectiveness of the different host defenses during the different phases of the primary viral infection (implantation, spread to target organs, and subsequent recovery of each of the infected tissues), as well as during resistance to reinfection. Furthermore, the activated host defenses can actually cause disease manifestations. The presence of multiple defenses against each infection helps explain why impairment of one or a few defenses does not entirely abrogate host resistance to viral infections. Several immune and non-immune host defenses may operate to control viral infections or, at times, add to the disease process.

Many of the immune defenses against viral invasion are fairly well understood, but the relative effectiveness of each requires additional research. In particular, as this chapter attempts to make clear, humoral and cell-mediated immunity are not independent, but interact intimately to influence the duration and magnitude of each type of immune response.

Humoral Immunity

B Lymphocytes

As described in Chapter 1, specific B lymphocytes respond to viral antigen introduced by immunization or infection. Binding of antigen to the cell surface immunoglobulin receptors, followed by interaction of the B cell with macrophages and helper T lymphocytes, causes the B cell to differentiate into clones of antibody-secreting plasma cells, each capable of secreting antigen-specific immunoglobulin of one of five major classes: IgG, IgM, IgA, IgD, and IgE (Fig. 50-1). Antibodies act against viruses primarily by binding to and neutralizing virions and by directing the lysis of infected cells by complement or killer leukocytes.

Antibody-Mediated Reactions

NEUTRALIZATION OF VIRION INFECTIVITY At least three immunoglobulin classes have been demonstrated to exert antiviral activity: IgG, IgM, and IgA. These antibodies can neutralize the infectivity of virtually all known viruses. Antibody binds to the virus extracellularly, either neutralizing it immediately or blocking its interaction with host cells. Antibody that has bound to virus can block the infection of a cell at one of three steps:

(1) attachment of virus to the cell surface, (2) penetration of virus into the cell, and (3) uncoating of virus inside the cell (Fig. 50-3). The mechanism of viral neutralization involves the binding of antibody to virus coat proteins; this usually alters the viral receptor for the target cell. More rarely, bound antibody may also interfere with penetration or uncoating. The exact mechanism of neutralization is unclear, but it probably involves changes in steric conformation of the virus surface. These antibody-virus interactions can take place independently of complement.

Antibody also can neutralize virus by causing aggregation (Fig. 50-4), thus preventing adsorption of virus to cells and decreasing the number of infectious particles. Antibody and complement acting together can inactivate certain viruses (in most cases, enveloped viruses). Antibody is most effective against virus in large fluid spaces (e.g., serum) and on moist body surfaces (e.g., the respiratory and gastrointestinal tracts), where the virus is exposed to antibody for a relatively long period before escaping into cells. Consequently, viruses that spread by viremia are effectively eliminated by low levels of circulating antibody. Much higher levels of antibody are needed to prevent the spread of viruses that do not travel in the blood plasma (such as herpesviruses and rabiesviruses), because these viruses spend only a brief period traversing the small extracellular spaces between cells in solid tissue.

Besides binding directly to virus, antibodies may enhance phagocytosis. Three types of antibody interactions with phagocytic cells are seen: direct binding of antibody to the surface of the phagocytic cells (cytophilic antibody), uptake of antigen-

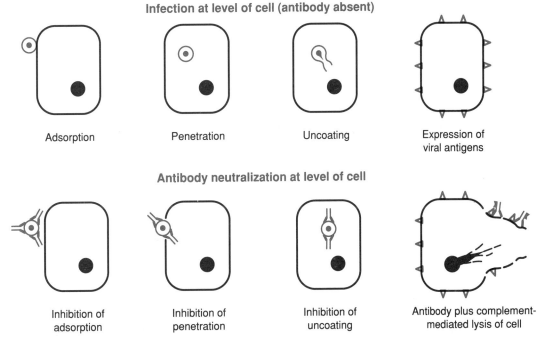

Infection at level of cell (antibody absent)

Adsorption   Penetration   Uncoating   Expression of
                                                           viral antigens

Antibody neutralization at level of cell

Inhibition of   Inhibition of   Inhibition of   Antibody plus complement-
adsorption   penetration   uncoating   mediated lysis of cell

FIGURE 50-3 Mechanisms of virus neutralization by antibody at the cellular level. At the cellular level, antibody can block the following steps associated with a virus infection: (1) virus attachment and adsorption to the cell surface, (2) penetration of the virus into the cells, and (3) actual uncoating of the antibody-virus complex once inside the cell. Antibody can also act at the cellular level by recognizing virus-specific antigens on the surface of infected cells. In the presence of complement, these virally infected cells can be destroyed.

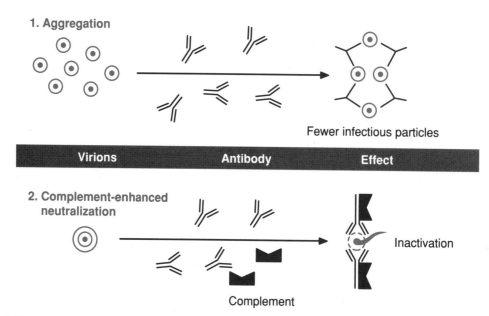

FIGURE 50-4 *Extracellular neutralization of virus by antibody. Antibody can reduce the number of infectious particles by linking virions and thereby causing aggregation. Antibody alone or with complement can also inactivate viruses.*

antibody complexes through the Fc receptor, and uptake of antigen-antibody-complement complexes through the C3b receptor (see Ch. 1). This phagocytosis of virions may result in inactivation of virus (see Ch. 49).

ANTIBODY EFFECTS ON VIRUS-INFECTED CELLS Antibody also can act on virus-infected cells by recognizing virus-specific antigens on the surface of infected cells (Fig. 50-3). Complement can then cause lysis of these cells. This complement-mediated lysis occurs both by the classic and the alternative complement pathways. Antibody-coated infected cells also can be destroyed by various effector cells via ADCC. Alternatively, however, some antibodies can mask viral antigens on the surface of infected cells, thereby removing or covering antigen on the surfaces of infected cells.

PHYSICAL BARRIERS TO ANTIBODY Before antibody can combine with and neutralize the virus, it must reach the site of virus replication. Barriers to the distribution of antibody include the cell membrane, which excludes antibody, and anatomic tissue barriers, which limit the distribution of macromolecules into certain organs such as the central nervous system and lungs.

IgG ANTIBODIES IgG is the most thoroughly studied antibody class and is responsible for most antiviral activity in serum. IgG antibodies reach infected (inflamed) sites by transduction (leakage) from capillaries. IgG is particularly protective in generalized viral infections that have a viremic phase (e.g., measles, polio, and hepatitis), perhaps because virions in serum are exposed to antibody. IgG antibodies are transferred passively from mother to offspring through the placenta and usually provide temporary protection against generalized viral infections during the first 6 to 9 months of life. Antibody is most protective when present before infection or during the spread of virus to target organs.

PRODUCTION AND THE ROLES OF ANTIBODY CLASSES After immunization or infection with viruses, various classes of antibody appear sequentially. For example, during primary infection or immunization, most antigens first elicit IgM (early antibody) responses; IgA and IgG responses follow within a few days. Reinfection, in contrast, stimulates production mainly of IgG, although some IgM and IgA are generated. When the primary antigenic stimulation is in the respiratory or gastrointestinal tract, IgA antibody is predominant, accompanied by some IgM. These antibodies are secreted locally at mucosal surfaces and are important in protecting the host against localized surface viral infections such as the common cold, influenza, and enteric viral infections. When viral replication is confined to a mucosal surface, resistance to infection is determined primarily by secretory IgA; serum IgG antibody provides less protection. Viral infections that begin on a mucosal surface and then spread hematogenously (e.g., measles, rubella, and polio) can be prevented at the mucosal stage by local secretory antibody and at the viremic stage by IgG antibodies. If serum IgG only is induced in a host, hematogenous spread can be prevented, but viral replication still may occur on the mucosal surface.

IgE ANTIBODIES AND IMMEDIATE HYPERSENSITIVITY

Recent information suggests that viruses that bind to IgE antibodies may trigger immediate hypersensitivity responses through the release of vasoactive mediators (see Ch. 1). These observations may explain many of the apparent allergic manifestations, such as wheezing and urticaria, that accompany some viral infections.

COMPLEMENT

Complement enhances the phagocytosis of many viruses. This enhanced phagocytosis is due to coating (opsonization) of virions by complement or by complement bound to antibody. Complement also can neutralize virus by enhancing either antibody-mediated steric changes on the virus or aggregation of the virus via antibody. In addition, complement can directly inactivate antibody-coated, enveloped virions.

HYPOGAMMAGLOBULINEMIA

A small minority of patients with impaired B-lymphocyte function (hypogammaglobulinemia limited to impairment of humoral immunity) have a significantly increased frequency of severe poliovirus and enterovirus infections of the nervous system (in addition to more frequent and severe infections with pyogenic bacteria). The risk of central nervous system invasion is related to the duration of viremia, as has been shown in immunosuppressed animals. The course of most viral infections is typically benign in most of these hypogammaglobulinemic patients, indicating that their weak antibody response and other defense mechanisms may be effective. The development of normal specific resistance to reinfection in hypogammaglobulinemic patients may result, in part, from their ability eventually to produce low levels of serum antibody to virus, as well as from the action of their intact cell-mediated immune system.

Cell-Mediated Immunity

Cell-mediated immunity (CMI) was once thought to be mediated solely by T lymphocytes; however, it is now clear that it is mediated by a variety of cell types, cell factors, or both. Virus-infected or virally transformed cells activate strong cell-mediated immune responses (Fig. 50-1). For some viral infections, cell-mediated immune reactions may be more important than antibody in early termination of viral infection and prevention of dissemination within the host. Recent evidence shows that cell-mediated immunity functions at the body surfaces, as well as internally. Cell-mediated immune responses to viral infections involve T lymphocytes, ADCC, macrophages, natural killer cells, lymphokines, and monokines (Figs. 50-5 and 50-6).

T Lymphocytes

Much evidence indicates that T lymphocytes are important in recovery from viral infections. Of the many functional subsets of T cells, those that express specific cytotoxic activity against virus-infected or transformed cells have aroused the most interest.

CYTOTOXIC T LYMPHOCYTES

The generation of virus-specific **cytotoxic T lymphocytes (CTLs)** is believed to be important in preventing viral multiplication (Fig. 50-5). Presumably, the T lympho-

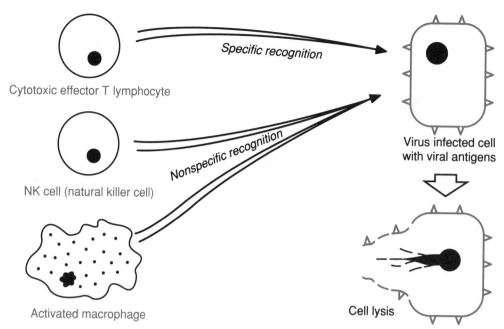

FIGURE 50-5 Lysis of virus-infected cells by cytotoxic effector cells. Cytotoxic effector cells that can destroy virus-infected cells include cytotoxic T cells, natural killer cells, and activated macrophages. Cytotoxic T lymphocytes can recognize and destroy virus-infected cells, and this recognition is virus specific and major histocompatibility complex (MHC) restricted. Activated macrophages and natural killer cells can also recognize virus-infected cells, but this is not virus specific or major histocompatibility complex restricted.

cytes prevent virus multiplication by destroying infected cells before mature, infectious virus particles can be assembled. This hypothesis assumes that viral antigens appear on the plasma membrane before the release of virus progeny, a view that is substantiated by studies of many, but not all, infections.

The generation of cytotoxic T cells is mediated by cell-associated antigens. Virus glycoproteins that can be recognized by cytotoxic T cells not only are synthesized in infected cells, but also can be derived by fusion of enveloped virions with the cell plasma membrane during the first stage of viral penetration. Therefore, even some noninfectious or inactivated viruses can induce a cytotoxic T-cell response.

Exposure to a virus-infected cell can cause the antigen-specific T lymphocytes to differentiate into cytotoxic effector T cells, which can lyse virus-infected or virally transformed cells. These cytotoxic T cells are specific not only for the viral anti-gen but also for self major histocompatibility antigens and will lyse virus-infected cells only if these cells also express the correct major histocompatibility complex (MHC) gene products.

Activation of cytotoxic and other T lymphocytes may be one of the earliest manifestations of an immune response. T-cell effector functions occur as early as 3 to 4 days after initiation of a viral infection. However, T-cell responses often decrease rapidly, within 5 to 10 days of elimination of the virus (although virus-specific memory T cells persist for long periods). In contrast, antibodies usually become measurable later in the viral infection (after 7 days) and persist at high levels for much longer (often for years).

Helper T cells and T cells that mediate delayed-type hypersensitivity may be as important as cytotoxic T cells in the immune response to a virus infection. Helper T cells are required for the generation of cytotoxic T cells and for optimal antibody production. In addition, helper T cells, T

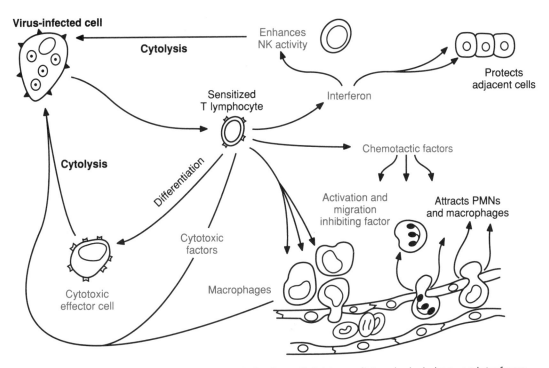

FIGURE 50-6 Cell-mediated events in viral infections. Soluble mediators include immune interferon, chemotactic factors, macrophage migration inhibitory factor, and lymphotoxin; other lymphokines and monokines are not depicted. Cytotoxic effector lymphocytes, macrophages, and natural killer cells play complex but important roles in host defense. PMNs, Polymorphonuclear leukocytes.

cells that mediate delayed-type hypersensitivity, and cytotoxic T cells produce a number of important soluble factors (lymphokines) that can recruit and influence other cellular components of the immune and inflammatory responses.

Animal studies indicate that impairing the T-cell defenses enhances infections by herpes simplex virus, poxviruses, and Sindbis virus and enhances the development of tumors induced by polyomavirus. Since the host retains some resistance to infections, T lymphocytes probably are not the sole defense against these viruses. Impairment of T lymphocytes also hinders T cell-dependent antibody production. In humans, T-cell impairment is associated mainly with more frequent and severe poxvirus and herpesvirus infections. Nevertheless, these infections still do not develop in most individuals with T-cell deficiencies, even though the prevalence of herpesviruses (and many other viruses) is great.

Antibody-Dependent Cell-Mediated Cytotoxicity

Effector leukocytes for ADCC have surface receptors that recognize and bind to the Fc portion of IgG molecules. When IgG binds to virus-specified antigens on the surface of an infected cell, the Fc portion becomes a target for effector cells capable of mediating ADCC. Binding of these effector cells to the Fc portion of IgG bound to the infected-cell surface antigens results in lysis of the infected cell. ADCC is a very efficient way of lysing virus-infected cells because it requires 10-fold less antibody than does antibody-complement lysis.

Lymphocytes, macrophages, and neutrophils are all capable of mediating ADCC against virus-infected cells. The lymphocytes with this ability appear to be heterogeneous. Natural killer cells, as well as null lymphocytes with Fc receptors for IgG, appear to be able to mediate ADCC activity.

Macrophages

Macrophages are important in both specific and nonspecific responses to viral infections (e.g., herpesvirus infections). Factors that modify macrophage activity can influence the outcome of an infection. Moreover, since macrophages are central to the induction of T and B lymphocyte responses, any effect on macrophages will influence B and T cells.

Macrophages confer protection against viruses through either an intrinsic or an extrinsic process. In the former, virions are disposed of within macrophages acting either as phagocytes or as nonpermissive host cells. In the latter case, macrophages retard or ablate virus multiplication in neighboring cells by destroying virus-infected cells or by producing soluble factors (interferons) that act on these cells. Phagocytosis of some viruses by macrophages decreases virus levels in body fluids (as during viremia) and thereby impedes virus spread. These effects are produced only if the virus is destroyed or contained by macrophages. If a virus replicates in macrophages, the infected macrophages may aid in transmission of the virus to other body cells. The permissiveness of macrophages for virus replication may depend on the age and genetic constitution of the host and on the specific condition of the macrophages.

Macrophage activation mediated either by products of infection (viral and cellular) or by soluble factors produced by T cells (e.g., gamma interferon) often enhance phagocytosis and the elimination of free virus particles. Another important effector mechanism of activated macrophages is their ability to recognize and destroy virus-infected and virus-transformed cells (Fig. 50-5). In addition, activated macrophages participate in virus inhibition by producing interferon and mediating ADCC.

Natural Killer Cells

Natural killer (NK) cells exhibit cytotoxic activity against a number of tumor cell lines, particularly against virus-infected or virus-transformed cells (Fig. 50-5). Natural killer or natural killer-like cells, which have been found in almost every mammalian species examined and even in some invertebrates, are identified as large granular lymphocytes that possess Fc receptors. They can mediate ADCC activity; their nonspecific cytotoxic activity is increased by interferon and interleukin-2 (IL-2); and they can produce interferon when stimulated with virus or virus-infected cells.

Although natural killer cells display cytotoxic activity against virus-infected or transformed cells, they show little or no cytotoxic activity against normal cells. Unlike that of cytotoxic T lymphocytes, natural killer cell killing is not human leukocyte antigen (HLA) restricted, and natural killer cells do not exhibit conventional immunologic specificity. There is evidence that natural killer cells play an important defensive role in virus infections in humans and animals.

Lymphokines and Monokines

Soluble factors from T lymphocytes **(lymphokines)** and macrophages **(monokines)** regulate the degree and duration of the immune responses generated by T lymphocytes, B lymphocytes, and macrophages (see Ch. 1). Interleukin-2 and gamma interferon are two such important factors produced by activated T cells. Interleukin-1 is a soluble factor produced by macrophages. All three of these factors are essential for the full differentiation and proliferation of cytotoxic T cells. The two interleukins are also important for antibody production by B lymphocytes.

Macrophages and T lymphocytes also produce several other important factors that act in both the immune and the inflammatory responses. Gamma interferon can activate macrophages to become cytotoxic toward virus-infected cells and can increase the level of phagocytosis and degradation. Lymphotoxins produced by T cells also may participate in the destruction of virus-infected cells. Virus can stimulate alpha interferon production from macrophages; this enhances natural killer cell function and inhibits virus multiplication in neighboring cells.

VIRUS-INDUCED IMMUNOPATHOLOGY

A host clearly has numerous mechanisms to recognize and eliminate the viruses that it encounters. However, some viruses persist despite these mechanisms, and then the immune responses may become detrimental to the host and cause immune-mediated disease. When an antigen (virus) persists, pathologic changes and diseases result from different types of immunologic interactions, including immediate hypersensitivity, antibody-mediated immune complex syndrome, and tissue damage caused by cell-mediated effector cells and antibody plus complement. Of these mechanisms, the immune complex syndrome during viral infections has been studied most intensively. Two major complications of deposition of immune complexes are vascular damage and nephritis. Some viral diseases in which immune complexes have been demonstrated are hepatitis B, infectious mononucleosis, dengue hemorrhagic fever, and subacute sclerosing panencephalitis.

Cytotoxic T cells also mediate immunopathologic injury in murine models of human infections (i.e., infections with lymphocytic choriomeningitis virus and poxviruses). Both cytotoxic T cells and T cells responsible for delayed-type hypersensitivity have also been implicated in the pathology associated with influenza pneumonia and coxsackievirus myocarditis of mice. A delicate balance between the removal of infected cells that are the source of viral progeny and injury to vital cells probably exists for T cells as well as for the other host immune components.

Viruses may sometimes circumvent host defenses. An important factor that may impair the function of sensitized T lymphocytes is apparent from the observation that T cells activated by reaction with antigen or mitogen lose their normal resistance to many viruses. Therefore, these activated T lymphocytes develop the capacity to support the replication of viruses, leading to impairment of T lymphocyte function.

ROLES OF IMMUNE FUNCTIONS DURING VIRAL INFECTIONS

On the basis of the mechanisms described here and in Chapter 49, a hypothetical model can be constructed that shows how the immune components defend against viruses (Fig. 50-1; Table 50-1).

Nonspecific Defenses

A primary infection in a nonimmune, susceptible host is countered first by the nonspecific defense mechanisms (see Ch. 49). The early nonspecific responses occur within hours and consist of interferon production, inflammation, fever, phagocytosis, and natural killer cell activity. These defenses may prevent or abort infection; if they do not, the virus is disseminated by local spread, viremia, or nerve spread. It then may seed to a number of target organs and thereby produce a generalized infection.

Specific Defenses

Antibody

The events that lead to a specific immune response begin almost immediately after exposure and result in the production of antiviral antibody and cell-mediated immunity in 3 to 10 days. The disseminated antibody response in serum is predominantly IgG (preceded by IgM); the local antibody response in secretions is predominantly secretory IgA (with some IgM). The persistence of IgA antibodies in secretions is much shorter (months) than the persistence of IgG antibody in serum (years). The role of IgE in secretions is unknown, but it may mediate immediate hypersensitivity and amplify the immune response during infection. Antibodies may neutralize virus directly or destroy virus-infected cells via ADCC or complement. Clearly, serum antibody confers protection against generalized infections (e.g., measles, polio, and type A hepatitis), in which virus must spread through the antibody-containing bloodstream; inoculation of small quantities of antibody into susceptible individuals prevents viral disease but may not prevent subclinical infection at mucosal surfaces.

In localized infections of mucosal surfaces, protection does not correlate with the presence of serum antibody, but it does correlate with the presence of local IgA antibody, as has been shown in human studies of viruses restricted to the respiratory tract (e.g., respiratory syncytial virus and influenza virus) or to the gastrointestinal tract (e.g., enteroviruses). Under some conditions in which serum antibody is present but local IgA is absent, hypersensitivity instead of protective immunity may occur (e.g., respiratory syncytial virus infection). Also, serum antibody may not protect against recurrence of latent infections, such as herpes zoster (shingles) and herpes simplex, both because the virus may be shielded by its intracellular location and because cell-mediated immunity may be the more important defense. Antibody may also cause undesirable effects in certain chronic infections. Examples in which small amounts of serum antibody complex with virus and deposit in the kidneys, thereby inducing immune complex disease, are listed in Table 50-1.

Therefore, serum IgM and IgG antibody seem to be effective in preventing infections of a generalized nature; however, in localized surface infections the presence of secretory IgA antibody appears to correlate much better with protection than the presence of circulating IgG antibody. In persistent infections, serum antibody may be responsible for certain long-term sequelae.

Cell-Mediated Immunity

Cell-mediated immunity is essential in recovery from and control of viral infections, especially infections involving oncogenic viruses or viruses that spread directly from cell to contiguous cell. In these situations antibody cannot reach the virus but virally induced antigens on the surface of the infected cell can be recognized by different effector cells (e.g., cytotoxic T cells) (Fig. 50-6).

If the virus reaches target organs, it is more difficult to control. The host defenses that may play important roles in target organs are initially inflammation, fever, and interferon and subsequently cell-mediated immunity.

In some situations, cell-mediated immunity may develop before antibody production begins. For example, cytotoxic effector T cells have been found in bronchial washings 3 to 4 days after initiation of intranasal infection in mice; at this time, antibody cannot yet be detected.

Cell-mediated immune responses can cause tissue damage; the lung lesions produced in influenza may be examples. The lethal effects of lymphocytic choriomeningitis virus in mice are mediated by cytotoxic effector T cells. The rash in many exanthems (such as measles) is thought to represent a cell-mediated attack on virus localized within cells of the dermis and its vasculature.

REFERENCES

Ada GL, Leung KN, Erty H: An analysis of effector T cell generation and function in mice exposed to influenza A or Sendai viruses. Immunol Rev 58:5, 1981

Baron S, Grossberg SE, Klimpel GR, Brunell PA: Mechanisms of action and pharmacology: the immune and interferon systems. In Galasso G (ed): Antiviral Agents and Viral Diseases of Man. Raven Press, New York, 1984

Doherty PC: Cell-mediated immunity in virus infections of the central nervous system. Ann NY Acad Sci 540:228, 1988

Herberman RB, Ortaldo JR: Natural killer cells: their role in defenses against disease. Science 214:24, 1981

Hirsch RL, Winkelstein JA, Griffin DE: The role of complement in viral infections. III. Activation of the classical and alternative complement pathways by Sindbis virus. J Immunol 124:2507, 1980

McChesney MB, Oldstone MBA: Viruses perturb lymphocyte functions: selected principles characterizing virus-induced immunosuppression. Annu Rev Immunol 5:279, 1987

Mogensen LA: Role of macrophages in natural resistance to virus infections. Microbiol Rev 43:1, 1979

Ogra PL, Leibovitz EE, Zhao RG: Oral immunization and secretory immunity to viruses. Curr Top Microbiol Immunol 146:73, 1989

Ogra PL, Morag A, Tiku ML: Humoral immune response to viral infections. In Notkins AL (ed): Viral Immunology and Immunopathology. Academic Press, San Diego, 1975

Oldstone MBA: Immune responses, immune tolerance and viruses. In Fraenkel-Conrat H, Wagner RR (eds): Comprehensive Virology. Vol 15. Plenum, New York, 1979

Rouse BT, Norley S, Martin S: Antiviral cytotoxic T lymphocyte induction and vaccination. Rev Infect Dis 10:16, 1988

Sissons JGP, Oldstone MBA: Antibody-mediated destruction of virus-infected cells. Adv Immunol 29:209, 1980

51 CONTROL

HARRY M. MEYER, JR.
DEBORAH J. HENDERSON
PAUL D. PARKMAN

GENERAL CONCEPTS

Immunoprophylaxis

Immunoprophylaxis against viral illnesses includes the use of vaccines or antibody-containing preparations to provide immune protection against a specific disease.

Active Prophylaxis

Active immunization involves administering a virus preparation that stimulates the body's immune system to produce its own specific immunity. Viral vaccines are of two types: those containing attenuated live viruses and those containing killed viruses.

Immune Response to Vaccines: Vaccination evokes an antibody response and stimulates T lymphocytes. Vaccine-induced immunity is assessed in terms of percentage of recipients protected and the duration and degree of protection. Most effective viral vaccines protect more than 90 percent of recipients and produce fairly durable immunity.

Vaccine Production: To develop a new vaccine, researchers must first identify the virus and then produce the virus or virus components in quantity under circumstances acceptable for vaccine preparation.

Adverse Reactions: Live attenuated virus vaccines typically cause some portion of the clinical spectrum of the natural disease. Inactivated virus vaccines can also cause

reactions, but the symptoms usually do not mimic the natural disease; the reaction is a general response to foreign proteins and viral antigens.

Passive Immunoprophylaxis

Passive immunity is conferred by administering antibodies formed in another host. Human immunoglobulins remain a mainstay of passive prophylaxis (and occasionally therapy) for viral illnesses; they are usually used to protect individuals who have been exposed to a disease and cannot be protected by vaccination.

Sanitation and Vector Control

Many viral diseases are controlled by reducing exposure to the virus by (1) eliminating nonhuman reservoirs, (2) eliminating the vector, and (3) improving sanitation.

Antiviral Chemotherapy

There are three types of antiviral agent: (1) virucidal agents, which directly inactivate viruses, (2) antiviral agents, which inhibit viral replication, and (3) immunomodulators, which boost the host immune response.

Interferons

Virus-infected cells can secrete the protein **interferon,** which protects normal cells from viral infection. Therapeutic administration of interferon has proven effective in only a few human viral illnesses.

INTRODUCTION

Viral diseases range from trivial infections to plagues that alter the course of history. Because of the enormous variations in viruses themselves and in their epidemiology and pathogenesis, there is no single, magic-bullet approach to control. Each virus presents its own set of problems. This chapter concerns methods useful to various degrees in controlling selected viral diseases. The most spectacular progress so far has involved immunoprophylaxis. Vector control and sanitation have contributed greatly. Also, a number of therapeutic antiviral agents are now available, including some for very serious infections such as human immunodeficiency virus type 1 (HIV-1) infection. In addition, we have just begun to discover the antiviral and immunomodulatory effects of the interferons in humans.

IMMUNOPROPHYLAXIS

Immunoprophylaxis against viral illnesses includes the use of vaccines or antibody-containing preparations to provide a susceptible individual with immunologic protection against a specific disease. Immunization against viral illnesses can be either active or passive. With **active immunity,** protection is achieved by stimulating the body's immune system to produce its own antibodies by immunization with a virus preparation. **Passive immunity** is conferred by antibodies formed in another host; for example, an antibody-containing gamma globulin preparation will protect a susceptible individual exposed to a viral illness.

Active Prophylaxis

The viral vaccines currently available for use in the United States are listed in Table 51-1. These products are of two types: those containing live viruses, and those containing viruses that have been killed. Live vaccines contain viruses that have been attenuated by laboratory manipulation. These attenuated viruses can infect and replicate in the recipient and produce a protective immune response without causing disease. Live attenuated viral vaccines usually confer lifelong immunity after one dose. However, because live viruses can multiply in the body, there is always the possibility that they may revert to a more pathogenic form. Adequate preclinical testing and extensive clinical studies must be performed to rule out this possibility. In addition, new recombinant technologies facilitate

TABLE 51-1   Viral Vaccines Available in the United States

Vaccine	Type
Hepatitis B	Inactivated viral antigen or recombinant DNA-derived protein
Influenza	Inactivated virus or viral components
IPV (inactivated poliovirus vaccine)	Inactivated viruses of all three serotypes
Measles	Live virus
MMR (measles, mumps, rubella)	Live viruses
Mumps	Live virus
OPV (oral poliovirus vaccine)	Live viruses of all three serotypes
Rabies	Inactivated virus
Rubella	Live virus
Smallpox	Live virus
Yellow fever	Live virus

direct alteration of viral genetic structure, thus permitting scientists to produce attenuated viruses in which the genetic regions likely to lead to pathogenetic reversion are modified or deleted.

Killed virus vaccines contain either *whole virus particles,* inactivated by chemical or physical means, or *some component(s) of the virus.* Although they cannot cause disease, they do not generally produce lifelong immunity following one dose; multiple doses are usually required. In addition, because killed virus does not multiply in the host, the inoculum itself must provide a sufficiently large concentration of viral antigens to induce the desired immune response. Application of a new recombinant DNA strategy to develop killed vaccines—identifying the specific protein component that can elicit the production of protective antibodies and cloning the gene encoding that protein—has made possible a safe and effective recombinant vaccine against hepatitis B virus.

Immune Response to Vaccines

Vaccination evokes an **antibody** response which is, in turn, a measure of the effectiveness of the vaccine in stimulating B lymphocytes. Antiviral antibodies are classified as IgA, IgM, or IgG and can be measured by various techniques. Some antibody categories (IgA and IgM) are normally more abundant in respiratory and intestinal secretions; others (mainly IgG) are more abundant in the circulatory system.

Vaccines also stimulate T lymphocytes, leading to **cell-mediated responses** that influence protection. Antiviral antibody assays are now routine laboratory procedures, but measuring cellular immunity in vitro usually requires research laboratory facilities. In general, despite the complexities of the immune system, resistance to the vaccine-preventable viral diseases correlates well with the presence of circulating antiviral antibodies, which are easily measured.

Effectiveness is a key concern with any vaccine. Here the standard for comparison is the immunity conferred by the natural disease. Both epidemiologic and laboratory methods are used to generate comparative data. Vaccine-induced immunity can be defined by the percentage of recipients protected, the projected duration of protection, and the degree of protection. Most viral vaccines considered effective protect more than 90 percent of recipients, and the immunity produced appears to be fairly durable. However, vaccines usually do not induce an immunologic response entirely comparable to that seen in the natural disease. Immunity to viral diseases should not be thought of as absolute. Vaccinees and persons immune from the natural disease sometimes experience subclinical reinfection if exposed. Often, upon revaccination or reinfection, a boost in IgG antibodies is observed with little or no detectable IgM response, suggesting prior protection. Therefore, the absence of measurable antibody may not mean that the individual is unprotected. Evaluating the degree of protection often involves measuring the frequency and extent to which subclinical reinfection can override vaccine-induced resistance.

Immune responses to viral vaccines may be modified by a number of factors related to the vaccine as well as to the host. As already discussed, the magnitude and duration of immunity differ significantly between live and killed vaccines. The immune response to vaccines can be enhanced by adding adjuvant substances such as aluminum salts (e.g., hepatitis B vaccine). The route of administration of a vaccine and the age of the recipient can also influence the immunogenicity of some vaccines. For example, maternal antibodies acquired transplacentally can interfere with responses to measles, mumps, and rubella (MMR) vaccine, as demonstrated by lower response rates when the vaccine is administered earlier than 15 months of age.

Vaccine Production

Vaccines share a number of general characteristics and have certain generic problems that have led to continuing improvements in vaccine development. Viruses are obligate intracellular parasites, and so, all virus vaccines contain substances derived from the cells or living tissues used in virus production. Technical advances have improved production methods. One can think of generations of vaccines: those prepared in the tissues of an inoculated animal are the **first generation** (e.g., smallpox vaccine from the skin of a calf), products from the inoculation of embryonated eggs are the **second generation** (e.g., inactivated influenza virus vaccine), and tissue culture-propagated vaccines are the **third generation** (e.g., poliomyelitis, measles, mumps, and rubella vaccines). The vaccine generation indicates the production methodology, sophistication, and relative purity. Third-generation vaccines usually contain the least host protein and other extraneous constituents, but they have been the most difficult to produce. Recent developments in biotechnology have afforded several basic techniques now being used in virus characterization and in the production of specific viral antigens that can be applied to the production of **subunit vaccines.** The new biotechnology serves as the cornerstone for a **fourth generation** of vaccines and has already provided a licensed recombinant yeast human hepatitis B vaccine.

To develop a new vaccine, researchers must first identify and then produce the virus (or virus components) in quantity under circumstances acceptable for vaccine preparation. Normally this means production of virus or virus components in cell cultures, embryonated eggs, or tissues of experimental animals or humans, or through nucleic acid recombinant technology. Interestingly, viral antigens in one hepatitis B vaccine are harvested and purified directly from the plasma of human carriers. Finding an acceptable production system can be a problem, especially in developing inactivated viral vaccines, because a high concentration of antigen is needed. As already mentioned, production of specific viral proteins by recombinant DNA procedures is providing a solution to many of these problems. A final consideration is the clinical importance of the virus. Normally, it must cause a disease of some severity and be capable of affecting a substantial proportion of the population before consideration is given to developing a vaccine. For example, group B coxsackieviruses can produce severe, sometimes fatal disease, but they do so rarely. Therefore, although developing a vaccine for any of the several group B serotypes is technically feasible, no one has proposed doing so.

Adverse Reactions

Reactions to live, attenuated virus vaccines typically mirror some portion of the clinical spectrum of the natural disease, as when attenuated polio vaccine causes the rare paralytic complications. Reactions to inactivated virus vaccines also can be caused by the viral components, but the adverse symptoms usually do not mimic the natural disease and the reaction is more a general response to foreign protein and viral antigens. Typically, local tenderness and inflammation occur at the injection site; systemic reactions commonly consist of fever, malaise, and myalgia. These reactions occur within the first 48 hours after administration of the inactivated vaccine, whereas the disease-mimicking symptoms caused by a live vaccine inoculation begin later, after many cycles of virus replication. Experience has shown that reactions to live or inactivated viral vaccines (e.g., allergic reactions and autoimmunity) are rarely attributable to mistakes in production; instead, these reactions generally reflect the inherent risk of the product, a function of the state of the art at any given time. It is important to distinguish between illnesses having a temporal association with vaccination and illnesses actually caused by vaccines. Although the reporting of temporal associations is an important first step in looking for causes of reactions, the documentation of cause-effect relationships generally requires careful study and statistical analysis.

Passive Immunoprophylaxis

The use of immunoglobulins remains a mainstay of passive prophylaxis (and occasionally of therapy) for viral illnesses. Passive immunoprophylaxis is most often recommended when exposure has occurred and time does not allow for vaccination or when no effective vaccine exists. Although once derived exclusively from animal sources, most immunoglobulins are now manufactured from human sources. Table 51-2 lists the types of immunoglobulins available in the United States.

Standard immunoglobulin is produced by pooling plasma from thousands of donors and contains antibodies to a number of common viruses. Manufacturers of standard immunoglobulin in the

TABLE 51-2   Approved Products Currently Used for Passive Immunization
and Immunotherapy Against Viral Disease in the United States

Product	Use
Immunoglobulin (Ig)	Congenital or acquired immunoglobulin deficiency; modification or prevention of measles; prevention of hepatitis A
Human Rabies Immunoglobulin (HRIg)	Postexposure prophylaxis (administered with vaccine)
Hepatitis B Immunoglobulin (HBIg)	Postexposure prophylaxis as in accidental needle-stick; high-risk neonatal immunization (administered with vaccine)
Vaccinia Immunoglobulin (VIg)	Therapy of progressive vaccinia, eczema vaccination, and vaccinia ophthalmicus
Varicella-zoster Immunoglobulin (VZIg)	Postexposure prophylaxis of high-risk individuals
Cytomegalovirus Immunoglobulin (CMVIg)[a]	Passive immunization of renal transplant recipients

[a] Not yet commercially available.

United States must demonstrate that their products contain antibodies to both poliovirus and measles virus. Specific immunoglobulins are produced from donors with high titers of antibodies to specific viruses, often chosen following immunization for these viruses.

SANITATION AND VECTOR CONTROL

Several early approaches to virus control deserve recognition, even though they are less dramatic than vaccination. One approach is the *avoidance of viral exposure*. For example, blood bank testing for hepatitis B surface antigen and for antibodies to HIV-1 is classified as avoidance.

Control of nonhuman viral reservoirs is another old, worthwhile approach. Unfortunately, few opportunities exist for practical application. The most notable successful use was the elimination of rabies in some countries through removal of stray dogs and quarantine of incoming pets. The control of animal rabies reservoirs continues to be valuable in countries where the virus cannot be eradicated because it is entrenched in sylvan reservoirs, such as foxes, raccoons, skunks, and bats.

Another approach of enormous contemporary and historic importance is *vector control*. Transmission of viral disease by the bite of an arthropod vector was first demonstrated by Walter Reed and his associates, with their discovery that yellow fever was transmitted by mosquitoes. At the turn of the century, yellow fever was a disease of major consequence in the Americas and Africa. By immediately applying Reed's discovery, Gorgas mounted the anti-*Aedes aegypti* campaign in Havana that marked the beginning of the conquest of epidemic yellow fever. In dealing with the arthropod-borne diseases such as St. Louis encephalitis, any procedure that reduces vector populations or limits the access of the arthropod to humans has potential value. These procedures include draining swamps, applying insecticide, screening homes, and using insect repellant or protective clothing.

The last of the older approaches is to *improve sanitation*. This method is applicable in a limited way to diseases whose epidemiology involves fecal-oral transmission. The well-known link between the discharge of raw sewage into tidal waters, contamination of shellfish, and type A hepatitis is an example of a situation readily reversible by improved sanitary practices.

ANTIVIRAL CHEMOTHERAPY

The development of effective antiviral agents had been slow and painstaking and has usually involved large-scale random testing and serendipity. The diverse nature of virus–host-cell interactions has precluded the development of a broad-spectrum antiviral agent. Until the recent rapid expansion of technologies available for virus manipulation, the development of a drug specific for a given virus was not considered technically feasible. Prophylactic use of drugs was not thought practical because of inherent drug toxicity. Therapeutic use also was not practical because of the long time needed for diagnosis. Economic factors have also dampened researchers' enthusiasm, since even the most promising compounds require years of laboratory and clinical testing, costing millions of dollars. Despite these obstacles, several useful drugs with proven therapeutic and prophylactic effectiveness have emerged and are approved (Table 51-3).

Antiviral chemotherapeutic agents can be divided into three categories: **virucidal agents, antiviral agents,** and **immunomodulators.** Virucidal agents directly inactivate intact viruses. Although some of these agents have limited usefulness, (e.g., treatment of warts with podophyllin, which destroys both virus and host tissues) most virucides have no demonstrated therapeutic usefulness. Antiviral agents inhibit viral replication at the cellular level, interrupting one or more steps in the life cycle of the virus. These agents have a limited spectrum of activity and, because most of them also interrupt host cell function, they are toxic to various degrees.

The demonstrated effectiveness of acyclovir against herpesvirus infections and of zidovudine against HIV has given recent impetus to the search for new antiviral agents. The concept of a targeted approach is now practical since information concerning the structure and replication of viruses and the spatial configuration and function of their proteins is available. Such data may be useful in identifying specific target sites for antiviral agents.

Immunomodulators that alter the host immune responses could, in principle, be protective. Many immunomodulators are being studied, some with promising results.

INTERFERONS

Since the mid-1930s, scientists have recognized that under certain circumstances one virus can interfere with another. In 1957, Isaacs and Linden-

TABLE 51-3   Approved Antiviral Agents

Product	Use[a]	Route
Acyclovir	Genital HSV infections	
	primary	IV, oral
	recurrent	Oral
	Mucocutaneous HSV infections in immunocompromised hosts	IV, oral, topical
Amantadine	Influenza A	Oral
	prophylaxis	
	treatment	
Adenine arabinoside	HSV encephalitis	IV
	HSV keratitis	Topical
Ganciclovir	Cytomegalovirus retinitis	IV
Interferon	Genital papilloma (refractory)	Intralesional
Iododeoxyuridine	HSV keratitis	Topical
Ribavirin	RSV bronchiolitis/pneumonia	Aerosol
Trifluorothymidine	HSV keratitis	Topical
Zidovudine	HIV infection	Oral

[a] HSV, Herpes simplex virus; RSV, respiratory syncytial virus.

man made a dramatic discovery that explained the mechanism of resistance. They found that virus-infected cells can elaborate a protein substance called **interferon,** which, when added to normal cells in culture, protects them from viral infection. Other microbial agents (such as rickettsiae and bacteria) and natural and synthetic polypeptides were later shown to induce interferon. Subsequent research established that interferons tend to have species specificity (mouse cell interferon protects mouse cells and not human cells) and are inhibitory to numerous viruses.

For many years it was not possible to obtain high yields of interferon to conduct major studies. However, the successful application of recombinant DNA technology and cell culture technology has solved the problem of interferon supply. Subsequently, interferon has been studied in extensive clinical trials with limited usefulness to date. Although broadly antiviral in some animal models, it has proven effective in few viral illnesses of humans and is currently approved in the United States for use in treating hairy cell leukemia, a selected group of individuals with Kaposi sarcoma, and refractory condyloma acuminata. A number of other studies are currently in progress, many to determine the effectiveness of the interferons in combination with other antiviral agents.

REFERENCES

Bauer DJ: A history of the discovery and clinical application of antiviral drugs. Br Med Bull 41:309, 1985

Centers for Disease Control. Recommendation of the Immunization Practices Advisory Committee (ACIP): general recommendation on immunization. Morbid Mortal Weekly Rep 38:205, 1989

Finter NB, Oldham RK (eds): Interferon: In Vivo and Clinical Studies. Elsevier, Amsterdam, 1985

Guinan ME: Oral acyclovir for treatment and suppression of genital herpes simplex virus infection—a review. J Am Med Assoc 255:1747, 1986

Hilleman MR: Newer directions in vaccine development and utilization. J Infect Dis 151:407, 1985

Mitsuya H, Broder S: Strategies for antiviral therapy in AIDS. Nature (London) 325:773, 1987

Newton AA: Tissue culture methods for assessing antivirals and their harmful effects. p. 23. In Field HJ (ed): Antiviral Agents: The Development and Assessment of Antiviral Chemotherapy. Vol 1. CRC Press, Boca Raton, FL, 1988

Quinnan G: Immunization against viral diseases. In Galasso GJ, Whitley RJ, Merigan TC (eds): Antiviral Agents and Viral Diseases of Man. Raven Press, New York, 1990

WHO Consultative Group on Poliomyelitis Vaccines: Report to World Health Organization, 1985

Zajac BA, West DJ, McAleer WJ et al: Overview of clinical studies with hepatitis B vaccine made with recombinant DNA. J Infect Dis, suppl. 13A:39, 1986

52

CHEMOTHERAPY OF VIRAL INFECTIONS

ERIK DE CLERCQ

GENERAL CONCEPTS

Basic Mechanisms
Antiviral drugs specifically inhibit one or more steps of virus replication without causing unacceptable side effects.

Approved Antiviral Drugs
The approved antiviral drugs and the viruses and diseases they treat are amantadine and rimantadine (influenza A virus), ribavirin (respiratory syncytial virus), idoxuridine and trifluridine (topical treatment of herpetic keratitis), vidarabine and acyclovir (systemic treatment of herpes simplex and varicella-zoster viruses), ganciclovir (cytomegalovirus), and retrovir (human immunodeficiency virus).

Future Antiviral Drugs
To overcome the limitations of current antiviral drugs, more effective compounds are being developed that

allow greater inhibition of viruses, greater selectivity for virus-specific functions, and fewer side effects and avoid induction of resistant mutants.

Main Targets for Antiviral Drugs
Specific events in virus replication identified as targets for antiviral agents are viral adsorption, penetration, uncoating, and viral nucleic acid synthesis as well as viral protein synthesis. Specificity for infected cells may occur when virus-specified enzymes activate drugs (e.g., herpes simplex virus and acyclovir).

Limitations of Antiviral Drugs
Limitations include a narrow antiviral spectrum, ineffectiveness against the latent virus, development of drug-resistant mutants, and side effects.

INTRODUCTION

We live in a time of rapid development of antiviral compounds. For selective chemotherapy of viral infections, a drug should inhibit virus replication

when used at concentrations not detrimental to the host. A number of antiviral drugs have been formally licensed and are widely used for the chemotherapy of specific viral infections. Other antiviral agents are being developed. These fall primarily in three classes: anti-herpesvirus, anti-retrovirus, and, to a lesser extent, anti-rhinovirus compounds. The mechanisms of action targeting virus-specific events are being studied. Antiviral chemotherapy offers a decisive approach to the control of virus, notwithstanding some current limitations.

BASIC MECHANISMS

Specificity against virus replication is the key issue in chemotherapy. Because of the close interaction between virus replication and normal cellular metabolism, it was originally thought too difficult to interrupt the virus replicative cycle without adversely affecting the host cell metabolism. It is now clear, however, that several events in the virus replicative cycle either do not occur in normal uninfected cells or are controlled by virus-specified enzymes that differ structurally and functionally from the corresponding host cell enzymes.

Quite schematically, the virus replicative cycle can be divided into 10 steps (Fig. 52-1): (1) adsorption, (2) penetration, (3) uncoating, (4) early transcription, (5) early translation, (6) replication of the viral genome, (7) late transcription, (8) late translation, (9) assembly, and (10) release of new virus particles. Adsorption, penetration, and uncoating are typical examples of replicative events that are specific for virus infection and do not occur in uninfected cells (see Ch. 42). Examples of virus replication steps controlled by virus-specified enzymes are the transcription of positive-sense RNA to DNA (catalyzed by the reverse transcriptase associated with retroviruses), the replication of DNA to DNA (catalyzed by the DNA polymerases of herpesviruses), and the proteolytic cleavage of viral precursor proteins (catalyzed by the protease of human immunodeficiency virus).

The various steps in the replicative cycle at which the virus deviates from normal host processes are potential targets for chemotherapeutic intervention. It is not yet possible to tailor new antiviral agents to virus-specific target molecules. The target molecules for some of the approved antiviral drugs have not been clearly defined.

APPROVED ANTIVIRAL DRUGS

Antiviral compounds that have been formally licensed for clinical use are amantadine, rimantadine, ribavirin, idoxuridine, trifluridine, vidarabine, acyclovir, ganciclovir, and retrovir (Fig. 52-2). The clinical indications and dosage regimens for these drugs are presented in Table 52-1. Their activity spectrum and mechanism of action are outlined in Tables 52-2 and 52-3.

Amantadine and Rimantadine

The clinical use of amantadine and rimantadine is restricted to the prophylaxis and early therapy of influenza A virus infections. Influenza prophylaxis is particularly indicated in immunodeficient patients, persons who are allergic to influenza vaccine, unvaccinated house contacts of high-risk patients, and residents of chronic care facilities where an outbreak of influenza A has been recognized. Amantadine is noted for its central nervous system side effects, such as hallucinations and disorientation, which lead, for example, to a risk of falling. Rimantadine causes fewer side effects than amantadine when used at the same dosage (200 mg/day, perorally).

Ribavirin

Although active against ortho- and paramyxoviruses, ribavirin (Virazole) is approved only for the treatment of respiratory syncytial virus (RSV) infection in infants. The drug is administered as a small-particle aerosol (particle diameter, 1 to 3 μm) so that it can reach the lower respiratory tract. Aerosolized ribavirin treatment results in more rapid cessation of viral shedding and resolution of clinical symptoms without signs of systemic toxicity.

Idoxuridine and Trifluridine

Because of their myelosuppressive, mutagenic, and teratogenic effects following systemic administration, idoxuridine and trifluridine are suitable only for topical use. Trifluridine is superior to idoxuridine when used in eyedrops for the topical

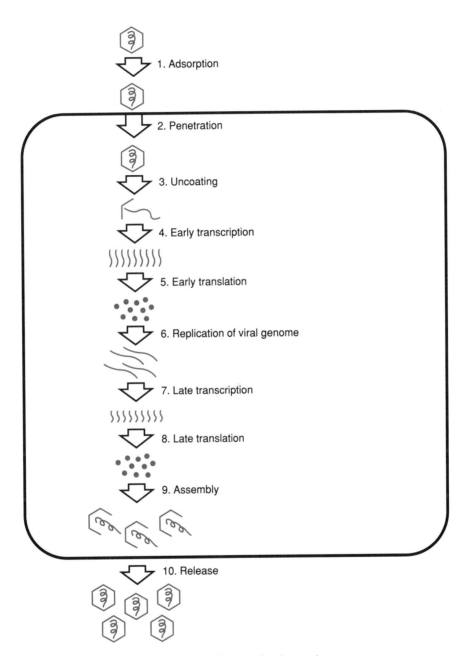

FIGURE 52-1 Virus replicative cycle.

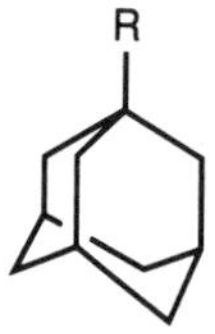

Amantadine: R = NH$_2$• HCl
Rimantadine: R = CH – NH$_2$• HCl
                                    |
                                  CH$_3$

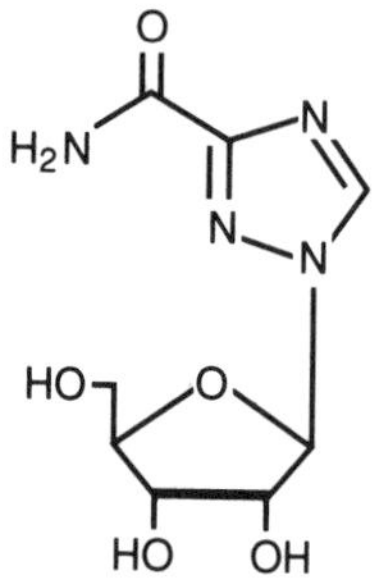

Ribavirin

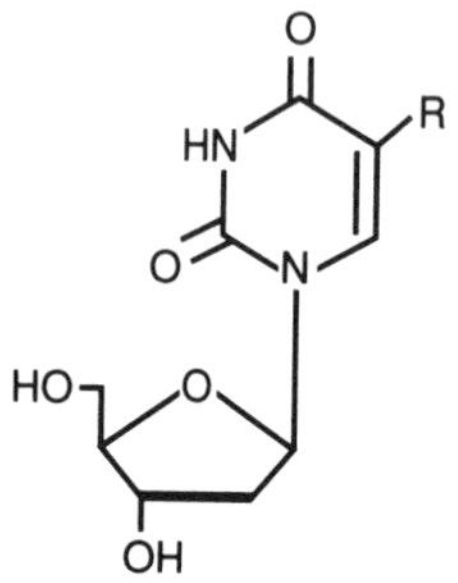

Idoxuridine: R = I
Trifluridine: R = CF$_3$

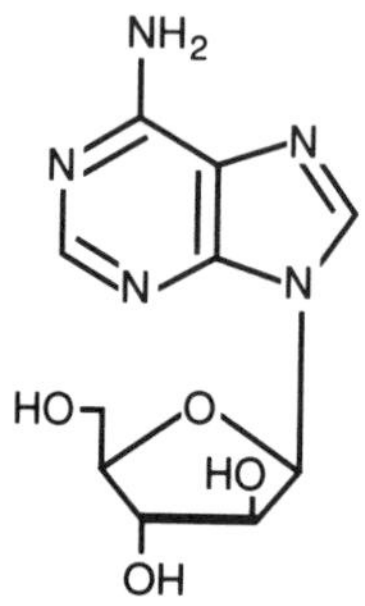

Vidarabine

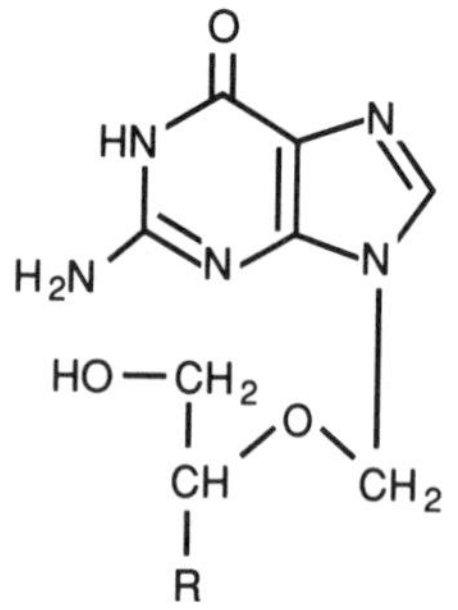

Acyclovir: R = H
Ganciclovir: R = CH$_2$OH

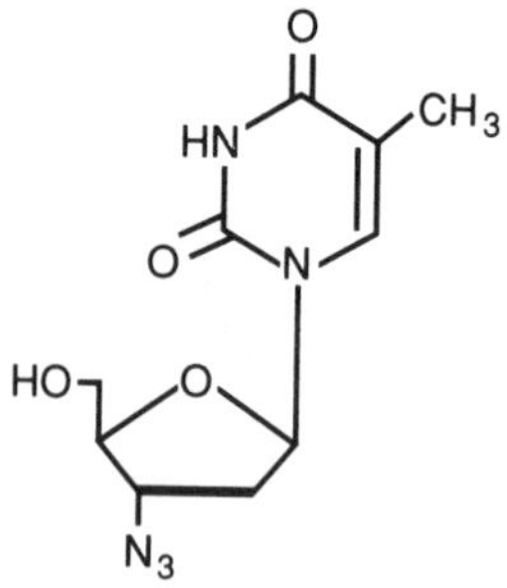

Retrovir

FIGURE 52-2 Approved antiviral drugs.

TABLE 52-1   Treatment, Dosage, and Indications for Use of Antiviral Drugs

Drug	Dosage	Indication
Antimyxovirus drugs		
Amantadine	200 mg/d, PO	Influenza A
Rimantadine	200 mg/d, PO	Influenza A
Ribavirin	20 mg/ml, aerosol (3–6 days), topical	RSV infection in infants
Antiherpesvirus drugs		
Idoxuridine	0.1% eyedrops, topical	Herpetic keratitis
Trifluridine	1% eyedrops, topical	Herpetic keratitis
Vidarabine	3% eye ointment, topical	Herpetic keratitis
	15 mg/kg/d (10 days), IV	Herpetic encephalitis
	15 mg/kg/d (10 days), IV	Neonatal herpes
	10 mg/kg/d (7 days), IV	VZV infection in immunocompromised patients
Acyclovir	3% eye ointment, topical	Herpetic keratitis
	5% cream (ointment), topical	Primary genital herpes
	1 g/d (5–10 days), PO	Primary genital herpes
	15 mg/kg/d (7 days), IV	HSV infection in immunocompromised patients
	30/mg/kg/d (10 days), IV	Herpetic encephalitis
	15–30 mg/kg/d (10 days), IV	Neonatal herpes
	800 mg/d, PO	Prophylaxis (recurring HSV infection in immuno-compromised patients)
	30 mg/kg/d (7 days), IV	VZV infection in immunocompromised patients
	4 g/d (7 days), PO	Herpes zoster
Ganciclovir	10 mg/kg/d (14–21 days), IV	CMV infection in immunocompromised patients
Antiretrovirus drugs		
Retrovir	Commonly used at 1200 mg/d (6 × 200 mg), PO	AIDS and AIDS-related complex

treatment of herpetic keratitis. Idoxuridine can be formulated for topical treatment of herpetic skin lesions.

Vidarabine

Vidarabine (Vira-A) is used for both topical and systemic treatment of herpesvirus infections. A serious drawback is the poor solubility of this drug in aqueous media, which means that intravenous administration requires a large volume of fluid. When vidarabine and acyclovir were compared for efficacy in treating herpetic encephalitis and varicella-zoster virus (VZV) infection in immunocompromised hosts, acyclovir proved clearly superior to vidarabine. Vidarabine has various toxic side effects (i.e., tremor, ataxia, seizures, myalgia, nausea, vomiting, and diarrhea).

Acyclovir

Acyclovir (Zovirax) represents a major breakthrough in the treatment of herpesvirus infections. The main indications for its use are primary genital herpes, herpetic encephalitis, and herpes simplex virus (HSV) and varicella-zoster virus infections in immunosuppressed patients. It can be used topically, intravenously, or perorally, although its oral absorption is only 20 percent. It is of little, if any, benefit in the topical treatment of recurrent herpes labialis. It is partly efficacious in preventing recurrent genital herpes, as well as in preventing herpes simplex virus and perhaps cytomegalovirus (CMV) infections in renal allograft recipients. Resistant mutants have been detected. Kidney failure may occur following intravenous administration.

TABLE 52-2   Activity Spectrum of Major Antiviral Compounds

Compound	Virus Family	Viruses[a]
Viral penetration inhibitors		
Amantadine,[b] Rimantadine[b]	Orthomyxoviridae	Influenza A virus
Viral nucleic acid synthesis inhibitors		
Ribavirin[b]	Orthomyxoviridae	Influenza A, B, and C viruses
	Paramyxoviridae	RSV, measles virus
	Arenaviridae	Lassa virus, Junin virus
Idoxuridine[b], Trifluridine[b]	Herpesviridae	HSV, VZV
Vidarabine[b]	Herpesviridae	HSV, VZV
Acyclovir[b]	Herpesviridae	HSV, VZV
Ganciclovir[b]	Herpesviridae	HSV, CMV, EBV
Retrovir[b]	Retroviridae	HIV
Foscarnet	Herpesviridae	HSV,[c] VZV, CMV
	Hepadnaviridae	HBV
	Retroviridae	HIV
Bromovinyldeoxyuridine	Herpesviridae	HSV-1, VZV, EBV
Bromovinylarabinofuranosyluracil		
Phosphonylmethoxyalkyl derivatives		
HPMPA, HPMPC[d]	Adenoviridae	Adenovirus
	Herpesviridae	HSV,[c] VZV, CMV, EBV
	Poxviridae	Vaccinia virus
	Hepadnaviridae	HBV
PMEA[e]	Herpesviridae	HSV,[c] VZV, CMV, EBV
	Hepadnaviridae	HBV
	Retroviridae	HIV
Viral adsorption inhibitors		
Sulfated polysaccharides	Herpesviridae	HSV,[c] CMV
	Retroviridae	HIV
Virus uncoating inhibitors		
Oxazolinyl isoxazole and piperazinyl pyridazine derivatives	Picornaviridae	Rhinovirus

[a] EBV, Epstein-Barr virus.
[b] Formally approved for human use.
[c] Including TK⁻ (thymidine kinase-deficient) mutants that have become resistant to acyclovir.
[d] HPMPA, HPMPC, Hydroxyphosphonylmethoxypropyl-adenine and-cytosine.
[e] PMEA, Phosphonylmethoxyethyladenine.

Ganciclovir

Ganciclovir (Cymevene) is the preferred drug for treating cytomegalovirus infections in patients with acquired immune deficiency syndrome (AIDS) or other immunodeficiencies. Since it has very poor oral bioavailability (3 percent), it must be given intravenously. Of the various clinical manifestations of cytomegalovirus infection in immunosuppressed patients, cytomegalovirus retinitis responds best to ganciclovir therapy, but recurs after treatment is stopped. The most frequent adverse side effects are neutropenia and thrombocytopenia.

Retrovir

Retrovir (Zidovudine, AZT) is licensed for patients infected with human immunodeficiency virus type 1 or 2 (HIV-1 or -2), the agent of AIDS. It appears

TABLE 52-3 Mechanism of Action of and Main Targets for Major Antiviral Compounds

Compound	Intracellular Activation Steps	Main Target for Antiviral Action
Amantadine, rimantadine	None	Uncoating and assembly
Ribavirin	Phosphorylation to 5'-triphosphate by cellular enzymes	Inhibition of 5' capping of viral mRNA
Idoxuridine	Phosphorylation to 5'-triphosphate by cellular enzymes	Incorporation into DNA
Trifluridine	Phosphorylation to 5'-monophosphate by cellular thymidine kinase	Inhibition of thymidylate synthase
Vidarabine	Phosphorylation to 5'-triphosphate by cellular enzymes	Incorporation into DNA and inhibition of HSV DNA polymerase
Acyclovir	Phosphorylation to monophosphate by HSV-specified thymidine kinase, and then to di- and triphosphate by cellular enzymes	DNA chain termination
Ganciclovir	Phosphorylation to triphosphate by cellular enzymes	Inhibition of viral DNA polymerase
Retrovir and other dideoxynucleosides	Phosphorylation to 5'-triphosphate by cellular enzymes	Inhibition of reverse transcriptase; DNA chain termination
Foscarnet	None	Inhibition of viral DNA polymerase
Bromovinyldeoxyuridine	Phosphorylation to 5'-diphosphate by HSV-1-specified thymidine kinase and then to 5'-triphosphate by cellular enzymes	Inhibition of viral DNA polymerase and incorporation into viral DNA
Phosphonylmethoxyalkyl-purines and -pyrimidines (HPMPA, HPMPC, PMEA)	Phosphorylation to diphosphoryl derivatives by cellular enzymes	Same plus DNA chain termination
Sulfated polysaccharides	None	Viral adsorption
Oxazolinyl isoxazole and piperazinyl pyridazine derivatives	None	Viral uncoating

to impede progression from the latent to the symptomatic infection and to lower the mortality rate and the frequency of opportunistic infections. The duration of the beneficial effects is being studied in view of the emergence of resistant mutants. It is well absorbed orally (60 percent) and readily crosses the blood-brain barrier. Serious side effects, particularly megaloblastic anemia and leukopenia, necessitate withdrawal of the drug in some patients.

FUTURE ANTIVIRAL DRUGS

The importance of virus infections and the early successes with some antiviral drugs have prompted a search for new agents. This search has focused on compounds that are active against herpesviruses, retroviruses, and rhinoviruses (Table 52-2). These antiviral drugs of the future are expected to be useful in clinical settings in which the approved antiviral drugs are not sufficiently efficacious.

MAIN TARGETS FOR ANTIVIRAL DRUGS

For rational drug design, the molecular targets (i.e., proteins or enzymes) should be identified first and then the drugs should be tailored on the basis of the molecular configuration and action of the target proteins. None of the antiviral drugs now available or considered for clinical use have been developed in this way. Instead, their antiviral activity was found first, often by chance, and their molecular targets determined later.

Antiviral compounds can be divided into two categories (Table 52-3): (1) those that can interact directly with their target and (2) those that must first be activated intracellularly by phosphorylation to the active (generally triphosphate) forms. Amantadine, rimantadine, foscarnet, sulfated polysaccharides, and the oxazolinyl isoxazole and piperazinyl pyridazine derivatives do not require such activation; they interact directly with their target (viral adsorption, penetration, or uncoating). In contrast, all nucleoside analogs, whether active as antiherpesvirus agents (such as acyclovir, ganciclovir, and bromovinyldeoxyuridine) or antiretrovirus agents (such as retrovir and other dideoxynucleoside analogs) must be activated through three consecutive phosphorylation steps before they can interact with their target enzyme, the herpesvirus DNA polymerase or retrovirus reverse transcriptase. The triphosphates of the nucleoside analogs then compete with the natural substrates of the DNA polymerase or reverse transcriptase reaction. They can inhibit the incorporation of the natural substrates (e.g., dTTP and dGTP) into the growing DNA chain or can themselves become incorporated into DNA. This has been clearly demonstrated with a number of nucleoside analogs, such as idoxuridine, bromovinyl-deoxyuridine, acyclovir, ganciclovir, and retrovir. The incorporation of acyclovir and retrovir into DNA leads to termination of chain elongation; therefore, these compounds act as chain terminators.

Antiviral selectivity may stem from the specific affinity of the antiviral compounds (or their activated forms) for their target protein (or enzyme). Alternatively, when phosphorylation is involved, antiviral selectivity may also evolve from the phosphorylation by a virus-encoded thymidine kinase. Herpes simplex virus and varicella-zoster virus encode such virus-specific thymidine kinase, and since acyclovir and bromovinyldeoxyuridine are excellent substrates for the viral enzymes but poor substrates for the cellular thymidine kinase, their preferential phosphorylation by virus-infected cells, as compared with uninfected cells, significantly contributes to their selectivity as antiherpetic agents.

LIMITATIONS OF ANTIVIRAL DRUGS

As mentioned above, clinical use of the currently available antiviral drugs is limited by toxic side effects. There are also some general limitations inherent in antiviral chemotherapy (Table 52-4). First, the more selective the antiviral drug, the narrower its antiviral activity spectrum. Second, since antiviral drugs target steps in virus replication, the latent phases characteristic of some viral

TABLE 52-4　Limitations Inherent in the Use of Antiviral Drugs

Limitation	Comment
Toxic side effects	Specific for each compound (for vidarabine, neurologic and gastrointestinal disorders; for ganciclovir, neutropenia and thrombocytopenia; for retrovir, anemia and leukopenia
Narrow activity spectrum	See Table 52-2
Latent phase of the virus infection	Not amenable to antiviral chemotherapy
Treatment effective only when started early in infection	
Emergence of drug-resistant virus strains	Acyclovir-resistant HSV mutants in AIDS patients

infections are not amenable to chemotherapy. This is particularly relevant for herpesvirus and retrovirus infections. Therefore, eradication of latent virus infections is not feasible currently. Third, antiviral drug treatment should be started early, before irreversible damage occurs. Such timely treatment is not possible without early and accurate diagnosis, which is difficult for many viral infections (such as infections of the respiratory tract). Fourth, perhaps inevitably for a specific antimicrobial agent, there is risk of emergence of drug-resistant virus strains. This has been most dramatically demonstrated with retrovir-treated AIDS patients from whom retrovir-resistant human immunodeficiency virus strains have been isolated. In the same patients treated with acyclovir for herpes simplex virus infections, acyclovir-resistant herpes simplex virus strains have been detected. The fact that these herpes simplex virus mutants and human immunodeficiency virus strains retained full susceptibility to other antiviral agents is reassuring. These findings indicate that attempts to develop new antiviral agents should continue unabated.

REFERENCES

Al-Nakib W: New promising drugs for the prophylaxis and therapy of rhinovirus infections. Curr Opin Infect Dis 2:415, 1989

Arvin AM: Current indications for the clinical use of acyclovir. Curr Opin Infect Dis 2:386, 1989

Balfour HH, Jr, Chace BA, Stapleton JT, et al: A randomized placebo-controlled trial of oral acyclovir for the prevention of cytomegalovirus disease in recipients of renal allografts. N Engl J Med 320:1381, 1989

Crumpacker CS: Drug resistance of herpes viruses: a clinical problem or not? Curr Opin Infect Dis 2:398, 1989

Crumpacker CS: Molecular targets of antiviral therapy. N Engl J Med 321:163, 1989

De Clercq E: Recent advances in the search for selective antiviral agents. Adv Drug Res 17:1, 1988

De Clercq E: Antiviral agents: facts and prospects. p. 45. In Reeves DS, Geddes AM (eds): Recent Advances in Infection. No. 3. Churchill Livingstone, Edinburgh, 1989

De Clercq E: Molecular targets of chemotherapeutic agents against the human immunodeficiency virus. p. 255. In Jackson GG, Schlumberger HD, Zeiler HJ (eds): Perspectives in Antiinfective Therapy. Friedrich Vieweg, Braunschweig/Wiesbaden, 1989

De Clercq E: New promising inhibitors of the human immunodeficiency virus. Curr Opin Infect Dis 2:401, 1989

Exley AR: Ganciclovir and foscarnet—current status and future prospects in the treatment of cytomegalovirus infection in the immunosuppressed patient. Curr Opin Infect Dis 2:393, 1989

Haseltine WA: Development of antiviral drugs for the treatment of AIDS: strategies and prospects. J Acquired Immune Defic Syndr 2:311, 1989

Langtry HD, Campoli-Richards DM: Zidovudine. A review of its pharmacodynamic and pharmacokinetic properties, and therapeutic efficacy. Drugs 37:409, 1989

O'Brien JJ, Campoli-Richards DM: Acyclovir. An updated review of its antiviral activity, pharmacokinetic properties and therapeutic efficacy. Drugs 37:233, 1989

Rossmann MG: The structure of antiviral agents that inhibit uncoating when complexed with viral capsids. Antiviral Res 11:3, 1989

Sim IS: Potential of new drugs in the prophylaxis and therapy of influenza A virus infections. Curr Opin Infect Dis 2:411, 1989

53

PICORNAVIRUSES

MARGUERITE YIN-MURPHY

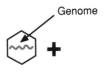

Genome

C = 32
30 nm

GENERAL CONCEPTS

Clinical Manifestations

Most infections are inapparent. Some picornaviruses cause mild illnesses; a few serotypes give rise to serious conditions of the central nervous system, heart, skeletal muscles, and liver.

Structure

The picornavirus virion is an icosahedral, nonenveloped, small (20 to 30 nm) particle. The capsid protein encases a sense RNA strand consisting of approximately 7,500 nucleotides. The RNA carries a covalently bound noncapsid viral protein (VPg) at its 5′ end and a polyadenylated tail at its 3′ end.

Classification and Antigenic Types

Classification is based on morphology, physicochemical and biologic properties, antigenic structures, and mode of replication. The four genera are the enteroviruses, rhinoviruses, cardioviruses, and aphthoviruses.

Multiplication

Picornaviruses multiply in the cytoplasm, and their RNA acts as a messenger to synthesize viral macromolecules. Viral RNA replicates in complexes associated with cytoplasmic membranes via two distinct, partially double-stranded RNAs—the "replicative intermediates." One complex uses the sense RNA strand, and the other uses the antisense RNA strand as template.

Pathogenesis

Enterovirus can replicate in epithelium of the nasopharynx and regional lymphoid tissue, conjunctiva, intestines, mesenteric nodes, and the reticuloendothelial system. Viremia may cause virus transfer to the spinal cord, brain, meninges, heart, liver, and skin. Some chronic enterovirus infections result in postviral fatigue syndrome. Rhinoviruses infect and replicate mainly in nasopharyngeal epithelium and regional lymph nodes.

Host Defenses

Interferon and virus-specific IgA, IgM, and IgG antibodies are important in host defense. Neutralizing antibody confers serotype-specific immunity.

Epidemiology

Picornaviruses are widely prevalent. Enteroviruses are transmitted by the fecal-oral route, via salivary and respiratory droplets, and in some cases via conjunctival secretions and skin lesion exudates. Cockroaches and flies may be vectors. Rhinoviruses are transmitted by saliva, respiratory discharge, and contaminated inanimate objects.

Diagnosis

Viruses must be isolated and identified in the clinical laboratory. Serology is used to confirm the virus as the cause of infection.

705

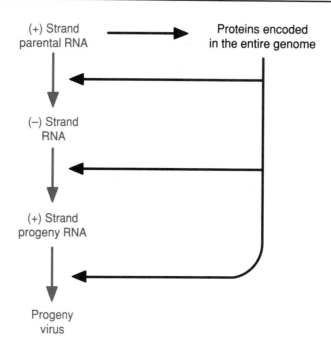

Control

Poliomyelitis can be prevented by Salk-type (inactivated) and Sabin-type (live) poliovirus vaccines. Control can be achieved via public education on transmission modes and personal hygiene. Adequate sewage disposal and uncontaminated water supplies are critical. There is no specific therapy.

ENTEROVIRUSES

Poliovirus

Poliovirus has tropism for epithelial cells of the alimentary tract and cells of the central nervous system. Infection is asymptomatic or causes a mild, undifferentiated febrile illness. Spinal and bulbar poliomyelitis occasionally occurs. Paralytic poliomyelitis is not always preceded by minor illness. Paralysis is usually irreversible, and there is residual paralysis for life.

Coxsackieviruses

Most infections are inapparent or mild. Rashes and vesicular lesions are most commonly caused by group A coxsackievirus, and pleurodynia and viral pericarditis/myocarditis by group B coxsackieviruses. Coxsackievirus A24 variant causes epidemic and pandemic outbreaks of acute hemorrhagic conjunctivitis. Occasionally, coxsackieviruses are associated with paralytic and encephalitic diseases. Coxsackieviruses are characterized by their pathogenicity for suckling mice. They are classified by neutralization tests as coxsackievirus group A (A1 to A24) and coxsackievirus group B (B1 to B6).

Echoviruses

Echoviruses have been associated with febrile and respiratory illnesses, rash, occasional conjunctivitis, and paralytic diseases.

New Enteroviruses

Enteroviruses types 68 and 69 cause respiratory illnesses; type 70 causes acute hemorrhagic conjunctivitis and occasionally paralysis; type 71 can cause meningitis and encephalitis. Type 72, also known as hepatitis A virus, gives rise to gastrointestinal disturbances and hepatitis.

RHINOVIRUSES

Rhinoviruses cause mainly respiratory infections. There are to date 115 serotypes. Immunity is type specific.

INTRODUCTION

The picornaviruses are small (20 to 30 nm) nonenveloped, single-stranded RNA viruses with cubic symmetry. Because they contain no essential lipids, they are ether resistant. They replicate in the cytoplasm, have four structural polypeptides, and are stabilized against thermal inactivation by molar $MgCl_2$. The picornaviruses that affect humans are divided into two subgroups: the **enteroviruses,** found primarily in the gut; and the **rhinoviruses,** found in the upper respiratory tract.

The enteroviruses, which share common nucleotide sequences, are further subdivided into the polioviruses, coxsackieviruses groups A and B, and echoviruses. Initially 67 distinct enterovirus immunotypes were recognized, but reclassification has reduced this number to 63. Since 1968, 5 new serotypes—namely, enterovirus types 68 to 72—were added to the list. One hundred fifteen distinct rhinovirus serotypes have now been identified.

Subclinical infections with the picornaviruses are common. These agents also can cause various disorders ranging from minor illness, respiratory infections, and skin rashes to myocarditis, pericarditis, aseptic meningitis, and paralytic disease.

CLINICAL MANIFESTATIONS

Human disease can be caused by members of both the enteroviruses (Fig. 53-1) and rhinoviruses (Fig. 53-2). Enteroviruses are implicated in many diseases including undifferentiated febrile illnesses, upper and lower respiratory tract infections, gastrointestinal disturbances, conjunctivitis,

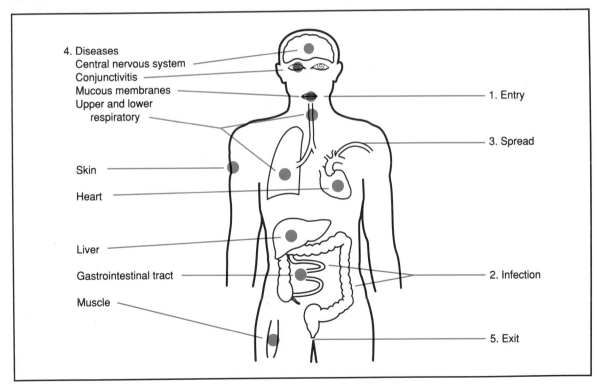

FIGURE 53-1 Pathogenesis of enterovirus infections.

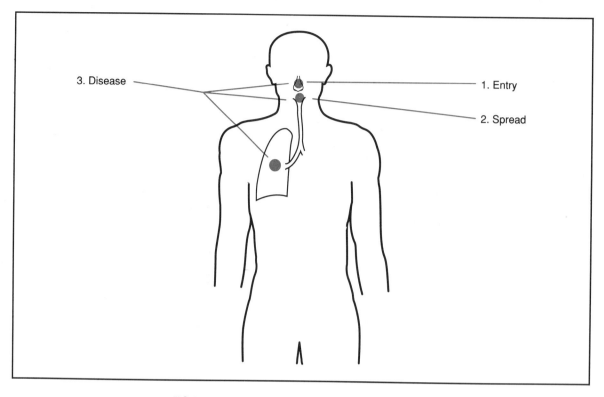

FIGURE 53-2 Pathogenesis of rhinovirus infections.

skin and mucous membrane lesions, and diseases of the central nervous system, muscles, heart, and liver. Less commonly, enteroviruses are associated with generalized neonatal infections, diabetes mellitus, pancreatitis, orchitis, and occasionally hemolytic-uremic syndrome and intrauterine infections. Recently, a new disease called wandering myoclonus was discovered in China (see below). Rhinoviruses cause mainly upper and lower respiratory tract illnesses (Table 53-1).

Laboratory tests are needed to establish the etiology of a suspected picornavirus infection because a particular serotype can give rise to more than one clinical syndrome and different serotypes can produce the same syndrome. Some illnesses caused by enteroviruses are clinically indistinguishable from those caused by other viruses.

STRUCTURE

The picornaviruses are nonenveloped (naked), small (20 to 30 nm) icosahedral virions resistant to lipid solvents and having a single sense-strand RNA genome (molecular weight, approximately 2×10^6 to 3×10^6) (Fig. 53-3). The RNA strand consists of approximately 7,500 nucleotides and is covalently bonded to a noncapsid viral protein (VP_g) at its 5' end and to a polyadenylated tail at its 3' end. This genome RNA serves as an mRNA and initiates the synthesis of virus macromolecules. Replication and assembly take place in the cytoplasm of infected cells. The viral RNA replicates via two distinct, partially double-stranded RNAs called the replicative intermediates (RIs). One complex uses the sense RNA strand and the other uses the antisense RNA strand as template. Functional proteins are produced mainly from a single large polyprotein (molecular weight, 2.4×10^5 to 2.5×10^5) followed by posttranslational cleavage. The coat protein is encoded by the 5' half; VPg, three proteases, and polymerases or polymerase factors are encoded downstream. The major neutralizing antigen that distinguishes picornavirus species and induces serotype-specific immunity resides mainly in the VP1 region. The viral capsid gives the picornaviruses their characteristic shape

TABLE 53-1   Clinical Picornavirus Syndromes

Virus	Disease (Virus Types)
Enteroviruses	
Polioviruses (types 1–3)	Undifferentiated febrile illnesses (1–3)
	Aseptic meningitis (1–3)
	Paralysis and encephalitic diseases (1–3)
Coxsackievirus group A (A1–A22, A24)[a]	Acute hemorrhagic conjunctivitis (CA24 variant)
	Herpangina (2–6, 8, 10, 22)
	Exanthem (4–6, 9, 16)
	Hand-foot-mouth disease (5, 10, 16)
	Aseptic meningitis (1–2, 4–7, 9, 10, 14, 16, 22)
	Paralysis and encephalitic diseases (occasional 4, 7, 9, 10)
	Hepatitis (4, 9)
	Upper and lower respiratory tract illnesses (9, 10, 16, 21, 24 variant)
	Lymphonodular pharyngitis (10)
	Infantile diarrhea (18, 20–22, 24 variant)
Coxsackievirus group B (B1–B6)	Undifferentiated febrile illnesses (1–6)
	Pleurodynia (1–5)
	Pericarditis, myocarditis (1–5)
	Aseptic meningitis types (1–6)
	Paralysis and encephalitic diseases (1–5)
	Severe systemic infection in infants, meningoencephalitis and myocarditis (1–5)
	Upper and lower respiratory tract illnesses (4, 5)
	Exanthem, hepatitis, diarrhea (5)
Echoviruses (1–9, 11–27, 29–33)[a]	Aseptic meningitis (many)
	Paralysis and encephalitic diseases (occasional 1, 2, 4, 6, 7, 9, 11, 14–16, 18, 22, 30)
	Exanthem (1–9, 11, 14, 16, 18, 19, 25, 30, 32)
	Hand-foot-mouth disease (19)
	Pericarditis and myocarditis (1, 6, 9, 19, 22)
	Upper and lower respiratory tract illnesses (4, 9, 11, 20, 22, 25)
	Neonatal diarrhea (11, 14, 18, 20, 32)
	Epidemic myalgia (1, 6, 9)
	Hepatitis (4, 9)
New enteroviruses (68–72)	Pneumonia and bronchiolitis (68, 69)
	Acute hemorrhagic conjunctivitis (70)
	Aseptic meningitis, meningoencephalitis, hand-foot-mouth disease (71)
	Hepatitis (72)
Rhinoviruses (1–115)	Upper and lower respiratory tract illnesses (1–115)

[a] Reclassification of coxsackievirus A23 as echovirus 9, echovirus 10 as reovirus, echovirus 28 as rhinovirus type 1A, and echovirus 34 as coxsackievirus A24.

and size (Fig. 53-3) and protects the infectious viral RNA from hostile environments and host ribonucleases. Enteroviruses can survive for long periods in organic matter and are resistant to the low pH in the stomach (pH 3.0 to 5.0). By contrast, rhinoviruses are labile at this pH range. Picornaviruses are inactivated by pasteurization, boiling, Formalin, and chlorine. Enteroviruses and rhinoviruses are distinguished by density gradient centrifugation. The buoyant density of enteroviruses

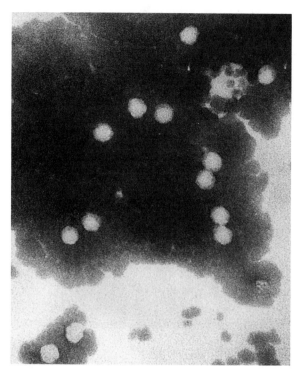

FIGURE 53-3   Electron micrograph of a poliovirus showing the characteristic nonenveloped, small (20 to 30 nm) icosahedral particles of a picornavirus.

is approximately 1.33 to 1.34 g/ml in CsCl, and that of human rhinoviruses is about 1.38 to 1.42 g/ml.

Picornaviruses may undergo antigenic variation during replication and may give rise to strains with altered virulence and disease patterns.

CLASSIFICATION AND ANTIGENIC TYPES

The family *Picornaviridae* comprises four genera: *Enterovirus* and *Rhinovirus,* which infect humans; *Apthovirus* (foot-and-mouth disease virus), which infects cloven-hoofed animals and occasionally humans; and *Cardiovirus,* which infects rodents. At the time of writing, 68 human enterovirus serotypes and 115 rhinovirus serotypes are known.

Picornaviruses do not have a common group-specific antigen. However, antigenic sharing is observed between a few species. Each species has a

type-specific antigen, which is identifiable by neutralization tests.

PATHOGENESIS

When the portal of entry for a picornavirus is the mouth or nose, the virus infects and replicates in the nasopharyngeal epithelium and regional lymphoid tissues to give rise to asymptomatic infections or respiratory illnesses. Because enteroviruses can resist stomach acid and bile, they can penetrate to the lower intestine, where they infect and multiply in the intestinal epithelium and mesenteric lymph nodes. Viremia may result; this leads to further multiplication of virus in the reticuloendothelial system. From there, the virus can be carried by the bloodstream to target organs such as the spinal cord, brain, meninges, heart, liver, and skin. From the central nervous system the virus can travel via neural pathways to skeletal and heart muscles. It can be transferred by fingers and inanimate objects, such as handkerchiefs and towels, to the eye, where it may replicate in the conjunctival epithelium and cornea.

HOST DEFENSES

Shortly after infection of the respiratory or alimentary tract, increasing amounts of interferon and subsequently virus-specific IgA-antibody are detected in the saliva and the respiratory and gut secretions. Interferon inhibits virus multiplication, and IgA complexes with extracellular virus. The complexing of virus by IgA not only inhibits the spread of virus to susceptible epithelial cells but also reduces the oral and fecal shedding of infectious virus.

The earliest serum antibody to appear in response to picornavirus infection is IgM. By about 2 weeks, IgM is overtaken by IgG. The IgG response peaks at about 2 to 3 weeks and remains at a plateau for a few weeks, before it begins to fall. The IgG elicited by some enterovirus infections remains detectable for several years. This neutralizing IgG confers serotype-specific immunity. Both IgG and IgM can complex with invading virus and prevent the spread of virus via the bloodstream to target organs. Virus-antibody complexes are eliminated by phagocytosis, digestion, and excretion.

EPIDEMIOLOGY

Picornaviruses are found worldwide, the enteroviruses primarily in alimentary tracts of humans and animals and the rhinoviruses only in respiratory tracts of humans and chimpanzees. Although enteroviruses are transmitted mostly by the fecal-oral route, they can also be transmitted by salivary and respiratory droplets. Some serotypes are spread by conjunctival secretions and exudates from skin lesions.

In temperate countries, outbreaks of enterovirus illnesses occur most frequently in summer and autumn, whereas rhinovirus infections appear more often in autumn and spring. In the tropics, there is no apparent seasonal occurrence. Enteroviruses in excreta that contaminate the soil are carried by surface waters to lakes, beaches, vegetation, and community water supplies. These sources may serve as foci of infection. Shellfish that feed in freshwater or seawater beds contaminated by excreta harbor enteroviruses. Cockroaches in sewage pipelines and flies that settle on excreta may act as transient vectors.

DIAGNOSIS

Enteroviruses and rhinoviruses may be isolated from pharyngeal swabs, saliva, and nasal aspirates, and some enteroviruses may be isolated from skin lesions, cerebrospinal fluid, spinal cord, brain, heart, and blood. Virus is present in respiratory and conjunctival secretions from a few days before onset of illness to about 1 week after. Virus excretion in feces may continue for several weeks or longer. However, the chance of virus isolation is greatest if appropriate specimens are sent to the laboratory at the onset of illness. Table 53-2 lists the virus isolation systems that are used. The most specific of the conventional laboratory tests used to identify picornavirus serotypes is the neutralization test.

Serodiagnosis for the whole range of picornaviruses is impractical because of the multiplicity of serotypes. A serologic test is performed primarily to confirm the causative role of virus isolated from clinical specimens (i.e., to exclude the coincidental presence of a passenger virus that does not con-

TABLE 53-2 Choice of Virus Isolation System

Virus	Tissue Cultures	Suckling Mice
Polioviruses	+	−
Coxsackievirus group A	(+)[a]	+
Coxsackievirus group B	+	+
Echoviruses	+	−(+)[b]
New enteroviruses	+	−
Rhinoviruses	+	−

[a] Only a few serotypes of coxsackievirus group A can be recovered from clinical specimens in tissue cell cultures.
[b] Only a few strains are positive.

tribute to the disease process). A fourfold or greater rise in the titer of neutralizing antibody to the isolate between sera collected during the acute and convalescent phases of the illness is regarded as diagnostic of a current or recent infection.

CONTROL

Control of picornavirus diseases depends largely on mass education of the public on the mode of virus transmission, stressing the importance of good personal hygiene, and on provision of a good sewage disposal system and uncontaminated water supply. Fecal and pharyngeal discharges are infectious; hence, they must be handled with care and disposed of safely. Vaccine is commercially available only for poliomyelitis.

There is no specific therapy. Treatment is symptomatic and supportive. Clinical studies show that ribavirin shortens respiratory illnesses and interferon nasal sprays have prophylactic value for common colds.

◀ ENTEROVIRUSES ▶

POLIOVIRUSES
Clinical Manifestations

Paralytic poliomyelitis can occur without antecedent minor illnesses. A patient may suffer aseptic meningitis with pains in the back and neck muscles for several days without progressing to paralytic poliomyelitis. The incubation period is about 3 to 5 days for minor illness and 1 to 2 weeks for central nervous system involvement, with a range of 3 to 35 days between ingestion of virus and onset of symptoms. Virus is present in the throat before onset of illness. It disappears from the throat in about 1 week but persists in the feces for weeks. Examination of cerebrospinal fluid in the early phase of central nervous system involvement reveals increased numbers of leukocytes. In confirming a poliovirus etiology, a patient's poliomyelitis immunization record, if available, is reviewed together with the history and clinical and laboratory findings.

The outcome of poliovirus infection is influenced by the virulence of the infecting strain, the size of the infecting dose, and the immune status of the host. Predisposing factors include recent or previous tonsillectomy, which not only removes the immunologically active tonsils but also exposes nerve endings to the virus. There have been reports of unimmunized persons who developed paralysis in the limb inoculated with alum-precipitated diphtheria-pertussis-tetanus (DPT) vaccines during outbreaks of poliomyelitis. Pregnant, immunodeficient, and immunocompromised persons are predisposed.

Pathogenesis

Humans are the only natural host of poliovirus. Polioviruses have a tropism for the epithelial cells lining the alimentary tract and for cells of the central nervous system. They attach to a specific receptor on these cells, which in humans is encoded by a gene on chromosome 19. Poliovirus infection is quite common in nonimmunized individuals, but only about 1 percent of these cases progress to the paralytic form of the disease. The histocompatibility antigens HLA-3 and HLA-7 are believed to be highly associated with an increased risk of paralysis. Primary replication of poliovirus takes place in the oropharyngeal and intestinal mucosa (the **alimentary phase**). From here, the virus spreads to the tonsils and Peyer's patches of the ileum and to deep cervical and mesenteric nodes, where it multiplies abundantly (the **lymphatic phase**). Subsequently, the virus is carried by the bloodstream to various internal organs and regional lymph nodes (the **viremic phase**). In most cases, no further virus spread occurs and there is asymptomatic or mild febrile undifferentiated illness such as fever, malaise, headache, nausea, gastrointestinal disturbances, and sore throat, or combinations of these.

In the rare cases in which disease progresses to the **neurologic phase,** the virus spreads hematogenously to the spinal cord or brain stem or to both. If only scattered nerve cells are destroyed, the patient may develop no visible sign of muscle weakness. More concentrated damage results in flaccid paralysis of the muscles innervated by the affected motor nerves. Muscle involvement peaks a few days after the paralytic phase begins. Some paralysis is usually irreversible, and residual paralysis remains for life. Paralytic disease is called **spinal poliomyelitis** if the weakness is limited to muscles innervated by the motor neurons in the spinal cord and **bulbar poliomyelitis** if the cranial nerve nuclei or medullary centers are involved. The areas most affected are the anterior horn cells of the spinal cord, the motor area of the cerebral cortex, and the motor nuclei of the medulla. The lesions feature neuronal necrosis, neurophagia, and loss of nerve cells. Areas of neuronal damage show leukocytic infiltration and perivascular cuffing. Round-cell infiltration is usually present in leptomeninges. Bulbar poliomyelitis is serious because it may result in swallowing dysfunction and in cardiac or respiratory failure. Comparative clinical aspects of poliomyelitis, Guillain-Barré syndrome, and transverse myelitis are presented in Table 53-3.

Epidemiology

Poliomyelitis affects all age groups. In areas with poor hygiene and poor sanitation, most infants are infected relatively early in life and acquire active immunity while still protected by maternal antibodies. Infants who escape early contact with poliovirus become susceptible to infection as maternal antibodies wane. With improving sanitation, infants may escape early contact with polioviruses and become susceptible for an outbreak of poliomyelitis when wild poliovirus is introduced into the

TABLE 53-3 Clinical Aspects of Poliomyelitis,
Guillain-Barré Syndrome, and Transverse Myelitis

Signs and Symptoms	Poliomyelitis	Guillain-Barré Syndrome	Transverse Myelitis
Fever at onset	Yes	No	+/−
Meningeal irritation	Usually	Usually not	No
Muscle Pain	Severe	Variable	No
Paralysis	Usually asymmetric	Symmetric ascending	Symmetric stationary
Progression of Paralysis	3–4 days	2 weeks	Few hours
Residual Paralysis	Usually	Usually not	Variable
Paresthesia	Rare	Frequent	Frequent
Sensation	Normal	May be diminished	Diminished
Tendon Reflexes	Diminished or absent	Diminished, may return in few days	Absent may return in 1–3 wks
Spinal fluid at onset	WBC high; protein normal to 25% increase	WBC normal or slight increase; protein very high	WBC normal or high; protein moderate
Case fatality	2–20%	5–10%	<1%

(From the World Health Organization: Global Poliomyelitis Eradication by the Year 2000. Manual for Managers of Immunization Programmes. WHO/EPI/Polio/89.1. 1989, with permission.)

community. The most susceptible are children less than 2 years old. In countries with a high poliomyelitis immunization coverage in their childhood vaccination program, an older age group is the most susceptible group.

Control

The Salk-type inactivated poliovirus vaccine (IPV) consists of a mixture of the three poliovirus serotypes grown in monkey kidney cell cultures and made noninfectious by Formalin treatment. It is given in two intramuscular injections spaced a month apart and requires periodic boosters to maintain an adequate serum neutralizing-antibody level. Its effectiveness depends on stimulation of serum neutralizing antibodies that block the spread of poliovirus to the central nervous system. It has some suppressive effect on replication of wild poliovirus in the highly vascularized oropharyngeal region, but it has no effect on replication in the gut or on viral transmission in the excreta.

The Sabin-type live attenuated oral poliovirus vaccine (OPV) that is commercially available is also trivalent, but monovalent vaccine can be obtained if requested. The viruses are attenuated by multiple passages in monkey kidney or human diploid cell cultures, and the vaccine potency is stabilized with molar magnesium chloride or sucrose. This vaccine mimics wild poliovirus infections by inducing serum neutralizing antibody, as well as interferon and virus-specific IgA antibody, in the pharynx and gut. Hence, the vaccine virus not only prevents paralytic poliomyelitis but also, when given in sufficient doses, can abort a threatening epidemic and has the potential of eradicating poliomyelitis. During an outbreak trivalent OPV is recommended, but as soon as the causative poliovirus serotype is known, monovalent OPV containing the responsible serotype should be administered without delay to susceptible individuals in the community to prevent an epidemic. The chief disadvantage of this vaccine is the occurrence of vaccine-associated paralysis. The risk of paralytic poliomyelitis associated with reversion to neurovirulence is exceedingly small, estimated at one case of paralysis for every 2 to 4 million doses of trivalent OPV distributed. In 1988, the World Health Assembly, the governing body of the World

Health Organization, set the goal of global eradication of poliomyelitis by the year 2000.

COXSACKIEVIRUSES

Coxsackieviruses are differentiated by their pathogenicity for suckling mice and by classification of their antigenicity. They are classified as coxsackievirus group A (A1 to A22, A24) and coxsackievirus group B (B1 to B6) (Table 53-2).

Pathogenesis

Subcutaneous and intracerebral inoculation of suckling mice with group A coxsackieviruses produces myositis in skeletal muscles and generalized paralysis. Group B coxsackieviruses produce focal muscle lesions, necrosis of fat pads between the shoulders, focal lesions in the brain, and spinal cord and spastic paralysis.

Little is known about the pathology of human coxsackievirus infections because very few patients die of them. Autopsies of neonates with generalized coxsackievirus B infection show focal myocarditis and inflammation. Fatal myocarditis in adults is also associated with focal necrosis. Findings in order of decreasing incidence include meningoencephalitis, hepatitis, and pancreatitis. Fatal cases of encephalomyelitis show involvement of the motor neurons in the brain stem and spinal cord. Coxsackievirus B affects both white and gray matter.

Clinical Manifestations

Humans are the only natural host for these agents. Disorders caused by coxsackieviruses are shown in Table 53-1. Most infection is inapparent or mild. Illnesses include acute nonspecific febrile disease and common cold-like or influenzalike respiratory diseases, pharyngitis, croup, and pneumonia.

Rashes and vesicular lesions are most commonly caused by group A viruses. Herpangina presents as small, scattered oral vesicles with red areolae in the posterior oropharynx, tonsils, tongue, and palate, which progress to shallow ulcers and heal within a week. Coxsackievirus A10 causes acute lymphonodular pharyngitis with solid white to yellow papules. Coxsackieviruses A16, A10, and A5 give rise to sporadic cases and outbreaks of hand-foot-mouth diseases characterized by fever, an oral vesicular exanthema, and sparse symmetric maculopapular eruptions that involve the hands, feet, mouth, buttocks, and occasionally other sites.

Coxsackieviruses also cause exanthematous diseases that may be mistaken for rubella and an aseptic meningitis that is clinically indistinguishable from meningitis caused by polioviruses and a list of other viruses. Occasionally, they cause paralytic and encephalitic diseases or other cerebral dysfunction.

Pleurodynia, also known as epidemic myalgia, devil's grip, and Bornholm disease, is caused primarily by group B coxsackieviruses. Onset is usually abrupt, with fever, headache, and stabbing pain in muscles of the chest and/or upper abdomen. The pain is intensified by respiration and movement and may persist for a few weeks. The disease is self-limiting, but relapses with recurrences of fever and other symptoms are common. Occasional complications include pleuritis and orchitis.

The most important cause of viral pericarditis and myocarditis in children and adults is coxsackievirus B. Patients develop fever, tachycardia, dyspnea, precordial pain, and occasionally pericardial friction rub. Electrocardiography and radiography are helpful in confirming the diagnosis. The prognosis for uncomplicated pericarditis is good, but when myocarditis is also present the situation is serious.

Neonatal myocarditis in the first month of life may result in severe and frequently fatal disease. The myocarditis is accompanied by involvement of various organs, especially the central nervous system and liver. Onset may be abrupt, with lethargy, feeding difficulties, fever, and often signs of cardiac or respiratory distress. The infant may die within days or may recover over the next few weeks. These infections are generally acquired from infected mothers or during a nursery outbreak.

Coxsackievirus A24 gives rise to extensive epidemics and pandemics of acute hemorrhagic conjunctivitis characterized by a short incubation period and high secondary attack rate. Lacrimation, chemosis, edema and hyperemia of the conjunctiva, and preauricular gland enlargement also occur. Follicular hypertrophy of the conjunctiva is more prominent in the upper than lower fornix. Small petechiae to large blotches of subconjunctival hemorrhage, although striking, are seen in only a few cases. Anterior uveitis is common. Corneal lesions cause pain and blurring of vision. Recovery occurs within 1 to 2 weeks without sequelae.

Diagnosis

Serodiagnosis is used to confirm a suspected case of coxsackievirus B myocarditis because by the time the cardiac involvement is recognized, virus excretion has usually ceased. The diagnostic fourfold or greater rise in neutralizing-antibody titer between paired sera or high antibody titers to a single serotype is commonly registered in children. In adults, antibody to more than one serotype is frequently observed. It is recommended that in the absence of a fourfold or greater rise in antibody titer, unchanging titers of 512 and above be regarded as suggestive of recent infection. Some patients maintain high antibody titers for years, which suggests that chronic infections do occur.

ECHOVIRUSES

The echoviruses (enteric, cytopathic, human, and orphan viruses) are grouped together because they produce cytopathogenic effects in cell cultures but generally are not pathogenic for mice (unlike the coxsackieviruses) and they differ antigenically from the polioviruses. They were first named "orphan viruses" because their relationship with disease was obscure. Echoviruses are identified by neutralization tests as serotypes 1 to 9, 11 to 27, and 29 to 33 (Table 53-2). They are similar in epidemiology and pathogenesis to other enteroviruses.

Clinical Manifestations

Echoviruses, like coxsackieviruses, are associated with various disorders including respiratory illnesses, febrile illnesses with or without rash, Bos-ton exanthema, aseptic meningitis, paralytic diseases, and occasional conjunctivitis (Table 53-1). Echovirus type 3 was responsible for epidemics of wandering myoclonus in China that most commonly affected young adults. The prominent features are migratory pains and tenderness in the trunk and musculatures of the limbs and severe sweating. Mortality is high (12 to 33 percent).

NEW ENTEROVIRUS TYPES

Enterovirus types 68 and 69 cause respiratory illnesses in infants and children. Enterovirus type 70 gives rise to an acute hemorrhagic conjunctivitis that is clinically similar to that caused by coxsackievirus A24 variant. Enterovirus type 71 causes meningitis and encephalitis. Enterovirus type 72 (hepatitis A virus) is discussed with hepatitis B virus in Chapter 70. It has distinctive biologic properties such as an affinity for liver cells, and it gives rise to persistent nonlytic infection in susceptible cell cultures. Furthermore, nucleotide sequence analysis shows that these viruses are more distantly related to enteroviruses than to aphthoviruses.

◀ RHINOVIRUSES ▶

The natural hosts of rhinoviruses are humans and chimpanzees. Rhinoviruses are present in the nose and pharynx, and, unlike enteroviruses, which are acid resistant and have an optimum growth temperature of 36 to 37°C, they are sensitive to pH 3.0 and have an optimum growth temperature of 33°C. Furthermore, not all strains are stabilized by molar magnesium chloride.

CLINICAL MANIFESTATIONS

Rhinovirus infections are among the most prevalent of acute respiratory illnesses in humans. More than 90 percent of susceptible individuals infected with rhinoviruses succumb to the infection. Although most rhinovirus infections manifest as mild common colds with rhinorrhea, nasal obstruction, fever, sore throat, coughs, and hoarseness lasting for a few days, serious lower respiratory tract illnesses in infants are common. Secondary bacterial infections with *Streptococcus pneumoniae* and *Haemophilus influenzae* may result in sinusitis and otitis media. The incubation period is a few days. Viral shedding begins several days after infection, peaks shortly after the onset of symptoms, and may persist for a few weeks. In the adult population, rhinovirus disorders create significant economic losses in terms of lost working hours.

PATHOGENESIS

Pathologic findings in the common cold consist of inflammatory changes with hyperemia, edema, and inflammation of the columnar epithelial cells lining the nasopharynx. Desquamation of these infected cells coincides with the peak of virus spread. Regeneration is completed within a few weeks.

EPIDEMIOLOGY

Volunteer experiments indicate that virus spreads from nasal secretions by contaminated hands and that autoinoculation of nasal and conjunctival mucosa is a more important mode of virus transmission than are respiratory droplets and aerosols.

HOST DEFENSES

Immunity to infection is type specific, as it is with the enteroviruses. Therefore, because of the multiple rhinovirus serotypes, control of rhinovirus infections and development of an effective vaccine are difficult. Furthermore, the localized nature of infections results in poor humoral antibody response, and the secretory antibody that is vital in conferring protection is not long lasting.

REFERENCES

Almond JW, Stanway G, Cann AJ, et al: New poliovirus vaccines: a molecular approach. Vaccine 2:177, 1984

Cora L, Kopecka H, Aymard M, Gizard M: Use of cRNA probes for the detection of enteroviruses by molecular hybridization. J Med Virol 24:11, 1988

Crainic R, Couillin P, Blondel B et al: Natural variation of poliovirus neutralization epitopes. Infect Immun 41:1217, 1984

Ferguson M, Magrath DI, Minor PD, Schild GC: WHO collaborative study on the use of monoclonal antibodies for the intratypic differentiation of poliovirus strains. Bull WHO 64:239, 1986

McCay J, Werner G: Different rhinovirus serotypes neutralized by antipeptide antibodies. Nature 329:736, 1987

Minor PD, Ferguson M, Evans DM et al: Antigenic structure of polioviruses of serotypes 1, 2 and 3. J Gen Virol 67:1283, 1986

World Health Organization: Expanded Programme on Immunization. Immunization policy. WHO/EPI/GEN/86/7 Rev 1. 1986/87

World Health Organization: Global Poliomyelitis Eradication by the Year 2000. Manual for Managers of Immunization Programmes. WHO/EPI/Polio/89.1. 1989

Wu J-J, Zhang Q-L, Hu B-Y, Chen M-Y: Isolation and identification of Coxsackievirus A24 variant from outbreak of acute haemorrhagic conjunctivitis, China. Virol Sin 1:45, 1990

Yin-Murphy M: Acute hemorrhagic conjunctivitis. In Melnick JL (ed): Progress in Medical Virology. Karger, Basel, 1984

Yin-Murphy M: Enterovirus and enterovirus infections. Ann Acad Med 16:683, 1987

Yousef GE, Mann GF, Smith DG et al: Chronic enteroviruses infection in patients with postviral fatigue syndrome. Lancet 1:146, 1988

Zhang LB, Jiang Y, Mo H et al: Studies on the etiology of "Zhi-Fang Disease." Chin J Virol 4:118, 1988

54
ALPHAVIRUSES (TOGAVIRIDAE) AND FLAVIVIRUSES (FLAVIVIRIDAE)

ALAN L. SCHMALJOHN
PHILIP K. RUSSELL

Envelope

Icosahedral
40-90 nm

GENERAL CONCEPTS

ALPHAVIRUSES

Clinical Manifestations

Disease occurs in either of two general forms, depending on the virus: one is typified by fever, malaise, headache, and/or symptoms of encephalitis (e.g., eastern, western, or Venezuelan equine encephalitis viruses) and the other by fever, rash, and arthralgia (e.g., chikungunya, Ross River, Mayaro, and Sindbis viruses).

Structure

The enveloped virions are spherical, 60 to 70 nm, in diameter, with a positive-sense, monopartite, single-stranded RNA genome, 11.7 kilobases long. The lipid-containing envelope has two (rarely three) surface glycoproteins that mediate attachment, fusion, and penetration. The icosohedral nucleocapsid contains capsid protein and RNA. The virions mature by budding through the plasma membrane.

Classification and Antigenic Types

The genus *Alphavirus* is one of three genera in the family Togaviridae; *Rubivirus* (rubella virus), the other togavirus pathogenic for humans, is discussed in Chapter 55. The 26 alphaviruses are classified on the basis of antigenic properties. All alphaviruses share antigenic sites on the capsid and at least one envelope glycoprotein, but viruses can be differentiated by several serologic tests, particularly neutralization assays.

Multiplication

Genomic RNA is capped and polyadenylated and serves as mRNA for nonstructural proteins (e.g., RNA-dependent RNA polymerase) which are encoded in the 5' two-thirds of the genome. Complementary (antisense) RNA, made from genomic RNA, serves as a template for progeny genomic RNA. A subgenomic mRNA representing the 3' one-third of the genome encodes the structural proteins.

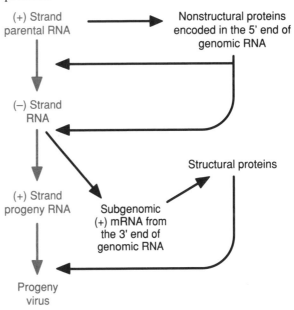

(+) Strand parental RNA → Nonstructural proteins encoded in the 5' end of genomic RNA

(−) Strand RNA

(+) Strand progeny RNA

Subgenomic (+) mRNA from the 3' end of genomic RNA

Structural proteins

Progeny virus

Pathogenesis

Infection is transmitted via infected mosquitoes. In the vertebrate host, virus disseminates after lytic infection of cells, resulting in viremia. Infection with seroconversion in the absence of clinical disease is common, but disease can be incapacitating and, in cases of encephalitis, occasionally fatal. Virus is eliminated by the immune system, but arthritis or central nervous system impairment may persist for weeks.

Host Defenses

Initial resistance is conferred by nonspecific defenses such as interferon. Antibodies are important in recovery and resistance, and T-cell responses are also probably relevant. Lasting protection is generally restricted to the same alphavirus and is associated with, but not solely attributable, to the presence of neutralizing antibodies.

Epidemiology

Viruses are maintained in nature by mosquito-vertebrate-mosquito cycles. Restricted interactions between viruses, vector species, and vertebrate hosts tend to confine the geographic spread of alphaviruses. Occasionally, a virus escapes its usual ecologic niche and causes widespread epizootics (Venezuelan equine encephalitis virus) or urban epidemics (chikungunya virus). Human infections are seasonal and are acquired in endemic areas.

Diagnosis

Diagnosis is suggested by clinical evidence and by known risk of exposure to virus; it is confirmed by virus isolation and identification or by a specific rise in antibody, particularly IgM.

Control

Disease surveillance and virus activity in natural hosts are used to determine whether control measures will be undertaken to reduce populations of vector mosquitoes or to vaccinate hosts, especially horses. Human vaccines, where available, are used only in individuals at particularly high risk of exposure, such as laboratory workers.

FLAVIVIRUSES

Clinical Manifestations

Major syndromes and the causative flaviviruses include encephalitis (St. Louis encephalitis, Japanese encephalitis, Powassan, and tick-borne encephalitis viruses), febrile illness with rash (dengue virus), hemorrhagic fever (Kyasanur Forest disease virus and sometimes dengue virus), and hemorrhagic fever with hepatitis (yellow fever virus).

Structure

Virions are spherical and 40 to 50 nm in diameter with a positive-sense, nonsegmented, single-stranded RNA genome of ca. 10.9 kilobases. The lipid-containing envelope has one surface glycoprotein that mediates attachment, fusion, and penetration, and an internal matrix protein. The nucleocapsid contains capsid protein and RNA. The virions mature at intracytoplasmic membranes.

Classification and Antigenic Types

Classification within the genus is based upon antigenic properties. Flaviviruses share one or more common antigenic sites but can be differentiated by several serologic tests, particularly neutralization assays.

Multiplication

Genomic RNA is capped (not polyadenylated) and serves as the mRNA for all proteins. Structural proteins are encoded at the 5' end of the genome, and nonstructural proteins (e.g., RNA-dependent RNA polymerase) are encoded at the 3' two-thirds. Complementary (negative-sense) RNA, made from genomic RNA, serves as a template for additional genomic RNA.

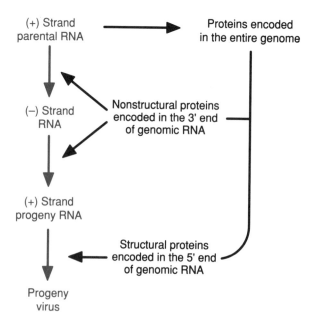

Pathogenesis

Infection is initiated by the bite of an infected mosquito or tick. Virus disseminates after lytic infection of cells, causing viremia. Infection and seroconversion in the absence of apparent disease are common, but case fatality rates can be high. Virus is eliminated (with rare exceptions) by the immune system. In dengue hemorrhagic shock syndrome, disease is thought to be exacerbated by preexisting antibodies to a related flavivirus (i.e., immune enhancement).

Host Defenses

Initial resistance is conferred by a variety of nonspecific defenses. Antibodies are demonstrably important in recovery and resistance, and T-cell responses are also evident. Lasting protection is generally restricted to the same flavivirus and is associated with neutralizing antibodies.

Epidemiology

Viruses are maintained in nature by transmission in mosquito-vertebrate-mosquito or tick-vertebrate-tick cycles. With yellow fever (usually sylvatic in monkeys) and dengue viruses, humans are important intermediate hosts during urban epidemics. Human infections are seasonal and are acquired in endemic areas.

Diagnosis

Diagnosis is suggested by clinical evidence and by known risk of exposure to virus; it is confirmed by virus isolation and identification. Alternatively, a specific rise in antibody titer may confirm diagnosis, but for individuals immune to more than one flavivirus, it may be difficult to serologically discriminate the more recent infection.

Control

Surveillance of disease activity and of virus in natural hosts is used to determine whether control measures will be undertaken to reduce populations of vector mosquitoes. A safe and effective live attenuated vaccine exists for yellow fever, and inactivated-virus vaccines are available for Japanese encephalitis and tick-borne encephalitis.

INTRODUCTION

At least 26 alphaviruses and 65 flaviviruses have been recognized, approximately one-third of which are medically important human pathogens. They vary widely in their basic ecology; each virus occupies a distinct ecologic niche, often with restricted geographic and biologic distribution. As shown in Tables 54-1 and 54-2, alphaviruses and flaviviruses can cause various syndromes, ranging from benign febrile illnesses to severe systemic diseases with hemorrhagic manifestations or major organ involvement. The neurotropic alphaviruses and flaviviruses can produce severe destructive central nervous system disease with serious sequelae. Several alphaviruses (chikungunya, Mayaro, and Ross River viruses) cause painful arthritis that persists for weeks or months after the initial febrile illness. Yellow fever virus has unique hepatotropic properties that cause a clinically and pathologically distinct form of hepatitis with a hemorrhagic diathesis. The dengue viruses, which cause more human illness than all other members of their family, may produce a serious, sometimes fatal, immunopathologic disease in which shock and hemorrhage occur.

Alphavirus is but one genus of the family Togaviridae, which also contains *Rubivirus* and *Pestivirus*. *Flavivirus,* formerly classified in the Togaviridae, now constitutes the only genus of the family Flaviviridae. *Rubivirus,* of which rubella virus is the only member, is covered separately in Chapter 55. *Pestivirus* includes animal pathogens (bovine viral diarrhea and hog cholera viruses) that are of considerable economic importance, but contains no known human pathogens. Pestiviruses have recently been found to be more similar to Flaviviridae than to Togaviridae in their replica-

TABLE 54-1 Principal Medically Important Alphaviruses[a]

Virus	Clinical Syndrome	Antigenic Properties	Vector[b]	Hosts	Distribution
Eastern equine encephalitis (EEE)	Encephalitis	EEE complex	Mosquito	Birds	Americas
Western equine encephalitis (WEE)	Encephalitis	WEE complex	Mosquito	Birds	North America
Venezuelan equine encephalitis (VEE)	Febrile illness, encephalitis	VEE complex (several subtypes)	Mosquito	Rodents, horses	Americas
Chikungunya (CHIK)	Febrile illness, rash, arthralgia	SF complex	Mosquito	Primates, humans	Africa, India, Southeast Asia
Mayaro (MAY)	Febrile illness, rash, arthralgia	SF complex	Mosquito	Primates, humans	South America, Trinidad
O'nyong-nyong (ONN)	Febrile illness, rash, arthralgia	SF complex (CHIK subtype)	Mosquito	Primates	Africa
Ross River (RR)	Febrile illness, rash, arthralgia	SF complex	Mosquito	Mammals, including humans	Australia, Pacific
Sindbis[c] (SIN)	Febrile illness, rash, arthralgia	WEE complex	Mosquito	Birds	Northern Europe, Africa, Asia, Australia
Semliki Forest[c] (SF)	Encephalitis	SF complex	Mosquito	Birds	Africa

[a] This does not include all alphaviruses of veterinary or occasional human disease importance, nor are all antigenic complexes represented. For complete listings and comprehensive reviews of classified alphaviruses, see references.
[b] For a given virus, a very limited number of mosquito species are epidemiologically relevant vectors.
[c] Sindbis and Semliki Forest viruses have been studied extensively in research laboratories. Semliki Forest virus is not well established as an epidemiologically important human pathogen, but a fatal human laboratory infection has occurred with a pathogenic strain.

tion and coding strategies, and may be reclassified accordingly. All alphaviruses and flaviviruses that cause disease in humans are arthropod-borne viruses (arboviruses). In the original classification scheme based on antigenic relationships, alphaviruses and flaviviruses were termed group A and group B arboviruses, respectively.

Most alphaviruses and flaviviruses survive in nature by replicating alternately in a vertebrate host and a hematophagous arthropod (mosquitoes or, for some flaviviruses, ticks). Arthropod vectors acquire the viral infection by biting a viremic host, and after an extrinsic incubation period during which the virus replicates in the vector's tissues, they transmit virus through salivary secretions to another verebrate host. Virus replicates in the vertebrate host, causing viremia and sometimes illness. The ability to infect and replicate in both vertebrate and arthropod cells is an essential quality of alphaviruses and flaviviruses. The principal vertebrate hosts are various species of wild mammals or birds. The natural zoonotic cycles that maintain the virus do not usually involve humans. However, a few viruses (yellow fever virus, dengue virus types 1, 2, 3, and 4 and chikungunya virus) can be transmitted in a human-mosquito-human cycle. As a result of being pathogenic for humans and capable of transmission in heavily populated areas, these viruses can cause widespread and serious epidemics. Because of their high transmission potential, they are major public health problems in many tropical and subtropical regions of the world, where appropriate mosquito vectors are present. Because some of these agents are danger-

TABLE 54-2   Principal Medically Important Flaviviruses[a]

Virus	Clinical Syndrome	Antigenic Properties	Vector[b]	Hosts	Distribution
Dengue (DEN)	Febrile illness, rash; hemorrhagic fever; shock syndrome	DEN complex four types: DEN-1, -2, -3, -4	Mosquito	Humans	Worldwide, especially tropics
Yellow fever (YF)	Hemorrhagic fever, hepatitis	Unique type, no complex assigned	Mosquito	Primates, humans	Africa, South America
St. Louis encephalitis (SLE)	Encephalitis	SLE complex	Mosquito	Birds	Americas
Japanese encephalitis (JE)	Encephalitis	SLE complex	Mosquito	Pigs, birds	India, China, Japan, Southeast Asia
Murray Valley encephalitis (MVE)	Encephalitis	SLE complex	Mosquito	Birds	Australia
West Nile (WN)	Febrile illness	SLE complex	Mosquito	Birds	Africa, Middle East, Europe
Rocio (ROC)	Encephalitis	Unassigned	Mosquito	Birds?	South America
Tick-borne encephalitis (TBE)[c]	Encephalitis	TBE complex[c]	Tick	Rodents	Europe, Asia
Omsk hemorrhagic fever (OMSK)	Hemorrhagic fever	TBE complex	Tick	Muskrats	Siberia
Kyasanur Forest disease (KFD)	Hemorrhagic fever	TBE complex	Tick	Rodents, primates	India
Powassan (POW)	Encephalitis	TBE complex	Tick	Rodents	North America

[a] This does not include all flaviviruses of veterinary or occasional human disease importance, nor are all antigenic complexes represented. For complete listings and comprehensive reviews of classified flaviviruses, see references.

[b] For a given virus, a very limited array of mosquito or tick species are epidemiologically relevant vectors.

[c] Instead of using the common name of TBE to denote a single virus, many will more precisely substitute either Russian spring-summer encephalitis (RSSE) or Central European encephalitis (CEE); thus, the tick-borne viruses listed would all be included in the RSSE antigenic complex.

ous human pathogens and are highly infectious, special containment and safety precautions in the laboratory are required.

◀ ALPHAVIRUSES ▶

PATHOGENESIS AND CLINICAL MANIFESTATIONS

Human illness caused by alphaviruses (Fig. 54-1) is exemplified by agents that produce three markedly different disease patterns. Chikungunya virus causes an acute (3- to 7-day) febrile illness with malaise, arthralgia, a rash, and occasionally arthritis. O'nyong'nyong, Mayaro, and Ross River viruses, which are closely related (antigenically) to chikungunya virus, cause similar or identical clinical manifestations; Sindbis viruses cause similar but milder diseases known as Ockelbo (in Sweden), Pogosta (in Finland), or Karelian fever (in the USSR). Virus introduced by the bite of an infected mosquito replicates and causes a viremia with concomitant fever and generalized malaise; the specific site of viral replication is unknown. The vire-

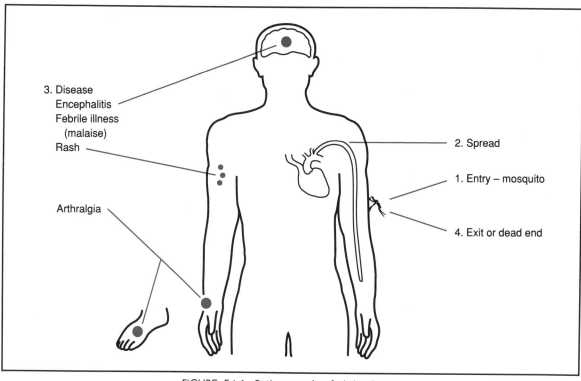

FIGURE 54-1 Pathogenesis of alphaviruses.

mia subsides in 3 to 5 days, and antiviral antibody appears in the blood within 1 to 4 days of onset of symptoms. A maculopapular rash frequently occurs, usually from the days 3 to 5. Arthralgia involving mainly the small joints (hands, wrists, feet, and ankles) occurs most commonly in adults; involved joints are red, swollen, and tender, and effusions may occur. Joint symptoms may last for weeks after the acute illness.

The pathogenesis of eastern and western equine encephalitis virus infections of humans (as well as of equines) similarly involves percutaneous introduction of virus by a vector (Fig. 54-1) and development of viremia; however, in eastern and western equine infections, the viremic phase often is asymptomatic and the infection may resolve without serious manifestations of disease. In some instances, however, central nervous system invasion by the virus results in viral replication in neural tissues, which produces cytolysis, inflammation, and clinical manifestations of encephalitis. The encephalitis may be severe, with high fever, delirium, and coma progressing to death. Convulsions,

motor dysfunction, and paralysis are common. Histopathologic findings are similar to those of most other acute viral encephalitides and include inflammatory cell infiltration, perivascular cuffing, and neuronal degeneration. All regions of the brain may be affected.

Venezuelan equine encephalitis virus infections of humans cause acute febrile illnesses, often with a superimposed central nervous system component. The systemic manifestations are often pronounced, whereas the central nervous system disease occurs only infrequently and usually is much less severe than in eastern and western equine encephalitis. Venezuelan equine encephalitis virus infection can cause severe, sometimes fatal, systemic disease with shock and coma. The fulminant disease may be due in part to lymphocytolysis by the virus.

STRUCTURE

Virions are spherical, 60 to 70 nm in diameter, with an icosohedral nucleocapsid enclosed in a lipid envelope. Alphavirus RNA is a single 42S strand of approximately 4×10^6 daltons that is capped and polyadenylated. The alphavirus genomes that have been sequenced in their entirety are approximately 11.7 kb long. Virion RNA is positive sense. It can function intracellularly as mRNA, and the RNA alone has been shown experimentally to be infectious. The single capsid protein (C protein) has a molecular weight of approximately 30,000. The alphavirus envelope consists of a lipid bilayer derived from the host cell plasma membrane and contains two viral glycoproteins (E1 and E2) with molecular weights of 48,000 to 52,000. A small third protein (E3) with a molecular weight of 10,000 to 12,000 remains virion associated in Semliki Forest virus but is dispatched as a soluble protein in most other alphaviruses. The only proteins in the envelopes of alphaviruses are the viral glycoproteins, which are anchored in the lipid at the hydrophobic C terminus.

CLASSIFICATION AND ANTIGENIC TYPES

Classification is based on antigenic relationships. Viruses have been grouped into seven antigenic complexes; typical species in four medically important antigenic complexes are Venezuelan equine encephalitis, eastern equine encephalitis, western equine encephalitis, and Semliki Forest viruses. Classified viruses are often subdivided into subtypes and varieties as new isolates are found that differ significantly (usually by neutralization tests) from the prototype. Recent molecular and genetic characterizations of several alphaviruses have repeatedly confirmed virus relationships established originally on serologic grounds.

The capsid protein induces antibodies, some of which are widely cross-reactive within the genus by complement fixation and fluorescent-antibody tests. Anti-capsid antibodies do not neutralize infectivity or inhibit hemagglutination. The E2 glycoprotein elicits and is thought to be the principal target of neutralizing antibodies; however, some neutralizing antibodies react with E1. Similarly, hemagglutination-inhibiting antibodies may react with either E2 or E1. Hemagglutination-inhibiting antibodies cross-react, sometimes extensively, among alphaviruses. Such cross-reactivity is attributable to the E1 glycoprotein, the amino acid sequences of which are more highly conserved among alphaviruses than those of E2. Neutralization assays are virus specific, and species or subtypes are defined principally on the basis of neutralization tests.

MULTIPLICATION

Alphaviruses attach to cells, probably via interactions between E2 and undefined cellular receptors. Entry is thought to take place in mildly acidic endosomal vacuoles, where glycoprotein spikes undergo conformational rearrangements and an acid-dependent fusion event (principally a function of E1) delivers genomic RNA to the cell cytoplasm. Viral replication occurs in the cytoplasm. Initial translation of virion RNA produces a polyprotein that is proteolytically cleaved into an RNA polymerase. Transcription of the virion RNA through an antisense RNA intermediate produces a 26S positive-sense mRNA, which encodes only the structural proteins, as well as additional 42S RNA, which is incorporated into progeny virions. Translation from the 26S mRNA (which represents the 3′ one-third of genomic RNA) produces a polyprotein that is cleaved proteolytically into three proteins: C, PE2, and E1; PE2 is subsequently cleaved into E2 and E3. Envelope proteins formed by posttranslational cleavage are glycosylated and translocated to the plasma membrane. Virion formation occurs by budding of preformed icosohedral nucleocapsids through regions of the plasma membrane containing E1 and E2 glycoproteins (Fig. 54-2).

HOST DEFENSES

Differences in susceptibility between individuals and species are not easily ascribed to specific immune responses, and a variety of nonspecific defense mechanisms may be important. Alphaviruses are efficient inducers of interferon, which probably plays a role in modulating or resolving infections. Antibodies are important in disease recovery and resistance. The appearance of neutralizing antibodies in serum coincides with viral clearance, and immune serum can diminish or prevent alpha-

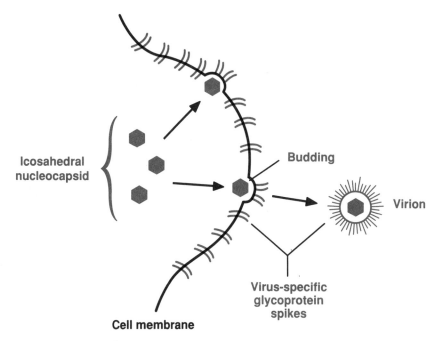

FIGURE 54-2 Morphogenesis of alphaviruses.

virus infection. Although their precise roles are not clearly established, T-cell responses are also demonstrable and may contribute substantially to immunity. Lasting protection is generally restricted to the same alphavirus and is associated with (but not solely attributable to) the presence of neutralizing antibodies. Cross-reactive immunity among different alphaviruses is sometimes observed in the absence of cross-neutralizing antibodies. In experimental animals, such immunity can be mediated by cytolytic nonneutralizing antibodies. The role of T cells is less clear but has been inferred from cytotoxic and other effector activities in vitro that may be alphavirus specific or cross-reactive.

EPIDEMIOLOGY

Eastern and western equine encephalitis viruses are important in the United States. Both are maintained in natural ecologic cycles involving birds and, principally, bird-feeding mosquitoes such as

Culiseta melanura. Eastern equine encephalitis (EEE) virus is enzootic in freshwater swamps in the eastern United States; it causes sporadic equine and rare human cases; small human outbreaks may occur (Fig. 54-3). Western equine encephalitis (WEE) virus is widespread in the United States and Canada and has been responsible for outbreaks of equine and human disease in western and southwestern states. Its principal vector, *Culex tarsalis,* is a common mosquito, especially in irrigated regions.

Eight or more antigenic subtypes of Venezuelan equine encephalitis (VEE) virus exist; they have differing virulence and epidemic potentials. Endemic subtypes of relatively low equine virulence exist in South and Central America and Florida. Endemic strains are ecologically restricted to cycles between small mammals and mosquitoes, and only occasional human cases have been described. Epidemic strains of Venezuelan equine encephalitis virus, however, may spread by an equine-mosquito cycle involving several mosquito

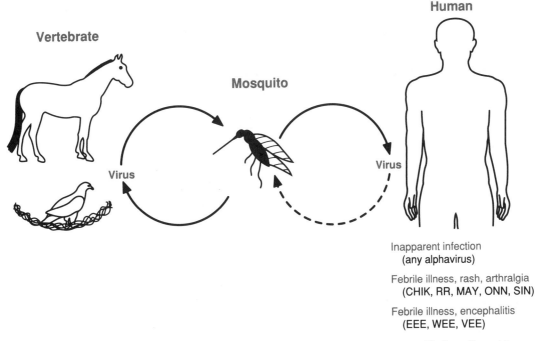

FIGURE 54-3 Alphavirus transmission. Virus abbreviations: Chik, chickungunya; RR, Ross River; May, Mayaro; ONN, O'nyong-nyong; SIN, Sindbis; EEE, eastern equine encephalitis; VEE, Venezuelan equine encephalitis.

species. In this manner, these strains have caused massive equine epizootics with associated human epidemics. An epizootic in 1969 to 1972 involved several Central American countries and spread through Mexico to Texas.

Chikungunya virus exists in Africa in a forest cycle involving baboons and other primates and forest species of mosquitoes. It can also be transmitted in a human-mosquito-human cycle by *Aedes aegypti*. This mode of transmission has caused massive epidemics in Africa, India, and Southeast Asia. The virus is endemic throughout much of south and Southeast Asia. The antigenically similar Mayaro virus exists in the Amazon Basin. Its cycle involves new world primates and hematophagous mosquitoes and causes outbreaks of human disease through exposure to the forest cycle. Ross River virus is endemic in Australia and has spread in epidemic form to several islands of the Western Pacific.

DIAGNOSIS

Diagnosis of alphavirus infection is suggested by clinical evidence and known risk of exposure to virus; it can be confirmed only by laboratory tests. Infection by one of the viruses of the chikungunya-Mayaro complex may be difficult to distinguish from many clinically similar illnesses such as rubella, dengue, phlebotomus fever, enterovirus infection, and scrub typhus. Encephalitis from one of the alphaviruses must be suspected on epidemiologic grounds and distinguished from other viral encephalitides by laboratory tests. Laboratory diagnosis can be established by isolating virus from the blood during the viremic phase or by antibody determination. A variety of serologic tests, especially neutralization, but also enzyme-linked immunosorbent assay (ELISA), hemagglutination inhibition, complement fixation, and reactivities with appropriate monoclonal antibodies, are used by public health laboratories to diagnose alphavirus infections. Testing by enzyme-linked immunosorbent assay for specific IgM is particularly useful in discriminating recent infection with one alphavirus from previous exposure to another alphavirus.

CONTROL

Control of alphavirus diseases in the United States is based on surveillance of disease and virologic activity in natural hosts and, when necessary, on control measures directed at reducing populations of vector mosquitoes. These measures include control of larvae and adult mosquitoes, sometimes by using ultra-low-volume aerial spray techniques. In some areas, insecticide resistance (e.g., resistant *C tarsalis*) is a major limitation to effective control. Inactivated vaccines are used to protect laboratory workers from eastern, western, and Venezuelan equine encephalitis. An effective live attenuated Venezuelan equine encephalitis vaccine has been

used extensively in equines as an epidemic control measure, and a similar vaccine is used to protect laboratory workers. Experimental human vaccines for chikungunya have been tested for safety and immunogenicity and may be available in the near future.

◀ FLAVIVIRUSES ▶

PATHOGENESIS AND CLINICAL MANIFESTATIONS

Flaviviruses vary widely in their pathogenic potential and mechanisms for producing human disease. Three examples are discussed here: St. Louis encephalitis, yellow fever, and dengue viruses (Fig. 54-4). In addition, hepatitis C virus may be a member of this virus group.

St. Louis encephalitis (SLE) virus infections are initiated by deposition of virus through the skin via

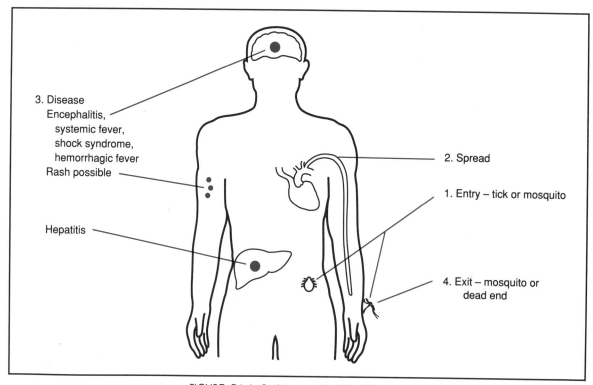

FIGURE 54-4 Pathogenesis of flaviviruses.

the saliva of an infected mosquito (Fig. 54-4). Virus replicates locally and in regional lymph nodes and results in viremia. In most human infections, no apparent disease occurs. The infection resolves, and lasting immunity is produced. In some infections (1:800 to 1:100, depending on the individual's age), central nervous system invasion occurs and viral replication in neural and glial tissue produces a severe inflammatory process. Neuronal degeneration accompanied by lymphocytic infiltrates may be widespread. Clinical manifestations of St. Louis encephalitis are fever, headache, stiff neck, convulsions, delirium, coma, tremors, and motor dysfunction; death may follow. In nonfatal cases, neurologic sequelae are common in older age groups. The pathogenic potential of St. Louis encephalitis virus and several other flaviviruses such as Japanese encephalitis (JE), Murray Valley encephalitis (MVE), and tick-borne encephalitis viruses depends entirely on their neurovirulence (i.e., their ability to invade and replicate in the central nervous system). The systemic phase of infection with these mosquito- and tick-borne encephalitic agents produces negligible illness.

In contrast to the encephalitis-producing agents, yellow fever virus produces severe systemic disease. Virus replicates in reticuloendothelial cells in many organs and in the parenchyma of the liver, adrenal glands, heart, and kidneys. High concentrations of virus are present in the blood and involved organs. Characteristic liver damage from infection of hepatic cells is midzonal necrosis and intracellular hyaline deposits called Councilman bodies. Liver function tests become markedly abnormal, and icterus is often severe. Cellular degeneration of kidney and cardiac cells produces an acute nephritis and myocarditis. Coagulation defects, probably resulting from both liver damage and disseminated intravascular coagulation, are major manifestations and are associated with the severe gastrointestinal hemorrhages characteristic of yellow fever. The clinical course of yellow fever is that of an acute illness lasting 1 week or more. The first phase consists of fever, myalgia, headache, nausea, and vomiting; it is often followed by a second phase involving severe toxicity, jaundice, gastrointestinal hemorrhage, anuria, and shock.

Death may occur within 5 to 10 days; case fatality rates are 10 to 50 percent.

Dengue viruses of all four serotypes cause three distinct syndromes: classic dengue fever, dengue hemorrhagic fever, and dengue shock syndrome. Although apparently caused by the same viruses, dengue and dengue hemorrhagic fever are pathogenetically, clinically, and epidemiologically distinct. Dengue viruses appear to replicate in macrophages at the site of the mosquito bite, in regional lymph nodes, and then throughout the reticuloendothelial system. Viremia is concurrent with clinical illness. Virus is present in the serum and in association with circulating monocytes. Severe leukopenia often is present. Fever, headache, myalgia, anorexia, and a maculopapular or petechial rash, which occurs on the days 3 to 5, are the major manifestations of dengue fever. Dengue fever lasts 3 to 9 days, is self limiting, and is rarely associated with hemorrhagic phenomenon or serious sequelae.

Dengue hemorrhagic fever results from additional pathogenetic processes not present in classic dengue fever; the most important are increased vascular permeability, hemoconcentration, thrombocytopenia, and disseminated intravascular coagulation. In dengue shock syndrome, lowered plasma volume secondary to increased vascular permeability causes clinical shock that, if uncorrected, may lead to acidosis, hyperkalemia, and death.

The specific pathogenetic mechanism that produces dengue hemorrhagic fever and dengue shock syndrome is not well understood, but strong evidence incriminates immunopathologic mechanisms. Ninety percent of dengue hemorrhagic fever cases occur in children experiencing multiple infections with dengue viruses. Four dengue serotypes can be discriminated by neutralization assays, and persons can be infected serially or even simultaneously by two different serotypes. Dengue type 2 virus is the most frequently isolated from patients with hemorrhage and shock, although the other serotypes (serotypes 1, 3, and 4) also may be involved. The immunologic processes that result from closely spaced infections with antigenically related viruses probably are responsible for the immunopathologic manifestations of dengue hemorrhagic fever. In infants, the presence of subprotective levels of maternal anti-dengue virus antibody has been reported to be a factor. Activation of complement and release of inflammatory mediators are usually found in patients with dengue shock syndrome. Immune complexes in circulation or on infected cell surfaces have been postulated to be the cause of this complement activation. A phenomenon called immune enhancement is thought to play a major role in pathogenesis. Both homologous and heterologous antibodies binding to dengue virus can markedly enhance infection of macrophages in vitro via cellular Fc receptors. Several antigenic determinants for infection-enhancing antibodies have been found on the envelope glycoprotein, and it has been postulated that cross-reacting antibodies from a previous dengue infection or maternal anti-dengue virus antibodies in infants enhance the entry of virus into macrophages. The increased viral replication in the macrophages then contributes to complement activation, vascular permeability, and clotting abnormalities through the release of products from infected macrophages. These products may be released by increased destruction of infected macrophages via cellular immune mechanisms.

The clinical course of dengue hemorrhagic fever is characterized by an initial stage of fever, rash, and anorexia, (lasting 3 to 5 days) followed by a shock phase in which hepatomegaly, hypotension, and a hemorrhagic diathesis occur. Complement activation and thrombocytopenia typically take place at the onset of the shock phase and reverse spontaneously after a period that ranges from hours to a few days.

In the great majority of flavivirus infections, the virus is cleared by the immune system. However, persistence in neurologic tissue has been noted, particularly with tick-borne encephalitis viruses.

STRUCTURE

Flavivirus virions are spherical, 40 to 50 nm in diameter, with a nucleoprotein capsid enclosed in a lipid envelope. The RNA is a single 40S (ca. 10.9 kilobases) positive-sense strand and is capped at the 5' end, but, unlike alphaviruses, has no poly (A) segment at the 3' end. The virion has a single capsid protein (C) that is approximately 13,000 daltons. The envelope consists of a lipid bilayer, a single envelope protein (E) of 51,000 to 59,000 daltons, and a small nonglycosylated protein (M) of approximately 8,500 daltons. Only E, which is glycosylated in most flaviviruses, is clearly demonstrable on the virion surface.

CLASSIFICATION AND ANTIGENIC TYPES

Classification within the genus is based upon antigenic relationships. Viruses have been grouped into several antigenic complexes typified, for example, by dissimilar viruses such as dengue, tick-borne encephalitis, St. Louis encephalitis, and yellow fever viruses. Although classification was not intentionally based upon vectors or diseases, the tick-borne flaviviruses important in human disease are aligned with tick-borne encephalitis virus in a single antigenic complex, whereas several encephalitogenic mosquito-borne viruses (St. Louis encephalitis, Japanese encephalitis, Kunjin, Murray Valley encephalitis, and West Nile viruses) make up another complex. Classified virus species are often subdivided into subtypes and varieties as new isolates are found that differ significantly from the prototype.

All flaviviruses are antigenically related by sharing common or similar antigenic determinants on C and E proteins. The single envelope glycoprotein, E, is the viral hemagglutinin; antibodies against E are involved in virus neutralization and hemagglutination inhibition. The antigenic determinants that induce neutralizing antibody are specific, and species or subtypes of flaviviruses are distinguished principally by neutralization tests. Hemagglutination inhibition tests reveal a broad range of cross-reactions among the flaviviruses. Monoclonal antibody studies reveal genus-, group-, and virus-specific epitopes on the envelope glycoprotein. The nonstructural proteins also are antigenic, and at least one nonstructural protein, NS-1, contains both virus-specific and cross-reactive epitopes.

MULTIPLICATION

The mechanism by which flaviviruses enter cells probably involves an interaction between the E protein and cellular receptors, followed by a post-attachment fusion event that occurs in acidic intracytoplasmic vacuoles. Naked genomic RNA is infectious if introduced into the cytoplasm. The genomic RNA is capped but not polyadenylated; it serves as the mRNA for all proteins. Structural proteins are encoded at the 5' end of the genome, and nonstructural proteins (e.g., NS-1 and RNA-dependent RNA polymerase) are encoded in the 3' two-thirds. Complementary (antisense) RNA, made from genomic RNA, serves as a template to generate genomic RNA. Replication occurs in the cytoplasm.

Virions are formed in perinuclear regions of the cytoplasm in association with Golgi or smooth membranes (Fig. 54-5). Virions appear within cytoplasmic vacuoles and apparently exit the cell as the vacuoles fuse with the plasma membrane. Unlike alphaviruses, no evidence of budding has been seen in flavivirus-infected cells, and the mechanisms of virion assembly and release remain obscure.

Flavivirus proteins arise by co- or posttranslational cleavage of the polyprotein encoded by the genome. The E protein mediates attachment and penetration; it also has hemagglutinating activity. The C protein associates with RNA to form a nucleocapsid, and the M protein is membrane associated and is thought to serve a matrix function, linking capsid and envelope. The nonstructural glycoprotein NS-1 is not incorporated into virions, but is found in the endoplasmic reticulum, at the cell surface, and in a soluble form. The function of this protein has not been defined but is probably associated with virion morphogenesis. Other nonstructural proteins form the RNA-dependent RNA polymerase.

HOST DEFENSES

Nonspecific host factors are responsible for heritable patterns of susceptibility and resistance in

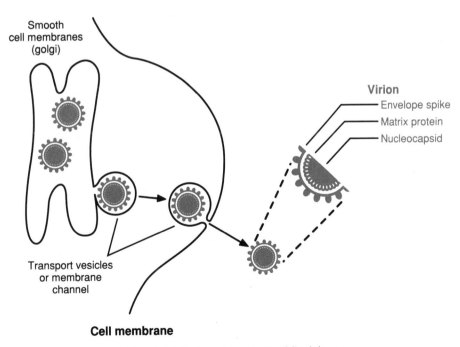

FIGURE 54-5 Morphogenesis of flaviviruses.

mice, and interferon may play a role in resolving infections. As with many viruses, neonates and children tend to be particularly susceptible; however, natural defenses against central nervous system invasion by St. Louis encephalitis virus are most effective in children and much less effective in the elderly, resulting in much higher disease-to-infection ratios in older persons. Antiviral antibody has an important protective role in host defenses against flaviviruses: recovery from infection usually coincides with the appearance of neutralizing antibodies, and prophylactically administered immune serum can prevent or diminish infection. Virus-specific cytotoxic and helper T-cell activities are also demonstrable. Heterologous immunity is not usually protective, even though prominent serologic cross-reactions by hemagglutination inhibition and complement fixation tests are present. Indeed, heterologous antibody increases the infectivity of dengue viruses for human macrophages in vitro.

Lasting protection is generally restricted to the immunizing flavivirus and is associated with neutralizing antibodies directed against the E protein. Antibodies directed against NS-1, in the presence of complement or Fc receptor-bearing cells, can mediate destruction of flavivirus-infected cells and thereby contribute to humoral immunity.

EPIDEMIOLOGY

The flaviviruses constitute a highly diverse genus, and their ecology is similarly varied and complex. Only the basic concepts are considered here. The mosquito-borne encephalitis viruses (St. Louis encephalitis, Japanese encephalitis, Murray Valley encephalitis, and West Nile viruses) exist primarily as viruses of birds and are transmitted by *Culex* mosquitoes which feed readily on birds (Fig. 54-6). St. Louis encephalitis virus is maintained in nature in an avian cycle; in temperate areas it is maintained through the winter in infected hibernating adult mosquitoes. In the United States, human epidemics of St. Louis encephalitis are preceded by increased virus dissemination among wild birds along with increased vector populations and vector infection rates. St. Louis encephalitis virus is

widespread in the United States and causes periodic outbreaks in California, Texas, the Ohio-Mississippi Valley, and the southeast. In Asia, Japanese encephalitis virus occupies an ecologic niche similar to St. Louis encephalitis virus in the western hemisphere, with one major difference: it infects swine, in which it causes high viremias. Because Asian vectors of Japanese encephalitis virus feed readily on swine, these animals are an efficient amplifying host for this virus. As a result, Japanese encephalitis epidemics in regions where swine are present have been frequent and severe. This virus is a major public health concern in Japan, China, India, and Southeast Asia.

The tick-borne flaviviruses are maintained by tick-mammal cycles and by transovarian transmission in ticks. Humans are infected with this subgroup of flavivirus through the bite of infected ticks.

Yellow fever virus in Africa and South America has two distinct epidemiologic patterns: **sylvan** and **urban.** In South America, sylvan (jungle) yellow fever is transmitted among canopy-dwelling monkeys and mosquitoes of the genera *Haemagogus* and *Sabethes.* Human disease occurs sporadically or in small outbreaks, initially only in persons exposed to forest mosquitoes. In previous years, urban yellow fever was transmitted in a highly efficient human-mosquito-human cycle by the urban mosquito *Aedes aegypti.* Epidemic yellow fever occurred in several U.S. cities (e.g., Philadelphia, New York, New Orleans) in the late 19th and early 20th centuries. However, in the Americas, yellow fever is now confined to the Amazon basin and adjacent savannah forest. In Africa, sylvan and rural yellow fever involves monkeys and several *Aedes* spp; the urban cycle involves *A aegypti.* Yellow fever epidemics with high mortality continue to occur with alarming frequency in tropical sub-Saharan Africa.

Dengue viruses are distributed through the tropics and are maintained principally by a human-mosquito-human cycle, although primate infections occur in Asia and probably in Africa. The principal vector is *A aegypti*, but other *Aedes* spp of the subgenus *Stegomyia* may be involved in Asia and the Pacific region. Epidemiologic pat-

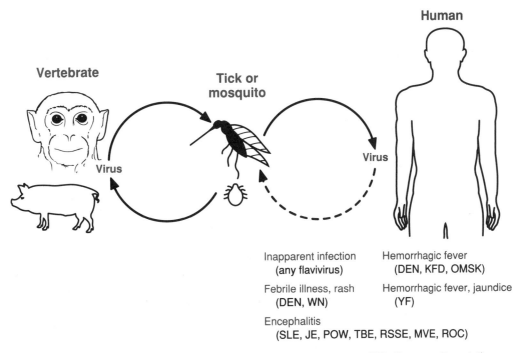

FIGURE 54-6 Flavivirus transmission. Virus abbreviations: DEN, dengue; KFD, Kyasanur Forest disease; OMSK, Omsk hemorrhagic fever; WN, West Nile; YF, yellow fever; SLE, St. Louis encephalitis; JE, Japanese encephalitis; POW, Powssan; RSSE, Russian spring-summer encephalitis; MVE, Murray Valley encephalitis; ROC, Rocio.

terns are highly varied but may be described as epidemic, endemic, or hyperendemic. Epidemics of dengue fever are relatively frequent in Caribbean and Pacific islands. Epidemics occur in non-immune populations when a dengue virus is introduced and vectors are present. Endemic regions in the western hemisphere in which one or more serotypes are continuously transmitted include Jamaica, Haiti, the Dominican Republic, Cuba, Puerto Rico, Columbia, Venezuela, El Salvador, Guatemala, and Mexico. In Africa, endemic dengue is present in Niger, Nigeria, Senegal, Kenya, and Somalia. India, Pakistan, and Bangladesh also have endemic and epidemic regions. In endemic regions, dengue fever occurs principally in children and often is unrecognized. In Southeast Asia, dengue viruses of all four serotypes are continuously transmitted, often at high rates. Under these conditions, epidemics of dengue hemorrhagic fever occur among children. Dengue hem-

orrhagic fever has become a major cause of death among children in hyperendemic regions, including Indonesia, Vietnam, Cambodia, Thailand, Malaysia, and Burma. In these countries, its incidence has been steadily increasing; annual rainy-season epidemics involve thousands of cases with a 3 to 10 percent case fatality rate.

DIAGNOSIS

Diagnosis of flavivirus infection is based on compatible epidemiologic and clinical features and can be confirmed only by laboratory tests (e.g., serology and virus isolation). When a patient develops symptoms of encephalitis, viruses are not easily demonstrable in the cerebrospinal fluid and are no longer present in the blood; they usually can be isolated only by brain biopsy or from the brain at autopsy. Thus, serologic tests showing an antibody rise are most practical for diagnosis.

Interpretation of serologic data obtained by hemagglutination inhibition, complement fixation, and fluorescent antibody tests is difficult in most tropical areas where several flaviviruses are endemic. In primary infections, the virus neutralization test provides virus-specific confirmation. If a patient has had previous flavivirus infections, cross-reactions make even neutralization test results difficult or impossible to interpret. Demonstration of specific IgM in the cerebrospinal fluid by antibody capture immunoassay can be an excellent way to diagnose flavivirus encephalitis. In yellow fever, dengue, and dengue hemorrhagic fever, virus is present in the blood for 4 or even 5 days after onset of fever. Virus isolation in mammalian or insect cell culture is the method of choice for diagnosis. The earlier the specimen is obtained for isolation, the higher the likelihood of success.

CONTROL

Control of disease caused by flaviviruses is based on vaccines for some viruses and on vector control. At present, formalinized (killed) virus vaccines are used to prevent Japanese encephalitis and tickborne encephalitis in endemic regions. The live attenuated 17D yellow fever vaccine is an extremely effective and safe vaccine and is widely used in South America and Africa.

Urban epidemics of yellow fever in the Americas were controlled by containment and, in some regions, eradication of the *A aegypti* vectors. Vector control is not feasible as a method of preventing jungle yellow fever; therefore, vaccines are widely used in affected regions.

No vaccines are yet available for dengue or dengue hemorrhagic fever, although experimental attenuated vaccines have been developed and experimental subunit vaccines have been made through recombinant DNA technologies. Vector control, including destruction of larval habitats and spraying of insecticide to kill adult mosquitoes, is the only means available to control dengue and dengue hemorrhagic fever.

St. Louis encephalitis is managed in the United States by vector control, including water drainage and aerial ultra-low-volume spraying of insecticides in populated areas with epidemic potential. No vaccine is available. Surveillance of St. Louis encephalitis virus activity in wild bird populations and vectors is used to monitor the risk of epidemics and to guide vector control requirements.

REFERENCES

Brinton MA, Heinz FX (eds): New Aspects of Positive-Strand RNA Viruses. American Society for Microbiology, Washington, DC, 1990

Collett MS: Recent advances in pestivirus research. J Gen Virol 70:253, 1989

Karabatsos N (ed): International Catalog of Arboviruses Including Certain Other Viruses of Vertebrates. American Society of Tropical Medicine and Hygiene, 1985

Monath T (ed): The Arboviruses: Epidemiology and Ecology. Vol 1–5. CRC Press, Boca Raton, FL, 1988

Schlesinger S, Schlesinger MJ (eds): The Togaviridae and Flaviviridae. Plenum, New York, 1986

U.S. Department of Health and Human Services: Biosafety in Microbiological and Biomedical Laboratories. 2nd Ed. HHS Publication no. 88-8395. U.S. Department of Health and Human Services, 1988

Westaway EG: Togaviridae: taxonomy. Intervirology 24:125, 1985

Westaway EG: Flaviviridae: taxonomy. Intervirology 24:183, 1985

55 TOGAVIRUSES: RUBELLA VIRUS

DEBORAH J. HENDERSON
PAUL D. PARKMAN

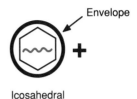

Envelope

Icosahedral
40-90 nm

GENERAL CONCEPTS

Clinical Manifestations

Postnatal **rubella** (German measles) is a generally mild, self-limited illness characterized by rash, lymphadenopathy, and low-grade fever. However, congenital rubella may cause a number of anomalies, depending on the organ system involved and gestational age.

Structure

Rubella virus is a spherical, 40 to 80-nm, positive-sense, single-stranded RNA virus with spikelike, hemagglutinin-containing surface projections. An electron-dense 30-nm core is surrounded by a lipoprotein envelope.

Classification and Antigenic Types

Rubella virus is the sole member of the genus *Rubivirus* in the family Togaviridae. Only one serotype has been identified. It contains three major structural polypeptides.

Multiplication

The multiplication of togaviruses is described in Chapter 54.

Pathogenesis

The disease is transmitted via direct or droplet contact with respiratory secretions. Rubella virus multiplies in cells of the respiratory system; this is followed by viremic spread to target organs. Congenital infection is transmitted transplacentally.

Host Defenses

Initially, the infection is limited by nonspecific defenses such as interferon. Neutralizing and hemagglutination-inhibiting antibodies and cell-mediated immunity develop promptly. Reinfection (usually asymptomatic) can occur.

Epidemiology

Rubella occurs worldwide with a seasonal distribution. There have been no major epidemics in the United States since vaccine licensure in 1969, and the incidence has decreased by 99 percent. Continued cases of congenital rubella are due to infection in unvaccinated, susceptible young women.

Diagnosis

Rubella is suggested by typical rash and lymphadenopathy. This diagnosis is confirmed by virus isolation and serologic studies.

Control

Rubella can be prevented by routine childhood immunization and by immunization of susceptible adolescents and adult populations with live attenuated rubella vaccine. Immunoglobulin is not very effective in prophylaxis of rubella in pregnant women, and it use is not recommended.

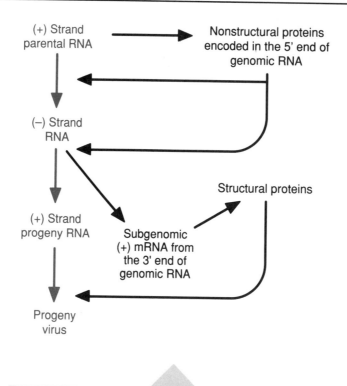

INTRODUCTION

Rubella (German measles) is a common mild disease characterized by a rash. It affects children and adolescents worldwide and can also affect young adults. When rubella virus infects susceptible women early in pregnancy, it may be transmitted to the fetus and may cause birth defects. Therefore, accurate diagnosis is critical in pregnancy. The rubella virus is a member of the genus *Rubivirus* in the family Togaviridae.

CLINICAL MANIFESTATIONS

Postnatal Infection

Postnatal rubella is often asymptomatic but may result in a generally mild, self-limited illness characterized by rash, lymphadenopathy, and low-grade fever. As is the case for many viral diseases, adults often experience more severe symptoms than do children. In addition, adolescents and adults may experience a typical mild prodrome

that is not seen in infected children; this occurs 1 to 5 days before the rash and characterized by headache, malaise, and fever.

The typical picture of rubella (Fig. 55-1) includes a maculopapular rash that appears first on the face and neck and quickly spreads to the trunk and upper extremities and then to the legs. The lesions tend to be discrete at first, but rapidly coalesce to produce a flushed appearance. The onset of rash is often accompanied by low-grade fever. Although the rash usually lasts 3 to 5 days (hence the term "3-day measles"), the associated fever rarely persists for more than 24 hours.

The earliest and perhaps the most prominent and characteristic symptom of rubella infection is lymphadenopathy of the postauricular, occipital, and posterior cervical lymph nodes; this is usually most severe during the rash but may occur even in the absence of rash.

Postnatal rubella usually resolves without complication. However, a number of studies report that as many as one-third of adult women with

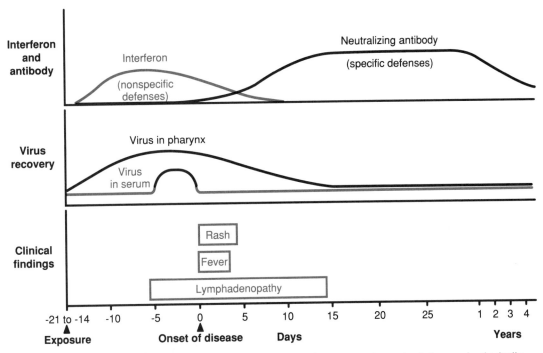

FIGURE 55-1 Clinical findings, virus shedding, and serologic response in postnatally acquired rubella.

rubella experience self-limited arthritis of the extremities and/or polyarthralgia; such effects are rare in children or men. Other complications of rubella, reported with much less frequency than arthritis, include encephalitis and thrombocytopenic purpura.

Congenital Infection

Rubella infection acquired during pregnancy can result in stillbirth, spontaneous abortion, or several anomalies associated with the congenital rubella syndrome. The clinical features of congenital rubella vary and depend on the organ system(s) involved and the gestational age at the time of maternal infection (Table 55-1). The classic triad of congenital rubella syndrome includes cataracts, heart defects, and deafness, although many other symptoms may be seen. Defects may occur alone or in combination and may be temporary or permanent. The risk of rubella-associated congenital defects is greatest during the first trimester of pregnancy, although some defects have been reported after maternal infections in the second trimester.

STRUCTURE

Rubella virus is a spherical 40- to 80-nm, positive-sense, single-stranded RNA virus consisting of an electron-dense 30-nm core surrounded by a lipoprotein envelope. The RNA has a molecular weight of about 3×10^6. The virus particles are spherical with spikey hemagglutinin-containing surface projections.

CLASSIFICATION AND ANTIGENIC TYPES

Rubella virus is the single member of the genus *Rubivirus* in the family Togaviridae. However, rubella virus is serologically distinct from other members of the Togaviridae, and, unlike most other togaviruses, is not known to be transmitted by an arthropod. Only one genetically stable serotype of rubella virus has been identified, although many isolates exist with minor different antigenic strain characteristics.

Rubella virus contains three major structural polypeptides: two membrane glycoproteins, E1

TABLE 55-1   Common Malformations Associated with Congenital Rubella Syndrome

Type of Defect	Examples
Ocular defects	Cataracts
	Microphthalmia
	Glaucoma
	Retinitis
Heart defects	Patent ductus arteriosis
	Peripheral pulmonaric artery stenosis
Hearing impairment	Cochlear deafness
	Central auditory imperception
Central nervous system impairment	Mental retardation
	Encephalitis
	Microcephaly
	Psychomotor retardation
Other	Intrauterine growth retardation
	Hepatosplenomegaly
	Hematologic abnormalities (thrombocytopenia, hemolytic anemia)
	Hepatitis
	Pneumonitis

and E2, and a single nonglycosylated RNA-associated capsid protein, C, within the virion. One of the envelope proteins, E1, is responsible for viral hemagglutination and neutralization. E2 has been found in two forms, E2a and E2b, and the differences among strains of rubella viruses have been correlated with differences in the antigenicity of E2.

PATHOGENESIS

Humans are the only known reservoir or rubella virus, with postnatal person-to-person transmission occurring via direct or droplet contact with the respiratory secretions of infected persons. Although the early events surrounding infection are incompletely characterized, the virus almost certainly multiplies in cells of the respiratory tract, extends to local lymph nodes, and then undergoes viremic spread to target organs (Fig. 55-2). Subsequent additional replication in selected target organs, such as the spleen and lymph nodes, leads to a secondary viremia with wide distribution of rubella virus. At this time (approximately 7 days after infection and 7 to 10 days before the onset of rash) the virus can be detected in the blood and respiratory secretions (Fig. 55-1). Viremia disappears shortly after the onset of rash; it is also associated with the appearance of circulating neutralizing antibodies. However, virus shedding from the respiratory tract may continue for up to 21 days following the onset of rash.

Rubella infection in the first 3 or 4 months of pregnancy provides opportunities during the period of maternal viremia for invasion of the placenta and subsequent fetal infection. Development of infection probably depends upon gestational age. It has been estimated that the fetus has a 40 to 60 percent chance of developing multiple rubella-associated defects if the mother is infected during the first 2 months of pregnancy, with the risk dropping to 30 to 35 percent during the third month of gestation and 10 percent during the fourth. This difference in both risk for and severity of fetal infection seen with gestational age may be associated with immature host defenses during the first trimester of pregnancy.

Fetal infection commonly results in birth defects; the virus can multiply in and damage virtually any organ system. Pathogenesis of the congenital defects is not fully understood; however, a number of mechanisms have been proposed. Cell culture

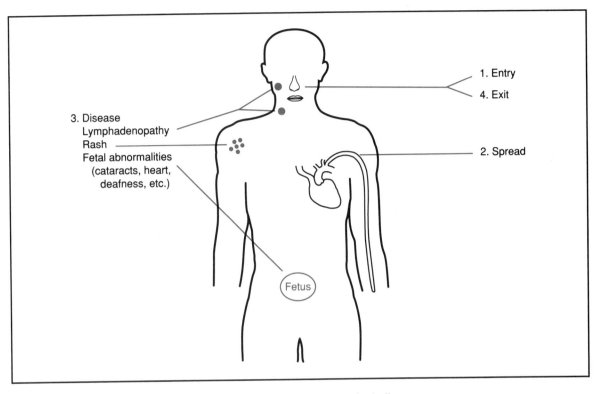

FIGURE 55-2 Pathogenesis of rubella.

studies show that the virus produces chromosomal abnormalities, slows cellular growth rates, and causes cell lysis and death in some cell types; these effects appear to produce the characteristic abnormalities of cell structure and function. In addition, rubella infection induces angiopathy of early placental and embryonic tissues, causing interference with the fetal blood supply and subsequent compromised growth and/or malformation of the fetus.

HOST DEFENSES

Postnatal infection rapidly induces the nonspecific defense systems such as interferon. Subsequently, specific immune response occurs and, in most cases, accounts for lifelong protection against reinfection. Neutralizing and hemagglutination-inhibiting antibodies appear shortly after the onset of rash and reach maximum levels in 1 to 4 weeks. Specific antibodies persist for as long as 14 years

after immunization. Cell-mediated immunity (CMI) also develops in convalescence and can be detected for years following infection. When exposed to rubella virus, individuals with neutralizing or hemagglutination-inhibiting antibodies are most often protected against the natural disease. However, reinfection with rubella virus has been documented in individuals with demonstrated natural immunity and, more commonly, in vaccinees. The vast majority of such reinfections are asymptomatic, detectable only by a boost in antibody titer; however, a few cases of reinfection-associated rash and arthritis have been reported.

EPIDEMIOLOGY

Rubella occurs worldwide. There have been no major epidemics in the United States since the licensure of the live attenuated rubella vaccine in 1969. However, limited sporadic outbreaks of rubella continue to occur each year, particularly in settings (such as schools) where susceptible individuals come into close contact. The incidence of infection shows the same prominent seasonal pattern as for other respiratory diseases. The incidence increases in winter, peaks in spring, and then subsides to extremely low levels in summer and fall.

Epidemiologic data suggest that maximum infectivity occurs from 3 days before the onset of rash until 3 days afterward. However, throat swabs from children with rubella have been reported to contain virus from as early as 10 days before the onset of rash to as late as 28 days afterward. In addition, asymptomatic individuals have been reported to transmit rubella.

In the prevaccine era, the disease usually affected children 5 to 9 years old. However, because rubella is less contagious than diseases such as measles and varicella, a significant proportion of the population (10 to 15 percent) escaped rubella infection in childhood. Widespread vaccine use

has reduced rubella incidence by more than 99 percent in all age groups (Fig. 55-3). However, a greater percentage of cases are now reported in unvaccinated young adults. In 1987, 48 percent of reported rubella infections were in persons older than 15 years of age. In addition, about 10 to 15 percent of young adults in the United States currently lack serologic evidence of earlier rubella infection, are unvaccinated, and hence are susceptible to rubella. These data are of particular concern as they apply to young woman of childbearing age, a potential source of congenital infection.

An average of 39 cases per year of congenital rubella were reported to the Centers for Disease Control between 1969 and 1979, falling rather dramatically to an average of only 7 cases per year between 1979 and 1988. In infants with congenital rubella, the virus commonly persists during the first year of life and occasionally even longer. Such infants thus serve as reservoirs of infection for health care personnel and other contacts.

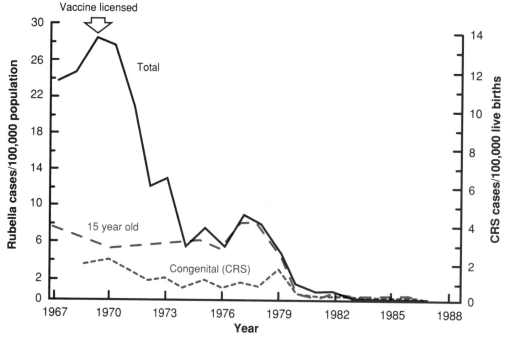

FIGURE 55-3 Incidence rates of reported rubella and congenital rubella syndrome (CRS) cases in the United States from 1967 to 1988. (From Centers for Disease Control: Rubella and congenital rubella—United States, 1985–1988. MMWR 38:11, 1989.)

DIAGNOSIS

The occurrence of the typical rash and lymphadenopathy may suggest the diagnosis of rubella. Laboratory diagnosis of rubella is typically made by using serologic studies (i.e., detection of IgM and/ or fourfold antibody rises). The presence of specific IgM antibodies indicates recent rubella infection. Specific IgG antibodies in healthy individuals demonstrate immunity to rubella. Virus can be readily recovered from respiratory tract secretions and, in infants with congenital infection, from urine, cerebrospinal fluid, and blood by viral interference or immunoperoxidase staining assays. Because virus isolation procedures are costly and require a relatively sophisticated virologic laboratory, they are used primarily for the diagnosis of congenital rubella.

Congenital rubella in the neonate is diagnosed by virus isolation or serologic testing. The affected neonate has circulating antibodies, including transplacentally acquired maternal IgG antibody and actively produced fetal and neonatal IgM antibody. Maternal IgG antibody is detectable in the neonate and wanes during the first 6 months of life. Therefore, the persistence of IgG antibody beyond 6 months or the demonstration of IgM antibody is diagnostic for congenital rubella infection.

CONTROL

Vaccines

Since 1969, several live attenuated rubella vaccines for the prevention of rubella have been licensed for use in the United States. The vaccine in current use is prepared from attenuated rubella virus (RA 27/3) and induces immunity by producing a modified rubella infection in susceptible recipients. When administered in a single subcutaneous dose, the live rubella virus vaccine is most commonly given at 15 months of age in combination with mumps and measles vaccines. Vaccine-induced infection is usually asymptomatic in children, but is associated more frequently with rubellalike symptoms in adults (most commonly in women over the age of 25). Vaccine-associated re-

actions include fever, lymphadenopathy, and arthritis and are usually mild and transient.

Although the levels of vaccine-induced antibody are lower than those produced by the natural disease, approximately 95 percent of vaccinees seroconvert between 14 and 28 days following vaccination. As with all attenuated vaccines, the duration of protection may be a matter of concern. In 1982, the Centers for Disease Control reported surveillance studies on individuals enrolled in a vaccine study in 1969. During the first 4 years after vaccination, there was approximately a 50 percent drop in the hemagglutination inhibition titer, with generally stable titers after that time. Nevertheless, measurable antibody levels persisted in 97 percent of vaccinees over the 10-year study period. The continued decline in reported cases of rubella in the United States indicates that immunity conferred by vaccination appears adequate to interrupt the transmission of disease.

The immunization strategy in the United States is aimed at minimizing the potential for exposure of pregnant women (i.e., their fetuses) to rubella by using vaccination programs designed primarily to provide widespread childhood immunity to rubella and to reduce the occurrence of disease in the community. A continued downward trend in cases of rubella has been reported by the Centers for Disease Control, with a record low of 221 cases in 1988. Still of concern, however, is the fact that approximately 10 to 20 percent of postpubertal women show no serologic evidence of immunity to rubella virus. Additional emphasis is therefore being placed on immunization of this population. Suggested strategies include proof of rubella immunity as a prerequisite for college entry, required vaccination of susceptible health care and military personnel, and vaccination of susceptible women after childbirth, miscarriage, or abortion.

Although the use of rubella vaccine is not recommended under any circumstances during pregnancy, data collected since 1971 indicate that vaccination within the first 3 months of conception poses little risk of congenital rubella syndrome and should not be an automatic reason for interruption of pregnancy. However, the theoretical risk for vaccine-induced congenital rubella infection remains, and women are advised not to become pregnant for 3 months following rubella immunization.

Immunoglobulin

No specific chemotherapeutic measures are available for the treatment of rubella. Immunoglobulin has been used in attempts to prevent rubella in pregnant women exposed to the virus. However, immunoglobulin does not appear to be highly effective; congenital infection has been observed in the infants of women given appropriately timed large doses. The failure of antibody to prevent infection and spread to the fetus may be due to intracellular spread or direct cell-to-cell spread of virus. Therefore, immunoglobulin is not routinely recommended for prophylaxis of rubella in early pregnancy.

REFERENCES

Bakshi SS, Cooper LZ: Rubella (review). Clin Dermatol 7:8, 1989

Centers for Disease Control: Rubella vaccination during pregnancy. MMWR 36:457, 1987

Centers for Disease Control: Rubella and congenital rubella—United States, 1985–1988. MMWR 38:11, 1989

Cochi SL, Edmonds LE, Dyer K et al: Congenital rubella syndrome in the United States, 1970–1985: on the verge of elimination. Am J Epidemiol 129:349, 1989

Green RH, Balsamo MR, Giles JP et al: Studies of the natural history and prevention of rubella. Am J Dis Child 110:348, 1965

Heggie AD, Robbins FC: Natural rubella acquired after birth. Am J Dis Child 118:12, 1969

Horstmann D, Schluederberg A, Emmons JE et al: Persistence of vaccine-induced immune responses to rubella: comparison with natural infection. Rev Infect Dis S7:S80, 1985

Orenstein WA, Bart KJ, Hinman AR et al: The opportunity and obligation to eliminate rubella from the United States. J Am Med Assoc 251:1988, 1984

Parkman PD, Hopps HE, Meyer HM: Rubella virus: isolation, characterization and laboratory diagnosis. Am J Dis Child 118:68, 1969

Preblud SR, Serdula MK, Frank JA et al: Current status of rubella in the United States, 1969–1979. J Infect Dis 142:776, 1980

56
BUNYAVIRUSES

ROBERT E. SHOPE

C = 122
80-120 nm

GENERAL CONCEPTS

Clinical Manifestations

Bunyaviruses cause fevers sometimes with rash. In addition, Crimean-Congo hemorrhagic fever virus may cause hemorrhage; Rift Valley fever virus may cause hemorrhagic hepatitis, encephalitis, or blindness; La Crosse virus and related viruses may cause encephalitis; and Hantaan virus and related viruses may cause hemorrhage and renal failure.

Structure

Bunyaviruses are spherical, enveloped particles 90 to 100 nm in diameter. They contain three segments of antisense (and sometimes ambisense) single-stranded RNA combined with nucleoprotein. Two external glycoproteins form surface projections. A virus-encoded transcriptase is present in the virion.

Classification and Antigenic Types

There are five genera—*Bunyaviruses, Phlebovirus, Nairovirus, Uukuvirus,* and *Hantavirus*—which include *35 serogroups* with at least 304 types and subtypes.

Multiplication

Bunyaviruses replicate in the cytoplasm. Their RNA genome is transcribed to mRNA. The host RNA sequence in some representative viruses primes viral mRNA synthesis. Bunyaviruses mature by budding into vesicles at or near the Golgi apparatus. Reassortment of RNA segments occurs between closely related members.

Pathogenesis

Fever accompanies viremia, which seeds the liver in Rift Valley fever and Crimean-Congo hemorrhagic fever. Encephalitis, retinitis, and renal involvement usually appear later in infection (after antibody formation). More specific mechanisms of pathogenesis are not known.

Host Defenses

Interferon is an early defense mechanism. Viremia ceases with the appearance of humoral antibody, which does not alter established encephalitis, retinitis, or renal lesions.

Epidemiology

The distribution of each disease is determined by the distributions of the vector and vertebrate host. Except for hantaviruses, biologic transmission is by a tick, mosquito, midge, or sand fly vector. Arthropods are infected for life. Transovarial transmission is common in arthropods . Wild or domestic vertebrates usually are needed to maintain the cycle. Humans are usually dead-end hosts for all these viruses except phleboviruses. There is a secondary nosocomial spread of Crimean-Congo hemorrhagic fever. Hantaan virus cycles among rodents, probably by aerosol or fomite transmission from infected rodent urine. Human infection is incidental.

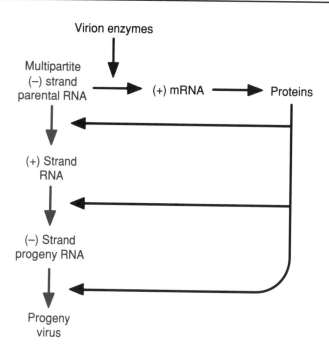

Diagnosis

Knowledge of the geographic site of exposure, season, and presence of arthropods leads to presumptive diagnosis in febrile cases. Diagnosis is confirmed by virus isolation, presence of specific IgM, or an antibody titer rise in paired sera.

Control

Control is often achieved by control of vector arthropods or vaccination (of humans for Crimean-Congo hemorrhagic fever and of sheep and cattle for Rift Valley fever). Control of the rodent host is important for hemorrhagic fever with renal syndrome.

INTRODUCTION

Bunyaviridae is a family of arthropod-borne or rodent-borne, spherical, enveloped RNA viruses. Bunyaviruses are responsible for a number of febrile diseases in humans and other vertebrates. They have either a rodent host or an arthropod vector and a vertebrate host.

CLINICAL MANIFESTATIONS

The Bunyaviridae are divided into arthopod-borne viruses **(arboviruses)** and rodent-borne viruses **(roboviruses).** Bunyaviruses cause several diseases

of human and domestic animals, including fever, hemorrhagic fever, renal failure, encephalitis, meningitis, blindness, and, in domestic animals, congenital defects. Most illnesses are self-limited fevers that last 1 to 4 days and are accompanied by headache, muscle aches, nausea, conjunctival injection, and generalized weakness. A few are more serious illnesses: **La Crosse encephalitis** is characterized by fever, convulsions, drowsiness, and focal neurologic signs; **Crimean-Congo hemorrhagic fever** is characterized by headache, pain in limbs, and, in severe cases, bleeding from multiple orifices; and **hemorrhagic fever with renal syn-**

drome (Korean hemorrhagic fever, nephropathia epidemica) is characterized by fever, hemorrhage, and acute renal failure. **Rift Valley fever** may mimic the febrile, encephalitic, or hemorrhagic illness of other bunyavirus infections, and the patient may also go blind as a result of retinal vasculitis. These illnesses are significant, currently uncontrolled human diseases. La Crosse virus causes most of the arbovirus encephalitis in North America. Also, more than 100,000 cases of hemorrhagic fever with renal syndrome occur annually in Asia and Europe. Rift Valley fever has explosive potential, as shown in Egypt in 1977, when an estimated 200,000 cases, with 598 deaths, were recorded.

STRUCTURE

Bunyaviruses are spherical, enveloped particles 90 to 100 nm in diameter. They contain single-stranded RNA, which, with the nucleoprotein, forms three nucleocapsid segments. The segments are large, medium, and small helical, circular structures. The RNA has a total molecular weight of 5×10^6. The nucleocapsid is surrounded by a lipid-containing envelope. Surface spikes are composed of two glycoproteins that confer properties of neutralization of infectivity and hemagglutination of red blood cells.

CLASSIFICATION AND ANTIGENIC TYPES

The family Bunyaviridae includes five genera containing 35 serogroups with at least 304 viruses, of which 51 in four genera are known to cause human disease (Table 56-1).

MULTIPLICATION

Replication occurs in the cytoplasm. In most bunyaviruses the genome is antisense. In some phleboviruses, the small RNA segment is ambisense (i.e., one portion is viral complementary in sense and the other portion is viral in sense). Genetic reassortment can occur during infection because the RNA is segmented (Fig. 56-1). Virus particles bud into the Golgi cisternae and are liberated from the cell by plasma membrane disruption and by fusion of intracellular vacuoles with the plasma membrane.

PATHOGENESIS

Except for members of the genus *Hantavirus,* bunyaviruses replicate in arthropods. The gut of the vector is infected initially, and after a few days or weeks the virus appears in the saliva; the arthropod then remains infective for life but is not ill. When the vector takes a blood meal, the infective saliva enters the small capillaries or lymphatics of the human or other vertebrate host (Fig. 56-2). The primary site of replication in humans is not known; it may be the vascular endothelium, the skin, or the regional lymph nodes. An incubation period of a few days ensues, after which the vertebrate host develops viremia. The infection is usually inapparent. Less often, the host becomes febrile, manifesting the more serious signs and symptoms that are characteristic of the infecting virus. Viremia subsides with the appearance of humoral antibody, and the host recovers unless a specific target organ is affected. This target organ—the liver in Rift Valley fever, the brain in La Crosse encephalitis, and the liver and vascular endothelium in Crimean-Congo hemorrhagic fever and hemorrhagic fever with renal syndrome—is damaged, and a specific disease occurs. Although the damage in most infections is believed to result from direct invasion by the virus and not from a host-mediated antigen-antibody or antigen-lymphocyte reaction, the pathogenesis of bunyaviruses in the vertebrate host has not been extensively studied. The damage to the kidneys in hemorrhagic fever with renal syndrome and to the brain and retina in Rift Valley fever occurs after humoral antibody is formed. These complications have been postulated to result from a host reaction.

HOST DEFENSES

The initial response to bunyavirus infection is the production of interferon. Bunyaviruses are sensitive to the action of interferon, so this response may play a protective role. Humoral antibody is also protective. The appearance of antibody, ei-

TABLE 56-1 Human Diseases Caused by Viruses of the Family Bunyaviridae

Genus and Group	Virus	Disease	Vector	Geographic Location	Case Fatality Rate (%)
Bunyavirus					
Anopheles A	Tacaiuma	Fever	Mosquito	South America	0
Bunyamwera	Bunyamwera	Fever	Mosquito	Africa	0
	Germiston	Fever	Mosquito	Africa	0
	Ilesha	Fever	Mosquito	Africa	0
	Shokwe	Fever	Mosquito	Africa	0
	Tensaw	Encephalitis	Mosquito	North America	0
	Wyeomyia	Fever	Mosquito	South America, Panama	0
Bwamba	Bwamba	Fever, rash	Mosquito	Africa	0
	Pongola	Fever	Mosquito	Africa	0
C	Apeu	Fever	Mosquito	South America	0
	Caraparu	Fever	Mosquito	South America	0
	Itaqui	Fever	Mosquito	South America	0
	Madrid	Fever	Mosquito	Panama	0
	Marituba	Fever	Mosquito	South America	0
	Murutucu	Fever	Mosquito	South America	0
	Nepuyo	Fever	Mosquito	South and Central America	0
	Oriboca	Fever	Mosquito	South America	0
	Ossa	Fever	Mosquito	Panama	0
	Restan	Fever	Mosquito	Trinidad	0
California	California encephalitis	Encephalitis	Mosquito	North America	0
	Guaroa	Fever	Mosquito	South America	0
	Inkoo	Fever	Mosquito	Scandinavia	0
	La Crosse	Encephalitis	Mosquito	North America	0.5–1
	Snowshoe hare	Encephalitis	Mosquito	North America, Asia	0
	Jamestown Canyon	Encephalitis	Mosquito	North America	0
	Tahyna	Fever	Mosquito	Europe	0
Guama	Catu	Fever	Mosquito	South America	0
	Guama	Fever	Mosquito	South America	0
Simbu	Shuni	Fever	Mosquito	Africa, Asia	0
	Oropouche	Fever	Midge	South America, Panama	0

744

		Disease	Vector	Distribution	
Phlebovirus					
Phlebotomus fever	Alenquer	Fever	Unknown	South America	0
	Candiru	Fever	Unknown	South America	0
	Chagres	Fever	Sand fly	Panama	0
	Naples	Fever	Sand fly	Europe, Africa, Asia	0
	Punta Toro	Fever	Sand fly	Panama	0
	Rift Valley fever	Fever, encephalitis, hemorrhagic fever, blindness	Mosquito	Africa	0.2–10
	Sicilian	Fever	Sand fly	Europe, Africa, Asia	0
	Toscana	Aseptic meningitis	Sand fly	Italy	0
Nairovirus					
Crimean-Congo	Crimean-Congo hemorrhagic fever	Hemorrhagic fever	Tick	Africa, Asia	2–50
Nairobi sheep disease	Nairobi sheep disease	Fever	Tick	Africa, Asia	0
Hantavirus					
Hantaan	Hantaan	HFRS[a]	Rodent	Asia	7
	Puumala	HFRS	Rodent	Europe	0.5
	Seoul	HFRS	Rodent	Asia, Europe	5
Genus unassigned	Bangui	Fever, rash	Unknown	Africa	0
	Bhanja	Fever, encephalitis	Tick	Africa, Europe, Asia	0
	Issk-kul	Fever	Tick	Asia	0
	Kasokero	Fever	Unknown	Africa	0
	Nyando	Fever	Mosquito	Africa	0
	Tamdy	Fever	Tick	Soviet Union	0
	Tataguine	Fever	Mosquito	Africa	0
	Wanowrie	Fever, hemorrhage	Tick	Middle East, Asia	0

[a] HFRS, Hemorrhagic fever with renal syndrome.

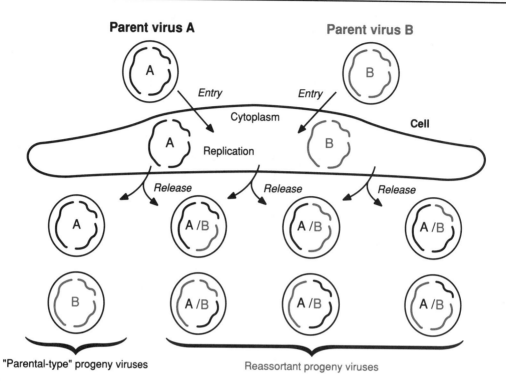

FIGURE 56-1   Genetic reassortment in bunyaviruses. Reassortment occurs when a cell is infected simultaneously with two different but closely related bunyaviruses. Each of the three RNA segments is a gene. Parent viruses A and B each donate three genes. These replicate in the cytoplasm, are packaged in different combinations, and are released as eight kinds of progeny viruses, two of which are identical to the parent strains and six have reassorted genes.

ther natural or passively administered, is associated with the disappearance of virus from the blood. The role of cell-mediated immunity has not been fully evaluated.

EPIDEMIOLOGY

Except for hantaviruses the life cycle of the bunyaviruses involves replication alternately in an arthropod (mosquito, tick, *Culicoides* midge, or phlebotomine sand fly) and in a vertebrate host, usually a small mammal. Humans may become ill when infected, but human blood rarely infects biting arthropods in the natural cycle; therefore, humans are usually dead-end hosts. In addition to the arthropod-vertebrate-arthropod cycle, some bunyaviruses, such as those in the California and phlebotomus fever groups, are transmitted trans-

ovarially in the arthropod and can therefore overwinter in the egg and be transmitted to humans in the late spring or early summer, when the adult arthropod emerges. Bunyaviruses are found throughout the world, but each serotype has a limited geographic distribution because it relies on one or, at best, a few arthropod species to maintain its natural cycle. Hantaviruses are maintained in rodent reservoirs and are not arthropod borne. Transmission to humans is believed to occur by inhalation of virus excreted in rodent urine and other body fluids (Fig. 56-3).

La Crosse Virus

The most serious disease of bunyavirus origin in the United States is La Crosse encephalitis. First recognized when there was a fatal case in La

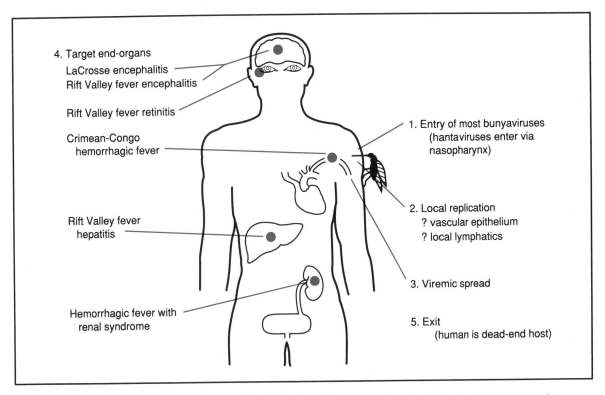

4. Target end-organs
LaCrosse encephalitis
Rift Valley fever encephalitis

Rift Valley fever retinitis

Crimean-Congo
hemorrhagic fever

Rift Valley fever
hepatitis

Hemorrhagic fever with
renal syndrome

1. Entry of most bunyaviruses
(hantaviruses enter via
nasopharynx)

2. Local replication
? vascular epithelium
? local lymphatics

3. Viremic spread

5. Exit
(human is dead-end host)

FIGURE 56-2 Pathogenesis of bunyavirus infections. Humans are dead-end hosts of most bunyaviruses; however, the blood of Crimean-Congo hemorrhagic fever patients may be highly infectious.

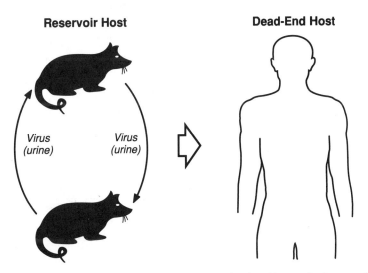

Reservoir Host

Dead-End Host

Virus
(urine)

Virus
(urine)

FIGURE 56-3 Hantavirus transmission. Hantaviruses are maintained in a rodent reservoir. The rodents are asymptomatic and transmit virus to other rodents and humans by way of infected urine and perhaps other body secretions. Humans are dead-end hosts. Hantaviruses cause hemorrhagic fever with renal syndrome in Europe and Asia.

Crosse, Wisconsin, in 1960, it is now diagnosed not only in the north central United States, but also in much of the eastern portion of the country and in Canada. The closely related California encephalitis, snowshoe hare, and Jamestown Canyon viruses are also occasionally implicated as agents of encephalitis. At least 1,000 cases have been reported since 1960, with a case fatality ratio of about 1:200. La Crosse encephalitis affects children; boys are infected more frequently than girls because boys are more often exposed. The vector of La Crosse virus is the woodland mosquito *Aedes triseriatus,* which breeds in tree holes. Consequently, the infection usually occurs after exposure in the woods when camping, or among children living in rural areas. Chipmunks and tree squirrels are amplifying hosts. Virus may also be transmitted from male to female mosquitoes venereally (Fig. 56-4).

Group C and Guama Viruses

The group C and Guama viruses cause self-limited febrile disease in humans in Central and South America. The disease lasts 2 to 4 days and may be severe enough to incapacitate even the most robust forest worker. Infection is usually transmitted by forest *Culex (Melanoconion)* mosquitoes. Forest rodents and marsupials are the vertebrate hosts, and infection in humans is dead end. Bunyamwera group virus illnesses occur in Africa and South America. These are transmitted by mosquitoes and are also self-limited febrile diseases.

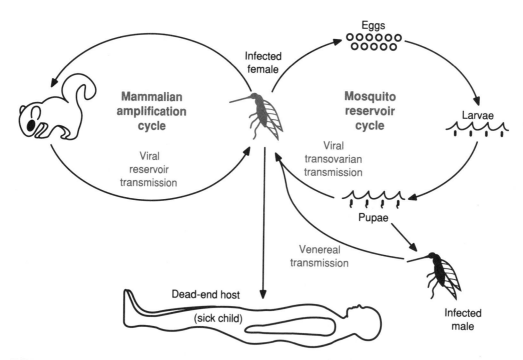

FIGURE 56-4 La Crosse encephalitis transmission cycle. La Crosse virus is maintained in the hardwood forest habitat and in discarded tires in the suburban habitat by transovarial transmission in *Aedes triseriatus* mosquitoes. An adult female mosquito is able to transmit virus to humans and to squirrels and chipmunks with her first blood meal. Squirrels and chipmunks become viremic and amplify the cycle when fed upon by infected *Aedes* mosquitoes. Uninfected female mosquitoes can also be infected by venereal transmission from male mosquitoes. Humans, mostly children, develop encephalitis and do not transmit the virus (dead-end hosts).

Phlebotomus Fever Viruses

Naples and Sicilian phlebotomus fevers are endemic in North Africa and southern Europe and from the Middle East to Pakistan. Humans and sand flies are believed to be the reservoirs. During World War II, severe epidemics of these diseases were recognized as febrile illnesses in troops in the Mediterranean theater. The sand fly *Phlebotomus papatasii* proved to be the vector. Subsequently, related viruses such as Candiru, Chagres, and Punta Toro viruses were discovered in the New World tropics, where a cycle of phlebotomine sand flies and forest rodents was responsible for maintaining the infection.

Oropouche Virus

Oropouche virus causes a major nonfatal febrile disease in Brazil, Trinidad, and Panama. Tens of thousands of cases have been recorded in epidemics. The vertebrate host is not yet known; *Culicoides* midges are implicated as vectors.

Crimean-Congo Hemorrhagic Fever Virus

Crimean-Congo hemorrhagic fever is a tick-transmitted viral disease found in Bulgaria, Yugoslavia, the Soviet Union, China, Iraq, United Arab Emirates, Pakistan, and sub-Saharan Africa. The vector tick is usually of the *Hyalomma* genus. Domestic and wild mammals may be amplifying and reservoir hosts. Human infection also occurs directly from contaminated blood of hospitalized patients; therefore, patients hospitalized with this disease should be isolated.

Rift Valley Fever Virus

Rift Valley fever appears as epizootics in sheep, cattle, camels, and goats in Africa. Massive outbreaks have been recognized in South Africa, Kenya, Uganda, Sudan, Egypt, and Mauretania. Human cases usually are restricted to veterinarians, butchers, and others in close contact with blood of domestic livestock. However, in Egypt in 1977 and again in Mauretania in 1987, widespread human epidemic disease was recognized. Transmission is via aerosolized infected blood and mosquitoes. Epizootics in the Rift Valley arise periodically after heavy rains. There is evidence that the virus is maintained in nature in the dried eggs of *Aedes* mosquitoes that hatch only in very moist years.

DIAGNOSIS

Illnesses caused by bunyaviruses are diagnosed by isolating the virus or by showing a fourfold or greater rise in antibody titer between acute- and convalescent-phase sera. The virus can be isolated from blood (or from brain, liver, and other organs postmortem) during the viremic phase, but not usually after the third day of fever. It is propagated in baby mice or mosquitoes or in vertebrate or invertebrate tissue cultures. Serologic tests used to diagnose bunyavirus infections include the enzyme-linked immunosorbent assay and complement fixation, fluorescent antibody, neutralization, and hemagglutination inhibition tests. The complement fixation and fluorescent antibody tests and the enzyme-linked immunosorbent assay (ELISA) are often group reactive; the neutralization and hemagglutination inhibition tests are type specific. Assessments of IgM may be especially useful in establishing an early diagnosis. Once isolated, virus is identified by the same tests with a reference immune serum.

Bunyavirus diseases usually are restricted to focal geographic areas because of the limited distribution of their vectors and vertebrate hosts. Awareness of their geographic distribution, seasonality, and clinical syndrome may help in establishing a diagnosis. For instance, hemorrhagic fever with renal syndrome should be strongly suspected in a person in Europe or Asia who has fever, proteinuria, thrombocytopenia, and elevated blood urea nitrogen, especially if the patient has been exposed to rodents. Definitive diagnosis, however, can be made only by laboratory tests.

CONTROL

Bunyavirus transmission is controlled by restricting the arthropod vector or vertebrate reservoir. Personal measures, such as the use of proper protective clothing, repellents, bed nets, and house screens, are effective but are often forgotten. Pesticides are used on a community-wide basis, as well as at the breeding sites of arthropods. Proper disposal of tires (a breeding site of the mosquito transmitting La Crosse encephalitis virus) is effective. Rodenticides are used in outbreaks of hemorrhagic fever with renal syndrome.

Rift Valley fever vaccines are used in Africa to immunize sheep and cattle and hence to stop the transmission cycle to humans. A human vaccine for Crimean-Congo hemorrhagic fever is used in the Soviet Union and Bulgaria.

Patients in the viremic phase of illness should be protected from arthropod bites by the use of pesticides, bed nets, and screening. Medical personnel who care for viremic patients should be careful in handling needles and surgical instruments to prevent accidental transmission by blood. When hemorrhage occurs, as in Crimean-Congo hemorrhagic fever, hospital personnel should wear a gown and mask to prevent aerosol infection. For other bunyavirus infections, no quarantine, isolation, or concurrent disinfection is needed other than the precautions noted above.

REFERENCES

Benenson AS (ed): Control of Communicable Diseases in Man. 15th Ed. American Public Health Association, Washington, DC, 1990

Gear JHS (ed): Handbook of Viral and Rickettsial Hemorrhagic Fevers. CRC Press, Boca Raton, FL, 1988

Monath TP (ed): The Arboviruses: Epidemiology and Ecology. CRC Press, Boca Raton, FL, 1988

Shope RE: Arborvirus. In Lennette EH, Balows A, Hausler WJ Jr, Shadomy HJ (eds): Manual of Clinical Microbiology. 4th Ed. American Society for Microbiology, Washington, DC, 1985

57

ARENAVIRUSES

CHARLES J. PFAU

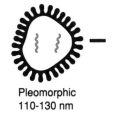

Pleomorphic
110-130 nm

GENERAL CONCEPTS

Clinical Manifestations

Most infections never go beyond "flu-like" illness, but sometimes these symptoms herald the onset of neurologic diseases or hemorrhagic fevers of varying severity.

Structure

The virus is round, oval, or pleomorphic, 110 to 130 nm in diameter, and enveloped. The genome consists of two distinct single-stranded viral RNA species, called L and S. Although the arenaviruses are considered to have antisense genomes, both segments actually are **ambisense:** the 3′ half is antisense, whereas the 5′ half is positive-sense. Cellular ribosomes appear to be incorporated into the virion.

Classification and Antigenic Types

Of the numerous arenaviruses known to infect animals, only four cause disease in humans: Lassa virus, Junin virus, Machupo virus, and lymphocytic choriomeningitis virus. All arenaviruses contain a set of internal cross-reacting antigens as well as species-specific envelope antigens.

Multiplication

Arenaviruses are thought to multiply like typical antisense RNA viruses (e.g., bunyaviruses).

Pathogenesis

Aerosol and respiratory spread are suspected. The gross pathology caused by these diseases is unimpressive and is of little help in explicating the pathogenetic mechanism.

Host Defenses

Interferon is induced by arenavirus infection, but is of questionable benefit. The humoral response is exceptionally slow. Cell-mediated immunity is probably of prime importance.

Epidemiology

The arenaviruses that affect humans exist in nature as benign infections in restricted rodent hosts; human disease is usually due to contact with rodent excreta.

Diagnosis

Differential clinical diagnosis is complex; the diagnosis is confirmed only by detecting a rise in antibody titers or by isolating the virus.

Control

Elimination of rodents is effective but often not practical; effective vaccines and antiviral agents (e.g., ribavirin) are becoming available.

751

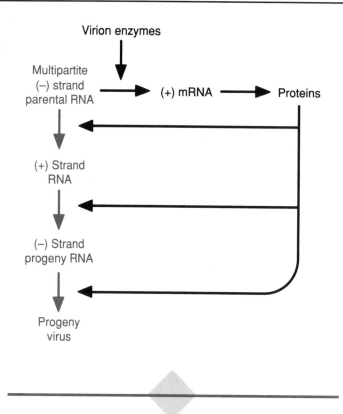

INTRODUCTION

The hallmark of arenaviruses is their tendency to cause persistent silent infections in their natural hosts (rodents) and severe, often lethal, disseminated disease in humans. Arenaviruses are pleomorphic enveloped particles that contain two RNA segments of virus origin and ribosomelike components. Suitable conditions for transmission of virus to humans occur in areas where humans ingest foods contaminated with rodent urine that contains virus. Persistent viremia and viruria in rodents result from a slow or insufficient immune response when immunologically immature fetuses or neonates are infected. In humans, the disease is acute.

There are four pathogens of humans, who are only accidental hosts. Three cause severe hemorrhagic fever with a mortality of about 15 percent among hospitalized patients in circumscribed areas (**Lassa virus** in West Africa, **Junin virus** in the Argentine pampas, and **Machupo virus** in Bolivia). The fourth, **lymphocytic choriomeningitis (LCM) virus,** is much more widely distributed, but causes milder infections, often neurologic.

CLINICAL MANIFESTATIONS

Only lymphocytic choriomeningitis, Junin, Machupo, and Lassa viruses have demonstrated natural disease potential. About 70 percent of human lymphocytic choriomeningitis virus infections are asymptomatic or so mild that they can not be distinguished from common respiratory or gastrointestinal illnesses. The more severe LCM infections present such a wide spectrum of manifestations that a typical case is difficult to describe. Nevertheless, headache, photophobia, listlessness, apathy, memory defects, confusion, and subtle mental difficulties are among the most common symptoms.

Even though this infection can be temporarily debilitating, it is rarely fatal, and even when neurologic involvement occurs, complete recovery is usually seen.

The clinical presentations of **Argentine hemorrhagic fever** (Junin virus), **Bolivian hemorrhagic fever** (Machupo virus), and **Lassa fever** (Lassa virus) are similar in several ways, yet sufficiently different to warrant brief mention. The incubation period is probably around 10 to 14 days (as is also true for lymphocytic choriomeningitis virus infections). Disease onset usually begins with insidious progression of general malaise and fever over a 2- to 4-day period. Progression beyond this stage is the norm for both Argentine and Bolivian hemorrhagic fevers, in contrast to Lassa fever. Hepatitis is unusual or mild in Argentine and Bolivian hemorrhagic fevers, whereas it is frequent and moderately severe in Lassa fever. With Lassa fever, marked elevations of serum glutamic oxaloacetic transaminase (SGOT) is associated with a poor prognosis. Hemorrhaging, neurologic signs and symptoms, and leukopenia and thrombocytopenia are much more common in Argentine and Bolivian hemorrhagic fever than in Lassa fever. Both increased hemoconcentration and urinary protein are associated with a high mortality in the two hemorrhagic fevers.

STRUCTURE

Arenaviruses appear in ultrathin sections as round, oval, or pleomorphic enveloped particles with a mean diameter of 110 to 130 nm. The viral envelope, which is acquired by budding through the host cell plasma membrane, carries club-shaped surface projections about 10 nm long. During morphogenesis, sandy-appearing granules resembling ribosomes are found within the unstructured interiors of nascent viruses. These particles give arenaviruses their name: *arena* is Latin for "sand." Highly purified arenaviruses appear to contain 18S and 28S host ribosomal RNAs. These RNAs have no required role in virus replication.

The viral RNA comes in two distinct segments or species, designated L and S. In general, arenavirus RNA is minus stranded. However, as with members of one genus of the Bunyaviridae (phleboviruses), an extraordinary situation exists with the S segment of lymphocytic choriomeningitis virus and of the New World arenavirus Pichinde virus. This molecule is **ambisense** (i.e., the 3′ half is of negative polarity and the 5′ half is positive); consequently, some viral proteins are encoded in subgenomic, virus-complementary mRNA species, whereas other proteins are encoded in subgenomic, virus-sense mRNA sequences. Most recently, the L segment of lymphocytic choriomeningitis virus has been shown also to be ambisense. Little is known about the genome structure of arenaviruses; this ambisense strategy of replication may well be shared by all.

CLASSIFICATION AND ANTIGENIC TYPES

All arenaviruses contain a distinctive set of internal cross-reacting antigens. Other antigens distinct for each species are primarily structures of the envelope. In the past, intraspecific differences were recognized by pathogenicity, but now they can also be determined by oligonucleotide fingerprints. Little is known about the molecular biology of arenvirus-cell interactions.

MULTIPLICATION

The multiplication of areanaviruses is not fully understood. They are thought to multiply like other viruses with multipartite antisense RNA genomes (e.g., the bunyaviruses).

PATHOGENESIS

The arenaviruses are not ordinarily contagious among humans, and they are nonpathogenic in their rodent hosts, but rodent-to-human infections can cause severe, sometimes fatal, disease (Fig. 57-1). This type of situation is not uncommon after interspecies transmission of viruses to humans, as with Marburg and Ebola viruses (see Ch. 41). However, it remains one of the central unresolved questions in arenavirus research. Perhaps infrequent exposure has prevented the weeding out of unsuitable immune response genes in

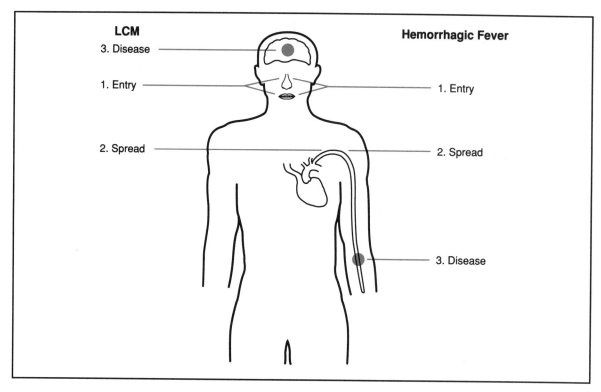

FIGURE 57-1   Pathogenesis of lymphocytic choriomeningitis (LCM) and hemorrhagic fevers.

populations that for 5,000 years have been subject to major epidemics caused by viruses. The explosive nature of some of the arenavirus diseases in clinical settings may indicate rapid attenuation of the viruses as human-to-human transmission occurs.

Although aerosol and respiratory spread are suspected, the portal of entry of arenaviruses and time course of their systemic distribution are uncertain. The onset of the hemorrhagic fevers caused by Lassa, Junin, and Machupo viruses may be insidious, with the disease presentation within 7 to 14 days after infection simply as pyrexia, headache, sore throat, and myalgia. Virus can be recovered from the blood and serum for up to 3 weeks after onset of the infection, and Lassa virus can be recovered from the urine for up to 5 weeks. Hemorrhagic phenomena, heralded by unremitting high fever, can begin after day 5 of illness and are followed by dehydration and hemoconcentration, shock syndrome, hemorrhagic manifestations, and cardiovascular collapse. The pantropic nature of these viruses is revealed by their presence in various dysfunctional organs.

Compared with the dramatic clinical course and mortality, the gross pathology is unimpressive and of little help in constructing a pathogenetic scheme. Complete autopsies have not been performed on patients with Lassa and Bolivian hemorrhagic fevers; however, autopsies performed on patients with Argentine hemorrhagic fever show a lack of deposited immunoglobulin and complement component C3 in the kidneys and small blood vessels. Mediators released from infected cells have a potential role in the pathogenesis of dysfunction of some target organs. Although lymphocytic choriomeningitis virus can produce severe human disease, characterized by prominent neurologic manifestations, pathologic lesions have not been studied extensively. However, in the mouse model the immune response against lymphocytic choriomeningitis virus (specifically in the

T cell compartment) is central to the development of fatal neurologic disease. Furthermore, mice infected with a lethal dose of this virus can invariably be saved by treatment with antibody to alpha/beta interferon.

HOST DEFENSES

Antibodies develop following overt human infection with arenaviruses and are detectable by enzyme-linked immunosorbent assay (ELISA), complement fixation, neutralization, and fluorescent antibody techniques. The humoral response is exceptionally slow, but ultimately a long-lasting and vigorous production of antibodies occurs. Usually, antibodies demonstrable by immunofluorescence are the first to appear, followed by complement-fixing antibodies. These complement-fixing antibodies are short-lived, with titers diminishing rapidly 6 to 12 months after onset. In contrast, neutralizing antibodies remain detectable for many years. Cell-mediated immunity is important in arenavirus infections of experimental animals; it is sometimes harmful, but is probably beneficial in human infections, at least for Lassa fever. In Lassa fever passive transfer of early-convalescent-phase human antibodies does not protect monkeys or guinea pigs, whereas late antibodies neutralize virus and are protective. Induction of alpha interferon has been found in patients with Argentine hemorrhagic fever. In general, arenaviruses are relatively resistant to the antiviral action of alpha/beta interferon. Interferon titers are significantly higher in fatal cases than in survivors (perhaps owing to higher levels of virus in the former). All evidence suggests that viral clearance in humans is complete and that chronic infection is not established. Reinfection with Lassa virus is possible, but appears to be uncommon.

EPIDEMIOLOGY

The arenaviruses exist in nature as benign infections in restricted rodent hosts (Fig. 57-2). The only exception is Tacaribe virus, which was isolated from *Artibeus* bats. In every case in which a human arenavirus disease has been studied, an interface between humans and rodents has been described;

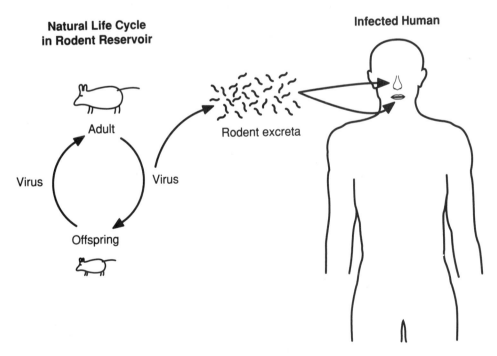

FIGURE 57-2 Transmission of arenaviruses from rodent reservoirs to humans.

the one common characteristic of these zoonotic infection patterns is human contact with rodent excreta. For example, Argentinian agricultural workers are exposed to Junin virus in maize fields when large numbers of reservoir rodents are disturbed by crop harvesting. In recent years, significant numbers of lymphocytic choriomeningitis infections have been attributed to silently infected pet hamsters and hamsters in biomedical laboratory colonies.

Frequent and explosive hospital-acquired infections in West Africa brought Lassa virus to the attention of the medical world 20 years ago. It is now clear that the virus is transmitted mostly at the village level and that most infections are mild or asymptomatic. For those sick enough to be admitted to the hospital, mortality is about 15 percent. Outside the hospital setting there can be an astonishingly high seroconversion rate (nearly 20 percent per year) and an even more perplexing reversion to seronegativity (about 6 percent). The case fatality rates associated with Junin and Machupo viruses range from 5 to 25 percent. Lymphocytic choriomeningitis virus, which is found worldwide in *Mus musculus* (the common field mouse), is considered to be the agent in about 5 percent of central nervous system infections of virus origin; these infections may be debilitating but are rarely fatal. The other arenaviruses—Amapari, Flexal, Ippy, Mobala, Mopeia, Latino, Parana, Pichinde, Tacaribe, and Tamiami—can cause infections in laboratory personnel, especially when high concentrations of virus are being processed.

DIAGNOSIS

Differential clinical diagnosis of the arenavirus hemorrhagic fevers is complex. The arenaviruses must be suspected if they are prevalent in geographic areas where infections have occurred and in regions known to harbor reservoir rodent species. Various diseases leading to sepsis, with disseminated intravascular coagulation and shock, can be confused with diseases caused by arenaviruses. Other viruses also must be considered along with lymphocytic choriomeningitis virus in differ-

ential diagnosis of aseptic meningitis. Junin and Machupo viruses are isolated primarily by intracerebral inoculation of newborn hamsters. Lassa virus is regularly isolated by inoculation of Vero cells. The most sensitive method for isolating lymphocytic choriomeningitis virus is intracerebral inoculation of weanling mice. If identification of specific viral antigens is the goal, antigen capture enzyme-linked immunosorbent assays (ELISA) are available.

All arenaviruses appear to share antigenic determinants in their ribonucleoproteins, as well as antigenically distinct determinants in their outer glycoproteins. Positive immunofluorescent staining of acetone-fixed infected cells is definitive for more than just family identification, since with limiting dilutions of antibody, Old World viruses (Lassa and lymphocytic choriomeningitis viruses) can be readily distinguished from New World viruses (Junin and Machupo viruses). Arenavirus species may be identified by their unique surface glycoproteins and infectivity neutralization.

CONTROL

A successful rodent control program in areas affected by Bolivian hemorrhagic fever has been described. Although elimination of rodents that shed virus has protected humans, it is not a reasonable long-term approach for other arenaviruses, because of the rodent ecology. A live attenuated Junin virus vaccine has now been tested in about 100 volunteers, with a resulting humoral and cell-mediated response frequency of more than 95 percent. Vaccines are still needed for the other pathogenic arenaviruses. Plasma from convalescent patients has become the single specific therapeutic adjunct for patients severely ill with Bolivian and Argentine hemorrhagic fevers. Use of plasma is not indicated yet for patients with Lassa fever. Physicians attending patients are convinced that such plasma is valuable if given during the first 8 days of disease, but more controlled trials are needed. At least seven seriologically distinct strains of Lassa virus have been isolated; animal studies suggest that effective therapy should involve geographic matching of immune plasma and virus strain. Early admission to the hospital, bed rest, oral hydration, sedation, and analgesia are important. In view of the frequency of Lassa virus transmission from person to person in a hospital setting, strict measures must be taken to isolate patients who have or are suspected to have the disease. Isolation of patients with the other pathogenic arenaviruses is also probably desirable.

Although several classes of antiviral compounds have been found with specific *in vitro* activity against arenaviruses, only ribavirin has been proven to be effective against Lassa fever in humans. It may be used at any point in the illness, as well as for postexposure prophylaxis.

REFERENCES

Bishop DHL (ed): The Arenaviridae. Plenum, New York, 1991

Howard CR: Arenaviruses. Elsevier, Amsterdam, 1986

Oldstone MBA: Arenaviruses—Genes, Proteins, and Expression. Springer-Verlag, Berlin, 1987

Oldstone MBA: Arenaviruses—Biology and Immunotherapy. Springer-Verlag, Berlin, 1987

Peters CJ: Arenaviruses. In Belshe R (ed): Textbook of Human Virology. 2nd Ed. PSG Publishing, Littleton, Mass, 1991

Pevear DC, Pfau CJ: Lymphocytic choriomeningitis virus. pgs 141–172. In Gilden DH, Lipton HL (eds): Clinical and Molecular Aspects of Neurotropic Virus Infection. Kluwer, Boston, 1989

58
ORTHOMYXOVIRUSES

ROBERT B. COUCH

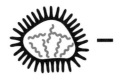

Helical, Pleomorphic
80-120 nm

GENERAL CONCEPTS

Clinical Manifestations

Classic influenza is a febrile illness of the upper and lower respiratory tract, characterized by sudden onset of fever, cough, myalgia, malaise, and other symptoms. Many patients do not exhibit the full syndrome. Pneumonia is the most common serious complication.

Structure

Influenza viruses are spherical or filamentous enveloped particles 80 to 120 nm in diameter. The helically symmetric nucleocapsid consists of a nucleoprotein and a multipartite genome of single-stranded antisense RNA in seven or eight segments. The envelope carries a hemagglutinin attachment protein and a neuraminidase.

Classification and Antigenic Types

Influenza viruses are divided into types A, B, and C on the basis of variation in the nucleoprotein antigen. In types A and B the hemagglutinin and neuraminidase antigens undergo genetic variation, which is the basis for the emergence of new strains; type C is antigenically stable.

Multiplication

The virus binds to host cells via the hemagglutinin. Transcription and nucleocapsid assembly take place in the nucleus. Progeny virions are assembled in the cytoplasm and bud from the cell membrane, killing the cell. In cells infected simultaneously with more than one parent virion, the genome segments may undergo reassortment.

Pathogenesis

The virus is transmitted in aerosols of respiratory secretions. It multiplies in the respiratory mucosa, causing cellular destruction and inflammation.

Host Defenses

Both a cell-mediated response and antibody develop after infection. Antibody provides long-lasting immunity against the infecting strain.

Epidemiology

Influenza epidemics occur each winter; worldwide pandemics appear irregularly. Changes in the hemagglutinin and neuraminidase surface antigens are responsible for the appearance of antigenically novel strains that evade host immunity.

Diagnosis

The diagnosis is suggested by the symptoms, particularly if an influenza epidemic is under way. Definitive diagnosis depends on detecting the virus or a rise in antibody titer.

Control

An inactivated virus vaccine is developed each year against the strains most likely to cause disease the next winter. The drug amantadine can be used for prophylaxis and treatment of influenza A infections.

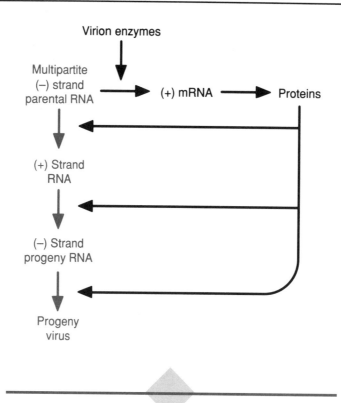

INTRODUCTION

The orthomyxoviruses (influenza viruses) constitute the genus *Orthomyxovirus,* which consists of three types (species): A, B, and C. These viruses cause influenza, an acute respiratory disease with prominent systemic symptoms. Pneumonia may develop as a complication and may be fatal, particularly in elderly persons with underlying chronic disease. Type A viruses cause periodic worldwide epidemics (pandemics); both types A and B cause recurring regional and local epidemics. Influenza epidemics have been recorded throughout history. In temperate climates, the epidemics typically occur in the winter and cause considerable morbidity in all age groups. An epidemic with associated mortality has occurred in most of the past 100 years. The worst of these was the 1918 pandemic, which caused about 20 million deaths worldwide and about 500,000 deaths in the United States.

CLINICAL MANIFESTATIONS

The classic influenza syndrome is a febrile illness of sudden onset, characterized by tracheitis and marked myalgias (Fig. 58-1). Headache, chills, fever, malaise, myalgias, anorexia, and sore throat appear suddenly. The fever rapidly climbs to 101 to 104°F (38.3 to 40.0°C), and respiratory symptoms ensue. A nonproductive cough is characteristic. Sneezing, rhinorrhea, and nasal obstruction are common. Patients may also report photophobia, hoarseness, nausea, vomiting, diarrhea, and abdominal pain. They appear acutely ill and are usually coughing. Minimal to moderate nasal obstruction, nasal discharge, and pharyngeal inflammation may be present. Lung examination is usually negative.

Most adults ill with an influenza virus infection do not display the classic syndrome described above. Moreover, the influenza syndrome is uncommon in children and is not seen in infants. A

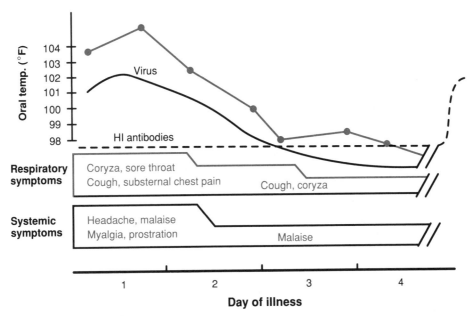

FIGURE 58-1   A case of acute uncomplicated influenza in a healthy 18-year-old college student.

given patient may exhibit symptoms including predominantly sneezing, nasal obstruction, and nasal discharge (common cold), nasal obstruction, discharge, and sore throat (upper respiratory illness); sore throat with erythema (pharyngitis); hoarseness (laryngitis); or cough (tracheobronchitis). Fever may be absent.

The respiratory and systemic symptoms of influenza generally last 1 to 5 days. Complications of influenza are many, but an influenza pneumonia, which can be extensive, and secondary bacterial pneumonia are the most common.

STRUCTURE

Influenza viruses are spherical and 80 to 120 nm in diameter, although filamentous forms may also occur. Figure 58-2 shows the structure of a type A or B influenza virus. The antisense RNA genome occurs in eight separate segments containing 10 genes. The segments are complexed with nucleoprotein to form a nucleocapsid with helical symmetry. The nucleocapsid is enclosed in an envelope consisting of a lipid bilayer and two surface glycoproteins, a **hemagglutinin** and a **neuraminidase.** Because influenza viruses are enveloped, they are readily inactivated by nonpolar solvents and by surface-active agents. The influenza C virus is less well studied, but is known to contain only seven RNA segments and a single surface glycoprotein.

CLASSIFICATION AND ANTIGENIC TYPES

Three influenza virus antigens—the nucleoprotein, the hemagglutinin, and the neuraminidase—are used in classification. The nucleoprotein antigen is stable and is used to differentiate the three influenza virus types. The nucleoprotein antigens of influenza viruses A, B, and C exhibit no serologic cross reactivity. The hemagglutinin and neuraminidase antigens, on the other hand, are variable. Antibody directed against these two surface antigens is responsible for immunity to infection.

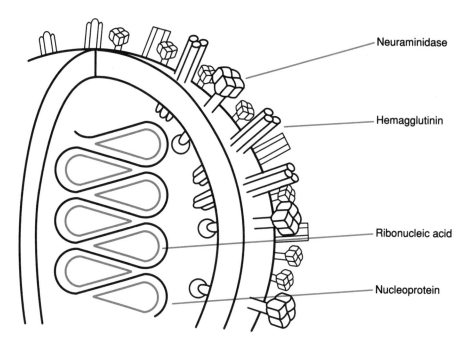

FIGURE 58-2 Diagrammatic representation of a segment of the influenza virus particle. Hemagglutinin and neuraminidase proteins protrude from the surface of the virus. The orientation of the nucleoprotein–RNA complex in the virion has not been fully elucidated.

MULTIPLICATION

Orthomyxovirus replication takes about 6 hours and kills the host cell. The viruses attach to permissive cells via the hemagglutinin subunit, which binds to cell membrane glycolipids or glycoproteins containing N-acetylneuraminic acid, the receptor for virus adsorption. The virus is then engulfed by pinocytosis into endosomes. The acid environment of the endosome causes the virus envelope to fuse with the plasma membrane of the endosome, uncoating the nucleocapsid and releasing it into the cytoplasm. The nucleocapsid is then transported to the nucleus, where the genome is transcribed by viral enzymes to yield viral mRNA. Unlike replication of other RNA viruses, orthomyxovirus replication depends on the presence of active host cell DNA. The virus scavenges cap sequences from the nascent mRNA generated in the nucleus by transcription of the host DNA and attaches them to its own mRNA. These cap sequences allow the viral mRNA to be transported to the cytoplasm, where it is translated by host ribosomes. The nucleocapsid is assembled in the nucleus. Virions acquire an envelope and undergo maturation as they bud through the host cell membrane. During budding, the viral envelope hemagglutinin is subjected to proteolytic cleavage by host enzymes. This process is necessary for the released particles to be infectious. Newly synthesized virions have surface glycoproteins that contain N-acetylneuraminic acid as a part of their carbohydrate structure, and thus are vulnerable to self-agglutination by the hemagglutinin. A major function of the viral neuraminidase is to remove these residues.

Gene Reassortment

Because the influenza virus genome is segmented, **genetic reassortment** can occur when a host cell is infected simultaneously with viruses of two different parent strains. If a cell is infected with two strains of type A virus, for example, some of the progeny virions will contain a mixture of genome segments from the two strains. This process of genetic reassortment probably accounts for the periodic appearance of the novel type A strains that cause influenza pandemics (see Epidemiology, below).

PATHOGENESIS

Influenza virus is transmitted from person to person primarily in droplets released by sneezing and coughing. Some of the inhaled virus lands in the lower respiratory tract, and the primary site of disease is the tracheobronchial tree, although the nasopharynx is also involved (Fig. 58-3). The neuraminidase of the viral envelope may act on the *N*-acetylneuraminic acid residues in mucus to produce liquefaction. In concert with mucociliary transport, this liquified mucus may help spread the virus through the respiratory tract. Infection of mucosal cells results in cellular destruction and desquamation of the superficial mucosa. The resulting edema and mononuclear cell infiltration of the involved areas are accompanied by such symptoms as nonproductive cough, sore throat, and nasal discharge. Although the cough may be striking, the most prominent symptoms of influenza are systemic: fever, muscle aches, and general prostration. Viremia is rare, so these systemic symptoms are not caused directly by the virus. Circulating interferon is a possible cause: administration of therapeutic interferon causes systemic symptoms resembling those of influenza.

Current evidence indicates that the extent of virus-induced cellular destruction is the prime factor determining the occurrence, severity, and duration of clinical illness. In an uncomplicated case, virus can be recovered from respiratory secretions for 3 to 8 days. Peak quantities of 10^4 to 10^7 infectious units/ml are detected at the time of maximal illness. After 1 to 4 days of peak shedding, the titer

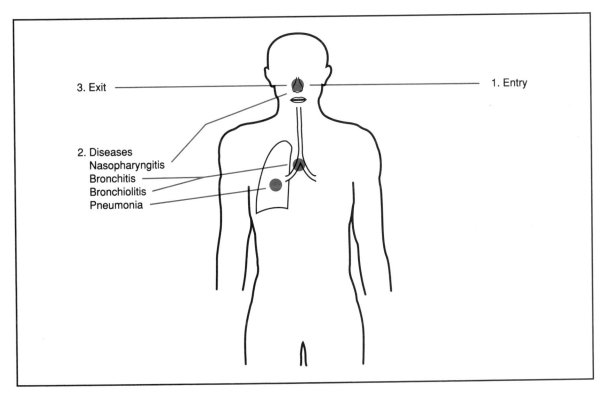

FIGURE 58-3 Pathogenesis of influenza.

begins to drop, in concert with the progressive abatement of disease.

Occasionally—particularly in patients with underlying heart or lung disease—the infection may extensively involve the alveoli, resulting in interstitial pneumonia, sometimes with marked accumulation of lung hemorrhage and edema. Pure viral pneumonia of this type is a severe illness with a high mortality. Virus titers in secretions are high, and viral shedding is prolonged. In most cases, however, pneumonia associated with influenza is caused by bacteria, principally pneumococci, staphylococci, and Gram-negative bacteria. These bacteria can invade and cause disease because the preceding viral infection damages the normal defenses of the lung.

HOST DEFENSES

The immune mechanisms responsible for recovery from influenza have not been clearly delineated. Several mechanisms probably act in concert. Interferon appears in respiratory secretions shortly after viral titers reach their peak level, and may play a role in the subsequent reduction in viral shedding. Antibody usually is not detected in serum or secretions until later in recovery or during convalescence; nevertheless, local antibody appears responsible for the final clearing of virus from secretions. T cells and antibody-dependent cell-mediated cytotoxicity also participate in clearing the infection.

Antibody is the primary defense in immunity to reinfection. IgG antibody, which predominates in lower respiratory secretions, appears to be the most important. The IgG in these secretions is derived from the serum, which accounts for the close correlation between serum antibody titer and resistance to influenza. IgA antibody, which predominates in upper respiratory secretions, is less persistent than IgG but also contributes to immunity.

Only antibody directed against the hemagglutinin is able to prevent infection. A sufficient titer of anti-hemagglutinin antibody will prevent infection. Lower titers of anti-hemagglutinin antibody lessen the severity of infection. Anti-hemagglutinin antibody administered after an infection is

under way reduces the number of infectious units released from infected cells, presumably because the divalent antibody aggregates many virions into a single infectious unit. Antibody directed against the neuraminidase also reduces the number of infectious units (and thus the intensity of disease), presumably by impairing the action of neuraminidase against N-acetylneuraminic acid residues in the virion envelope and thus promoting virus aggregation. Antibody directed against nucleoprotein has no effect on virus infectivity or on the course of disease.

Immunity to an influenza virus strain lasts for many years. Recurrent cases of influenza are caused primarily by antigenically different strains.

EPIDEMIOLOGY

A community experiences an influenza epidemic every year. Figure 58-4 shows the course of a typical epidemic of type A influenza in an urban community. In the initial phases of an epidemic, infection and illness appear predominantly in school-aged children, as indicated by a sharp rise in school absences, physician visits, and pediatric hospital admissions. These children bring the virus into the home, where preschool children and adults acquire infection. Infection and illness in adults are reflected in industrial absenteeism, adult hospital admissions, and an increase in mortality from influenza-related pneumonia. The epidemic generally lasts 3 to 6 weeks, although the virus is present in the community for a variable number of weeks before and after the epidemic. The highest attack rates during type A epidemics are in children 5 to 9 years old, although the rate is also high in preschool children and adults. Influenza B epidemics exhibit a similar pattern, except that the attack rates in preschool children and adults usually are lower and the epidemic may not cause an increase in mortality over the expected number of deaths ("excess mortality").

Although influenza virus types A and B (and probably C) cause illness every winter, an epidemic does not always develop. The constellation of factors that precipitate an epidemic are not fully understood, but the most important is a population susceptible to the circulating strains. Influenza can

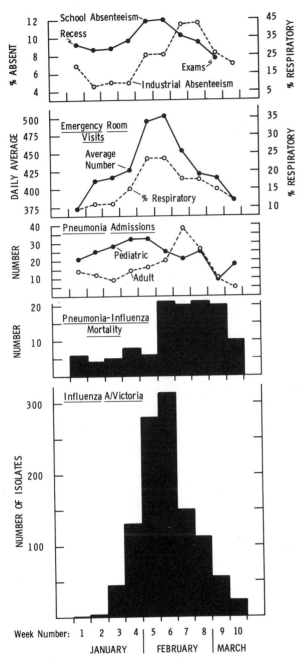

FIGURE 58-4 Correlation of nonvirologic indices of epidemic influenza with the number of isolates of influenza A/Victoria virus according to week in Houston during 1976. (Industrial absenteeism is indicated by the percentage with respiratory complaints.) (From Glezen WP, Couch RB: Interpandemic influenza in the Houston area, 1974–76. N Engl J Med 298:598, 1978, with permission.)

recur despite the development of immunity because type A and B viruses are proficient at altering their surface antigens and thus at generating strains that evade the existing immunity. Influenza strains are constantly appearing to which part or all of the human population is susceptible.

Influenza epidemics are of two types. Yearly epidemics are caused by both type A and type B viruses. The rare, severe influenza **pandemics** are always caused by type A virus. Two different mechanisms of antigenic change are responsible for producing the strains that cause these two types of epidemic. A *major* change in one or both of the surface antigens—a change that yields an antigen showing no serologic relationship with the antigen of the strains prevailing at the time—is called **antigenic shift.** Changes of this magnitude have been demonstrated in type A virus only and produce the strains responsible for influenza pandemics. Repeated *minor* antigenic changes, on the other hand, which generate strains that retain a degree of serologic relationship with the currently prevailing strain, are called **antigenic drift.** Antigenic drift occurs in both type A and type B influenza viruses and is responsible for the strains that cause yearly influenza epidemics. When persons are reinfected with drift viruses, the serum antibody responses to the surface antigens that are shared with earlier strains to which the person has been exposed are frequently stronger and of greater avidity than are the responses to the new antigens. This phenomenon, which has been called "original antigenic sin," is sometimes useful in serologic diagnosis.

Antigenic *drift* represents selection for naturally occurring variants under the pressure of population immunity. The completely novel antigens that appear during antigenic *shift,* in contrast, are acquired by gene reassortment. The donor of the new antigens is probably an animal influenza virus. Type A viruses have been identified in pigs, horses, and birds, and animal influenza viruses possessing antigens closely related to those of human viruses have been described. Thirteen distinct hemagglutinin and nine neuraminidase antigens are known. Since continued surveillance of animal influenza viruses in recent years has failed to discover new antigens, these may represent the full variety of major influenza virus surface antigens (subtypes).

Since the initial isolation of influenza viruses from swine in 1931 and from humans in 1933, the emergence and prevalence of human antigenic strains have been monitored. Table 58-1 shows the current classification and years of prevalence of the human viruses. New subtypes that arise spread around the world along transportation routes. A new virus can seed a population during the "off season" and may cause localized outbreaks, but epidemics generally do not begin until after school opens in the fall or during the succeeding winter.

DIAGNOSIS

A diagnosis of influenza is suggested by the clinical picture of sudden onset of fever, malaise, headache, marked muscle aches, sore throat, nonproductive cough, and coryza. When a syndrome resembling influenza occurs in the winter in an adult (the etiologies of illnesses of this type are more complex in children), an influenza virus is a likely cause. If an epidemic of febrile respiratory disease is known to be under way in the community, the diagnosis is yet more likely. Definitive diagnosis, however, relies on detecting either the virus or a significant rise in antibody titer between acute-phase and convalescent-phase sera.

Influenza virus is usually isolated from respiratory secretions by being grown in tissue cultures or chick embryos. Virus growth in tissue cultures is detected by testing for hemadsorption: red cells are added to the culture and adhere to virus budding from infected cells. If the culture tests positive, serologic tests with specific antisera may be used to identify the virus. In the chick embryo culture method, fluid from the amniotic or allantoic cavity of chick embryos is tested for the presence of newly formed viral hemagglutinin; the virus in positive fluids is then identified by hemagglutination inhibition tests with specific antisera. Finally, a rise in serum antibody titer between acute-phase and convalescent-phase sera can be identified by various tests, of which complement fixation, hemagglutination inhibition, and immunodiffusion (using specific viral antigens) are the most common. None of these techniques will identify all infections.

CONTROL

Prevention

Inactivated influenza virus vaccines have been used for about 40 years to prevent influenza. The viruses for the vaccine are grown in chick embryos, inactivated by formalin, purified to some extent, and adjusted to a dosage known to elicit an antibody response in most individuals. A given vaccine contains the strains of types A and B viruses that are judged most likely to produce epidemics during the following winter. The vaccine is administered parenterally in the fall; one or two doses are

TABLE 58-1 Classification of Human Influenza Viruses[a]

Type	Subtype	Years of Prevalence	Selected Variants*
A	H1N1	1918–1957	A/Puerto Rico/8/34
			A/FM/1/47
	H2N2 (Asian)	1957–1967	A/Singapore/1/57
	H3N2	1968–	A/Hong Kong/1/68
			A/Shanghai/16/89
	H1N1	1977–	A/USSR/90/77
			A/Taiwan/1/86
B	none defined	1940–	B/Yamagata/6/88
C	none defined	1949–	C/JHB/2/66

[a] Variants (drift) are monitored by using a reference strain described by subtype/geographic origin/strain number/year of isolation.

required, depending on the immune experience of the population with related antigens. Protection against illness has varied from 50 to 90 percent in civilian populations and from 70 to 90 percent in military populations. Local and systemic reactions to the vaccine are minor and occur in the first day or two after vaccination. During the national swine flu immunization of 1976 in the United States, an increased risk of developing Guillain-Barré syndrome accompanied vaccination; however, this correlation has not been detected since. Annual use of inactivated influenza virus vaccine is currently recommended in the United States for persons at risk of developing pneumonia from the disease and for their close associates. Live attenuated vaccines are being developed as alternatives to inactivated vaccine.

The synthetic drug amantadine hydrochloride effectively prevents infection and illness caused by type A, but not by type B, viruses. The drug interferes with virus uncoating. It prevents about 50 percent of infections and about 67 percent of illnesses under natural conditions. When administered for 10 days to household contacts of a person with influenza, it protects up to 80 percent of the persons from illness. Side effects are limited primarily to the central nervous system.

Treatment

Amantadine is the only specific antiviral treatment available for influenza. As in the case of prophylaxis, amantadine is effective only against type A virus. When administration is started early in the course of illness, the drug hastens the disappearance of fever and other symptoms.

REFERENCES

Beare AS (ed): Basic and Applied Influenza Research. CRC Press, Boca Raton, FL

Couch RB: Influenza: its control in persons and populations. J Infect Dis 153:431, 1986

International Conference on Asian Influenza. Am Rev Respir Dis 83:1, 1961

International Conference on Hong Kong Influenza. Bull WHO 41:335, 1969

Kilbourne ED: Influenza. Plenum, 1987

Krug RM (ed): The Influenza Virus. Plenum, New York, 1989

59

PARAMYXOVIRUSES

GISELA ENDERS

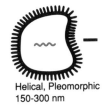

Helical, Pleomorphic
150-300 nm

GENERAL CONCEPTS

PARAMYXOVIRUSES

The family Paramyxoviridae consists of three genera: *Paramyxovirus*, which includes the parainfluenza viruses and mumps virus; *Pneumovirus*, which includes respiratory syncytial virus; and *Morbillivirus*, which includes the measles virus.

Structure

All paramyxoviruses are enveloped particles 150 to 300 nm in diameter. The tubelike, helically symmetrical nucleocapsid contains a monopartite, single-stranded, antisense RNA genome and an RNA-directed RNA polymerase. In parainfluenza viruses, viral protein spikes on the envelope have hemagglutinating and neuraminidase activities. Respiratory syncytial virus lacks both these activities, and measles virus lacks neuraminidase but has hemagglutinating activity.

Multiplication

The multiplication of all paramyxoviruses is similar to that of orthomyxoviruses except that the paramyxovirus genome is monopartite.

PARAINFLUENZA VIRUSES

Clinical Manifestations

Parainfluenza viruses cause mild or severe upper and lower respiratory tract infections, particularly in children.

Classification and Antigenic Types

Human parainfluenza viruses are divided into types 1, 2, 3, and 4; type 4 consists of A and B subtypes.

Pathogenesis

Transmission is by droplets or direct contact. The virus disseminates locally in the ciliated epithelial cells of the respiratory mucosa.

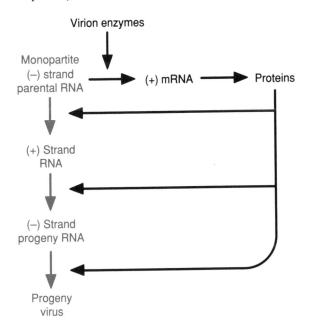

Host Defenses

Nonspecific defenses, including interferon, are followed by the appearance of secretory and humoral antibodies and cell-mediated immune responses.

Epidemiology

Parainfluenzavirus diseases occur worldwide; they are usually endemic but sometimes epidemic. Primary infections occur in young children; reinfection is common but results in milder disease.

Diagnosis

Clinical symptoms are nonspecific. Laboratory diagnosis is made by isolating the virus, by detecting viral antigen, or by detecting a rise in antibody titer.

Control

No vaccine is available.

RESPIRATORY SYNCYTIAL VIRUS

Clinical Manifestations

This virus causes upper and lower respiratory tract disease; the latter is most frequent in young children and is also significant in the elderly.

Classification and Antigenic Types

Respiratory syncytial viruses are divided into types A and B.

Pathogenesis

Transmission is by droplets or direct contact. The virus infects the ciliated epithelial cells of the respiratory mucosa and disseminates locally. Disease is caused partly by immunopathologic antibody-dependent cellular cytotoxicity.

Host Defenses

Nonspecific immune defenses, including interferon, are followed by the appearance of secretory and serum antibody and cell-mediated responses. Reinfection occurs, but the frequency and severity of disease decrease with age.

Epidemiology

This disease is found worldwide; in temperate climates, epidemics occur in winter and early spring and affect mainly infants and young children.

Diagnosis

Clinical symptoms are nonspecific; laboratory diagnosis

is made by isolating the virus or by detecting viral antigen, IgM, or IgA or a rising titer of IgG.

Control

There is no vaccine. Aerosolized ribavirin can be used for treatment if necessary. In hospital wards, infected patients may be isolated.

MUMPS VIRUS

Clinical Manifestations

Mumps is a systemic febrile infection of children and young adults. Swelling of the salivary glands, especially the parotid glands, is characteristic; meningitis is common, and encephalitis may occur. In adults, orchitis or oophoritis is not uncommon.

Classification and Antigenic Type

The single serotype of mumps virus shares antigens with parainfluenza viruses, particularly type 1.

Pathogenesis

The virus is spread in droplets. Primary infection consists of viremia and involvement of glandular and nervous tissue, resulting in inflammation and cell death.

Host Defenses

Interferon and other initial defenses are followed by specific cellular and humoral immune responses, which confer lifelong immunity.

Epidemiology

Mumps is found worldwide. It is endemic in cities but intermittent in rural areas, reappearing there every 2 to 7 years as an epidemic. Incidence peaks from January to May.

Diagnosis

In typical cases, the clinical picture is diagnostic. Atypical cases are diagnosed by isolating the virus, by detecting viral antigen in saliva or cerebrospinal fluid, or by detecting specific IgM or a rising titer of IgG.

Control

Vaccination with live attenuated mumps virus vaccine gives long-lasting immunity, but reinfection may occur.

MEASLES VIRUS

Clinical Manifestations

Measles sets in abruptly with coryza, conjunctivitis, fever, and rash. The typical maculopapular rash appears

1 to 3 days later. Complications include otitis, pneumonia, and encephalitis. Subacute sclerosing panencephalitis is a rare late sequela.

Classification and Antigenic Type

There is only a single antigenic type.

Pathogenesis

The virus causes viremia and multiplies in cells of the lymphatic and respiratory systems, the skin, and sometimes the brain.

Host Defenses

Interferon and other initial defenses are followed by specific cellular and humoral immune responses, which confer long-lasting immunity.

Epidemiology

Measles occurs worldwide in an endemic or epidemic pattern. Incidence peaks in the late winter and early summer.

Diagnosis

In typical cases, the clinical picture is diagnostic. Atypical cases are diagnosed by isolating the virus or by detecting specific IgM or a rising titer of IgG.

Control

Active vaccination with a live attenuated virus vaccine gives long-lasting protection. Passive prophylaxis with measles immunoglobulin is used to prevent disease in susceptible, exposed individuals.

INTRODUCTION

The family Paramyxoviridae consists of three genera: *Paramyxovirus, Pneumovirus,* and *Morbillivirus* (Table 59-1). All members of the genus *Paramyxovirus* share similar properties. *Pneumoviruses* lack hemagglutinin and neuraminidase activity. They also differ from other paramyxoviruses in morphology (diameter of nucleocapsid and surface projections). *Morbillivirus* is distinguished by the absence of neuraminidase in the virions and by presence of common envelope and nucleocapsid antigens in the species listed in Table 59-1.

PARAINFLUENZA VIRUSES

CLINICAL MANIFESTATIONS

Parainfluenza viruses cause approximately 30 to 40 percent of all acute respiratory infections in infants and children. The spectrum of disease ranges from a mild, afebrile common cold to severe, potentially life-threatening croup, bronchiolitis, and pneumonia. These viruses are the most common identifiable agents of croup and are sur-

TABLE 59-1 Human Paramyxoviruses

Genus	Species	Distinguishing Properties
Paramyxovirus	Parainfluenza virus types 1, 2, 3, 4A, and 4B, mumps virus	Contains neuraminidase and hemagglutinin; distinctive antigens
Pneumovirus	Respiratory syncytial virus	Lacks neuraminidase and hemagglutinin; morphology; distinctive antigens
Morbillivirus	Measles virus	Lacks neuraminidase; distinctive antigens

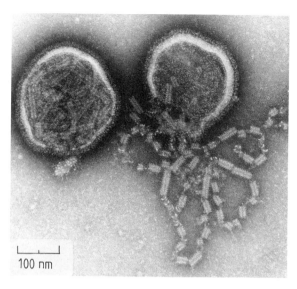

100 nm

FIGURE 59-1 Parainfluenza virus type 1, Sendai strain. An intact virion and a disintegrating particle with free nucleocapsid fragments. (Courtesy of June Almeida, The Wellcome Research Laboratories, Beckenham, England.)

passed only by respiratory syncytial virus as the cause of severe lower respiratory tract disease in infants. Reinfection, causing milder upper respiratory illness, is common in older children and adults.

STRUCTURE

The virions are enveloped particles with an average diameter of 120 to 300 nm. The complete virion consists of a nucleocapsid and an envelope (Fig. 59-1). The 18-nm-wide nucleocapsid is a tubelike structure with helical symmetry. It contains one piece of single-stranded antisense RNA (molecular weight about 5×10^6 to 6×10^6), the nucleoprotein, and an RNA-dependent RNA polymerase, which is necessary for transcription of viral RNA. The envelope is a double-layered membrane covered with spikes. It contains lipoproteins and glycoproteins, as well as glycolipids derived mainly from the host cell. Also, a nonglycosylated membrane protein is attached to the inner side of the envelope. The surface glycoproteins that form the spikes contain the hemagglutination, neuraminidase, cell fusion, and hemolysis activities of the virus. Hemagglutination and neuraminidase activities are located at different sites on the same glycoprotein molecule (HN). The fusion activity is found in a separate fusion (F) glycoprotein. The F protein lyses the cell membrane, leading to cell fusion and formation of syncytia.

CLASSIFICATION AND ANTIGENIC TYPES

Among the paramyxoviruses four human parainfluenza serotypes are now recognized: 1, 2, 3, and 4. Type 4 occurs in two subtypes (A and B), which possess common internal but different capsid antigens.

MULTIPLICATION

Parainfluenza viruses attach to the host cell by the hemagglutinin, which binds to the host cell neuraminic acid receptor, and then penetrate the cell by fusion with the cell membrane mediated by the F protein. The viral genome is a single-stranded antisense RNA that cannot act as mRNA. The virion contains an RNA polymerase that transcribes the genome to yield sense RNA strands that both direct viral protein synthesis and are copied into antisense genomic RNA strands, which are integrated in the new virions. For envelopment, the virus-specific glycoproteins accumulate in the cell membrane. Assembly is completed by budding of the nucleocapsid through the cell membrane studded with glycoproteins.

PATHOGENESIS

The parainfluenza viruses generally initiate localized infections in the upper and lower respiratory tracts without causing systemic infection (Fig. 59-2), although viremia may occur. Local and serum antibodies develop after primary infection. The resulting immunity is not adequate to prevent reinfection, but does provide some protection against disease.

These viruses first infect the ciliated epithelial cells of the nose and throat. Infection may extend to the paranasal sinuses, the middle ear, and occasionally to the lower respiratory tract. Progeny viruses spread among cells both extracellularly and

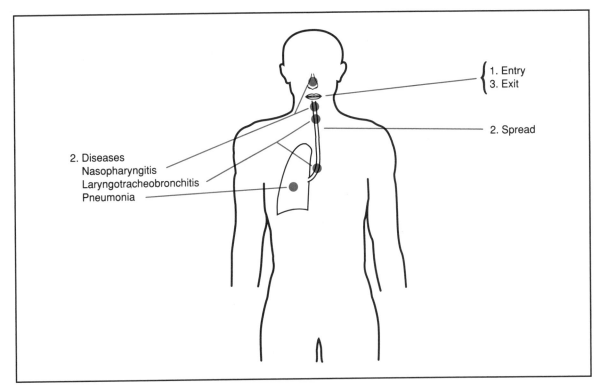

FIGURE 59-2 Pathogenesis of paramyxovirus and respiratory syncytial virus infections.

intracellularly. Virus is shed in the respiratory secretions for 3 to 16 days. Shedding starts shortly
before the onset of disease and ends with development of local antibody. The main pathogenic
change is an inflammatory response in the superficial layers of the mucous membranes.

The most characteristic and important clinical
syndromes associated with parainfluenza virus infection are croup, bronchiolitis, and pneumonia.
The most severe manifestation of infection with
type 1 and 2 viruses is croup, whereas type 3 virus
causes all three syndromes. Croup caused by parainfluenza virus is not distinguishable from that
caused by other viruses such as respiratory syncytial virus or measles virus.

HOST DEFENSES

Nonspecific defenses (including interferon) may
contribute to resistance against human parainfluenza viruses. The immunologic events during and
after natural infection with parainfluenza viruses

in infants and children are not well understood.
Type-specific secretory and humoral immune responses occur, but protection does not last, since
reinfection with the same serotype may occur
within 3 months to several years after primary infection. The degree of resistance to reinfection
and, even more, to clinical disease seems to depend
mainly on the concentration of secretory IgA antibodies that possess neutralizing activity. Neutralizing IgA is found in infants and young children only
for a short time after primary infection. Serum
antibodies usually are not significant in resistance
to reinfection with the nonsystemic respiratory viruses, but their presence in high titers may restrict
local virus multiplication and disease manifestation. Passive maternal antibodies do not protect
against infection; however, they appear to prevent
disease manifestations with types 1 and 2 virus, but
not type 3 virus, in infants. Also, maternal antibodies may suppress the immune response following
primary infection.

EPIDEMIOLOGY

The parainfluenza viruses are distributed world-wide, causing infection and illness in young children. These virus infections are endemic, sometimes reaching epidemic proportions. The source of human parainfluenza virus infection is the respiratory tract of humans; the incubation period ranges from 2 to 6 days. In primary infection, the duration of contagion ranges from 3 to 16 days. During reinfections, the contagious periods become progressively shorter. Parainfluenza viruses are transmitted by direct person-to-person contact and by the airborne route through large droplets. Only a small inoculum is required to infect. However, parainfluenza viruses are labile and do not persist in the environment. They are spread mainly by infants and preschool children with only mild signs of infection. Serologic surveys show that most 5-year-old children have antibodies for types 1, 2, and 3 virus.

DIAGNOSIS

Diagnosis based on clinical manifestations is not possible. Laboratory diagnosis can be made by isolating the virus in tissue culture. More rapid diagnosis involves fluorescent-antibody staining of nasopharyngeal cells, or detection of viral antigens and/or antibodies in sonicated nasopharyngeal specimens by indirect radioimmunoassay (RIA) and enzyme-linked immunosorbent assay (ELISA).

Serologic evidence of infection may be obtained by demonstrating a significant rise in antibody titer between two serum samples. Serodiagnosis by these means is hampered by the heterotypic anamnestic responses to previous parainfluenza and mumps virus infection. A rapid and usually reliable type-specific serodiagnosis of acute infection can be made when significant levels of the transient IgM antibodies are found in a single serum sample.

CONTROL

Cross-infection with parainfluenza virus types 1 and 3 is common in hospital wards and day care centers. It can be prevented by strict isolation. Re-

cent techniques that allow rapid diagnosis facilitate such control.

Active immunization against parainfluenza viruses is desirable but not yet available. Experimental killed vaccines are not effective. Experimental live virus vaccines have failed to induce protective secretory antibody levels. Passive prophylaxis with human immunoglobulin in exposed infants is not indicated, because it may dampen an active serum antibody response. Ribavirin has been documented to exhibit activity in vitro against parainfluenza virus, and recent reports indicate that it has clinical efficacy in humans.

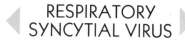

RESPIRATORY SYNCYTIAL VIRUS

CLINICAL MANIFESTATIONS

Most respiratory syncytial virus infections lead to illnesses ranging from mild upper respiratory disease to life-threatening lower respiratory tract illness (e.g., bronchiolitis and pneumonitis) in infants and young children, among whom respiratory syncytial virus is the most important serious lower respiratory tract pathogen. It is also an important cause of otitis media in young children. It can infect the middle ear directly or predispose to bacterial superinfection. Older children and adults usually have common cold symptoms. In the elderly, respiratory syncytial virus can again be a significant lower respiratory tract pathogen.

STRUCTURE

Respiratory syncytial virus has a linear single-stranded RNA of about 5×10^6 daltons, which encodes 10 proteins. The RNA is surrounded by a helical nucleocapsid, which in turn is surrounded by an envelope of pleomorphic structure. Virions range from 100 to 350 nm in diameter. Respiratory syncytial virus has neither hemagglutinin nor neuraminidase activity. The virion contains distinct proteins. Two of the proteins are the large glycoprotein (G) and the fusion protein (F) that form external projections on the surface of the virus envelope. The membrane protein (M) is located on the inner side of the envelope. The major nucleocapsid protein (N) and phosphoprotein (P) form the nucleocapsid of the virion.

CLASSIFICATION AND ANTIGENIC TYPES

Respiratory syncytial virus belongs to a separate genus, *Pneumovirus*, because of its distinctive surface projections, nucleocapsid diameter, molecular weight of the N and P proteins, lack of hemagglutinin and neuraminidase activity, and differences in number and order of its genes. Its host range is limited in vivo to humans and chimpanzees.

MULTIPLICATION

After absorption, penetration, and uncoating, the respiratory syncytial virus genome serves as a template for the production of 10 different mRNA species and a full-length, positive-sense complementary RNA (cRNA). The mRNAs serve as the template for translation of viral proteins. The full-length, cRNA serves as a template for transcription of virion RNA. Within 10 to 24 h after infection, projections of viral proteins appear on the cell surface, and virions bud through the cell membrane incorporating part of the cell membrane into their envelope.

PATHOGENESIS

Respiratory syncytial virus generally initiates a localized infection in the upper or lower respiratory tract or both (Fig. 59-2). The degree of illness varies with the age and immune status of the host.

Initially, the virus infects the ciliated mucosal epithelial cells of the nose, eyes, and mouth. Infection generally is confined to the epithelium of the upper respiratory tract, but may involve the respiratory tract. The virus spreads both extracellularly and by fusion of cells to form syncytia. Thus humoral antibodies that do not penetrate intracellularly cannot completely restrict infection. The virus is shed in respiratory secretions usually for

about 5 days and sometimes for as long as 3 weeks. Shedding begins with the onset of symptoms and declines with the appearance of local antibody.

The most important clinical syndromes caused by respiratory syncytial virus are bronchiolitis and pneumonia in infants, croup and tracheobronchitis in young children, and tracheobronchitis and pneumonia in the elderly. Conjunctivitis, otitis media, and various exanthems involving the trunk or face or both are occasionally seen in primary and secondary infections.

Bronchiolitis is inflammatory, and pneumonia is interstitial. The pathogenesis of bronchiolitis may be immunologic or directly viral.

HOST DEFENSES

Nonspecific defenses such as virus-inhibitory substances in secretions and interferon production probably contribute to resistance to and recovery from respiratory syncytial virus infection. Age, immunologic competence, and physical condition also appear to be important. Data on the development, persistence, and effectiveness of specific cell-mediated and secretory immunity in first and repeat infections are still fragmentary. Although secretory and serum antibody responses occur, immunity does not protect completely against reinfection and repeat illness, which may occur as early as a few weeks after recovery from the first infection.

Resistance to reinfection and repeat illness seems to depend mainly on the presence of neutralizing antibody activity on the mucosal surfaces. There is increasing evidence that humoral antibody contributes to protection from lower but not upper respiratory tract infection.

EPIDEMIOLOGY

Respiratory syncytial virus is distributed worldwide, causing infection and illness in infants and young children. The infection is endemic, reaching epidemic proportions every year. In temperate climates, these epidemics occur each winter and last 4 to 5 months, with peaks mainly from January to March. Estimates for urban settings suggest that about one-half of the susceptible infants undergo primary infection in each epidemic. The infection is almost universal by the second birthday. Reinfection may occur as early as a few weeks after recovery, but usually takes place during subsequent annual outbreaks, with a rate of 10 to 20 percent per epidemic throughout childhood. In adults, the frequency of reinfection is lower.

The source of human respiratory syncytial virus infection is the respiratory tract of humans. The incubation period for the disease is about 4 days. As noted above, primary infections are contagious from about 5 days to 3 weeks, with greatest virus shedding in the first 4 to 5 days after onset of symptoms. The contagious periods become progressively shorter during reinfections. The virus is transmitted by direct person-to-person contact and by the airborne route through droplet spread. It is probably introduced into families by schoolchildren undergoing reinfection. Secondary spread is to younger siblings and parents. In hospital and institutional settings, mildly symptomatic infected adults also spread the infection. Respiratory syncytial virus readily infects infants during the first few months of life despite the presence of maternal serum antibodies. Thus, the age at which first infection takes place depends primarily on the opportunity for exposure. Sex and socioeconomic factors appear also to influence the outcome of infection.

DIAGNOSIS

In infants with lower respiratory tract disease, respiratory syncytial virus infection can be strongly suspected on the basis of the time of year, the presence of a typical outbreak, and the family epidemiology. Aside from this virus, only parainfluenza virus type 3 attacks infants with any frequency during the first few months of life.

Definite diagnosis of infection (of practical importance in ruling out bacterial involvement) rests on the virology laboratory. The diagnosis is made within 4 to 8 days by isolating the virus from nasal secretions in tissue culture or within hours by using fluorescent antibody staining of infected nasal epithelial cells or by antigen detection in the secretion by enzyme-linked immunosorbent assay and radioimmunoassay.

Serologic evidence of respiratory syncytial virus infection may be obtained by detecting either seroconversion or a significant antibody rise in IgG antibodies between acute- and convalescent-phase sera. Since respiratory syncytial virus IgM can remain positive for several months, a positive result does not confirm a current infection. Recent studies have shown that IgA determination is more sensitive for diagnosis than is detection of IgM antibodies.

CONTROL

It is nearly impossible to prevent respiratory syncytial virus transmission in the home setting. In hospital wards, cross-infection may be restricted by isolation and sanitation. Vaccines are being studied, but active immunization is not likely to be achieved in the near future. Treatment of infections has recently become available. Aerosolized ribavirin can decrease the titer of virus excreted and speed improvement in clinical symptoms and arterial oxygenation.

◄ MUMPS VIRUS ►

CLINICAL MANIFESTATIONS

Mumps is a common acute disease of children and young adults that is characterized by a nonpurulent inflammation of the salivary glands, especially the parotids. Severe manifestations may include meningitis and encephalitis at any age and orchitis or oophoritis in adults. Most disease manifestations are benign and self-limiting. Both symptomatic and asymptomatic mumps virus infections usually induce lifelong immunity.

STRUCTURE

Mumps virus shares many properties with the other paramyxoviruses. The single antisense RNA strand is surrounded by a helical nucleocapsid made of a nucleocapsid protein (NP). The RNA-dependent RNA polymerase is located in the nucleocapsid, which has a unit length of 1 μm and a diameter of 17 nm. The coiled nucleocapsid is surrounded by a lipid-containing envelope, which gives the virion a diameter of 120 to 200 nm. Five major structural proteins, HN, F, NP, P, and M, have been identified in the virus. The envelope contains the matrix (M) protein and two surface glycoproteins, the hemagglutinin-neuraminidase (HN) and the cell-fusing (F) and hemolytic protein. The F and HN proteins form two different kinds of projections and are the targets for protective antibodies.

CLASSIFICATION AND ANTIGENIC TYPE

Mumps virus belongs to the genus *Paramyxovirus* and exhibits most characteristics of the Paramyxoviridae. It occurs only in a single serotype and shares minor common envelope antigens with other *Paramyxovirus* species.

MULTIPLICATION

The replication of mumps virus is not understood in great detail. Like other paramyxoviruses, mumps virus initiates infection by attaching to cel-

lular mucoprotein receptors and penetrating the cell by fusion. Following uncoating, the antisense viral RNA is transcribed by the RNA-dependent RNA polymerase of the virus into a sense RNA strand, which directs the synthesis of viral proteins. The order in which the structural genes are transcribed has been established in mumps virus, as in other paramyxovirus. The first proteins that are detectable in the infected cell are the internal proteins of the mature virus, NP and P. The final step of maturation is budding of the virus from the cell membrane at about 20 h postinfection.

PATHOGENESIS

Mumps virus causes a systemic generalized infection that is spread by viremia with involvement of glandular and nervous tissues as target organs (Fig. 59-3). The infecting virus probably enters the body through the pharynx or the conjunctiva. Local multiplication of the virus at the portal of entry and possibly a primary viremia precedes a secondary viremia, lasting 2 to 3 days. The incuba-

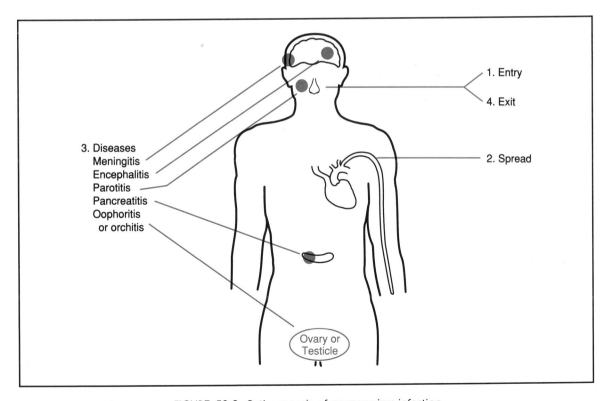

FIGURE 59-3 Pathogenesis of mumps virus infection.

tion period usually is 18 to 21 days, but may extend from 12 to 35 days. Recognizable symptoms do not appear in 35 percent of infected individuals. The virus is carried to the main target organs (various salivary glands, testes, ovaries, pancreas, and brain). Viral replication takes place in the ductal cells of the glands. It is not known how the virus spreads to the central nervous system. Studies in experimental animals suggest that indirect spread occurs by passage of infected mononuclear cells across the epithelium of the plexus to the epithelial cells of the plexus choroideus. Alternatively, direct spread of virus is possible.

Shedding of the virus in salivary gland secretions begins about 6 days before onset of symptoms and continues for another 5 days, even though local secretory IgA and humoral antibodies become detectable during that time. Insignificant shedding occurs in conjunctival secretions and urine. During the first 2 days of illness, the virus may be recovered from blood. In cases of meningitis or early-onset encephalitis, virus can be detected in cerebrospinal fluid and cells during the first 6 days after onset of disease. The virus may persist in tissues for 2 to 3 weeks after the acute stage, despite the presence of circulating antibodies. The main pathogenic changes induced by mumps virus infection in the salivary glands and the pancreas are inflammatory reactions. When the testes are involved, swelling, interstitial hemorrhage, and focal infarcts (leading to atrophy of the germinal epithelium) may occur. Infection of the pancreas disturbs endocrine and exocrine functions, leading to diabetic manifestations and increased serum amylase levels. Mumps virus infection of the pancreas has been reported to be associated with onset of juvenile diabetes; however, a causal relationship has not been established.

The pathologic reaction to mumps virus infection of brain tissues is generally an aseptic meningitis. Less often, the infection involves the brain neurons (as in early-onset mumps encephalitis). Histopathologic findings are widespread and include neuronolysis and ependymitis, which may lead to deafness and obstructive hydrocephalus in children. One human case of chronic central nervous system mumps virus infection has been de-

scribed. The late-onset (postinfectious) type of mumps encephalitis is attributed to autoimmune reactions. Histopathologic findings are characterized by perivascular accumulation of mononuclear leukocytes, demyelinization, and overgrowth of glial cells, with relative sparing of the neurons. These findings resemble those seen in postinfectious measles, rubella, and varicella encephalitis.

The most characteristic clinical feature of mumps virus infection is the edematous, painful enlargement of one or both of the parotid glands. Commonly, the submandibular salivary glands are involved and, less frequently, the sublingual glands. Pancreatitis is uncommon as a severe illness. Epididymo-orchitis develops in 23 percent of infected postpubertal males and may lead to atrophy of the affected testicles, although rarely to total sterility. Oophoritis develops in 5 percent of infected postpubertal women. Mumps meningitis occurs in up to 10 percent of patients with or without parotitis. Encephalitis has been reported to occur in 1 in 400 cases of mumps. Transient high-frequency deafness is the most common complication (4 percent), and permanent unilateral deafness occurs infrequently (0.005 percent).

HOST DEFENSES

Mumps virus infection is followed rapidly by interferon production and then by specific cellular and humoral immune responses. Interferon limits virus spread and multiplication, and its production ceases as virus levels decrease and humoral antibodies and cell-mediated immunity appear. Little is known about cell-mediated immunity to mumps virus; in contrast, the humoral antibody response is well understood.

IgM class-specific antibodies to mumps antigens develop rapidly within the first 3 days after onset of symptoms and persist for approximately 2 to 3 months. The IgG antibodies appear a few days later and persist for life. Circulating antibodies are responsible for the lifelong protection against recurrent disease, but reinfection may occur. Parainfluenza virus infections, particularly with type 1 virus, cause a rise of mumps antibody titers, contributing to the lifelong stability of the mumps antibody. Protective mumps antibody of the IgG class is transplacentally transferred to the newborn and persists in declining titers during the first 6 months of life.

EPIDEMIOLOGY

Mumps occurs worldwide. In urban areas, the infection is endemic with a peak incidence between January and May. Local outbreaks are common wherever large numbers of children and young adults are concentrated (institutions, boarding schools, and military camps). Epidemics occur every 2 to 7 years. In rural areas, mumps tends to die out until enough susceptible individuals have accumulated and the virus is reintroduced. Humans are the only known hosts.

Infection is transmitted by salivary gland secretions, mainly just before and shortly after clinical onset. In asymptomatic infections, peak contagion occurs within a similar period. Mumps virus is transmitted usually by direct and close person-to-person contact and less often by the airborne route. School children (6 to 14 years old) are the main source of spread. Mumps infection is acquired later in childhood than are other paramyxovirus infections; 95 percent of individuals have antibody by age 15. As already mentioned, 35 percent of these infections are subclinical. In remote areas, a much lower percentage of children may be infected.

Active vaccination in the United States has reduced the incidence of reported mumps and mumps complications by more than 90 percent.

DIAGNOSIS

Typical cases of mumps involving the salivary glands can usually be diagnosed without laboratory tests. An etiologic diagnosis of other clinical manifestations without parotitis (e.g., meningitis, encephalitis, orchitis, and oophoritis) requires laboratory confirmation. Acute infections can be diagnosed by isolating the virus from saliva or urine (or cerebrospinal fluid when appropriate), usually in tissue culture over several days or, more rapidly, by detecting specific antigen in infected specimens by immunofluorescence, enzyme-linked immunosorbent assay, or radioimmunoassay. Serologic evidence of acute infection can be obtained early by demonstrating IgM antibodies in the first serum specimen and later by detecting a significant IgG antibody rise in paired sera.

CONTROL

In view of the long period of virus shedding and the 35 percent rate of subclinical infection, isolating patients with typical symptoms does little to prevent spread. Passive prophylaxis with mumps immunoglobulin prior to viremia is used for individuals at high risk, such as children with underlying disease, those in hospital wards, postpubertal males, and pregnant women. New serologic techniques (e.g., enzyme-linked immunosorbent assay) assess immunity in 4 hours so that immunoglobulin is given only to exposed seronegative (susceptible) individuals.

Active immunization against mumps is recommended for all children at 15 months of age. A combined live virus vaccine is available for mumps, measles, and rubella. The mumps component contains attenuated virus grown in chick embryo tissue culture. It is well tolerated and safe and usually is effective only when maternal antibodies are absent. The vaccine-induced antibody titers are initially much lower than those following natural infection. This antibody protects against clinical disease but not against reinfection. Long-term vaccine-induced immunity seems to be maintained by inapparent (and sometimes also by apparent) reinfection with mumps wild-type virus and infections with other parainfluenza viruses.

No specific drugs or therapeutic measures are available for treatment of mumps virus infection. Management is purely symptomatic. Fortunately, disease manifestations generally are self-limited, and death is rare.

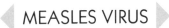

MEASLES VIRUS

CLINICAL MANIFESTATIONS

Measles virus usually causes, in the nonvaccinated population, an acute childhood disease characterized by coryza, conjunctivitis, fever, and rash. The disease usually is benign but can be dangerous, causing pneumonia and acute encephalitis. Defective measles virus persisting after natural infection may later cause subacute sclerosing panencephalitis and possibly other chronic neurologic diseases. A live vaccine has markedly reduced the incidence of disease in developed countries, but measles remains a major health problem in developing countries.

STRUCTURE

Measles virus has the structure of the family Paramyxoviridae, consisting of spherical, enveloped particles with a central helical nucleocapsid. The diameter of the pleomorphic particles varies between 100 and 250 nm. The nucleocapsid contains the genome, a single piece of single-stranded antisense RNA (molecular weight 7×10^6), three structural proteins, and an RNA-dependent RNA polymerase. The envelope, covered with spikes, contains a bimolecular lipid layer of cellular origin with the matrix protein (M) attached on its inside. The spikes are formed by two transmembranous proteins. One kind of polypeptide in the envelope is involved in hemagglutination (H), and the other kind in hemolytic and cell fusion (F) activities. All of the six different structural components of the virus can serve as antigens. Virion infectivity is lost readily when the envelope is disrupted spontaneously and when the virus is treated with lipid solvents or subjected to one of several chemical and physical reactions.

CLASSIFICATION AND ANTIGENIC TYPE

Measles virus is a member of the genus *Moribillivirus* (Table 59-1). It differs from other paramyxoviruses in lacking neuraminidase and in having hemagglutination activity restricted to monkey erythrocytes. Measles virus and the other moribiliviruses occur only as one cross-reactive antigenic type.

The natural disease is limited to humans and monkeys. In vitro, the host range of measles virus is human, monkey, and canine kidney cell cultures and embryonated eggs.

MULTIPLICATION

Measles virus multiplies like the other members of the family Paramyxoviridae. Attachment of particles to the cell surface is followed by fusion of the virus envelope and the cytoplasmic membranes and penetration of the nucleocapsid structures into the cytoplasm. The antisense RNA is transcribed by the nucleocapsid-associated polymerase. The order of genes in terms of their products is nucleoprotein (NP), phosphoprotein (P), M, FH, and a gene directing the synthesis of a large (L) protein. The P gene also gives rise to a nonstructural protein named C. The virion RNA serves not only as a template for production of RNA, but also for replication of intact RNA via a sense-stranded intermediate. After the accumulation of new genomic RNA and the different structural proteins in the cell cytoplasm, maturation takes place by budding of the virus from the cell. The cell membrane is modified by attachment of N-linked carbohydrate chains of cellular origin before virus transmembranous proteins appear at the cell surface.

The release of viral particles from single cells varies from a few hours, if the cells succumbs rapidly to cytopathology, to an unlimited time in chronic, steady-state infections. Development of chronic infections and disease may be caused by highly defective virus variants that do not express any viral antigen at the cell surface.

PATHOGENESIS

Measles virus causes a systemic infection, disseminated by viremia, with acute disease manifestations involving the lymphatic and respiratory systems, the skin, and sometimes the brain (Fig. 59-4). Inapparent infections are rare. Measles virus may persist for years and occasionally causes subacute sclerosing panencephalitis and autoimmune and chronic active hepatitis.

Measles virus enters the host through the oropharynx and possibly through the conjunctiva. Local virus multiplication in the respiratory tract and the regional lymph nodes is followed by a primary viremia with virus spread to the rest of the reticuloendethelial system, where extensive replication takes place. A second viremia, which occurs

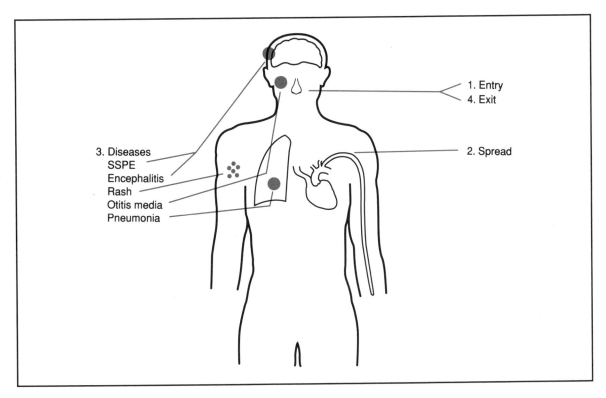

FIGURE 59-4 Pathogenesis of measles (rubeola) virus infection.

5 to 7 days later, disseminates virus to the mucosa of the respiratory, gastrointestinal, and urinary tracts, to the skin, and to the central nervous system. With development of serum antibodies, free virus is quickly cleared from the blood and body fluids, but virus persists for various periods in lymphoid, lung, and bladder tissue. In subacute sclerosing panencephalitis patients, measles virus antigen and measles virus RNA are identified regularly in the brain and lymph nodes and peripheral lymphocytes, but infectious virus can be "rescued" only occasionally by cocultivation of brain and lymph node explant cultures with measles-susceptible cells.

The main pathologic change attributable to viral replication in the main target organs is an inflammatory response. Virus-infected cells contain virus antigens and inclusions in the cytoplasm and nuclei. Infected cells may fuse to form giant cells. The pathology and pathogenesis of postinfectious (allergic) measles encephalitis are the same as those of other exanthematous viral diseases.

The temporary loss of delayed skin hypersensitivity during measles may be due to virus multiplication in T and B lymphocytes. The maculopapular rash is a consequence of the interaction between virus-infected endothelial cells and immune T cells. The simultaneous onset of rash and appearance of serum antibodies suggests an antibody-dependent cellular cytotoxic cause of the exanthem. In cases of dysfunction of T cells, no rash is seen and relentless progression of the infection may lead to giant-cell pneumonia with fatal outcome. Abnormal encephalograms are common during measles, suggesting frequent viral invasion of the brain.

Clinically, measles is characterized by upper respiratory tract symptoms during the prodromal stage and by the maculopapular rash during the eruptive phase. After an incubation period of 9 to 12 days, the prodromal stage starts with malaise, fever, coryza, cough, and conjunctivitis. At the end of this stage, the pathognomonic Koplik spots (red spots with bluish-white specks in their centers) appear in the oral mucosa opposite the second molars. The rash appears 1 or 2 days later, first on the head and then spreading down the body and limbs, including the palms and soles. Initially it is erythematous and maculopapular and later becomes confluent. Uncomplicated illness lasts 7 to 10 days. Otitis media caused by bacterial superinfection is the most frequent complication. Primary viral or secondary bacterial pneumonia is the most common complication responsible for hospitalization and death. Purely viral complications are croup, bronchiolitis, and the fatal giant-cell pneumonia; these often occur without rash in immunocompromised children.

A rare, severe form is **hemorrhagic (black) measles.** Also severe is the atypical **measles syndrome** (high fever; urticarial, purpuric rash resembling varicella that begins peripherally with centripedal spread; and atypical pneumonia). This syndrome is an allergic response to measles infection in adolescents and young adults who were inadequately immunized (mainly with killed measles vaccine) in childhood. **Measles encephalomyelitis** has a frequency of 0.1 percent with a mortality of 20 percent. Permanent sequelae (neurologic disorders, epilepsy, and personality changes) occur in 20 to 40 percent of cases. **Subacute sclerosing panencephalitis (SSPE)** is a rare, chronic, usually lethal encephalitis that develops in children and adolescents some years after the original attack of measles. **Mild (modified) measles** develops in children who possess low levels of maternally derived or injected antibodies.

HOST DEFENSES

Little natural resistance to measles virus infection exists. Nonspecific substances, such as interferon, appear to contribute to early limitation of virus spread. Interferon may be detected until virus-specific antibodies appear. The cell-mediated immune response is associated with recovery from primary infection and also with resistance to reinfection at the portal of entry. The humoral immune response helps to eliminate extracellular virus during primary infection and to prevent systemic spread at reinfection.

The humoral immune response occurs in the three immunoglobulin classes. Lifelong persistence of serum antibodies may be due to persistence of viral antigen. Maternal IgG antibodies completely protect the infant for 6 months; between 6 and 12 months of age, subclinical infection or modified disease may occur.

In patients with subacute sclerosing panencephalitis, strikingly high titers of measles oligoclonal antibody (IgG) are present in serum and cerebrospinal fluid.

EPIDEMIOLOGY

Measles occurs throughout the world, in all races and all climates, with humans as the only host. The main factors accounting for the epidemiologic pattern are universal susceptibility to infection in the absence of antibody, extreme contagiousness, population density, and standard of living.

Sporadic cases occur throughout the year, with peak incidence in the late winter and early summer months. Epidemics occur every 2 to 4 years in developed urban areas with a nonimmunized population and every 4 to 8 years in rural areas, when the number of susceptible persons reaches about 40 percent of the population. The epidemics last 3 to 4 months, until the number of susceptible persons falls below 20 percent. Local outbreaks occur in crowded institutional settings, even when less than 2 percent of the population is susceptible.

The source of infection is the virus-containing respiratory tract secretions, either airborne or transmitted by fomites. The contagious period lasts about 6 days, beginning with the prodromal symptoms and persisting until about 2 days after rash develops, at which time antibodies first appear.

In developed societies, measles infects children between 4 and 7 years of age. In underdeveloped societies, measles occurs before age 4. By age 7 to 12 years, in all but the most isolated areas, nearly all children have had measles and possess specific antibodies.

In countries such as the United States, in which vaccine is used extensively, the incidence of reported disease and its complications have dropped more than 95 percent. As a result of this decreased transmission, a transitory shift to older teenagers has occurred. The incidence of measles encephalitis is almost twice as great in teenagers as in younger children. Subacute sclerosing panencephalitis follows natural measles at an estimated rate of 6 to 20 cases for every 10^6 children developing measles. The risk of subacute sclerosing panencephalitis from live measles vaccine is $\frac{1}{10}$ of that of natural infection.

DIAGNOSIS

Clinical diagnosis of measles is easy when the characteristic symptomatology is present. Laboratory diagnosis helps during uncharacteristic exanthems, atypical measles, pneumonia, or encephalitis after a rash, as well as in suspected cases of giant-cell pneumonia and of subacute sclerosing panencephalitis.

Laboratory diagnosis can be made until about 2 days after onset of rash by demonstrating multinucleated giant cells or fluorescent antibody-staining cells in nasal secretions, urine, and skin biopsies. Isolation of measles virus in tissue culture is difficult and therefore not suitable for routine diagnosis.

Use of the newer solid-phase techniques (enzyme-linked immunosorbent assay and radioimmunoassay) permits serodiagnosis of acute measles infection with a single serum specimen, taken as early as 5 days after the rash appears, by demonstrating significant levels of IgM antibodies or significant IgG titer rises. A specific serologic diagnosis of subacute sclerosing panencephalitis can be made by demonstrating extremely high IgG antibody levels in serum and cerebrospinal fluid.

CONTROL

Quarantine is futile, because by the time the rash signals the disease, shedding has been in progress for 2 or 3 days. Passive prophylaxis with measles immunoglobulin is recommended for exposed, susceptible individuals, especially those at high risk (e.g., patients with cancer, immunosuppressed and immunodeficient patients, infants younger than 1 year of age, and pregnant women). To completely prevent measles infection, viremia must be prevented by an appropriate dose of immunoglobulin given within 3 days of exposure. Administration of immunoglobulin between days 5 and 9 after exposure cannot prevent the secondary viremia, but will modify the disease and allow immunity to develop. Disease also can be modified within 3 days of exposure by reducing the dose of immunoglobulin. Immunoglobulin may protect recipients for about 4 weeks.

Active immunization with the combined measles-mumps-rubella live-virus vaccine is recommended for all healthy 15-month-old children. Vaccine-induced antibody develops in about 95 percent of the seronegative recipients and usually persists in declining titers for more than 18 years. Natural exposure to virus may cause an antibody booster response. Revaccination is now recommended at the age of 4 to 6 years to reach primary vaccine failures (5 percent) and for adolescents entering college. Furthermore, live-virus vaccine also should be given to anyone who does not have a history of measles or has not received live virus vaccine after the age of 15 months.

No specific treatment for measles, measles encephalitis, or subacute sclerosing panencephalitis is available. Management is symptomatic and supportive. Bacterial superinfection should be treated with appropriate antimicrobial agents, but prophylactic antibiotics to prevent superinfection have no known value and are contraindicated.

REFERENCES

Chonmaitree T, Howie VM, Truant AL: Presence of respiratory viruses in middle ear fluids and nasal wash specimens from children with acute otitis media. Pediatrics 77:698, 1986

Enders-Ruckle G: Frequency, serodiagnosis and epidemiological features of subacute sclerosing panencephalitis (SSPE) and epidemiology and vaccination policy for measles in the Federal Republic of Germany. Dev Biol Stand 41:195, 1978

Fox JP, Hall CE: Infections with other respiratory pathogens: influenza, parainfluenza, mumps and respiratory syncytial virus: mycoplasma pneumoniae. p. 335. In Fox JP, Hall CE (eds): Viruses in Families. PSG Publishing, Littleton, MA, 1980

Glezen WP, Taber LH, Frank AL et al: Risk of primary infection and reinfection with respiratory syncytial virus. Am J Dis Child 140:543, 1986

Hall CB, Geiman JM, Biggar R et al: Respiratory syncytial virus infections within families. N Engl J Med 294:414, 1976

Jabbour J, Duenas D, Sever JL et al: Epidemiology of subacute sclerosing panencephalitis. J Am Med Assoc 220:959, 1972

Kingsbury DW, Bratt MA, Choppin PW et al: Paramyxoviridae. Intervirology 10:137, 1978

Lennette EH, Halonen P, Murphy FA: Laboratory Diagnosis of Infectious Disease, Principles and Practice. Springer-Verlag, New York, 1988

Miller CH: Live measles vaccine: a 21 year follow up. Br Med J 295:22, 1987

Taber LH, Knight V, Gilbert BE et al: Ribavirin aerosol treatment of bronchiolitis associated with respiratory syncytial virus infection in infants. Pediatrics 72:613, 1983

ter Meulen VT, Carter MJ: Measles virus persistency and disease. Prog Med Virol 30:44, 1984

Vaheri A, Julkunen J, Koskiniemi ML: Chronic encephalomyelitis with specific increase in intrathecal mumps antibodies. Lancet 2:685, 1982

Wolinsky JS, Waxham MN, Server AC: Protective effects of glycoprotein-specific monoclonal antibodies on the course of experimental mumps virus meningoenzephalitis. J Virol 53:727, 1985

Yanagihara R, McIntosh K: Secretory immunological response in infants and children to parainfluenza virus types 1 and 2. Infect Immun 30:23, 1980

60
CORONAVIRUSES

DAVID A. J. TYRRELL

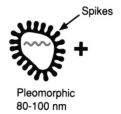

Spikes

Pleomorphic
80-100 nm

GENERAL CONCEPTS

Clinical Manifestations
Coronaviruses cause acute, mild upper respiratory infection (common cold).

Structure
Spherical or pleomorphic enveloped particles contain single-stranded sense (+) RNA associated with a matrix protein. The envelope bears club-shaped glycoprotein projections.

Classification and Antigenic Types
Coronaviruses are classified on the basis of the crown- or halolike appearance of the envelope glycoproteins and on characteristic features of chemistry and replication. Human coronaviruses fall into one of two serotypes: OC43-like and 229E-like.

Multiplication
The virus enters the host cell, and the uncoated genome is transcribed and translated. The mRNAs form a unique "nested set" sharing a common 3' end. New virions form by budding.

Pathogenesis
Transmission is usually via airborne droplets to the nasal mucosa. Virus replicates locally in cells of the ciliated epithelium, causing cell damage and inflammation.

Host Defenses
The appearance of antibody in serum and nasal secretions is followed by resolution of the infection. Immunity disappears within 2 years.

Epidemiology
Incidence peaks in the winter, taking the form of local epidemics lasting a few weeks or months. The same serotype may return to an area after several years.

Diagnosis
Colds caused by coronaviruses cannot be distinguished clinically from other colds. Laboratory diagnosis is made on the basis of antibody titers in paired sera. The virus is difficult to isolate. Nucleic acid hybridization tests are now being introduced.

Control
Treatment of common colds is symptomatic; no vaccines or specific drugs are available. Hygiene measures reduce the rate of transmission.

INTRODUCTION

Coronaviruses are found in many mammalian species. The coronaviruses resemble each other in morphology and chemical structure. For example, coronaviruses of humans and cattle are antigenically related. There is no evidence, however, that human coronaviruses can be transmitted by animals. In animals, various coronaviruses invade many different tissues and cause a variety of diseases, but in humans they have only been proved to cause mild upper respiratory infections—i.e., common colds. On rare occasions, gastrointestinal coronavirus infection has been associated with outbreaks of diarrhea in children, but these enteric viruses are not well characterized and are not discussed in this chapter.

CLINICAL MANIFESTATIONS

Coronaviruses invade the respiratory tract via the nose. After an incubation period of about 3 days, they cause the symptoms of a common cold, including nasal obstruction, sneezing, runny nose, and occasionally cough (Figs. 60-1 and 60-2). The disease resolves in a few days. Virus is shed in nasal secretions. There is no clear evidence that the respiratory coronaviruses cause systemic disease or invade the gut or lower airways.

STRUCTURE

Coronavirus virions are spherical to pleomorphic enveloped particles (Fig. 60-3). The envelope is studded with projecting glycoproteins and sur-

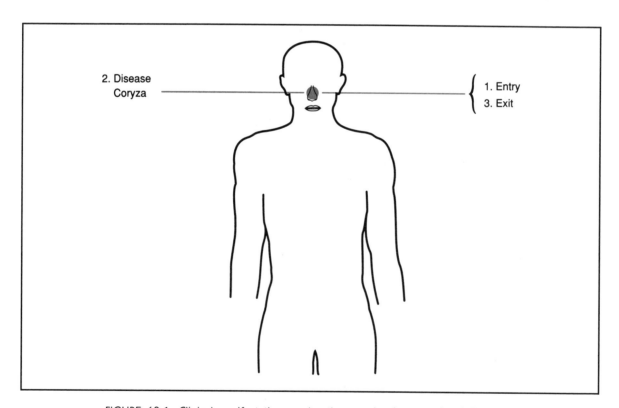

FIGURE 60-1   Clinical manifestations and pathogenesis of coronavirus infections.

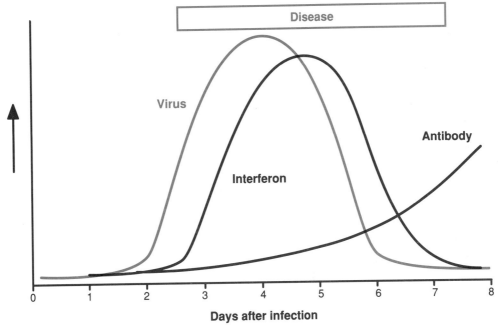

FIGURE 60-2 Immunopathogenesis of coronavirus infections.

rounds a core consisting of a matrix protein associated with a single strand of positive-sense RNA (molecular weight, 6×10^6). The envelope glycoproteins are responsible for attachment to the host cell and carry the main antigenic epitopes, particularly the epitopes recognized by neutralizing antibodies.

CLASSIFICATION AND ANTIGENIC TYPES

The coronaviruses were originally grouped into the family Coronaviridae on the basis of the crown- or halolike appearance given by the glycoprotein-studded envelope on electron microscopy. This classification has since been confirmed by unique features of the chemistry and replication of these viruses. Human coronaviruses fall into one of two groups — 229E-like and OC43-like — which differ in both antigenic determinants and requirements for virus isolation. There is little antigenic cross-reaction between these two types. They cause independent epidemics of indistinguishable disease.

MULTIPLICATION

After the virus enters the host cell and uncoats, the genome is transcribed and then translated. A unique feature of replication is that all the mRNAs

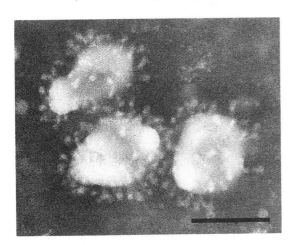

FIGURE 60-3 Electron micrograph showing human coronavirus 229E. Bar, 100 nm. (Courtesy of H. Davies, Clinical Research Center, Harrow, London.)

form a "nested set" with common 3'ends; only the unique portions of the 5' ends are translated. The shortest mRNA codes for the nucleoprotein, and the others each direct the synthesis of a further segment of the genome. The proteins are assembled at cell membranes and genomic RNA is incorporated as the mature particle forms, usually by budding through internal cell membranes.

PATHOGENESIS

Studies in both organ cultures and human volunteers show that coronaviruses are extremely fastidious and grow only in differentiated respiratory epithelial cells. Infected cells become vacuolated, show damaged cilia, and may form syncytia. Cell damage triggers the production of inflammatory mediators, which increase nasal secretion and cause local inflammation and swelling. These responses stimulate sneezing, obstruct the airway, and raise the temperature of the mucosa.

HOST DEFENSES

Although mucociliary activity is designed to clear the airways of particulate material, coronaviruses can successfully infect the superficial cells of the ciliated epithelium. Only about one-half of infected individuals develop symptoms, however. Interferon can protect against infection, but its importance is not known. Because coronavirus infections are common, many individuals have specific antibodies in their nasal secretions, and these antibodies can protect against infection. Most of these antibodies are directed against the surface projections and neutralize the infectivity of the virus. Cell-mediated immunity and allergy have not been extensively studied, but may play a role.

EPIDEMIOLOGY

The epidemiology of coronavirus colds has not been extensively studied. Waves of infection pass through communities during the winter months and often cause small outbreaks in families, schools, etc. (Fig. 60-4). Immunity does not persist, and subjects may be reinfected, sometimes within a year. The pattern thus differs from that of rhinovirus infections, which peak in the fall and spring and generally elicit long-lasting immunity. About 20 percent of colds are due to coronaviruses.

The rate of transmission of coronavirus infections has not been studied in detail. The virus is usually transmitted via inhalation of contaminated droplets, but it may also be transmitted by the hands to the mucosa of the nose or eyes.

DIAGNOSIS

There is no reliable clinical method to distinguish coronavirus colds from colds caused by rhinoviruses or less common agents. For research pur-

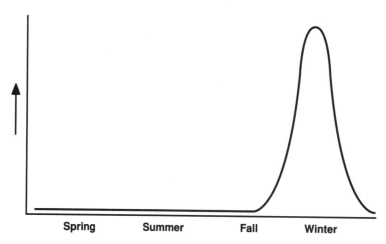

FIGURE 60-4 Seasonal incidence of coronavirus infections.

poses, virus can be cultured from nasal swabs or washings by inoculating organ cultures of human fetal or nasal tracheal epithelium. The virus in these cultures is detected by electron microscopy or other methods. The most useful method for laboratory diagnosis is to collect paired sera (from the acute and convalescent phases of the disease) and to test by enzyme-linked immunosorbent assay (ELISA) for a rise in antibodies against OC43 and 229E. Complement fixation tests are insensitive; other tests are inconvenient and can be used only for one serotype. Direct hybridization tests for viral nucleic acid are being developed and may be available soon.

CONTROL

Treatment of coronavirus colds is symptomatic. Transmission is reduced by practicing hygienic measures. No specific drugs or vaccines are available.

REFERENCES

Gwaltney JM, Jr: Virology and immunology of the common cold. Rhinology 23:265, 1985

Myint S, Siddell S, Tyrrell D: The use of nucleic acid hybridization to detect human coronaviruses. Arch Virol 104:335, 1989

Sanchez CM, Jimenez G, Laviada MD et al: Antigenic homology among coronaviruses related to transmissible gastroenteritis virus. Virology 174:410, 1990

Schmidt OW, Allan ID, Cooney MK et al: Rises in titers of antibody to human coronaviruses OC43 and 229E in Seattle families during 1975–1979. Am J Epidemiol 123:862, 1986

Soaan W, Cavanagh D, Horzinek MC: Coronaviruses: structure and genome expression. J Gen Virol 69:2939, 1988

61 RHABDOVIRUSES: RABIES VIRUS

FRANCES L. REID-SANDEN
DANIEL B. FISHBEIN

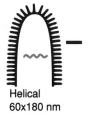

Helical
60x180 nm

GENERAL CONCEPTS

Clinical Manifestations
Rabies virus causes acute infection of the central nervous system. Five stages are recognized in humans: incubation, prodrome, acute neurologic period, coma, and death. The incubation period is exceptionally variable, ranging from 5 days to longer than 2 years.

Structure
Rabies virus is a bullet-shaped, single-stranded, negative-sense enveloped RNA virus. The virus genome encodes five proteins.

Classification and Antigenic Types
Classification is based on the structure of the virus particle. The genus *Lyssavirus* includes rabies virus and three rabies-like viruses.

Multiplication
Viral RNA uncoats in the cytoplasm of infected cells, and the genome is transcribed by virion-associated RNA-dependent RNA polymerase. RNA is then translated into individual viral proteins. Replication occurs with synthesis of positive-stranded RNA templates for producing progeny negative-stranded RNA.

Pathogenesis
Rabies virus replicates in muscle tissue, remaining sequestered at or near the entry site during incubation. It then enters the peripheral nervous system, migrates rapidly to the brain, and then spreads centrifugally to nu-

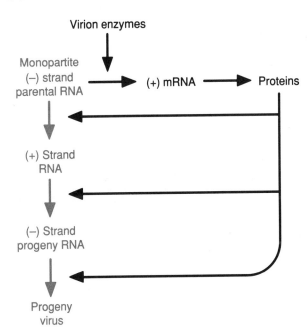

merous organs. The exact pathogenic mechanism is not fully understood.

Host Defenses
Susceptibility to infection is associated with the animal species, inoculum size, location and severity of exposure, and host immune status. Antibody is protective only if present before virus enters the nerves.

791

Epidemiology

Rabies occurs in nearly all countries. Disease in humans is almost always due to a bite by an infected mammal. Nonbite exposures (e.g., aerosols) rarely cause rabies in humans.

Diagnosis

Early diagnosis is difficult. Rabies should be suspected in cases of unexplained encephalitis with a history of animal bite. Unvaccinated persons are often negative for virus-neutralizing serum antibody until late in the infection. Virus isolation from saliva or immunofluorescence-positive skin biopsy establishes diagnosis.

Control

Control is by vaccination of susceptible animal species, particularly dogs and cats.

INTRODUCTION

The family Rhabdoviridae consists of more than 100 negative-sense, nonsegmented viruses that infect a wide variety of hosts, including vertebrates, invertebrates, and plants. Common to all members of this family is a unique, bullet-shaped morphology. Human pathogens of medical importance are found in the genera *Lyssavirus* and *Vesiculovirus.*

Only **rabies virus,** medically the most significant member of the genus *Lyssavirus,* is reviewed in this chapter.

CLINICAL MANIFESTATIONS

Five stages of rabies are recognized in humans: incubation, prodrome, acute neurologic period, coma, and death (or, rarely, recovery) (Fig. 61-1).

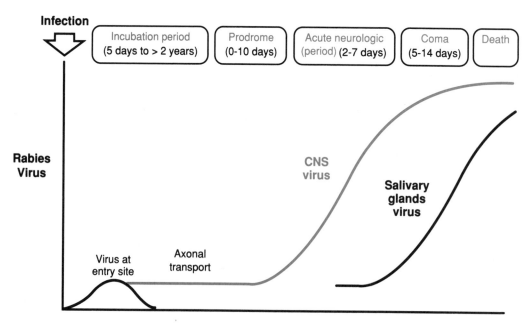

FIGURE 61-1 Pathogenesis of rabies.

No specific antirabies agent is useful once clinical symptoms develop.

The incubation period in rabies, usually 30 to 60 days but ranging from as few as 5 days to longer than 2 years, is more variable than in any other acute infection. Incubation periods are somewhat shorter in children and in individuals bitten close to the central nervous system (e.g., the face).

Clinical symptoms are first noted during the prodromal period, which lasts from 2 to 10 days. These symptoms are often nonspecific (general malaise, chills, fever, and fatigue) or suggest involvement of the respiratory system (sore throat, cough, and dyspnea), gastrointestinal system (anorexia, dysphagia, nausea and vomiting, abdominal pain, and diarrhea), or central nervous system (headache, vertigo, anxiety, apprehension, irritability, and nervousness). More remarkable abnormalities (agitation, photophobia, priapism, increased libido, insomnia, nightmares, and depression) may also occur, suggesting encephalitis, psychiatric disturbances, or other diagnoses. Pain or paresthesia at the site of virus inoculation, which occurs in about 50 percent of patients, is fairly specific and should suggest the diagnosis of rabies.

The acute neurologic period begins with objective signs of central nervous system dysfunction. The disease is classified as **furious rabies** if hyperactivity (i.e., hydrophobia) predominates and as **dumb rabies** if paralysis dominates the clinical picture. Fever, paresthesia, nuchal rigidity, muscle fasciculation, focal and generalized convulsions, hyperventilation, and hypersalivation occur in both forms of the disease.

At the end of the acute neurologic phase, periods of rapid, irregular breathing begin; paralysis and the coma phase follow. Respiratory arrest occurs soon thereafter, unless the patient is receiving ventilatory assistance, which may prolong survival for days, weeks, or longer, with death due to other complications.

Although life support measures can prolong the course of rabies, rarely will they affect the outcome of disease. The possibility of recovery, however, must be recognized, and when resources permit, every effort should be made to support the patient.

STRUCTURE

The rabies virus is a negative-sense, single-stranded RNA virus measuring approximately 60 nm by 180 nm. It is composed of an internal protein core (nucleocapsid), containing the nucleic acid, and an outer envelope, a lipid-containing bilayer covered with transmembrane glycoprotein spikes (Fig. 61-2).

The virus genome encodes five proteins associated with either the ribonucleoprotein complex or the viral envelope (Fig. 61-3). The L (transcriptase), N (nucleoprotein), and NS (transcriptase-associated) proteins are associated with the RNP complex. These aggregate in the cytoplasm of rabies-infected cells and compose **Negri bodies,** the characteristic histopathologic finding of rabies virus infections. The M (matrix) and G (glycoprotein) proteins are associated with the lipid envelope. The G protein forms the protrusions that cover the outer surface of the virion envelope and is the only rabies virus protein known to induce and react with the protective virus-neutralizing antibody.

CLASSIFICATION AND ANTIGENIC TYPES

The genus *Lyssavirus* includes rabies virus and the immunologically similar rabies-like viruses: Lagos bat, Mokola, and Duvenhage viruses. Cross-protection studies demonstrate that animals immunized with rabies vaccines are protected when challenged with most (but not all) rabies-like viruses.

Rabies viruses may be categorized as either fixed (adapted by passage in animals or cell culture) or street (wild type). The use of monoclonal antibodies to differentiate wild-type rabies viruses has been extremely helpful in identifying virus strains originating in major host species in different parts of the world.

MULTIPLICATION

The replication of rabies virus is similar to that of all negative-stranded RNA viruses. The virus attaches to the host cell membrane, penetrates the

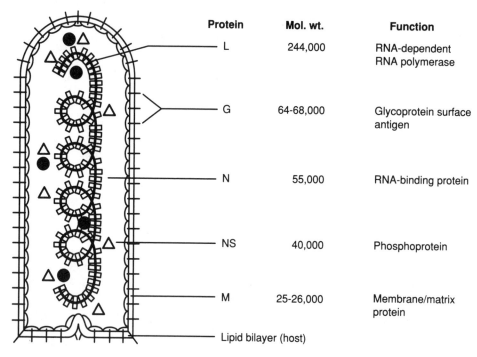

Protein	Mol. wt.	Function
L	244,000	RNA-dependent RNA polymerase
G	64-68,000	Glycoprotein surface antigen
N	55,000	RNA-binding protein
NS	40,000	Phosphoprotein
M	25-26,000	Membrane/matrix protein
Lipid bilayer (host)		

FIGURE 61-2   Virion structure of rabies virus.

Rabies virus RNA genome

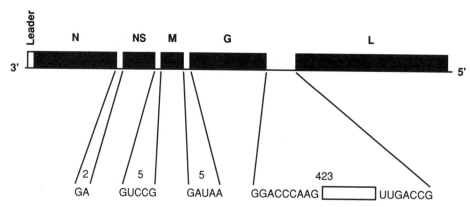

Nucleotides of intergenic regions

FIGURE 61-3   Genome of rabies virus (ERA strain). This contains single-stranded RNA (12 kilobases); N, NS, M, G, and L genes; a leader sequence at the 3' end; and four intergenic regions.

cytoplasm by fusion or pinocytosis, and is uncoated to the core. The core initiates primary transcription of all five complementary monocistronic messenger RNAs by using the virion-associated RNA-dependent RNA polymerase. Each RNA is then translated into an individual viral protein. After protein has been synthesized, replication of the genomic RNA continues with the synthesis of a full-length, positive-stranded RNA, which acts as a template for the production of progeny negative-stranded RNA.

PATHOGENESIS

Rabies virus is most commonly transmitted through a bite and is capable of infecting, to different degrees, all warm-blooded animals. The virus replicates in muscle tissue after entering the host and remains at or near the site of introduction for most of the incubation period. However, the exact site of virus sequestration remains unknown, since neither antigen nor virus can be found in any organ during this phase.

The virus then enters the peripheral nervous system, apparently via the neuromuscular junction, and moves rapidly to the brain; symptoms develop shortly thereafter. The virus then begins to pass centrifugally to many tissues and organs.

The cytopathology of rabies in the central nervous system of animals is strain dependent. In general, gross examination of the brain shows mild congestion of the meningeal vessels; microscopic examination usually demonstrates slight perivascular cuffing, limited tissue necrosis, and, rarely, neuronophagia.

HOST DEFENSES

The animal species, inoculum size, location and severity of exposure, and host immune status have been associated with susceptibility to infection and with different lengths of incubation periods.

The association between rabies virus neutralizing antibody, principally IgG, and protection is well known. However, vaccine-induced antibody is protective only if present before the virus enters the nerves. Interferon production, which is induced during rabies virus infection, has been reported to abort the disease if it occurs shortly after infection. In one clinical trial, however, all the subjects died despite experimental treatment with high doses of alpha interferon.

Recently it has been demonstrated that animals immunized with purified ribonucleoprotein complexes resisted lethal challenge with rabies virus. Subsequent studies have shown that mice immunized with genetically engineered N protein from the CVS strain of rabies virus survived lethal rabies virus challenge, although the role of N protein in protection is not clear.

EPIDEMIOLOGY

Rabies has been recognized since the 23rd century B.C. Today, it is found in most (but not all) countries. Virtually all human rabies is caused by the bite of a rabid animal (Fig. 61-4 and Table 16-1). The risk of rabies is highest in countries where dog rabies remains highly endemic, including most of Africa, Asia, and Latin America. In the United States and Europe, the disease was controlled in domestic animals in the 1940s and 1950s and now occurs primarily in terrestrial wildlife. During the 1980s, reported cases of domestic animal rabies in the United States accounted for only about 10 percent of all animal rabies recorded. Skunks have been the most frequently reported rabid animals in the United States since 1960. An epizootic of raccoon rabies in the mid-Atlantic region in the late 1970s led to this animal's status as the next most frequently rabid, with bats the third most common.

Human rabies is almost always attributable to a bite (any penetration of the skin by the teeth). Nonbite exposures (contamination of an open wound or a mucous membrane via scratches, licks, and inhalation of aerosol) rarely cause rabies in humans. In the United States, nonbite exposures were reported as the source of infection for only 5 (3 percent) of the 163 cases reported from 1950 through 1988. Of these five cases, four were attributable to exposure to aerosols containing highly concentrated live rabies virus: two in spelunkers and two in rabies research laboratory workers. The fifth case occurred in the recipient of a cornea

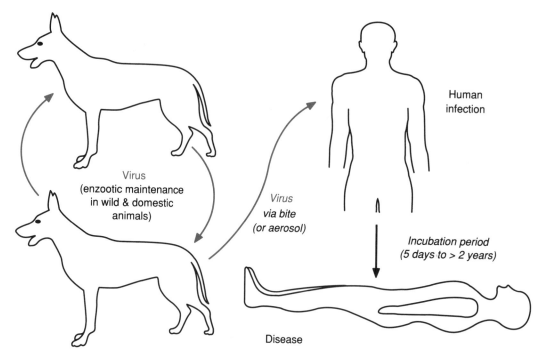

FIGURE 61-4 Life cycle of rabies.

transplanted from a patient dying of unsuspected rabies encephalitis. An increasing proportion of the remaining patients in the United States have had no known exposure to the disease; since 1960, 22 percent of rabies patients have given no exposure history. This may be attributable to failure to question the patient. The initial suspicion of rabies occurred at postmortem examination in three of the last five reported cases in the United States.

DIAGNOSIS
Differential Diagnosis

The diagnosis of rabies is usually suggested by epidemiologic and clinical findings and confirmed in the laboratory. The diagnosis is not difficult if there is a history of exposure and once the full spectrum of symptoms and signs has appeared. A careful but rapid assessment of the epidemiologic and clinical features of less typical cases is essential before special laboratory tests are performed. Every patient with neurologic signs or symptoms or unexplained encephalitis should be asked about

animal exposure in a rabies-endemic area inside or outside the country of residence. The failure to suspect rabies in three of the last five U.S. rabies deaths may have been because no exposure history had been sought.

Early in the course of illness, rabies can mimic numerous infectious and noninfectious diseases. Many other encephalitides, such as those caused by herpesviruses and arboviruses, resemble rabies; other infectious diseases that may resemble rabies include tetanus, cerebral malaria, rickettsial diseases, and typhoid. Paralytic infectious illnesses that can be confused with rabies include poliomyelitis, botulism, and simian herpes type B encephalitis. Differentiation from rabies often requires the above-mentioned special tests.

Noninfectious diseases that may be confused with rabies include a number of neurologic syndromes, especially acute inflammatory polyneuropathy (Guillain-Barré syndrome), as well as allergic postvaccinal encephalomyelitis secondary to vaccination with nervous-tissue rabies vaccines, intoxication with poisons or drugs, withdrawal

TABLE 61-1   Rabies Postexposure Prophylaxis Guide

Animal Species	Condition of Animal at Time of Attack	Treatment of Exposed Person[a]
Dogs and cats	Healthy and available for a 10-day observation	None, unless animal develops symptoms of rabies[b]
	Rabid or suspected rabid	RIG and HDCV
	Unknown (escaped)	Consult public health officials. If indicated, give RIG and HDCV
Skunks, raccoons, foxes, bats, and other carnivores	Regard as rabid unless proven negative by laboratory tests[c]	RIG and HDCV
Livestock, rodents, and lagomorphs (rabbits and hares)		Consider individually. Local and state public health officials should be consulted about the need for rabies prophylaxis. Bites of squirrels, hamsters, guinea pigs, gerbils, chipmunks, rats, mice, other rodents, rabbits, and hares almost never call for anti-rabies prophylaxis.

These recommendations are only a guide. In applying them, take into account the animal species involved, the circumstances of the exposure, the vaccination status of the animal, and the presence of rabies in the region. Local or state public health officials should be consulted if questions arise about the need for rabies prophylaxis.

[a] *All bites and wounds should be thoroughly cleansed with soap and water immediately.* If antirabies treatment is indicated, both rabies immune globulin (RIG) and human diploid-cell rabies vaccine (HDCV) should be given as soon as possible, regardless of the interval from exposure. Local reactions to vaccines are common and do not contraindicate continuing treatment. Discontinue vaccine if the immunofluorescence test of the animal is negative.

[b] During the usual holding period of 10 days, begin treatment with rabies immune globulin and human diploid-cell rabies vaccine at the first sign of rabies in a dog or a cat that has bitten someone. The symptomatic animal should be killed immediately and tested.

[c] The animal should be killed and tested as soon as possible. Holding for observation is not recommended.

from alcohol, acute porphyria, and rabies hysteria. Guillain-Barré syndrome may be mistaken for the paralytic form of rabies, and vice versa.

Laboratory Diagnosis

The detection of rabies antigen, antibody, or the isolation of virus establishes the diagnosis of rabies. Because any individual test may not be positive in a patient with rabies, serial serum specimens for detection of rabies antibodies, saliva specimens for culture of virus, and skin biopsy for direct immunofluorescence testing for virus antigen are sometimes necessary.

The most rapid way to diagnose rabies antemor-tem in humans is to perform a direct immunofluo-rescence test on a skin biopsy from the nape of the neck for evidence of rabies antigen. The direct immunofluorescence test is the most sensitive and specific method of detecting rabies antigen in skin and other fresh tissue, although the results may occasionally be negative in early stages of the disease. Enzyme digestion of Formalin-fixed tissues may enhance the reactivity of the test; however, sensitivity is unacceptably low.

The diagnosis can also be established if virus is isolated from saliva after inoculating mice or neuroblastoma cells; this is generally most successful during the first 2 to 3 weeks of illness. The detection of rabies neutralizing antibody in the serum of unvaccinated persons is also diagnostic. The presence of antibody in cerebrospinal fluid also confirms the diagnosis, but it appears 2 to 3 days later than serum antibody and is therefore less useful early in the disease. Although the serum antibody response after vaccination cannot be differentiated from that due to disease, vaccination does not produce cerebrospinal fluid antibody (except in some patients with postvaccinal allergic encephalomyelitis). In such persons, rabies is diagnosed only by demonstrating the presence of rabies virus or viral antigen.

Only three recoveries from rabies, all in the 1970s, have been well documented. Although rabies virus was not isolated and antigen was not demonstrated in any of the patients, the large

TABLE 61-2   Criteria for Rabies Immunization

Criteria for Preexposure Immunization
(Preexposure immunization consists of three 1-ml IM doses of HDCV or three 0.1-ml ID doses of HDCV, one each on days 0, 7, and 21 or 28. Administration of routine booster doses depends on risk category.)

Risk Category	Nature of Risk	Typical Populations	Preexposure Regimen
Continuous	Virus present continuously; specific exposures may go unrecognized	Rabies research lab workers.[a] Rabies biologics production workers.	Primary preexposure immunization. Serology every 6 months. Boost when titer falls below acceptable level.[a]
Frequent	Exposure usually episodic, with source usually recognized	Rabies diagnostic lab workers,[a] spelunkers, veterinarians, and animal control workers in rabies epizootic areas. Certain international travelers.	Primary preexposure immunization. Booster or serology every 2 years.
Infrequent (greater than population at large)	Exposure nearly always episodic, with source recognized	Veterinarians and animal control workers in low rabies enzootic areas. Veterinary students.	Primary preexposure immunization. No routine booster or serology.
Rare (population at large)	Exposure always episodic with source recognized	U.S. population at large	No preexposure immunization

Postexposure Wound Treatment
(Postexposure wound treatment should begin with immediate thorough cleansing with soap and water.)

Persons not previously immunized: RIG, 20 IU/kg of body weight, one-half infiltrated at bite site (if possible), remainder gluteal area; five doses of HDCV, 1.0 ml IM, one each on days 0, 3, 7, 14, and 28.

Persons previously immunized[b]: Two doses of HDCV, 1.0 ml IM, one each on days 0 and 3. RIG should not be given.

[a] Judgment of relative risk is the responsibility of laboratory supervisor. Preexposure booster immunization is one 1-ml IM dose of HDCV. Acceptable antibody level is neutralization at 1 : 5 serum dilution by rapid fluorescence forms inhibition test (RFFIT). Boost if antibody titer falls below this level.

[b] Preexposure immunization with HDCV; prior postexposure prophylaxis with HDCV; or previous immunization with any other type of rabies vaccine and a documented history of antibody response to the earlier vaccination.

rabies neutralizing antibody titer in serum samples and the presence of neutralizing antibodies in cerebrospinal fluid strongly supported the diagnoses.

CONTROL

Animal rabies is best prevented by vaccinating susceptible species, particularly dogs and cats. Mass dog vaccination programs in the United States and Europe were largely responsible for a dramatic reduction in canine and human rabies during the 1950s. In these countries, the number of reported cases in wild animals is currently about 10-fold greater than that in domestic animals; wild animals therefore constitute the greatest risk to human beings. Oral vaccination of wild animals with attenuated and recombinant rabies vaccines by the use of vaccine-containing bait offers hope of controlling the disease in susceptible wild populations.

Human rabies is best prevented by avoiding exposures to the disease. When an exposure is suspected, the patient's physician and local health department authorities should determine whether an exposure actually occurred and whether a risk of rabies exists in the geographic area (Table 61-2). If treatment (postexposure prophylaxis) is deemed necessary, it should be initiated promptly. Postexposure prophylaxis (the combination of local wound cleansing, rabies immune globulin, and rabies vaccine) will abort the infection, but there is no cure for clinical disease.

Preexposure immunization may be offered to persons at high risk, such as veterinarians, animal handlers, certain laboratory workers, and persons spending time (e.g., 1 month or more) in foreign countries where rabies is a constant threat. Persons such as spelunkers whose vocational or recreational pursuits bring them into frequent contact with potentially rabid animals should also be considered for preexposure prophylaxis. The criteria for preexposure prophylaxis are given in Table 61-2.

REFERENCES

Baer GM, Bridbord K, Hui FW et al (ed): Research towards rabies prevention. Rev Infect Dis 10:S573, 1988

Centers for Disease Control: Rabies prevention—United States, 1984. Recommendation of the Immunization Practices Advisory Committee (ACIP). MMWR 33:393,407, 1984

Centers for Disease Control: Rabies surveillance—United States, 1987. CDC Surveillance Summaries. MMWR 37:1, 1988

Centers for Disease Control: Health Information for International Travel 1988. HHS publication no. (CDC) 88-8280:111, 1988

Dietzschold B, Wang H, Rupprecht CD et al: Induction of protective immunity against rabies by immunization with rabies virus ribonucleoprotein. Proc Natl Acad Sci USA 84:9165, 1987

Esposito JJ: Live poxvirus-vectored vaccines in wildlife immunization programmes: the rabies paradigm. Res Virol (Netherlands) 140:480, 1989

Kaplan C, Turner GS, Warrell DA: Rabies: The Facts. 2nd Ed. Oxford University Press, Oxford, 1986

Koprowski H, Plotkin SA (ed): World's Debt to Pasteur. Alan R Liss, New York, 1985

Reid-Sanden FL, Sumner JW, Smith JS et al: Expression of rabies virus nucleoprotein (N) gene by recombinant baculovirus. Proc Annu Meet SE Am Soc Microbiol, Jekyll Island, 1988

Sumner J, Esposito J, Bellini WJ: Expression of rabies virus nucleoprotein gene by recombinant pox viruses. Abstr Annu Meet Am Soc Microbiol, Miami, 1988

Wagner RR (ed): The Rhabdoviruses. Plenum, New York, 1987

World Health Organization Expert Committee on Rabies: Seventh Report. WHO Technical Report Series no. 709. World Health Organization, Geneva, 1984

62 HUMAN RETROVIRUSES

ANTHONY S. FAUCI
ZEDA F. ROSENBERG

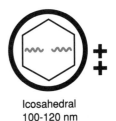

Icosahedral
100-120 nm

GENERAL CONCEPTS

HUMAN T-CELL LEUKEMIA VIRUSES

Clinical Manifestations

Human T-cell leukemia viruses (HTLVs) are associated with three presentations: (1) **asymptomatic infection** (most common); (2) **adult T-cell leukemia** (ATL) (pre-adult T-cell leukemia, chronic, acute, and lymphoma forms); and (3) **tropical spastic paraparesis,** a neurologic disease.

Structure

HTLVs are spherical particles, 100 nm in diameter, made up of an external lipid bilayer/glycoprotein envelope covering an internal protein core. The core contains several copies of **reverse transcriptase** (the enzyme that transcribes RNA to DNA) bound to two identical single-stranded RNA molecules. The RNA codes for internal core proteins *(gag)*, external envelope proteins *(env)*, reverse transcriptase (polymerase) *(pol)*, and regulatory proteins *(tax, rex)*. The lengths of the HTLV-1 and HTLV-2 proviral genomes are about 9.0 and 8.9 kilobases, respectively.

Classification and Antigenic Types

Three types of HTLV are recognized: HTLV-1, HTLV-2, and HTLV-5. HTLVs are classified on the basis of (1) isolation from and ability to infect mature T cells and (2) the presence of reverse transcriptase and cross-reacting internal core proteins. The coding re-

gions of HTLV-1 and HTLV-2 share about 60 percent homology.

Multiplication

After the virion enters the cell, viral reverse transcriptase transcribes the viral RNA into DNA, which integrates into the host cell genome. The integrated viral DNA may remain inactive or be transcribed into progeny viral RNA and into messenger RNA that is translated to produce the viral structural and regulatory proteins. Progeny virions assemble at the cell surface and acquire an envelope by budding off.

Pathogenesis

HTLV-1 and HTLV-2 infect T cells. The viral transactivator protein *(tax)* turns on the expression of cellular proteins and may lead to uncontrolled proliferation of target cells. The long incubation period (10 to 40 years) between infection and the development of leukemia suggests that additional events are required for leukemogenesis. The pathogenic mechanisms of tropical spastic paraparesis are unknown.

Host Defenses

HTLV-specific antibodies, cytotoxic T cells, and interferon have been identified in individuals with persistent infection, but their roles in protection and pathogenesis are unclear.

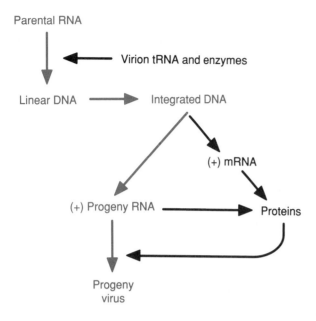

Epidemiology

HTLV-1 is endemic in southwestern Japan, the Caribbean basin, southeastern United States, southern Italy, and sub-Saharan Africa. Up to 15 percent of normal blood donors in endemic areas of Japan and the Caribbean basin are positive for antibodies to HTLV-1; in nonendemic areas, fewer than 1 percent are positive. Data for HTLV-2 are incomplete. HTLVs can be transmitted by transfusion of blood from infected donors, by sexual contact, and from mothers to babies via breast milk.

Diagnosis

HTLV diseases are diagnosed by the presence of HTLV-specific antibodies and by clinical manifestations. The polymerase chain reaction detects the HTLV genome in infected cells and distinguishes between HTLV-1 and HTLV-2 infection. Pre-adult T-cell leukemia is diagnosed on the basis of leukocytosis and abnormal lymphocytes. Acute adult T-cell leukemia-lymphoma is characterized by the presence of pleomorphic neoplastic cells with mature T-cell markers. Chronic adult T-cell leukemia is diagnosed on the basis of skin lesions, low levels of circulating leukemic cells, and the absence of visceral involvement. Tropical spastic paraparesis is characterized by a meningeal inflammatory process,

largely limited to the spinal cord, with progressive weakness in the lower extremities.

Control

Infection is prevented by (1) screening blood products for HTLV antibodies and (2) education to prevent transmission by sexual contact or the sharing of needles. Glucocorticoids have been of limited value in treating some cases of tropical spastic paraparesis. Various combined chemotherapy regimens have been tried for adult T-cell leukemia with limited success.

HUMAN IMMUNODEFICIENCY VIRUS
Clinical Manifestations

Human immunodeficiency virus (HIV) is associated with three presentations: (1) **asymptomatic infection;** (2) **acute infection** with symptoms that may include fever, sweats, myalgia or arthralgia, sore throat, lymphadenopathy, nausea, vomiting, diarrhea, headaches, and rash; and (3) **acquired immune deficiency syndrome (AIDS),** characterized by progressive immune deficiency accompanied by a wide range of opportunistic infections, neoplasms, and neurologic abnormalities, including progressive dementia and peripheral neuropathy.

Structure

HIV is similar overall to HTLV, although the genome is larger (approximately 10 kilobases). As with HTLV, the HIV genome codes for core structural proteins, envelope proteins, reverse transcriptase, and a set of regulatory proteins more complex than those of HTLV.

Classification and Antigenic Types

Techniques of identification are similar to those used for HTLV. Two antigenic types (HIV-1 and HIV-2) are distinguished by antibody reactivity to envelope glycoproteins.

Multiplication

HIV recognizes host cells by binding to the CD4 cell membrane receptor. Multiplication within the host cell is similar to that of HTLV.

Pathogenesis

HIV infects CD4-bearing cells (T4 lymphocytes and monocyte-macrophages). Infection may be latent or chronic low level. Activation leads to the development of immune dysfunction as a result of direct and indirect killing of T4 cells and functional impairment of viable T4 cells. Macrophages may be the primary target cells in brain infection. The pathogenic mechanisms of neurologic disease are not known.

Host Defenses

Persistent infection stimulates humoral and cell-mediated immune responses and interferon production, but the role of these responses in preventing pathogenesis or disease progression is not known.

Epidemiology

HIV infection occurs worldwide and is endemic in central Africa. In the United States and other developed countries, infection is found primarily in homosexual and bisexual men, intravenous drug users, hemophiliacs, transfusion recipients, sexual partners of infected persons, and infants born to infected mothers. Transmission occurs through sexual contact, exposure to contaminated blood or blood products, and perinatally.

Diagnosis

HIV infection is determined by demonstrating HIV-specific antibodies, which usually appear 8 to 12 weeks after infection. The polymerase chain reaction detects the HIV genome in infected cells. Detection of the p24 core antigen in serum also indicates HIV infection. AIDS is diagnosed mainly on the basis of specific opportunistic infections or cancers coinciding with a T4 cell defect in the absence of other known causes of immunodeficiency. In addition, HIV infections with neuropsychiatric manifestations or severe wasting are classified as AIDS.

Control

Infection is prevented by screening blood products for HIV and by education to prevent transmission by sexual contact and sharing of needles. Azidothymidine (AZT) and other antiviral agents are used for prophylaxis against progression to disease and for treatment. Opportunistic infections and neoplasms are treated individually. Immunostimulatory substances are used in treatment.

INTRODUCTION

Over the last 10 years, scientists have uncovered a new class of human pathogens, the **human retroviruses,** which are associated with adult T cell leukemia, tropical spastic paraparesis, and acquired immune deficiency syndrome (AIDS). The mechanisms by which the human retroviruses cause disease involve an intimate relationship between the virus and the human immune system. The wealth of knowledge about animal retroviruses and about the function of the human immune system has laid the foundation for rapid progress in understanding the intricacies of infection with the human retroviruses.

HUMAN T-CELL LEUKEMIA VIRUSES

CLINICAL MANIFESTATIONS

Infection with human T-cell leukemia virus type 1 (HTLV-1) results in a spectrum of clinical manifestations ranging from asymptomatic infection to lymphoproliferative and neurologic disorders (Fig. 62-1). Most HTLV-1-infected individuals are asymptomatic, with normal white blood cell and differential counts. However, some asymptomatic individuals may present with moderate lymphocytosis and aberrant lymphocytes. Approximately half of these latter individuals will progress to a

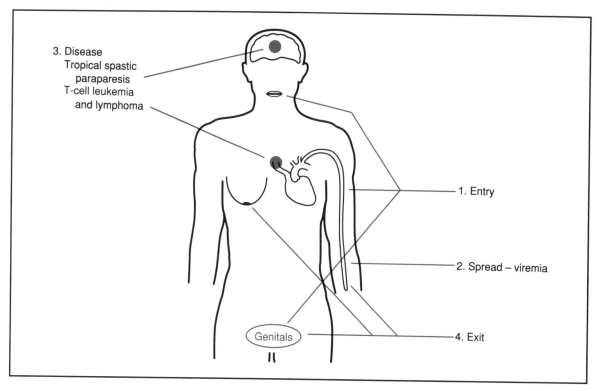

FIGURE 62-1   Clinical manifestations and pathogenesis of HTLV-1 and HTLV-2 infections.

chronic form of **adult T-cell leukemia (ATL),** characterized by small numbers of leukemic cells in the peripheral blood, by skin lesions, and by a lack of involvement of other organ systems. Approximately 15 to 20 percent of adult T-cell leukemia cases follow a chronic course. T cell lymphomas occur and may involve a variety of organ systems. The most common malignant sequela of HTLV-1 infection is acute adult T-cell leukemia, which follows an aggressive course characterized by polylobular malignant T cells, hypercalcemia, leukemic cell infiltrates of the dermis and epidermis, and immunosuppression leading to opportunistic infections.

Infection with HTLV-1 may also result in a slowly progressive encephalomyelopathy called **tropical spastic paraparesis** or **HTLV-1-associated myelopathy.** The predominant clinical manifestation is progressive weakness and partial paralysis of the lower extremities. The clinical fea-

tures may mimic those of multiple sclerosis. In fact, there is some speculation that an HTLV-related virus is involved in multiple sclerosis. There have also been reports that HTLV-1 is associated with large granular lymphocytic leukemia and malignant hypereosinophilic syndrome. However, these claims have not been substantiated.

Two other HTLVs, HTLV-2 and HTLV-5, have been identified. The relation of these viruses to human disease is unclear. HTLV-2 has been associated with two cases of hairy-cell leukemia and has been reported in one case of T-cell prolymphocytic leukemia and one of T-cell chronic lymphocytic leukemia. HTLV-5 has been isolated from a patient with Tac antigen-negative cutaneous T cell lymphoma-leukemia **(mycosis fungoides).** HTLV-5 DNA sequences have been found in the tumor cells of an additional seven patients with mycosis fungoides.

STRUCTURE

HTLVs are members of the retrovirus family, which are distinguished from other viruses by the presence of **reverse transcriptase,** an enzyme that transcribes RNA into DNA. Most retroviruses are spherical particles, approximately 100 nm in diameter, consisting of an internal protein core surrounded by an envelope of glycoproteins embedded in a lipid bilayer. The core contains several copies of reverse transcriptase bound to two identical single-stranded RNA molecules. The genomic viral RNA (Fig. 62-2) is flanked on each end by a long terminal repeat (LTR) that contains sequences for the integration of the virus into the cellular DNA and the regulation of virus expression. In the viruses that cause chronic leukemias, the viral genes encode the core proteins *(gag),* envelope proteins *(env),* replication enzymes *(pol),* and regulatory proteins *(tax* and *rex).* Some animal retroviruses, in contrast, are acutely transforming. The *env* gene of these viruses is truncated and replaced with a cellular gene *(onc)* that causes acute transformation of the target cells.

The envelope of HTLV consists of two glycoproteins of molecular weights approximately 20,000 and 46,000. Three *gag* proteins (molecular weights of 9,000, 15,000, 24,000 to 26,000) constitute the viral core. Unlike most animal retroviruses, the genome of HTLV codes for two nonstructural proteins, *tax* and *rex,* which do not transform cells but are involved in the regulation of HTLV expression.

CLASSIFICATION AND ANTIGENIC TYPES

A virus is classified as an HTLV by the presence of reverse transcriptase and by its isolation from and infection of mature T cells. In vitro, HTLV infection of T cells results in their **transformation** (i.e., in the continuous proliferation of the cells in the absence of exogenous growth factors). The genomes of HTLV hybridize only weakly with the genomes of other animal retroviruses. HTLV-1, HTLV-2, and HTLV-5 are the antigenic types recognized currently. HTLV-3 was redesignated as human immunodeficiency virus type 1 (HIV-1). There is also a related virus called HIV-2. The HTLVs share cross-reacting internal core proteins, which differ slightly in molecular weight. The HTLV-1 and HTLV-2 proviral genomes are approximately 9.0 and 8.9 kilobases in length, respectively, and have approximately 60 percent overall homology. Although the long terminal repeat sequences of these two viruses are quite dissimilar, specific regulatory regions in the long terminal repeat are highly conserved. The other highly (more than 80 percent) homologous region of the genomes of HTLV-1 and HTLV-2 is the *tax* gene. The genome of HTLV-5 is less well characterized. The DNA of HTLV-5 hybridizes only weakly to HTLV-1 and does not hybridize to HTLV-2. The different HTLVs are distinguished by using **polymerase chain reaction (PCR)** techniques to amplify HTLV sequences and by hybridization with specific viral probes.

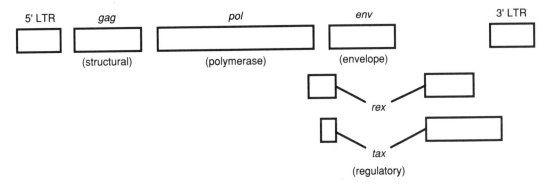

FIGURE 62-2 HTLV genome (proteins encoded).

MULTIPLICATION

Retroviruses have a common mode of viral replication that is based on the function of the reverse transcriptase molecules (Fig. 62-3). The initial event in retroviral infection is the attachment of the virus to the cell membrane. The specific cellular receptor(s) for HTLV has not yet been identified, but recent experiments have shown that a receptor is encoded by a gene on human chromosome 17. After binding to the cell membrane, the virion enters the cell and is uncoated to release the viral RNA. The reverse transcriptase, which is complexed to the viral RNA, transcribes the RNA into DNA. The virion-associated integrase then enables the viral DNA to integrate into the host cell genome. The integrated viral DNA, now called a **provirus,** can either remain inactive or be transcribed into viral RNA and into messenger RNA that is translated into viral structural and regulatory proteins. Progeny viral RNA and structural proteins assemble at the cell surface and bud from the cell membrane. Since the provirus is duplicated along with the cellular DNA during the replication cycle of the cell, infection of the cell will persist throughout the lifespan of the clone.

PATHOGENESIS

The HTLVs appear to induce disease in a fundamentally different way from other oncogenic animal retroviruses. The acutely transforming animal retroviruses cause malignant transformation by the insertion of their *onc* genes into the cellular DNA. Although the *onc* genes were originally derived from cellular growth genes, they are no longer under cellular control, but rather under the control of the viral promoter. The chronic oncogenic animal retroviruses appear to provoke leukemogenesis when the provirus inserts near a cellular *onc* gene. As a result, the cellular gene comes under the control of the viral promoter, thereby enhancing its expression. Therefore, the virally transformed animal leukemic cells have proviral copies integrated at specific sites in the cellular DNA. In contrast, the HTLVs do not possess an *onc* gene, nor do they integrate in the same site in

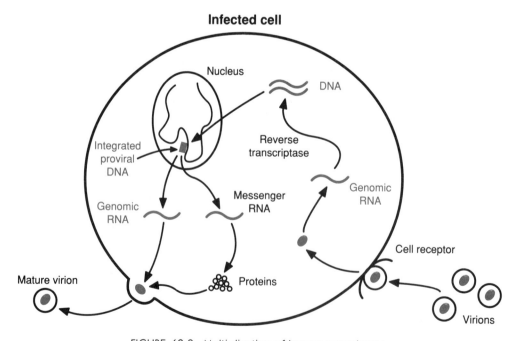

FIGURE 62-3 Multiplication of human retroviruses.

different tumors (i.e., they show random integration).

HTLVs possess two unique genes, *tax* and *rex*, which are required for viral replication and efficient transcription of the HTLV genome. The *rex* gene encodes a protein of molecular weight 26,000 to 27,000 that is localized in the nucleus and is required for the accumulation of unspliced *gag* mRNA and for efficient expression of the *gag* gene products. The *tax* gene product is a nuclear protein of molecular weight 37,000 to 40,000 that transactivates viral gene expression. The exact mechanism of *tax*-induced transactivation is unknown, but it has been suggested that the *tax* gene product may activate a constitutively expressed cellular transcription factor that binds to the viral promoter and indirectly enhances viral gene expression. Although expression of the *tax* gene can lead to cancer in some strains of transgenic mice, the resulting tumors are neurofibromas and do not demonstrate a direct effect of *tax* on leukemogenesis.

One mechanism by which the HTLV *tax* gene product may play a role in leukemogenesis is by activating cellular genes that are involved in T-cell growth (Fig. 62-4). Mitogen- or antigen-stimulated T cells produce a factor, **interleukin-2 (IL-2),** that binds to a receptor on the surface of activated T cells and induces T-cell multiplication. Primary tumor cells from patients infected with HTLV-1 and from T-cell lines that have been transformed in vitro with HTLV-1 or HTLV-2 express large numbers of receptors for IL-2 on their surface. In addition, cells transfected with HTLV-1 *gag-tax* genes release high levels of IL-2 receptors constitutively. Therefore, it has been hypothesized that the *tax* gene product is responsible for stimulating the production of IL-2 receptors through the induction of host transcription factors that bind to the IL-2 receptor gene. Research has identified in the IL-2 receptor gene a region that is essential for *tax*-mediated regulation of gene expression. It has also been suggested that the *tax* protein can transactivate the IL-2 gene itself, although less strongly

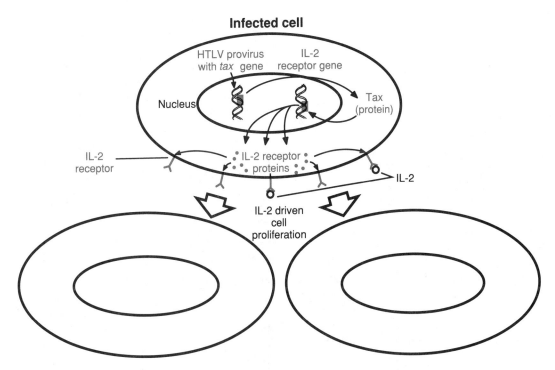

FIGURE 62-4 Pathogenesis of HTLV-induced leukemia.

than the IL-2 receptor gene. HTLV can also stimulate T-cell growth without actually infecting the cell. Exposure of T cells to inactivated HTLV-1 or to partially purified viral proteins can result in mitogenic stimulation and proliferation of the T cells in the absence of exogenous IL-2.

Two features of infection indicate that HTLV-induced leukemogenesis must involve additional pathogenetic events. The first is the long incubation period between infection with HTLV and the appearance of leukemic cells: it is thought that leukemia may take several decades to develop. The second feature is the monoclonal nature of the malignant cells in adult T-cell leukemia patients. Although HTLV integrates randomly into the cellular DNA of target T cells, the adult T-cell leukemia cells in an individual patient arise from a single HTLV-infected cell. Therefore, although HTLV may polyclonally stimulate the growth of T cells via either *tax*-mediated mechanisms or mitogenic stimulation, the outgrowth of leukemic cells presumably depends on as yet unidentified secondary events.

Infection with HTLV-1 also results in immunosuppression. In vitro, HTLV-1 infection not only alters helper T-cell function by causing increased proliferation, but also induces nonspecific polyclonal immunoglobulin production by B cells regardless of the type of antigen-presenting cell. Infection of cytotoxic T-cell clones leads to reduction or loss of cytotoxic function. Cells expressing HTLV-1 have abnormal expression of major histocompatibility complex (MHC) antigens (cell surface proteins essential for the functional interaction of immune cells). Inappropriate expression of these antigens on infected T cells would impede or abolish their normal function. In addition, the HTLV-1 envelope and major histocompatibility complex proteins share certain antigenic determinants, so the immune system may be tricked into thinking that the HTLV-infected cell is self and need not be eliminated by the cytotoxic T-cell response.

The pathogenesis of the second major clinical manifestation of HTLV-1 infection, tropical spastic paraparesis, is unknown. Several animal retroviruses, particularly members of the lentivirus sub-family, can infect the central nervous system and cause chronic neurologic disease in animals. The damage to the central nervous system is generally considered to result not from direct infection of neuronal cells but rather from the release of toxic factors by cells infected with HTLV-1. Another hypothesis is that neural tissue is damaged by the host immune system via an autoimmune mechanism. Like adult T-cell leukemia, tropical spastic paraparesis occurs with very low frequency in HTLV-1-infected individuals. Even rarer is the occurrence of both diseases in the same individual. Possible explanations for these observations include the existence of distinct adult T-cell leukemia-inducing strains and tropical spastic paraparesis-inducing strains of HTLV-1 or genetic determinants or host cell factors that contribute to variable disease expression.

HOST DEFENSES

A hallmark of HTLV infection is its persistence. Once an individual is infected with HTLV, the virus remains in that individual for life. Specific antibodies are produced against a variety of HTLV proteins, including *env, gag,* and *tax.* Cytotoxic lymphocytes that recognize viral proteins have also been identified. In patients with tropical spastic paraparesis, antibody against HTLV-1 is synthesized intrathecally. The role of HTLV-specific antibodies and T-cell cytotoxicity in the prevention of new infections or in disease progression is unclear. It is also unclear whether interferon, which is produced by HTLV-1-infected cells in culture, is beneficial in HTLV infections. HTLV-1 is not lysed by human serum, although human complement can lyse other animal retroviruses. The persistence of HTLV infection in vivo indicates that completely effective immune responses do not occur naturally.

EPIDEMIOLOGY

HTLV-1 infection occurs, with varying degrees of prevalence, in several regions of the world (Table 62-1). The highest prevalence is in southwestern Japan, where six endemic areas have been identified. The prevalence of anti-HTLV-1 antibodies in

TABLE 62-1   Geographic Distribution of HTLV

Southwestern Japan
Caribbean basin
Southwestern United States
Sub-Saharan Africa
Southern Italy

inhabitants of these areas ranges from 6 to 37 percent. The Caribbean is another region where HTLV-1 is endemic, with an overall seropositivity rate of 4 percent. Between 19 and 48 percent of family members of HTLV-1-infected individuals in these two endemic areas are seropositive. In both regions, the prevalence of anti-HTLV-1 antibodies increases with age, from 2 percent in young children to 30 percent in adults in their mid-forties. Although fewer data are available for Africa, HTLV-1 infection is also endemic there, with seropositivity rates ranging from 4 to 7 percent. HTLV infection is also found in defined populations (e.g., predominantly in intravenous drug users and homosexuals in developed countries such as the United States and Italy). It is not clear whether the HTLV type in these populations is HTLV-1 or HTLV-2.

The predominant modes of transmission of HTLV infection are by sexual contact, via contaminated blood or blood products, and from mother to child via breast milk. Studies in Japan have shown that between 48 and 82 percent of recipients of seropositive blood seroconverted. The rising prevalence with age of antibodies to HTLV-1 is consistent with sexual transmission of HTLV-1.

One unique characteristic of HTLV-1 infection is the extremely long incubation period between initial infection and the occurrence of disease. The incubation period for adult T-cell leukemia can range from years to decades and may be as long as 40 years; the incubation period for tropical spastic paraparesis is thought to be shorter but is still several years. Antibodies to HTLV-1 are found in the vast majority of patients with adult T-cell leukemia and tropical spastic paraparesis. However, the incidence of T-cell cancers or tropical spastic paraparesis in HTLV-1-infected individuals is extremely low. Studies on the incidence of adult T-cell leukemia in Japan estimate that fewer than 0.1 percent of HTLV-1-infected individuals develop adult T-cell leukemia each year. Adult T-cell leukemia is usually found in individuals older than 40 years.

DIAGNOSIS

The determination of HTLV infection is usually made on the basis of a positive anti-HTLV antibody test. The enzyme-linked immunosorbent assay (ELISA) is the most common screening test for the presence of anti-HTLV antibodies. A positive assay is confirmed by direct radioimmunoprecipitation assays or Western immunoblots. Owing to immunogenic cross-reactivity, these tests do not distinguish between HTLV-1 and HTLV-2 infection. The polymerase chain reaction assay, which is based on the amplification of viral DNA segments, is used to distinguish between these two viruses. Since the interval between HTLV infection and the appearance of antibodies is not known, the polymerase chain reaction can also be used to diagnose HTLV infection in antibody-negative individuals.

The presence of modest leukocytosis with abnormal-appearing lymphocytes in an asymptomatic, HTLV-infected individual is indicative of pre-adult T-cell leukemia. Acute adult T-cell leukemia-lymphoma is characterized by the presence of pleomorphic neoplastic cells with mature T-lymphocyte markers. Since adult T-cell leukemia cells express high levels of Tac antigen (a protein chain that is part of the IL-2 receptor), diagnosis should include staining for the Tac antigen. Clinical features may include dermal or epidermal infiltrates, hypercalcemia, osteolytic bone lesions, hepatosplenomegaly, and increased susceptibility to opportunistic infections. Chronic (smoldering) adult T-cell leukemia is diagnosed on the basis of skin lesions, low levels of circulating leukemic cells, and an absence of visceral involvement. Not all cases of adult T-cell leukemia are associated with HTLV-1 infection.

Tropical spastic paraparesis is characterized by a meningeal inflammatory process largely limited to the spinal cord, with progressive weakness in the lower extremities and sensory abnormalities. HTLV-1 can be isolated from the blood and cerebrospinal fluid of many patients with tropical spastic paraparesis.

CONTROL

Control of HTLV infection and disease involves three approaches: therapy, education and public health, and vaccination (Table 62-2). Treatment of HTLV-1 infection and its sequelae is extremely difficult. Current treatment regimens for adult T-cell leukemia involve combination chemotherapy protocols which have not significantly increased survival. The elimination of Tac-positive cells by anti-Tac antibodies coupled to toxin is being considered as an experimental therapy. Glucocorticoids have been used in treating tropical spastic paraparesis, but with only limited success. In vitro, **azidothymidine (AZT)** and **dideoxycytidine (DDC)** inhibit the infectivity of HTLV-1 in T4 cells and reduce the growth of HTLV-1-infected T cells. The effect of these agents on HTLV in vivo is unknown.

Although there is no treatment for HTLV infection, asymptomatic HTLV-infected individuals should be routinely screened for evidence of disease progression and counselled on ways to avoid spreading the infection. Methods to prevent the spread of HTLV infection include screening of blood products for antibodies to HTLV-1 and HTLV-2, educating people about prevention of HTLV transmission via sexual intercourse and the sharing of needles, and advising mothers to refrain from breast-feeding.

There is no vaccine against HTLV infection or disease. The development of vaccines for retrovirus infections in general has proven extremely difficult. One important consideration in the design of a candidate vaccine is that the introduction of

TABLE 62-2 Control of HTLV

Identification of infected individuals
Education to prevent spread via sexual intercourse, needles, transfusions, and mother's milk
Production of vaccines (under evaluation)
Therapy (limited)

viral genetic material in the form of killed or attenuated viruses may result in the integration of the viral genome into the host cell DNA. Therefore, many of the approaches to human retrovirus vaccines have involved natural or recombinant protein preparations. Several experimental HTLV-1 vaccines have been designed that use the envelope portion of the virus as the immunogen. One HTLV-1 recombinant hybrid envelope product has been tested in cynomolgus monkeys. The monkeys that developed anti-HTLV-1 envelope antibody titers of 20 or higher were protected from challenge with HTLV-1 producing cells. Control monkeys and those with antibody titers below 20 developed signs of infection between 2 and 6 weeks after inoculation. Rabbits have been successfully immunized with vaccinia virus-*env* constructs. These products have not been tested in humans.

Because the development of adequate therapeutic approaches and vaccines may take many years, the most effective strategy to reduce the number of individuals with HTLV infection and disease is education.

◀ HUMAN IMMUNODEFICIENCY VIRUS ▶

CLINICAL MANIFESTATIONS

Initial infection with HIV may result in an acute syndrome with symptoms including fever, sweats, myalgia or arthralgia, sore throat, lymphadenopathy, nausea, vomiting, diarrhea, headaches, and rash (Fig. 62-5). During the acute infection there may be a drop in the number of circulating T4 lymphocytes. It is not known what proportion of new HIV infections present with an acute syndrome. Following initial infection, there is a long and variable asymptomatic period. During this period there may be a slow, progressive decline in T4-cell numbers and an increase in T8 cells. Some individuals may maintain relatively constant, normal levels of T4 cells during the asymptomatic period.

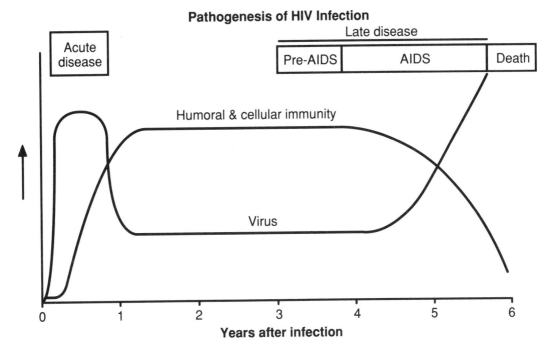

FIGURE 62-5 Pathogenesis of HIV infection.

Acquired immune deficiency syndrome (AIDS) is a late manifestation of infection with HIV (Fig. 62-6). AIDS is characterized by a marked depletion of T4 cells, resulting in a reversal of the T4/T8-cell ratio (normally 1.5:1 to 2.0:1) (Fig. 62-7). The progressive immune deficiency is accompanied by a wide range of life-threatening opportunistic infections and neoplasms, the most common being *Pneumocystis carinii* pneumonia and Kaposi sarcoma, respectively. Another manifestation of HIV infection is the **AIDS-dementia complex (AIDS encephalopathy).** This syndrome is characterized by neurologic abnormalities, including progressive dementia and peripheral neuropathy, and may occur in the absence of opportunistic diseases.

STRUCTURE

The general structure of HIV is similar to that of HTLV (see above); the virus consists of an external lipid bilayer glycoprotein envelope (including envelope proteins gp120 and gp41), an internal protein core (proteins p15, p17, and p24), and viral RNA complexed with reverse transcriptase. The HIV genome is approximately 10 kilobases, which is larger than that of HTLV. In addition to the structural *gag, pol,* and *env* genes and the regulatory *tat* (analogous to HTLV *tax*) and *rev* (analogous to HTLV *rex*) genes, the HIV-1 genome contains at least four regulatory genes (*nef, vif, vpu,* and *vpr*). HIV-2 does not have sequences for *vpu,* but does encode a novel gene, *vpx,* that is also found in the simian immunodeficiency virus.

CLASSIFICATION AND ANTIGENIC TYPES

HIV is classified as a retrovirus because it contains reverse transcriptase. Infection of cultured T4 cells with HIV results in syncytium formation and cell death. Two major antigenic types (HIV-1 and HIV-2) have been identified and are readily distinguished by differences in antibody reactivity to the envelope glycoprotein. The two HIV types share approximately 40 percent genetic identity. There is some disagreement about whether they are equally pathogenic. Both apparently cause AIDS,

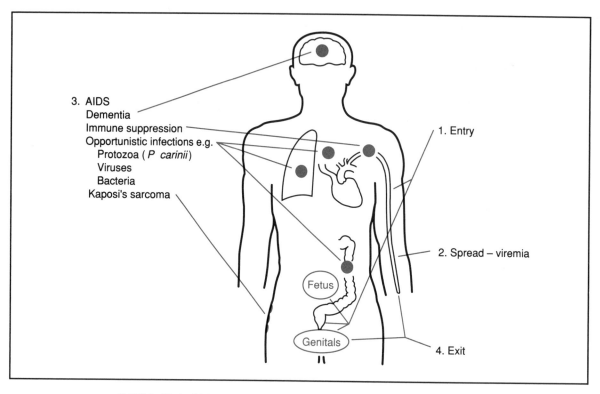

FIGURE 62-6 Clinical manifestations and pathogenesis of HIV infection.

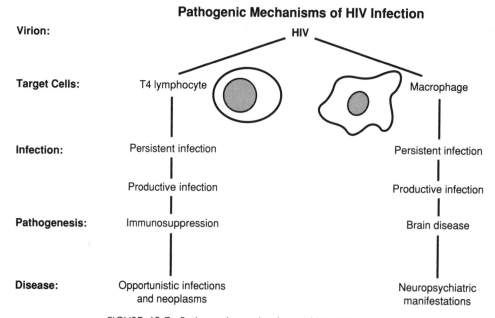

FIGURE 62-7 Pathogenic mechanisms of HIV infection.

but some researchers think that HIV-2 is less efficient in causing disease.

Different isolates of HIV-1 and HIV-2 exhibit considerable genomic variation and antigenic heterogeneity. The most variable regions of the genome are in the *env* gene. This type of variation is also observed in HIV isolates obtained from individuals over the course of their infection. HIV strains often display differences in replicative capacity and cytopathicity. The significance of these variations for the disease process is unclear, although some data suggest that HIV isolates with higher replicative and cytopathic ability are more common in individuals who have progressive disease.

MULTIPLICATION

The first step in HIV infection is the high-affinity binding of the gp120 envelope glycoprotein to the CD4 receptor. The CD4 receptor is present on the surface of several cell types, including T4 cells and monocyte-macrophages. Following attachment to the CD4 receptor, HIV multiplication proceeds in a manner similar to that of HTLV (see above). In contrast to HTLV infection, however, the final step in HIV replication often involves the budding of massive numbers of virions from the cell surface, resulting in cell lysis.

PATHOGENESIS

The high-affinity binding of the HIV envelope glycoprotein to the CD4 receptor is a crucial step in the pathogenesis of HIV, since the major cell expressing CD4 is the T4 lymphocyte (often a helper cell). The T4 cell plays a central role in all aspects of immune system function, so that death or impairment of this cell results in widespread immune dysfunction. There are several potential ways that HIV can damage T4 cells. (1) HIV replication may kill T4 cells as a result of destruction of the cell membrane by budding viruses or viral proteins. (2) The production of large quantities of viral genetic material and proteins may interfere with normal cell metabolism. (3) HIV may also infect and destroy the progenitor cells that are responsible for the propagation of the lymphoid cell pool.

In addition to direct cytopathicity, HIV infection may indirectly cause T4-cell death by several means. The first involves the formation of the giant cells of syncytia that are often seen in HIV-infected cell cultures in vitro. Syncytium formation results from binding of the HIV envelope protein that is expressed on the surface of an infected T cell to the CD4 receptors on the surface of uninfected T4 cells. One HIV-infected T4 cell may thus bind to many uninfected T4 cells. The membranes of these bound cells fuse to form a syncytium, which usually dies shortly after formation. Another mechanism of indirect cell killing may involve autoimmune phenomena in which anti-HIV immune responses are targeted to uninfected T4 cells that either have free envelope protein bound to their membrane or present processed envelope antigens. In addition, since both the HIV envelope protein and the class II major histocompatibility complex antigens bind to the CD4 receptor, their common binding sites may represent cross-reacting antigens. Therefore, anti-HIV antibodies may react with uninfected T4 cells that express class II major histocompatibility complex molecules.

HIV-infected individuals may exhibit immune dysfunction prior to a depletion of their T4 cells. HIV may induce these functional abnormalities by a variety of pathways not necessarily involving a spreading infection of T4 cells. For example, by binding to the CD4 receptor, HIV or its envelope protein can interfere with the CD4-mediated monocyte–T-cell interactions that are necessary for antigen-specific responses. In addition, cross-linking of the CD4 molecules by the envelope protein may render the cell nonresponsive to subsequent antigenic stimulation.

During the long asymptomatic period of HIV infection, the virus resides in a latent or low-level chronic form within T4 cells and, to a lesser extent, within monocytes-macrophages. The mechanisms by which the virus is maintained in this relatively quiescent state are unclear. Similarly, little is known about the events that provoke activation. In vitro, a number of factors have been identified that are associated with the activation of HIV expression. These factors include antigens, mitogens, cotransfection, or coinfection of heterologous viruses, and cytokines. It is thought that HIV up regulation by these factors involves the induction of cellular proteins that bind to the promotor region of the HIV DNA and boost its expression.

The monocyte-macrophage is a target cell for HIV infection both in vivo and in vitro. Infection of these cells may occur through the CD4 receptor or via phagocytosis. In contrast to T4 cells, monocyte-macrophages appear to be resistant to both cell lysis and syncytium formation. Moreover, the virus can replicate intracellularly in monocyte-macrophages, with virions budding into intracytoplasmic vesicles. As a result, viral antigens may not be expressed on the cell surface, potentially enabling the monocyte-macrophages to escape immune surveillance and to transport the infection to other organ systems, particularly the lungs and brain. Although the mechanisms by which HIV induces neuropsychiatric abnormalities are unknown, the macrophage is thought to play an important role. HIV infection in the brain appears to be largely restricted to macrophages, which may indirectly damage neuronal tissue by releasing neurotoxic factors or factors that induce inflammation. HIV may also interfere with the binding of neurotropic factors to their receptors on neurons. Another mechanism of HIV-induced neuropathology may involve autoimmune phenomena.

Clearly, some fraction of the neurologic abnormalities in HIV-induced disease is due to the wide range of opportunistic infections and tumors that afflict AIDS patients. Although other retroviruses can directly cause cancers, HIV does not transform cells in vivo or in vitro. The multitude of tumors found in AIDS patients may result from widespread immunosuppression and/or the induction of factors that induce cellular proliferation, as may be the case with Kaposi sarcoma. HIV proviral DNA has not been found in any of these tumors.

HOST DEFENSES

A broad range of immune responses to HIV has been observed in all stages of HIV infection. Antibodies to both the structural and regulatory proteins of HIV generally appear several weeks to

months after initial infection; however, this response is occasionally delayed for years. During the progression of HIV infection, antibody titers to the p24 core antigen decline, while antibody titers to the envelope protein remain relatively constant. HIV-infected individuals produce low titers of virus-neutralizing antibodies, and these decline as disease progresses. Antibodies that mediate antibody-dependent cellular cytotoxicity (ADCC) have also been observed in the sera of AIDS patients. Cell-mediated responses to HIV include T-cell proliferation and cytotoxicity mediated by both T cells and natural killer (NK) cells. Interferon has been found in some AIDS patients, but coinfecting opportunistic viruses may be responsible. Since it is thought that HIV ultimately causes a slowly progressive, persistent infection in all infected individuals, the role of immune responses in preventing HIV-induced disease is unclear. The emergence of genetic variants of HIV in vivo during the disease may be one way that HIV evades both humoral and cellular immune responses.

EPIDEMIOLOGY

HIV-1 infection has been reported throughout the world in both developed and developing countries. In the United States and other developed countries, HIV infection is found predominantly in homosexual and bisexual men and intravenous drug users. Hemophiliacs, transfusion recipients, sexual partners of infected persons, and infants born to infected mothers are also at high risk. In many parts of Africa and the Caribbean, HIV-1 is found predominantly in heterosexuals, transfusion recipients, and infants born to infected mothers. HIV-2 is found predominantly in West Africa, Portugal, and Brazil. Both HIV-1 and HIV-2 are spread through sexual contact, exposure to contaminated blood or blood products, and perinatally from an infected mother to her offspring. It is estimated that as of 1990, between 800,000 and 1.3 million individuals in the United States are infected with HIV. It is not known what proportion of these individuals will develop AIDS. The median incubation period is thought to be approximately 10 years.

DIAGNOSIS

HIV infection is determined by the presence of HIV-specific antibodies, which usually occur 6 to 12 weeks after infection. An HIV enzyme-linked immunosorbent assay is commonly used as the initial screening assay. An individual is considered to be infected with HIV if a positive assay is confirmed by a positive Western blot or a similar, more specific assay. Diagnosis of HIV-2 infections requires HIV-2-specific assays. There are sporadic reports of individuals in whom anti-HIV antibodies did not develop for several years after infection. Detection of virus nucleic acid by the polymerase chain reaction may be used to diagnose HIV infection in antibody-negative individuals.

AIDS is diagnosed predominantly on the basis of opportunistic infections or cancers indicative of a T4 cell defect in the absence of a known cause of immunodeficiency. Neuropsychiatric manifestations are also indicative of AIDS. Although neurologic complications may arise from opportunistic infections of the central nervous system, tumors, and vascular problems, AIDS may present in the absence of these conditions as an HIV encephalopathy that is diagnosed by clinical findings of cognitive or motor dysfunction that interferes with daily activities. AIDS may also be diagnosed in an HIV-infected individual on the basis of unexplained weight loss with either chronic diarrhea or chronic weakness and fever, known as **HIV wasting syndrome.**

CONTROL

Strategies for the control of HIV infection and disease are similar to those for HTLV infection: therapy, education and public health, and vaccination. Therapeutic categories for HIV include antiviral therapies, immune modulators, and therapies to treat and prevent opportunistic diseases. Azidothymidine, a nucleoside analog, is currently the only anti-HIV agent that has been shown to significantly improve survival in AIDS patients. Additional nucleoside analogs, as well as other potential

antiviral agents, are undergoing clinical trials. A combination of antiviral agents may prove to be the most effective treatment for AIDS since it may allow the use of lower doses of drugs to minimize toxicity. Owing to the persistence of HIV infection, lifelong antiviral treatment will probably be necessary. In addition to the antiviral agents, several immunomodulatory agents are undergoing clinical trials. With regard to treatment of opportunistic infections, the use of aerosolized pentamidine has brought about a major advance in preventing *P carinii* pneumonia. Since *P carinii* pneumonia is the most common cause of death in AIDS patients, aerosolized pentamidine can greatly improve survival in these patients.

Intensive educational efforts are needed to prevent transmission of HIV by sexual intercourse, intravenous drug use, and exposure to blood or blood products. Sexual abstinence, monogamous sexual relationships with uninfected partners, the use of condoms, and abstinence from intravenous drug use or the use of clean needles are necessary for the control of HIV through sexual intercourse and intravenous drug use. Transmission of HIV can be prevented in health care workers and other medical settings by the application of universal precautions (i.e., treating all blood as potentially infected by HIV). HIV infection via blood products is prevented by screening donated blood for anti-HIV antibodies and by excluding donors at high risk of HIV infection. HIV-infected women of childbearing age should be counseled about the 30 to 40 percent risk of transmitting HIV infection perinatally.

One important obstacle to the development of a vaccine against HIV is that the relation of immunity to HIV infection is not understood. The experience gained in developing a vaccine against an animal retrovirus, feline leukemia virus, suggests that immunity to the viral envelope protein is crucial for prevention of infection. Efforts have therefore been made to develop HIV vaccines that use the precursor HIV glycoprotein (gp160) or its external subunit (gp120) as immunogens. These envelope subunit vaccines are being evaluated in phase 1 clinical trials for safety and immunogenicity in uninfected volunteers. In addition, phase 1 trials are being conducted with inactivated HIV preparations in symptomatic HIV-infected individuals. Although the usual use of a vaccine is to prevent infection with a microorganism, it is hoped that an HIV vaccine will also prevent the development of AIDS in individuals already infected with HIV.

REFERENCES

Blattner WA: Retroviruses. In Evan AS (ed): Viral Infections of Humans. Plenum, New York, 1989

Centers for Disease Control: Revision of the CDC surveillance case definition for acquired immunodeficiency syndrome. MMWR 36:3S, 1987

Ehrlich GD, Poiesz BJ: Clinical and molecular parameters of HTLV-1 infection. Clin Lab Med 8:65, 1988

Fauci AS: The human immunodeficiency virus: infectivity and mechanisms of pathogenesis. Science 239:617, 1988

Nerurkar LS, Wong-Staal F, Gallo RC: Human retroviruses, leukemia, and AIDS. In Henderson ES, Lister TA (ed): Leukemia. 5th Ed. WB Saunders, Philadelphia, 1990

Rosenblatt JD, Chen ISY, Wachsman W: Infection with HTLV-I and HTLV-II: evolving concepts. Semin Hematol 25:230, 1988

Rosenberg ZF, Fauci AS: The immunopathogenesis of HIV infection. Adv Immunol 47:377, 1989

Wong-Staal F, Gallo RC: Human T-lymphotropic retroviruses. Nature (London) 317:395, 1985

63 ROTAVIRUSES, REOVIRUSES, AND ORBIVIRUSES

ALBERT Z. KAPIKIAN
ROBERT E. SHOPE

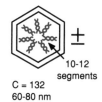

10-12
segments
C = 132
60-80 nm

GENERAL CONCEPTS

ROTAVIRUSES

Clinical Manifestations

Rotaviruses cause enteric disease with symptoms characterized by diarrhea, vomiting, abdominal discomfort, and fever, or any combination. The virus affects mainly infants and young children. Diarrhea ranges from mild to severe and can cause fatal dehydration.

Structure

The 70-nm-diameter wheel-shaped particles consist of a double-layered icosahedral capsid enclosing a core particle that contains 11 segments of double-stranded RNA, each segment representing one gene.

Classification and Antigenic Types

Rotavirus is a genus in the family Reoviridae. Rotaviruses have three important antigenic specificities: group, subgroup, and serotype. Group A rotaviruses are major pathogens in humans and animals. Seven serotypes of human group A rotaviruses are defined by neutralization. Of the non-group A rotaviruses (groups B through G), only groups B and C have been detected in humans; they are not an important cause of disease in infants and young children.

Multiplication

The virus enters the cell by endocytosis or by direct membrane penetration if activated by protease. Replication occurs in the cytoplasm. Removal of the outer shell of the capsid in lysosomes activates the viral RNA polymerase. Newly assembled subviral particles acquire the outer capsid proteins by budding through the endoplasmic reticulum, and are released by cell lysis.

Pathogenesis

Transmission is by the fecal-oral route (and possibly the respiratory route). Reversible damage to the proximal small intestine appears as shortened villi and as sparse, irregular microvilli with a patchy, irregular but predominantly intact mucosa and as mononuclear cell infiltration of the lamina propria.

Host Defenses

The mechanism of immunity is not firmly established. In animals, antibody in the intestinal lumen is crucial; in humans, serum antibodies correlate with protection.

Epidemiology

Group A rotaviruses are ubiquitous and infect most individuals by the third year of life. They are the single most important cause of severe diarrhea in infants and young children worldwide, accounting for about 30 to 50 percent of cases requiring hospitalization or treatment. In temperate climates, incidence peaks in the winter; in the tropics, the disease occurs year-round.

Diagnosis

Clinical findings are nonspecific. Diagnosis depends on detecting virus in feces (e.g., by immunoassay) or on demonstrating a serum antibody response.

817

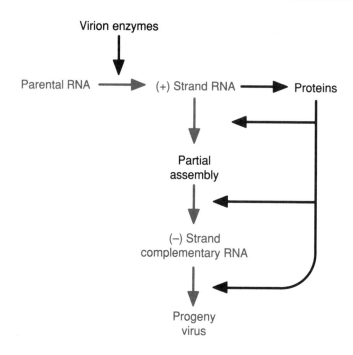

Control

Dehydration is treated by fluid and electrolyte replacement. Vaccine development is under way.

REOVIRUSES

Reovirus infections occur frequently, but most are mild or subclinical. The role of these viruses in human disease is not clear, but they are not considered to be important agents of human disease.

ORBIVIRUSES

Clinical Manifestations

The four human orbiviruses cause fevers. The most important is **Colorado tick fever,** a diphasic fever with headache, severe muscle pain, and arthralgia. Children may develop hemorrhage or encephalitis.

Structure

The spherical virions (diameter, 60 to 80 nm) are similar to those of rotaviruses except that the genome contains 10 or (in Colorado tick fever virus) 12 RNA segments.

Classification and Antigenic Types

The genus *Orbivirus* contains 109 serotypes in 13 serogroups; four serotypes cause human disease.

Multiplication

Multiplication is as for rotaviruses and takes place in both the arthropod vector and the vertebrate host. Gene segment reassortment occurs among closely related orbivirus serotypes.

Pathogenesis

Colorado tick fever virus chronically infects the tick *Dermacentor andersoni*, which transmits it to humans. The virus infects bone marrow cells, arresting development of several blood cell types and sometimes causing thrombocytopenia. In young children, the virus may invade the central nervous system and cause encephalitis.

Host Defenses

Colorado tick fever elicits interferon and humoral antibody; the role of these and other defenses is not known.

Epidemiology

The distribution of Colorado tick fever, in the Rocky Mountains and western United States, matches that of its tick vector. The virus propagates in a rodent-tick cycle, with humans as secondary hosts.

Diagnosis

Diagnosis depends on isolation of virus from erythrocytes or detection of viral antigen on erythrocytes by immunofluorescence. Antibody appears in convalescent-phase serum.

Control

Control is by avoidance of tick bites.

INTRODUCTION

The family Reoviridae is composed of six genera: *Orthoreovirus, Orbivirus, Rotavirus, Phytoreovirus, Fijivirus,* and *Cypovirus.* Certain *Orthoreovirus, Orbivirus,* and *Rotavirus* species infect humans; *Phytoreovirus* and *Fijivirus* species infect plants and insects; and the cypoviruses (the cytoplasmic polyhedrosis viruses) infect insects. This chapter concerns only the members of the Reoviridae known to infect humans.

Although the orthoreoviruses (referred to commonly as reoviruses), orbiviruses, and rotaviruses are similar in morphology, diameter (about 70 nm), and possession of a segmented, double-stranded RNA genome, they differ in epidemiology, association with disease, and ability to be cultured. In addition, the three groups are distinct antigenically.

Rotaviruses are major agents of severe diarrhea in infants and young children in developed and developing countries. Such diarrhea can lead to dehydration that may be fatal if rehydration fluids are not available. Reovirus infections are quite common in humans, although they tend to be mild or subclinical. The extent of their role as agents of illness in humans is unclear. Four orbiviruses have been associated with human disease. The most serious of these diseases is Colorado tick fever, characterized by diphasic fever, headache, muscle pain, anorexia, leukopenia, and weakness; some cases are complicated by encephalitis, hemorrhage, thrombocytopenia, or pericarditis; death is rare.

◄ ROTAVIRUSES ►

Diarrheal diseases are a major cause of morbidity in infants and young children in developed countries and a major cause of morbidity and mortality in developing countries. For example, in a family study of some 25,000 illnesses in the United States, infectious gastroenteritis was the second most common disease and accounted for 16 percent of all illnesses. The impact of diarrheal illnesses on infants and young children in developing countries is staggering. An estimate of the number of diarrheal episodes in children younger than 5 years of age in Asia, Africa, and Latin America for a 1-year period indicated that more than 450 million cases of diarrhea occurred and that 1 to 4 percent were fatal, resulting in the deaths of 5 to 18 million children. A later study in the same areas estimated 3 to 5 billion cases of diarrhea and 5 to 10 million diarrhea-associated deaths in 1 year, ranking diarrhea first among infectious diseases in the categories of both frequency and mortality, with the burden greatest in infants and young children. Despite the importance of this disease, the agents of a large proportion of diarrheal illnesses of infants and young children were not known until relatively recently. It was assumed that viruses were important because the bacterial agents known at that time could be recovered from only a small proportion of cases during nonepidemic periods. In 1973, rotaviruses were discovered in duodenal biopsies obtained from hospitalized infants and young children with acute gastroenteritis. Subsequently, the agent was detected in stools by electron microscopy, and laboratories all over the world soon began to detect the virus in stools of a large proportion of pediatric patients with gastroenteritis. Efficient and practical tests were developed to detect rotavirus from clinical specimens, thus facilitating the study of this agent, which replicated inefficiently in cell cultures. Soon, the major role of rotavirus in diarrheal disease was established. The other major pathogens associated with diarrheal disease in infants and young children (predominantly in developing countries), the enterotoxigenic *Escherichia coli* strains, are discussed in Chapter 25. In addition, the 27-nm Norwalk group of viruses that is associated with epidemic gastroenteritis in older children and adults is discussed in Chapter 65.

CLINICAL MANIFESTATIONS

Rotaviruses induce a clinical illness characterized by vomiting, diarrhea, abdominal discomfort, fever, and dehydration (or a combination of some of these symptoms) that occurs primarily in infants and young children and may lead to hospitalization for rehydration therapy. Fever and vomiting frequently precede the onset of diarrhea. Although milder gastroenteric illnesses that do not require hospitalization are also common, most studies of clinical manifestations of rotavirus-induced gastroenteritis rely on data from hospitalized patients. The duration of hospitalization ranges from 2 to 14 days with a mean of 4 days. The highest attack rate is usually among infants and young children 6 to 24 months old, and the next highest in infants less than 6 months old. Normal neonates infected with rotavirus do not usually develop clinical manifestations. Deaths from rotavirus gastroenteritis may occur from dehydration and electrolyte imbalance. In older children and adults, rotavirus gastroenteritis occurs infrequently, although subclinical infections are common.

Rotaviruses also induce chronic symptomatic diarrhea in immunodeficient children, with an occasional fatal outcome. In addition, rotavirus infections can be especially severe and sometimes fatal in individuals of any age who are immunosuppressed for bone marrow transplantation. Rotavirus infections have also been associated with necrotizing enterocolitis and hemorrhagic gastroenteritis in neonates in special-care units. Rotaviruses have also been found in stools of patients with a variety of other conditions, but the association appears to be temporal rather than etiologic.

STRUCTURE

Rotaviruses have a distinctive wheel-like shape (Fig. 63-1). Complete particles have a double-layered capsid and measure about 70 nm in diameter. When the outer layer is absent, they measure about 55 nm. Within the inner capsid is the 37-nm core, which contains the RNA genome. The term **rotavirus** is derived from the Latin word *"rota,"* meaning wheel, and was suggested because the

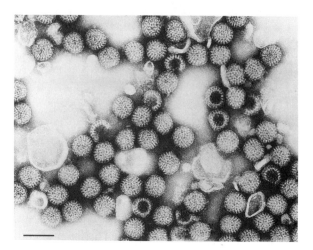

FIGURE 63-1   Human rotavirus particles from a stool filtrate. Particles appear to have a double-shelled capsid. Occasional "empty" particles are seen. (Adapted from Kapikian AZ, Kim HW, Wyatt RG et al: Reovirus-like agent in stools: association with infantile diarrhea and development of serologic tests. Science 185:1049, 1974, with permission.)

sharply defined circular outline of the outer capsid resembles the rim of a wheel placed on short spokes radiating from a wide hub. Morphologically, rotaviruses resemble the reoviruses and orbiviruses. However, the sharply defined circular outline of the outer capsid of rotavirus differs from the amorphous outer capsid of orbiviruses. Reoviruses also have a distinct outer capsid, although it is not characteristically as sharply defined as that of the rotaviruses.

The rotavirus genome contains 11 segments of double-stranded RNA, in contrast to the reoviruses and orbiviruses, both of which contain 10 segments (except Colorado tick fever virus, an orbivirus with 12 segments of double-stranded RNA). Rotavirus RNA segments 1, 2, 3, and 6 encode inner capsid polypeptides VP1, VP2, VP3, and VP6, respectively, whereas RNA segments 4 and 7, 8, or 9 encode the major outer capsid polypeptides VP4 and VP7, respectively. The biochemical properties of human rotaviruses have not been studied extensively because, until recently, these agents were difficult to propagate in cell culture. Rotaviruses and orbiviruses are ether stable, but acid labile, whereas reoviruses are acid and ether stable. Studies of the effect of various disinfectants on simian rotavirus infectivity demonstrated that 95 percent (vol/vol) ethanol was most effective for rotavirus inactivation in the laboratory setting, where disinfection may be necessary.

CLASSIFICATION AND ANTIGENIC TYPES

Rotaviruses are distinct serologically from the three reovirus serotypes and from all orbiviruses with which they have been tested. Most human rotaviruses share a common group antigen and are designated group A rotaviruses, but other antigens separate the group A rotaviruses into serotypes and subgroups. Seven human rotavirus serotypes have been defined by neutralization of one of the outer capsid proteins, VP7. Group A rotaviruses can also be separated into two distinct subgroups by various assays. The neutralization and subgroup specificities are encoded by different genes. Rotaviruses also have been detected in stools of the young of numerous animals with diarrhea. Rotaviruses of humans and animals characteristically share a common group antigen, but strains may differ in serotype specificity by neutralization. However, several animal rotavirus strains (simian, canine, feline, equine, murine, porcine, and lapine strains) share serotype specificity with human rotavirus type 3, and two porcine rotavirus strains are antigenically similar to human rotavirus type 4. In addition, a few human and animal rotavirus strains have been detected (by electron microscopy) that do not share the common group antigen; these have been designated as non-group A rotaviruses. The non-group A viruses are divided into groups B, C, D, E, F, and G on the basis of distinct group antigens. The group A rotaviruses are the most important agents of severe diarrhea in infants and young children and are prevalent worldwide. The group B and C rotaviruses have a more limited distribution and are not considered to be an important cause of infantile diarrhea. Group B rotavirus has been responsible for large outbreaks of severe gastroenteritis in China, which predominantly involved adults, but the impor-

tance of the group B rotaviruses outside China has not been defined. Groups D, E, F, and G have not been detected in humans. Unless otherwise noted, the description of rotaviruses in this chapter deals with the group A rotaviruses exclusively.

Human rotaviruses are rather fastidious agents, and for many years they could not be efficiently cultivated from clinical specimens. Recently, efficient cell culture propagation of human rotavirus strains directly from clinical material has become possible by altering the conditions of propagation.

MULTIPLICATION

Rotaviruses replicate exclusively in the cytoplasm. The virion enters the cell by endocytosis (or direct membrane penetration if activated by protease), and the outer shell of the double capsid is removed in lysosomes with the liberation of 50-nm subviral particles, thus activating the viral RNA polymerase (transcriptase). RNA positive-sense transcripts induce the production of proteins and are also a template for the production of antisense strands, which remain associated with the positive-sense strand. About 8 hours after infection, viroplasmic inclusions of dense granular material, representing newly synthesized proteins and RNA, accumulate in the cytoplasm. Viral RNA is packaged into core particles, and viral capsid proteins assemble around the cores. These particles accumulate in vesicles of the endoplasmic reticulum and leave the viroplasm by budding through the membrane of the endoplasmic reticulum, where they acquire the outer capsid protein. The budding process (plus transient acquisition of an envelope) is unique to rotaviruses among members of the family Reoviridae. Particles are released by cell lysis.

PATHOGENESIS

Rotaviruses are transmitted by the fecal-oral route (Fig. 63-2). Other routes of transmission, such as water-borne or airborne (respiratory) routes, have also been suggested. From clinical studies, the incubation period of rotavirus diarrheal illness was estimated to be less than 48 hours. Large numbers of virus particles are shed in the stool following multiplication in epithelial cells of the small intes-

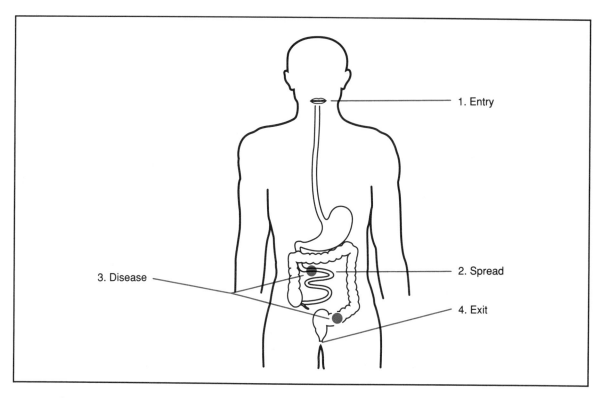

FIGURE 63-2 Pathogenesis of rotavirus infection. Virus entry is via the oral route, with virus replication and pathology in proximal small intestine, resulting in diarrhea and/or vomiting.

tine. Shedding may persist for 10 days or more after the illness, but peak shedding appears to occur within 8 days of illness. Studies in adult volunteers have demonstrated that oral administration of a rotavirus-containing suspension can induce a diarrheal illness in certain individuals. Also, human rotavirus induces a gastrointestinal illness following administration by the alimentary route in various newborn, colostrum-deprived animal models. Histopathologic studies of tissue from the small intestine of humans with rotavirus infection show shortening and blunting of villi on a patchy, irregular, but predominantly intact mucosa, and mononuclear cell infiltration of the lamina propria. Electron microscopy shows sparse and irregular microvilli with denudation of epithelial cells in some areas, distended cisternae of the endoplasmic reticulum that contain virus particles, and

mitochondrial swelling. D-Xylose absorption was impaired, and some patients had depressed disaccharidase levels.

HOST DEFENSES

The mechanism of immunity is not firmly established. Serum antibody in volunteers was found to correlate with resistance to rotavirus-induced illness, whereas the relationship of intestinal fluid neutralizing activity to resistance was not clear. In animal models, resistance to rotavirus-induced illness correlates with rotavirus antibody present in the intestinal lumen, and not with circulating serum antibody. Serotype-specific immunity may be of importance in protecting against illness with individual serotypes. Little is known about other host defenses during rotavirus infection.

EPIDEMIOLOGY

Despite the frequency of rotavirus diarrhea in developed countries, mortality is low. For example, it was recently estimated that the 1- to 4-year age group in the United States would experience annually more than 1 million cases of severe diarrhea and up to 150 deaths. In contrast, it was estimated that in developing countries infants and young children under 5 years of age would experience annually more than 18 million moderately severe or severe cases of rotavirus diarrhea and that 873,000 children from 1 to 4 years of age would die from rotavirus diarrhea.

Rotaviruses are recognized as the major agents of severe gastroenteritis of infants and young children in most areas of the world. These agents also have been associated with milder episodes of gastroenteritis that do not require hospitalization. The efficient transmission of rotavirus is evident by the presence of rotavirus antibody in most children by the age of 3 years. This high prevalence of antibody is maintained into adulthood, probably a result of frequent reinfection. Important sources of rotavirus infection for infants are individuals of any age who shed this virus. Community outbreaks of rotavirus infection occur infrequently, probably because previous rotavirus exposure leads to protective immunity. Although rotavirus gastroenteritis occurs infrequently in adults, large outbreaks of severe gastroenteritis in adults have been associated with a group B rotavirus in China. The importance of non-group A rotaviruses outside China has not been defined.

Rotaviruses have been associated with about 30 to 50 percent of hospitalized cases of diarrheal illness in infants and young children in various countries in the temperate climates. A striking feature of rotaviral illness in these climates is its seasonal distribution. It usually occurs in the cooler months of the year when, cumulatively, more than 50 percent of diarrheal illnesses are associated with rotaviruses (Fig. 63-3). The reason for this temporal distribution is not known. This striking seasonal pattern has not been observed uniformly in all settings. In tropical climates, rotavirus infections have been detected throughout most of the year, although less pronounced peaks can occur. In studies of newborns in nurseries, most neonates with rotavirus infections are asymptomatic. A mechanism for this relative lack of susceptibility to illness in neonates in nurseries has yet to be explained satisfactorily. However, a 3-year study showed that such neonatal infections induced significant protection against postneonatal rotavirus diarrheal illness (but not infection) throughout the study period.

Rotaviruses also cause diarrhea in many newborn animals, such as calves, mice, piglets, foals, lambs, rabbits, deer, antelopes, apes, turkeys, chickens, goats, kittens, and puppies. No evidence exists that animal rotaviruses are transmitted to humans under natural conditions, but human rotavirus has been shown to induce a diarrheal illness in certain animals under experimental conditions.

DIAGNOSIS

Because the clinical manifestations of rotavirus gastroenteritis are not distinct enough to permit a specific diagnosis, specimens must be examined in the laboratory. This is necessary even in temperate climates during the cooler months of the year, when more than 50 percent of hospitalizations due to diarrhea may be associated with rotavirus.

Laboratory diagnosis of rotavirus infections requires identifying the virus in feces or rectal swab specimens or demonstrating a fourfold or greater increase in antibody to a rotavirus antigen between acute- and convalescent-phase sera. Numerous methods to detect rotavirus in stool and rectal swab specimens have been described. These include electron microscopy, radioimmunoassay, counterimmunoelectro-osmophoresis, centrifuging of clinical material onto tissue culture cells followed by immunofluorescence, inoculation of tissue cultures, latex agglutination, reverse passive hemagglutination assay, polyacrylamide gel electrophoresis, dot hybridization, and enzyme-linked immunosorbent assay (ELISA). ELISA has now become the mainstay in most laboratories, because it is practical, rapid, and efficient and does not require sophisticated laboratory equipment. Commercial ELISA kits are now available; certain ones

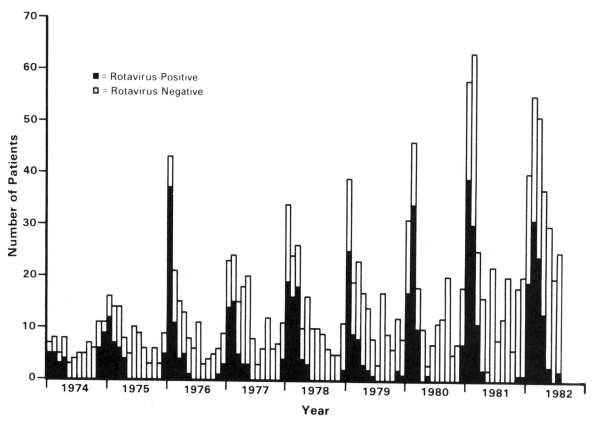

FIGURE 63-3 Temporal distribution of human rotavirus infections in 1,537 infants and young children hospitalized with gastroenteritis at Children's Hospital National Medical Center, Washington, DC, January 1974 (partial) through July 1982, as demonstrated by electron microscopy, immunoelectron microscopy, and rotavirus-confirmatory enzyme-linked immunosorbent assay. (From Brandt CD, Kim HW, Rodriquez WJ et al: Pediatric viral gastroenteritis during eight years of study. J Clin Microbiol 18:71, 1983, with permission.)

should be used with caution if confirmatory reagents (i.e., positive and negative controls) are not included in the kit, since nonspecific reactions may yield false-positive results. When the number of specimens is limited, the most rapid method of rotavirus diagnosis in a hospital setting is by examination of a stool specimen by negative-stain electron microscopy. This can be accomplished in a few minutes. Non-group A human rotaviruses that do not share the common group antigen cannot be detected by conventional serologic assays; however, they can be detected by electron microscopy because they are morphologically identical to conventional rotaviruses.

Serologic evidence of rotavirus infection can be detected by various techniques, such as ELISA immunofluorescence, neutralization, and complement fixation.

CONTROL

The primary aim of treatment of rotavirus gastroenteritis is the replacement by the intravenous or oral route of fluids and electrolytes lost by vomiting or diarrhea. Oral rehydration is more readily available and has gained widespread use worldwide as a life-saving treatment. In patients with severe dehydration and shock, intravenous rehydration is indicated for efficient replacement of fluid loss. Virus-specific chemotherapy is not available. Ribavirin was found to inhibit animal rotaviruses in vitro, but was not effective against murine rotavirus in the mouse model. Human milk that contains rotavirus antibody is effective when given orally to treat immunodeficient patients with chronic rotavirus infection. Human immune serum globulin (γ-globulin) that contains rotavirus antibody was given prophylactically (orally) to low-birth-weight infants in a nursery in which recurrent rotavirus infections occurred. Treatment resulted in delayed rotavirus excretion and milder symptoms. In addition, cow colostrum that contains rotavirus antibody was given prophylactically to infants and young children daily, as a single or divided dose orally, and was shown to induce significant protection against rotavirus diarrhea. However, colostrum or milk concentrate from cows that were immunized with human rotavirus did not have a therapeutic effect when administered to children who already had rotavirus diarrheal illness, although virus shedding was decreased.

The importance of rotavirus as a cause of diarrheal illness in infants and young children throughout the world indicates that an effective vaccine is needed to prevent rotavirus-induced illness. An attenuated monovalent bovine rotavirus strain (serotype 6) or an attenuated monovalent rhesus rotavirus strain (serotype 3) has been administered orally to infants and young children as experimental vaccines. Their efficacy has been variable. Thus, other candidate vaccines are being evaluated with the aim of achieving serotype-specific immunity by combining the VP7 specificity of serotypes 1, 2, 3, and 4 into a single vaccine.

Because rotaviruses are highly contagious and can spread by the fecal-oral route, careful attention to hand washing, disinfection, and disposal of contaminated material may limit its spread, especially in nurseries and hospitals where nosocomial infections occur frequently.

REOVIRUSES

The family name Reoviridae is derived from the prototype "reovirus" strain of the genus *Orthoreovirus,* the first genus of this family to be identified. The name reovirus was proposed in 1959 to describe a group of viruses previously classified as enteric cytopathic human orphan (ECHO) virus type 10, but which was found to differ from the other echoviruses in several important aspects (e.g., size). In addition, the acronym "reo" was suggested to denote that these agents were isolated from the *r*espiratory and *e*nteric tracts and had not been associated with any disease (*o*rphan virus). Important features of the orthoreoviruses (or "reoviruses") include a diameter of 70 nm; a double capsid; ether and acid stability; a genome of 10 segments of double-stranded RNA; three serotypes designated types 1, 2, and 3; and the ability to infect humans as well as various other animals. The three serotypes share a common complement fixation antigen but can be distinguished by hemagglutination inhibition and neutralization techniques. Reoviruses grow efficiently from clinical specimens in various cell cultures, including monkey kidney cells.

Reoviruses are ubiquitous agents. Strains identical serologically to the human reovirus serotypes have been recovered from a wide variety of animals, including mice, chimpanzees, dogs, cats, cattle, sheep, swine, horses, and monkeys. Avian reoviruses also have been isolated; however, with one possible exception, these are antigenically distinct from the three reovirus serotypes described previously. In addition, a reovirus possessing certain characteristics of the mammalian and avian reoviruses has been recovered from a bat.

Reovirus infections occur often in humans, but most are mild or subclinical. The virus is detected efficiently in feces. It may also be recovered from nasal or pharyngeal secretions, urine, blood, cerebrospinal fluid, and various organs obtained at autopsy. Despite the ease with which reoviruses are detected in clinical specimens, their role in human disease remains uncertain. Reovirus infections have been observed in patients with various conditions such as fever, exanthema, upper and lower respiratory tract illnesses, gastrointestinal illness (including steatorrhea), hepatitis, pneumonitis, keratoconjunctivitis, neonatal cholestasis, meningitis, encephalitis, myocarditis, and Burkitt's lymphoma. Their role as agents of such illnesses remains unclear since convincing evidence of an etiologic association remains elusive. Thus, it is generally considered that although reoviruses can readily infect humans, they are not important agents of human disease.

ORBIVIRUSES

CLINICAL MANIFESTATIONS

Orbiviruses cause fever. Table 63-1 shows the four human pathogens, their diseases, vectors, and geographic distribution. The most serious of these is **Colorado tick fever virus,** which will be emphasized in the rest of this chapter. Colorado tick fever virus causes diphasic fever in about half the infected individuals. Colorado tick fever is manifested by headache, chills, muscle pain (especially in the back and legs), and photophobia. Children may have hemorrhagic illness or encephalitic signs (including disorientation and stiff neck). Pericarditis has been reported. The case fatality rate is estimated at 0.2 percent. Most patients recover within 2 weeks, but occasionally convalescence is prolonged.

Kemerovo virus is a tick-borne virus that was isolated from cerebrospinal fluid of two patients in western Siberia in 1962 during a small outbreak of febrile disease. Orungo virus was found in the blood of febrile patients in tropical Africa and is believed to cause small epidemics. Changuinola virus was isolated from a patient with fever in Panama. Little more is known about the disease potential of these three viruses.

STRUCTURE

Orbiviruses have spherical virions that contain 10 (or, for Colorado tick fever virus, 12) segments of double-stranded RNA, exhibit icosahedral symmetry, and have a diameter of 60 to 80 nm. The total molecular weight is about 12×10^6. Orbivirus infectivity is destroyed at pH 3.0. Orbiviruses have at least seven structural and two nonstructural polypeptides.

CLASSIFICATION AND ANTIGENIC TYPES

The genus *Orbivirus* consists of at least 109 serotypes of arthropod-borne viruses. They form 13 serogroups and at least 6 ungrouped viruses. The major group-reactive polypeptide is P7, which reacts broadly by the complement fixation test. The major type-specific polypeptide is P2, a surface component principally responsible for the neutralization reaction.

MULTIPLICATION

Orbiviruses replicate in the cytoplasm. They replicate in arthropods as well as in vertebrates and are transmitted by arthropods, thus differing from ro-

TABLE 63-1   Orbiviruses Associated with Human Disease

Virus	Disease in Humans	Vector	Location
Colorado tick fever	Fever, rarely pericarditis, encephalitis, or hemorrhage	Tick	Western North America
Kemerovo	Fever, meningitis	Tick	Western Siberia
Orungo	Fever	Mosquito	Nigeria, Uganda, Senegal, Central African Republic
Changuinola	Fever	Phlebotomine sandfly	Panama, northern South America

taviruses and reoviruses. The virion outer shell must be removed to activate the RNA-dependent RNA polymerase. RNA segment reassortment between closely related orbiviruses accounts for genetic diversity and may lead to rapid changes in properties of viruses.

PATHOGENESIS

Colorado tick fever virus replicates in *Dermacentor andersoni* ticks that are infected in the larval stage when they feed on blood of the golden-mantled ground squirrel or other rodents (Fig. 63-4). After a period of days or weeks, the virus appears in the tick's saliva. The tick, which remains infectious for life, feeds on humans during its adult stage. The virus does not pass transovarially in the tick.

In humans, Colorado tick fever virus, possibly after infecting the regional lymph nodes, replicates in the bone marrow cells, arresting the maturation of the polymorphonuclear leukocytes, eosinophils, and basophils and sometimes causing severe thrombocytopenia. Erythrocytes presumably are infected as erythroblasts and are later detected in large numbers as antigen-containing red blood cells in the peripheral blood. The virus is found only briefly in serum. Antibody appears about 2 weeks after the onset of symptoms, but virus can still be isolated from peripheral blood cells for up to 6 weeks.

In 3 to 15 percent of infected children under 10 years of age, Colorado tick fever virus invades the central nervous system and causes encephalitis. Virus has been isolated from the cerebrospinal fluid of some of these patients.

HOST DEFENSES

There have been very few studies of the host defenses against Colorado tick fever virus. Nonimmune persons appear to be uniformly susceptible. Symptoms subside when humoral antibody appears, although exacerbations are reported; the role of cell-mediated immunity is not known. The

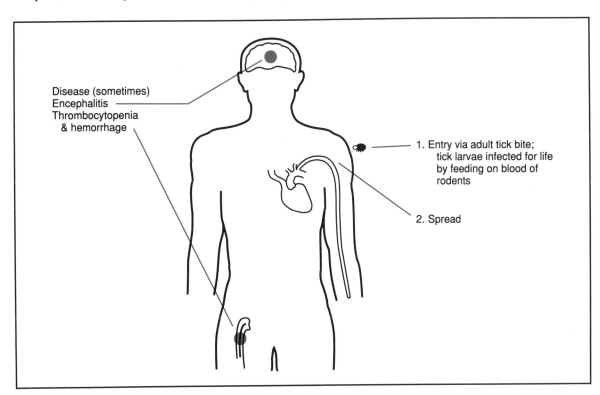

Disease (sometimes)
Encephalitis
Thrombocytopenia
& hemorrhage

1. Entry via adult tick bite; tick larvae infected for life by feeding on blood of rodents

2. Spread

FIGURE 63-4 Pathogenesis of Colorado tick fever.

virus induces interferon, but it is not known whether interferon is important in host defense.

EPIDEMIOLOGY

The distribution of Colorado tick fever is the same as that of its principal tick vector, *D andersoni*. The disease is found in California, Colorado, Idaho, Montana, Nevada, Oregon, Utah, Washington, Wyoming, British Columbia, and Alberta; 200 to 400 cases are reported each year. Campers, hikers, and foresters are commonly infected. Infections occur mainly in April, May, and June, when adult ticks are abundant. The virus overwinters in nymphal ticks, which feed on and infect small rodents in the spring. The rodents become viremic and in turn infect larval ticks. The larvae metamorphose during the summer; they overwinter as infected nymphs and do not transmit virus to humans until reaching the adult stage, which may be 1 or 2 years after infection. Foci of infected ticks occur primarily in ecologic zones favorable to large populations of ground squirrels and other small rodents.

DIAGNOSIS

Colorado tick fever should be suspected in individuals in western North America with diphasic fever, leukopenia, and a history of exposure to ticks 3 to 6 days before onset of disease. Diagnosis depends on isolation of the virus, demonstration of antigen in the red blood cells, or demonstration of a fourfold rise or fall in antibody titer from the acute to the convalescent phase. Virus is readily isolated from erythrocytes by inoculating them into tissue culture or intracerebrally into baby mice. Antibody is washed from red cells or removed by trypsin treatment to enhance the chance of isolation. Red cells may still be positive up to 6 weeks after infection. Antigen also can be detected in red cells by the immunofluorescence technique. Within 1 week of onset of symptoms, antibody appears in the serum as determined by indirect immunofluorescence. Neutralizing antibody appears somewhat later. The complement fixation test does not become positive until about 3 weeks after onset of illness. A travel history can aid the physician and the laboratory in diagnosis. Because of the long duration of

viremia, definitive diagnosis of Colorado tick fever has been made in persons returning home far from the endemic area where the infection was acquired.

CONTROL

Colorado tick fever can be prevented by avoiding tick-infested areas, by wearing long-sleeved tight-fitting clothing, by checking the body for ticks every 3 hours while camping or hiking and removing them, and by using tick repellents such as diethyltoluamide. Theoretically, campgrounds should be located away from the habitat of the golden-mantled ground squirrel and other rodents; however, these creatures are favorites of campers, and such a measure would not be popular. No vaccine or specific treatment for the disease is available.

REFERENCES

Carlson JAK, Middleton PJ, Szymanski M et al: Fatal rotavirus gastroenteritis. Analysis of 21 cases. Am J Dis Child 132:477, 1978

Cook SM, Glass RI, LeBaron CW, Ho M-S: Global seasonality of rotavirus infections. Bull WHO 68:171, 1990

Davidson GP, Whyte PBD, Daniels E et al: Passive immunization of children with bovine colostrum containing antibodies to human rotavirus. Lancet 2:709, 1989

Emmons RW: Ecology of Colorado tick fever. Annu Rev Microbiol 42:49, 1988

Estes MK, Cohen J: Rotavirus gene structure and function. Microbiol Rev 53:410, 1989

Kapikian AZ, Chanock RM: Rotaviruses. p. 1353. In Fields BN, Knipe DM (eds): Virology. Vol. 2. Plenum, New York, 1990

Kapikian AZ, Flores JF, Midthun K et al: Strategies for the development of a rotavirus vaccine against infantile diarrhea with an update on clinical trials of rotavirus vaccines. Adv Exp Biol Med 257:67, 1989

Matsui SM, Mackow ER, Greenberg HB: Molecular determinants of rotavirus neutralization and protection. Adv Virus Res 36:181, 1989

Perez-Schael I, Garcia D, Gonzalez M et al: Prospective study of diarrheal diseases in Venezuelan children to evaluate the efficacy of rhesus rotavirus vaccine. J Med Virol 30:219, 1990

Rodriguez WJ, Kim HW, Arrobio JO et al: Clinical features of acute gastroenteritis associated with human reovirus-like agent in infants and young children. J Pediatr 91:188, 1977

Santosham M, Burns B, Nadkarni V et al: Oral rehydration therapy for acute diarrhea in ambulatory children in the United States. A double-blind-comparison of four different solutions. Pediatrics 76:159, 1985

Sharpe AH, Fields BN: Pathogenesis of viral infections. Basic concepts derived from the reovirus model. N Engl J Med 312:486, 1985

Tyler KL, Fields BN: Reoviruses. p. 1307. In Fields BN, Knipe DM (eds): Virology. Vol. 2. Plenum, New York, 1990

Yolken RH, Bishop CA, Townsend TR et al: Infectious gastroenteritis in bone-marrow transplant recipients N Engl J Med 306:1009, 1984

64 PARVOVIRUSES

JOHN R. PATTISON
GARY PATOU

C = 12
18-26 nm

GENERAL CONCEPTS

Clinical Manifestations

Individuals with **erythema infectiosum** have a fever and a rubelliform rash that begins on the face and spreads to the trunk and limbs. In patients with a preexisting hemolytic anemia (e.g., sickle cell anemia), the disease can cause **aplastic crisis** (transient bone marrow erythroid aplasia). In women, disease late in pregnancy can cause spontaneous abortion and edematous anemic stillbirth **(hydrops fetalis).**

Structure

Parvoviruses are nonenveloped, icosahedral particles 18 to 26 nm in diameter. The DNA is positive sense and single-stranded. There are two or three capsid proteins.

Classification and Antigenic Types

Parvoviruses are classified by size, morphology, and genomic organization. A single antigenic type is associated with human disease.

Multiplication

Replication takes place in the nucleus of dividing cells. The single-stranded DNA genome forms an intermediate double-stranded form, which replicates to form progeny positive and negative single-stranded DNA.

Positive and negative strands are packaged separately in viral capsids in equal numbers.

Pathogenesis

The disease is transmitted by the respiratory route. The virus replicates in committed erythroid precursor cells in the bone marrow, leading to erythroid aplasia. Aplastic anemia develops in patients with underlying hemolytic anemia, and rash and arthralgia develop at the time specific antibody appears.

Host Defenses

Specific IgM and IgG antibodies develop in response to infection.

Epidemiology

Erythema infectiosum is found worldwide. Outbreaks occur predominantly in spring, mainly in school children and young adults, with peaks of activity at 4- to 5-year intervals.

Diagnosis

Diagnosis is by detecting viral DNA in serum and a rise in parvovirus-specific IgM or IgG.

Control

No specific antiviral therapy or vaccine is yet available.

INTRODUCTION

The parvoviruses (*parvo* meaning small) are a group of very small DNA viruses that are ubiquitous and infect many species of animals. The small amount of DNA contained in the viruses does not carry sufficient genetic information to direct its own replication in host cells. As a result, parvoviruses have unusual requirements for replication, such as a helper virus or rapidly dividing cells, and are divided into two groups on the basis of these requirements. The parvoviruses that multiply only in cells coinfected with a helper adenovirus constitute the genus *dependovirus* (previously called the adeno-associated viruses [AAVs]). These viruses have not been shown to cause disease in humans. The second group of parvoviruses, constituting the genus *Parvovirus,* do not require a helper virus for replication; however, they multiply only in cells that are in the process of replicating their own DNA. The diseases caused by autonomous parvoviruses reflect their requirement for actively dividing cells. The human autonomous parvovirus, B19 virus, replicates in erythroid precursor cells and hence produces aplastic crisis in predisposed individuals with underlying hemolytic anemia or immunodeficiency. Other clinical manifestations of B19 virus infection are due to the host immune response to the virus.

CLINICAL MANIFESTATIONS
Erythema Infectiosum

Erythema infectiosum, also known as **fifth disease,** is the commonest clinical manifestation of B19 virus infection. Clinical symptoms develop in a biphasic fashion. Some 7 to 8 days after infection, a prodromal influenzalike illness develops, characterized by headache, malaise, chills, and pyrexia. Individuals are then asymptomatic for a week. The second phase of illness occurs 17 to 18 days after infection, with the development of a mild febrile illness and a maculopapular rash. The first sign of illness is marked erythema of the cheeks ("slapped-cheeks" appearance) followed by a rash on the trunk and limbs. The rash initially has a discrete erythematous maculopapular appearance and then becomes reticular, disappearing in 1 to 3 weeks. Erythema infectiosum often resembles the rash of rubella. A rash does not always occur following B19 virus infection, and the only manifestation of the second phase of the illness may be a mild, influenzalike illness. Joint involvement occurs in most women and much less frequently in men and children. The commonest presentation is of an acute-onset, symmetric arthritis involving the small joints of the hands, wrists, ankles, and knees. Recovery usually occurs within 2 to 4 weeks. B19 arthropathy may also occur in the absence of the rash. Transient lymphopenia, neutropenia, and thrombocytopenia are complications of B19 virus infection, but are rarely severe enough to cause problems.

Aplastic Crisis

An acute, self-limiting **aplastic crisis** occurs following B19 virus infection in individuals with underlying hemolytic anemias such as sickle cell anemia, hereditary spherocytosis, β-thalassemia intermedia, pyruvate kinase deficiency, and autoimmune hemolytic anemia. Patients develop acute symptoms of severe anemia with a critically low hemoglobin level, reticulocytopenia, and occasionally leukopenia and thrombocytopenia. Bone marrow examination shows a complete absence of erythroid precursors. The anemia is self-limiting, but blood transfusion support is required until the bone marrow recovers. Reticulocytes then reappear in the peripheral blood, and hemoglobin concentrations return to the steady state for this patient group. Individuals who have hemolytic anemias and have recently been transfused may escape the aplastic crisis complication of B19 virus infection.

Fetal Loss and Hydrops Fetalis

During B19 virus infection an intense viremia develops. In a pregnant woman host the virus may cross the placenta and establish infection in the fetus. The fetus is unable to control and eradicate B19 virus, and accordingly viral replication may continue for several weeks. In the first and second trimesters of pregnancy, B19 virus infection is associated with an increased risk of **fetal abortion** and nonimmune **hydrops fetalis.** Severe anemia (akin to the aplastic anemia seen in patients with hemolytic anemia) and edema occur up to 12 weeks after maternal infection. Infection in the third trimester of pregnancy has been less intensively studied, but a macerated stillbirth fetus has been reported at 39 weeks of gestation. The overall incidence of B19 virus-induced fetal loss is not precisely known but appears to be about 9 percent of affected pregnancies. Most pregnancies continue to term with the delivery of normal babies.

STRUCTURE

Human B19 virus is a nonenveloped, icosahedral virus with a diameter of 18 to 26 nm. The virus capsid is composed of two (possibly three) structural proteins. Structural proteins VP-1 and VP-2 have molecular weights of 83,000 and 58,000, respectively, and account for 60 to 80 percent of the virion mass. The virus has a positive single-stranded DNA genome 5.5 kilobases long. It is very hardy and viral infectivity is resistant to ether, chloroform, deoxyribonuclease (DNase) and ribonuclease (RNase) treatment.

CLASSIFICATION AND ANTIGENIC TYPES

Both genera in the family Parvoviridae, *Dependovirus* and *Parvovirus,* contain members capable of infecting humans, but only one parvovirus strain causes disease. Dependoviruses are defective parvoviruses that require a helper virus, such as an adenovirus, for replication. They have not been shown to cause disease in humans. Parvoviruses are **autonomous** (capable of independent replication). The parvovirus known as B19 virus, which exists as a single serotype, causes disease in humans. Parvoviruslike particles have been observed by electron microscopy in feces, but their pathogenic potential is uncertain. Definitive classification of these agents awaits their biochemical characterization.

MULTIPLICATION

B19 virus replicates in the nucleus of infected cells. B19 DNA synthesis is assumed to be similar to that of other autonomous parvoviruses and involves the formation of double-stranded replicative intermediates. Progeny DNA is formed by strand displacement and depends on some function found only in the late S phase of the cell cycle. Single positive and negative strands are packaged separately within newly synthesized capsids. Nonstructural proteins cause lysis of the cell, with release of progeny virus.

PATHOGENESIS

B19 virus is transmitted most commonly via the respiratory route, although blood-borne transmission following whole blood or factor VIII transfusion has been reported (Fig. 64-1). Virus is detectable in throat secretions for some 5 days, starting 1 week after infection (Fig. 64-2). It is not known whether the virus has a site of replication in the respiratory tract.

The manifestation of clinically apparent disease following parvovirus infection depends on two interacting factors: the survival time of the circulating erythrocytes in the host and the immune response to the virus. The virus replicates in erythroid precursor cells, causing lysis of these susceptible cells and transient loss of all erythrocyte precursors from the bone marrow. In hematologically normal hosts this leads to a transient reticulocytopenia without a significant fall in the number of circulating erythrocytes. In patients with hemolytic anemia, however, the life span of erythrocytes is much shorter than normal, so that the loss of erythroid precursors in the marrow leads to a rapid fall in the circulating erythrocyte population and to development of the aplastic crisis of B19 infection.

Six to seven days after acquisition of the virus a viremia develops, coincident with the prodromal influenzalike illness. The second phase of B19 disease depends on the immune response to the virus. Erythema infectiosum and arthralgia develop 17 to 18 days after the acquisition of the virus and at the time of the appearance of specific IgM and IgM-virus immune complexes. The virus is no longer detectable, and the rash is probably due to the antibody response to the virus. The mechanism of the occurrence of B19 infection without the development of a rash is not understood.

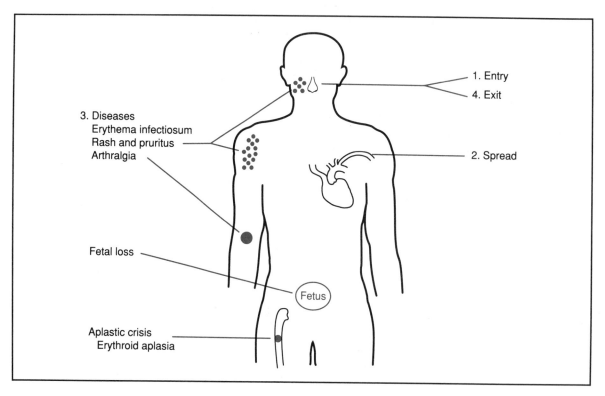

FIGURE 64-1   Clinical manifestations and pathogenesis of B19 virus infection.

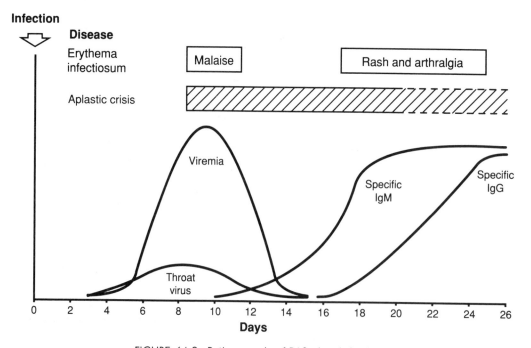

FIGURE 64-2   Pathogenesis of B19 virus infection.

Fetal disease develops when the virus crosses the placenta and establishes infection in the fetal erythroid precursors. Since the fetus cannot mount an adequate immune response, B19 infection becomes chronic and leads to erythroid aplasia and anemia, with consequent fetal loss early in pregnancy and hydrops fetalis and stillbirths following infection later in pregnancy. Chronic B19 virus infection accompanied by chronic anemia has occurred occasionally in immunodeficient patients suffering from leukemia or acquired immune deficiency syndrome (AIDS).

HOST DEFENSES

B19-specific IgM is first detectable as the viremia wanes, 9 to 10 days after the onset of infection, and peak levels develop within 1 week. Much of the early antibody is complexed with virus in immune complexes. Specific IgG is not detectable until 2 weeks after the onset of infection, and peak levels develop more slowly over the following 2 weeks. The role of cell-mediated immunity following B19 infection is unknown.

EPIDEMIOLOGY

B19 infection is found worldwide and occurs throughout the year, although in temperate zones infection is most common in the spring. In addition, there are longer-term cycles of virus activity with peaks of activity every 4 to 5 years. B19 infection is most commonly acquired between the ages of 4 and 10 years, with outbreaks of erythema infectiosum occurring in junior schools in the spring. Sixty percent of adults have specific IgG, indicating past infection with B19 virus.

DIAGNOSIS

B19 virus is not cultivatable in conventional cell culture, although bone marrow suspension and fetal liver culture support very limited viral replication. For this reason, the early diagnosis of B19 infection is established by detection of B19 antigen or DNA in serum or throat secretions. Parvovirus particles are visualized by electron microscopy within 24 hours of the onset of symptoms in 30 percent of patients. Later the diagnosis is established by demonstrating a specific IgM response or the development of specific IgG in an individual known to lack specific IgG prior to the illness (seroconversion). Since normal individuals are viremic and shed virus prior to the onset of characteristic symptoms, the diagnosis is established by antibody testing. Patients with hemolytic anemia may develop aplastic crisis while still viremic, and so antigen and DNA detection tests, along with the antibody test, may be used. To establish the diagnosis of fetal infection, fetal serum should be tested for B19 DNA, as the fetus may fail to make an IgM response and IgG, if present, may reflect passively acquired maternal antibody.

B19 antigen may be detected in serum by countercurrent immunoelectrophoresis, radioimmunoassay, and enzyme immunoassay, although only the last two are sensitive enough to detect B19 antigen in throat secretions. DNA–DNA dot blot hybridization is a very sensitive test for detecting B19 DNA in any infected body fluid.

Anti-B19 antibody is detected by countercurrent immunoelectrophoresis or immune electron microscopy, although the most widely used tests are IgM and IgG capture radioimmunoassays or enzyme immunoassays. B19 IgM persists for 2 to 3 months after the onset of symptoms; IgG is detectable for much longer and probably persists for life, although it may fall below the level of detection by currently available assays.

CONTROL

There is no specific antiviral therapy or vaccine for B19 infection, and most individuals do not require symptomatic therapy. Patients with aplastic crisis require erythrocyte transfusion support until the bone marrow recovers. Administration of normal human immunoglobulins to immunodeficient, B19-infected patients may produce transient amelioration of viremia and anemia.

Most persons infected with B19 virus are asymptomatic when viral shedding is maximal, and therefore control of infection is difficult. Patients presenting with erythema infectiosum are no longer infectious and do not require isolation. Patients with aplastic crisis may be infectious at the time of presentation and should not be cared for near other high-risk-at-risk hematology, immunodeficient, or pregnant patients.

REFERENCES

Anderson MJ, Higgins PG, Davis LR et al: Experimental parvovirus infection in man. J Infect Dis 152:257, 1985

Anderson MJ, Pattison JR: The human parvovirus. Arch Virol 82:137, 1985

Clewley JP: Biochemical characterization of a human parvovirus. J Gen Virol 65:241, 1984

Cotmore S, Tattersall P: Characterization and molecular cloning of a human parvovirus genome. Science 226:1161, 1984

Coulombiel L, Morinet F, Mielot F, Tchernia G: Parvovirus infection, leukaemia, and immunodeficiency. Lancet 1:101, 1989

Reid DM, Reid TM, Brown T, Rennie J: Human parvovirus-associated arthritis: a clinical and laboratory description. Lancet 1:422, 1985

Schwarz TF, Roggendorf M, Hottentrager B et al: Human parvovirus B19 infection in pregnancy. Lancet 2:566, 1988

Serjeant GR, Topley JM, Mason K et al: Outbreak of aplastic crisis in sickle cell anemia associated with parvovirus-like agent. Lancet 2:595, 1981

65 NORWALK VIRUS AND CALICIVIRUSES

NEIL R. BLACKLOW

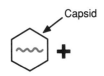

Capsid

C = 32 (holes)
35-40 nm

GENERAL CONCEPTS

Clinical Manifestations

Norwalk virus and calicivirus infections cause acute diarrhea and vomiting (gastroenteritis), abdominal cramps, myalgias, malaise, headache, nausea, and low-grade fever.

Structure

Norwalk virus is a round, nonenveloped, 27-nm virion. It is not cultivatable in vitro, and the nucleic acid is not known. It has the single structural protein characteristic of a calicivirus. Human calicivirus virions are similar but slightly larger and have surface cup-shaped indentations.

Classification and Antigenic Types

The caliciviruses are grouped on the basis of morphology, size, protein profile, and buoyant density. Norwalk virus, a few other Norwalk-like viruses, and human calicivirus are antigenically distinct.

Multiplication

Nucleic acids and replicative cycles are unknown.

Pathogenesis

Infection is by oral ingestion. Viruses grow in the small intestine, causing transient lesions of intestinal mucosa, and are shed in feces.

Host Defenses

Antibodies against Norwalk virus are not protective, but represent risk factors or markers for illness. Antibody against human calicivirus correlates with resistance to illness.

Epidemiology

About half of the outbreaks of acute infectious nonbacterial gastroenteritis in the United States are due to Norwalk virus. The disease occurs worldwide and is common in older children and adults. Outbreaks occur in camps, schools, nursing homes, etc., and are associated with contaminated water and uncooked foods.

Diagnosis

The diagnosis is suggested by acute gastroenteritis in a community outbreak setting. It may be confirmed by antigen detection or observation of an antibody rise; these techniques are available only in research laboratories.

Control

No antiviral therapy or vaccine is available.

INTRODUCTION

The caliciviruses are small, nonenveloped RNA viruses that have characteristic cup-shaped depressions on a spherical capsid surface; hence their name, which is derived from *calyx* or chalice. Caliciviruses have a distinctive structure, sometimes described as a star of David, and are also distinctive in their size (27 to 35 nm), in having only a single major polypeptide, and in the functions of the single-stranded RNA genome. They produce mucocutaneous and respiratory tract lesions in several animal species, including swine, pinnipeds, and cats, and they have been grown in cell culture, purified, and characterized.

Human caliciviruses have not been cultivated in vitro, and so no human strains are as well characterized as the animal caliciviruses. Human viruses with morphologic and biophysical features similar to those of animal caliciviruses, however, are often observed in patients with diarrheal illness. The best known of the human agents is Norwalk virus, which is a major cause of epidemics of self-limited diarrhea and vomiting in school children and adults. Resistance to the infection is unrelated to serum antibody.

CLINICAL MANIFESTATIONS

Norwalk virus produces a classic clinical picture of acute diarrhea and/or vomiting (gastroenteritis) in older children and adults. This common illness has an abrupt onset and is accompanied by a varying combination of signs and symptoms, including abdominal cramps, myalgias, malaise, headache, nausea, and low-grade fever. The disease usually resolves spontaneously within 24 to 48 hours. Fatalities are very rare and are confined to elderly or debilitated individuals. Human calicivirus produces a clinical syndrome similar to that of Norwalk virus, but, similar to rotavirus gastroenteritis, also causes diarrhea and vomiting in infants and young children.

STRUCTURE

Norwalk virus is a small (diameter, 27 nm), round, nonenveloped virus with an amorphous surface structure possessing a feathery, ragged outline.

Because it has not been cultivated in cell culture, the nature of its nucleic acid is unknown. It is recognized in human stool specimens only by immune electron microscopic or immunoassay techniques. Norwalk virus, purified from feces, contains a single structural protein with a molecular weight of about 60,000. The only defined group of animal viruses known to possess this protein profile is the single-stranded, RNA-containing calicivirus group.

Human calicivirus is described as being round and slightly larger than Norwalk virus in feces (31 to 35 nm in diameter). It has cup-shaped indentations on the virion surface, which make the virus indistinguishable from well-characterized caliciviruses of animals. Human calicivirus contains a single structural protein of a similar molecular weight to that of Norwalk virus; also, it has not been cultivated and serially passaged in cell culture.

CLASSIFICATION AND ANTIGENIC TYPES

On the basis of their morphology, size, protein profile, and buoyant density, Norwalk virus and human calicivirus are classified in the family Caliciviridae. This classification is not based on characterization of their nucleic acids, since this has not been done. Several viruses are described that share with Norwalk virus the characteristics of morphology, size, density, noncultivatability in vitro, and association with epidemics or family outbreaks of acute gastroenteritis. Like Norwalk virus, these viruses are named after the location of the outbreak from which they are derived (Norwalk, Ohio; Hawaii; Snow Mountain, Colorado; Taunton, England; Otofuke and Sapporo, Japan). At least three of these viruses (Norwalk, Hawaii, and Snow Mountain) are antigenically distinct on the basis of immune electron microscopy studies. Less is known about these Norwalk-like viruses than about Norwalk virus. Immune electron microscopy studies indicate that human calicivirus is also antigenically distinct from Norwalk virus. However, some patients recovering from human calicivirus gastroenteritis mount antibody responses to Norwalk virus in addition to calicivirus; this suggests that the two viruses share some immunologic properties.

MULTIPLICATION

Because these viruses have not been cultivated in vitro, their nucleic acids and replicative cycles are unknown.

PATHOGENESIS

These viruses are ingested orally from contaminated water or foods or are spread from person to person by the fecal-oral route (Fig. 65-1). Norwalk virus was first discovered in diarrheal stool specimens from patients infected during an epidemic of gastroenteritis that occurred in Norwalk, Ohio, in 1968. The disease was reproduced in adult volunteers, who developed a transient mucosal lesion of the proximal small intestine. Norwalk virus infection seems to spare the large intestine, and so fecal leukocytes are not present in the stool. Delayed gastric emptying occurs during this infection.

HOST DEFENSES

Although most adults have serum antibodies to Norwalk virus, the antibodies do not protect them from the disease. In fact, they may be a marker or risk factor for illness. When Norwalk virus was given to volunteers, one of two types of immune responses occurred. One group of individuals, who lacked appreciable serum or intestinal antibodies, persistently failed to develop illness or to mount antibody responses on initial exposure to the virus and after rechallenge up to 3 years later. A second group of volunteers, who had systemic or local antibodies, developed gastroenteritis on initial exposure and were again susceptible when rechallenged 3 years later. After the illness, these individuals usually developed a short-term immunity that lasted for about 12 weeks. Further studies are needed to ascertain whether genetic susceptibility or the need for repetitive past exposures to the virus play a role in the pathogenesis of Norwalk virus infection. For human calicivirus, the pres-

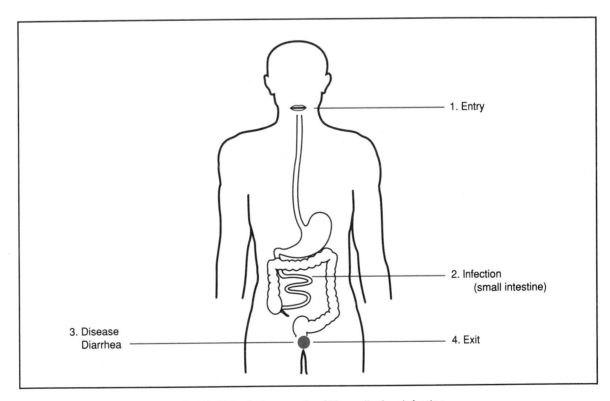

FIGURE 65-1 Pathogenesis of Norwalk virus infection.

ence of serum antibody correlates with resistance to illness, unlike the pattern of clinical immunity seen with Norwalk virus.

EPIDEMIOLOGY

Norwalk virus produces nearly 50 percent of all outbreaks of acute infectious, nonbacterial gastroenteritis in the United States. This common syndrome is characterized by 1 to 2 days of diarrhea or vomiting or both and is the second most common cause of illness in American families, after respiratory tract disease. In developed areas, the illness typically occurs in older children and adults and spares preschool children.

Seroprevalence studies indicate that Norwalk virus infection occurs worldwide. Two-thirds of Americans have serum antibodies, which are uncommon in children and are acquired during early adulthood. The results of antibody studies correlate with the rarity of Norwalk virus infection as a cause of gastroenteritis in infants and young children in the United States. Disease outbreaks among older children and adults occur in camps, schools, nursing homes, cruise ships, and areas with contaminated drinking or swimming water. The ingestion of raw shellfish or other uncooked foods, such as salads or cake frosting, that have been handled in an unsanitary manner may lead to the disease. Outbreaks of Norwalk virus infection occur throughout the year.

Infection is transmitted by the fecal-oral route. Although no evidence proves that the virus is also spread by the respiratory route, it might be transmitted via aerosolized virus-containing vomitus, in light of the very rapid secondary spread of infection during outbreaks.

Human calicivirus infection shares the epidemiologic pattern described above for Norwalk virus. However, unlike Norwalk virus, it also produces gastroenteritis in infants and preschool children, for example, in day care centers.

DIAGNOSIS

The diagnosis is suggested by acute diarrhea and/or vomiting in a community outbreak setting. Norwalk virus may be identified in stool specimens, and antibody can be measured in serum samples by

immune electron microscopic or immunoassay techniques (enzyme-linked immunosorbent assay, radioimmunoassay). Because these diagnostic methods require the use of human clinical materials (stools and sera), they can be performed in only a few research laboratories that possess the needed reagents. Immunoassay is preferable to immune electron microscopy for the examination of large numbers of specimens that are required for epidemiologic studies. Human calicivirus is diagnosed by techniques similar to those used for Norwalk virus.

CONTROL

No specific antiviral therapy is available for Norwalk or human calicivirus gastroenteritis. Prospects for vaccine development seem poor because of the complex pattern of clinical immunity to Norwalk virus. The development of a vaccine that produces long-lasting immunity seems unlikely because such immunity has been found to be absent in rechallenged volunteers. The inability to cultivate Norwalk virus and human calicivirus and to purify them extensively from feces also precludes vaccine development. Hand washing and careful monitoring of water purification are the most important measures in the control of infection.

REFERENCES

Blacklow NR, Cukor G: Viral gastroenteritis. N Engl J Med 304:397, 1981
Cubitt WD, Blacklow NR, Herrmann JE et al: Antigenic relationships between human caliciviruses and Norwalk virus. J Infect Dis 156:806, 1987
Greenberg HB, Valdesuso JR, Kalica AR et al: Proteins of Norwalk virus. J Virol 37:994, 1981
Johnson PC, Mathewson JJ, DuPont HL, Greenberg HB: Multiple-challenge study of host susceptibility to Norwalk gastroenteritis in US adults. J Infect Dis 161:18, 1990
Kaplan JE, Gary GW, Baron RC et al: Epidemiology of Norwalk gastroenteritis and the role of Norwalk virus in outbreaks of acute nonbacterial gastroenteritis. Ann Intern Med 96:756, 1982
Nakata S, Chiba S, Terashima H, Nakao T: Microtiter solid-phase radioimmunoassay for detection of human calicivirus in stools. J Clin Microbiol 17:198, 1983
Schaffer FL. Caliciviridae. Intervirology 14:1, 1980

66

PAPOVAVIRUSES

JANET S. BUTEL

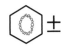

C = 72
45-55 nm

GENERAL CONCEPTS

POLYOMAVIRUS

Clinical Manifestations

Polyomaviruses exhibit asymptomatic persistent infections in humans. They induce tumors in laboratory rodents. JC virus causes progressive multifocal leukoencephalopathy in humans.

Structure

Polyomaviruses are icosahedral, 45-nm-diameter particles, with three capsid proteins and no envelope. They contain a 5-kbp circular, double-stranded DNA genome. The genome structure is similar for all members of the polyomavirus group and consists of two or three replicative genes (tumor antigens) encoded on one strand and three structural genes (capsid antigens) encoded on the other strand.

Classification and Antigenic Types

Classification is based on the structure of the virus particle. Human and animal polyomaviruses are antigenically distinct; only one serotype is known for each virus. The prototype is simian virus 40 (SV40) from monkeys.

Multiplication

Viral DNA uncoats in the nuclei of infected cells. Early viral genes are expressed and host cells are stimulated to enter the S phase, providing cellular enzymes that are utilized for viral DNA synthesis. Late viral genes are expressed, and progeny virions are assembled in nuclei. Cell lysis occurs later. Virus particles usually stay asso-

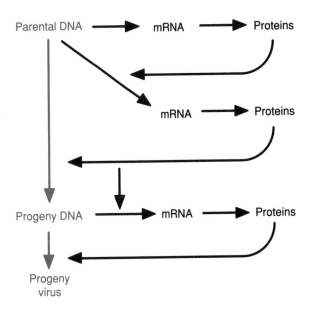

ciated with cell debris. The papovaviruses have oncogenic potential (the papillomaviruses in their natural hosts and the polyomaviruses under experimental conditions).

Pathogenesis

Human polyomaviruses establish persistent infections in the kidneys; these infections may reactivate in immunosuppressed hosts and during some normal pregnancies. Progressive multifocal leukoencephalopathy is a rare demyelinating disease of the central nervous system of some immunosuppressed patients. It is caused by replication of JC virus in oligodendrocytes. Although oncogenic in rodents, polyomaviruses are not believed to cause any human cancers.

Host Defenses

Infections are persistent and induce production of humoral antibodies and cytotoxic T cells. Virus reactivation occurs in immunosuppressed persons. Impaired cell-mediated immunity is the background for the development of progressive multifocal leukoencephalopathy. Interferon is weakly induced by papovaviruses, which vary in their sensitivity to the antiviral action of interferon. Transformation by polyomaviruses can be inhibited by interferon.

Epidemiology

BK and JC viruses are widespread. Infections occur during childhood, and 70 to 80 percent of adults have antibodies. The route of transmission is unknown, but may be respiratory. Human viruses have no animal reservoirs.

Diagnosis

Clinical presentation and the presence of antibodies are the best means of diagnosis.

Control

There are no known control measures.

PAPILLOMAVIRUS

Clinical Manifestations

Clinical manifestations include benign papillomatous lesions of skin and mucous membranes (common warts, plantar warts, flat warts, anogenital warts, epidermodysplasia verruciformis, and laryngeal papillomas). Cervical intraepithelial neoplasia and cervical cancer are associated with human papillomavirus infection.

Structure

Papillomaviruses are similar to polyomaviruses, except that the particles are 55 nm in diameter, the DNA is 8 kbp in size, and the genome structure is more complex. All viral genes are encoded on one strand of DNA.

Classification and Antigenic Types

Classification is based on the structure of the virus parti-
cle. Reagents are not available for serotyping; human papillomavirus types are distinguished by DNA hybridization assays. There are more than 50 human types.

Multiplication

Replication is dependent on the differentiated state of epithelial cells. Viral DNA remains latent (not integrated) in basal cells of benign lesions. Replication occurs in differentiating cells. Capsid proteins and virus particles are found only in terminally differentiated epidermal cells. Viral DNA is integrated in cancer cells, which contain no replicating virus.

Pathogenesis

Different human papillomavirus types cause specific lesions. The pathogenic mechanisms are not well understood. A few specific types, notably human papillomavirus types 16 and 18, are associated with the development of premalignant and malignant genital lesions. Cofactors are required for cancer development.

Host Defenses

The roles of humoral and cell-mediated immune responses in disease pathogenesis or prevention are not known. Warts tend to regress spontaneously.

Epidemiology

Papillomaviruses are widely distributed. Transmission occurs by contact. Genital warts are sexually transmitted. Laryngeal papillomas may be due to human papillomavirus acquired during birth from a mother with genital warts. Prevalence data are incomplete, and there are no serologic assays to distinguish the different types.

Diagnosis

Clinically, nucleic acid hybridization may be used to detect viral DNA in tissue samples. Serologic methods are needed to identify specific human papillomavirus types.

Control

Instruments should be sterilized after examination of patients with human papillomavirus infections. The public should be educated about this disease to prevent sexual transmission. Most warts regress spontaneously. Available treatments include local destructive methods and application of caustic agents. Interferons are effective against laryngeal papillomas, common warts, and anogenital warts.

INTRODUCTION

The term "papovavirus" was derived from the first two letters of the names of three members of this group: *pa*pillomavirus, mouse *po*lyoma virus, and simian *va*cuolating virus (SV40). Members of this group can induce tumors in susceptible hosts and transform the morphologic characteristics of cells in culture.

STRUCTURE

Papovaviruses are small, nonenveloped, icosahedral viruses that contain circular, double-stranded DNA. Virus particles range in diameter from 45 to 55 nm. Papovaviruses contain a limited amount of genetic information (six or seven genes); the DNA has a molecular weight of 3×10^6 to 5×10^6. Two or three polypeptides are used to construct the icosahedral capsid that packages the genomic DNA. Cellular histones are incorporated into virions in close association with viral DNA, probably to aid in condensing the DNA inside the capsid.

CLASSIFICATION AND ANTIGENIC TYPES

Papovaviruses are divided into two genera, *Polyomavirus* and *Papillomavirus*, on the basis of physicochemical and biologic properties (Table 66-1).

TABLE 66-1 Properties of Papovaviruses

Characteristics	Subgroup (Genus)	
	Polyomavirus	*Papillomavirus*
Virion		
Capsid symmetry	Cubic	Cubic
Presence of envelope	No	No
Diameter	45 nm	55 nm
Genome		
Type of nucleic acid	DNA	DNA
Structure	Circular, double-stranded	Circular, double-stranded
Size	3×10^6 mol. wt.; 5 kbp	5×10^6 mol. wt.; 8 kbp
Coding of information	On both strands	On one strand
Oncogenic potential		
Tumors in natural hosts	No	Yes
Result of natural infection	Inapparent	Benign wart
Persistence of infectious virus in tumors	No	Sometimes
Transform cells in vitro	Yes	Rarely
Individual members		
Infect humans	JC, BK viruses	Human papillomaviruses, >50 types
Important animal isolates	Polyoma virus (mouse), SV40 (monkey)	Bovine, rabbit papillomaviruses

Polyomaviruses

Polyomaviruses, which are smaller than papillomaviruses, are about 45 nm in diameter and have a genome of approximately 3×10^6 daltons (approximately 5,200 bp). These viruses tend to induce persistent, apparently harmless infections in their natural hosts. They have attracted the attention of research scientists because they induce tumors when injected into rodents. In addition, because of their small genetic content, the polyomaviruses have served as simple model systems for exploring the molecular events in transformation and other mammalian cell biologic processes. One of the SV40 early gene products, the large tumor antigen (T antigen), is required for viral DNA replication during productive infection and for initiation and maintenance of the transformed phenotype. Two polyomaviruses, BK virus and JC virus, are found in humans. The human and animal polyomaviruses all are antigenically distinct. Only one serotype is known for each agent.

The genome of simian virus 40 (SV40), a polyomavirus that has been intensively studied, is diagrammed in Figure 66-1. The genetic structure of the human viruses in this genus, JC and BK viruses, closely resembles that of SV40. The polyoma virus of mice differs only in that it codes for an additional early gene product. The entire nucleotide sequences of several papovavirus DNAs have been determined. About half of the SV40 genome encodes nonstructural proteins that are expressed before viral DNA synthesis begins. The products of that region are designated **early functions.** The early proteins also are referred to as **tumor antigens** because they were first detected in virus-induced tumors by using sera from tumor-bearing animals. The other half of the viral genome codes for virion structural proteins, which are called **late functions** because they are expressed after viral DNA synthesis begins. The structural proteins make up the protein coat of the virus particles.

These viruses make maximum use of their limited amount of genetic information. Some of the virus-encoded proteins are encoded partly by shared regions of the DNA (e.g., VP2 and VP3; small t and large T antigens). Other proteins are

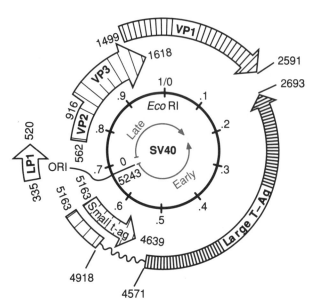

FIGURE 66-1 Physical and functional map of the SV40 genome (genus *Polyomavirus*). The thick circle represents the circular SV40 DNA genome. The unique *Eco*RI site is shown at map unit 0/1. Nucleotide numbers begin and end at the origin (ORI) of viral DNA replication (0/5243). Arrowheads point in the direction of transcription. The boxed arrows indicate the coding regions of mRNA, with the encoded protein designated within each arrow. Hatched areas within boxed arrows indicate that virus-specified polypeptides or portions thereof are encoded in different reading frames. The beginning and end of each open reading frame is indicated by nucleotide numbers. The genome is divided into early and late regions, which are expressed before and after the onset of viral DNA replication, respectively. Only the early region is expressed in transformed cells. (Modified from Butel JS, Jarvis DL: The plasma-membrane-associated form of SV40 large tumor antigen: biochemical and biological properties. Biochim Biophys Acta 865:171, 1986, with permission.)

translated from different reading frames from overlapping regions of the DNA (e.g., VP2 and VP1) (Fig. 66-1).

The two known human polyomaviruses have been studied extensively. BK virus was isolated from the urine of a recipient of a renal allograft who was undergoing immunosuppressive therapy, whereas JC virus was recovered from the brain tissue of a patient with progressive multifocal leukoencephalopathy, a rare demyelinating disease. The two viruses are antigenically distinct from each other and from other members of the *Polyomavirus* genus, but the early proteins (tumor antigens) induced by BK and JC viruses have some of the same antigenic determinants as those of SV40.

Papillomaviruses

The papillomaviruses are slightly larger than the polyomaviruses, with a more complex circular DNA genome (Table 66-1). In contrast to the polyomaviruses, the papillomaviruses induce tumors in their natural hosts. Papillomaviruses have been found in many species, including humans, rabbits, cows, and dogs. They are associated with a variety of benign papillomatous lesions of the skin and squamous mucosa.

The genome organization of the papillomaviruses differs significantly from that of the polyomaviruses (Fig. 66-2). Studies have been impeded by the lack of a tissue culture system that is able to support papillomavirus replication in vitro. However, recombinant DNA technology has been used to clone several papillomavirus genomes. Nucleotide sequence analyses have revealed as many as 10 open reading frames with molecular characteristics of probable structural genes. Two are "late" open reading frames that encode capsid proteins; others are "early" open reading frames that are probably involved in viral replication and/or cellular transformation.

Papillomaviruses cannot be cultured in vitro, and no serologic reagents are available to distinguish human isolates. Human papillomavirus types are distinguished on the basis of DNA homology. Each type shares less than 50 percent homology with all other recognized types under stringent DNA hybridization conditions. More than 50 different types have been identified, each of which

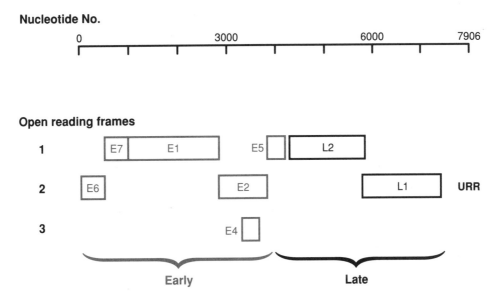

FIGURE 66-2 Map of the human papillomavirus type 16 genome (genus *Papillomavirus*). The DNA is circular, but is shown linearized in the upstream regulatory region (URR). The upstream regulatory region contains the origin of replication and enhancer and promoter sequences. Early (E1 – 7) and late (L1,2) open reading frames are shown. All the open reading frames are on the same strand of viral DNA.

tends to be associated with specific pathologic conditions.

Papillomavirus isolates from different animal species are serologically distinct. Antisera prepared against intact virus particles are type specific and will not react with tissues infected by another type of papillomavirus, but antisera against virions disrupted by detergent cross-react with capsid antigens of all papillomaviruses, including those from other species. This reflects the presence in papillomavirus structural proteins of conserved sequences that are not exposed on the surface of virus particles.

VIRUS MULTIPLICATION AND CELL TRANSFORMATION

Papovaviruses undergo two types of interactions with host cells (Fig. 66-3). **Permissive cells** sup-

port viral replication, which results in the synthesis of progeny virus and cell death (lysis). **Nonpermissive cells** do not support viral replication but can be transformed. When cells are transformed, the cells survive, the cellular phenotype is altered, and no progeny virus is produced. Most of our knowledge of viral replication and cell transformation is based on studies with SV40 and mouse polyoma virus. The expression of SV40-specific events in lytic and in transforming infections is compared in Table 66-2.

Polyomaviruses

The polyomaviruses have a narrow host range. Permissive cells are derived from the natural host of each isolate (monkey cells for SV40, mouse cells for polyoma virus, and human cells for BK and JC viruses). Not all cell types from the susceptible species will support viral replication.

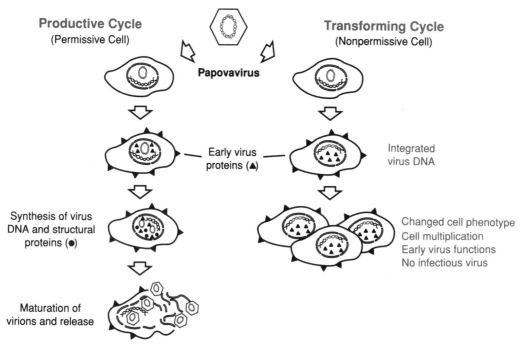

FIGURE 66-3 Schematic comparison of two types of interaction between a papovavirus and a host cell. The productive cycle that results in the synthesis of progeny virions is diagrammed on the left. The transforming cycle that is characterized by partial viral gene expression and cellular phenotypic changes is represented on the right. (Modified from Benyesh-Melnick M, Butel JS: Oncogenic viruses. p. 439. In Busch H (ed): The Molecular Biology of Cancer. Academic Press, San Diego, 1974, with permission.)

TABLE 66-2 Expression of Virus-Induced Events in
SV40 Productive and Transforming Infections

Event	Cytolytic Cycle[a]	Transformed Cells[a]
Synthesis of viral mRNA (early)	+	+
Synthesis of tumor antigens	+	+
Synthesis of transplantation antigen	+	+
Induction of host cell enzymes	+	+
Stimulation of host cell DNA synthesis	+	+
Integration of viral DNA into cellular chromosome	0	+
Synthesis of viral DNA	+	0
Synthesis of viral mRNA (late)	+	0
Synthesis of virus capsid antigens	+	0
Formation of virus particles	+	0
Cell death	+	0

[a] +, Present; 0, absent.

The infecting virion first attaches to specific receptors on permissive cells, then penetrates the plasma membrane and is transported to the nucleus, where the viral DNA is uncoated and released. During the early phase of the lytic cycle, the virus drives the cell into the S phase, thereby providing cellular enzymes associated with DNA metabolism, such as thymidine kinase and DNA polymerase. The virus uses the cellular enzymes for its own replication, as the polyomavirus genetic content is too limited to encode all the necessary replicative functions. The induction of host cell synthetic processes depends on the expression of the early portion of the viral genome. (The synthesis of SV40 large T antigen is required in that system.)

The early proteins (tumor antigens) are synthesized soon after infection and reach detectable levels about 12 to 15 hours after infection. Viral DNA synthesis begins shortly after that time. The large T antigen is a prerequisite for viral DNA replication. It binds to viral DNA at the site of initiation of DNA synthesis and is essential for viral replication in permissive cells. DNA replication proceeds bidirectionally from the unique origin site. The expression of late viral genes occurs after DNA synthesis begins. Early RNA is transcribed from half of one strand of viral DNA (E strand), whereas late viral RNA is transcribed from the other half of the genome, using the opposite strand of DNA (L strand) as a template (Fig. 66-1).

T-antigen binding initiates transcription of late viral RNA, in addition to initiating viral DNA replication.

The structural viral proteins VP1, VP2, and VP3 are synthesized from late viral mRNA and are transported into the nucleus. Progeny virions are assembled and accumulate in the nucleus, becoming detectable by 24 hours after infection. The host cells are killed eventually. As a group, the papovaviruses have the longest (slowest) growth cycle of the DNA viruses. Cell lysis usually does not occur until 40 to 48 hours after infection. Progeny virus particles are frequently not efficiently released from cell debris.

An important biologic property of the polyomaviruses is their ability to transform cells (i.e., to convert normal cells into tumor cells). Because transformation requires cell survival and multiplication, it is not compatible with lytic (productive) infections. Transforming infections are basically abortive and may result either from viral infection of nonpermissive cells or from the infection of permissive cells with defective viral genomes (Fig. 66-3). Permanent transformation by a polyomavirus is very rare (see Ch. 47).

The virus-induced early events that are expressed in permissive cells also occur in nonpermissive cells (Table 66-2). Host enzymes are induced, tumor antigens are synthesized, and cellular DNA synthesis is stimulated. However, no free viral DNA synthesis occurs, and late viral genes that encode capsid proteins are not expressed. The viral genome becomes integrated in the cellular chromosome. Integration of viral sequences into host cell DNA is random and can occur at many different sites. In general, only one or a very few viral DNA copies are present in an individual transformed cell. The entire viral genome need not be retained in transformed cells, but an intact early region is required because the transforming protein (the large T antigen) must be synthesized continuously for a cell to remain transformed.

Viral transformation and tumor induction involve two or more separate viral functions. One event is responsible for cell immortalization (unlimited cell proliferation), whereas another event mediates structural and behavioral changes characteristic of the transformed phenotype. The large T antigen is the critical gene product in the SV40 system. In transformed cells, the large T antigen localizes predominantly in the nucleus, although a small fraction (no more than 5 percent) is associated with the plasma membrane, where it is involved in virus-specific transplantation antigen reactions. In the mouse polyoma virus system, two early proteins have a role in carrying out the two transforming functions. Immortalization of primary cells is mediated by the large T antigen, which is localized in the nucleus. However, those cells remain phenotypically normal. In contrast, the polyoma virus middle T antigen (which associates with the plasma membrane) transforms immortalized cells, but is not able to alter primary cells. SV40 T antigen seems to mediate both transforming functions that are separated into two proteins in the polyomavirus system.

Transformation is a stable, inherited change in cell properties. The most prominent phenotypic modifications associated with SV40-transformed cells include altered morphology (more rounded); altered growth patterns (increased growth rate, decreased requirement for serum growth factors, loss of contact inhibition, and enhanced ability to grow in semisolid medium [anchorage independence]); biochemical changes (increased metabolic rate, increased glycolysis, changes in properties of the cell membrane, synthesis of new antigens in the cell); and tumorigenicity (production of tumors when transformed cells are injected into appropriate test animals).

Papillomaviruses

Papillomaviruses have a high tropism for epithelial cells of the skin and mucous membranes. Replication of the viruses depends strongly on the differentiated state of the cell. When present, progeny virions can be detected only in nuclei of cells in the upper layers of the infected epidermis (Fig. 66-4). Viral nucleic acid is presumably maintained in basal cells at low copy numbers, where it replicates in synchrony with the cell cycle. Vegetative viral DNA synthesis occurs predominantly in the stratum spinosum and the stratum granulosum, and capsid protein expression is restricted to the uppermost layer of terminally differentiated epidermal cells. Virus particles can be detected easily in some types of warts (e.g., hand and plantar warts), but may not be found in other types of lesions (e.g., those of the larynx, external genitalia, and cervix). Certain events in the viral life cycle presumably depend on cellular factors present in specific differentiated states of epithelial cells. This dependence of viral replication on cell differentiation probably is responsible for the failure of researchers to obtain a reproducible tissue culture system that is permissive for papillomavirus replication or transformation.

Regulation of gene expression in papillomaviruses appears much more complex than in polyomaviruses. Viral DNA remains episomal (free) in benign lesions, whereas it is integrated into host chromosomal DNA in malignant cells (e.g., cervical carcinoma). The E6 and E7 open reading frames are the transforming genes; both seem to be required for cell transformation.

The papillomaviruses induce benign tumors (warts) of the epithelium in their natural hosts. A few types are associated with carcinoma development. This expression of oncogenic potential in natural hosts is in marked contrast to the actions of the polyomaviruses, which do not cause tumors in natural hosts. The papillomaviruses have a narrow

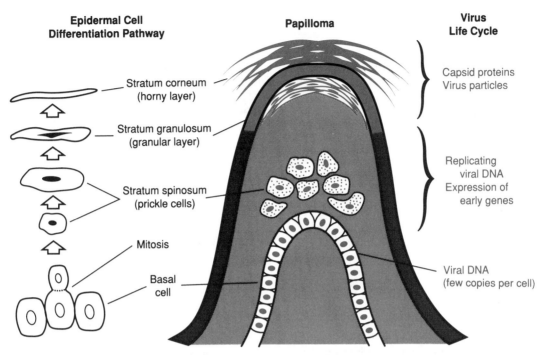

**Epidermal Cell
Differentiation Pathway**

Papilloma

**Virus
Life Cycle**

Stratum corneum
(horny layer)

Capsid proteins
Virus particles

Stratum granulosum
(granular layer)

Stratum spinosum
(prickle cells)

Replicating
viral DNA
Expression of
early genes

Mitosis

Basal
cell

Viral DNA
(few copies per cell)

FIGURE 66-4 Schematic representation of a skin wart (papilloma). The papillomavirus life cycle is tied to epithelial cell differentiation. The terminal differentiation pathway of epidermal cells is shown on the left. Events in the virus life cycle are noted on the right. Late events in viral replication (capsid protein synthesis and virion morphogenesis) occur only in terminally differentiated cells.

host range; no interspecies transmission has been documented.

POLYOMAVIRUSES

CLINICAL MANIFESTATIONS

The polyomaviruses establish persistent, harmless infections in their natural hosts. BK virus has not been proven to cause any clinical disease.

JC virus is presumed to cause **progressive multifocal leukoencephalopathy,** a rare disease due to an opportunistic JC virus infection of individuals with impaired immunity. Large numbers of virus particles are present within the nuclei of glial cells in the brain lesions of patients with progressive multifocal leukoencephalopathy. The onset of the disease is insidious. Early signs include abnormalities of speech and vision and alterations in mental function. The disease is progressive, culminating in coma and death, usually within 6 months of onset.

PATHOGENESIS

Both human polyomaviruses are ubiquitous among humans, with the initial infection occurring during childhood. Primary infections must include a viremic phase, because both BK and JC viruses persist in the kidneys of healthy individuals after the primary infection and may reactivate when the host immune response is impaired. It is not known whether JC virus reaches the brain during primary infection and persists there in a latent form until reactivated by immunosuppression, or whether it invades the brain (by viremia?) after reactivation of a persistent infection at a distant site, such as the kidneys. Even in cases of severe immunosuppression, progressive multifocal leukoencephalopathy rarely develops. The distinctive features of this disease are the presence of altered oligodendrocytes containing many papovavirus particles in their nuclei and the presence of giant astrocytes with hyperchromatic nuclei. Demyelination occurs because JC virus causes a lytic infection of the oligodendrocytes. In advanced lesions, oligodendrocytes are absent because of cell necrosis.

BK virus is often activated in renal transplant patients and in others who have received immunosuppressive agents, and it is excreted in the urine. Several cases of papovavirus-associated obstruction of the ureter have been described in renal allograft recipients. In addition, BK virus has been recovered from the urine of patients with hereditary immunodeficiency diseases, such as the Wiskott-Aldrich syndrome. Both BK and JC viruses may be reactivated and excreted in urine during normal pregnancies.

SV40 seems to localize in the urinary tract of its natural host, the rhesus monkey, but tumor induction in the monkey has not been observed. Early lots of live poliomyelitis vaccines that had been produced in monkey cells were contaminated with SV40. Many persons inadvertently received such SV40-contaminated vaccines 25 years ago; however, none have been reported to have developed SV40-related tumors. Although wild mice harbor polyoma virus, tumors do not result from natural infections. The virus probably is transmitted through urine, feces, and saliva. The oncogenic potential of the polyomaviruses can be demonstrated only by experimental inoculation of certain heterologous newborn animals (hamsters for SV40; mice, rats, and hamsters for polyoma virus).

HOST DEFENSES

The polyomavirus members of the papovavirus group produce asymptomatic, persistent infections in their natural hosts. They elicit an antibody response that can be detected serologically by, for example, neutralization or hemagglutination inhibition assays. BK and JC viruses have often been isolated from immunosuppressed individuals, indicating that their expression is under the control of the immunologic system. Impaired cell-mediated immunity is associated with virus reactiva-

tion and appears to be a determining factor in the development of progressive multifocal leukoencephalopathy. In contrast, patients with progressive multifocal leukoencephalopathy commonly have normal levels of serum antibody to JC virus.

The immune response of animals with tumors induced by polyomaviruses or SV40 has been studied extensively. Tumor-bearing animals develop antibodies against the virus-specific tumor antigens involved in the maintenance of the transformed phenotype. In addition, cellular immunity develops against virus-induced, tumor-specific transplantation antigens that are located at the cell membrane. This immunity renders the animals resistant to challenge with tumor cells. These rodent model systems afford an opportunity for understanding more about the immune response to neoplastic cells in humans.

EPIDEMIOLOGY

Seroepidemiologic studies have shown that BK and JC viruses occur worldwide. Infections occur early in childhood, and 70 to 80 percent of adults have antibodies to these viruses. Little is known about the routes of infection, but the spread in early childhood and the high infection rates suggest respiratory transmission. Although a low percentage of pregnant women shed BK or JC virus in their urine, especially during the third trimester, there is no indication of transplacental transmission and congenital infection by either virus. Both JC and BK viruses appear to be strictly human viruses, with no animal reservoirs.

SV40 infection of humans is rare, even though many persons were exposed to the virus when they received contaminated poliovirus vaccines.

DIAGNOSIS

Primary isolation of human polyomaviruses is too difficult to be attempted outside of specialized research laboratories. Viral DNA can be detected in suspect tissues by nucleic acid hybridization, and tissues and body fluids may be examined by electron microscopy to detect papovavirus particles. The hemagglutination-inhibition test is useful for serodiagnosis of JC and BK virus infections.

CONTROL

No control measures for human polyomavirus infections are currently available. As they are not linked to important human disease, there is no incentive to attempt to prevent infections in the general population. No effective treatments exist for progressive multifocal leukoencephalopathy. Reduction in immunosuppression would appear to offer the best opportunity for slowing the progression of this disease.

◀ PAPILLOMAVIRUSES ▶

CLINICAL MANIFESTATIONS

A variety of benign papillomatous lesions of the skin and squamous mucosa are caused by human papillomaviruses. These include common and plantar warts, flat warts, anal and genital condylomata acuminata, cervical flat warts, macular pityriasis-like lesions in patients with epidermodysplasia verruciformis, oral papillomas, and juvenile laryngeal papillomas. The laryngeal papillomas can be dangerous because they occur in young children and tend to cause acute respiratory obstruction and because they often recur.

Papillomavirus infections may be subclinical. The most common clinical changes in both males and females are condylomata acuminata (anogenital warts). Papillomavirus infections occur throughout the lower female genital tract. Multiple sites are often involved, including on the cervix, in the vagina, and in the vulvar region. In addition, lesions called cervical flat warts or cervical intraepithelial neoplasia are associated with human papillomavirus infection. These lesions are believed to reflect mild to moderate cervical dysplasia and are typified by large round cells called koilocytes. In men, anal condylomas and penile warts occur separately or together.

Epidermodysplasia verruciformis is a rare cutaneous disease characterized by disseminated lesions resembling flat warts and reddish macules.

Most papillomavirus-induced lesions are entirely benign and are not correlated with malignant transformation. However, certain human papillomavirus-associated anogenital lesions may progress to squamous cell carcinomas. In addition, epidermodysplasia verruciformis patients may develop skin carcinomas, and rare cases of laryngeal papillomatosis become malignant.

PATHOGENESIS

Papillomaviruses induce benign papillomas of the skin and squamous mucosa. Viruses are transmitted by contact and enter the body through minute abrasions in the skin. Cell growth control is disrupted, resulting in thickening of the epidermis with hyperplasia in the stratum spinosum and some degree of hyperkeratosis. Basophilic intranuclear inclusion bodies often occur in the stratum granulosum. The basement membrane remains intact.

Different human papillomavirus types cause distinct pathologic lesions (Table 66-3), although exceptions do occur. A few specific types are strongly associated with the development of premalignant and malignant genital disease. Most precancerous cervical intraepithelial neoplasias, as well as cervical, penile, and vulvar cancers, carry human papillomavirus DNA. On the basis of the relative occurrence of viral DNA in certain cancer tissues, human papillomavirus types are believed to vary in oncogenic potential. Types 16 and 18 are considered to pose a high cancer risk; type 31, intermediate risk; and types 6 and 11, low risk. Many other types are considered benign. For this reason, it will become important to identify the specific type present in a clinical lesion.

Laryngeal papillomas in children are caused by human papillomavirus types 6 and 11. It is believed the infection is acquired during passage through an infected birth canal, because infants with laryngeal papillomas are often born to mothers with genital condylomas.

Viral DNA is commonly found in epithelial cells surrounding a given lesion. Cofactors are most probably involved in the progression of high-risk human papillomavirus lesions to carcinomas. Suspected cofactors include irradiation, carcinogenic products of tobacco smoke, and genital infection by herpes simplex virus.

TABLE 66-3   Association of Human Papillomavirus
Types with Clinical Lesions

Human Papillomavirus Type	Clinical Lesion	Suspected Oncogenicity[a]
1	Plantar warts	Benign
2	Common warts	Benign
3, 10	Flat warts, EV[b]	Rare
5, 8, 9, 12, 14, 15, 17, 19–25	Macular lesions in EV	Some progress to carcinomas
6, 11	Anogenital condylomas; laryngeal papillomas; dysplasias and intraepithelial neoplasias	Low
7	Hand warts in butchers	Benign
13, 32	Oral focal hyperplasia (Heck's disease)	Possible progression
16, 18, 31, 33, 35, 39	Cervical intraepithelial neoplasia; invasive cervical cancer; Bowen's disease of vulva; laryngeal and esophageal carcinomas	High correlation with genital and oral cancers
37	Keratoacanthoma	Benign

[a] Based on presence of viral DNA in tumor tissue.
[b] EV, Epidermodysplasia verruciformis.

HOST DEFENSES

Host immune responses to papillomavirus infections are not well understood. In general, warts persist for variable periods and then regress. The host is probably immune to reinfection with the same virus. The respective roles of humoral and cellular immunity in this response are not known. Cell-mediated immunity is probably important, as immunosuppressed patients experience an increased incidence of warts. Among immunocompetent individuals, about one-third of the warts will regress within 2 months of appearance, two-thirds will disappear within a year, and all will be gone within 5 years.

Papovaviruses are generally poor inducers of interferon and vary greatly in their susceptibility to its antiviral action.

EPIDEMIOLOGY

Papillomaviruses are widely distributed in humans. Epidemiologic studies have been limited by the lack of suitable assays and the existence of multiple virus types.

Transmission of human papillomavirus occurs by direct contact with another infected person, by autoinoculation (e.g., common warts spread by scratching), or by indirect contact (e.g., plantar warts acquired in showers). Genital warts are sexually transmitted. Estimates of the rate of papillomavirus genital infections in the general population, based on studies of small groups, have ranged from 2 to 13 percent for women in western Europe to more than 30 percent for women in Latin America.

Strong epidemiologic evidence suggests that a sexually transmitted infectious agent is involved in the etiology of cervical cancer. This is compatible with the notion that human papillomavirus is a factor in the development of genital cancers. At least 80 to 90 percent of dysplastic cervical lesions (cervical intraepithelial neoplasia) and cervical cancers have been reported to contain human papillomavirus DNA. A recent study involving Latin American women concluded that infection with type 16 or 18 significantly increased the risk of cervical cancer. The prevalence of type 16 infections is about 10 times that of type 18 infections.

Preliminary results suggest that progression of precancerous lesions to cancer is higher with type 16 than with other types.

DIAGNOSIS

Papillomavirus infections are usually clinically recognizable. Because in vitro culture methods are not available, diagnostic procedures are based on biochemical assays. Molecular hybridization may be used to detect viral DNA in samples, and serologic reagents may detect capsid antigens in tissues. The latter is not very useful, as the number of antigen-producing cells in a lesion is usually small. Because of the differing oncogenic potential of human papillomavirus types, it is important that methods be developed to identify specific virus types in clinical lesions.

CONTROL

Cross-infection can be prevented by avoiding sharing of towels, shower shoes, and dressings. Correct sterilization of all instruments used for examining and treating patients with human papillomavirus infection is very important. Papillomaviruses are stable, and infectivity can survive improper sterilization procedures. General principles for the control of sexually transmitted diseases apply to human papillomavirus infection, including health education to avoid casual sex, to use condoms, and to seek medical attention for lesions.

There is no generally effective treatment for all warts. Most warts regress spontaneously, but patients will seek treatment for cosmetic purposes or because of discomfort. Available treatment modalities consist of locally destructive techniques, such as cautery, surgical excision, and cryotherapy with liquid nitrogen. Caustic agents (podophyllin, trichloroacetic acid) may be applied directly to lesions. Interferons have given good clinical responses against laryngeal papillomas and skin and anogenital warts. Antiviral drugs, such as idoxuridine and acyclovir, are ineffective. Condylomata and laryngeal papillomas tend to recur after treatment.

The aim of treatment of dysplastic lesions is to prevent invasive cancer. Local destructive methods are used.

The high prevalence of papillomavirus infections and their association with cancer make these viruses candidates for vaccine development. However, successful vaccine development requires a better understanding of both the host immune response to human papillomavirus infection and the epidemiology of different virus types.

REFERENCES

Bishop JM: The molecular genetics of cancer. Science 235:305, 1987

Broker TR: Structure and genetic expression of papillomaviruses. Obstet Gynecol Clin North Am 14:329, 1987

Butel JS, Jarvis DL: The plasma-membrane-associated form of SV40 large tumor antigen: biochemical and biological properties. Biochim Biophys Acta 865:171, 1986

Gissmann L: Papillomaviruses and their association with cancer in animals and in man. Cancer Surv 3:161, 1984

Norkin LC: Papovaviral persistent infections. Microbiol Rev 46:384, 1982

Reeves WC, Brinton LA, García M et al: Human papillomavirus infection and cervical cancer in Latin America. N Engl J Med 320:1437, 1989

Tevethia SS, Butel JS: SV40 tumor antigen: importance of cell surface localization in transformation and immunological control of neoplasia. p. 231. In Greene MI, Hamaoka T (eds): Development and Recognition of the Transformed Cell. Plenum, New York, 1987

Tooze J (ed): Molecular Biology of Tumor Viruses. 2nd ed. Part 2: DNA Tumor Viruses. Cold Spring Harbor Laboratory, Cold Spring Harbor, NY, 1981

World Health Organization: Genital human papillomavirus infections and cancer. Memorandum from a WHO meeting. Bull WHO 65:817, 1987

67 ADENOVIRUSES

WALTER DOERFLER

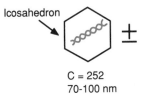

Icosahedron

C = 252
70-100 nm

GENERAL CONCEPTS

Clinical Manifestations

Adenoviruses cause acute respiratory disease (usually), pneumonia (occasionally), acute follicular conjunctivitis, epidemic keratoconjunctivitis, and cystitis, and gastroenteritis (occasionally). In infants, pharyngitis and pharyngeal-conjunctival fever are common.

Structure

The icosahedral capsid (70 to 100 nm) is made up of 252 capsomeres: 240 **hexons** forming the faces and 12 **pentons** at the vertices. Each penton bears a slender **fiber.** The double-stranded linear DNA is associated with two major core proteins and carries a 55-kDa protein covalently attached to its 5′ end.

Classification and Antigenic Types

More than 80 antigenic types of adenoviruses have been identified that infect mammals (mastadenoviruses) and birds (aviadenoviruses); 41 human adenovirus types plus 6 candidate types are known.

Multiplication

Infection may be productive, abortive, or latent. In productive infections, the viral genome is transcribed in the nucleus, mRNA is translated in the cytoplasm, and virions self-assemble in the nucleus. In latent infections and in transformed and tumor cells, viral DNA is integrated into the host genome. Virus-host DNA recombinants are also found in productive infections.

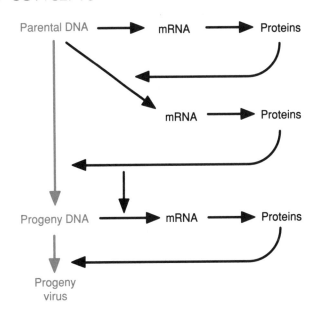

Pathogenesis

Infection is usually transmitted in droplets of respiratory or ocular secretions. Persistent infection occurs in the tonsils. Some adenovirus types are oncogenic in newborn rodents and can transform cells. A few transformed human cell lines exist. Human oncogenesis has not been found but may nevertheless occur (e.g., by a "hit-and-run" mechanism).

Host Defenses

Most adolescents and adults have circulating neutralizing antibodies; immunity is widespread. Cytotoxic T lymphocytes destroy adenovirus-infected cells.

Epidemiology

Infection is common in children. Epidemics do not occur in the general population, but outbreaks of acute respiratory disease occur in military recruits. Serious complications are very rare.

Diagnosis

Adenovirus infection is suggested clinically by fever, upper respiratory tract infections, and conjunctivitis; the diagnosis is confirmed by a rise in antibody titers and by virus isolation.

Control

There is no treatment. Whole-virus vaccines are not used because of the risk of oncogenesis. Other vaccines, including recombinant vaccines, are under development, but adenoviruses do not represent a serious health hazard.

INTRODUCTION

The adenoviruses are common pathogens of humans and animals. Moreover, several strains have been the subject of intensive research and are used as tools in mammalian molecular biology. More than 80 serologically distinct types of adenovirus have been identified, including 41 to 47 types that infect humans. The family Adenoviridae is divided into the mammalian adenoviruses (**mastadenoviruses**) and the avian adenoviruses (**aviadenoviruses**). The adenoviruses are named after the human adenoids, from which they were first isolated.

Several adenoviruses cause human diseases. In addition, a few types of human adenoviruses induce undifferentiated sarcomas in newborn hamsters and other rodents and can transform certain rodent and human cell cultures. There is currently no evidence that adenoviruses are oncogenic in humans, but the possibility remains of great interest.

CLINICAL MANIFESTATIONS

The main target for human adenoviruses is the respiratory tract. Various adenoviruses can also cause acute follicular conjunctivitis, epidemic keratoconjunctivitis, and, less frequently, cystitis and gastroenteritis (Fig. 67-1). In infants, the most common clinical manifestations of adenovirus infections are acute febrile pharyngitis and pharyngeal-conjunctival fever. In military recruits, acute respiratory disease is the predominant form of adenovirus disease, with adenovirus pneumonia as a not infrequent complication. Except for outbreaks in military groups and occasionally among children, adenovirus infections do not occur epidemically. The virus is probably transmitted via droplets of respiratory or ocular secretions.

STRUCTURE

The adenovirus particle consists of an icosahedral protein shell surrounding a protein core that contains the linear, double-stranded DNA genome (Fig. 67-2). The shell, which is 70 to 100 nm in diameter, is made up of 252 structural capsomeres. The 12 vertices of the icosahedron are occupied by units called **pentons,** each of which has a slender projection called a **fiber.** The 240 capsomeres that make up the 20 faces and the edges of the icosahedron are called **hexons** because they form hexagonal arrays. The shell also contains some additional, minor polypeptide elements. The core particle is made up of two major proteins (polypeptide V and polypeptide VII) and a minor arginine-rich protein (μ). A 55 kDa protein is covalently attached to the 5′ ends of the DNA.

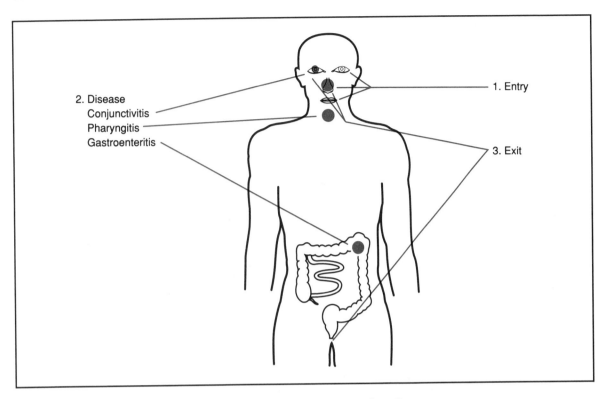

FIGURE 67-1 Pathogenesis of adenovirus diseases.

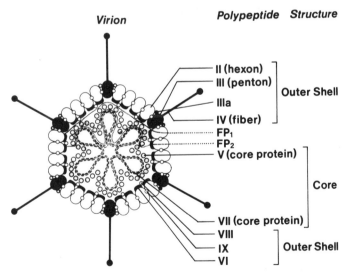

FIGURE 67-2 Structural model of the adenovirus virion. The Roman numerals refer to the standard designations of the viral structural proteins according to their decreasing molecular masses. FP stands for fracture plane in freeze etching. (From Brown DT, Westphal M, Burlingham BT et al: Structure and composition of the adenovirus type 2 core. J Virol 16:366, 1975, with permission.)

Figure 67-3 shows the genetic map of a typical adenovirus, adenovirus type 2 (Ad2). The genome is divided into **early functions** (E1A, E1B, E2A, E2B, E3, and E4 regions), which are expressed first during viral replication, and **late functions** (L1 to L5 regions), which are usually expressed after the early functions and after the beginning of viral DNA replication. The late genes encode the viral structural proteins. In the case of Ad2, DNA replication begins 6 to 8 hours after infection of cultured human cells. The VA segment of the genome codes for small RNAs (VAI and VAII RNAs) about 160 nucleotides long, which are not translated but regulate the translation of viral mRNAs. The VA RNAs are transcribed by eukaryotic RNA polymerase III. The genome also codes for a tripartite RNA leader sequence that is spliced onto all the late viral mRNAs. Both strands of the double-stranded DNA code for specific viral functions

(Fig. 67-3). The termini of the DNA molecule carry inverted repeat sequences so that denatured single strands can form circular DNA molecules.

CLASSIFICATION AND ANTIGENIC TYPES

At present, 41 types of human adenoviruses as well as 6 candidate types (42 through 47) have been identified (Table 67-1). The genomes of the different adenoviruses are genetically distinct and vary somewhat in size.

MULTIPLICATION

Host cells differ in permissivity for adenovirus types (Table 67-2). In permissive cells, the virus multiplies productively and kills the host cell. Other cells are semipermissive, allowing replication at low efficiency, whereas in still others repli-

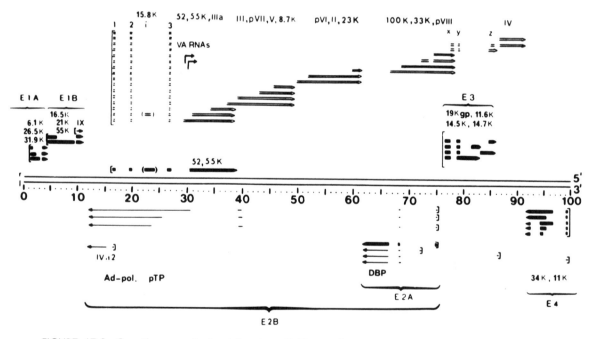

FIGURE 67-3   Genetic map of adenovirus type 2. The coding capacities of individual genome segments are indicated by the sizes of polypeptides (K represents 1,000 Da) or by the designations of the virion structural proteins (Roman numerals; see Fig. 67-2). The double-stranded DNA molecule with its 3′ and 5′ ends and a scale in map units are in the center of the graph. (From Akusjärvi G, Pettersson U, Roberts RJ: Structure and function of the adenovirus-2 genome. In Doerfler W (ed): Adenovirus DNA. Martinus Nijhoff, Boston, 1986, with permission.)

TABLE 67-1   Human Adenovirus Types

Subgenus	Serotype
A	12, 18, 31
B	3, 7, 11, 14, 16, 21, 34, 35
C	1, 2, 5, 6
D	8, 9, 10, 13, 15, 17, 19, 20, 22–30, 32, 33, 36–39
E	4
F	40, 41
Candidate types	42–47

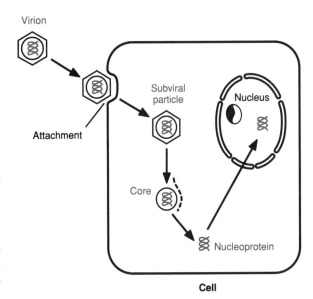

FIGURE 67-4   Early events in the interaction of the adenovirion with a host cell. The figure shows a model based on biochemical studies that depicts the major steps in viral penetration and uncoating. (From Lonberg-Holm K, Philipson L: Early events of virus-cell interaction in an adenovirus system. J Virol 4:323, 1969, with permission.)

cation is blocked and the infection is abortive. As discussed below, in some abortive infections all or part of the genome may be integrated into the host DNA, resulting in a latent infection, which may lead to oncogenic transformation.

Productive Infection

The virion enters host cells either by attaching to the cytoplasmic membrane and then being engulfed into the cytoplasm in a membrane-bound vesicle (**viropexis**) or by directly penetrating the cytoplasmic membrane. The viral DNA is gradually uncoated and enters the nucleus of the cell, most probably as a nucleoprotein complex that still contains viral core proteins (Fig. 67-4).

The viral DNA is transcribed and replicates in the nucleus of the host cell. The viral mRNA undergoes processing in the nucleus and/or during transport through the nuclear membrane into the cytoplasm, where it is translated by polysomes into viral proteins. These proteins return to the nucleus, where new virions self-assemble. The mass of newly synthesized virus particles can assume crystal-like arrangements. The bulk of the virions may not be easily released from the nucleus and the

TABLE 67-2   Adenovirus-Host Cell Interactions

Type of Interaction	Functional Definition	Biologic System
Productive infection	Complete replication of infectious virions	Cultured human cells
Abortive infection	Synthesis of viral gene products without production of infectious virions	Cultured hamster or monkey cells
Semipermissive infection	Complete replication with low yields of infectious virions	Cultured rat cells
Malignant transformation	Associated with integration of viral DNA and differential viral and cellular gene expression	Cultured hamster and rat cells
Tumor induction	Associated with integration of viral DNA and differential viral and cellular gene expression	Newborn hamsters (mice)
Viral latency	Persistence of viral genome	Human tonsils

cell. There is evidence that extracellular adenovirus type 12 virions have a considerably higher specific infectivity than intracellular virions. During active viral release, the newly synthesized virions may receive properties conferring high infectivity toward the host cells.

The initiation of adenovirus DNA replication is atypical in that the β-hydroxyl group of a serine residue in the precursor to the terminal protein (pTP), an 80- to 87-kDa poly-peptide, acts as a primer in DNA replication. Viral DNA replication can proceed bidirectionally and by single-strand displacement from either end of the DNA duplex. The adenovirus-encoded DNA polymerase, pTP, the adenovirus E2A protein, and several host proteins catalyze viral DNA replication.

Most of the adenovirus genes (Fig. 67-3) are transcribed by the host DNA-dependent RNA polymerase II in a complex transcriptional program. This program is regulated by the nucleotide sequences and the structure of the viral promoters and by a host of cell-encoded transcription factors that recognize specific upstream and downstream nucleotide sequence motifs in the promoters. Genes in the E1A region of the adenovirus genome are the first to be transcribed. One protein product of this gene region is a transactivator that is essential for the activation of all other viral genes. This immediate-early viral function can also activate or inactivate certain cellular genes.

The jointly controlled E2A and E2B regions code for proteins that are essential for viral DNA replication. Among the E3-encoded functions, one is a 25,000 (19,000)-molecular-weight glycoprotein responsible for the interaction with cell membrane-associated proteins (major histocompatibility complex). The E3 region-encoded functions may be unnecessary for viral replication in cell culture, but essential for the interaction with the intact defense system of an organism. The late viral L1 region can also be transcribed early in the infection cycle, probably to a limited extent. Genes encoded in the L1 region of Ad5 DNA are essential for virion assembly.

All the late viral functions are under the control of the major late promoter (MLP) components, which are located at about 17, 20, and 27 map units on the viral genome. The gene encoding the fiber structural protein can also be controlled by the x, y, and z leaders (Fig. 67-3).

The regulation of promoter activity in all biologic systems is dominated by the interaction of promoter sequence motifs with specific factors. Viral promoters are conditioned to the factors present in specific host cells. **Enhancers** and **silencers** are quantitative modulators of promoter function. Both act independently of position and orientation and can exert their influence over relatively long distances. Enhancers strengthen promoter activity, whereas silencers have a negative effect, abrogating or diminishing promoter function. Enhancer and silencer elements are species specific.

The VAI and VAII RNAs (Fig. 67-3) are transcribed by RNA polymerase III. VAI RNA is an important translational activator of host cell and viral messenger RNAs (mRNAs) late after infection. It prevents activation of a protein kinase that is responsible for the phosphorylation and ensuing inhibition of the eIF-2 translation factor. This kinase can be induced by interferon. VAI RNA thus can be considered as a viral defense mechanism against interferon.

Abortive Infection

Virus interaction with a host cell can be blocked at many different steps, thus leading to an incomplete or abortive cycle. Depending on the permissivity of the host cell, different types of adenovirus-host cell interactions can be distinguished (Table 67-2). Many cultured human epithelioid cell lines are productively infected by human adenoviruses. Rat cells are semipermissive (e.g., for Ad5), and permit viral replication only at low efficiency. The outcome of an adenovirus infection depends on the animal species, cell type, and virus type involved. For example, hamster cells are abortively infected with Ad12. The viral DNA is transported to the nucleus, where part of it is integrated into the host cell genome. Most of the early viral genes are transcribed, but the late genes remain silent in the host cells. Ad12 DNA replication in hamster cells cannot be detected with the most sensitive techniques. The major late promoter of Ad12 DNA is inactive in both uninfected and

Ad12-infected hamster cells, whereas it functions in infected human cells. Ad2 cannot replicate in monkey cells; in this case, the translation of some of the late viral mRNAs is amiss. The adenovirus genome persists, perhaps for a very long time, in cells of the human tonsils. It is not known how adenovirus replication in this human organ is restricted.

PATHOGENESIS

Adenovirus disease results from localized virus multiplication at the portals of entry (Fig. 67-1). The pathogenesis of localized infections is presented in Chapter 45.

Integration of Adenovirus DNA into the Host Genome

Latency and persistence of, as well as oncogenicity by, DNA viruses are frequently associated with integration of all or part of the viral genome into the host cell DNA. Integration of adenovirus DNA has been demonstrated in abortively infected cells, in adenovirus-transformed cells, and in Ad12-induced tumor cells. In productively infected human cells, recombination between adenovirus DNA and host cell DNA has also been observed. However, it is not known whether this recombination can lead to stable integration, because in the productive infection cycle the host cells are eventually killed. There is evidence that early in productively infected human cells Ad12 DNA becomes preferentially integrated into chromosome 1.

Soon after infection, the viral genome may be inserted into selective sites of the cellular genome. The initial steps of viral malignant transformation could involve insertional mutagenesis at a certain number of selective cellular sites. From the viewpoint of the geneticist, this model of viral oncogenesis is still one of the more attractive possibilities. Moreover, after being inserted initially at a limited number of sites and eliciting decisive mutagenic events (e.g., deletions), the viral DNA could perhaps be transposed to other loci in the host genome or could be lost.

Analyses of several different integration sites in transformed cell lines suggest that transcriptionally active regions of the host cellular genome, which have a characteristic chromatin structure, are most apt to recombine with foreign (viral) DNA. Adenovirus DNA frequently recombines with cellular DNA via its termini, and terminal viral nucleotides are often deleted from the integrated viral DNA molecule. In general, considerable variability is observed in the structure of the site of integration. No specific cellular DNA sequence has been found at the site of viral DNA insertion in established cell lines. Cellular DNA can be deleted at the insertion site, or the cellular site can be preserved to the last nucleotide. Ad12 DNA is frequently integrated intact in the DNA of nonpermissive hamster cells. However, Ad2 DNA is usually integrated in fragments in hamster cells permissive for Ad2.

The adenovirus system has also served as a model for studying the function of sequence-specific promoter methylations in mammalian cells. Upon integration of the adenovirus genome into the host cell genome, a highly specific pattern of methylation is de novo imposed on the integrated viral genome during many cell generations. There is evidence from analyses in many different biologic systems that sequence-specific promoter methylations can cause long-term gene inactivation.

Ad12-transformed hamster cells or Ad12-induced hamster tumor cells maintained in culture can eventually lose the integrated copies of viral DNA. This loss suggests that adenoviruses may cause transformation by a "hit and run" mechanism.

Malignant Transformation and Oncogenesis

Cells from a number of rodent species can be transformed in culture by adenoviruses. The frequency of malignant transformation is extremely low, and this has prohibited quantitative studies in this system. A transformed human cell line has also been described. Some adenoviruses, such as Ad2 and Ad5, are not oncogenic in animals at all. Tumorigenic potential has been attributed to the capacity of some adenoviruses (e.g., Ad12) to turn off the expression of genes of the major histocompatibility complex and thus to allow the transformed cells to overcome host defenses and grow into solid tumors. Most of the adenovirus-induced tumors, tumor cell lines, and transformed cell lines have one or several copies of the viral genome integrated into the chromosomes. The tumor or transformed state is also associated with the differential expression of the integrated viral genes. The early viral genes are often the predominant genes expressed. It is thought that the E1 region of the viral genome is particularly important in eliciting the transformed state. However, the continued presence of the viral genome, or of parts of it, is not essential for maintenance of the transformed state.

The so-called oncogenes represent a set of cellular genes that are involved in many different ways in growth control. Oncogenes in adenovirus-induced tumor or transformed cells have received surprisingly little attention. The few studies on this topic have reported occasional changes of oncogene activity, particularly for the *myc* gene. Moreover, the E1A proteins can bind tightly to the product of the retinoblastoma gene, which is considered to be an anti-oncogene. It has been suggested that the fixation of the anti-oncogene product, retinoblastoma, by the E1A proteins might contribute to the transformation of cells. The interplay of several viral and cellular factors may eventually alter the cellular growth control and weaken or overcome the host defenses in such a way that an adenovirus-transformed rodent cell can grow into a solid tumor.

Since many human tumors do not contain even traces of adenovirus genes or gene products, the possibility that adenoviruses cause human tumors is low. New, more sensitive techniques are now available. Moreover, the "hit and run" hypothesis has not been ruled out. Since even experimentally induced tumors lose the viral genome and retain oncogenicity, this possible mechanism of transformation of human cells is still being studied.

Persistence of Adenoviruses in Human Tonsils

Adenoviruses were first isolated from human adenoids, and the persistence of these viruses or their DNA in the human adenoids has been studied. It is not known whether adenoviruses or their genomes can persist in other human organ systems. When the adenoids are removed during acute adenovirus infection, intact viral genomes are present. In contrast, when adenoid tissue obtained during a symptom-free interval or from a chronically infected carrier is analyzed, only a small number of cells seem to harbor the viral genome, which may not be intact. In some cases, in situ hybridization is needed to show that individual cells in the adenoids contain the viral DNA and/or adenovirus-specific RNA. These cells do not produce infectious virus. It is not known to what extent adenovirus virions continue to replicate in the adenoids throughout adult life.

HOST DEFENSES

In adolescents and adults a high prevalence of circulating neutralizing antibodies contributes to widespread immunity against adenovirus infections. Cytotoxic T lymphocytes also recognize and destroy adenovirus-infected cells. Interferon is induced by adenoviruses in vitro but fails to inhibit many adenovirus types (e.g., VA RNA). Nevertheless, interferon has been effective in the treatment of adenovirus conjunctivitis.

EPIDEMIOLOGY

Adenovirus infections are widely distributed in human populations. The highest susceptibility is found among children from 6 months to 2 years of age and extends to the group 5 to 9 years old. Types 2, 1, 3, 5, 7, and 6 (in that order) are most frequently isolated from adenovirus-infected children, with types 1 and 2 constituting some 60 percent of all isolates. Nevertheless, adenovirus infections are responsible for only 2 to 5 percent of acute respiratory infections in children.

Adenoviruses also infect military recruits in the United States (and perhaps other countries). Adenovirus types 4, 7, and 3 cause acute respiratory diseases, including pneumonia, in this population.

Adenoviruses have been isolated from severely immunocompromised patients, such as those with acquired immune deficiency syndrome (AIDS). Many of these isolates, including the adenovirus candidate types 42 to 47, are found in the urine of AIDS patients.

DIAGNOSIS

Infection with an adenovirus may be suspected on the basis of a characteristic clinical presentation. The diagnosis can be confirmed by demonstrating a rise in antibody titer between acute-phase and convalescent-phase sera.

CONTROL

Since adenoviruses are excellent antigens, vaccination could be very effective. However, viral vaccines usually have not been used because adenoviruses are involved in tumorigenesis in animals and in cell culture. Moreover, adenovirus infections only rarely cause serious complications. Nevertheless, efforts are under way to produce vaccines by recombinant DNA technology. Purified hexon or fiber preparations induce high levels of neutralizing antibodies, and vaccines based on these proteins have been tested successfully.

REFERENCES

Akusjärvi G, Pettersson U, Roberts RJ: Structure and function of the adenovirus-2 genome. In Doerfler W (ed): Adenovirus DNA. Martinus Nijhoff, Boston, 1986

Brown DT, Westphal M, Burlingham BT et al: Structure and composition of the adenovirus type 2 core. J Virol 16:366, 1975

Doerfler W: The fate of the DNA of adenovirus type 12 in baby hamster kidney cells. Proc Natl Acad Sci USA 60:636, 1968

Doerfler W: DNA methylation and gene activity. Annu Rev Biochem 52:93, 1983

Doerfler W (ed): The Molecular Biology of Adenoviruses. Vol. 109 to 111. Springer Verlag, Berlin, 1983/1984

Doerfler W: Complexities in gene regulation by promoter methylation. Nucleic Acids Mol Biol 3:92, 1989

Doerfler W, Gahlmann R, Stabel S et al: On the mechanism of recombination between adenoviral and cellular DNAs: the structure of junction sites. Curr Top Microbiol Immunol 109:193, 1983

Doerfler W, Stabel S, Ibelgaufts H et al: Selectivity in integration sites of adenoviral DNA. Cold Spring Harbor Symp Quant Biol 44:551, 1979

Flint J, Shenk T: Adenovirus E1A protein: paradigm viral transactivator. Annu Rev Genet 23:141, 1989

Ginsberg H (ed): Adenoviruses. Plenum Press, New York, 1985

Kuhlmann I, Achten S, Rudolph R et al: Tumor induction by human adenovirus type 12 in hamsters: loss of the viral genome from adenovirus type 12-induced tumor cells is compatible with tumor formation. EMBO J 1:79, 1982

Lonberg-Holm K, Philipson L: Early events of virus-cell interaction in an adenovirus system. J Virol 4:323, 1969

Rowe WP, Huebner RJ, Gilmore LK et al: Isolation of a cytopathogenic agent from human adenoids undergoing spontaneous degeneration in tissue culture. Proc Soc Exp Biol Med 84:570, 1953

Trentin JJ, Yabe Y, Taylor G: The quest for human cancer viruses. Science 137:835, 1962

68

HERPESVIRUSES

MARK MIDDLEBROOKS
RICHARD J. WHITLEY

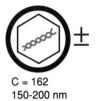

C = 162
150-200 nm

GENERAL CONCEPTS

GENERAL BIOLOGY OF HUMAN HERPESVIRUSES

Of the more than 100 known herpesviruses, 6 infect only humans: herpes simplex virus type 1 (HSV-1), herpes simplex virus type 2 (HSV-2), varicella-zoster virus (VZV), cytomegalovirus (CMV), Epstein-Barr virus (EBV), and human herpesvirus 6 (HHV-6). A simian virus called B virus occasionally infects humans. All herpesviruses can establish latent infection within specific tissues, which are characteristic for each virus.

Structure

Herpesviruses have a unique four-layered structure: a core containing the large, double-stranded DNA genome is enclosed in an icosapentahedral protein capsid, which is surrounded by an amorphous tegument, which is encased in a glycoprotein-bearing lipid bilayer envelope.

Classification

Herpesviruses are divided into three groups: The **α herpesviruses** (HSV-1, HSV-2, and VZV), with a short replicative cycle, cytopathology, and a broad cell host range; **β herpesviruses** (CMV), with a long replicative cycle and restricted host range; and **γ herpesviruses** (EBV and probably HHV-6), with a very restricted host range.

Multiplication

Transcription, genome replication, and capsid assembly occur in the host cell nucleus. Genes are replicated in a specific order: (1) immediate-early genes, which encode regulatory proteins; (2) early genes, which encode enzymes for replicating viral DNA; and (3) late genes, which encode structural proteins. The tegument and envelope are acquired as the virion buds out through the nuclear envelope or endoplasmic reticulum. Virions are transported to the cell membrane via the Golgi complex, and the host cell dies as mature virions are released. Alternatively, in specific cell types, the virus may be maintained in a latent state. The latent viral genome may reactivate at any time; the mechanism of reactivation is not known.

Diagnosis

CMV retinitis is diagnosed clinically. Diagnosis of all other herpesvirus infection relies on isolation of the virus through culturing and/or on detection of viral genes or gene products.

Control of Herpesvirus Infections

Prevention: A vaccine against VZV awaits licensing. Vaccines against HSV-1, HSV-2, and CMV are under development. Passive immunization with immunoglobulin or hyperimmune globulin is used either to prevent infection or as an adjunct to antiviral therapy.

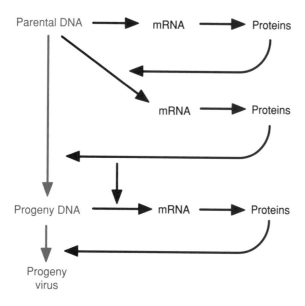

Parental DNA → mRNA → Proteins

mRNA → Proteins

Progeny DNA → mRNA → Proteins

Progeny
virus

Treatment: Infections with HSV-1, HSV-2, and VZV are currently the most amenable to therapy; acyclovir is the drug of choice. Ganciclovir is used to treat CMB retinitis. B virus appears to respond to either of these drugs. There is as yet no treatment for EBV or HHV-6 infections.

HERPES SIMPLEX VIRUSES

Clinical Manifestations

HSV-1 and HSV-2 have approximately 50 percent genomic homology but share most other characteristics. Mucocutaneous manifestations of HSV infection include gingivostomatitis, herpes genitalis, herpetic keratitis, and dermal whitlows. Neonatal HSV infection and HSV encephalitis also occur.

Pathogenesis

The virus replicates initially in epithelial cells, producing a characteristic vesicle on an erythematous base. It then ascends sensory nerves to the dorsal root ganglia, where it can establish latency. During reactivated infection, the virus spreads distally from the ganglion to initiate new cutaneous and/or mucosal lesions.

Host Defenses

Interferon and humoral and cellular immunity are important defenses. HSV infections are more severe in immunocompromised hosts.

Epidemiology

HSV-1 transmission is primarily oral, and HSV-2 primarily genital. Transmission requires intimate contact.

VARICELLA-ZOSTER VIRUS

Clinical Manifestations

Primary VZV infection causes **varicella (chickenpox).** Reactivation of latent virus (usually in adults) causes **herpes zoster (shingles),** a vesicular rash with a dermatomal distribution and acute neuritis.

Pathogenesis

VZV virus is usually transmitted by droplets and replicates initially in the oropharynx. In seronegative individuals, viremia and chickenpox ensue. Latency is established in dorsal root ganglia, and reactivated infection travels down sensory nerves.

Host Defenses

As with HSV, interferon and cellular and humoral immunity are important defenses. Reactivated virus can cause disseminated disease in immunocompromised individuals.

Epidemiology

VZV is highly contagious; about 95 percent of adults show serologic evidence of infection.

CYTOMEGALOVIRUS

Clinical Manifestations

CMV causes three clinical syndromes. (1) **Congenital CMV infection** (when symptomatic) causes hepatosplenomegaly, chorioretinitis, rash, and central nervous system involvement. (2) In about 10 percent of older children and adults, primary CMV infection causes a mononucleosis with fever, malaise, atypical lymphocytosis, and pharyngitis. (3) Immunocompromised hosts (transplant recipients and human immunodeficiency virus [HIV]-infected individuals) may develop life-threatening disseminated disease involving the lungs, gastrointestinal tract, liver, retina, and central nervous system.

Pathogenesis

CMV replicates mainly in the salivary glands and kidneys and is shed in saliva and urine. Replication is slow, and the virus induces characteristic multinucleated giant cells with intranuclear inclusions.

Epidemiology

Transmission is via intimate contact with infected secretions. CMV infections are among the most prevalent viral infections worldwide.

EPSTEIN-BARR VIRUS

Clinical Manifestations

EBV causes classic mononucleosis. In immunocompromised hosts, the virus causes lymphoproliferative cancer.

Pathogenesis

EBV replicates in epithelial cells of the oropharynx and in B lymphocytes.

Epidemiology

EBV is transmitted by intimate contact, particularly via the exchange of saliva.

HUMAN HERPESVIRUS 6

Clinical Manifestations

HHV-6 is associated with **exanthem subitum (roseola)** and with rejection of transplanted kidneys.

Pathogenesis

The pathogenesis is poorly understood.

Epidemiology

Antibodies to this virus are present in almost everyone by age 5.

B VIRUS

Clinical Manifestations

In humans, B virus causes an encephalitis that is usually fatal; survivors have brain damage.

Pathogenesis

B virus is transmitted to humans by the bite of infected rhesus monkeys and is transported up neurons to the brain.

Epidemiology

The reservoir for the disease is latent infection in rhesus monkeys, particularly those from Southeast Asia and India. In stressed or unhealthy animals, the virus may reactivate and appear in saliva.

INTRODUCTION

Herpesviruses infect both vertebrate and nonvertebrate species, and more than 100 types have been at least partially characterized. Only the six types routinely isolated from humans are discussed here. These six, called the **human herpesviruses,** are herpes simplex virus type 1 (HSV-1), herpes simplex virus type 2 (HSV-2), varicella-zoster virus (VZV), cytomegalovirus (CMV), Epstein-Barr virus (EBV), and human herpesvirus (HHV-6). A primate herpesvirus known as B virus also occasionally infects humans and may cause life-threatening disease.

The human herpesviruses share three significant biologic properties. First, like all herpesviruses, they have a genome that codes for a series of enzymes involved in nucleic acid processing. These enzymes, which are structurally diverse, are of interest because they offer unique targets for antiviral agents. Second, the synthesis of both viral DNA and the capsid is initiated in the nucleus. Finally, all herpesviruses establish latent infections in tissues that are characteristic for each virus.

This chapter summarizes first the structure, classification, replication, and detection of all human herpesviruses and then considers the specific viruses and the diseases they cause.

GENERAL BIOLOGY OF HERPESVIRUSES

STRUCTURE

The members of the family Herpesviridae are large, enveloped viruses with a unique, four-layered structure. The double-stranded DNA genome is located in a central core of unknown structure. Herpesvirus DNA varies in molecular weight from about 8×10^7 to 15×10^7 (about 120 to 230 kilobase pairs), depending on the species. The DNA core is surrounded by a protein capsid, 100 to 110 nm in diameter, which consists of 162 capsomers in an icosapentahedral array. Tightly adherent to the capsid is a layer called the **tegument** which appears to consist of amorphous material. The tegument is loosely surrounded by a lipid bilayer envelope consisting mainly of polyamines, membrane lipids, and glycoproteins. This envelope is derived usually from the nuclear envelope, but occasionally from endoplasmic reticulum. The envelope glycoproteins give each virus distinctive properties and carry the unique viral antigens to which the host responds.

On the basis of the arrangement of unique and repeated DNA sequences, the herpesviruses are divided into six genomic groups, three of which contain the human herpesviruses.

CLASSIFICATION AND ANTIGENIC TYPES

The herpesviruses are grouped into three subfamilies, the α, β, and γ **herpesviruses,** which presumably reflect phylogenetic relatedness.

α Herpesviruses

The α herpesviruses consist of HSV-1, HSV-2, and VZV. These viruses are characterized by an extremely short replication cycle (hours), prompt destruction of the host cell, and the ability to replicate in a wide variety of host cells. They characteristically establish latent infection in sensory nerve ganglia.

β Herpesviruses

CMV is a β herpesvirus. In contrast to the α herpesviruses, the β herpesviruses infect a restricted range of host cells. Their replication cycle is long (days), and infection progresses slowly in cell culture systems. A characteristic of these viruses is their ability to induce host cells to enlarge. These viruses establish latent infections in secretory glands, cells of the reticuloendothelial system, and the kidneys.

γ Herpesviruses

The γ herpesviruses, such as EBV, have the most limited host cell range of any herpesviruses. In vitro, they replicate in lymphoblastoid cells and cause lytic infections in certain cells. Latent virus has been demonstrated in lymphoid tissue. HHV-6 is probably best classified as a γ herpesvirus, even though its host range resembles that of β herpesviruses.

MULTIPLICATION AND LATENCY

Multiplication

Herpesvirus replication is a multistep process. After the virus enters the cell, the DNA is uncoated and carried to the nucleus. The first genes to be transcribed, called the **immediate-early genes,** code for regulatory proteins. Expression of the immediate-early genes is followed by expression of the **early genes** and then the **late genes.**

The viral core and capsid are assembled in the nucleus, and the tegument and envelope are acquired as the virion buds through the nuclear envelope or (sometimes) the endoplasmic reticulum. Release of mature virions is accompanied by death of the host cell. The replication of all herpesviruses is quite inefficient since only a small proportion of the virus particles produced are infective.

Latency

A unique characteristic of herpesviruses is their ability to establish latent infection in specific host cells. The latent viral genome may be either extrachromosomal or integrated into the host DNA. Cells containing latent herpesviruses have recently been shown to express specific viral products. HSV-1, HSV-2, and VZV all establish latency in neurons of the dorsal root ganglia. EBV maintains latency in B lymphocytes and cells of the salivary glands. The sites of latency for CMV, HHV-6, and B virus have not been identified.

Latent virus may be reactivated and enter a replicative cycle at any time. The mechanism of reactivation is not understood. Stimuli associated with reactivation of latent HSV include stress, menstruation, and exposure to ultraviolet light; how these factors act at the dorsal root ganglia is not clear. Reactivation of herpesviruses may be clinically asymptomatic or may lead to mild or severe disease.

DIAGNOSIS

Except for CMV retinitis, which can be identified clinically, definitive diagnosis of herpesvirus infections requires either isolation of the virus or detection of viral gene products. For virus isolation, susceptible cell lines are inoculated with swabs of clinical specimens and observed for characteristic cytopathic effects. This technique is most useful with HSV-1, HSV-2, and VZV because of their short replicative cycle; identification of CMV by cell culture is slow. EBV does not cause cytopathic changes in cell culture systems and therefore can be identified in culture only by transformation of cord blood lymphoctyes.

Newer, more rapid diagnostic techniques involve detection of viral gene products. Fluorescent antibodies against immediate-early or late genes may be applied to tissue cultures after 24 to 72 hours of incubation; a positive result is the appearance of intranuclear fluorescence. A method involving monoclonal antibodies to an immediate-early gene product has been most useful for identifying CMV. Alternatively, fluorescent antibodies may be applied directly to cell monolayers or scrapings of clinical lesions, with intranuclear fluorescence again indicating the presence of replicating virus.

Diagnostic techniques that are still under development include DNA amplification and in situ or dot-blot hybridization. DNA amplification by the polymerase chain reaction (PCR) is of interest because of its ability to detect small amounts of specific genomic material. This test may be too sensitive to be diagnostically useful, however, because amplification of small amounts of contaminant DNA could give false-positive results.

In addition to these new tests for viral DNA and gene products, improved serologic assays are be-

coming available. However, because they rely on comparison of acute-phase and convalescent-phase sera, these tests are only useful for making retrospective diagnoses.

Finally, the diagnosis of CMV retinitis deserves special mention because it is made clinically on the basis of characteristic retinal changes. The detection of CMV viruria or viremia supports the diagnosis but is not necessary.

◀ HERPES SIMPLEX ▶ VIRUSES

Of all the herpesviruses, HSV-1 and HSV-2 are the most closely related, with approximately 50 percent genomic homology. These two viruses can be distinguished most reliably by DNA composition; however, differences in antigen expression and biologic properties also serve as methods for differentiation.

CLINICAL MANIFESTATIONS AND PATHOGENESIS

A critical factor for transmission of HSV, regardless of virus type, is intimate contact between a person who is shedding virus and a susceptible recipient. After inoculation onto the skin or mucous membrane and an incubation period of 4 to 6 days, HSV replicates in epithelial cells (Fig. 68-1). Cell lysis and local inflammation ensue, resulting in characteristic vesicles on an erythematous base. Regional lymphatics and lymph nodes become involved: viremia and visceral dissemination may develop depending upon the immunologic competence of the host. In all hosts, the virus generally ascends the peripheral sensory nerves to reach the dorsal root ganglia. Replication within neural tissue is followed by spread of the virus to other mucosal and skin surfaces via the peripheral sensory nerves. Virus replicates further in epithelial cells, reproducing the lesions of the initial infection, until infection is contained through host immunity.

Latency is established when HSV reaches the dorsal root ganglia after retrograde transmission

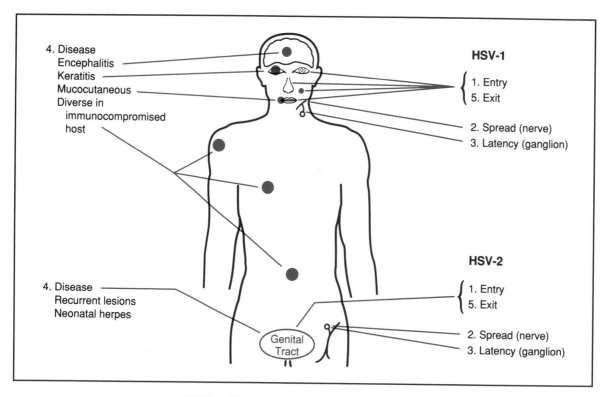

FIGURE 68-1 Pathogenesis of HSV infections.

via sensory nerve pathways. In its latent form, intracellular HSV DNA cannot be detected routinely unless specific molecular probes are used.

Mucocutaneous Infections

Gingivostomatitis

Mucocutaneous infections are the most common clinical manifestations of HSV-1 and HSV-2. **Gingivostomatitis,** which is usually caused by HSV-1, occurs most frequently in children younger than 5 years of age. HSV-1 gingivostomatitis is characterized by fever, sore throat, pharyngeal edema, and erythema, followed by development of vesicular or ulcerative lesions on the oral and pharyngeal mucosa. Recurrent HSV-1 infections of the oropharynx are most frequently manifested as **herpes simplex labialis** (cold sores) and usually appear on the vermilion border of the lip. Intraoral lesions as a manifestation of recurrent disease are uncommon.

Genital Herpes

Genital herpes is most frequently caused by HSV-2. Primary infection in women usually involves the vulva, vagina, and cervix (Fig. 68-2). Initial infection in men is most often associated with lesions on the glans penis, prepuce, or penile shaft. Primary disease in individuals of either sex is associated with fever, malaise, anorexia, and bilateral inguinal adenopathy. Women frequently have dysuria and urinary retention as a result of urethral involvement. As many as 10 percent of individuals develop an aseptic meningitis with primary infection. Sacral radiculomyelitis may occur in both men and women, resulting in neuralgias, urinary retention, or obstipation. Complete healing of primary infection may take several weeks. The first episode of genital infection is less severe in individuals who have had previous HSV infections at other sites, such as herpes simplex labialis.

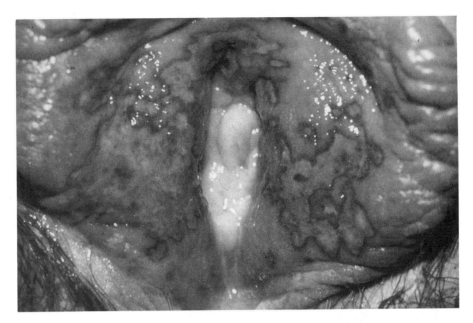

FIGURE 68-2 Genital herpes lesions of the vulva.

Recurrent genital infections in either men or women is particularly distressing. The frequency of recurrence varies significantly among individuals. It has been estimated that one-third of individuals with genital herpes have virtually no recurrences, one-third have approximately three recurrences per year, and one-third have more than three per year. Recent seroepidemiologic studies have found that between 25 and 65 percent of individuals in the United States in 1988 had antibodies to HSV-2 and that seroprevalence is dependent upon the number of sexual partners.

Herpetic Keratitis

Herpes simplex keratitis is usually caused by HSV-1 and is accompanied by conjunctivitis in many cases. It is the most common infectious cause of blindness in the United States. The characteristic lesions of herpes simplex keratoconjunctivitis are dendritic ulcers best detected by fluorescein staining. Deep stromal involvement has also been reported and may result in visual impairment.

Other Skin Manifestations

HSV infections can manifest at any skin site. Common among health care workers are lesions on abraded skin of the fingers, known as **herpetic whitlows** (Fig. 68-3). Similarly, because of physical

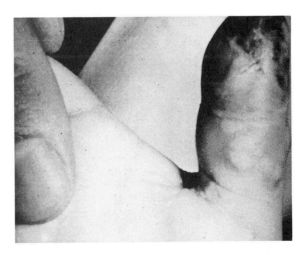

FIGURE 68-3 Herpetic whitlow involving the thumb.

contact, wrestlers may develop disseminated cutaneous lesions known as **herpes gladiatorum.**

Neonatal Herpes Simplex Virus Infection

Neonatal HSV infection occurs in approximately 1 in 3,500 deliveries in the United States each year. Approximately 70 percent of cases are caused by HSV-2 and usually result from contact of the fetus with infected maternal genital secretions at the time of delivery. Manifestations of neonatal HSV infection can be divided into three categories: (1) skin, eye and mouth disease; (2) encephalitis; and (3) disseminated infection. As the name implies, skin, eye, and mouth disease consists of cutaneous lesions and does not involve other organ systems (Fig. 68-4). Central nervous system involvement includes encephalitis or disseminated infection and generally results in a diffuse encephalitis. The cerebrospinal fluid formula characteristically reveals an elevated protein and a mononuclear pleocytosis. Disseminated infection involves multiple organ systems and can produce disseminated intravascular coagulation, hemorrhagic pneumonitis, encephalitis, and cutaneous lesions. Diagnosis

is particularly difficult in the absence of skin lesions. The mortality for each disease classification varies from zero for skin, eye, and mouth disease to 15 percent for encephalitis and 60 percent for disseminated infection. In addition to the high mortality associated with these infections, morbidity is significant: only about 40 percent of children with encephalitis or disseminated disease develop normally, even with the administration of appropriate antiviral therapy.

Herpes Simplex Encephalitis

Herpes simplex encephalitis is characterized by hemorrhagic necrosis of the temporal lobe (Fig. 68-5). Disease begins unilaterally and then spreads to the contralateral temporal lobe. It is the most common focal, sporadic encephalitis in the United States today and occurs in approximately 1 in 150,000 individuals. Most cases are caused by HSV-1. The actual pathogenesis of herpes simplex encephalitis requires further clarification, although it is believed that primary or recurrent virus can reach the temporal lobe by ascending neural pathways, such as the trigeminal tracts or the olfactory nerves.

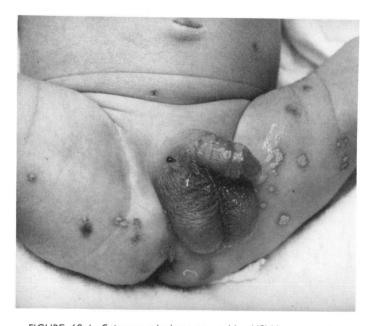

FIGURE 68-4 Cutaneous lesions caused by HSV in a neonate.

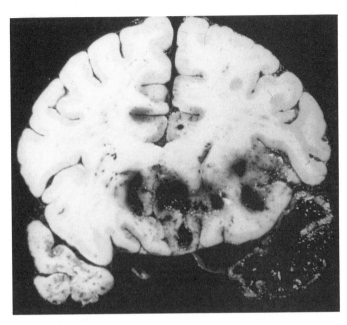

FIGURE 68-5 Hemorrhagic necrosis of the temporal lobe due to HSV encephalitis.

Clinical manifestations of herpes simplex encephalitis include headache, fever, altered consciousness, and abnormalities of speech and behavior. Focal seizures may also occur. The cerebrospinal fluid formula is variable, but usually consists of a pleocytosis with both polymorphonuclear leukocytes and monocytes present. The protein concentration is characteristically elevated, and the glucose level is usually normal. Brain biopsy is needed for a definitive diagnosis, since other pathogens may produce a clinically similar illness. The mortality and morbidity are high, even when appropriate antiviral therapy is administered. At present, the mortality is approximately 30 percent 1 year after treatment. In addition, approximately 70 percent of survivors have significant neurologic sequelae.

HERPES SIMPLEX VIRUS INFECTIONS IN THE IMMUNOCOMPROMISED HOST

HSV infections in immunocompromised hosts are clinically more severe, may be progressive, and require more time for healing than those in immunocompetent individuals. Manifestations of HSV infections in immunocompromised hosts include pneumonitis, esophagitis, hepatitis, colitis, and disseminated cutaneous disease. Individuals infected with human immunodeficiency virus (HIV) may have extensive perineal or orofacial ulcerations. HSV infections are also severe in individuals who are burned.

EPIDEMIOLOGY

HSV is transmitted only by intimate contact. Therefore, HSV-1 is usually transmitted by kissing or other contact with saliva, while HSV-2 infection is usually a consequence of sexual contact. Nosocomial spread of HSV-2 has been documented, particularly in intensive care units for neonates.

◀ VARICELLA-ZOSTER ▶ VIRUS

CLINICAL MANIFESTATIONS AND PATHOGENESIS

VZV is one of the most common human viruses. It is usually transmitted by droplet spread, with replication in the oropharynx (Fig. 68-6). Replication

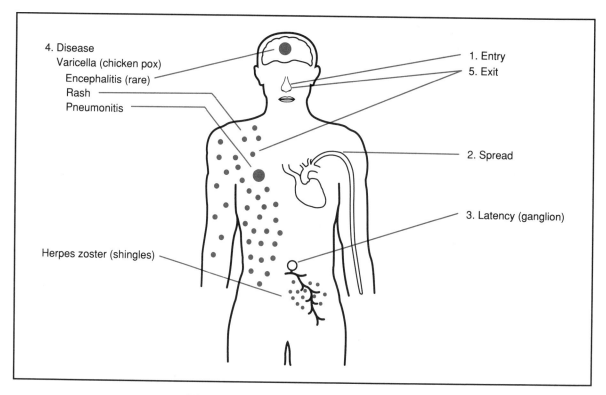

FIGURE 68-6 Pathogenesis of VZV infections.

of virus in the oropharynx of a susceptible or sero-negative individual leads to primary viremia, with subsequent development of a vesicular rash. VZV replication in vitro is similar to that of HSV, although the period of replication is somewhat prolonged.

Varicella

Varicella (chickenpox), is the manifestation of primary VZV infection. This infection occurs most commonly in young children of preschool age and has a characteristic disseminated vesicular rash, which appears after an incubation period of 14 to 17 days. The rash begins on the face and trunk and spreads to the extremities. The lesions of chickenpox are initially vesicles, which become pustular, crusted, and then scabbed prior to healing. The average duration of lesion formation is 3 to 5 days in the normal child; however, it can be longer in adolescents and adults or in immunocompromised

persons. At the time of primary infection, VZV may establish latency in dorsal root ganglia.

Herpes Zoster

The recurrent form of VZV is **herpes zoster (shingles).** This form of infection, which is a reactivation of latent virus, typically manifests as a localized vesicular rash with a dermatomal distribution. The rash initially appears within the dermatome as erythema, which is soon followed by the development of vesicles (Fig. 68-7). In some individuals, vesicles coalesce into bullous lesions. New vesicles may form for 5 to 7 days and then evolve through the sequence of healing described for the lesions of varicella. The average time to healing ranges from 10 to 21 days, depending upon the age and immune status of the individual.

Characteristic of herpes zoster is the appearance of both acute neuritis and post-herpetic neuralgia. Acute neuritis is present in most individuals

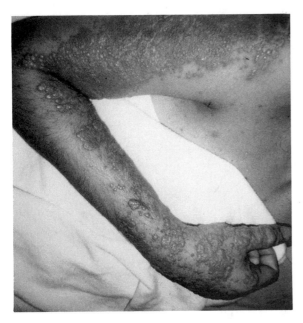

FIGURE 68-7 The vesicular rash of herpes zoster.

with localized zoster, the exception being young children. Post-herpetic neuralgia develops in as many as 50 percent of adults, depending upon age. The treatment of acute neuritis and post-herpetic neuralgia can be problematic for individual patients.

VARICELLA-ZOSTER VIRUS INFECTIONS IN THE IMMUNOCOMPROMISED HOST

Serious complications of chickenpox in immunocompetent children are rare, but secondary bacterial infection can be problematic. Adults and immunocompromised children have a higher incidence of visceral disease. Immunocompromised children, particularly those with acute lymphoblastic leukemia, are at increased risk for progressive disease, specifically those involving the liver and lungs. As many as one-third of these children will suffer visceral disease, with a mortality of 15 percent in the absence of antiviral therapy.

Herpes zoster in immunocompromised hosts is associated with cutaneous dissemination and visceral complications. In the absence of antiviral therapy, as many as 25 percent of individuals with lymphoproliferative cancers will have cutaneous dissemination and 10 percent will develop visceral complications, with an overall mortality of approximately 8 percent.

EPIDEMIOLOGY

VZV is spread by droplet transmission from a person who is shedding virus to a susceptible host. By adulthood, 90 to 95 percent of individuals have serologic evidence of infection with VZV.

The epidemiology of herpes zoster is more complicated. It does not appear that herpes zoster can be transmitted from one individual to another. However, spread of virus from the vesicles of herpes zoster may lead to the development of varicella in a susceptible host. Approximately 1 percent of individuals older than 50 years experience zoster.

◄ CYTOMEGALOVIRUS ►

CLINICAL MANIFESTATIONS

CMV infection can result in one of three distinct clinical syndromes. **Congenital CMV infection** is common in the United States, appearing in approximately one percent of all live births. Approximately 1 in 10,000 children will have severe symptomatic congenital CMV infection, as evidenced by hepatosplenomegaly, chorioretinitis, a petechial/purpuric skin rash, and involvement of the central nervous system (ventriculomegaly, intracranial calcifications, etc.) (Fig. 68-8). Some children who excrete the virus at birth, but have no other symptoms, may later have impaired hearing. An additional 10 to 25 percent of children acquire CMV infection early in life, either through contact with infected maternal genital secretions or by acquisition from breast milk. Symptomatic congenital disease is most frequent when the mother has a primary CMV infection during gestation and is extremely uncommon when the infection is acquired after the neonatal period.

The second manifestation of CMV infection is a **mononucleosis syndrome.** This occurs in approximately 10 percent of primary CMV infections in

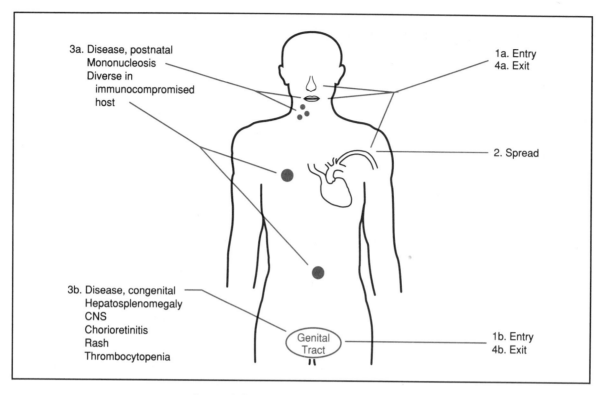

FIGURE 68-8 Pathogenesis of CMV infections.

older children and adults; the remaining 90 percent are associated with asymptomatic primary infection. Mononucleosis in these patients is heterophile negative but otherwise similar to classic EBV mononucleosis. Patients characteristically have fever, malaise, atypical lymphocytosis, pharyngitis, and, rarely, cervical adenopathy or hepatitis. CMV mononucleosis is distinguished from EBV mononucleosis by the absence of EBV-specific antibodies to either nuclear or viral capsid antigens.

The third clinical manifestation is CMV infection in severely immunocompromised individuals. In contrast to symptomatic congenital CMV and CMV mononucleosis, which are most commonly manifestations of primary CMV infection, immunocompromised hosts may experience life-threatening disease from either primary or reactivated CMV infection. In these patients, infection can involve the lungs, gastrointestinal tract, liver, retina, and central nervous system (Fig. 68-9). Individuals at high risk for severe CMV infection (especially CMV pneumonia) include organ transplant recipients, particularly bone marrow transplant recipients, and individuals with human immunodeficiency virus infection.

PATHOGENESIS

CMV replication is most prominent in cells of glandular origin, particularly in the salivary glands and the kidneys. As a result, large quantities of virus can be shed in the saliva and urine. The replicative cycle of CMV in these organs is more prolonged than that of other herpesviruses and produces characteristic multinucleated giant cells with Cowdry's type A intranuclear inclusion bodies. Intracytoplasmic inclusion bodies may also be present, but are less easily demonstrated. These giant cells can be found in the parotid gland, and similar cells are excreted in the urine.

CMV can cause persistent infection in various tissues, including those of the salivary glands, breasts, kidneys, endocervix, seminal vesicles, and peripheral blood leukocytes. This persistent infec-

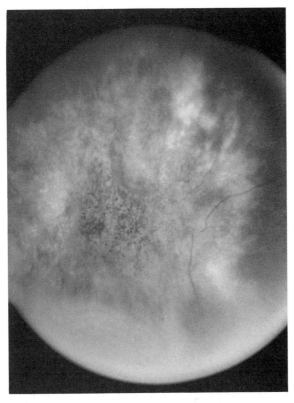

FIGURE 68-9   CMV retinitis.

tion leads to chronic viral excretion by the involved organ. Transmission is through contact with infected secretions. The average incubation period is 4 to 6 weeks. The kidneys of organ donors can be a source of CMV in the recipient. Peripheral blood leukocytes have been implicated in the transmission of CMV via blood transfusion.

EPIDEMIOLOGY

CMV infections are among the most prevalent viral infections worldwide. As with other herpesviruses, transmission is by intimate contact. Large quantities of virus can be excreted in saliva and urine for prolonged periods. Transmission of virus from mother to child occurs by one of several routes, including cervical secretions, infected breast milk, and saliva. Conversely, a child can transmit infection to the mother through infected secretions or urine. Moreover, transmission of CMV by children in the day care environment has introduced new

occupational risks, particularly for seronegative women of child-bearing age. Hence, the susceptible women are at risk for developing primary CMV infection during gestation and delivering a child with symptomatic congenital CMV infection.

Reactivation of CMV infection in immunosuppressed individuals is particularly problematic, as noted above. The extent of immunosuppression is a major determinant of the severity of disease. In addition, seronegative individuals who receive organs from persons seropositive for CMV can develop a life-threatening primary CMV infection.

EPSTEIN-BARR VIRUS

CLINICAL MANIFESTATIONS

The most significant clinical manifestations of EBV infection are those associated with **classic mononucleosis.** This form of mononucleosis is the most common in humans. The predominant findings are malaise, myalgia, pharyngitis, cervical adenopathy, splenomegaly, and atypical lymphocytosis. The diagnosis is confirmed by demonstrating heterophile antibodies or type-specific antibodies to EBV nuclear antigen and viral capsid antigen.

EBV has been incriminated as a cause of lymphoproliferative disease in highly immunocompromised individuals. The development of lymphoproliferative cancer in heart and bone marrow transplant recipients is believed to be associated with the presence of EBV.

PATHOGENESIS

EBV has a particular tropism for B lymphocytes. Replication has been documented in the parotid gland, as well as other lymphatic tissues. Evidence of lytic disease, as evidenced by the formation of multinucleated giant cells, is not apparent with infection caused by EBV.

EPIDEMIOLOGY

EBV is transmitted by intimate contact. Exchange of saliva provides a major route for horizontal transmission of infection. Excretion of virus from other sites does occur, but does not appear to be a major vector for transmission of infection.

HUMAN HERPESVIRUS 6

CLINICAL MANIFESTATIONS

HHV-6 is associated with **exanthem subitum (roseola).** This illness is characterized by 3 to 5 days of fever, followed by the appearance of a maculopapular "slapped-cheek" rash. HHV-6 is also associated with rejection of transplanted kidneys.

PATHOGENESIS

The reservoir and mode of transmission of HHV-6 are not well understood. High prevalence of antibodies early in life would implicate transmission within the home from oropharyngeal secretions; however, this has not yet been documented.

EPIDEMIOLOGY

The epidemiology of HHV-6 infection is poorly understood at the present time. Loss of transplacental antibodies, followed by acquisition of antibodies early in life, implies horizontal transmission within the home environment. Almost everyone has antibodies by the age of 5 years.

B VIRUS

CLINICAL MANIFESTATIONS

A major concern following exposure to B virus is the development of an almost uniformly fatal encephalitis in most individuals. Fewer than 30 cases have ever been documented; the mortality is approximately 75 percent. Survivors of B virus infection of the central nervous system have been left with a broad spectrum of neurologic impairment. Recurrent cutaneous disease has been noted, but generally only in patients who initially had a severe encephalitis.

PATHOGENESIS

Fortunately, B virus infections in humans are uncommon, because humans are not the natural reservoir of this infection. Instead, the virus is found routinely in rhesus monkey colonies. Infection is transmitted to humans by the bite of an infected animal. Virus replicates locally in a fashion very similar to that of HSV infection. An important difference, however, is that there is a predisposition for rapid neuronal transport of virus to the central nervous system, with ensuing encephalitis in most cases.

EPIDEMIOLOGY

B virus is resident in rhesus monkeys, particularly those obtained from Southeast Asia and India. In a manner similar to human herpesvirus infections, crowding and stress of monkeys lead to virus reactivation and excretion in saliva. Improper animal-handling techniques can cause human exposure to this virus. Strict adherence to guidelines for the handling of rhesus monkeys is advised.

CONTROL OF HERPESVIRUS INFECTION

PREVENTION

There are no licensed vaccines for treatment of herpesviruses. Only one is currently in use and is pending licensure; it is directed against VZV. This live, attenuated vaccine is intended for use in immunocompetent children only. Experimental vaccines for HSV-1, HSV-2, and CMV will be entering phase 1 and phase 2 trials by mid-1990. Vaccines engineered for the control of EBV, HHV-6, and B virus are in the early stages of development.

Passive immunization with immune or hyperimmune serum has been used either to prevent infection or as an adjunct to therapy. The administration of VZV immunoglobulin to immunocompromised children exposed to VZV is routinely used to prevent, or at least attenuate, chickenpox in these high-risk individuals. More recently, CMV immunoglobulin has been used, along with antiviral drugs, to treat life-threatening infection in immunocompromised patients, with reported success.

TREATMENT

Infections due to HSV-1, HSV-2, and VZV are the most amenable to therapy with antiviral drugs. Vidarabine and acyclovir are useful for the management of specific infections caused by these viruses. Acyclovir is the treatment of choice for mucocutaneous HSV infections in the immunocompromised host, herpes simplex encephalitis, neonatal HSV infections, and VZV infections in the immunocompromised hosts. Intravenous administration is preferred for therapy against life-threatening disease. Immunocompromised individuals with mucocutaneous HSV infections that are not life threatening may be given oral acyclovir. Intravenous acyclovir must be used with caution because it may crystallize in the renal tubules when given too rapidly or to dehydrated patients.

In June 1989, ganciclovir was licensed for the treatment of CMV retinitis in immunocompromised individuals. Treatment with ganciclovir is associated with potential hematologic toxicity, notably neutropenia and thrombocytopenia. Dose reductions are required if evidence of toxicity appears. B virus infections of humans have been treated with both acyclovir and ganciclovir, with some reports of success; however, no controlled studies have been performed. There is no form of therapy for infection due to EBV or HHV-6.

REFERENCES

Bloom JN, Palestine AG: The diagnosis of cytomegalovirus retinitis. Ann Intern Med 109:963, 1988

Corey L, Spear P: Infections with herpes simplex viruses. N Engl J Med 314:686, 1986

Corey L, Spear P: Infections with herpes simplex viruses. N Engl J Med 314:749, 1986

Drew WL: Cytomegalovirus infection in patients with AIDS. J Infect Dis 158:449, 1988

Goldsmith SM, Whitley RJ: Herpes simplex encephalitis. In Lambert HP (ed): Infections of the Central Nervous System. BC Decker, Philadelphia, in press

Goldsmith S, Whitley RJ: Antiviral therapy. In Gorbach SL, Bartlett JG, Blacklow NR (eds): Infectious Diseases in Medicine and Surgery. WB Saunders, Philadelphia, in press

Ho M: Cytomegalovirus. p. 1159. In Mandell GL, Douglas RG, Bennett JE (eds): Principles and Practice of Infectious Diseases. 3rd Ed. Churchill Livingstone, New York, 1990

Nalesnik NA: Pathology of posttransplant lymphoproliferative disorders occurring in the setting of cyclosporine A-prednisone immunosuppression. Am J Pathol 133:173, 1988

Roizman B: Herpesviridae: a brief introduction. p. 1787. In Fields BN, Knipe DM, Chanock E, et al (eds): Virology. 2nd Ed. Raven Press, New York, 1990

Schooley RT, Dolin R: Epstein-Barr virus (infectious mononucleosis). p. 1172. In Mandell GL, Douglas RG, Bennett JE (eds): Principles and Practice of Infectious Diseases. 3rd Ed. Churchill Livingstone, New York, 1990

Straus S: Introduction to herpesviridae. p. 1139. In Mandell GL, Douglas RG, Bennett JE (eds): Principles and Practice of Infectious Diseases. 3rd Ed. Churchill Livingstone, New York, 1990

Whitley RJ. Cercopithecine herpes virus 1 (B virus). p. 2063. In Fields BN, Knipe DM, Chanock E et al (eds): Virology. 2nd Ed. Raven Press, New York, 1990

69

POXVIRUSES

DERRICK BAXBY

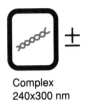

Complex
240x300 nm

GENERAL CONCEPTS

Clinical Manifestations

Smallpox has been eradicated. The remaining human poxvirus infections cause skin lesions with limited constitutional involvement. Human cowpox and parapox infections are usually localized and relatively unimportant; human monkeypox is a severe generalized infection with involvement of organs such as the lungs.

Structure

Poxviruses are brick-shaped (240 nm by 300 nm) and have a complex internal structure including a double-stranded DNA genome and associated enzymes. Naturally released virions have an additional outer membrane not found on infective virions extracted artificially from infected cells.

Classification and Antigenic Types

Genera are identified by genetic and serologic properties. Species within genera (e.g., *Orthopoxvirus, Parapoxvirus*) are very closely related antigenically and are recognized by biologic and/or DNA characteristics. Some poxviruses (e.g., molluscum contagiosum and tanapox viruses) are not yet formally classified.

Multiplication

Viral DNA is not infectious per se; virion-associated enzymes are important for replication. An important practical development is the production of recombinant poxvirus vectors (especially vaccinia virus) that express foreign genes and can be used for immunization against other pathogens.

Pathogenesis

Infection is usually caused by invasion through broken skin and in most cases remains localized. Human monkeypox is acquired by contact or by airborne transmission to the respiratory mucosa. Initial viremia during the incubation period spreads infection to internal organs; a second viremia then spreads the virus to the skin.

Host Defenses

The first line of defense is unbroken skin. The initial response after infection involves interferon and inflammation. Cell-mediated and humoral responses to viral antigens are important for recovery and subsequent immunity. The immune response to antigens on the membrane of naturally released virions is particularly important.

Epidemiology

With smallpox now eradicated, all natural human poxvirus infections except molluscum are zoonoses. Despite their names, the reservoir hosts of cowpox and monkeypox viruses are not known with certainty.

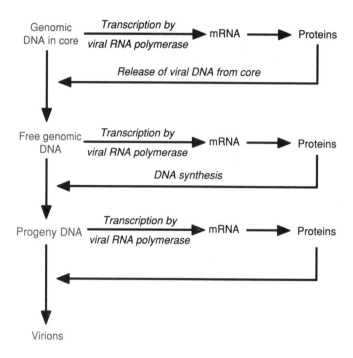

Diagnosis

The diagnosis is often suggested by the presence of skin lesions and a history of contact with human or animal cases. Diagnosis is confirmed by electron microscopy and/or virus isolation.

Control

Vaccination is not appropriate because human infections are mild. Some infections are occupational hazards and are probably unavoidable, despite care in handling infected animals.

INTRODUCTION

The last endemic case of smallpox occurred in 1977, total eradication was confirmed in 1980, and the official account of the disease and its eradication has appeared. Consequently, smallpox is not discussed below. However, its importance should not be forgotten. It helped to shape history, and it made history by being the first disease to be controlled by immunization and the first to be eradicated. A typical case is shown in Fig. 69-1, and Table 69-1 lists the features that made smallpox an ideal candidate for eradication. Features 9 and 10 meant that the disease spread slowly; features 3 and 11 to 13 meant that the source of infection of virtually all cases was another clinically ill individual. The disease was controlled and then eradicated by vigorous surveillance and containment, backed up by vaccination.

The remaining poxvirus infections of humans are relatively insignificant (Table 69-2). Furthermore, even such important animal diseases as sheeppox and camelpox are less important than animal infections caused by other pathogens.

CLINICAL MANIFESTATIONS

Poxvirus infections are characterized by the production of skin lesions. With most poxviruses there is typically just a primary lesion, but with human

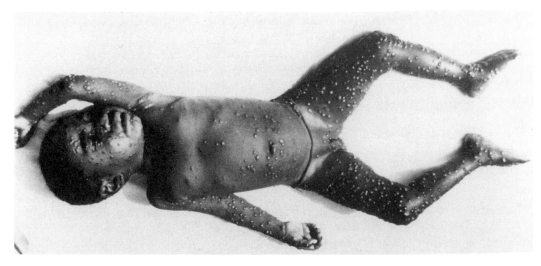

FIGURE 69–1   Smallpox in a child, demonstrating the characteristic centrifugal distribution of the lesions. (Courtesy of WHO Smallpox Eradication Unit.)

monkeypox and molluscum generalized lesions develop (Fig. 69-2). In human cowpox and parapox infections the lesion develops at the site of inoculation (usually the hand), and infection may be spread to other sites such as the face and/or genitals by scratching. When seen by the physician, cowpox and parapox lesions are usually hemorrhagic crusting ulcers, but early in infection the

TABLE 69-1   Features of Smallpox That Made it Eradicable

Effective vaccine
One stable serotype
No animal reservoir
Severe disease with high morbidity and mortality
Feasibility demonstrated by elimination from developed countries
Potential savings in developed nonendemic countries that are no longer required to vaccinate and monitor
No cultural and social barriers to case tracing and control
Easily diagnosed
Long incubation period
Low communicability
Infectious only after incubation period
No persistent infection
Subclinical infection rare and not a source of infection
Long-term immunity conferred by infection

former are usually vesicular and the latter nodular. The lesions of molluscum, usually multiple, are firm, pearly, flesh-colored nodules.

Parapox and molluscum infections cause very little constitutional disturbance. Human cowpox, particularly in young children, usually causes pyrexia and marked lymphadenopathy, and patients often require hospitalization. Rare encephalitic complications of cowpox have been reported, and erythema multiforme is a complication of parapox infections. Infection in immunocompromised or eczematous individuals is more severe and usually results in generalized illness.

Smallpox vaccination has been associated with serious complications. However, routine use of smallpox vaccine has been discontinued, and any future use of recombinant vaccinia virus vaccines will involve attenuated strains, thus reducing the chances of complications.

Although human monkeypox is rare and geographically localized, it is a serious generalized infection, which clinically resembles mild smallpox (Figs. 69-1 and 69-2). A febrile prodrome precedes the development of a vesicular or pustular rash, typically centrifugal in distribution. Detailed examination of more than 300 cases in Zaire showed an overall mortality of 10 percent, reaching 15 to 20 percent in unvaccinated children. Res-

TABLE 69-2 Poxviruses Pathogenic for Humans[a]

Virus (Reservoir)	Disease	Comments
Molluscum contagiosum virus (humans)	Skin nodules, often multiple, often long lasting	Often sexually transmitted
Milker's nodes virus (cattle), Orf virus (sheep, goats)	Skin lesions similar to cowpox; usually painless	Occupational hazards of those in contact with infected animals
Cowpox virus (not known)	Localized hemorrhagic ulcer with pyrexia; painful	Restricted to Europe, bovine infection rare; domestic cats most commonly detected host
Monkeypox virus (squirrels?)	Resembles human smallpox (15 percent mortality)	>400 cases since 1970 in West Africa; limited human-to-human spread
Tana poxvirus (monkeys)	Localized skin nodules with pyrexia	Human cases reported from West Africa
Vaccinia virus (no general natural host)	Rare complications of vaccination	Routine vaccination now discontinued; possible use of attenuated recombinants
Smallpox virus (humans)	Generalized infection with pustular rash	Total eradication confirmed in 1980

[a] The order of listing is intended to indicate current global importance, rather than clinical importance in the individual.

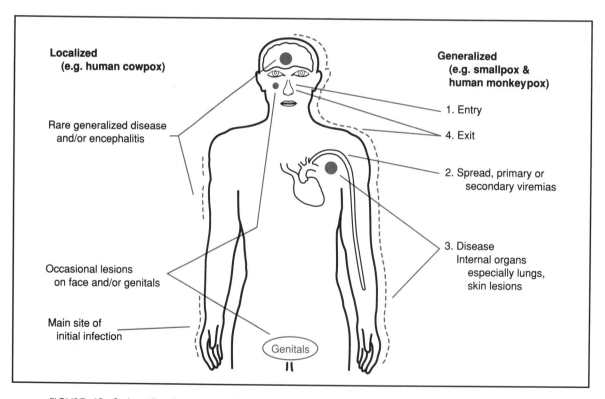

FIGURE 69-2 Localized and generalized poxvirus infections. Numbers indicate progression of infection.

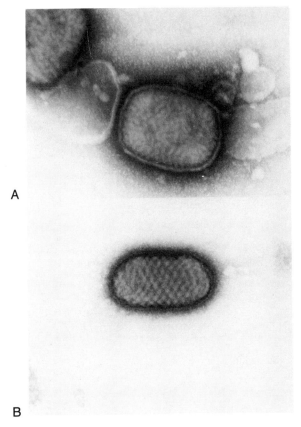

A

B

FIGURE 69-3   Electron micrographs of negatively stained naturally released virions of (A) vaccinia virus and (B) parapoxvirus. (X 100,000.)

piratory complications were seen in about 12 percent of unvaccinated patients.

STRUCTURE

Poxvirus virions are large and brick shaped. Orthopoxviruses are approximately 240 nm by 300 nm, with short surface tubules 10 nm wide. Parapoxviruses are narrower (160 nm) and have one long tubule that winds around the virion; in electron micrographs, superimposition of the top and bottom surfaces gives a criss-cross appearance (Fig. 69-3). Virions extracted artificially from infected cells are infectious and are generally used in studies on poxviruses. However, virions released naturally from infected cells acquire an additional envelope, which is easily lost during manipulation (Fig. 69-4). These naturally released virions possess extra antibody neutralization sites not present on the artificially extracted forms (Fig. 69-4). Internally, virions have a dumbbell-shaped core and two lateral bodies (Fig. 69-5). The genome consists of one molecule of double-stranded DNA (molecular weight, 8×10^7 to 24×10^7), and the core contains enzymes for virus uncoating and genome replication.

CLASSIFICATION AND ANTIGENIC TYPES

Poxviruses are assigned to genera on the basis of close genetic and serologic relationships (Table 69-3). The viruses are antigenically complex. Surface and soluble antigens show extensive cross-reaction between species in a genus but not between genera. This means that antigenic typing, as used for other virus groups, is not appropriate. Poxviruses have traditionally been assigned to species on the basis of biologic criteria. Genome analysis is now used and has generally confirmed biologic work, although some strains (e.g., rabbitpox and buffalopox viruses) are now regarded as variants of vaccinia virus. Some poxviruses (e.g., molluscum and tanapox viruses) are not yet formally classified.

MULTIPLICATION

Poxvirus replication takes place in cytoplasmic inclusions. Infecting virions are partly uncoated by cellular enzymes and then fully uncoated by viral enzymes released from the virion core. The viral DNA is not infectious per se, and other core enzymes (including a DNA-dependent RNA polymerase) play essential roles in the replication cycle. The replication cycle can be divided into functions controlled by early (prereplicative) gene products and those controlled by late (postreplicative) gene products. Most virions (80 to 90 percent) remain within cells and therefore lack the outer envelope found on naturally released virions (Fig. 69-4).

Knowledge of the molecular biology of poxvirus replication has led to the development of recombinant vaccinia virus strains that code for the products of foreign genes inserted into the vaccinia virus genome (Fig. 69-6). Such recombinants are infectious and are being widely used to study gene expression, as candidate vaccines (e.g., against rabies and rinderpest), and for the production of biopharmaceuticals such as factor VIII.

Intracellular and Extracellular Poxviruses

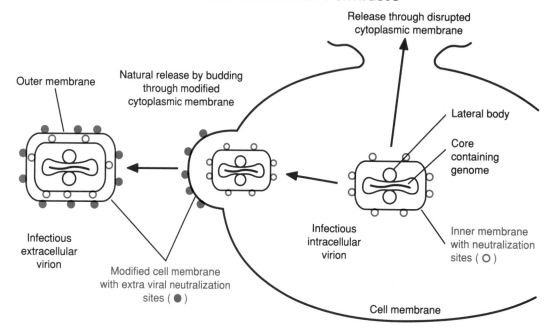

FIGURE 69–4 Intracellular and extracellular poxviruses.

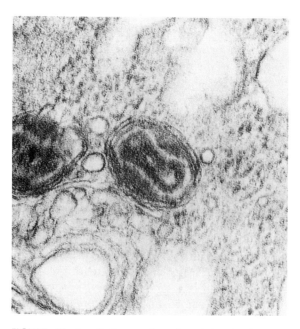

FIGURE 69–5 *Orthopoxvirus* (vaccinia virus). Thin section showing internal structure. (× 100,000.)

PATHOGENESIS

The pathogenesis of localized poxvirus infections is simple. Virus invades through local skin lesions, replicates at the site of inoculation, and causes dermal hyperplasia and leukocyte infiltration. With cowpox, and to a lesser extent with parapox, there is limited lymphatic spread; this causes lymphadenopathy and elicits an immune response. The lesion of molluscum is circumscribed by a connective tissue capsule, and the dermis, although distorted, is not usually broken.

Human monkeypox is usually acquired via the respiratory tract, and during a 12-day incubation period viremia distributes infection to internal organs, which are damaged by virus infection. Spread to the skin initiates the clinical phase, and the lesions progress through the classic stages of macule to papule to vesicle to pustule to crust. Lymphadenopathy, usually involving the cervical and inguinal areas, is often marked.

TABLE 69-3   Poxviruses of Vertebrates

Genus	Species and Members
Orthopoxvirus[a]	Smallpox, monkeypox, vaccinia, cowpox, camelpox, mouse-pox, raccoonpox viruses
Parapoxvirus[b]	Orf (contagious pustular dermatitis), milker's nodes (pseudo-cowpox), bovine papular stomatitis viruses
Capripoxvirus	Sheeppox, goatpox, lumpy skin disease viruses
Avipoxvirus	Fowlpox, canarypox, pigeonpox, sparrowpox viruses, etc.
Leporipoxvirus	Myxoma, hare fibroma, rabbit fibroma, squirrel fibroma viruses
Suipoxvirus	Swinepox virus
Unclassified[c]	Tana and Yaba poxviruses; molluscum contagiosum virus

[a] Whitepox viruses, indistinguishable from smallpox virus and apparently isolated from wild animals, are considered to represent laboratory contamination with smallpox virus. Strains similar to cowpox virus have been isolated from captive carnivores. Strains previously referred to as rabbitpox and buffalopox are regarded as variants of vaccinia virus.

[b] Unclassified parapoxviruses have been isolated from camels, squirrels, and kangaroos.

[c] Tana and Yaba poxviruses are serologically related.

HOST DEFENSES

With the exception of human monkeypox, which is usually acquired via the respiratory route, human poxvirus infections are acquired by inoculation into the skin or contact with broken skin (Fig. 69-2). Consequently, unbroken skin presents the first line of defense. Interferon, nonspecific inflammation, and probably pyrexia play a role in limiting infection during the early stages.

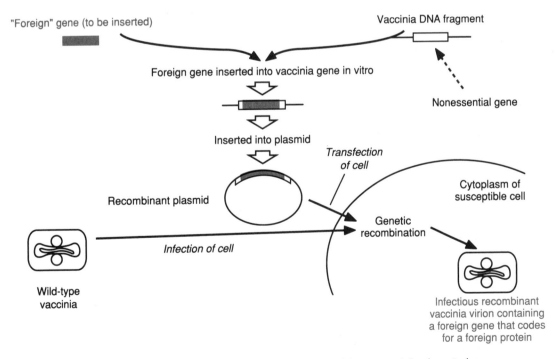

FIGURE 69-6   Strategy for the production of recombinant vaccinia virus strains.

Infection induces humoral and cellular immune responses to naturally released virions and to viral antigens on the surface of virus-infected cells. Responses to the extra antigens on the envelope of naturally released virions (Fig. 69-4) are particularly important, determining the speed and extent of recovery and the prevention or attenuation of future infection.

In general, the immune response is related to the severity of infection; the immunity elicited by a mild infection may be insufficient to prevent reinfection, as is often the case with human parapox infections.

EPIDEMIOLOGY

With the exception of molluscum, which is a specifically human disease, human poxvirus infections are acquired from animal reservoirs (Table 69-2). In some cases the reservoir is known and distributed worldwide, as in the case of ovine and bovine parapoxviruses. Human infection with these viruses is an occupational hazard of those working with the infected reservoir hosts.

Monkeypox is restricted to West Africa, and squirrels are more important as reservoir hosts than monkeys. Cowpox virus is restricted to Europe. Bovine cowpox is rare, and the domestic cat is the most commonly reported host. Conclusive information about the reservoir host of cowpox virus is lacking, but it is generally assumed to be a small wild mammal. Cases occur without known contact with cats or cattle, and indirect spread via barbed wire or brambles is possible.

Limited natural person-to-person spread of monkeypox has been observed, but not further than four or five generations. Parapox and cowpox infections are occasionally spread directly from person to person. Person-to-person spread of molluscum is traditionally associated with physical contact sports (e.g., wrestling) and the sharing of towels. There is increasing evidence, however, that sexual transmission of molluscum is important.

Vaccinia virus is traditionally regarded as a laboratory virus with no natural reservoir. However, buffalopox virus is now considered a variant of vaccinia virus and appears to have established itself in India after the cessation of smallpox vaccination. Because of the potential use of recombinant vaccinia virus vaccines, it is important to remember that such strains may become established in animal populations and/or interact with genetically related viruses circulating in them.

DIAGNOSIS

In many cases, the nature of the lesions and a careful history that establishes contact with an infected reservoir animal or another infected person will permit a satisfactory diagnosis. Difficulties may arise if no such contact is established. This is perhaps most common with human cowpox, since most cases are not traced to a particular source and a clinical diagnosis of anthrax is sometimes made.

Electron microscopy of vesicle or scab material is an effective means of rapid diagnosis; poxviruses and herpesviruses are readily distinguished, and the characteristic morphology of parapoxviruses can be recognized (Fig. 69-4). Immunofluorescence of infected cell cultures will differentiate morphologically similar poxviruses from different genera (e.g., *Orthopoxvirus* and *Tanapoxvirus*). Although molluscum contagiosum virus has yet to be cultivated, the other poxviruses are easily isolated in tissue culture and/or chicken embryos. Cultivation then allows identification by biologic and serum neutralization tests.

CONTROL

Control of the common human poxvirus infections depends on knowledge of their epidemiology. In particular, persons caring for sick livestock should take precautions, but the extent of occupational exposure is such that infection and reinfection are inevitable. Control of infections such as cowpox, which has an unknown reservoir, is virtually impossible. Person-to-person transmission of these infections, and also of molluscum, is reduced by improving hygiene. Monkeypox is a special case. The World Health Organization considers that the benefits of vaccination do not outweigh the risks and expense. Control of this disease depends on health education and on breaking the link with the animal reservoir; this last should be achieved by the use of forest land near villages for agriculture.

In conclusion, it is significant that the strategies used for smallpox eradication are being assessed for the control and eradication of other diseases such as measles and that smallpox vaccine, through genetic engineering, may play an important role in the control of other infections.

REFERENCES

Baxby D: Poxvirus infections in domestic animals. p. 17. In Darai GM (ed): Virus Diseases in Laboratory and Captive Animals. Martinus Nijhoff, Boston, 1988

Baxby D: Human poxvirus infection after the eradication of smallpox. Epidemiol Infect 100:321, 1988

Bennett M, Gaskell CJ, Baxby D et al: Feline cowpox virus infection. J Sm Anim Pract 31:167, 1990

Brown ST, Nalley JF, Kraus SJ: Molluscum contagiosum. Sex Transm Dis 8:227, 1981

Dumbell KR: Poxviridae. p. 395. In Porterfield JS (ed): Andrewes' Viruses of Vertebrates. 5th Ed. Balliere Tindall, London, 1989

Esposito JJ, Knight JC: Orthopoxvirus DNA: a comparison of restriction profiles and maps. Virology 143:230, 1985

Fenner F, Henderson DA, Arita I et al: Smallpox and Its Eradication. World Health Organization, Geneva, 1988

Fenner F, Wittek R, Dumbell KR: The Orthopoxviruses. Academic Press, San Diego 1989

Jezek Z, Arita I, Szczeniowski M et al: Human tanapox in Zaire: clinical and epidemiological observations on cases confirmed by laboratory studies. Bull WHO 63:1027, 1985

Jezek Z, Fenner F: Human Monkeypox. Karger, Basel, 1988

Johanneson JV, Krogh HK, Solberg I et al. Human orf. J Cutaneous Pathol 2:265, 1975

Kaplan C: Vaccinia virus: a suitable vehicle for recombinant vaccines? Arch Virol 106:127, 1989

70 HEPATITIS VIRUSES

ARIE J. ZUCKERMAN

GENERAL CONCEPTS

INTRODUCTION
Hepatitis is an inflammation of the liver and is caused by several distinct viruses.

HEPATITIS A VIRUS
Clinical Manifestations
Frequently hepatitis A virus infection is asymptomatic or anicteric in children and shows a range of gastrointestinal symptoms (bile in urine, pale stools, jaundice, and fulminant hepatic failure with coma).

Structure, Classification, and Antigenic Types
The organism consists of unenveloped cubic particles 27 nm in diameter and containing a linear genome of single-stranded RNA. Hepatitis A virus is classified as enterovirus type 72. There is one major antigenic type.

Multiplication
Hepatitis A virus multiplies by the same mechanism as that for picornaviruses (see Ch. 53).

Pathogenesis
The primary site of replication is the intestinal epithelium. Viremia and multiplication in the liver follow.

Host Defenses
There are both humoral and cell-mediated defenses.

Epidemiology
Spread is by the fecal-oral route. Hepatitis A is common throughout the world and hyperendemic in countries with poor socioeconomic conditions.

Diagnosis
Hepatitis A is diagnosed by the presence of the anti-hepatitis A virus antibody of the IgM class.

Control
Hepatitis A is best controlled by simple hygienic measures and sanitary disposal of excreta. Injection of normal human immunoglobulin sometimes prevents infection. Vaccines are under development.

HEPATITIS B VIRUS
Clinical Manifestations
The various types of hepatitis cannot be distinguished with accuracy on clinical grounds.

Structure
Double-shelled, 42-nm particles constitute the complete virus, which contains a double-stranded DNA. There is excess surface antigen protein in the form of 22-nm particles and tubules.

Classification and Antigenic Types
Hepatitis B virus is a hepadna virus, with four principal

phenotypes, having at least 10 subtypes. Several variants and mutants have been described.

Multiplication

Hepatitis B virus is unusual in that it multiplies by reverse transcription via an RNA intermediate.

Pathogenesis

From the site of inoculation the virus travels in the bloodstream to the liver, where it multiplies, may set up chronic infection, and may induce hepatocellular carcinoma.

Host Defenses

Humoral and cell-mediated immune responses may be involved in defense and pathogenesis.

Epidemiology

The principal modes of transmission are by blood-to-blood contact and by the sexual route. Perinatal transmission is very important in some regions of the world.

Diagnosis

The markers of hepatitis B virus for diagnosis include HBsAg, anti-HBs, anti-HBc antibody, and HBV DNA.

Control

Hepatitis B vaccines may prevent the disease.

NON-A, NON-B HEPATITIS VIRUS

Clinical Manifestations

Non-A, non-B hepatitis virus has the same disease manifestations as the other hepatitis viruses.

Structure, Classification, and Antigenic Types

There are at least two types, one of which is referred to as hepatitis C virus. This non-A, non-B hepatitis virus is unclassified, but it may be a member of the flavivirus group and may have at least two serotypes.

Multiplication, Pathogenesis, and Host Defenses

Mechanisms of multiplication, pathogenesis, and host defenses are not yet established.

Epidemiology

Transmission is mainly by contact with blood and blood products. The epidemiology is essentially similar to that for hepatitis B virus.

ENTERICALLY TRANSMITTED NON-A, NON-B HEPATITIS VIRUS

Enterically transmitted non-A, non-B hepatitis virus is also referred to as hepatitis E virus. It is spread via con-

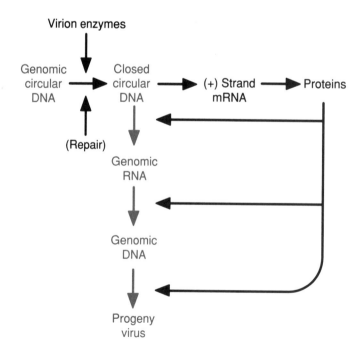

taminated water and is frequently found in parts of Asia, the Middle East, and North and East Africa, as well as in travelers returning from these areas. It is associated with high mortality when contracted during pregnancy.

DELTA HEPATITIS VIRUS

Delta hepatitis virus is a defective single-stranded RNA virus consisting of a core of delta antigen encapsulated by a protein coat derived from hepatitis B surface antigen. Delta hepatitis virus requires the helper function of hepatitis B virus. There is one serotype. Delta hepatitis is endemic in some regions. Superinfection in a carrier of hepatitis B virus may result in reactivation of chronic liver damage and may be associated with high mortality.

INTRODUCTION

Viral hepatitis is a major public health problem, occurring endemically in all parts of the world. The general term **viral hepatitis** applies to liver infections caused by several unrelated viruses (Table 70-1). Two types of hepatitis were initially recognized: hepatitis A and hepatitis B. **Hepatitis A** is a self-limiting, sometimes severe disease transmitted mainly by the fecal-oral route. The agent, **hepatitis A virus,** is a picornavirus. **Hepatitis B** is transmitted mainly parenterally, by blood and other body fluids; clinically it resembles hepatitis A, but it may evolve into a chronic form. It is caused by **hepatitis B virus,** a hepadna virus. In the 1960s, it became clear that many cases of viral hepatitis are caused by neither of these pathogens. Such cases are collectively referred to as **non-A, non-B hepatitis.** There are at least two types of non-A, non-B hepatitis: one transmitted parenterally, like hepatitis B, and the other transmitted enterally, like hepatitis A. One of the two viruses associated with parenteral non-A, non-B hepatitis has been isolated and named **hepatitis C virus.** Finally, an especially

TABLE 70-1 Distinguishing Characteristics of Viral Hepatitis

Virus	Classification	Transmission	Mean Incubation Period	Type	Distribution
Hepatitis A	Enterovirus[a]	Fecal-oral	4 weeks	Acute or inapparent	Worldwide
Enterically transmitted non-A, non-B	Unclassified	Fecal-oral	About 6 weeks	Acute or inapparent	Regional SE Asia, India, Middle East, Africa, Mexico
Hepatitis B	Hepadna virus	Blood	3 months	Acute or persistent	Worldwide
Parenterally transmitted non-A, non-B	Unclassified	Blood	2 weeks–6 months	Acute or persistent	Worldwide
Delta agent	RNA genome, hepatitis B capsid	Blood	Not known and variable	Acute or persistent	Areas worldwide

[a] Picornavirus family.

severe form of hepatitis occurs when a carrier of hepatitis B is coinfected by an agent called **delta hepatitis virus.**

Viral hepatitis is a systemic infection characterized particularly by inflammation and necrosis of the liver. The disease ranges in severity from inapparent to fulminating; at least half the cases of both type A and type B hepatitis are subclinical. A mild case of hepatitis consists of general malaise with various influenzalike symptoms. In more severe disease, signs and symptoms of liver damage ensue: icterus (jaundice), dark urine, swelling and tenderness of the liver, and high serum titers of transaminases and other indicators of hepatocyte necrosis. A small proportion of hepatitis B and parenteral non-A, non-B cases evolve into a chronic form, which may be either a benign carrier state or low-grade active disease.

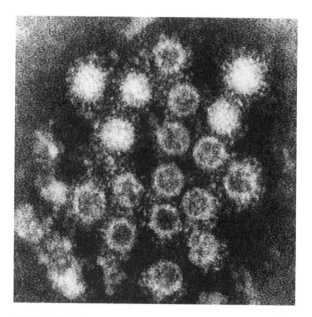

FIGURE 70-1 Hepatitis A virus particles found in fecal extracts by immunoelectron microscopy. Both full and empty particles are present. Particles are surrounded by a halo of hepatitis A antibody. The virus is 27 to 29 nm in diameter. (X 300,000.)

HEPATITIS A VIRUS

CLINICAL MANIFESTATIONS

Clinically, hepatitis A conforms to the general picture described above. Most cases are asymptomatic. The full disease consists of a 3- to 5-week incubation period (mean, 28 days) followed by an acute phase during which influenzalike malaise is accompanied by evidence of hepatic inflammation. The mortality is low, but patients may be incapacitated for weeks. The disease is always self-limiting. Hepatitis A is usually mild and anicteric in children. The ratio of icteric to anicteric cases varies from one epidemic to another.

STRUCTURE, CLASSIFICATION, AND ANTIGENIC TYPES

Like other picornaviruses (see Ch. 53), hepatitis A virus is a small, nonenveloped, single-stranded RNA virus (Fig. 70-1). It is relatively resistant to ether, to heating at 60°C for 1 hour, and to acidic conditions (down to pH 3), but it can be inactivated by Formalin or chlorine. It can remain viable for fairly long periods in the environment (for example, on kitchen cutting boards). Hepatitis A virus has been classified as **enterovirus type 72.** Only one serotype has been identified.

MULTIPLICATION

The multiplication of picornaviruses is discussed in Chapter 53. Hepatitis A virus has been cultured in both primary and continuous cell cultures of primate origin.

PATHOGENESIS

Hepatitis A virus enters the body by ingestion. It infects the intestinal epithelium, multiplies there, and eventually spreads (probably in the bloodstream) to the liver, which is the principal target organ. Beginning as early as 10 to 14 days after infection, virus is shed copiously in the feces. Fecal shedding continues into the early acute phase of the illness and usually ceases at about the time jaundice develops. Hepatitis A antigen has been demonstrated by immunofluorescence in the cytoplasm of hepatocytes in experimentally infected chimpanzees; following intravenous inoculation, the antigen appears only in the liver.

The liver is the only organ that shows pathologic changes during hepatitis A. Several changes occur: conspicuous focal activation of sinusoid lining cells; accumulation of lymphocytes and histiocytes in the parenchyma (predominantly in the periportal areas), often replacing hepatocytes lost by cytolytic necrosis; occasional coagulative necrosis in the form of acidophilic bodies; and focal degeneration.

HOST DEFENSES

Antibody to hepatitis A virus develops late in the incubation period. Specific hepatitis A IgM is detectable in the serum within 1 week of the onset of dark urine, peaks about 1 week later, and declines slowly over the next 40 to 60 days. Specific IgG antibody appears shortly after IgM and peaks in 60 to 80 days. This antibody is protective and persists for many years.

EPIDEMIOLOGY

Hepatitis A (also called **infectious** or **epidemic hepatitis**) is endemic throughout the world and causes frequent minor or major outbreaks. The actual incidence is difficult to estimate, not only because of the high proportion of subclinical and anicteric infections, but also because of uneven surveillance and differing patterns of disease. The degree of underreporting is believed to be very high.

Hepatitis A is spread by the fecal-oral route, most commonly by person-to-person contact or via food or water. Epidemics are encouraged by conditions of overcrowding and poor sanitation. In developed countries the disease occurs mainly in small clusters, often with only a few identified cases. Common-source outbreaks are most frequently due to water or food contaminated by a food handler who is shedding virus in the feces during the incubation period. Waterborne transmission is not common in industrialized communities; more often, outbreaks can be traced to uncooked food or food that has been handled after being cooked.

Two developments have permitted a study of the epidemiology of hepatitis A: (1) identification of virus particles in fecal extracts by immunoelectron microscopy (Fig. 70-1) and (2) identification of viral antigen and specific antibodies. The latter achievement made it possible to develop serologic tests for hepatitis A and to determine the susceptibility of humans and other primates to the infection. Hepatitis A has been transmitted to certain nonhuman primates shown to be free of homologous antibody (some species of marmosets and, particularly, the chimpanzee), thus providing an animal model and an initial source of reagents.

Serologic tests for hepatitis A have been used to study the incidence and distribution of the disease in various countries. These studies have shown not only that the virus is endemic throughout the world, but also that chronic viral shedding does not occur and that the disease is very rarely transmitted by blood transfusion. No evidence of progression to chronic liver disease has been found.

DIAGNOSIS

Clinically, hepatitis A resembles other types of viral hepatitis. Various serologic tests are used to make the diagnosis, including immunoelectron microscopy, complement fixation, immune adherence hemagglutination, radioimmunoassay, and enzyme immunoassay. Immune adherence hemagglutination, widely used in the past, is only moderately specific and sensitive. A solid-phase radioimmunoassay is convenient and has proved very sensitive and specific. Extremely sensitive enzyme immunoassay techniques have also been developed. Because isolation of the virus in tissue culture requires prolonged adaptation, that technique is not yet suitable for diagnosis.

CONTROL

There is no specific treatment for hepatitis A. Spread of the disease can be reduced by simple hygienic measures and by the sanitary disposal of excreta. Prophylactic administration of normal human immunoglobulin containing 2 IU of hepatitis A antibody/kg of body weight before exposure to the virus or early in the incubation period will prevent or attenuate clinical illness. This dose is sometimes doubled for individuals at particularly high risk, such as pregnant women and patients with liver disease. Immunoglobulin does not always prevent infection, however; inapparent or subclinical hepatitis with fecal shedding of virus may occur and may induce active immunity. Hepatitis A vaccines are being evaluated in clinical studies.

HEPATITIS B VIRUS

CLINICAL MANIFESTATIONS

Clinically, acute hepatitis B is a typical viral hepatitis. The incubation period is highly variable, ranging from 4 to 26 weeks. Although hepatitis B is often more severe than hepatitis A, most cases end in complete recovery. A few, however, progress to one of two chronic conditions: **chronic persistent hepatitis** or **chronic active hepatitis.** Patients with chronic persistent hepatitis are usually asymptomatic, but may show mild elevation of serum alanine transaminase. This syndrome, which occurs in 8 to 10 percent of cases of hepatitis B, is apparently benign and does not result in liver fibrosis. About 25 percent of patients with chronic hepatitis show

the active form of the disease. Jaundice may be present, and serum alanine transaminase is elevated. Liver biopsy reveals liver cell necrosis. Progressive cirrhosis leads to liver failure in a high proportion of patients. Moreover, patients with chronic active hepatitis show a strong predisposition for developing hepatocellular carcinoma.

A case of hepatitis B is considered chronic if the surface antigen of the virus persists for more than 6 months (Fig. 70-2). Infections early in life usually result in a carrier state, whereas only 5 to 10 percent of adult infections produce carriers.

STRUCTURE

The hepatitis B virus is a 42-nm, enveloped hepadna virus (Fig. 70-3) with a circular DNA genome. The envelope encloses an icosahedral core particle that contains the genome in association with an endogenous DNA-dependent DNA polymerase. The DNA is about 3,200 nucleotides long and has a molecular weight of 2.3×10^6. It is double stranded except for a single-stranded gap of

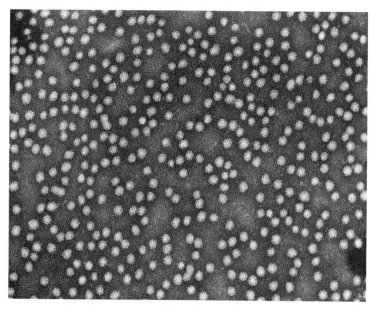

FIGURE 70-2 Purified preparation of approximately 22-nm spherical HBsAg particles. Such preparations are being used as subunit small particle hepatitis B vaccines. ($\times$ 126,000.)

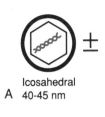

Icosahedral
A 40-45 nm

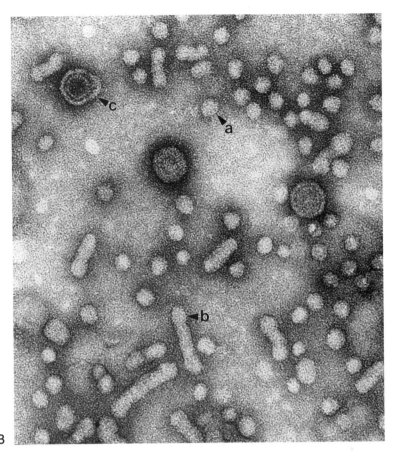

B

FIGURE 70-3 (*A*) Structure of the hepadna viruses. (*B*) Electron micrograph of serum containing hepatitis B virus after negative staining. The three morphologic forms are shown intermingled in this photograph: a, small pleomorphic spherical particles 20 to 22 nm in diameter; b, tubular forms; c, 42-nm double-shelled virus. (X 252,000.) (Fig. B from Zuckerman AJ: Human Viral Hepatitis. Elsevier-North Holland, Amsterdam, 1975, with permission.)

about 600 to 2,100 nucleotides. The viral DNA polymerase appears to repair this gap, but the relevance of the gap to viral replication is not clear.

In addition to the 42-nm complete virion, the blood of patients with hepatitis B contains two other types of viral particle: small, pleomorphic spherical particles about 22 nm in diameter and long, tubular forms (Fig. 70-3). These particles represent excess viral components, which are released into the circulation.

Three serologic markers are detectable in the blood of patients with hepatitis B (Fig. 70-4). **Hepatitis B surface antigen** (HBsAg), originally called Australia antigen, is associated with the 22-nm spherical particle. It elicits production of a corresponding antibody, **surface antibody** (anti-HBs). The second antigen, associated with the virion core, is called the **core antigen** (HBcAg) and elicits production of **core antibody** (anti-HBc). The third marker of hepatitis B infection is a soluble core-associated antigen known as **e antigen** (HBeAg). This antigen and its corresponding anti-HBe antibody correlate closely with the number of virus particles and the relative infectivity of serum containing HBsAg: the presence of anti-HBe indicates relatively low infectivity.

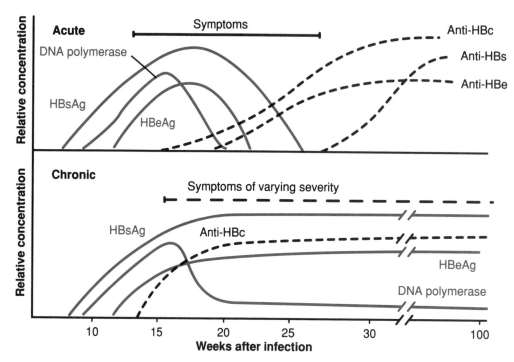

FIGURE 70-4 Sequence of development of viral antigens and antibodies in acute and chronic hepatitis B.

CLASSIFICATION AND ANTIGENIC TYPES

Hepatitis B virus is classified as a member of the hepadna viruses (hepatitis DNA viruses), which include human hepatitis B virus, woodchuck hepadna virus, ground squirrel hepadna virus, and duck hepadna virus.

There are at least 10 subtypes of human hepatitis B virus, based on serologic analysis of HBsAg. HBsAg generally carries a common group-specific determinant *a* and usually at least two mutually exclusive subdeterminants *d* or *y*, and *w* or *r*. The subtypes are the phenotypic expressions of distinct genotype variants of the virus. Four principal phenotypes are recognized: *adw, adr, ayw,* and *ayr.* However, other complex permutations of these subdeterminants and new variants have been described, and all apparently are on the surface of the same physical particles. An important escape mutant of hepatitis B virus (i.e., a mutant with an altered antigenic phenotype that allows it to escape immune surveillance) has also been described recently. This escape mutant may be important in the context of prophylactic immunization.

The major subtypes have differing geographic distributions and are of epidemiologic significance.

MULTIPLICATION

A mode of replication via an RNA intermediate is now accepted for the entire hepadna virus group. The viral genome consists of two strands of DNA, a complete antisense strand and an incomplete sense strand, held in a circular configuration by base pairing over approximately 250 nucleotide pairs at the 5′ ends. An identical motif of 11 base pairs is located near the 5′ ends of both strands, and these direct repeats appear to be important in DNA replication. The template for sense-strand DNA synthesis appears to be the antisense strand, and the template for antisense-strand DNA synthesis is RNA, requiring reverse transcriptase activity.

PATHOGENESIS

Hepatitis B formerly was also called **serum hepatitis** because it is transmitted parenterally. The virus can be transmitted by various body fluids (blood, saliva, menstrual and vaginal discharges, serous exudates, semen, and breast milk), but blood is the most infectious. From the site of inoculation the virus travels in the bloodstream to the liver, where it infects cells and multiplies. It is not known why some cases resolve and some become chronic. Factors that correlate with chronic disease include anicteric or mild infection, a long incubation period, immunosuppression, genetic predisposition, and infection early in childhood. It is also not clear whether the hepatitis B virus acts alone or as a cocarcinogen in the pathogenesis of liver cancer.

Large quantities of HBsAg persist in hepatocytes of apparently healthy carriers, which suggests that the virus damages hepatocytes by some indirect mechanism rather than directly. There is evidence that the pathogenesis of liver damage in hepatitis B involves an autoimmune response. For example, cell-mediated immunity to hepatitis B antigens has been demonstrated in most patients during the acute phase of the disease and in a significant proportion of patients with active chronic disease, but not in asymptomatic chronic carriers. This observation suggests that cell-mediated immunity may be important not only in terminating the infection, but also, under certain circumstances, in promoting liver damage and in the genesis of autoimmune responses. Evidence also suggests that progressive liver damage may result from an autoimmune reaction directed against hepatocyte membrane antigens, initiated in many cases by infection with hepatitis B virus.

HBsAg–antibody complexes are found in the sera of some patients during both the incubation and acute phases of the illness. Immune complexes have been found by electron microscopy in the sera of all patients with fulminant hepatitis, but only infrequently in nonfulminant cases. Immune complexes have also been identified in a number of patients with virtually all the recognized chronic sequelae of hepatitis B. Deposits of such immune complexes have been found in the cytoplasm and plasma membrane of hepatocytes and on or in the nuclei. Immune complexes are important in the pathogenesis of various diseases characterized by severe damage to blood vessels (e.g., polyarteritis nodosa). It is not clear why only a small proportion of hepatitis B patients with circulating immune complexes develop vasculitis or polyarteritis.

HOST DEFENSES

As mentioned above, both humoral and cell-mediated responses to various hepatitis B viral antigens are induced during infection. These are not always protective; in some instances, they may be involved in autoimmune pathogenesis. The immune response is directed against at least the three antigens HBsAg, HBcAg, and HBeAg. The response to HBsAg is known to be protective and is used as the basis for vaccination.

Cellular immune responses are generally important in determining the clinical features and course of viral infections. As mentioned above, cell-mediated immunity to hepatitis B antigens appears during the acute phase of the disease and appears important in recovery; however, cell-mediated immunity during chronic active disease may cause autoimmune damage.

Exogenous interferon may be effective in treating some patients with chronic hepatitis, but as yet endogenous interferon production has not been detected during natural hepatitis B infection. More studies to define the role of interferon are needed.

EPIDEMIOLOGY

Hepatitis B virus can be transmitted by various body fluids, particularly by blood. Thus, the infection can be spread by inadequately sterilized syringes and instruments, by transfused blood and blood products, by sexual and other close contact, and possibly by blood-sucking arthropods. Hepatitis B can be transmitted from mother to child antenatally (rare) or perinatally (common); in some parts of the world, such as Southeast Asia and Japan, perinatal transmission is very common. Almost all infected neonates become carriers. Table

TABLE 70-2   Prevalence of Hepatitis B in
Various Areas

Area	Percentage of Population Positive for HBsAg	Percentage of Population Positive for Anti-HBs Antibody	Neonatal Infection	Childhood Infection
Northern, Western, and Central Europe; North America; Australia	0.2–0.5	4–6	Rare	Infrequent
Eastern Europe, the Mediterranean, the USSR, Southwest Asia, Central and South America	2–7	20–55	Frequent	Frequent
Parts of China, Southeast Asia, tropical Africa	8–20	70–95	Very frequent	Very frequent

70-2 gives the prevalence of hepatitis B in various parts of the world.

All three serologic markers (HBsAg, HBcAg, and HBeAg) can be detected by sensitive techniques such as radioimmunoassay and enzyme immunoassay. These markers have proved extremely useful for unraveling the global epidemiology of the disease. Because blood donors are now routinely screened for surface antigen, transmission of hepatitis B by contaminated blood and blood products is now uncommon. However, the survival of the disease is ensured by the vast reservoir of carriers, estimated to number at least 300 million. The prevalence of carriers ranges from an extreme low of 0.1 percent or less among blood donors in North America and Northern Europe to 20 percent or sometimes even 35 percent of the population in some parts of Africa, in Asia, and in the Pacific regions.

DIAGNOSIS

Hepatitis B virus can be demonstrated directly in serum samples by using electron microscopy, by detecting virus-associated DNA polymerase, or by assaying viral DNA. None of these techniques is practical for a general diagnostic laboratory, however, so diagnosis usually relies on serologic techniques (Table 70-3).

TABLE 70-3   Interpretation of Results of Serologic
Tests for Hepatitis B

HBsAg	HBeAg	anti-HBe	Anti-HBc IgM	Anti-HBc IgG	Anti-HBs	Interpretation
+	+	−	−	−	−	Incubation period
+	+	−	+	+	−	Acute hepatitis B or persistent carrier state
+	+	−	−	+	−	Persistent carrier state
+	−	+	+/−	+	−	Persistent carrier state
−	−	+	+/−	+	+	Convalescence
−	−	−	−	+	+	Recovery
−	−	−	+	−	−	Infection with hepatitis B virus without detectable HBsAg
−	−	−	−	+	−	Recovery with loss of detectable anti-HBs
−	−	−	−	−	+	Immunization without infection, repeated exposure to antigen without infection, or recovery from infection with loss of detectable anti-HBc

Figure 70-4 shows the sequence in which hepatitis B-associated antigens and antibodies appear in the sera of patients. HBsAg, which is easily detected by radioimmunoassay or enzyme immunoassay, usually appears during the late incubation period, 2 to 8 weeks before biochemical evidence of liver damage or the onset of jaundice, and persists through the acute illness. It decreases sharply when anti-HBs antibody appears and clears from the circulation during convalescence unless chronic disease develops. Next to appear is the virus-associated DNA polymerase activity, which coincides with damage to liver cells, as indicated by elevated serum transaminases. This polymerase activity persists for days or weeks in acute cases and for months or years in some persistent carriers. IgM antibody to the core antigen appears in the serum after the onset of clinical symptoms and declines slowly after recovery. The titer of anti-HBc antibody appears to correlate with the amount and duration of virus replication; persistently high titers of anti-HBc IgM suggest chronic infection. IgG against HBcAg remains detectable for many years and provides evidence of past infection. Antibody to the surface antigen is the last serum factor to appear.

CONTROL

There is no specific treatment for hepatitis B; however, the disease may be prevented by either passive or active immunization.

Passive Immunization

Hepatitis B immunoglobulin administered before or shortly after exposure to hepatitis B virus confers temporary passive immunity. This immunoglobulin is prepared from the pooled plasma of volunteer donors with high titers of anti-HBs. Hepatitis B immunoglobulin is given in response to acute exposure to hepatitis B virus, for example, if contaminated blood is inoculated, ingested, or splashed on mucous membranes or conjunctiva. The optimal dose has not been established; doses in the range of 250 to 500 IU have proved effective. The immunoglobulin should be administered as soon as possible after exposure, preferably within 48 hours; it should not be administered if more than 7 days have elapsed since exposure. A second dose is generally given 30 days later.

Hepatitis B immunoglobulin ideally should be administered immediately after birth to all babies born to infected mothers or in endemic areas, since hepatitis B contracted during infancy usually develops into a carrier state. If the immunoglobulin is administered within 12 hours after birth, the chance that the infant will become a carrier is reduced by 70 percent. More recent studies with combined passive and active immunization indicate an efficacy approaching 90 percent.

Active Immunization

Hepatitis B virus has not yet been grown in tissue culture, so other routes have been used to develop vaccines. The 22-nm spherical surface antigen particle has been purified from the plasma of asymptomatic carriers and used as a vaccine (Fig. 70-2). Trials with high-risk groups have shown this vaccine to be effective and safe. There is no risk of transmitting the agents of acquired immune deficiency syndrome (AIDS) and other infections via plasma-derived vaccines that meet current World Health Organization standards. More recently, hepatitis B vaccine has been produced by recombinant DNA technology, using antigen expressed in yeast. Local reactions to hepatitis vaccination are minor, occurring in fewer than 20 percent of individuals and consisting of slight swelling and redness at the inoculation site. Fever of up to 38°C has been observed, but is rare.

Indications for Hepatitis B Immunization

Groups at high risk of contracting hepatitis B should be immunized. These groups are listed in Table 70-4. Infants born in endemic areas should be universally immunized; and those born to carrier mothers should receive both immunoglobulin prophylaxis and vaccination. In developed countries, selected high-risk groups should be immunized. These groups include individuals who need repeated transfusions of blood or blood products, patients who are undergoing prolonged inpatient

TABLE 70-4   Indications for Immunization against
Hepatitis B

Health care personnel

Health care personnel in frequent contact with
blood or needles

Staff in residential institutions with a known high
risk of hepatitis

Personnel in hemodialysis, hemophilia, and other
centers treating patients with blood or blood
products

Laboratory workers handling infected material

Health care personnel on assignment in areas
where there is a high prevalence of hepatitis B
infection

Dentists and ancillary dental personnel with direct
patient contact

Patients

Patients on first entry into residential institutions
with a known high incidence of hepatitis B

Patients treated by maintenance hemodialysis

Patients likely to require numerous blood transfusions and/or treatment with blood products

Contacts of patients with hepatitis B

Spouses and other sexual contacts and families

Others

Infants born to infected mothers (vaccine and hepatitis B immunoglobulin administered within 12
hours of birth)

Health care workers accidentally pricked with needles used on patients with hepatitis B (vaccine
alone or in combination with hepatitis B immunoglobulin)

Individuals requiring immediate protection

For example, infants born to HBsAg-positive
mothers, transfer of individuals into a "high-risk"
setting or after accidental inoculation (vaccine
and hepatitis B immunoglobulin at a different
site)

Immunocompromised patients and the elderly

Patients with a poor immune response, should be
immunized before hemodialysis or transplantation

Other groups at risk

Promiscuous individuals

Parenteral drug abusers

Staff at refugee and immigration centers where
hepatitis B is common

Sometimes prisoners and staff of custodial institutions, ambulance, rescue and selected police
personnel

Military personnel in some countries

treatment, patients who require repeated venous
access or other penetrating procedures, immunodeficient individuals, and patients with cancer.
Viral hepatitis is an occupational hazard among
health care workers and the staff of some semiclosed institutions, such as homes for the mentally
retarded. Intravenous drug users, homosexual
men, and prostitutes are often infected. Individuals working or living in endemic areas (particularly developing tropical and subtropical countries) are at risk; infants and children, in particular,
should be immunized. Women in such areas
should also be immunized because of the high frequency of mother-to-infant transmission.

PARENTERALLY TRANSMITTED NON-A, NON-B HEPATITIS VIRUS

After specific serologic tests for hepatitis A, B, and
D were developed, surveys of posttransfusion hepatitis in the United States and elsewhere gave
strong evidence for the existence of another type
of parenterally transmitted hepatitis. Parenteral
non-A, non-B hepatitis appears to be associated
with at least two viruses.

CLINICAL MANIFESTATIONS

Parenteral non-A, non-B hepatitis resembles hepatitis B clinically. The disease is most often subclinical or anicteric, but severe hepatitis with jaundice
does occur, and the infection is a significant cause
of fulminant hepatitis. There is considerable evidence that the infection is followed in many patients (and in experimentally infected chimpanzees) by prolonged viremia and the development
of a persistent carrier state. Chronic liver damage
may occur in as many as 50 percent of patients.
There is also preliminary information of an association with hepatocellular carcinoma.

STRUCTURE AND CLASSIFICATION

The viruses causing parenteral non-A, non-B hepatitis have not been fully characterized, and their

mode of replication and antigenic composition remains unclear, despite intensive efforts. Clinical, experimental, and epidemiologic studies in several laboratories indicate that non-A, non-B hepatitis is caused by at least two infectious agents. First, multiple attacks of parenteral non-A, non-B hepatitis have been observed in individual patients. Also, cross-challenge experimental transmission studies in chimpanzees indicate the existence of at least two distinct viruses. Short-incubation (2 to 5 weeks) and long-incubation (5 to 10 weeks or longer) forms of the disease have been described; however, this variation can be explained as easily by differences in the infective dose as by multiple pathogens. Final confirmation awaits the availability of specific laboratory tests and the identification and characterization of the virus(es).

Various types of virus particles have been found in the serum, urine, some implicated blood products, hepatocytes, and Küpffer cells, but independent confirmation has not been obtained. One virus, which appears to be associated with a large proportion of non-A, non-B hepatitis cases, has been cloned in three laboratories by recombinant DNA techniques and named **hepatitis C virus.** Specific antibody to this virus has been detected in the sera of a well-documented panel of convalescent non-A, non-B hepatitis patients, as well as in a proportion of blood donors and patients with acute and chronic liver disease in several countries. Published data are not yet comprehensive, but the availability of specific laboratory tests for parenteral non-A, non-B hepatitis is an important development.

In hepatocytes from a number of British patients who received liver transplants for sporadic non-A, non-B fulminant hepatitis, viruslike particles with envelope surface projections were seen budding into cell vacuoles. Rod-shaped inclusions were also detected in the nuclei of these cells. Identical particles were seen in two successive liver grafts at regrafting for fulminant hepatic failure. Ultrastructural features resembled those of the RNA-containing arboviruses, but serologic studies with arboviruses and transmission in mice proved negative. These findings, together with the recent report of isolation of an RNA-containing virus resembling a togavirus in cases of parenteral non-A, non-B hepatitis, suggest that viruses resembling arboviruses (flavivirus) but not transmitted by an insect vector may be a cause of parenteral non-A, non-B hepatitis, including the sporadic, fulminant form.

ANTIGENIC TYPES

Hepatitis C virus is the term used in the United States to designate the agent that causes tubular changes in the reticuloendothelium of hepatocytes in experimental transmission to nonhuman primates (the "tubule-forming" agent). In Japan, the 29 clones of hepatitis C virus can be divided into three groups according to the antigenicity of their translation products against antibodies obtained from acute and chronic hepatitis C infection. Hepatitis C virus shows no homology with any other known human virus.

A "non-tubule-forming," parenterally transmitted virus has been identified experimentally, epidemiologically, and clinically. This virus has been designated tentatively by some as non-A, non-B, non-C hepatitis.

EPIDEMIOLOGY

Parenteral non-A, non-B hepatitis has been found in every country in which it has been sought; it shares a number of epidemiologic features with hepatitis B. This form of hepatitis is most commonly recognized as a complication of blood transfusion, and in countries (such as the United States) where all blood donations are screened for HBsAg by very sensitive techniques, non-A, non-B hepatitis may account for as many as 90 percent of all cases of posttransfusion hepatitis. Outbreaks of non-A, non-B hepatitis have also been reported after the administration of clotting factors VIII and IX. Non-A, non-B hepatitis has occurred in hemodialysis and similar specialized units, among intravenous drug users, and after accidental inoculation by contaminated needles and other sharp objects. Mother-to-infant transmission occurs occasionally.

Surrogate Tests

Until specific tests for parenteral non-A, non-B hepatitis become widely available, several nonspecific (surrogate) tests have been recommended for screening units of blood.

The Transfusion-Transmitted Viruses Study Group found that units of blood positive for anti-HBc were associated with a two- to threefold greater risk of non-A, non-B hepatitis in recipients than were units without anti-HBc. This finding was confirmed more recently by a study suggesting that 54 percent of posttransfusion non-A, non-B cases would be prevented by excluding anti-HBc-positive donors, with a donor loss of only 4 percent.

The indicator that has received the most attention, however, is the serum aminotransferase level in blood donors. Several studies have shown that the risk of non-A, non-B posttransfusion hepatitis is directly related to the serum alanine aminotransferase level of the donor. It was concluded that excluding blood units with serum alanine aminotransferase levels about 53 IU/L would prevent 29 percent of posttransfusion hepatitis cases, with a loss of only 1.6 percent of donor units. This method is thus better than screening for anti-HBc, since the corrected efficacy of anti-HBc screening was slightly lower than that for serum alanine aminotransferase screening, and twice as many units would be lost. However, the sensitivity of the serum alanine aminotransferase test is only 26 percent, and, despite its high specificity, the predictive value is only 42 percent. Thus, almost two of three units of blood with an elevated serum alanine aminotransferase level will not transmit hepatitis. Serum alanine aminotransferase levels vary with age, sex, alcohol use, and geographic region.

DIAGNOSIS

Laboratory diagnosis of infection with hepatitis C virus is based on a recombinant viral antigen (C100-3) and used in a "capture" assay for circulating antibody. Anti-C100-3 antibody appears to be directed toward nonstructural viral epitopes,

and the antibody generally develops weeks or months after acute infection. This antibody is useful as a marker of chronic persistent viremia. The sensitivity and specificity of the test have not been established, and confirmatory tests that are essential are not yet available.

There are no specific laboratory tests yet for the other forms of non-A, non-B hepatitis.

CONTROL

Control of the infection will ultimately depend on measures currently used for hepatitis B, namely, establishing the epidemiology of the infection with precision, screening blood and blood products, making an accurate laboratory diagnosis, performing preventive immunization, and developing specific antiviral therapy.

◀ ENTERICALLY TRANSMITTED NON-A, NON-B HEPATITIS VIRUS ▶

An enteric hepatitis that resembles hepatitis A but is serologically distinct has been reported from the Indian subcontinent, Central and Southeast Asia, the Middle East, North Africa, and Mexico, as well as in travelers returning from these regions. The infection is acute and self-limiting and occurs predominantly in young adults. The incubation period is 30 to 40 days. The disease is more severe in pregnant women, in whom it is associated with a high mortality (10 to 20 percent), especially during the last trimester of pregnancy. The infection is spread by the ingestion of contaminated water and probably food, but secondary clinical cases appear to be uncommon. Electron-microscopic studies suggest that the virus is about 32 nm in diameter, with a "degraded" particle 27 nm in diameter. Morphologic and biophysical data suggest that this virus is a member of the calicivirus group (see Ch. 65). Serologic tests are under development, and molecular cloning of the agent is under way.

◀ DELTA HEPATITIS VIRUS ▶

The delta hepatitis virus is a defective virus that is able to replicate only with the help of hepatitis B viral products. Delta hepatitis thus occurs solely as a coinfection with hepatitis B. The resulting dual disease is generally more severe than hepatitis B; 5 percent or more of patients with fulminant hepatitis B have serologic evidence of delta virus coinfection. Severe, rapidly progressive chronic active hepatitis is often associated with delta hepatitis coinfection. Moreover, a sudden, severe exacerbation of disease in a hepatitis B carrier often indicates delta virus superinfection. The delta agent consists of a 35- to 37-nm particle that resembles the hepatitis B virus and, indeed, shares its surface antigen protein coat. However, the very small RNA genome of the delta agent (molecular weight approximately 5×10^5) does not hybridize with the DNA of hepatitis B virus. The genome is contained in a core particle that bears the delta antigen. Only one serotype of delta hepatitis virus has been recognized.

Sensitive laboratory techniques, including immunofluorescence, radioimmunoassay, and enzyme immunoassay, have been developed to detect delta antigen and anti-delta antibody. Epidemiologic studies indicate that the disease occurs in many countries and is most common in persistent carriers of HBsAg and in individuals at risk for repeated exposure to hepatitis B. The infection is transmitted by contaminated blood and blood products. Serologic evidence of infection is found most often in hemophiliacs and other persons chronically exposed to blood and in intravenous drug users. The infection may also be transmitted by nonpercutaneous routes.

REFERENCES

Deinhardt F, Zuckerman AJ: Immunization against hepatitis B. Report on a WHO meeting on hepatitis in Europe. J Med Virol 17:209, 1985

Gerety RJ: Recombinant hepatitis B vaccines. p. 1017. In Zuckerman AJ (ed): Liver Disease. Alan R Liss, New York, 1988

Kuo G, Choo Q-L, Alter HJ et al: An assay for circulating antibodies to a major etiologic virus of human non-A, non-B hepatitis. Science 244:362, 1989

Lemon SM: Type A viral hepatitis. N Engl J Med 313:1059, 1985

Ramalingaswame V, Purcell RH: Waterborne non-A, non-B hepatitis. Lancet 1:571, 1988

Reyes, GR, Purdy MA, Kim JP et al: Isolation of a cDNA from the virus responsible for enterically transmitted non-A, non-B hepatitis. Science 247:1335, 1990

Rizzetto M, Penzetto A, Bonino F et al: Hepatitis delta virus infection: clinical and epidemiological aspects. p. 389. In Zuckerman AJ (ed): Liver Disease. Alan R Liss, New York, 1988

Tiollais P, Pourcel C, Dejean A: The hepatitis B virus. Nature 317:489, 1985

World Health Organization. Prevention of Primary Liver Cancer. WHO Technical Report Series no. 691. World Health Organization, Geneva, 1983

Zuckerman AJ: Tomorrow's hepatitis B vaccine. Vaccines 5:165, 1987

Zuckerman AJ: Viral hepatitis. Gastroenterology 12:56, 1988

71 SUBACUTE SPONGIFORM VIRUS ENCEPHALOPATHIES

CLARENCE J. GIBBS, JR.

GENERAL CONCEPTS

Clinical Manifestations

Subacute progressive degenerative diseases of the central nervous system are always fatal with progressive dementia, myoclonus, ataxia, pyramidal and extrapyramidal signs, spiking slow waves on the electroencephalogram, no cerebrospinal fluid pleocytosis, and no changes in clinical chemistry or hematologic values.

Structure

In recent years we have come to recognize all these diseases as the transmissible cerebral amyloidoses, with their infectivity associated with the modification of the same host precursor protein into insoluble amyloid fibrils. These fibrils appear as rods by electron microscopy or as crystalline deposits in the form of extracellular amyloid plaques by light microscopy. The structure is mainly unknown but may be a normal host membrane sialoglycoprotein that crystallizes into rods and/or fibrils on extraction. There is no identifiable nucleic acid, no foreign protein, and no antigenicity. The agent is highly resistant to most organic and inorganic chemicals, ultraviolet light, and cobalt-60 radiation; is heat stable; is nonantigenic (no foreign protein); and has no viruslike structure by electron microscopy.

Classification

Classification is based on clinical signs, histopathologic lesions, and detection of a specific sialoglycoprotein of 27 to 30 kDa (PrP$^{27-30}$).

Multiplication

The replication process is presently unknown. Hypotheses include (1) autocatalytic alteration of a normal host precursor protein to a β-pleated insoluble and protease-resistant form, and (2) induction of different posttranslational modification of a normal host protein.

Pathogenesis

The development of the natural disease is unknown. Infection can be caused by iatrogenic transmission via corneal transplant, implants of contaminated electrodes, injection of contaminated human pituitary gland-derived growth hormone, and transplantation of contaminated dura mater. Between 10 and 12 percent of Creutzfeldt-Jakob disease cases are of familial origin (autosomal dominant pattern); kuru is transmitted by ritualistic cannibalism. In general, the pathology is that of noninflammatory, transmissible, cerebral amyloidosis including slowly progressive vacuolation of neurons of the gray matter and to a lesser extent astrocytes (status spongiosis), astrocytic gliosis, neuronal dropout, and periodic acid-Schiff positive amyloid plaques composed of precursor protein (PrP).

Epidemiology

Medical practice has changed as a result of the recognition of the routes of transmission and the resistance to inactivation of these unconventional viruses.

Host Defenses

None of the defense mechanisms known to control conventional viral diseases is effective against spongiform encephalopathy viruses. Antibody is not produced during the infection, and the course of infection is not altered by suppression or potentiation of the host immune response. Also, interferon is undetectable and administration of exogenous interferon or interferon inducers is not protective. The diseases are always fatal.

SCRAPIE

Epidemiology

Scrapie is a prototype animal disease in which the mechanism of spread in nature is uncertain. Bovine spongiform encephalopathy and transmissible mink encephalopathy result from feeding scrapie-infected animal renderings.

Diagnosis

Clinically, scrapie is manifested as a chronic fatal ataxia of sheep and goats with progressive ataxia, tremor, wasting, and severe pruritis.

Control

Destroying affected animals is effective.

KURU

Epidemiology

The mechanism of spread is contamination of the population during ritual cannibalistic consumption of the brains of their dead relatives as a rite of respect and mourning.

Diagnosis

This disease is manifested as cerebellar ataxia and a shivering-like tremor that progresses to complete motor incapacity with dysarthria and total loss of speech and death in less than 1 year from onset.

Control

Cessation of the practice of ritualistic cannibalism has resulted in disappearance of the disease.

CREUTZFELDT-JAKOB DISEASE

Epidemiology

In the United States, South America, Europe, Australia, and Asia the prevalence approaches one per million, with an annual incidence and mortality of about the same magnitude since the average duration of the disease is 6 to 12 months. There has been occasional temporal and spatial clustering of nonfamilial cases in small population centers in Israel, Czechoslovakia, Hungary, England, and Chile. Conjugal and iatrogenic transmission have been described.

Diagnosis

This disease is manifested as a rapidly progressive global dementia, characterized by myoclonus, marked progressive motor dysfunction, and paroxysmal bursts of high-voltage slow waves on electroencephalogram.

Control

Iatrogenic transmission may be prevented by strict measures of decontamination of surgical instruments and sterilization of biologic materials and transplantation tissues by using sodium hydroxide, sodium hypochlorite, and autoclaving.

INTRODUCTION

Subacute progressive degenerative diseases of the nervous system are important because they appear to be caused by infectious agents that are smaller than conventional viruses and composed mainly of protein related to a cell protein. Few, if any, of these diseases are curable. Although some are genetically determined, most occur sporadically and a history of the disease does not appear in close relatives. Therefore, it was surprising to discover that several of these chronic idiopathic disorders of humans, i.e., kuru (a heredofamilial disease restricted in distribution to the Eastern Highlands of Papua New Guinea), the sporadic and familial

TABLE 71-1   Subacute Spongiform Virus
Encephalopathies

Victims	Disease
Humans	Kuru
	Creuztfeldt-Jakob disease
	Gerstmann-Straussler-Schenker syndrome
Animals	Scrapie
	Transmissible mink encephalopathy
	Chronic wasting disease of mule deer
	Chronic wasting disease of captive elk
	Bovine spongiform encephalopathy
	Spongiform encephalopathy of zoo ungulates (eland, kudu, Arabian oryz, gemsbok, nyala)
	? "Downer" cattle in the United States

types of Creutzfeldt-Jakob disease (a presenile dementia with worldwide distribution), and the Gerstmann-Straussler-Schenker syndrome, were caused by infectious agents.

In humans, kuru and the transmissible viral dementias are in a group of slow infections termed **subacute spongiform virus encephalopathies** because of their strikingly similar histopathologic lesions (Table 71-1). In animals, scrapie of sheep and goats, transmissible mink encephalopathy, and the chronic wasting disease of captive mule deer, elk, and zoo ungulates have similar histopathology, pathogenesis, and properties of their infectious agents. They all belong to the same group of atypical diseases caused by **unconventional viruses (prions).**

We are at a challenging time in the study of the subacute spongiform encephalopathies and the unconventional viruses that cause them. The monomer of the scrapie-altered form of the normal scrapie precursor protein (PrP^{33-35}) and its cleavage product, the scrapie amyloid protein (PrP^{27-30}) (Figs. 71-1 and 71-2), seems to be the infectious agent directing its own synthesis by autonucleation and autopatterning of configurational change in the normal host precursor protein. Polymerization of fibril crystallization of this infectious scrapie amyloid monomer (PrP^{27-30}) forms the scrapie-associated fibrils and scrapie–kuru–Creutzfeldt-Jakob disease–Gerstmann-Straussler-Schenker syndrome plaques.

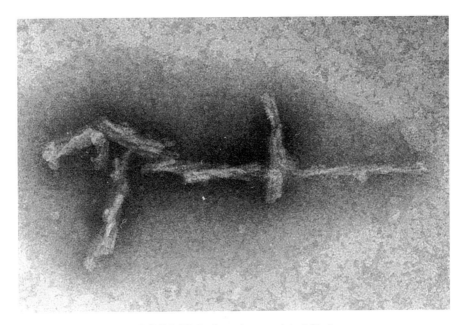

FIGURE 71-1   Scrapie-associated fibril.

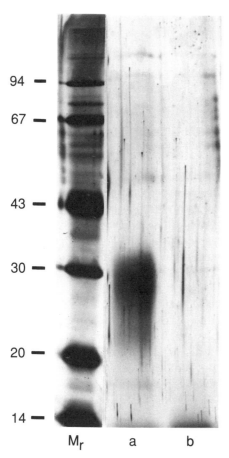

FIGURE 71-2   Spongioform encephalopathy specific sialoglycoprotein, 27 to 30 kDa. Mr, markers of mass; a, infected hamster brain; b, normal hamster brain.

UNCONVENTIONAL VIRUSES

CLINICAL MANIFESTATIONS

The **unconventional viruses** have also been called **slow viruses** because the asymptomatic incubation period may extend over many years (Table 71-1). The criteria established for slow infections have four cardinal features: (1) a prolonged incubation period (several months to several years), (2) a progressive clinical course of disease always leading to death, (3) pathologic lesions limited to a single organ system, and (4) a limited natural host range.

Three diseases of humans (Table 71-2) and six diseases of animals are recognized as belonging to the subacute spongiform virus encephalopathies.

STRUCTURE

The pursuit of the transmissibility and viral etiology of kuru and the presenile dementia of the Creutzfeldt-Jakob disease type has led to the definition of the unconventional viruses as a new group of microbes. Because of their very atypical physical, chemical, and biologic properties, this new definition has stimulated a worldwide quest to elucidate their structures, epidemiology, and clinical manifestations and to resolve the paradoxes involving the basic tenets of microbiology. We currently believe that these viruses are infectious proteins resulting from a modification of a host precursor protein (PrP) to an infectious form consisting of an insoluble cross-β-pleated configuration by a process that may involve autonucleation and autopatterning.

The structure of the unconventional viruses is implied by their spectrum of resistance and sensitivity to inactivating agents. These viruses are resistant, even when partially purified, to all nucleases, β-propriolactone, EDTA, and sodium deoxycholate. They are moderately sensitive to high concentrations of phenol ($>$60 percent); chloroform; ether; urea (6 to 8 M); periodate (0.1 M); 2-chloroethanol; alcoholic iodine; chloroform-butanol; hypochlorite; alkali; chaotropic ions such as thiocyanate, guanadinium, and tricho-

Future physicochemical studies should resolve the details of the process of configurational change by which a normal host protein is changed to the infectious self-inducing, insoluble, protease-resistant amyloidlike infectious virus.

This chapter is devoted to the three slow infections of the human nervous system (kuru, Creutzfeldt-Jakob disease, and Gerstmann-Straussler-Schenker syndrome) and one of animals, scrapie, the prototype infection of the spongiform encephalopathies.

TABLE 71-2   Brain Lesions and Clinical Manifestations
of Subacute Spongiform Virus Encephalopathies

Disease	Location	Histopathology	Amyloid Plaques	Clinical Manifestations
Kuru	Predominantly cerebellar	Spongiform change, normal loss, gliosis	Variable, contain PrP	Progressive ataxia, rigidity, intention tremor, variable others
Creutzfeldt-Jakob disease	Diffuse	Same	Same	Progressive dementia and myoclonus, triphasic EEG discharges, variable others
Gerstmann-Straussler-Schenker syndrome	Global	Same	Global, consistent, contain PrP	Familial, progressive cerebellar ataxia, dysarthria, variable others

loracetate; proteinase K; and trypsin (when partially purified). However, such treatments inactivates only 99 to 99.9 percent of the infectious particle, leaving behind highly resistant infectivity. Sodium hydroxide and sodium hypochlorite cause medically acceptable inactivation. The viruses are relatively resistant to ultraviolet light frequencies that affect nucleic acids and aromatic amino acids. However, they are sensitive to frequencies that are thought to affect polypeptides. Moreover, they show remarkable resistance to ionizing radiation, which would indicate a target size of less than 100 kDa. These atypical properties have led to speculation that the infectious agents lack a nucleic acid and they may be self-replicating protein.

CLASSIFICATION

There are other persistent infections of the human central nervous system that are caused by classic viruses (see Ch. 96). These viruses can be visualized as distinct morphologic structures by electron microscopy; they induce specific antigen-antibody reactions; they usually induce histopathologic lesions more generally associated with virus infections; and they have an RNA or DNA genome. Both conventional and unconventional viruses are capable of inducing subacute progressive degenerative diseases of the central nervous system many months to years after the initial infection. Examples of nervous-system slow infections caused by conventional viruses include subacute sclerosing panencephalitis caused by measles virus; progressive multifocal leukoencephalopathy caused by papovaviruses (see Ch. 66); rubella virus-induced encephalopathy (see Ch. 55); cytomegalovirus encephalopathy (see Ch. 68); and herpes simplex virus (see Ch. 68); adenovirus (see Ch. 67); Russian spring-summer encephalitis virus (see Ch. 54), HTLV-1, and human immunodeficiency virus (HIV) encephalitides (see Ch. 62). Unlike these conventional viruses, the unconventional viruses are truly slow in their replication. Oligomers or microfilaments of this amyloid subunit, PrP, may nucleate this subunit's own polymerization, crystallization, and precipitation as insoluble arrays of amyloid fibrils. Thus, a proteolytic cleavage and configurational change of PrP followed by oligomeric assembly produces an infectious fibril-amyloid-enhancing factor, which may be considered an unconventional virus.

PATHOGENESIS

The basic histopathologic lesions in all of these diseases are progressive vacuolations in the dendritic and axonal processes, cell bodies of neurons, and, to a lesser extent, astrocytes and oligodendrocytes. Extensive astroglial hypertrophy and proliferation and spongiform change or status spongiosus of gray matter (Fig. 71-3) and extensive neuronal dropout and loss also occur.

These atypical infections differ from other diseases of the human brain subsequently demonstrated to be slow infections in that they do not evoke a virus-associated inflammatory response in the brain (i.e., no perivascular cuffing or leukocytic infiltration) or a pleocytosis or marked rise in the protein level in cerebrospinal fluid. Furthermore, there is no immune response to the causative virus and there are no recognizable virions. Instead, there are ultrastructural alteration in the plasma membrane lining the vacuoles, piled-up neurofilaments in swollen nerve cells, and strange arrays of tubules in postsynaptic processes that look like particles in cross-section.

EPIDEMIOLOGY

Medical practices have changed because of the routes of transmission of these unconventional viruses and their high resistance to physical and chemical inactivation. They are resistant to high concentrations of formaldehyde or gluteraldehyde, psoralens and most other antiviral and antiseptic substances, ultraviolet light, ionizing radiation, ultrasonication, and heat. In addition, iatrogenic transmission occurs through contaminated surgical electrodes, surgical instruments, corneal transplants, human growth hormone from pituitary glands, dura mater from cadavers, and possibly dentistry. This has led to changes in autopsy-room and operating-theater techniques throughout the world as well as to the precautions used in handling older and demented patients. Many of the gentle organic disinfectants, including detergents and the quaternary ammonium salts (often used for disinfection), and even hydrogen peroxide, formaldehyde, ether, chloroform, iodine, phenol, acetone, and ethylene oxide, are inadequate for sterilization of the unconventional viruses. Formaldehyde-fixed unconventional virus-infected brain tissue is much more resistant to inactivation by autoclaving than is unfixed infected brain tissue.

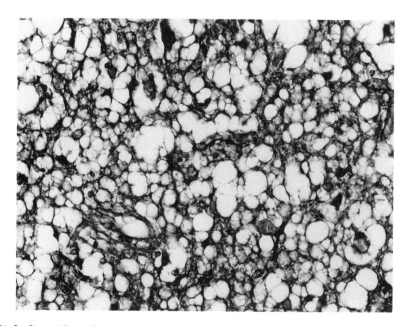

FIGURE 71-3 Spongiform (intracellular vacuolation) change in the cortical gray matter of the brain.

SCRAPIE

Scrapie is a chronic, fatal ataxia of sheep and goats. It is widespread in Europe, Asia, and America. When the disease was introduced, in sheep imported from England, into Australia, New Zealand, and South Africa, it was eradicated by extermination of the affected flocks. In Europe, sheep breeders have recognized the disease for more than two centuries and knew that it occurred in their scrapie-free flocks only after introduction of new breeding stock from scrapie-affected flocks.

Affected animals show progressive ataxia, tremor, wasting, and frequently severe pruritis that causes them to rub their hindquarters and flanks against any upright post. This has led to the name scrapie.

CLINICAL MANIFESTATIONS

In the natural disease, onset is insidious, without any recognizable antecedent fever or other acute manifestations. Early signs include apprehension, restlessness, hyperexcitability, and aggressiveness, and some animals even manifest apparent dementia. Early in the disease, fine tremors of the head and neck are observed. As the disease progresses, the tremors become more generalized, involving the whole body and producing a shivering effect as disturbances in locomotion become evident. In advanced stages, the animals become stuporous and manifest visual impairment, excessive salivation, urinary and fecal incontinence, and wasting lasitude. The host range includes sheep, goats, and mice. Field studies and experimental observations indicate a genetic influence of disease occurrence in sheep. In mice, there is genetic control of the length of the incubation period and of the distribution of pathologic lesions.

PATHOLOGY

Natural scrapie in sheep and goats is characterized by the presence of vacuolated neurons and extensive astrogliosis. In the experimentally transmitted disease, the neuronal vacuolation proceeds to a frank spongiform change. In sheep the presence of amyloid plaques in the brain is rare, whereas in mice the presence of amyloid plaques is dependent on the strain of scrapie virus being studied and the genetic line of the mice. Of interest is the alteration of the plasma membrane in vivo, resulting in the fusion of neurons with other neurons or astrocytes.

KURU

CLINICAL MANIFESTATIONS

Kuru is characterized by cerebellar ataxia and a shivering-like tremor that progresses to complete motor incapacity with dysarthria and total loss of speech and death usually in less than 1 year from onset (Fig. 71-4). The clinical course of kuru is remarkably uniform. The disease first manifests as the insidious onset of ataxia, which becomes progressively more severe and is soon accompanied by a fine tremor involving the trunk, head, and extremities. Both involuntary tremor and ataxia increase and progress until the patient is unable to walk or stand unaided. The course of the disease is conveniently divided into three stages: ambulatory, sedentary, and terminal. Occasionally patients complain of headache and limb pains.

The first stage is usually self-diagnosed before anyone else in the village, including doctors trained in the West, is aware that the patient is developing the disease. The early signs are subjective unsteadiness of gait and stance with postural instability and truncal tremor, titubation, and some degree of dysarthria. Speech deteriorates as the disease progresses, and eye movements become ataxic with some convergent strabismus.

The second stage of the disease is characterized primarily by the inability of the patient to walk without complete support. Tremors and ataxia become more severe, and rigidity of limbs frequently develops. This is associated with widespread clonus, coarse athetoid and choreiform movements, and an exaggerated startle response. The Babinski sign is negative, but ankle clonus is present. Emotional lability become apparent, as does mental slowing, but severe dementia is conspicuously absent.

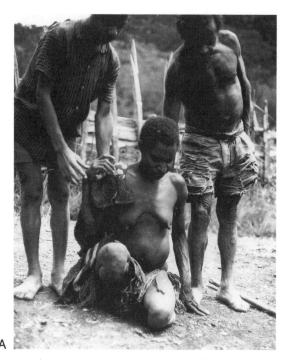

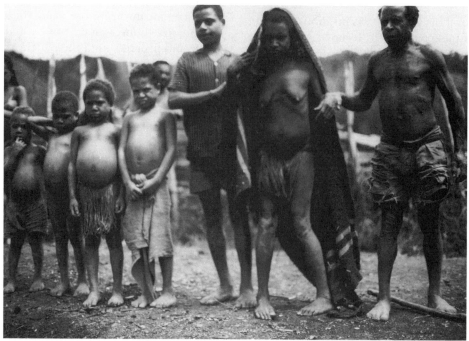

FIGURE 71-4 *(A & B)* Woman with stage 2 kuru. She had marked tremor and severe cerebellar ataxia. Although able to sit, she could not rise, stand, or walk without full assistance. Unlike patients with Creutzfeldt-Jakob disease, this patient did not manifest signs of dementia or myoclonic jerking. She is shown in her village with her husband and her children.

In the third stage, the patient is unable to sit up without support and the ataxia, tremors, and dysarthria are severe. Some patients develop signs of extrapyramidal deficits of posture and movement, and urinary and fecal incontinence develops. Ultimately during these advanced stages, deep decubitus ulcers appear, hypostatic pneumonia develops, and the patient dies in a stage of terminal inanition.

PATHOLOGY

The neuropathologic lesions are widespread and consist mainly of marked proliferation and hypertrophy of astrocytes, mild status spongiosus of the gray matter, and diffuse neuronal degeneration, mostly in the cerebellum. The status spongiosus is true intracellular vacuolization and is caused by the coalescing of vacuoles in pre- and postsynaptic processes of the neurons and, to a lesser extent, in astrocytes and oligodendrocytes. Most of the human cases have periodic acid-Schiff- positive, doubly birefringent, amyloid plaques mainly in the molecular layer of the cerebellum.

Since the start of kuru investigations in 1956, more than 2,500 cases have been recorded. All of these have ended in death within less than 2 years, with few exceptions of somewhat more prolonged disease. Kuru mortality has declined continuously over the past 30 years, and the disease no longer appears in children, adolescents, or young adults. More than 200 patients died annually during the early years of investigation, but now only 5 to 10 patients, all older than 35 years of age, still die of the disease each year.

Etiologically, kuru was first thought to be an epidemic of an infectious disease. However, a degenerative rather than an infectious process was suggested by the absence of fever or antecedent acute disease, the absence of pleocytosis or elevated protein in the cerebrospinal fluid, and the lack of changes in clinical chemistry values or hematologic findings. Early isolation studies were negative. However, in 1959 the striking similarity in the neuropathology of scrapie in sheep and goats with that of the pathology in the brains of patients who had died of kuru suggested that since scrapie was a transmissible disease associated with an incubation period of 3 to 5 years, studies of the etiology of kuru should be reinitiated and should be based on the inoculation and long-term holding of a wide variety of species of animals including chimpanzees and smaller nonhuman primates. In 1965, after 1.5 years of incubation, chimpanzees inoculated intracerebrally with suspensions of human brain from kuru patients developed the disease. This established for the first time that infection was the etiologic mechanism of subacute progressive degenerative diseases of the nervous system.

It has been demonstrated that the kuru, like scrapie, is caused by a viruslike agent that is filterable through 220-nm-pore-size membranes, is stable during storage at $-70°C$ for many years, retains its infectivity following lyophylization, is highly thermostable, has the same high resistance as scrapie to UV, cobalt-60 radiation, and sonication, and resists inactivation with more organic and inorganic chemicals.

◄ CREUTZFELDT-JAKOB ► DISEASE

Creutzfeldt-Jakob disease (CJD) is a relatively rare presenile dementia that occurs worldwide and has a prevalence of approximately one death per million per annum. Although usually sporadic, it has a familial pattern in about 10 to 12 percent of the cases, presenting as an autosomal dominant form of inheritance. It is not recognized as a dominantly contagious or a communicable disease; however, it is caused by a highly pathogenic agent with the same extraordinary biologic, physical, and chemical properties characteristic of the agents of scrapie and the other spongiform encephalopathies. Of particular note is its resistance to inactivation by formaldehyde, ultraviolet light, cobalt radiation, heat, and most other inorganic and organic compounds. Inactivation requires a combination of treatment with 1N NaOH and autoclaving. As with kuru, this disease has been transmitted to chimpanzees, smaller nonhuman primates, and rodents.

CLINICAL MANIFESTATIONS

In most cases, Creutzfeldt-Jakob disease appears as a process primarily of the cortical gray matter of the brain. The disease usually presents after age 45 as a variable period of vague symptoms including nervousness, behavioral changes, visual problems, fatigue, weight loss, anxiety, sleeplessness, malaise, headache, and vague psychic disturbances, progressing in a few weeks or months to complications in higher cortical functions and a state of frank dementia including memory loss, intellectual function, and impaired judgment. There are cerebellar, extrapyramidal, or pyramidal symptoms followed by mutism, rigidity, and death. Most patients show intermittent myoclonus. The other major sign is the development of abnormalities in the electroencephalogram. In advanced cases, patients have periodic bursts of repetitive, high-voltage, tri- and polyphasic sharp discharges. Thus, the diagnosis consists mainly in the detection of rapidly progressive dementia, myoclonus, and electroencephalogram abnormalities. As with kuru, there is no cerebrospinal fluid pleocytosis or consistent abnormality in clinical chemistry or hematologic findings.

During the early stages of Creutzfeldt-Jakob disease, the differential disagnosis may include Alzheimer's disease, cerebral vascular disease, pugilistic and dialysis dementia, brain tumors (glioblastomas and meningioma), brain abscess, progressive supranuclear palsy, stroke or senile dementia.

Certain cases of Creutzfeldt-Jakob disease present clinically as progressive cerebellar ataxia with amyloid plaques in the brain. In these cases the disease usually lasts longer than in the classic cases. In clinical symptomatology they more closely resemble kuru, mainly because of the severe ataxia, yet they are considered a subgroup of Creutzfeldt-Jakob disease and have been identified as Gerstmann-Straussler-Schenker syndrome (GSS). A higher percentage of these cases are of the genetically determined familial type. In such families, several mutations resulting in several different amino acid substitutions have been found in the human homolog of scrapie precursor protein PrP^{33-35C}. These cases exhibit an autosomal dominant pattern with nearly complete penetrance. A proline-leucine substitution at PrP codon 102 is linked to the disease in two families with Gerstmann-Straussler-Schenker syndrome. These results clearly support the single autosomal dominant gene pattern of occurrence in familial Creutzfeldt-Jakob disease and Gerstmann-Straussler-Schenker syndrome, even though the disease is transmissible to experimental animals. Creutzfeldt-Jakob disease became the first human infectious disease in which a single gene was demonstrated to control the susceptibility and occurrence of the disease.

PATHOLOGY

Histopathologically, Creutzfeldt-Jakob disease is characterized mainly as global spongiform degeneration with severe astrogliosis. In 10 to 15 percent of cases, periodic acid-Schiff-positive, doubly birefringent, amyloid plaques occur, much like those seen in kuru and Gerstmann-Straussler-Schenker syndrome. Brains are completely devoid of inflammatory responses such as perivascular cuffing. In Gerstmann-Straussler-Schenker syndrome, "kuru-like" amyloid-containing plaques are more numerous than in Creutzfeldt-Jakob diseae. There tends to be noticeable degeneration of white matter tracts along with the neuronal loss, gliosis, and spongiform degeneration. Both Creutzfeldt-Jakob disease and Gerstmann-Straussler-Schenker syndrome have been documented in the same family, and histopathologic lesions of Creutzfeldt-Jakob disease and Alzheimer's disease have been found simultaneously in the brain of an individual. The dual diseases can be differentiated by immunohistochemical reactions with antibodies prepared to PrP: the Creutzfeldt-Jakob disease plaques react, while the Alzheimer's disease plaques do not, but the Alzheimer's disease plaques do react with antibodies to β-amyloid protein.

EPIDEMIOLOGY

Creutzfeldt-Jakob disease occurs worldwide. The prevalence varies markedly with time and place throughout North America and Western Europe and approaches one per million, with an annual incidence and a mortality of about the same magnitude. There have been occasional reports on the temporal and spatial clustering of nonfamilial cases in small populations in Israel, Czechoslovakia, Hungary, Chile, and England. Approximately 10 to 12 percent of more than 1,000 case studies are of the familial form, and there have been two reports of conjugal disease in which the husband and wife died of Creutzfeldt-Jakob disease within a few years of each other.

Person-to-person transmission of Creutzfeldt-Jakob disease has occurred in a recipient of a corneal transplant from a donor who retrospectively was diagnosed as having had Cruetzfeldt-Jakob disease. Two patients with chronic focal epilepsy developed Creutzfeldt-Jakob disease within 2 years after implantation of in-depth silver electrodes that had previously been implanted into the brain of a patient with Creutzfeldt-Jakob disease. Recently, two patients developed the disease 19 and 31 months, respectively, after receiving dura mater grafts.

Eight patients have been reported to have developed Creutzfeldt-Jakob disease at early ages, 4 to 19 years after their last dose of human pituitary gland-derived growth hormone. From 0.5 to 1 percent of autopsied brain specimens in many academic services show Creutzfeldt-Jakob disease because of the high bias toward performing brain autopsies in patients whose final diagnosis requires pathologic confirmation. In general, between 10,000 and 15,000 pituitaries are contained in the preparation of one lot of growth hormone. Therefore, it is most fortuitous that the procedures used in the preparation of the hormone reduce the contamination to a low level, thereby preventing a major iatrogenic outbreak among young people.

Gerstmann-Straussler-Schenker syndrome is exceedingly rare, with fewer than 30 cases reported in the literature since its first description in 1936. The incidence is less than two per hundred million. Most cases are familial and exhibit an autosomal dominant pattern with nearly complete penetrance.

ETIOLOGY

Creutzfeldt-Jakob disease and Gerstmann-Straussler-Schenker syndrome are transmissible to chimpanzees and Old and New World monkeys

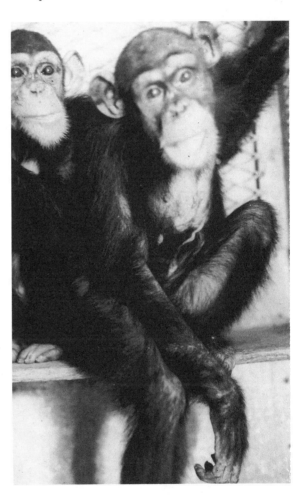

FIGURE 71-5 Female chimpanzee that developed Creutzfeldt-Jakob disease 12.5 months after inoculation with a brain suspension from a chimpanzee that had died of the disease. The chimpanzee showed tremor, incoordination, myoclonic jerking, fasiculation, right-sided neglect of limbs, and confusion (as manifested by inattention, listlessness, lethargy, and irritability).

and occasionally to domestic cats, guinea pigs, golden Syrian hamsters, and mice. Incubation periods from the time of inoculation to the onset of clinical disease vary with the strain of the virus and the experimental host. Pathology in experimental animals is indistinguishable from that induced by other members of the subacute spongiform virus encehalopathies group (Fig. 71-5).

REFERENCES

Bernoulli C, Siegfried J, Baumgartner C et al: Danger of accidental person-to-person transmission of Creutzfeldt-Jakob disease by surgery. Lancet 1:478, 1977

Bolis CL, Gibbs CJ, Jr: Proceedings of an international roundtable on bovine spongiform encephalopathy: summary report and recommendations. J Am Vet Med Assoc 196:1673, 1990

Diringer H, Gelderblom H, Helmert H et al: Scrapie infectivity, fibrils and low molecular weight protein. Nature 306:476, 1983

Gajdusek DC: Subacute spongiform encephalopathies: transmissible cerebral amyloidoses caused by unconventional viruses. p. 2289. In Fields BN, Knope DM (eds): Virology. 2nd Ed. Raven Press, New York, 1990

Gibbs CJ, Jr, Gajdusek DC: Atypical viruses as the cause of sporadic, epidemic, and familial chronic diseases in man: slow viruses and human diseases. p. 161. In Pollard M (ed): Perspectives in Virology: The Gustav Stern Symposium. Vol. 10. Raven Press, New York, 1978

Masters CL, Harris JO, Gajdusek DC et al: Creutzfeldt-Jakob disease: patterns of worldwide occurrence and the significance of familial and sporadic clustering. Ann Neurol 5:177, 1979

Merz PA, Rohwer RG, Kascsak, R et al: An infection specific particle from the unconventional slow virus diseases. Science 225:437, 1984

Prusiner SB, Hsiao KK, Bredesen DE et al: Prion disease. p. 543. In McKendall RR (ed): Handbook of Clinical Neurology. Vol. 12. Viral Disease. Elsevier, New York, 1989

III

MYCOLOGY

Of the approximately 100,000 recognized species of fungi, about 200 are known to cause human infections. In addition, some fungi have economic importance as plant and animal pathogens. Fungal diseases of healthy humans tend to be relatively benign, but the few life-threatening fungal diseases are extremely important. Fungal diseases are an increasing problem due to the use of antibacterial and immunosuppressive agents. Individuals with an altered bacterial flora or compromised defense mechanisms (e.g., AIDS patients) are more likely than healthy people to develop opportunistic fungal infections such as candidiasis. Consequently, opportunistic fungal pathogens are increasingly important in medical microbiology.

Fungi are eukaryotes. They possess a nucleus enclosed by a nuclear membrane, a rigid cell wall, endoplasmic reticulum, and mitochondria like those of plant and animal cells. These structures differ substantially from those of bacteria. Host defenses against fungi are similar to those utilized against bacterial diseases, except that the cell-mediated response is extemely important. Nonspecific immunity and cell-mediated immunity seem to be the most important means by which humans resist or eliminate fungal pathogens. It is the purpose of this section to provide a basic understanding of fungi and the diseases they cause.

Michael R. McGinnis

72 INTRODUCTION TO MYCOLOGY

MICHAEL R. McGINNIS

GENERAL CONCEPTS

Fungi

The fungi are a group of eukaryotic microorganisms, some of which are capable of causing superficial, cutaneous, subcutaneous, or systemic disease.

Physiology

Fungi are heterotrophic and essentially aerobic, with limited anaerobic capabilities, and can synthesize lysine by the L-α-adipic acid biosynthetic pathway.

Structure

Fungi possess chitinous cell walls, plasma membranes containing ergosterol, 80S rRNA, and microtubules composed of tubulin.

Morphology

Yeasts are single-celled forms that reproduce by budding, whereas molds form multicellular hyphae. Dimorphic fungi grow as yeasts or spherules in vivo, as well as in vitro at 37°C, but as molds at 25°C. Dimorphism is regulated by factors such as temperature, CO_2 concentration, pH, and the levels of cysteine or other sulfhydryl-containing compounds.

Progagules

Conidia are asexual propagules (reproductive units) formed in various manners. **Spores** may be either asexual or sexual in origin. Asexual spores are produced in sac-like cells called sporangia and are called sporangiospores. Sexual spores include ascospores, basidiospores, oospores, and zygospores, which are used to determine phylogenetic relationships.

Classification

Asexual structures are referred to as anamorphs; sexual structures are known as teleomorphs; and the whole fungus is known as the holomorph. Two independent, coexisting classification systems, one based on anamorphs and the other on teleomorphs, are used to classify fungi.

INTRODUCTION

Fungi are eukaryotic microorganisms. A fungus can occur in the form of a yeast, in the form of a mold, or as a combination of both forms. Some fungi are capable of causing superficial, cutaneous, subcutaneous, and systemic disease. **Yeasts** are microscopic fungi consisting of single cells that reproduce by budding. **Molds,** in contrast, occur in long filaments known as **hyphae,** which grow by apical extension. Hyphae can be sparsely septate to regularly septate and possess a variable number of nuclei. Regardless of their shape or size, fungi are all heterotrophic and digest their food externally by releasing hydrolytic enzymes into their immediate surrounding (**absorptive nutrition**). Other characteristics of fungi are the ability to synthesize lysine by the L-α-adipic acid biosynthetic pathway and possession of a chitinous cell wall, plasma membranes containing the sterol ergosterol, 80S rRNA, and microtubules composed of tubulin.

PHYSIOLOGY

Fungi can use a number of different carbon sources to meet their carbon needs for the synthesis of carbohydrates, lipids, nucleic acids, and proteins. Oxidation of sugars, alcohols, proteins, lipids, and polysaccharides provides them with a source of energy. Differences in their ability to utilize different carbon sources, such as simple sugars, sugar acids, and sugar alcohols, are used, along with morphology, to differentiate the various yeasts. Fungi require a source of nitrogen for synthesis of amino acids for proteins, purines and pyrimidines for nucleic acids, glucosamine for chitin, and various vitamins. Depending on the fungus, nitrogen may be obtained in the form of nitrate, nitrite, ammonium, or organic nitrogen; no fungus can fix nitrogen. Most fungi use nitrate, which is reduced first to nitrite (with the aid of nitrate reductase) and then to ammonia.

Nonfungal organisms, including bacteria, synthesize the amino acid lysine by the *meso-α,ϵ-*diaminopimelic acid pathway (DAP pathway), whereas fungi synthesize lysine by the unique L-α-adipic acid pathway (AAA pathway). Use of the DAP pathway is one of the reasons why microorga-

nisms previously considered to be fungi, such as the myxomycetes, oomycetes, and hyphochytrids, are no longer classified as fungi. The DAP and AAA biosynthetic pathways for lysine synthesis represent dichotomous evolution.

STRUCTURE
Cell Wall

The rigid cell wall of fungi (see Fig. 73-2A) is a stratified structure consisting of chitinous microfibrils embedded in a matrix of small polysaccharides, proteins, lipids, inorganic salts, and pigments that provides skeletal support and shape to the enclosed protoplast. **Chitin** is a (β1-4)-linked polymer of *N*-acetyl-D-glucosamine (GlcNAc). It is produced in the cytosol by the transfer of GlcNAc from uridine diphosphate GlcNAc into chains of chitin by chitin synthetase, which is located in the cytosol in organelles called chitosomes. The chitin microfibrils are transported to the plasmalemma and subsequently integrated into new cell wall.

The major polysaccharides of the cell wall matrix consist of noncellulosic glucans such as glycogen-like compounds, mannans (polymers of mannose), chitosan (polymers of glucosamine), and galactans (polymers of galactose). Small amounts of fucose, rhamnose, xylose, and uronic acids may be present. **Glucan** refers to a large group of D-glucose polymers having glycosidic bonds. Of these, the most common glucans composing the cell wall have the β-configuration. Polymers with (β1-3)- and (β1-6)-linked glucosyl units with various proportions of 1-3 and 1-6 linkages are common. Insoluble β-glucans are apparently amorphous in the cell wall. The cell walls of dimorphic fungi contain (α1-3)-glucans in appreciable amounts. In *Paracoccidioides brasiliensis,* the hyphal cell wall consists of a single, 80- to 150-nm layer composed of chitin and β-glucan. In contrast, the 200- to 600-nm-thick yeast cell wall has three layers. The inner surface is chitinous, containing some β-glucan, and the outer layer contains α-glucan. It has been suggested that the (α1-3)-glucan occurs in a microfibrillar form in *P brasiliensis* and *Histoplasma capsulatum.*

Many fungi, especially the yeasts, have soluble peptidomannans as a component of their outer cell wall in a matrix of α- and β-glucans. Mannans, galactomannans, and, less frequently, rhamnomannans are responsible for the immunologic response to the medically important yeasts and molds. **Mannans** are polymers of mannose or heteroglucans with α-D-mannan backbones. Structurally, mannan consists of an inner core, outer chain, and base-labile oligomannosides. The outer-chain region determines its antigenic specificity. Determination of mannan concentrations in serum from patients with disseminated candidiasis has proven a useful diagnostic technique.

Cryptococcus neoformans produces a capsular polysaccharide composed of at least three distinct polymers: glucuronoxylomannan, galactoxylomannan, and mannoprotein. On the basis of the proportion of xylose and glucuronic acid residues, the degree to which mannose has side-chain substituents, and the percentage of *O*-acetyl attachments of the capsular polysaccharides, isolates of *C neoformans* can be separated into four antigenic groups designated A, B, C, and D. The capsule is antiphagocytic, serves as a virulence factor, persists in body fluids, and allows the yeast to avoid detection by the host immune system.

In addition to chitin, glucan, and mannan, cell walls may contain lipid, protein, chitosan, acid phosphatase, α-amylase, protease, melanin, and inorganic ions such as phosphorus, calcium, and magnesium. The outer cell wall of dermatophytes contains glycopeptides that may evoke both immediate and delayed cutaneous hypersensitivity. In the yeast *Candida albicans,* for example, the cell wall contains approximately 30 to 60 percent glucan, 25 to 50 percent mannan (mannoprotein), 1 to 2 percent chitin (located primarily at the bud scars in the parent yeast cell wall), 2 to 14 percent lipid, and 5 to 15 percent protein. The proportions of these components vary greatly from fungus to fungus. Table 72-1 summarizes the relationship between cell wall composition and taxonomic grouping of the fungi.

Plasma Membrane

Fungal plasma membranes are similar to mammalian plasma membranes, differing in having the nonpolar sterol ergosterol, rather than cholesterol, as the principal sterol. The plasma membrane regulates the passage of materials into and out of the cell by being selectively permeable. Membrane sterols provide structure, modulation of membrane fluidity, and possibly control of some physiologic events.

The plasma membrane contains primarily lipids and protein, along with small quantities of carbohydrates. The major lipids are the amphipathic phospholipids and sphingolipids that form the lipid bilayer. The hydrophilic heads are toward the surface, and the hydrophobic tails are buried in the

TABLE 72-1 Cell Wall Composition and Taxonomic Classification
of Representative Medically Important Fungi

Principal Cell Wall Polymers	Taxonomic Group	Examples
Chitin-chitosan	Zygomycetes	*Rhizopus arrhizus*
Chitin-glucan	Ascomycetes (mycelial)	*Pseudallescheria boydii*
	Basidiomycetes (mycelial)	*Schizophyllum commune*
	Fungi Imperfecti	*Phialophora verrucosa*
Glucan-mannan	Ascomycetes (yeasts)	*Saccharomyces cerevisiae*
	Fungi Imperfecti (yeasts)	*Candida albicans*
Chitin-mannan	Basidiomycetes (yeasts)	*Filobasidiella neoformans*

interior of the membrane. Proteins are interspersed in the bilayer, with peripheral proteins being weakly bound to the membrane. In contrast, integral proteins are tightly bound. The lipoprotein structure of the membrane provides an effective barrier to many types of molecules. Molecules cross the membrane by either diffusion or active transport. The site of interaction for most antifungal agents is the ergosterol in the membrane. Polyene antifungal agents such as amphotericin B bind to ergosterol to form complexes that permit the rapid leakage of the cellular potassium, other ions, and small molecules. The loss of potassium results in the inhibition of glycolysis and respiration.

Several antifungal agents interfere with ergosterol synthesis. The first step in the synthesis of both ergosterol and cholesterol is demethylation of lanosterol. The necessary enzymes are associated with fungal microsomes, which contain an electron transport system analogous to the one in liver microsomes. Cytochrome P_{450} catalyzes the 14-α-demethylation of lanosterol, an essential step in the synthesis of ergosterol. The imidazole and triazole antifungal agents interfere with cytochrome P_{450}-dependent 14-α-demethylase, which inhibits the formation of ergosterol. This results in plasma membrane permeability changes and inhibition of growth. Ergosterol may also be involved in regulating chitin synthesis. Inhibition of ergosterol synthesis by antifungal agents can result in a general activation of chitin synthetase zymogen, resulting in excessive chitin production and abnormal growth.

Microtubules

Fungi possess microtubules composed of the protein tubulin. This protein consists of a dimer composed of two protein subunits. Microtubules are long, hollow cylinders approximately 25 nm in diameter that occur in the cytoplasm as a component of larger structures. These structures are involved in the movement of organelles, chromosomes, nuclei, and Golgi vesicles containing cell wall precursors.

Microtubules are the principal components of the spindle fibers, which assist in the movement of chromosomes during mitosis and meiosis. When cells are exposed to antimicrotubule agents, the movement of nuclei, mitochondria, vacuoles, and apical vesicles is disrupted. Griseofulvin, which is used to treat dermatophyte infections, binds with microtubule-associated proteins involved in the assembly of the tubulin dimers. By interfering with tubulin polymerization, griseofulvin stops mitosis at metaphase. The destruction of cytoplasmic microtubules interferes with the transport of secretory materials to the cell periphery, which may inhibit cell wall synthesis.

The fungal nucleus is bounded by a double nuclear envelope and contains chromatin and a nucleolus. Fungal nuclei are variable in size, shape, and number. The DNA and associated proteins occur as long filaments of chromatin, which condenses during nuclear division. The number of chromosomes varies with the particular fungus. Within the cell, 80 to 99 percent of the genetic material occurs in chromosomes as chromatin, and approximately 1 to 20 percent in the mitochondria. In some isolates of *Saccharomyces cerevisiae*, up to 5 percent of their DNA can be found in nuclear plasmids. When the DNA helix unwinds, one strand serves as the template for the synthesis of rRNA, tRNA, and mRNA. mRNA passes into the cytoplasm and attaches to one of the ribosomes, which are complexes of RNA and protein that serve as sites for the synthesis of protein.

MORPHOLOGY

Yeasts

Yeasts are fungi that grow as single cells that reproduce by budding (see Figs. 73-4 and 73-5). Yeast taxa are distinguished on the basis of the presence or absence of capsules, the size and shape of the yeast cells, the mechanism of daughter cell formation (conidiogenesis), the formation of pseudohyphae and true hyphae, and the presence of sexual spores, in conjunction with physiologic data. Morphology is used primarily to distinguish yeasts at the genus level, whereas the ability to assimilate and ferment various carbon sources and to utilize nitrate as a source of nitrogen are used in conjunction with morphology to identify species.

Yeasts such as *C albicans* and *Cryptococcus neoformans* produce budded cells known as **blastoconidia.** The formation of blastoconidia involves three basic steps: bud emergence, bud growth, and conidium separation. During bud emergence, the outer cell wall of the parent cell thins. Concurrently, new inner cell wall material and plasma membrane are synthesized at the site where new growth is occurring. New cell wall material is formed locally by activation of the polysaccharide synthetase zymogen. The process of bud emergence is regulated by the synthesis of these cellular components as well as by the turgor pressure in the parent cell. Mitosis occurs, as the bud grows, and both the developing conidium and the parent cell will contain a single nucleus. A ring of chitin forms between the developing blastoconidium and its parent yeast cell. This ring grows in to form a septum. Separation of the two cells leaves a **bud scar** on the parent cell wall. The bud scar contains much more chitin than does the rest of the parent cell wall. When the production of blastoconidia continues without separation of the conidia from each other, a **pseudohypha,** consisting of a filament of attached blastoconidia, is formed. In addition to budding yeast cells and pseudohyphae, yeasts such as *C albicans* may form true hyphae.

Molds

Molds are characterized by the development of hyphae (see Fig. 73-3), which result in the colony characteristics seen in the laboratory. Hyphae elongate by a process known as **apical elongation,** which requires a careful balance between cell wall lysis and new cell wall synthesis. Because molds are often differentiated on the basis of conidiogenesis, structures such as conidiophores and conidiogenous cells must be carefully evaluated. Some molds produce special sac-like cells called **sporangia,** the entire protoplasm of which becomes cleaved into spores called **sporangiospores.** Sporangia are typically formed on special hyphae called **sporangiophores.**

Dimorphism

A number of medically important fungi express themselves phenotypically as two different morphologic forms, which correlate with the saprophytic and parasitic modes of growth. Such fungi are called **dimorphic** fungi. Some researchers restrict the term to pathogens that grow as a mold at room temperature in the laboratory and as a budding yeast or as spherules either in tissue or at 37°C. In contrast, others use **dimorphic** for any fungus that can exist as two different phenotypes, regardless of whether it is pathogenic. We prefer to use the term "dimorphic" to describe fungi that typically grow as a mold in vitro and as either yeast cells or spherules in vivo (Table 72-2). Examples of medically important dimorphic fungi include *Blastomyces dermatitidis* (hyphae and yeast cells) and *Coccidioides immitis* (hyphae and spherules).

A number of external factors contribute to the expression of dimorphism. Increased incubation temperature is the single most important factor. Increased carbon dioxide concentration, which probably affects the oxidation-reduction potential, enhances the conversion of the mycelial form to the tissue form in *C immitis* and *Sporothrix schenckii.* pH affects the development of the yeast form in some fungi, and cysteine or other sulfhydryl-containing compounds affects it in others. Some fungi require a combination of these factors to induced dimorphism. Several medically significant dimorphic fungi are discussed below.

Blastomyces dermatitidis

The conversion of the mycelial form of *Blastomyces dermatitidis* to the large, globose, thick-walled, broadly based budding yeast form requires only increased temperature. Hyphal cells enlarge and undergo a series of changes resulting in the transformation of these cells into yeast cells. The cells enlarge, separate, and then begin to reproduce by budding. The yeast cell wall contains approximately 95 percent (α1-3)-glucan and 5 percent (β1-3)-glucan. In contrast, the mycelial cell wall contains 60 percent (β1-3)-glucan and 40 percent (α1-3)-glucan.

Candida albicans

Candida albicans may form a budding yeast, pseudohyphae, germ tubes, true hyphae, and chlamy-

TABLE 72-2 Overview of Major Medically Important Fungi

Group (Criteria Based on Morphology and Disease)	Disease	Etiologic Agents	Diagnostic In Vivo Form	Diagnostic In Vitro Form	Natural Habitat
I. Molds					
Black fungi	Chromoblastomycosis	*Cladosporium carrionii*	Chestnut brown, thick-walled, muriform cells 10 μm in diameter	Branching chains of single-celled conidia	Woody plant material
		Fonsecaea pedrosoi	Same	Series of single-celled conidia giving rise to series of secondary conidia	Same
	Phaeohyphomycosis	*Exophiala jeanselmei*	Hyaline to brown yeastlike cells, pseudohyphalike filaments, septate hyphae, in various combinations	Single-celled conidia in balls at the apices of annellides	Woody plant material
		Wangiella dermatitidis	Same	Single-celled conidia in balls at the apices of phialides and annellides	Soil and similar environments
		Xylohypha bantiana	Brown septate hyphae	Sparsely branched, long chains of single-celled conidia	Woody plant material
Dermatophytes	Tinea capitis	*Microsporum canis*	Hyphae in scaly erythematous lesions, arthroconidia within and around hair (ectothrix)	Macro- and microconidia	Animals (zoophilic)
		Trichophyton tonsurans	Hyphae in scaly erythematous lesions, arthroconidia within hair (endothrix)	Conidia of various sizes and shapes	Humans (anthropophilic)

Disease	Organism	Tissue form	Conidia	Natural habitat
Tinea corporis	*Microsporum gypseum*	Hyphae in stratum corneum	Macro- and micro-conidia	Soil (geophilic)
	Trichophyton mentagrophytes	Same	Same	Humans and other animals
	Trichophyton rubrum	Same	Same	Humans
Tinea cruris	*Epidermophyton floccosum*	Hyphae in stratum corneum	Club-shaped conidia	Humans
Tinea pedis	*Trichophyton mentagrophytes*	Hyphae in stratum corneum	Macro- and micro-conidia	Humans and other animals
	Trichophyton rubrum	Same	Same	Humans
Dimorphic morphology				
Blastomycosis	*Blastomyces dermatitidis*	Round to oval yeasts 8–15 μm in diameter having broad-based budded daughter cells	Small, round, smooth single-celled conidia	Unknown, probably woody plant material
Coccidioidomycosis	*Coccidioides immitis*	Spherules 30–60 μm containing single-celled endospores 2–5 μm in diameter	Alternating barrel-shaped arthroconidia 2.5–4 by 3–6 μm	Soil
Histoplasmosis	*Histoplasma capsulatum*	Oval, intracellular yeasts 2.5–3.5 μm in diameter	Tuberculate macroconidia and smooth-walled microconidia	Soil enriched by bat, starling, or chicken droppings
Paracoccidioidomycosis	*Paracoccidioides brasiliensis*	Multiple budding yeasts, round budded cells 2–10 μm attached to mature cells 30–60 μm in diameter	Typically sterile	Unknown, probably woody plant material
Sporotrichosis	*Sporothrix schenckii*	Round to oval yeasts 3–5 μm in diameter	Conidia developing from sympodial conidiophores and from the hyphae	Woody plant material

Continued

TABLE 72-2 *(continued)*

Group (Criteria Based on Morphology and Disease)	Disease	Etiologic Agents	Diagnostic In Vivo Form	Diagnostic In Vitro Form	Natural Habitat
Opportunistic infections	Aspergillosis	*Aspergillus flavus*	Septate, dichotomously branching hyphae 2.5–3.5 μm in diameter	Chains of conidia from phialides	Decaying plant material and soil
		Aspergillus fumigatus	Same	Same	Same
	Mycetoma	*Madurella mycetomatis*	Granules in tissue and draining sinuses	Usually sterile, some isolates form phialides	Soil and woody plant material
	Zygomycosis	*Absidia corymbifera*	Sparsely septate, irregularly branching hyphae varying from 6–50 μm in diameter	Branched sporangiophores, random rhizoids, sporangia	Decaying plant material and soil
		Rhizomucor pusillus	Same	Branched sporangiophores, primitive rhizoids, sporangia, thermotolerant	Same
		Rhizopus arrhizus	Same	Unbranched sporangiophores opposite rhizoids, sporangia	Same

II. Yeasts				
Candidiasis	Candida albicans	Oval yeasts 3–4 μm in diameter, pseudohyphae, septate hyphae, in various combinations	Oval budding yeasts, pseudohyphae, septate hyphae, in various combinations	Human gut and oral cavity
	Candida tropicalis	Same	Same	Human skin
Cryptococcosis	Cryptococcus neoformans	Round yeasts 5–15 μm in diameter, blastoconidia attached by narrow necks to parent cells, with or without a capsule	Round yeasts, typically with a capsule	Fruit, pigeon manure, and plants
Pityriasis versicolor	Malassezia furfur	Lipophilic, oval to bottle-shaped yeasts 2–5 μm in diameter, truncate short hyphae 2–3 μm in diameter, in combinations of various amounts	Oval to bottle-shaped yeasts with unipolar budding	Stratum corneum of humans
Torulopsosis	Torulopsis glabrata	Oval yeasts 2.5–5 μm in diameter	Oval yeast	Humans

dospores. A number of investigators are interested in germ tube formation because it represents a transition between a yeast and a mold. Generally, either low temperature or pH favors the development of a budding yeast. Other substances such as biotin, cysteine, serum transferrin, and zinc stimulate dimorphism in this yeast.

Approximately 20 percent of the *C albicans* yeast cell wall is mannan, whereas the mycelial cell wall contains a substantially smaller amount of this sugar. *Candida albicans* has three serotypes, designated A, B, and C. These are distinguished from each other on the basis of their mannans. The antigenic determinant for serotype A is its mannoheptaose side chain. In serotype B, it is the mannohexaose side chain. Serotype B tends to be more resistant to 5-fluorocytosine than is serotype A. Glucans with (β1-3)- and (β1-6)-linked groups compose about 50 to 70 percent of the yeast cell wall. It has been suggested that these glucans may impede the access of amphotericin B to the plasma

membrane. Overall, dimorphism in *C albicans* is not clearly understood.

Coccidioides immitis

Coccidioides immitis is a unique dimorphic fungus because it produces spherules containing endospores in tissue, and hyphae at 25°C. Increased temperature, nutrition, and increased carbon dioxide are important for the production of sporulating spherules. A uninucleate arthroconidium begins to swell and undergo mitosis to produce additional nuclei. Once mitosis stops, initiation of spherule septation occurs. The spherule is segmented into peripheral compartments with a persistent central cavity. Uninucleate endospores occurring in packets enclosed by a thin membranous layer differentiate within the compartments. As the endospores enlarge and mature, the wall of the spherule ruptures to release the endospores (Fig. 72-1). Pairs of closely appressed endo-

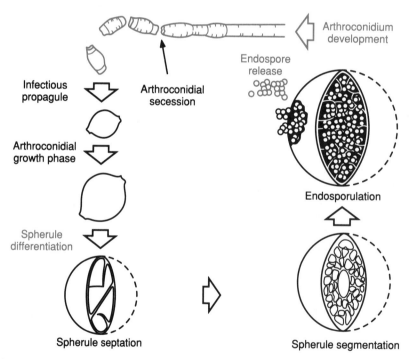

FIGURE 72–1 Development of the spherule of *Coccidioides immitis* from an arthroconidium. (From Cole GT, Kendrick B: Biology of Conidial Fungi. Academic Press, San Diego, 1981, with permission.)

spores that have not completely separated from each other may resemble the budding yeast cells of *B dermatitidis*.

Histoplasma capsulatum

Dimorphism in *Histoplasma capsulatum* involves three stages. In the first stage, induced by an increase in temperature, respiration ceases and the level of cytochromes decreases. During the second stage of the mycelial-to-yeast conversion, cysteine or other sulfhydryl-containing compounds are required. Shunt pathways are initiated that restore the appropriate cytochrome levels, which supply the needed ATP. Cysteine is also required for the yeast form to grow. The final stage is characterized by normal cytochrome levels and respiration as the yeast grows and reproduces. The conversion of terminal or intercalary hyphal cells to a yeast form requires 3 to 14 days. In tissue, *H capsulatum* proliferates within giant cells.

Yeast cells of *H capsulatum* have been divided into two chemotypes. Chemotype 1, which correlates with serotypes 1, 2, and 3, contains large amounts of (β1-3)-glucans and small amounts of chitin. Chemotype 2 contains (α1-3)-glucans, a little (β1-3)-glucan, and more chitin. Chemotype 2 correlates with serotypes 1 and 4. It is difficult to assess the importance of the chemotypes, because only a few isolates have been studied.

Paracoccidioides brasiliensis

A great deal of work has been done with the mycelial-to-yeast conversion of *Paracoccidioides brasiliensis*. In tissue the yeast is characterized by multiple budding. Series of smaller yeast daughter cells attached by narrow tubular necks are formed around a large central cell. Hyphal cells first swell and then separate from each other. The separated cells begin to bud, resulting in a yeast growth. As with *H capsulatum,* growth stops briefly as a result of increased temperature. At 37°C, synthesis of (β1-3)-glucan decreases and the hyphal cell wall softens. The hyphal cells then separate, and (α1-3)-glucans are formed as a layer on the outer cell wall surface of the yeast cells.

The yeast cell wall of *P brasiliensis* has three layers and is approximately 200 to 600 nm thick. The inner surface has chitin and some (β1-3)-glucan. The outer cell wall layer consists of (α1-3)-glucans. In contrast, the mycelial cell wall consists of one layer that is 80 to 150 nm thick, composed of chitin and (β1-3)-glucans. The (α1-3)-glucan of *P brasiliensis* is an important virulence factor. Only the yeast form has this glucan. When the α-linked glucan is absent, pathogenicity is attenuated; regeneration of α-glucan results in increased virulence.

Sporothrix schenckii   The last dimorphic fungus to be considered is *Sporothrix schenckii*. In this species, mycelial-to-yeast conversion is enhanced by increased carbon dioxide, increased temperature, and nutrition. The yeast form readily appears at 37°C and 5 percent carbon dioxide. It has been suggested that some product of carbon dioxide fixation may be required for development of the yeast form. Unlike the other dimorphic fungi capable of producing a yeast form, *S schenckii* initially produces yeast cells by direct budding from hyphae. In addition, the cell wall chemistry of the hyphal and yeast forms is similar. Glucans having (β1-3)-, (β1-4)-, and (β1-6)-linkages are present in addition to chitin. Rhamnomannan is the major antigenic determinant. The yeast cell wall is thought to contain more peptidorhamnomannan than the hyphal cell wall.

PROPAGULES (SPORES AND CONIDIA)

Spores can be produced either asexually or sexually. Asexual spores are always formed in a sporangium following mitosis and cytoplasmic cleavage. The number of sporangiospores and their arrangement in the sporangium are used to differentiate the various zygomycetes. Sexual spores (Table 72-3) occur following meiosis. **Ascospores** (see Ch. 73, Fig. 5A) are formed in a saclike cell (called an ascus) by free-cell formation, **basidiospores** form on basidia (see Ch. 73, Fig. 5B), and **zygospores** form within zygosporangia. **Oospores** are sexual spores that are produced by one group

TABLE 72-3   Classification of Fungi

Phyla	Criteria for Classification	
	Sexual[a]	Asexual[b]
Chytridiomy-cota	Oospores	Spores and conidia
Zygomycota	Zygospores	Spores and conidia
Ascomycota	Ascospores	Conidia
Basidiomycota	Basidiospores	Conidia
Fungi Imperfecti	Absent[b]	Conidia

[a] Sexual propagules (meiosis).
[b] Asexual propagules (mitosis).

of fungi that will not be considered because they are medically unimportant. Sexual spores are rarely seen in clinical isolates because most fungi are **heterothallic** (i.e., sexually self-sterile). Typically, only one of the two mating types is isolated from a particular clinical specimen. When homothallic isolates are recovered in the clinical laboratory, they often produce sexual spores because they are sexually self-fertile.

Conidia are always asexual in origin (see Fig. 73-6) and develop in any manner that does not involve cytoplasmic cleavage. The ontogeny of conidia (conidiogenesis) and their arrangement, color, and septation are used to differentiate the various genera of molds. Some fungi have melanin in the cell wall of the conidia, the hyphae, or both. Such fungi are considered to be **dematiaceous.** Many of the name changes that have been recently proposed reflect a better understanding of conidiogenesis.

CLASSIFICATION

In mycology, fungi are classified on the basis of their ability to reproduce sexually, asexually, or by a combination of both (Table 72-3). Asexual reproductive structures, which are referred to as **anamorphs,** are the basis for one of the sets of criteria. Because the criteria are based upon asexual morphologic forms, this system does not reflect phylogenetic relationships. It exists so that we can communicate in a simple and consistent manner by using names based upon similar morphologic structures. The second set of criteria is based upon sexual reproductive structures, which are referred to as **teleomorphs.** Ascospores, basidiospores, oospores, and zygospores, as well as any specialized structures associated with their development, are the basis of the second set of criteria. These criteria reflect phylogenetic relationships because they are based upon structures that form following meiosis. The term **holomorph** is used to describe the whole fungus, which consists of its teleomorph and anamorphs.

For example, the dimorphic fungus *Blastomyces dermatitidis* produces two anamorphs, one consisting of hyphae and one-celled conidia at 25°C and one consisting of budding yeast cells at 37°C. The name *B dermatitidis* summarizes these two anamorphs. When two sexually compatible isolates of *B dermatitidis* are mated under the appropriate conditions, a sexual fruiting body, called a gymnothecium, containing ascospores will develop. The name that is used for this sexual form or teleomorph is *Ajellomyces dermatitidis.* When one wishes to refer to the whole fungus, the name for the teleomorph is used because it reflects phylogenetic relationships. It is important to note that the name *B dermatitidis* can be used whenever one wishes to refer to the hyphal or yeast forms of this fungus.

REFERENCES

Bartnicki-Garcia S: Cell wall chemistry, morphogenesis, and taxonomy of fungi. Annu Rev Microbiol 22:87, 1968

Bhattacharjee JK: α-Aminoadipate pathway for the biosynthesis of lysine in lower eukaryotes. Crit Rev Microbiol 12:131, 1985

Cole GT, Samson RA: Patterns of Development in Conidial Fungi. Pittman, London, 1979

Fleet GH: Composition and structure of yeast cell walls. p. 24. In McGinnis MR (ed): Current Topics in Medical Mycology. Vol. 1. Springer-Verlag, New York, 1985

McGinnis MR: Laboratory Handbook of Medical Mycology. Academic Press, San Diego, 1980

McGinnis MR, Borgers M (eds): Current Topics in Medical Mycology. Springer-Verlag, New York, 1989

Rippon JW: Dimorphism in pathogenic fungi. Crit Rev Microbiol 8:49, 1980

San-Blas G: *Paracoccidioides brasiliensis:* cell wall glucans, pathogenicity, and dimorphism. p. 235. In McGinnis MR (ed): Current Topics in Medical Mycology. Vol. 1. Springer-Verlag, New York, 1985

Shepherd MG: Morphogenetic transformation of fungi. p. 278. In McGinnis MR (ed): Current Topics in Medical Mycology. Vol. 2. Springer-Verlag, New York, 1988

Yoshida Y: Cytochrome P-450 of fungi: primary target for azole antifungal agents. p. 388. In McGinnis MR (ed): Current Topics in Medical Mycology. Vol. 2. Springer-Verlag, New York, 1988

73 BASIC BIOLOGY OF FUNGI

GARRY T. COLE

GENERAL CONCEPTS

Yeasts and Molds

These fungi grow as **saprophytes, parasites,** or both by using specific proteolytic, glycolytic, or lipolytic enzymes to extracellularly break down substrates and to absorb the products of digestion through the fungal cell envelope.

Cell Wall

The fungal cell wall gives shape and form, protects against mechanical injury, prevents osmotic lysis, and provides passive protection against the ingress of potentially harmful macromolecules.

Filamentous Fungi and Filamentous Bacteria

Fungi are different from the Actinomycetes, a group of prokaryotic filamentous bacteria having peptidoglycans in their cell walls and an absence of nuclear membranes and organelles, but the two groups of microorganisms are usually considered together in texts.

Hyphal and Yeast Morphogenesis

Hyphal extension growth occurs apically by a sophisticated organization of tip-growth-related organelles and cytoskeletal elements. Hyphal wall and yeast cell wall polysaccharide synthetases are active at sites where growth is occurring and inactive when no growth is occurring. Morphogenesis is a balance between wall synthesis and wall lysis.

Sexual Reproduction

Sexual reproduction occurs by the fusion of two haploid nuclei (**karyogamy**), followed by meiotic division of the diploid nucleus. The union of two hyphal protoplasts (**plasmogamy**) may be followed immediately by karyogamy, or it may be separated in time.

Asexual Reproduction

Asexual reproduction occurs via division of nuclei by mitosis. With the absence of meiosis, other mechanisms associated with the nuclear cycle result in recombination of hereditary properties and genetic variation.

INTRODUCTION

Macroscopic fungi such as morels, mushrooms, puffballs, and the cultivated agarics available in grocery stores represent only a small fraction of the diversity in the kingdom Fungi. The molds, for example, are a large group of microscopic fungi that include many of the economically important plant parasites, allergenic species, and opportunistic pathogens of humans and other animals. They are characterized by filamentous, vegetative cells called **hyphae.** A mass of hyphae forms the **thallus** (vegetative body) of the fungus, composed of **mycelium.** The more phylogenetically primitive molds (e.g., water molds, bread molds, and other sporangial—saclike—forms) produce **cenocytic** filaments (multinucleate cells without cross-walls), while the more advanced forms produce hyphae with cross-walls **(septa)** that subdivide the filament into uninucleate and multinucleate compartments. The septum, however, still provides for cytoplasmic communication, including intercellular migration of nuclei. Many fungi occur not as hyphae but as unicellular forms called **yeasts,** which

reproduce vegetatively by budding. Some of the opportunistic fungal pathogens of humans are **dimorphic,** growing as a mycelium in nature and as a vegetatively reproducing yeast in the body. *Candida* is an example of such a dimorphic fungus (Fig. 73-1). It can undergo rapid transformation from the yeast to the hyphal phase in vivo, which partly contributes to its success in invading host tissue.

The true fungi obtain their carbon compounds from nonliving organic substrates **(saprophytes)** or living organic material **(parasites)** by absorption of nutrients through their cell wall. Small molecules (e.g., simple sugars and amino acids) accumulate in a watery film surrounding the hyphae or yeast and simply diffuse through the cell wall. Macromolecules and insoluble polymers (e.g., proteins, glycogen, starch, and cellulose), on the other hand, must undergo preliminary digestion before they can be absorbed by the fungal cell. This process involves release of specific proteolytic, glycolytic, or lipolytic enzymes from the hypha or yeast, extracellular breakdown of the substrate(s), and diffusion of the products of digestion through the fungal cell envelope (Fig. 73-2). Fungal pathogens

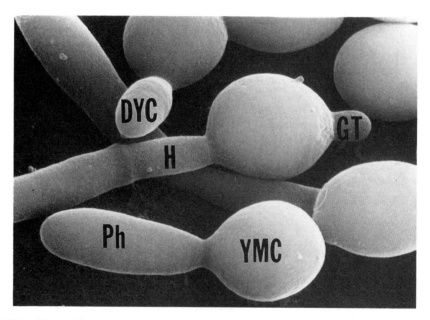

FIGURE 73-1 Dimorphism in *C albicans*. DYC, Daughter yeast cell; GT, germ tube; H, hypha; Ph, pseudohypha; YMC, yeast mother cell. (X8,980.) (From Cole GT, Kendrick B: Biology of Conidial Fungi. Vol. 1. Academic Press, San Diego, 1981, with permission.)

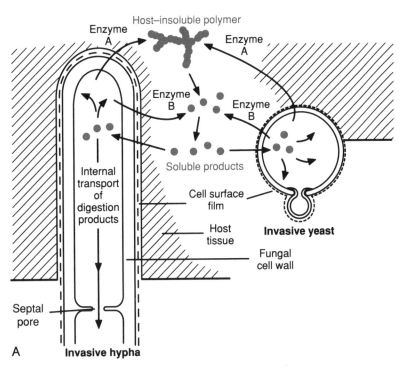

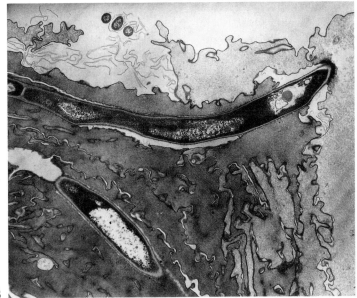

FIGURE 73-2   *(A)* Extracellular digestion and absorptive nutrition in fungi. *(B)* Invasive hyphae of *C albicans* in stratified epithelial tissue of mouse stomach. (×4,250.)

rely on these digestive enzymes to penetrate natural host barriers.

CELL WALLS

Not all species of fungi have cell walls, but in those that do, cell wall synthesis is an important factor in determining the final morphology of fungal elements. Thus, our knowledge of fungal morphogenesis has evolved in parallel with our understanding of fungal cell wall biosynthesis. The fungal wall also protects cells against mechanical injury and blocks the ingress of toxic macromolecules. This filtering effect may be especially important in protecting fungal pathogens against certain fungicidal products of the host. The fungal cell wall is also essential to prevent osmotic lysis. Even a small lesion in the cell wall can result in extrusion of cytoplasm as a result of the internal (turgor) pressure of the protoplast. The composition of fungal cell walls is relatively simple and includes substances not typically found in animal and plant hosts (e.g., chitin). On this basis, it may be possible to identify pathogen-specific molecular targets from investigations of the biosynthesis of fungal wall components. Such targets may prove pivotal for the successful development of antifungal drugs that are not toxic to mammalian cells.

FILAMENTOUS FUNGI AND FILAMENTOUS BACTERIA

Fungi, like bacteria, are ecologically important as decomposers as well as parasites of plants and animals. Both groups of microbes often inhabit the same ecosystem and thus compete for the same food supply. Associated with this competition is the production by both the fungi and bacteria of secondary products that function as microbial growth inhibitors or toxins. These compounds constitute a rich library of antimicrobial agents, many of which have been developed as pharmacologic antibiotics (e.g., penicillin from *Penicillium chrysogenum*, nystatin from *Streptomyces noursei*, amphotericin B from *S niveus*).

The superficial morphologic similarities between actinomycetes (filamentous bacteria) and molds suggest that the two groups have undergone parallel evolution. Despite the production of branching filaments and moldlike spores, the actinomycetes are clearly prokaryotes, whereas fungi are eukaryotes. Moreover, the sexual reproduction of bacteria, which typically occurs by transverse binary fission, should not be confused with asexual processes of budding and fragmentation associated with mitotic nuclear division in fungi. Most of the molds that produce septate vegetative hyphae reproduce exclusively by asexual means, giving rise to airborne propagules called **conidia.** On the other hand, elaborate mechanisms of sexual reproduction are also demonstrated by members of the Eumycota. Four distinct kinds of meiospores (products of karyogamy-meiosis-cytokinesis) are recognized: oospores (oomycetes), zygospores (zygomycetes), ascospores (ascomycetes), and basidiospores (basidiomycetes).

A summary of these and other diagnostic features of the fungi is presented in Table 73-1.

TABLE 73-1   Summary of Diagnostic Features of Fungi

---

1. *Heterotrophic* (no photosynthetic nutrition).
2. *Thallus* (vegetative body of fungus) on or in the substratum; may be plasmodial, ameboid, pseudoplasmodial, unicellular (e.g., *yeast*), or filamentous (*mycelial*).
3. Absorptive nutrition, typically by *extracellular, enzymatic digestion* (ingestion rare).
4. Occurrence ubiquitous as saprobes, parasites, symbionts, or hyperparasites (fungi parasitic on another fungi).
5. *Cell wall* present in nonplasmodial forms; well defined and typically contains *chitin* (polymer of *N*-acetylglucosamine subunits joined by glycosidic bonds), β1-3 and β1-6-*glucans*; cellulose and β1-4-glucans present in the oomycetes (water molds).
6. *Eukaryotic* (distinct from *actinomycetes* which are filamentous bacteria and prokaryotic); uninucleate or multinucleate, *haploid* or *diploid*; mycelium may be *homokaryotic* (nuclei genetically alike), *heterokaryotic* (genetically different nuclei present in same mycelium), or *dikaryotic* (pair of closely associated nuclei usually derived from different parent cells).
7. *Asexual* or *sexual* reproduction; spore-producing bodies (*sporocarps*) microscopic or macroscopic, showing limited tissue differentiation.

HYPHAL AND YEAST MORPHOGENESIS

Hyphal growth occurs by extension at the tips. This polarization is at least partially determined by directional movement and accumulation of vesicles that carry wall precursors and wall synthetases to the site of exocytosis at the apical dome of the hypha (Fig. 73-3). Despite the apparent simplicity of hyphal morphogenesis, ultrastructural investigations have shown a sophisticated organization of tip-growth-related organelles and cytoskeletal elements. There is evidence that intussusception and polymerization of chitin microfibrils occur at the apical dome of the hypha and that the biosynthesis of this major cell wall product is controlled by the

activity of membrane-bound chitin synthetase. The zymogen form of chitin synthetase has been detected in microvesicles called chitosomes, which appear to transport this enzyme to the hyphal tip. The chitosomes may arise from Golgi-like bodies or by a process of self-assembly of subunits freely within the cytoplasm or within larger vesicular bodies. Activation of chitin synthetase occurs upon fusion of the chitosome with the plasmalemma and may be due to the interaction of a membrane-bound protease and the zymogen. Chitin microfibrillogenesis is initiated at these sites of fusion.

Evidence has also been presented, primarily from studies of the yeast *Saccharomyces cerevisiae*, that biosynthesis of skeletal polysaccharides is catalyzed by polysaccharide synthetases (e.g., chitin synthetase and β1-3-glucan synthetase), which are uniformly distributed within the plasmalemma. These wall-synthesizing, cell–membrane-bound enzymes occur in either zymogen or active forms. The model of yeast morphogenesis (Fig. 73-4) suggests that the synthetase is active at sites where the wall is growing and inactive where it is quiescent. One possibility is that microvesicles transport activating factors (e.g., proteases, ATP, and GTP) to the plasmalemma at specific sites of wall biosynthesis (zones of bud emergence and of septal formation). These two concepts of regulation of wall biosynthesis in fungal hyphae and yeasts have been supported by considerable bodies of evidence, and it is likely that both are correct.

Extension growth of hyphal tips and yeast buds logically requires a balance between processes of insertion of newly synthesized polymeric material and modification of the existing microfibrillar matrix to accommodate expansion and further intussusception of wall polymers. In other words, a balance between wall synthesis and wall lysis, or plasticization, is essential for maintaining the orderly processes of hyphal tip elongation and bud emergence. The presence of lytic enzymes in the fungal wall has been reported, including β1-3-glucanase, *N*-acetyl-β-D-glucosaminadase, and chitinase. Localization of such activity may be mediated by macrovesicles. These organelles, like microvesicles, are probably derived from Golgi-

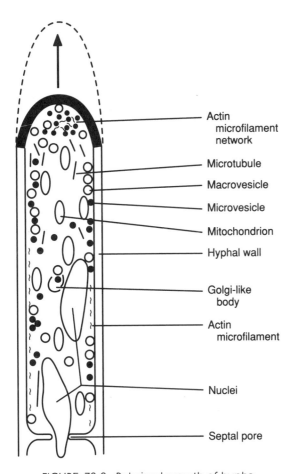

Actin microfilament network

Microtubule

Macrovesicle

Microvesicle

Mitochondrion

Hyphal wall

Golgi-like body

Actin microfilament

Nuclei

Septal pore

FIGURE 73-3   Polarized growth of hypha.

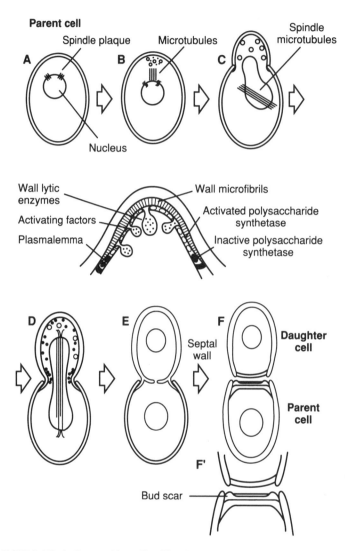

FIGURE 73-4 Stages (A to F) of bud emergence and yeast cell cycle.

like bodies and are directed to the hyphal tip or yeast bud and fuse with the plasmalemma, thereby delivering their contents to the site of wall synthesis.

REPRODUCTION

Sexual reproduction in the fungi typically involves fusion of two haploid nuclei **(karyogamy),** followed by meiotic division of the resulting diploid nucleus (Fig. 73-5A). In some cases, sexual spores are produced only by fusion of two nuclei of different mating types, which necessitates prior conjugation of different thalli. This condition of sexual reproduction is known as **heterothallism,** and the nuclear fusion is referred to as **heterokaryosis.** Normally plasmogamy (union of two hyphal protoplasts which brings the nuclei close together in the same cell) is followed almost immediately by karyogamy. In certain members of the Basidiomyco-

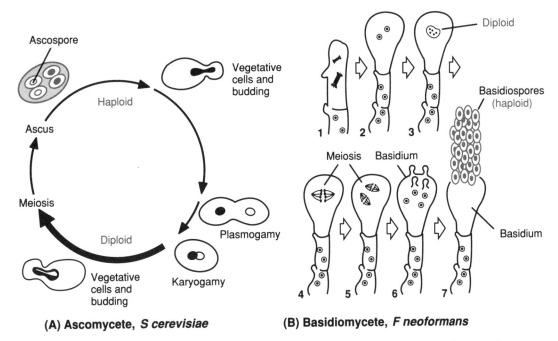

(A) Ascomycete, _S cerevisiae_   **(B) Basidiomycete, _F neoformans_**

FIGURE 73-5 _(A)_ Life cycle of _S cerevisiae._ _(B)_ Basidiospore formation by _Filobasidiella neoformans,_ sexual state of _Cryptococcus neoformans._ (1 and 2) Dikaryon formation. (3) Nuclear fusion (karyogamy). (4 and 5) Meiosis. (6) Basidiospore formation. (7) Mitosis and basidiospore proliferation.

tina, however, these two processes are separated in time and space, with plasmogamy resulting in a pair of nuclei (dikaryon) contained within a single cell. Karyogamy may be delayed until considerably later in the life history of the fungus. Meanwhile, growth and cell division of the binucleate cell occur. The development of a dikaryotic mycelium results from simultaneous division of the two closely associated nuclei and separation of the sister nuclei into two daughter cells (Fig. 73-5B). An alternative mechanism of sexual reproduction in the fungi is **homothallism,** in which a nucleus within the same thallus can fuse with another nucleus of that thallus (i.e., **homokaryosis).** An understanding of these nuclear cycles is fundamental to investigations of fungal genetics.

As mentioned above some fungi are classified as strictly asexually reproducing forms. These include the large group of asexual (imperfect) yeasts (e.g., _Candida_ species) and conidial fungi (e.g., _Coc-_

cidioides immitis). Most members of this group have permanently lost their ability to produce meiospores. A few undergo rare sexual reproduction, and perhaps for some species we have yet to discover their sexual (perfect) stage. The most common methods of asexual reproduction, in addition to simple budding in yeasts, are blastic development of conidia from specialized hyphae (conidiogenous cells), fragmentation of hyphae into conidia, and conversion of hyphal elements into conidia or chlamydospores (thick-walled resting spores) (Fig. 73-6).

Despite the absence of meiosis during the life cycle of these imperfect fungi, recombination of hereditary properties and genetic variation still occur by a mechanism called **parasexuality.** The major events of this process (Fig. 73-7) include the production of diploid nuclei in a heterokaryotic, haploid mycelium that results from plasmogamy and karyogamy; multiplication of the diploid along

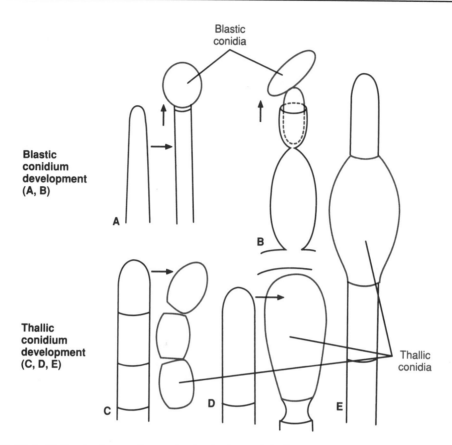

FIGURE 73-6 Methods of asexual reproduction in the conidial fungi. *(A)* Terminal blastic conidium. *(B)* Repetitive blastic conidium formation from specialized conidiogenous cell (phialide). *(C)* Conidium formation by hyphal fragmentation. *(D)* Conidium formation by conversion of apical segment of hypha into single, asexual propagule. *(E)* Conversion of hyphal element into an intercalary chlamydospore.

with haploid nuclei in the heterokaryotic mycelium; sorting out of a diploid homokaryon; segregation and recombination by crossing over at mitosis; and haploidization of the diploid nuclei. Sexual and parasexual cycles are not mutually exclusive. Some fungi that reproduce sexually also exhibit parasexuality.

An extensive foundation of knowledge on the basic biology of fungi is at hand, including fungi that cause superficial, deep-seated, and systemic infections of humans and other animals. Much less

is known, however, of the intricacies of interactions between these largely opportunistic pathogens and their hosts. Many areas of research in medical mycology are still in their infancy and offer formidable challenges and potential rewards. The current application of methods of recombinant DNA technology to problems of fungus-host interactions, especially the identification of pathogenicity genes, holds promise for significant contributions to our knowledge of medically important fungi.

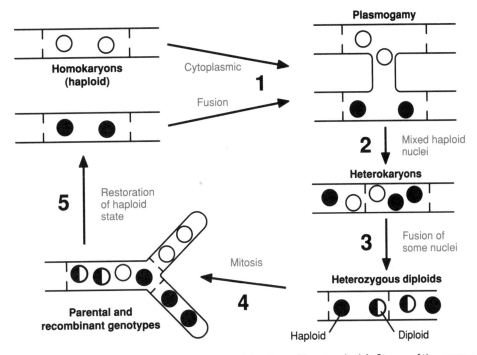

FIGURE 73-7 The parasexual cycle (genetic recombination without meiosis). Stages of the parasexual cycle are numbered as follows. (1) Hyphal conjugation (plasmogamy). (2) Heterokaryosis. (3) Nuclear fusion (karyogamy). (4) Mitotic recombination and nondisjunction. (5) Haploidization and nuclear segregation leading to homokaryosis.

REFERENCES

Cabib E, Bowers B, Sburlati A, et al: Fungal cell wall synthesis: the construction of a biological structure. Microbiol Sci 5:370, 1988

Cole GT, Hoch HC: The Fungal Spore and Disease Initiation in Plants and Animals. Plenum, New York, 1991

Evans EGV, Richardson MD: Medical Mycology: A Practical Approach. Oxford University Press, Oxford, England, 1989

Leal-Morales CA, Bracker CE, Bartnicki-Garcia S: Localization of chitin synthetase in cell-free homogenates of *Saccharomyces cerevisiae:* chitosomes and plasma membrane. Proc Natl Acad Sci USA 85:8516, 1988

Rippon JW: Medical Mycology: The Pathogenic Fungi and the Pathogenic Actinomycetes. 3rd Ed. WB Saunders, Philadelphia, 1988

Spencer JFT, Spencer DM, Bruce IJ: Yeast Genetics: A Manual of Methods. Springer-Verlag, New York, 1989

74

DISEASE MECHANISMS OF FUNGI

GEORGE S. KOBAYASHI

GENERAL CONCEPTS

Entry

Fungi rarely cause disease in healthy immunocompetent hosts. Disease results when fungi accidentally penetrate host barriers or when immunologic defects or other debilitating conditions exist that favor fungal entry and growth.

Adaptation and Propagation

Fungi often develop both virulence mechanisms (e.g., enzymes and capsule) and morphologic forms (e.g., yeasts, hyphae, and spherules) that facilitate their multiplication within the host.

Dissemination

Dissemination of fungi in the body indicates a breach or deficiency of host defenses (e.g., endocrinopathies and immune disorders).

Host Factors

Innate resistance to fungi is based primarily upon cutaneous and mucosal physical barriers. Severity of disease depends on factors such as inoculum, magnitude of tissue destruction, ability of the fungus to multiply in the tissue, and the immune status of the host.

Fungal Factors

Enzymes such as keratinase and phenol oxidase, the presence of a capsule in *Cryptococcus neoformans*, dimorphism, and other factors contribute to fungal pathogenesis, which involves a complex interplay of many fungal and host factors.

INTRODUCTION

Fungi are ubiquitous in nature and exist as free-living saprobes that derive no obvious benefits from parasitizing humans or animals. Since they are widespread in nature and are often cultured from diseased body surfaces, it is frequently difficult to assess whether a fungus found during disease is a pathogen or a transient environmental contaminant. Before a specific fungus can be confirmed as the cause of a disease, the same fungus must be isolated from serial specimens and fungal elements morphologically consistent with the isolate must be observed in tissues taken from the lesion.

In general, fungal infections and the diseases they cause are accidental. A few fungi have developed a commensal relationship with humans and are part of the indigenous microbial flora. Although a great deal of information is available concerning the molecular basis of bacterial pathogenesis, little is known about mechanisms of fungal pathogenesis.

Infection is defined as entry into body tissues followed by multiplication of the organism. The infection may be clinically inapparent or may result in disease due to cellular injury from competitive metabolism, elaboration of toxic metabolites, replication of the fungus, or an immune response. Immune responses may be transient or prolonged and may be cell mediated, humoral (with production of specific antibody to components of the infecting organism), or both. Successful infection may result in **disease,** defined as a deviation from or interruption of the normal structure or function of body parts, organs, or systems (or combinations thereof) that is marked by a characteristic set of symptoms and signs and whose etiology, pathology, and prognosis are known or unknown.

ENTRY

Fungi infect the body through several portals of entry (Table 74-1). The first exposure to fungi that most humans experience occurs during birth, when they encounter the yeast *Candida albicans* while passing through the vaginal canal. During this process the fungus colonizes the buccal cavity and portions of the upper and lower gastrointestinal tract of the newborn, where it maintains a lifelong residence as a commensal.

Another fungus, *Malassezia furfur,* is common in areas of skin rich in sebaceous glands. How it colonizes the skin is not known, but both *M furfur* and *C albicans* are the only fungi that exist as commensals of humans and are considered part of the indigenous flora. Only under certain unusual circumstances have they caused disease. Other fungi that have been implicated in human diseases come from exogenous sources, where they exist as saprobes on decaying vegetation or as plant parasites.

Fungi rarely cause disease in healthy, immunocompetent hosts, even though we are constantly exposed to infectious propagules. It is only when fungi accidentally penetrate barriers such as intact skin and mucous membrane linings, or when immunologic defects or other debilitating conditions exist in the host, that conditions favorable for fungal colonization and growth occur. When *C albicans,* for example, is implicated in disease processes, it may indicate that the patient has a coexisting immune, endocrine, or other debilitating disorder. In most cases, the underlying disorder must be corrected to effectively manage the fungal disease.

TABLE 74-1   Summary of Disease Mechanisms of Fungi

Source of Fungus	Clinical Classification	Mechanism of Entry
Endogenous	Opportunistic	Iatrogenic (indwelling lines, catheters, etc.)
Exogenous	Superficial	Trauma (personal hygiene?)
	Cutaneous	Trauma
	Subcutaneous	Trauma
	Systemic	Inhalation
	Opportunistic	Inhalation (iatrogenic, trauma)

ADAPTATION AND PROPAGATION

Although most fungal diseases are the result of accidental encounters with the agent, many fungi have developed mechanisms that facilitate their multiplication within the host. For example, the dermatophytes that colonize skin, hairs, and nails elaborate enzymes that digest keratin. *Candida albicans* as a commensal organism exists in a unicellular yeastlike morphology, but when it invades tissues it becomes filamentous; conversely, the systemic fungi *Histoplasma capsulatum*, *Blastomyces dermatitidis*, *Paracoccidioides brasiliensis*, and *Coccidioides immitis* exist as molds in nature and change to a unicellular morphology when they cause disease. Other properties, such as capsule production by *Cryptococcus neoformans* and the adherence properties of *Candida* species to host tissues, also contribute to their pathogenicity.

DISSEMINATION

Disseminated fungal diseases usually indicate a breach in host defenses. Such a breach may be caused by endocrinopathies or immune disorders, or it may be induced iatrogenically. Effective management of the fungal infection requires a concerted effort to uncover and correct the underlying defects.

HOST FACTORS

The high degree of innate resistance of humans to fungal invasion is based primarily on the various protective mechanisms that prevent fungi from entering host tissues. Fungal growth is discouraged by the intact skin and factors such as naturally occurring long-chain unsaturated fatty acids, pH, competition with the normal bacterial flora, epithelial turnover rate, and the desiccated nature of the stratum corneum. Other body surfaces, such as the respiratory tree, gastrointestinal tract, and vaginal vault, are lined with mucous membranes (epithelium) bathed in fluids that contain antimicrobial substances, and some of these membranes are lined with ciliated cells that actively remove foreign materials. Only when these protective barriers are breached can fungi gain access to, colonize, and multiply in host tissues. Fungi gain access to host tissues by traumatic implantation or inhalation. The severity of disease caused by these organisms depends upon the size of the inoculum, magnitude of tissue destruction, the ability of the fungi to multiply in tissues, and the immunologic status of the host.

FUNGAL FACTORS

Most of the fungi that infect humans and cause disease are classified by tissue or organ levels that are primary sites of colonization. These are discussed below.

Superficial Fungal Infections

Superficial fungal infections involve only the outermost layers of the stratum corneum of the skin (*Phaeoannelomyces werneckii* [syn. *Exophiala werneckii*] and *M furfur*) or the cuticle of the hair shaft (*Trichosporon beigelii* and *Piedraia hortai*). These infections usually constitute cosmetic problems and rarely elicit an immune response from the host (except occasionally *M furfur* infections). Recently *T beigelii* and *M furfur* were implicated as opportunistic agents of disease, particularly in immunosuppressed or otherwise debilitated patients. Patients are accidentally infected with these common organisms via indwelling catheters or intravenous lines. Virtually nothing is known concerning the pathogenic mechanisms of these fungi.

Dermatophyte Infections

The **dermatophytes** are fungi that colonize skin, hair, and nails. These fungi possess greater invasive properties than those causing superficial infections, but they are limited to the keratinized tissues. They cause a wide spectrum of diseases that range from a mild scaling disorder to one that is generalized and highly inflammatory. Studies have shown that the disease-producing potential of these agents depends on various parasite and host factors, such as the species of organism, immunologic status of the host, type of clothing worn, and type of footwear used. Trauma plays an important role in infection. These organisms gain entry and establish themselves in the cornified layers of traumatized or macerated skin and its integument and multiply by producing keratinase to metabolize the insoluble, tough, fibrous protein. The reason why these agents spread no deeper is not known, but it has been speculated that factors such as cell-mediated immunity and the presence of transferrin in serum inhibit fungal propagation to the deeper tissue layers. Some dermatophytes have evolved a commensal relationship with the host and are isolated from skin in the absence of disease. Little is known about specific pathogenic mechanisms of the dermatophytes, but they do not cause systemic disease.

Subcutaneous Mycoses

The fungi that have been implicated in the **subcutaneous mycoses** are abundant in the environment and have a low degree of infectivity. These organisms gain access to the subcutaneous tissues through traumatic implantation. Again, little is known about mechanisms of pathogenesis. Histopathologic evidence indicates that these organisms survive in the subcutaneous tissue layers by producing proteolytic enzymes and maintaining a facultative anaerobic existence because of the lowered redox potential of the damaged tissue. In **eumycotic mycetoma** there is extensive tissue damage and production of purulent fluid, which exudes through numerous intercommunicating sinus tracts. Microabscesses are common in **chromoblastomycosis,** but the clinical manifestation of disease indicates a vigorous host response to the organism, as seen by the intense tissue reaction that characterizes the disease (pseudoepitheliomatous hyperplasia).

Although most of the fungi implicated in this category of disease exist in a hyphal morphology, the agents of chromoblastomycosis and sporotrichosis are exceptions. Chromoblastomycosis is caused by a group of fungi that have several features in common. They are all darkly pigmented (**dematiaceous**) and exhibit a polymorphism consisting of three distinct morphologies: the organism may exist in a mycelial state, a yeastlike state, or as a thick-walled spherical cell that divides by cleavage. The latter cell morphology, called a

sclerotic cell or **Medlar body,** is the pathologic morphology seen in tissue sections. However, transition to the sclerotic morphology may not be a crucial requirement for pathogenesis. Several dematiaceous fungi cause a disease called **phaeohyphomycosis,** which clinically consists of a broad group of diseases characterized by the presence of various darkly pigmented yeastlike to hyphal elements, but not sclerotic cells, in pathologic specimens. Alternatively, the immune reaction of the host may dictate the morphology that the organism assumes. Again, there is no information about mechanisms or the role of morphogenesis in the pathogenesis of this group of fungi.

Sporotrichosis is caused by *Sporothrix schenckii,* which grows as a mold in nature or when cultured at 25°C, but as yeastlike cells when found in tissues. The clinical manifestations of disease caused by *S schenckii* vary, depending on the immune status of the patient. The classic condition, subcutaneous lymphangitic sporotrichosis, is characterized by numerous nodules, abscesses, and ulcerative lesions that develop along the lymphatics that drain the primary site of inoculation. The disease does not extend beyond the regional lymph nodes that drain the site of the original infection. Alternatively, infection may result in solitary lesions or pulmonary disease. Clinical manifestations of pulmonary infections vary depending on the immune status of the patient. The immunocompetent individual has a high degree of innate resistance to disease, and when infection occurs the organism is often a secondary colonizer of old infarcted or healed cavities of the lungs. If the patient is immunocompromised, dissemination can occur. There is no information about mechanisms of pathogenesis of this dimorphic fungus.

Systemic Mycoses

Of all the fungi that have been implicated in human disease, only the five agents that cause the **systemic mycoses** have the innate ability to cause infection and disease in humans and other animals. The primary site of infection is the respiratory tract. Conidia and other infectious particles are inhaled and lodge on the mucous membrane of the respiratory tree or in the alveoli, where they encounter macrophages and are phagocytosed. To successfully colonize the host these organisms must be able to survive at the elevated temperature of the body and either elude phagocytosis, neutralize the hostility they encounter, or adapt in a manner that will allow them to multiply.

Several factors contribute to infection and pathogenesis of these organisms. Of the five systemic agents, four, *H capsulatum, B dermatitidis, P brasiliensis,* and *C immitis,* are dimorphic, changing from a mycelial to a unicellular morphology when they invade tissues. The change from mycelial to yeast morphology in *H capsulatum* appears critical for pathogenicity. Several physiologic changes occur in the fungus during the transition, which is induced by the temperature shift to 37°C. The triggering event is a heat-related insult: the temperature rise causes a partial uncoupling of oxidative phosphorylation and a consequent decline in the cellular ATP level, respiration rate, and concentrations of electron transport components. The cells enter a period of dormancy, during which spontaneous respiration is maintained at a decreased level. Then there is a shift into a recovery phase, during which transformation to yeast morphology is completed. Mycelial cells of *H capsulatum* that are unable to undergo this morphologic transition are avirulent. Similar observations have been made when mycelia of *B dermatitidis* and *P brasiliensis* are shifted from 25°C to 37°C, and it has been implied that transformation to the yeast morphology is critical for infection.

Coccidioides immitis is also dimorphic, but its parasitic phase is a spherule. Little is known about the role of morphologic transformation in infection and disease of this organism. Dimorphism does not appear to play a role in *C neoformans* pathogenesis, since the organism is an encapsulated yeast both at 25°C and in host tissues. The sexual phase of *C neoformans, Filobasidiella neoformans,* is known, and the organism assumes a filamentous morphology, producing small basidiospores. It has been suggested that these propagules are relevant in infection.

In addition to adjustment to the elevated temperature of the host, the infectious propagules must deal with the hostile cellular environment of the lungs. Studies with mutants of *C neoformans* have shown that the acidic mucopolysaccharide capsule is important in pathogenesis. Acapsular variants of the yeast are either avirulent or markedly deficient in pathogenicity. Since these mutants were obtained by mutagenesis, it is difficult to rule out the contribution of other genetic defects to their decreased pathogenicity. However, at the cellular level, the capsular polysaccharide inhibits phagocytosis of the yeast. Encapsulated *C neoformans* cells are highly resistant to phagocytosis by human neutrophils, whereas acapsular variants are effectively phagocytosed. The active component of the capsular polysaccharide has been identified as glucoronoxylomannan. In addition, the capsular polysaccharide is poorly immunogenic in humans and laboratory animals, and the glucoronoxylomannan component persists for extended periods in the host.

In addition to the capsular polysaccharide, elaboration of phenyl oxidase (an enzyme that catalyzes the oxidation of various phenols to dopachrome) by *Cryptococcus neoformans* appears to be a determinant of virulence, although the role of this enzyme in virulence is unknown. The infectious propagules of *H capsulatum, B dermatitidis, P brasiliensis,* and *Coccidioides immitis* are readily phagocytosed by alveolar macrophages. To survive phagocytosis and to multiply, these fungi must neutralize the effects of the phagocytes. The production of reactive oxygen metabolites by phagocytic cells is an important host defense against microorganisms. Studies have shown that the yeast phase of *H capsulatum* fails to trigger release of reactive oxygen metabolites in unprimed murine macrophages despite extensive phagocytosis. How they avoid destruction by the fungicidal mechanisms within lysosomes is unclear. Arthroconidia of *C immitis* inhibit phagosome-lysosome fusion and survive within normal murine peritoneal macrophages. Phagosome-lysosome fusion takes place after *H capsulatum* infection, but the yeast cells survive in the phagolysosome. It has been speculated that the fungus neutralizes the fungicidal components of the lysosome by a mechanism not yet elucidated.

There is very little information about mechanisms of fungal pathogenicity, in contrast to what is known about molecular mechanisms of bacterial pathogenesis. Fungal pathogenesis is complex and involves the interplay of many factors. Studies to elucidate these mechanisms are needed because of the increasing incidence of opportunistic infections.

REFERENCES

Beaman L, Benjamini E, Pappagianis D: Role of lymphocytes in macrophage-induced killing of *Coccidioides immitis* in vitro. Infect Immun 34:347, 1981

Cox RA: Immunosuppression by cell wall antigens of *Coccidioides immitis.* Rev Infect Dis 10:S415, 1988

Domer J, Elkins K, Ennist D, Baker P: Modulation of immune responses by surface polysaccharides of *Candida albicans.* Rev Infect Dis 10:S419, 1988

Eissenberg LG, Goldman WE: *Histoplasma capsulatum* fails to trigger release of superoxide from macrophages. Infect Immun 55:29, 1987

Eng RHK, Bishburg E, Smith AM, Kapila R: Cryptococcal infections in patients with acquired immune deficiency syndrome. Am J Med 81:19, 1986

Finlay BB, Falkow S: Common themes in microbial pathogenicity. Microbiol Rev 53:210, 1989

Kwon-Chung KJ, Rhodes JC: Encapsulation and melanin formation as indicators of virulence in *Cryptococcus neoformans.* Infect Immun 51:215, 1986

Maresca B, Kobayashi GS: Dimorphism in *Histoplasma capsulatum:* a model for the study of cell differentiation in pathogenic fungi. Microbiol Rev 53:186, 1989

Medoff G, Kobayashi G, Painter AA, Travis SJ: Morphogenesis and pathogenicity of *Histoplasma capsulatum.* Infect Immun 55:1355, 1987

Medoff G, Painter AA, Kobayashi GS: Mycelial to yeast phase transitions of the dimorphic fungi *Blastomyces dermatitidis* and *Paracoccidioides brasiliensis.* J Bacteriol 169:4055, 1987

Moulder JW: Comparative biology of intracellular parasitism. Microbiol Rev 49:298, 1985

Rotrosen D, Calderone RA, Edwards JE, Jr: Adherence of *Candida* species to host tissues and plastic surfaces. Rev Infect Dis 8:73, 1986

Wolf JE, Kirchberger V, Kobayashi GS, Little JR: Modulation of the oxidative burst by *Histoplasma capsulatum.* J Immunol 138:582, 1987.

75 SPECTRUM OF MYCOSES

THOMAS J. WALSH
DENNIS M. DIXON

GENERAL CONCEPTS

CLASSIFICATION OF MYCOSES

The clinical nomenclatures used for the mycoses are based on the (1) site of the infection, (2) route of acquisition of the pathogen, and (3) type of virulence exhibited by the fungus.

Classification Based on Site

Mycoses are classified as superficial, cutaneous, subcutaneous, or systemic (deep) infections depending on the type and degree of tissue involvement and the host response to the pathogen.

Classification Based on Route of Acquisition

Infecting fungi may be either exogenous or endoge-

nous. Routes of entry for exogenous fungi include airborne, cutaneous, or percutaneous. Endogenous infection involves colonization by a member of the normal flora or reactivation of a previous infection.

Classification Based on Virulence

Primary pathogens can establish infections in normal hosts. Opportunistic pathogens cause disease in individuals with compromised host defense mechanisms.

EPIDEMIOLOGY

The primary pathogens have relatively well-defined geographic ranges; the opportunistic fungi are ubiquitous.

INTRODUCTION

Fungal infections (mycoses) cause a wide range of diseases in humans. Mycoses range in extent from superficial infections involving the outer layer of the stratum corneum of the skin to disseminated infection involving the brain, heart, lungs, liver, spleen, and kidneys. The range of patients at risk

for invasive fungal infections continues to expand; it includes, for example, patients with the acquired immune deficiency syndrome (AIDS), those immunosuppressed by therapy for cancer and organ transplantation, and those undergoing major operations. As the population at risk continues to expand, so does the spectrum of opportunistic fungal pathogens. Many of the deeply invasive mycoses are difficult to diagnose early and difficult to treat. New approaches to diagnosis and treatment of invasive fungal infections are the subjects of intensive research.

CLASSIFICATION OF MYCOSES ON THE BASIS OF SITE

Fungal infections are classified by the site of infection, route of acquisition, and type of virulence. When classified by the site of infection, fungal infections are designated as **superficial, cutaneous, subcutaneous,** or **deep.** Superficial mycoses are limited to the stratum corneum and elicit essentially no inflammation. Cutaneous infections involve the integument and its appendages, including hair and nails. Cutaneous infection may involve the stratum corneum or deeper layers of the epidermis. Inflammation of the skin is elicited by the organism or its products. Subcutaneous mycoses

include a range of infections initiated in subcutaneous tissues, usually at the point of traumatic inoculation. An inflammatory response develops in the subcutaneous tissue and frequently extends into the epidermal structures. Deep mycoses commonly involve the heart, lungs, abdominal viscera, bones, and/or central nervous system (Fig. 75-1). The most common portals of entry are the respiratory tract, gastrointestinal tract, and blood vessels (Fig. 75-2).

Superficial and Cutaneous Mycoses

Superficial mycoses include the following fungal infections and their agents: black piedra *(Piedraia hortai),* white piedra *(Trichosporon beigelii),* pityriasis versicolor *(Malassezia furfur),* and tinea nigra *(Phaeoannellomyces werneckii).* Pityriasis versicolor is a common superficial mycosis, which is characterized by hypopigmentation or hyperpigmenta-

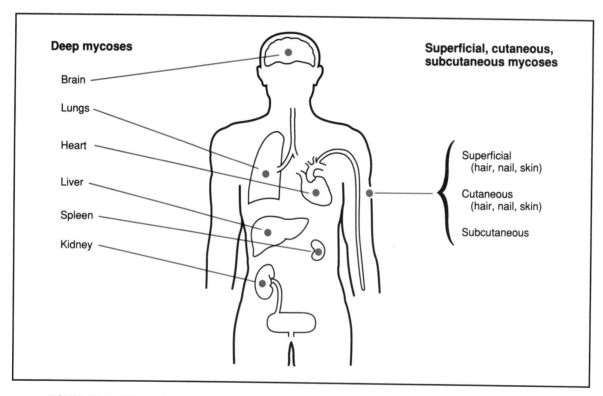

FIGURE 75-1 Principal tissue sites of deep mycoses in comparison with those of the superficial, cutaneous, and subcutaneous mycoses.

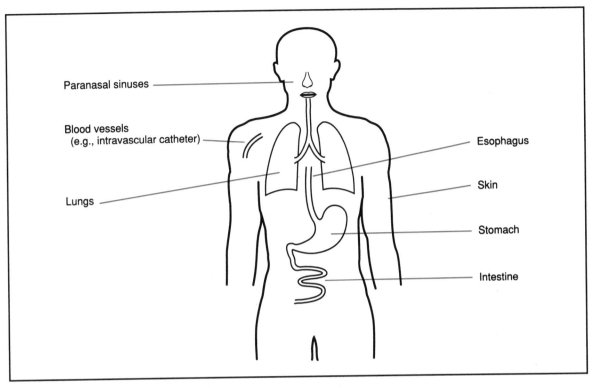

FIGURE 75-2 Portals of entry of pathogenic and opportunistic fungi that cause deep mycoses.

tion of the skin of the neck, shoulders, chest and back. Pityriasis versicolor is due to *M furfur* that involves only the superficial keratin layer. Black piedra is a superficial mycosis due to *Piedraia hortai* and is manifested by a small, firm, black nodule surrounding the hair shaft. By comparison, white piedra, due to *T beigelii*, is characterized by a soft, friable, beige nodule of the distal ends of hair shafts. Tinea nigra most typically presents as a silver nitrate-like stain on the palm of the hand.

Cutaneous mycoses may be classified as **dermatophytoses** or **dermatomycoses**. Dermatophytoses are caused by fungi classified in the genera *Epidermophyton*, *Microsporum*, and *Trichophyton*, which attack hair, nail, or skin. Dermatomycoses are cutaneous infections due to other fungi, the most common of which are *Candida* species. The dermatophytoses are characterized by an anatomic site specificity that correlates closely with the genus involved. For example, *Epidermophyton floc-*

cosum infects only skin and nails but usually does not infect hair shafts and follicles, whereas *Trichophyton* species may infect hair, skin, and nails.

Subcutaneous Mycoses

There are four general types of subcutaneous mycoses: chromoblastomycosis, phaeohyphomycosis, mycetoma, and sporotrichosis. All appear to be caused by traumatic inoculation of the etiologic fungi into the subcutaneous tissue. **Chromoblastomycosis** is a subcutaneous mycosis characterized by verrucoid lesions of the skin (usually of the lower extremities). Histologic examination reveals the characteristic muriform cells (cells having cross-walls in two directions). Chromoblastomycosis is generally limited to the subcutaneous tissue, with no involvement of bone, tendon, or muscle. By comparison, **mycetoma** is a suppurative and granulomatous subcutaneous mycosis, which destroys contiguous bone, tendon, and skeletal muscle. It is characterized by the presence of draining sinus tracts from which small but grossly visible pigmented grains or granules are extruded. These grains are microcolonies of the infectious agent.

Chromoblastomycosis and mycetoma are caused by a specific group of fungi. The most common fungi that cause chromoblastomycosis are *Fonsecaea pedrosoi, F compacta, Cladosporium carrionii,* and *Phialophora verrucosa.* The agents of mycetoma are more diverse but may be either fungi (eumycotic mycetoma) or actinomycete bacteria (actinomycotic mycetoma). The most common agent of eumycotic mycetoma in the United States is *Pseudallescheria boydii,* and the most common cause of actinomycotic mycetoma is *Nocardia brasiliensis.*

Fungi having a brown to black pigment are known as **dematiaceous** (melanized fungi). These fungi produce a range of infections from superficial to deep (visceral) infection characterized by the presence of dematiaceous hyphal and/or yeastlike cells in tissue. Infections caused by dematiaceous fungi with hyphal to yeast forms in tissue are termed **phaeohyphomycoses.**

Sporotrichosis is the fourth general class of subcutaneous mycoses. This infection is due to *Sporothrix schenckii* and involves the subcutaneous tissue at the point of traumatic inoculation. The infection usually spreads along the cutaneous lymphatic channels of the extremity involved.

Deep Mycoses

Deep mycoses are caused by primary pathogenic and opportunistic fungal pathogens. Primary pathogenic fungi are able to establish infection in a normal host, whereas opportunistic pathogens require a compromised state (e.g., due to cancer, organ transplantation, surgery, or AIDS) to establish infection. The primary deep pathogens usually gain access to the host via the respiratory tract. Opportunistic fungi that cause deep mycosis invade via the respiratory tract, alimentary tract, or intravascular devices.

The primary systemic fungal pathogens include *Coccidioides immitis, Histoplasma capsulatum, Blasto-*

myces dermatitidis, and *Paracoccidioides brasiliensis.* The major opportunistic fungal pathogens include *Cryptococcus neoformans, Candida* species, *Aspergillus* species, members of the order Mucorales, *Trichosporon beigelii,* and *Fusarium* species.

As defined above, fungal dimorphism is the morphologic and physiologic conversion of several specific fungi from one phenotype to another when such fungi change from one environment to another. The major dimorphic fungi include *C immitis, H capsulatum, B dermatitidis, P brasiliensis,* and *S schenckii* and other opportunistic fungi such as *Candida albicans.* Various environmental host factors regulate fungal dimorphism; these include amino acids, temperature, carbohydrates, and trace elements (e.g., zinc). In the primary pathogens and *S schenckii,* the morphologic transformation is from a hyphal form to a yeastlike form (or spherule in *C immitis*) in tissue (Fig. 75-3). However, the dimorphism of *Candida albicans* is somewhat different in that the organism transforms from a budding yeast-like (blastoconidia) form to a filamentous form via a transitional structure called a **germ tube** (Fig. 75-4). Other filamentous structures such as pseudohyphae may also be present.

CLASSIFICATION OF MYCOSES ON THE BASIS OF ROUTE OF ACQUISITION

When classified on the basis of the route of acquisition, a fungal infection may be designated as **exogenous** or **endogenous.** Exogenous pathogens may be transmitted by airborne, cutaneous, or percutaneous routes. An endogenous fungal infection may be acquired by colonization or by reactivation of a fungus from a latent infection.

CLASSIFICATION OF MYCOSES ON THE BASIS OF VIRULENCE

Fungi are classified by virulence as primary pathogens or as opportunistic pathogens.

Primary Mycoses

Most cases of primary deep mycosis are asymptomatic or clinically mild infections occurring in

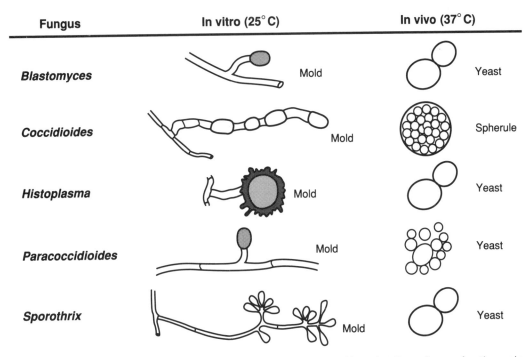

Fungus	In vitro (25° C)		In vivo (37° C)	
Blastomyces		Mold		Yeast
Coccidioides		Mold		Spherule
Histoplasma		Mold		Yeast
Paracoccidioides		Mold		Yeast
Sporothrix		Mold		Yeast

FIGURE 75-3 Diagrammatic representation of the saprophytic and invasive tissue forms of pathogenic fungi. These diagrams are conceptual and do not represent relative sizes of these organisms.

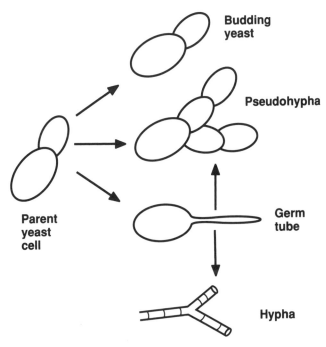

FIGURE 75-4 Germination of *Candida albicans*.

normal patients living or traveling in endemic areas. However, patients exposed to a high inoculum of organisms of patients with altered host defenses may suffer life-threatening progression.

The arthroconidia of *Coccidioides immitis* are inhaled and convert in the lungs to spherules. Most cases of coccidioidomycosis are clinically occult or mild infections in patients who inhale infective arthroconidia. However, some patients have progressive pulmonary infection and may also suffer dissemination to the brain, bone, and other sites. *Coccidioides* meningitis is a life-threatening infection that requires lifelong treatment.

Histoplasmosis (due to *Histoplasma capsulatum* var. *capsulatum*) causes a primary pulmonary infection in a budding-yeast form. Dissemination to the hilar and mediastinal lymph nodes, spleen, liver, bone marrow, and brain may be life-threatening in infants and immunocompromised patients. Histoplasmosis (like tuberculosis) elicits a granulomatous reaction in tissue. These granulomatous foci may reactivate and cause dissemination of fungi to other tissues. These patterns of primary infection and reactivation are similar to those of *Mycobacterium tuberculosis* (see Ch. 33). Histoplasmosis is also associated with a chronic inflammatory process known as fibrosing mediastinitis, in which scar tissue (formed in response to *H capsulatum*) encroaches on vital structures in the mediastinum.

Blastomycosis is a primary pulmonary infection caused by *Blastomyces dermatitidis* in a yeast form. The organism elicits a granulomatous reaction often associated with marked fibrosis. The clinical pattern of pulmonary blastomycosis is one of chronic pneumonia. Dissemination occurs most commonly to the skin, bone, and, in males, the prostate.

Opportunistic Mycoses

Candidiasis, caused most commonly by *Candida albicans* but also by other *Candida* spp, is the most common of the opportunistic fungal infections. It is classified as either superficial or deep. Superficial candidiasis may involve the epidermal and mucosal surfaces, including those of the oral cavity, pharynx, esophagus, stomach, intestines, urinary bladder, and vagina. The alimentary tract and intravascular catheters are the major portals of entry for deep (or visceral) candidiasis. The kidneys, liver, spleen, brain, eyes, heart, and other tissues are the major organ sites involved in deep or visceral candidiasis. The principal risk factors predisposing to deeply invasive candidiasis are protracted courses of broad-spectrum antibiotics, cytotoxic chemotherapy, corticosteroids, and vascular catheters.

Invasive aspergillosis, caused by *Aspergillus* species, most frequently involves the lungs and paranasal sinuses. The fungus may disseminate from the lungs to involve the brain, kidneys, liver, heart, and bones. The main portal of entry for aspergillosis is the respiratory tract; however, injuries to the skin may also introduce the organism into susceptible hosts. Quantitative and functional defects in circulating neutrophils are key risk factors for development of invasive aspergillosis. For example, neutropenia due to cytotoxic chemotherapy and systemic corticosteroids are common predisposing factors for invasive aspergillosis.

Zygomycosis caused by *Rhizopus*, *Rhizomucor*, or *Absidia* species may cause invasive sinopulmonary infections. An especially life-threatening form of zygomycosis, known as the rhinocerebral syndrome, occurs in diabetics with ketoacidosis. Neutropenia and corticosteroids are other major risk factors for zygomycosis. *Aspergillus* species and members of the Mucorales have a strong propensity for invading blood vessels.

Cryptococcosis is an opportunistic fungal infection that most frequently causes pneumonia and/or meningitis. Defective cellular immunity, especially that associated with AIDS, is the most common risk factor.

Phaeohyphomycosis is an infection of the deep tissues, especially the brain, and is caused by brown- to black-pigmented fungi. It is uncommon and life-threatening and occurs in hosts with various immunocompromised states. The term *phaeohyphomycosis* may also be applied to infections due to dematiaceous fungi in cutaneous and subcutaneous tissues.

Hyalohyphomycosis is an opportunistic fungal infection caused by any one of a variety of normally saprophytic fungi with hyaline hyphal elements. For example, *Fusarium* species infect neutropenic patients and can cause pneumonia and disseminated cutaneous lesions.

EPIDEMIOLOGY

The epidemiology of dimorphic primary pathogens contrasts with that of the opportunistic fungal pathogens. The primary pathogens have a relatively well-defined geographic range of endemic infection and cause disease in both immunocompetent and immunocompromised hosts. However, the opportunistic fungi (e.g., *Aspergillus* species) are ubiquitous, and the frequency of infection depends on the population of compromised hosts.

REFERENCES

Drutz DJ (ed): Systemic fungal infections: diagnosis and treatment, part 1. p. 779. In: Infectious Diseases Clinics of North America. Vol. 2. WB Saunders, Philadelphia, 1988

Drutz DJ (ed): Systemic fungal infections: diagnosis and treatment, part 2. p. 1. In: Infectious Diseases Clinics of North America. Vol. 3. WB Saunders, Philadelphia, 1989

Emmons CW, Binford CH, Utz JP et al: Medical Mycology. 3rd ed. Lea & Febiger, Philadelphia, 1977

Howard DH: Fungi Pathogenic for Humans and Animals. Marcel Dekker, New York, 1983

McGinnis, MR. Laboratory Handbook of Medical Mycology. Academic Press, San Diego, 1980

Odds FC: Candida and Candidosis. A Review and Bibliography. 2nd Ed. Bailliere Tindall, Philadelphia, 1988

Rippon JW: Medical Mycology. The Pathogenic Fungi and the Pathogenic Actinomycetes. WB Saunders, Philadelphia, 1988

Szaniszlo PJ, Harris JL: Fungal Dimorphism: With Emphasis on Fungi Pathogenic for Humans. Plenum, New York, 1985

Walsh TJ, Dixon DM: Nosocomial aspergillosis: environmental microbiology, hospital epidemiology, diagnosis, and treatment. Eur J Epidemiol 5:131, 1989

Walsh TJ, Pizzo PA: Nosocomial fungal infections: a classification for hospital-acquired fungal infections and mycoses arising from endogenous flora or reactivation. Annu Rev Microbiol 42:517, 1988

76 ANTIFUNGAL AGENTS

DENNIS M. DIXON
THOMAS J. WALSH

GENERAL CONCEPTS

Definition

An **antifungal agent** is a drug that selectively eliminates fungal pathogens from a host with minimal toxicity to the host.

Polyene Antifungal Drugs

Amphotericin B, nystatin, and pimaricin interact with sterols in the cell membrane (ergosterol in fungi, cholesterol in humans) to form channels through which small molecules leak from the inside of the fungal cell to the outside.

Azole Antifungal Drugs

Fluconazole, itraconazole, and ketoconazole inhibit cytochrome P_{450}-dependent enzymes involved in the biosynthesis of ergosterol, which is required for fungal cell membrane structure and function.

Antimetabolite Antifungal Drugs

5-Fluorocytosine acts as an inhibitor of both DNA and RNA synthesis via the intracytoplasmic conversion of 5-fluorocytosine to 5-fluorouracil.

INTRODUCTION

The development of antifungal agents has lagged behind that of antibacterial agents. This is a predictable consequence of the cellular structure of the organisms involved. Bacteria are prokaryotic and hence offer numerous structural and metabolic targets that differ from those of the human host. Fungi, in contrast, are eukaryotes, and consequently most agents toxic to fungi are also toxic to the host. Furthermore, because fungi generally grow slowly and often in multicellular forms, they are more difficult to quantify than bacteria. This difficulty complicates experiments designed to evaluate the in vitro or in vivo properties of a potential antifungal agent.

Despite these limitations, numerous advances have been made in developing new antifungal agents and in understanding the existing ones. This chapter summarizes the more common antifungal agents. Three groups of drugs are emphasized: the polyenes, the azoles, and one antimetabolite. Table 76-1 summarizes the most important antifungal agents and their most common uses.

959

TABLE 76-1 The Major Antifungal Agents and Their Common Uses

| | Clinical Application | | | | | | | | |
| | Systemic Mycoses | | | | Opportunistic Mycoses | | | | |
Drug	Coccidioidomycosis	Histoplasmosis	Blastomycosis	Paracoccidioidomycosis	Aspergillosis	Candidiasis	Cryptococcosis	Dermatophytoses	Other
Polyenes									
Amphotericin B	+	+	+	+	+	+	+	−	
Nystatin	−	−	−	−	−	mc[a]	−	−	
Pimaricin	−	−	−	−	−	−	−	−	Mycotic keratitis
Imidazoles									
Clotrimazole	−	−	−	−	−	mc	−	+	
Miconazole	−	−	−	−	−	mc	−	+	Pseudallescheriasis
Ketoconazole	+[b]	+[b]	+[b]	+[b]	−[c]	+[d]	−	+	
Triazoles									
Itraconazole	+[b]	+[b]	+[b]	+[b]	+	mc	+	+	Sporotrichosis
Fluconazole	+[e]	?[f]	?	?	−	+	+	+	
Antimetabolite									
5-Fluorocytosine[g]	−	−	−	−	+	+	+	−	Phaeohyphomycosis

[a] mc, Mucocutaneous but not systemic candidiasis.

[b] In immunocompetent hosts.

[c] Resistance has been reported, as has antagonism of amphotericin B.

[d] Both mucocutaneous and some forms of systemic candidiasis, but the latter is controversial.

[e] Selected cases.

[f] ?, Insufficient data.

[g] **Used only in combination with amphotericin B.**

POLYENE ANTIFUNGAL DRUGS

The polyene compounds are so named because of the alternating conjugated double bonds that constitute a part of their macrolide ring structure (Fig. 76-1). The polyene antibiotics are all products of *Streptomyces* species. These drugs interact with sterols in cell membranes (ergosterol in fungal cells; cholesterol in human cells) to form channels through the membrane, causing the cells to become leaky (Fig. 76-2). The polyene antifungal agents include nystatin, amphotericin B, and pimaricin.

Amphotericin B is the mainstay antifungal agent for the life-threatening mycoses and for most other mycoses, with the possible exception of the dermatophytoses. Discovered by Gold in 1956, it can truly be said to represent a gold standard. Its broad spectrum of activity includes most of the medically important molds and yeasts, including dimorphic pathogens such as *Coccidioides immitis*, *Histoplasma capsulatum*, *Blastomyces dermatitidis*, and *Paracoccidioides brasiliensis*. It is the drug of choice in treating most opportunistic mycoses caused by fungi such as *Candida* species, *Cryptococcus neoformans*, *Aspergillus* species, and the zygomycetes. Resistance to this agent is rare, but is noteworthy for *Pseudallescheria boydii* and certain isolates of *Candida lusitaniae* and *Candida guilliermondii*.

The drug must be administered intravenously and is associated with numerous side effects, ranging from phlebitis at the infusion site and chills to renal toxicity, which may be severe. A major advance in the use of this agent has resulted from an understanding of the mechanism of its renal toxicity, which is presumed to involve tubuloglomerular feedback. The suppression of glomerular filtration can be reduced by administering sodium chloride.

Nystatin was the first successful antifungal antibiotic to be developed, and it is still in general use. It is representative of the polyene antifungal agents developed after it: the promise of its broad-spectrum antifungal activity is offset by host toxicity. Therefore, it is limited to topical use, where it has activity against yeasts such as the *Candida* species.

Pimaricin (natamycin), another polyene, is used topically to treat superficial mycotic infections of the eye. It is active against both yeasts and molds.

AZOLE ANTIFUNGAL DRUGS

The azole antifungal agents have five-membered organic rings that contain either two or three nitrogen molecules (the **imidazoles** and the **triazoles** respectively). The clinically useful imidazoles are clotrimazole, miconazole, and ketoconazole. Two important triazoles are itraconazole and fluconazole. In general, the azole antifungal agents are thought to inhibit cytochrome P_{450}-dependent enzymes involved in the biosynthesis of cell membrane sterols.

Ketoconazole has become the gold standard of the azoles. It can be administered both orally and topically and has a range of activity including infections due to *H capsulatum* and *B dermatitidis*, for which it is often used in nonimmunocompromised patients. It is also active against mucosal candidiasis and a variety of cutaneous mycoses, including dermatophyte infections, pityriasis versicolor, and cutaneous candidiasis. It is not indicated for treatment of aspergillosis or of systemic infections caused by yeasts.

The new triazole agents have expanded the coverage offered by the conventional imidazoles. Itraconazole is useful against aspergillosis and sporotrichosis. Fluconazole is becoming important in the treatment of deep-seated candidiasis and cryptococcosis. Side effects are not as common with the azoles as with amphotericin B, but life-threatening liver toxicity can arise with long-term use. Other side effects include nausea and vomiting.

5-FLUOROCYTOSINE

In contrast to the situation with antibacterial agents, few antimetabolites are available for use against fungi. The best example is 5-fluorocytosine, a fluorinated analog of cytosine. It inhibits both DNA and RNA synthesis via intracytoplasmic conversion to 5-fluorouracil. The latter is converted to two active nucleotides: 5-fluorouridine triphosphate, which inhibits RNA processing, and

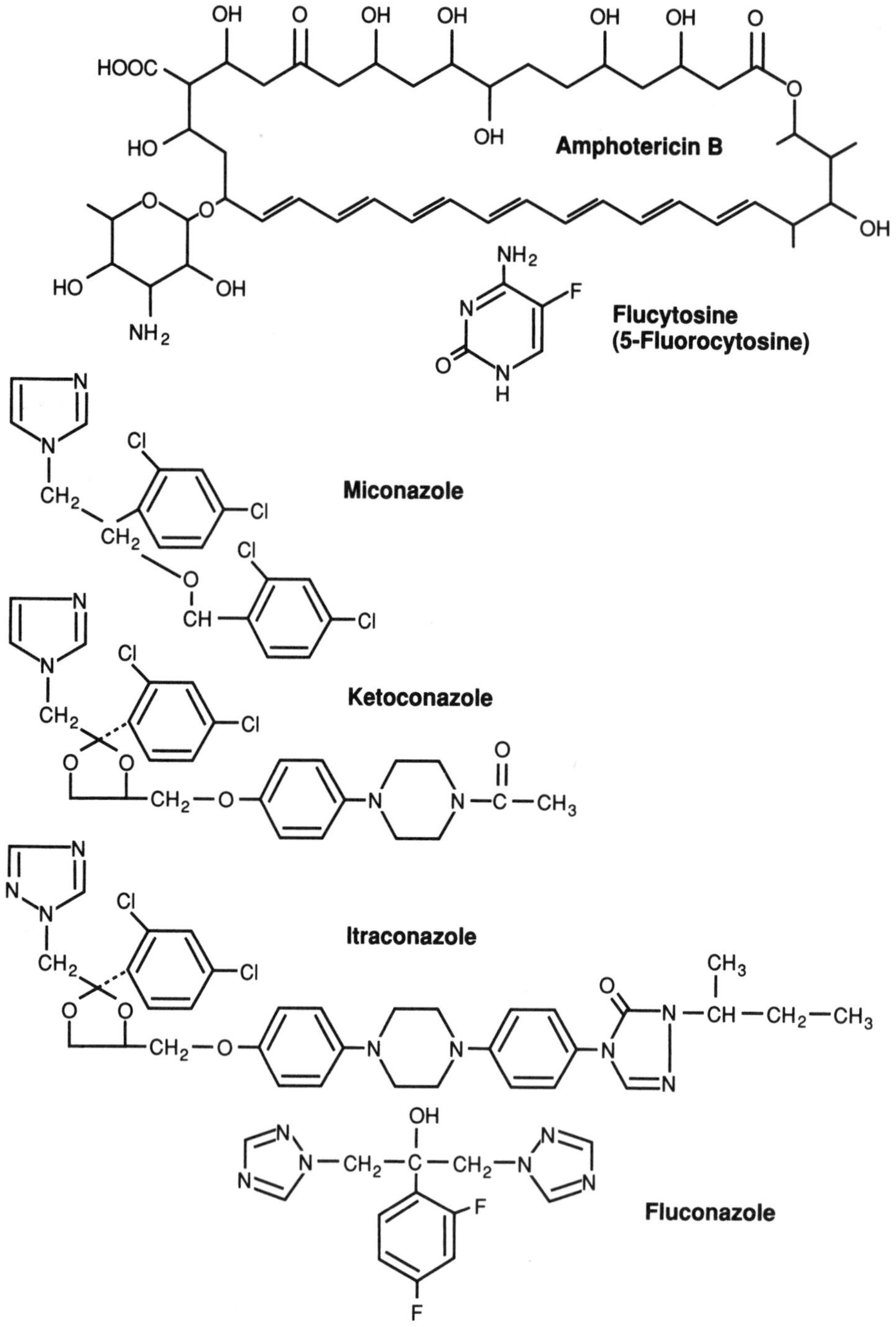

FIGURE 76-1 Structures of some common antifungal agents.

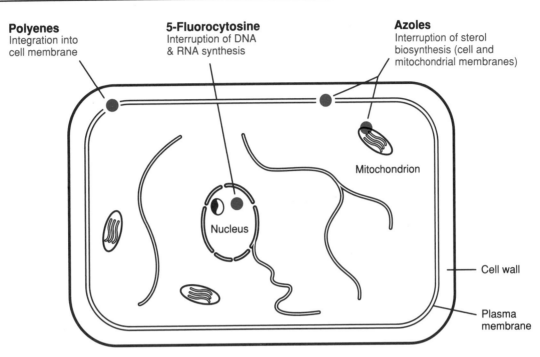

Polyenes
Integration into
cell membrane

5-Fluorocytosine
Interruption of DNA
& RNA synthesis

Azoles
Interruption of sterol
biosynthesis (cell and
mitochondrial membranes)

Mitochondrion

Nucleus

Cell wall

Plasma
membrane

FIGURE 76-2 *Generalized fungal cell depicting the sites of action of the common antifungal agents.*

5-fluorodeoxyuridine monophosphate, which inhibits thymidylate synthetase and hence the formation of the deoxythymidine triphosphate needed for DNA synthesis. As with other antimetabolites, the emergence of drug resistance is a problem. Therefore, 5-fluorocytosine is seldom used alone. In combination with amphotericin B it remains the treatment of choice for cryptococcal meningitis and is effective against a number of other mycoses, including some caused by the dematiaceous fungi and perhaps even by *C albicans.*

OTHER ANTIFUNGAL AGENTS

Griseofulvin is an antifungal antibiotic produced by *Penicillium griseofulvum.* It is active in vitro against most dermatophytes and has been the drug of choice for chronic infections caused by these fungi (e.g., nail infections with *Trichophyton rubrum*) since it is orally administered and presumably incorporated into actively growing tissue. It is still used in such instances but is being challenged by some of the newer azole antifungal agents.

Potassium iodide given orally as a saturated suspension is uniquely used to treat cutaneous and lymphocutaneous sporotrichosis. This compound, interestingly, is not active against *Sporothrix schenckii* in vitro. It appears to act by enhancing the transepidermal elimination process in the infected host.

SELECTION OF ANTIFUNGAL AGENTS

Preliminary selection of an antifungal agent for clinical use can be made on the basis of the specific fungal pathogen involved. This is true in part because the emergence of resistance to antifungal agents is relatively rare, with the exception of 5-fluorocytosine and the yeasts in particular. Also, in vitro susceptibility testing with the fungi is not yet standardized, and the results of in vitro tests do not always compare to results obtained in vivo. Therefore, experimental models of animal infection have been developed and have proven useful.

With the advent of the polyenes, azoles, and 5-

fluorocytosine, previously fatal infections can now be treated. However, as modern medicine continues to extend life through aggressive therapy of other life-threatening diseases such as cancer, there is an increasing population at risk for opportunistic fungal infections. Such patients represent a special challenge because they often are left with little host immune function. Therefore, chemotherapeutic agents should be fungicidal and not just fungistatic. The search continues for fungicidal agents that are nontoxic to the host. Research is also directed toward immunomodulating agents that can reverse the defects of native host immunity.

REFERENCES

Dixon DM: In vivo models: evaluating antifungal agents. Methods Find Exp Clin Pharmacol 9:729, 1987

Espinel-Ingroff A, Shadomy S: In vitro and in vivo evaluation of antifungal agents. Eur J Clin Microbiol 8:352, 1989

Fromtling RA (ed): Recent Trends in the Discovery, Development and Evaluation of Antifungal Agents. Prous, Barcelona, 1987

Fromtling RA: Overview of medically important antifungal imidazole derivatives. Clin Microbiol Rev 1:187, 1988

Galgiani JN: Antifungal susceptibility tests. Antimicrob Agents Chemother 31:1867, 1987

Graybill JR: New antifungal agents. Eur J Clin Microbiol 8:402, 1989

Heidemann JF, Gerkens JF, Spickard WA: Amphotericin B nephrotoxicity in humans decreased by salt repletion. Am J Med 75:476, 1983

Scholer HJ, Polak A: Resistance to systemic antifungal agents. p. 393. In Byron LE (ed): Antimicrobial Drug Resistance. Academic Press, San Diego, 1984

Vanden Bossche H: Biochemical targets for antifungal azole derivatives: hypothesis on the mode of action. p. 313. In McGinnis MR (ed): Current Topics in Medical Mycology. Vol. 1. Springer-Verlag, New York, 1985

Walsh TJ: Recent advances in the treatment of fungal infections. Methods Find Exp Clin Pharmacol 9:769, 1987

IV

PARASITOLOGY

Medical parasitology traditionally has included the study of three major groups of animals: parasitic protozoa, parasitic helminths (worms), and those arthropods that directly cause disease or act as vectors of various pathogens. A parasiste is a pathogen that simultaneously injures and derives sustenance from its host. Some organisms called parasites are actually commensals, in that they neither benefit nor harm their host (for example, *Entamoeba coli*). Althought parasitology had its origins in the zoologic sciences, it is today an interdisciplinary field, greatly influenced by microbiology, immunology, biochemistry, and other life sciences.

Parasitic infections of humans number in the billions and range from relatively innocuous to fatal. The diseases caused by these parasites constitute major human health problems throughout the world. (For example, approximately 30 percent of the world's population is infected with the nematode *Ascaris lumbricoides*.) The incidence of many parasitic diseases (e.g., schistosomiasis, malaria) have increased rather than decreased in recent years. Other parasitic illnesses have emerged as a result of the AIDS epidemic (e.g., cryptosporidiosis, *Pneumocystis carinii* pneumonia, and strongyloidiasis). The migration of parasite-infected people, including refugees, from areas with high prevalence rates of parasitic infection also has added to the health problems of certain countries.

A misconception about parasitic infections is that they occur only in tropical areas. Although most parasitic infections are more prevalent in the tropics, many people in temperate and subtropical areas also become infected, and visitors to tropical countries may return with a parasite infection.

The unicellular parasites (protozoa) and multicellular parasites (helminths, arthropods) are antigenically and biochemically complex, as are their life histories and the pathogenesis of the diseases they cause. During their life, parasitic organisms typically go through several developmental stages that involve changes not only in structure but also in biochemical and antigenic composition. Some helminth larval stages have little resemblance to the adult stages (for example, those of tapeworms and flukes). Some parasitic protozoa also change greatly during their life history; for example, *Toxoplasma gondii* is an intestinal coccidian in cats but in humans takes on a different form and localizes in deep tissues. Certain of these infections can convert from a well-tolerated or asymptomatic condition to life-threatening disease. Many parasitic infections are transmitted from animals to humans (zoonotic infections); the human disease may or may not resemble the disease caused in the lower animal host.

This section of the book has two types of chapters. Several general chapters deal with the structure and classification of parasites and the mechanisms of parasitic dieseases. The remaining chapters describe the specific human parasites and the diseases they cause. Emphasis is placed throughout on the basic biology of the pathogens and their host-parasiste relationships. Thus, descriptions of the basic properties of the pathogens, the pathogenesis of the diseases they cause, host defenses, and epidemiology are highlighted. Practical information on clinical manifestations, diagnosis, and control has been included in the chapters on specific pathogens. Most chapters treat a group of related pathogens (for example, trematodes, cestodes). Other chapters are more limited in scope because of the expertise of the authors and the difficulty involve in including these species the groups discussed in the other chapters.

This section gives the reader a broad, in-depth coverage of medically important parasites. Such an unusually comprehensive coverage is essential to give students the awareness and understanding necessary for proper diagnosis, treatment, and prevention of the parasitic infections. The most important element in diagnosing a parasitic infection is often the physician's suspicion that a parasite may be involved — a possibility that is too often overlooked. This kind of awareness requires a knowledge of the biology of the parasites. Diagnosis of parasitic infections requires laboratory support, since the signs and symptoms usually are nonspecific. A variety of methods and specimens are used for diagnosis. Since the most common parasites are enteric, microscopic examination of fecal specimens is done more often than any other laboratory procedure in the diagnosis of parasitic disease. Culturing has little application in the diagnosis of most parasitic infections, although it has been employed, for example, for *Trichomonas vaginalis* and *Entamoeba histolytica* infections. Immunodiagnostic tests are useful in several infections, including extraintestinal amebiasis, visceral larva migrans, and trichinosis.

Because the laboratory is so important in diagnosis, its personnel must be well trained. Continuing training and refresher courses should be encouraged and supported. In the United States, excellent short courses in diagnostic parasitology are available in various state and federal health laboratories and at the Centers for Disease Control (CDC) in Atlanta. These laboratories also offer a variety of diagnostic services in parasitology, including specialized serologic tests. Medical scientists in the United States should be aware of the Parasitic Disease Drug Service at CDC, from which they may obtain drug information and certain drugs not readily available. Announcements of regional workshops and continuing education programs in parasitology can be found in various journals, for example the *American Society for Microbiology News*.

Leroy J. Olson

77 PROTOZOA: STRUCTURE, CLASSIFICATION, GROWTH, AND DEVELOPMENT

ROBERT G. YAEGER

GENERAL CONCEPTS

Protozoa

Protozoa are one-celled animals found worldwide in most habitats. Most species are free-living, but all higher animals are infected with one or more species of protozoa. Infections range from asymptomatic to life threatening, depending on the species and strain of the parasite and the resistance of the host.

Structure

Protozoa are microscopic unicellular eukaryotes that have a relatively complex internal structure and carry out complex metabolic activities. Some protozoa have structures for propulsion or other types of movement.

Classification

On the basis of light and electron microscopic morphology, the protozoa are currently classified into six phyla. Most species causing human disease are members of the phyla Sarcomastigophora and Apicomplexa.

Life Cycle Stages

The stages of parasitic protozoa that actively feed and multiply are frequently called **trophozoites;** in some protozoa, other terms are used for these stages. **Cysts** are stages with a protective membrane or thickened wall. Protozoan cysts that must survive outside the host usually have more resistant walls than cysts that form in tissues.

Reproduction

Binary fission, the most common form of reproduction, is asexual; multiple asexual division occurs in some forms. Both sexual and asexual reproduction occur in the Apicomplexa.

Nutrition

All parasitic protozoa require preformed organic substances—that is, nutrition is holozoic as in higher animals.

INTRODUCTION

The Protozoa are considered to be a subkingdom of the kingdom Protista, although in the classical system they were placed in the kingdom Animalia.

More than 50,000 species have been described, most of which are free-living organisms; protozoa are found in almost every possible habitat. The fossil record in the form of shells in sedimentary rocks shows that protozoa were present in the Precambrian era. Anton van Leeuwenhoek was the first person to see protozoa, using microscopes he constructed with simple lenses. Between 1674 and 1716, he described, in addition to free-living protozoa, several parasitic species from animals, and *Giardia lamblia* from his own stools. Virtually all humans have protozoa living in or on their body at some time, and many persons are infected with one or more species throughout their life. Some species are considered commensals, i.e., normally not harmful, whereas others are pathogens and usually produce disease. Protozoan diseases range from very mild to life threatening. Individuals whose defenses are able to control but not eliminate a parasite infection become **carriers** and constitute a source of infection for others. In geographic areas of high prevalence, well-tolerated infections are often not treated to eradicate the parasite because eradication would lower the individual's immunity to the parasite and result in a high likelihood of reinfection.

Many protozoan infections that are inapparent or mild in normal individuals can be life-threatening in immunosuppressed patients, particularly patients with acquired immune deficiency syndrome (AIDS). Evidence suggests that many healthy persons harbor low numbers of *Pneumocystis carinii* in their lungs. However, this parasite produces a frequently fatal pneumonia in immunosuppressed patients such as those with AIDS. *Toxoplasma gondii*, a very common protozoan parasite, usually causes a rather mild initial illness followed by a long-lasting latent infection. AIDS patients, however, can develop fatal toxoplasmic encephalitis. *Cryptosporidium* was described in the 19th century, but widespread human infection has only recently been recognized. *Cryptosporidium* is another protozoan that can produce serious complications in patients with AIDS.

Acanthamoeba species are free-living amebas that inhabit soil and water. Cyst stages can be airborne. Serious eye-threatening corneal ulcers due to *Acanthamoeba* species are being reported in individuals who use contact lenses. The parasites presumably are transmitted in contaminated lens-cleaning solution. Amebas of the genus *Naegleria*, which inhabit bodies of fresh water, are responsible for almost all cases of the usually fatal disease primary amebic meningoencephalitis. The amebas are thought to enter the body from water that is splashed onto the upper nasal tract during swimming or diving. Human infections of this type were predicted before they were recognized and reported, based on laboratory studies of *Acanthamoeba* infections in cell cultures and in animals.

The lack of effective vaccines, the paucity of reliable drugs, and other problems, including difficulties of vector control, prompted the World Health Organization to target six diseases for increased research and training. Three of these were protozoan infections—malaria, trypanosomiasis, and leishmaniasis. Although new information on these diseases has been gained, most of the problems with control persist.

STRUCTURE

Most parasitic protozoa in humans are less than 50 μm in size. The smallest (mainly intracellular forms) are 1 to 10 μm long, but *Balantidium coli* may measure 150 μm. Protozoa are unicellular eukaryotes. As in all eukaryotes, the nucleus is enclosed in a membrane. In protozoa other than ciliates, the nucleus is **vesicular**, with scattered chromatin giving a diffuse appearance to the nucleus, and all nuclei in the individual organism appear alike. One type of vesicular nucleus contains a more or less central body, called an **endosome** or **karyosome.** The endosome lacks DNA in the parasitic amebas and trypanosomes. In the phylum Apicomplexa, on the other hand, the vesicular nucleus contains one or more nucleoli that contain DNA. The ciliates have both a micronucleus and macronucleus, which appear quite homogeneous in composition.

The organelles of protozoa have functions similar to the organs of higher animals. The plasma membrane enclosing the cytoplasm also covers the projecting locomotory structures such as pseudopodia, cilia, and flagella. The outer surface layer of some protozoa, termed a **pellicle,** is sufficiently rigid to maintain a distinctive shape, as in the trypanosomes and *Giardia*. However, these organisms can readily twist and bend when moving through their environment. In most protozoa the cytoplasm is differentiated into **ectoplasm** (the outer, transparent layer) and **endoplasm** (the inner layer containing organelles); the structure of the cytoplasm is most easily seen in species with projecting pseudopodia, such as the amebas. Some protozoa have a cytostome or cell "mouth" for ingesting fluids or solid particles. Contractile vacuoles for osmoregulation occur in some, such as *Naegleria* and *Balantidium*. Many protozoa have

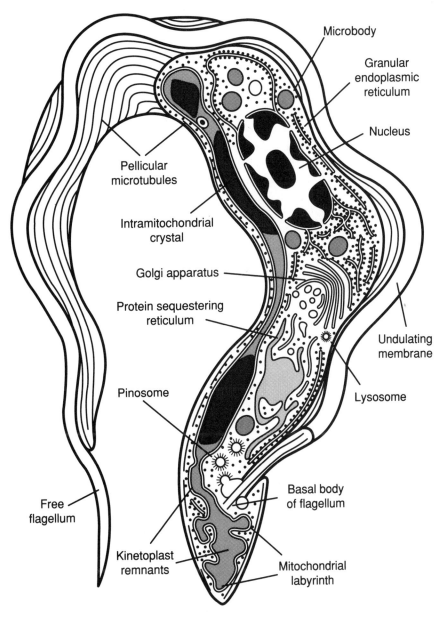

FIGURE 77-1 Fine structure of a protozoan parasite, *Trypanosoma evansi*, as revealed by transmission electron microscopy of thin sections. (Adapted from Vickerman K: Protozoology. Vol. 3. London School of Hygiene and Tropical Medicine, London, 1977, with permission.)

subpellicular microtubules; in the Apicomplexa, which have no external organelles for locomotion, these provide a means for slow movement. The trichomonads and trypanosomes have a distinctive undulating membrane between the body wall and a flagellum. Many other structures occur in parasitic protozoa, including the Golgi apparatus, mitochondria, lysosomes, food vacuoles, conoids in the Apicomplexa, and other specialized structures. Electron microscopy is essential to visualize the details of protozoal structure.

From the point of view of functional and physiologic complexity, a protozoan is more like an animal than like a single cell. Figure 77-1 shows the structure of the bloodstream form of a trypanosome, as determined by electron microscopy.

CLASSIFICATION

In 1985 the Society of Protozoologists published a taxonomic scheme that distributed the Protozoa into six phyla. Two of these phyla—the Sarcomastigophora and the Apicomplexa—contain the most important species causing human disease. This scheme is based on morphology as revealed by light, electron, and scanning microscopy. *Dientamoeba fragilis,* for example, had been thought to be an ameba and placed in the family Entamoebidae. However, internal structures seen by electron microscopy showed that it is properly placed in the order Trichomonadida of flagellate protozoa. In some instances, organisms that appear identical under the microscope have been assigned different species names on the basis of such criteria as geographic distribution and clinical manifestations; a good example is the genus *Leishmania,* for which subspecies names are often used. Biochemical methods have been employed on strains and species to determine isoenzyme patterns or to identify relevant nucleotide sequences in RNA, DNA, or both. Extensive studies have been made on the kinetoplast, a unique mitochondrion found in the hemoflagellates and other members of the order Kinetoplastida. The DNA associated with this organelle is of great interest. Cloning is widely used in taxonomic studies, for example to study differences in virulence or disease manifestations in isolates of a single species obtained from differ-

ent hosts or geographic regions. Antibodies (particularly monoclonal antibodies) to known species or to specific antigens from a species are being employed to identify unknown isolates. Eventually, molecular taxonomy may prove to be a more reliable basis than morphology for protozoan taxonomy, but the microscope is still the most practical tool for identifying a protozoan parasite. Table 77-1 lists the medically important protozoa.

LIFE CYCLE STAGES

During its life cycle, a protozoan generally passes through several **stages** that differ in structure and activity. **Trophozoite** (Greek for ''animal that feeds'') is a general term for the active, feeding, multiplying stage of most protozoa. In most parasitic species this is the stage associated with pathogenesis. In the hemoflagellates the terms **amastigote, promastigote, epimastigote,** and **trypomastigote** designate trophozoite stages that differ in the absence or presence of a flagellum and in the position of the kinetoplast associated with the flagellum. A variety of terms are employed for stages in the Apicomplexa, such as **tachyzoite** and **bradyzoite** for *Toxoplasma gondii.* Other stages in the complex asexual and sexual life cycles seen in this phylum are the **merozoite** (the form resulting from fission of a multinucleate **schizont**) and sexual stages such as **gametocytes** and **gametes.** Some protozoa form **cysts** that contain one or more infective forms. Multiplication occurs in the cysts of some species so that excystation releases more than one organism. For example, when the trophozoite of *Entamoeba histolytica* first forms a cyst, it has a single nucleus. As the cyst matures nuclear division produces four nuclei and during excystation four uninucleate metacystic amebas appear. Similarly, a freshly encysted *Giardia lamblia* has the same number of internal structures (organelles) as the trophozoite. However, as the cyst matures the organelles double and two trophozoites are formed. Cysts passed in stools have a protective wall, enabling the parasite to survive in the outside environment for a period ranging from days to a year, depending on the species and conditions. Cysts formed in tissues do not usually have a heavy protective wall and rely upon carnivorism for

TABLE 77-1 Classification of Parasitic Protozoa
and Associated Diseases

Phylum		Subphylum	Representative Genera	Major Diseases Produced in Human Beings	Chapter
Sarcomastigophora (with flagella, pseudopodia, or both)		Mastigophora (flagella)	*Leishmania*	Visceral, cutaneous and mucocutaneous infection	82
			Trypanosoma	Sleeping sickness Chagas disease	
			Giardia	Diarrhea	80
			Trichomonas	Vaginitis	
		Sarcodina (pseudopodia)	*Entamoeba*	Dysentery, liver abscess	79
			Dientamoeba	Colitis	
			Naegleria and *Acanthamoeba*	Central nervous system and corneal ulcers	81
Apicomplexa (apical complex)			*Babesia*	Babesiosis	
			Plasmodium	Malaria	83
			Isospora	Diarrhea	80
			Sarcocystis	Diarrhea	
			Cryptosporidium	Diarrhea	
			Toxoplasma	Toxoplasmosis	84
Ciliophora (with cilia)			*Balantidium*	Dysentery	80
Unclassified		—	*Pneumocystis*	Pneumonia	85

transmission. **Oocysts** are stages resulting from sexual reproduction in the Apicomplexa. Some apicomplexan oocysts are passed in the feces of the host, but the oocysts of *Plasmodium,* the agent of malaria, develop in the body cavity of the mosquito vector.

REPRODUCTION

Reproduction in the Protozoa may be asexual, as in the amebas and flagellates that infect humans, or both asexual and sexual, as in the Apicomplexa of medical importance. The most common type of asexual multiplication is binary fission, in which the organelles are duplicated and the protozoan then divides into two complete organisms. Division is longitudinal in the flagellates and transverse in the ciliates; amebas have no apparent anterior-posterior axis. **Endodyogeny** is a form of sexual division seen in *Toxoplasma* and some related organisms. Two daughter cells form within the parent cell, which then ruptures, releasing the smaller progeny which grow to full size before repeating the process. In **schizogony,** a common form of asexual division in the Apicomplexa, the nucleus divides a number of times, and then the cytoplasm divides into smaller uninucleate merozoites. In *Plasmodium, Toxoplasma,* and other apicomplexans, the sexual cycle involves the production of gametes (**gamogony**), fertilization to form the zygote, encystation of the zygote to form an oocyst, and the formation of infective sporozoites (**sporogony**) within the oocyst.

Some protozoa have complex life cycles requiring two different host species; others require only a single host to complete the life cycle. A single infective protozoan entering a susceptible host has the potential to produce an immense population. However, reproduction is limited by events such as death of the host or by the host's defense mechanisms, which may either eliminate the parasite or balance parasite reproduction to yield a chronic infection. For example, malaria can result when only a few sporozoites of *Plasmodium falciparum* — perhaps ten or fewer in rare instances — are introduced by a feeding *Anopheles* mosquito into a person with no immunity. Repeated cycles of schizogony in the bloodstream can result in the infection of 10 percent or more of the erythrocytes — about 400 million parasites per milliliter of blood.

NUTRITION

The nutrition of all protozoa is **holozoic;** that is, they require organic materials, which may be particulate or in solution. Amebas engulf particulate food or droplets through a sort of temporary mouth, perform digestion and absorption in a food vacuole, and eject the waste substances. Many protozoa have a permanent mouth, the cytostome or *micropore,* through which ingested food passes to become enclosed in food vacuoles. **Pinocytosis** is a method of ingesting nutrient materials whereby fluid is drawn through small, temporary openings in the body wall. The ingested material becomes enclosed within a membrane to form a food vacuole.

Protozoa have metabolic pathways similar to those of higher animals and require the same types of organic and inorganic compounds. In recent years, significant advances have been made in devising chemically defined media for the in vitro cultivation of parasitic protozoa. The resulting organisms are free of various substances that are present in organisms grown in complex media or isolated from a host and which can interfere with immunologic or biochemical studies. Research on the metabolism of parasites is of immediate interest because pathways that are essential for the parasite but not the host are potential targets for

antiprotozoal compounds that would block that pathway but be safe for humans. Many antiprotozoal drugs were used empirically long before their mechanism of action was known. The sulfa drugs, which block folate synthesis in malaria parasites, are one example. The rapid multiplication rate of many parasites increases the chances for mutation; hence, changes in virulence, drug susceptibility, and other characteristics may take place. Chloroquine resistance in *Plasmodium falciparum* and arsenic resistance in *Trypanosoma rhodesiense* are two examples.

Competition for nutrients is not usually an important factor in pathogenesis because the amounts utilized by parasitic protozoa are relatively small. Some parasites that inhabit the small intestine can significantly interfere with digestion and absorption and affect the nutritional status of the host; *Giardia* and *Cryptosporidium* are examples. The destruction of the host's cells and tissues as a result of the parasites' metabolic activities increases the host's nutritional needs. This may be a major factor in the outcome of an infection in a malnourished individual. Finally, extracellular or intracellular parasites that destroy cells while feeding can lead to organ dysfunction and serious or life-threatening consequences.

REFERENCES

Beaver PC, Jung RC (eds): Animal Agents and Vectors of Human Disease. 5th Ed. Lea & Febiger, Philadelphia, 1985

Englund PT, Sher A (eds): The Biology of Parasitism. A Molecular and Immunological Approach. Alan R Liss, New York, 1988

Goldsmith R, Heyneman D (eds): Tropical Medicine and Parasitology. Appleton and Lange, East Norwalk, CT, 1989

Lee JJ, Hutner SH, Bovee EC (eds): An Illustrated Guide to the Protozoa. Society of Protozoologists, Lawrence, KS, 1985

Trager W: Living Together, The Biology of Animal Parasitism. Plenum, New York, 1986

78 PROTOZOA: PATHOGENESIS AND DEFENSES

JOHN RICHARD SEED

GENERAL CONCEPTS

Resistance

Resistance is the ability of a host to defend itself against a pathogen. Resistance to protozoan parasites involves three interrelated mechanisms: nonspecific factors, cellular immunity, and humoral immunity.

Pathology

Protozoal infection results in tissue damage leading to disease. In chronic infections the tissue damage is often due to an immune response to the parasite and/or to host antigens; alternatively, it may be due to toxic protozoal products and/or to mechanical damage.

Escape Mechanisms

Escape mechanisms are strategies by which parasites avoid the killing effect of the immune system in an immunocompetent host. Escape mechanisms used by protozoan parasites include the following.

Antigenic Masking: Antigenic masking is the ability of a parasite to escape immune detection by covering itself with host antigens.

Blocking of Serum Factors: Some parasites acquire a coating of antigen-antibody complexes or noncytotoxic antibodies that sterically blocks the binding of specific antibody or lymphocytes to the parasite surface antigens.

Intracellular Location: The intracellular habitat of some protozoan parasites protects them from the direct effects of the host's immune response. By concealing the parasite antigens, this strategy also delays detection by the immune system.

Antigenic Variation: Some protozoan parasites change their surface antigens during the course of an infection. Parasites carrying the new antigens escape the immune response to the original antigens.

Immunosuppression: Parasitic protozoan infections generally produce some degree of host immunosuppression. This reduced immune response may delay detection of antigenic variants. It may also reduce the ability of the immune system to inhibit the growth of and/or to kill the parasites.

INTRODUCTION

Resistance to parasitic protozoa appears to be similar to resistance against other infectious agents, although the mechanisms of resistance in protozoan infections are not yet as well understood. Resistance can be divided into two main groups of mechanisms: (1) nonspecific mechanism(s) or factor(s) such as the presence of a nonspecific serum component that is lethal to the parasite; and (2) specific mechanism(s) involving the immune system (Fig. 78-1). Probably the best studied nonspecific mechanisms involved in parasite resistance are the ones that control the susceptibility of red blood cells to invasion or growth of plasmodia, the agents of malaria. Individuals who are heterozygous or homozygous for the sickle cell hemoglobin trait are considerably more resistant to *Plasmodium falciparum* than individuals with normal hemoglobin. Similarly, individuals who lack the Duffy factor on their red blood cells are not susceptible to *P vivax*. Possibly both the sickle cell trait and absence of the Duffy factor have become established in malaria-endemic populations as a result of selective pressure exerted by malaria. Epidemiologic evidence suggests that other inherited red blood cell abnormalities, such as thalassaemia and glucose-6-phosphate dehydrogenase deficiency, may contribute to survival of individuals in various malaria-endemic geographical regions. A second well-documented example of a nonspecific factor involved in resistance is the presence in the serum of humans of a trypanolytic factor that confers resistance against *Trypanosoma brucei brucei,* an agent of trypanosomiasis (sleeping sickness) in animals. There is evidence that other nonspecific factors, such as fever and the sex of the host, may also contribute to the host's resistance to various protozoan parasites. Although nonspecific factors can play a key role in resistance, usually they work in conjunction with the host's immune system (Fig. 78-1).

Different parasites elicit different humoral and/or cellular immune responses. In malaria and trypanosome infections, antibody appears to play a major role in immunity. In both *T cruzi* and *T brucei gambiense* infections (human sleeping sickness), antibody-dependent cytotoxicity reactions against the parasite have been reported. Although antibody has been shown to be responsible for

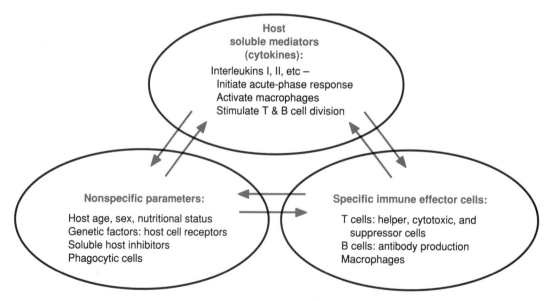

FIGURE 78-1 Some interrelationships between host factors involved in resistance to protozoan infections.

clearing the African trypanosomes from the blood of infected animals, recent evidence suggests that the survival time of infected mice does not necessarily correlate with the ability of the animal to produce trypanosome-specific antibody. In other words, resistance, as measured by survival time, may not solely involve the specific humoral immune system. Recent data suggest that cellular immunity is required for resistance to malaria. For example, vaccine trials with a sporozoite antigen indicated that both an active cellular response and sporozoite-specific antibody may be needed for successful immunization.

Cellular immunity is believed to be the single most important defense mechanism in leishmaniasis and toxoplasmosis. In animals infected with *Toxoplasma,* the activated macrophage has been shown to play an important role in resistance. Accordingly, resistance to the protozoan parasites most likely involves nonspecific factors as well as specific humoral and/or cellular mechanisms.

Unlike most viral and bacterial infections, protozoan diseases are often chronic, lasting months or years. When associated with a strong host immune response, this type of chronic infection is apt to result in a high incidence of immunopathology. The question also arises of how these parasites survive in an immunocompetent animal. The remainder of this chapter treats the mechanisms responsible for pathology, particularly immunopa-

thology, in protozoan disease, and the mechanisms by which parasites evade the immune responses of the host. Finally, because of the very rapid advances in our knowledge of the host-parasite relationship (due primarily to the development of techniques in molecular biology) it is necessary to briefly mention the potential for developing vaccines to the pathogenic protozoa.

PATHOLOGY

The immunopathology of a variety of parasitic protozoan diseases has been described. For the most part, the protozoa elicit humoral responses in which antigen-antibody complexes in the region of antibody excess activate Hageman blood coagulation factor (Factor XII), which in turn activates the coagulation, fibrinolytic, kinin, and complement systems. It has been suggested that this type of immediate hypersensitivity is responsible for various clinical syndromes in African trypanosomiasis, including blood hyperviscosity, edema, and hypotension. Similar disease mechanisms would be expected in other protozoan diseases involving a strong humoral immune response (Table 78-1).

Immune complexes have been found circulating in serum and deposited in the kidneys and other tissues of humans and animals infected with protozoans. These parasite antigen-antibody complexes, plus complement, have been eluted from

TABLE 78-1 Some Pathologic Mechanisms in Protozoal Diseases

Mechanism	Possible Examples
Toxic parasite products:	
High molecular weight (e.g., hydrolytic enzymes)	Presumably all parasitic protozoal infections
Low molecular weight	African trypanosomiasis
Immediate-type hypersensitivity	Malaria
	African trypanosomiasis
Delayed-type hypersensitivity	Leishmaniasis
	Amebiasis
	Toxoplasmosis
Autoimmunity	American trypanosomiasis
Immunosuppression	Malaria
	African trypanosomiasis
	Possibly many protozoal infections
Mechanical tissue damage	Malaria

kidney tissue in cases of malaria and African trypanosomiasis. Antigen and antibody have been directly visualized in the glomeruli of infected animals by light and electron microscopy. Inflammatory cell infiltrates accompany these deposits, and signs of glomerulonephritis are usually seen. African trypanosomes and presumably their antigens are also found in a variety of extravascular locations. Immune complexes, cellular infiltrates, and tissue damage have been detected in these tissues.

Another important form of antibody-mediated pathology is autoimmunity. Autoantibodies to a number of different host antigens (for example, red blood cells, laminin, collagen, and DNA) have been demonstrated. These autoantibodies may play a role in the pathology of parasitic diseases in two ways. First the antibodies may exert a direct cytotoxic effect on the host cells; for example, autoantibodies that coat red blood cells produce hemolytic anemia. Alternatively, autoantibodies may be pathogenic through a buildup of antigen-antibody complexes in the kidneys or other tissues, leading to glomerulonephritis or other forms of immediate hypersensitivity. A particularly good example of a protozoan infection in which autoimmunity appears to be an important contributor to pathogenesis is *T cruzi* infection. In this case, there is substantial evidence that host and parasite share cross-reacting antigens. Antibodies and cytotoxic lymphocytes to these antigens appear to be harmful to host tissue. This type of experimental data, combined with the fact that the parasite itself seems not to cause the tissue pathology, lead one to conclude that autoimmunity may play a key role in pathogenesis.

Cellular hypersensitivity is also observed in protozoan diseases (Table 78-1). For example, in leishmaniasis (caused by *Leishmania tropica*), the lesions appear to be caused by a cell-mediated immune response and have many if not all of the characteristics of granulomas observed in tuberculosis or schistosomiasis. In these lesions, a continuing immune response to pathogens that are able to escape the host's defense mechanisms causes further influx of inflammatory cells, which leads to sustained reactions and continued pathology at the sites of antigen deposition. During a

parasitic infection, various host cell products (cytokines, lymphokines, etc.) are released from activated cells of the immune system. These mediators influence the action of other cells and may be directly involved in pathogenesis. An example is tumor necrosis factor (TNF), which is released by lymphocytes. TNF may be involved in the muscle wasting observed in the chronic stages of African trypanosomiasis. However, in contrast to its apparent role in pathology, TNF also has been thought to contribute to resistance to malaria by inhibiting the growth of plasmodia. It is important to recognize that mediators involved in resistance to protozoan parasites may also lead to pathology during a chronic infection (Fig. 78-1). There appears to be a delicate balance between the factors involved in resistance to infectious agents and those which ultimately produce pathology and clinical disease.

Numerous authors have suggested that toxic products produced by parasitic protozoa are responsible for at least some aspects of pathology (Table 78-1). For example, the glycoproteins on the surface of trypanosomes have been found to fix complement. This activation of complement presumably results in the production of biologically active and toxic complement fragments. In addition, trypanosomes are known to release proteases and phospholipases when they lyse the host cell. These enzymes can produce host cell destruction, inflammatory responses, and gross tissue pathology. Furthermore, it has been hypothesized that the trypanosomes contain a B-cell mitogen that may alter the immune response of the host by eliciting a polyclonal B cell response that leads to immunosuppression. Parasitic protozoa have also been reported to synthesize (or contain) low-molecular-weight toxins. For example, the trypanosomes produce several indole catabolites; at pharmacologic doses, some of these catabolites can produce pathologic effects, such as fever, lethargy, and even immunosuppression. Similarly, enzymes, B-cell mitogen, etc., are presumably released by many if not all of the other parasitic protozoa. There has been limited work on the role of these protozoal products in pathogenesis. However, parasitic protozoa are not known to produce toxins with potencies comparable to those of the classic bacterial toxins (such as the toxins responsible for anthrax and botulism).

Immune Escape

Parasite escape mechanisms may include a number of different phenomena (Table 78-2). In **antigenic masking,** the parasite becomes coated with host components and so fails to be recognized as foreign. In **blocking,** noncytotoxic antibody combines with parasite antigens and inhibits the binding of cytotoxic antibodies or cells. The parasite may pass part of its life cycle in an intracellular location, for example, in erythrocytes or macrophages, in which it is sheltered from intracellular digestion and from the cytotoxic action of antibody and/or lymphocytes. Some parasites practice **antigenic variation,** altering their surface antigens during the course of an infection and thus evading the host's immune responses. Finally, the parasite may cause **immunosuppression,** reducing the host's immune response either to the parasite specifically or to foreign antigens in general. These strategies are discussed in more detail below.

Masking and Mimicry

Various species of trypanosomes have host immunoglobulins associated with their cell surfaces. There are several reports that these antibodies are not bound to the trypanosomes through their variable regions, but presumably through the Fc portion of their molecule. These antibodies may mask the parasite—that is, prevent immune recognition by the host. However, no evidence other than the presence of immunoglobulins on the surface of the trypanosomes supports this hypothesis. *Mimicry,* in which the parasite has the genetic information to synthesize antigens identical to those of its host, has not been demonstrated in parasitic protozoa.

Blocking

It has been hypothesized that in some cases antigen-antibody complexes in serum of infected animals bind to the parasite's surface, mechanically blocking the actions of cytotoxic antibodies or lymphocytes and directly inhibiting the actions of lymphocytes. This type of immune escape mechanism has been proposed for tumor cells and for the parasitic helminths. Since the trypanosomes carry immunoglobulins on their cell surfaces, they may use a similar mechanism; however, no direct evidence has yet been reported.

Intracellular Location

Many protozoan parasites grow and divide within host cells. For example, *Plasmodium* parasites grow first in hepatocytes then in red blood cells. *Leishmania* and *Toxoplasma* organisms are capable of growing in macrophages; one genus of parasitic protozoa, *Theilera,* not only multiplies in lympho-

TABLE 78-2 Some Proposed Immune Escape
Mechanisms Used by Protozoan Parasites

Mechanisms	Possible Examples
Antigenic variation	African trypanosomes
	Plasmodium
	Giardia
Masked or shared host antigens	African trypanosomes
Blocking	No documented examples
Intracellular sites	American trypanosomes
	Plasmodium
	Leishmania
	Toxoplasma
Immunosuppression	African trypanosomes
	American trypanosomes

cytes but appears even to stimulate the multiplication of the infected lymphocytes. Although some parasites, such as *Plasmodium,* are restricted to a limited number of host cell types, others, such as *Trypanosoma cruzi* and *Toxoplasma,* appear to be able to grow and divide in a variety of different host cells.

An intracellular refuge may protect a parasite from the harmful or lethal effects of antibody or cellular defense mechanisms. For example, *Plasmodium* may be susceptible to the actions of antibody only during the brief extracellular phases of its life cycle (the sporozoite and merozoite stages). It should be remembered that *Plasmodium* actually resides in a membrane-bound vacuole in the host cell. Thus, plasmodia are shielded from the external environment by at least two host membranes (the outer cell membrane and an inner vacuole membrane). Although intracellular plasmodia are very well protected from the host's immune response early in their growth, this strategy does create physiologic problems for the parasite. For example, the parasite must obtain its nutrients for growth through three membranes (two host and one parasite), and must eliminate its waste products through the same three membranes. Plasmodia solve this problem by appropriately modifying the host cell membranes. Parasitic proteins are incorporated into the red blood cell outer membrane. The host eventually responds to these antigens, and this response ultimately leads to the increased removal of infected host cells.

The existence of extracellular phases in the malaria life cycle is important, since immunization against these stages is the rationale for the development of our current vaccine candidates. The protective antigens on these extracellular stages have been purified as potential antigens for a vaccine. However, this approach has problems. For example, the sporozoite stage is exposed to protective antibody for only a brief period, and even a single sporozoite that escapes immune elimination will lead to an infection. Second, the antigenic variability of different isolates and the ability of different strains to undergo antigenic variation are not fully known. Therefore, the effectiveness of the vaccine candidates must still be demonstrated. However,

there is optimism that in the next 10 years, a recombinant or synthetic sporozoite surface peptide vaccine against falciparum malaria will be developed.

A number of parasitic protozoa reside in macrophages. Although these organisms are protected from external immune threats, they must still evade digestion by the macrophage. Three strategies have been suggested. First, the parasite may prevent the fusion of lysosomes with the phagocytic vacuole. The actual mechanism responsible for this inhibition is not yet understood, but it has been shown to occur in cells infected with *Toxoplasma.* A second mechanism is represented by the ability of *Trypanosoma cruzi* to escape from the phagocytic vacuole into the cytoplasm of the macrophage. Finally, it is possible that some parasites can survive in the presence of lysosomal enzymes, as can the leprosy bacillus. One of the best-studied examples of a protozoan parasite able to survive in the phagolysosome is *Leishmania.* It has been suggested that the resistance of this parasite to the host's hydrolytic enzymes is due to surface components that inhibit the host's enzymes and/or to the presence of parasitic enzymes that hydrolyze the host's enzymes. As previously noted, at least one protozoan parasite, *Theilera,* is capable of growing directly in lymphocytes. Therefore, this parasite may escape the host's immune response by growing inside the very cells required for the response.

Antigenic Variation

Three major groups of parasitic protozoa are known to be able to change the antigenic properties of their surface coat. The African trypanosomes can completely replace the antigens in their glycocalyx each time the host exhibits a new humoral response. The best evidence suggests these changes in surface coat are phenotypic and possibly induced by an external environmental factor. These alterations in serotype are one important way in which the African trypanosomes escape their host's defense mechanisms. Although less well characterized, similar changes are reported to occur in *Plasmodium, Babesia,* and *Giardia.*

It has been estimated that African trypanosomes

have approximately 1,000 different genes coding for surface antigen. These genes are located on various chromosomes; however, to be expressed, the gene must be located at the end of a chromosome (telomeric site). The rate at which variation occurs in a tsetse-fly-transmitted population appears quite high. It has been shown that 1 in 10^2 cells appears to be capable of switching its surface antigen. The order in which the surface coat genes are expressed is not predictable. Much information is available on the nucleotide sequence of the genes coding the coat proteins; however, neither the factor(s) that induces a cell to switch its surface antigens nor the specific genetic mechanisms involved in the switch have been determined. Apparently, the antibody response does not induce the genetic switch, but merely selects variants with new surface antigens out of the original population. Considerably less information is available on the phenomenon of antigenic variation in malaria or babesiosis. However, antigenic variation could be a major problem in reference to the development of a blood stage (merozoite) vaccine for malaria. Finally, antigenic variation has been found in *Giardia lamblia*. At present, neither the number of different genes coding for *Giardia* surface proteins nor the actual biologic importance of this variability is known. However, antigenic variation may assist *Giardia* in escaping the host's immune response.

Immunosuppression

Immunosuppression of the host has been observed with almost every parasitic organism carefully examined to date. In some cases the suppression is specific, involving only the host's response to the parasite. In other cases the suppression is much more general, involving the response to various heterologous and nonparasite antigens. It has not yet been proven that this immunosuppression allows the parasites to survive in a normally immunocompetent host. However, one can postulate that immunosuppression could permit a small number of parasites to escape immune surveillance, thus favoring establishment of a chronic infection. This mechanism might be particularly effective in parasites that undergo antigenic variation, since it could allow the small number of parasites with new surface antigens to go undetected initially. Immunosuppression experimentally induced by various extraneous agents has certainly been shown to produce higher parasitemias, higher infection rates, or both. Therefore, the hypothesis that parasite-induced immunosuppression increases the chance for a parasite to complete its life cycle makes sense.

It should be noted that immunosuppression can be pathogenic in itself. A reduced response to heterologous antigens could favor secondary infections. Humans suffering from malaria or trypanosomiasis have been shown to be immunosuppressed to a variety of heterologous antigens. Secondary infections may often be involved in death from African trypanosomiasis.

A variety of mechanisms have been suggested to explain the immunosuppression observed in protozoan infections. The most common mechanisms proposed are (1) the presence in the infected host of parasite or host substances that nonspecifically stimulate the growth of antibody-producing B cells, rather than stimulating the proliferation of specific anti-parasite B-cells; (2) proliferation of suppressor T-cells and/or macrophages that inhibit the immune system; and (3) production by the parasite of specific immune suppressor substances.

REFERENCES

Aggarwal A, Nash TE: Antigen variation of *Giardia lamblia* in vivo. Infect Immun 56:1420, 1988

Blackwell JM: Protozoan infections. In Wakelin DM, Blackwell JM (eds): Genetics of Resistance to Bacterial and Parasitic Infections. Taylor & Francis, Philadelphia, 1988

Capron A, Dessaint JP: Molecular basis of host-parasite relationship: towards the definition of protective antigens. Immun Rev 112:27, 1989

Denis M, Chadee K: Immunopathology of *Entamoeba histolytica* infections. Parasitol Today 4:247, 1988

Dyer M, Tait A: Control of lymphoproliferation by *Theilera anulata*. Parasitol Today. 3:309, 1987

Englund PT, Sher A (eds): The Biology of Parasitism. Alan R Liss, New York, 1989

Frenkel JK: Pathophysiology of toxoplasmosis. Parasitol Today 4:273, 1988

Hadley TJ, Klotz FW, Miller LH: Invasion of erythrocytes by malaria parasites: A cellular and molecular overview. Ann Rev Microbiol 40:457, 1986

Mock BA, Nacy CA: Hormonal modulation of sex differences in resistance to *Leishmania major* systemic infections. Infect Immun 56:3316, 1988

Tizard I, Nielsen KH, Seed JR, Hall JE: Biologically active products from African trypanosomes. Microbiol Rev 42:661, 1978

Turner M: Antigenic variation in the parasitic protozoa. In Birbeck TH, Penn CW (eds): Antigenic Variation in Infectious Diseases. IRL Press, Oxford, UK, 1986

Wakelin D: Immunity to Parasites: How Animals Control Parasitic Infections. Edward Arnold, London, UK, 1984

79 INTESTINAL PROTOZOA: AMEBAS, *DIENTAMOEBA*

WILLIAM A. SODEMAN, JR.

GENERAL CONCEPTS

ENTAMOEBA HISTOLYTICA

Clinical Manifestations

Patients have acute or chronic diarrhea, which may progress to dysentery. Extraintestinal disease may present as a complication or as a primary problem (e.g., liver, lung or brain abscess, or skin or perianal infection).

Structure

The trophozoite is 10 to 60 μm in diameter, ameboid, actively motile, and often erythrophagocytic. In stained specimens, the nucleus has a central karyosome with finely beaded peripheral chromatin. The cyst form is rounded, 10 to 20 μm in diameter, with one to four nuclei showing the characteristic appearance. A chromatoidal bar with rounded or square ends may be seen.

Classification and Antigenic Types

Pathogenic strains can be grown at 37°C but not at room temperature and fall into specific enzyme assay groups.

Multiplication and Life Cycle

Multiplication in the host occurs by binary fission. Nuclear replication produces four nuclei during cyst maturation. During excystation the cyst divides to form four cells which immediately divide again to yield eight tiny amebae.

Pathogenesis

The colon may be colonized without invasion of mucosa. Invasion of the mucosa produces ulcers that sometimes progress by direct extension or by metastasis. Metastatic infection first involves the liver. Extension or metastasis from the liver may involve the lung, brain, or other viscera.

Host Defenses

Gastric acid and rapid intestinal transit are nonspecific defenses. Humoral antibody and cell-mediated immunity play limited roles in preventing dissemination.

Epidemiology

Fecal-oral transmission of cysts involves contaminated food or water. Amebas can be transmitted directly by sexual contact involving the anus.

Diagnosis

Acute diarrhea is particularly associated with blood in stool and/or with a visceral abscess. The condition may be confirmed by identification of *E histolytica* in the stool or in abscess aspirates. Parasite can be cultured. Positive serologic tests, particularly tests showing a rising antibody titer, may provide indirect evidence of infection.

Control

Prevention is largely a matter of personal and public hygiene. There is no effective immunization or prophylaxis. Various drugs are used to treat the different clinical syndromes.

DIENTAMOEBA FRAGILIS

Clinical Manifestations

Dientamoeba fragilis causes acute and chronic diarrhea without mucosal invasion or extraintestinal involvement.

Structure

The trophozoite is 3 to 20 μm in diameter, ameboid, and actively motile. There is no cyst form. Stained nuclei show clumping of chromatin around the central karyosome with an otherwise clear nucleoplasm.

Multiplication and Life Cycle

Multiplication in the host occurs by binary fission. Survival outside the host is limited, and multiplication outside of host has not been described.

Pathogenesis

Fecal-oral transmission involves contaminated food or water.

Host Defenses

Dientamoeba fragilis does not seem to stimulate an immune response in the host, and reinfection occurs.

Epidemiology

Transmission is through contaminated food or water, much as with *E histolytica*. Possibly the parasite is also transmitted in *Enterobius* eggs.

Diagnosis

In patients with acute gastroenteritis, diagnosis can be confirmed by identifying *D fragilis* in stool. The parasite can also be cultured.

Control

Prevention is a matter of safe sanitation and good personal hygiene. Effective treatment is available.

INTRODUCTION

Amebas are unicellular organisms common in the environment; many are parasites of vertebrates and invertebrates. Relatively few species inhabit the human intestine and only *Entamoeba histolytica* is identified as a human intestinal pathogen. A second pathogen of the human colon is *Dientamoeba fragilis*, which looks like an ameba under the light microscope, and was classified as a true ameba for many years, but which is now classified as a flagellate. Because *D fragilis* does not invade tissues, the mechanism by which it produces symptomatic diarrhea remains obscure. *Entamoeba histolytica*, on the other hand, although it often lives as a harmless commensal in the digestive tract, harbors the capacity to penetrate the intestinal mucosa and cause ulceration. The infection sometimes spreads by direct extension or metastasis to other organs, such as the liver or the lung.

ENTAMOEBA HISTOLYTICA

CLINICAL MANIFESTATIONS

Figures 79-1 and 79-2 present an overview of the life cycle of the ameba and the pathogenesis of amebic infections. Pathogenic and nonpathogenic strains of *E histolytica* may inhabit the human digestive tract. Even pathogenic strains may live in the lumen as benign commensals. If mucosal invasion occurs, it may be limited to a few simple superficial erosions or it may progress to total involvement of the colonic mucosa with ulceration. Table 79-1 presents a World Health Organization classification of the clinical syndromes and related pathophysiologic mechanisms of *E histolytica* infections. The clinical manifestations vary with the extent of involvement. Mucosal erosion causes diarrhea, which increases in severity with increasing

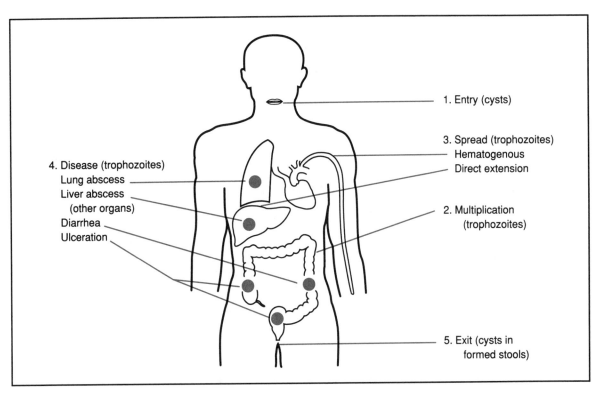

FIGURE 79-1 Pathogenesis of *E histolytica* infection.

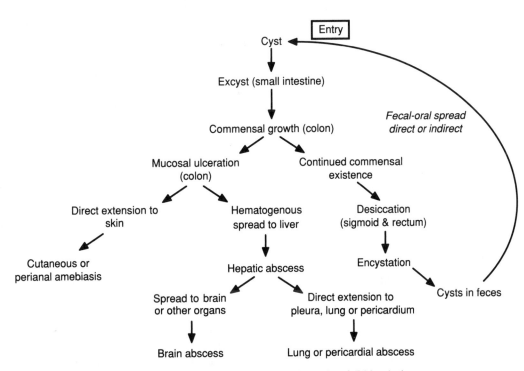

FIGURE 79-2 Multiplication and life cycle of *E histolytica*.

TABLE 79-1   Classification of Amebiasis

WHO Clinical Classification of Amebiasis Infection (Modified)	Pathophysiologic Mechanisms
Asymptomatic infection	Colonization without tissue invasion
Symptomatic infection	Invasive infection
Intestinal amebiasis	
A. Amebic dysentery	Fulminant ulcerative intestinal disease
B. Nondysentery gastroenteritis	Ulcerative intestinal disease
C. Ameboma	Proliferative intestinal disease
D. Complicated intestinal amebiasis	Perforation, hemorrhage, fistula
E. Post-amebic colitis	Mechanism unknown
Extraintestinal amebiasis	
A. Nonspecific hepatomegaly	Intestinal infection with no demonstrable invasion
B. Acute nonspecific infection	Amebas in liver but without abscess
C. Amebic abscess	Focal structural lesion
D. Amebic abscess, complicated	Direct extension to pleura, lung, peritoneum, or pericardium
E. Amebiasis cutis	Direct extension to skin
F. Visceral amebiasis	Metastatic infection of lung, spleen, or brain

area of involvement. Symptoms are also affected by the site of the infection. The more distal the lesion in the colon, the greater the likelihood and severity of symptoms; thus, small rectal lesions are more likely to be symptomatic than larger cecal lesions. Rectal bleeding is only slightly less common than diarrhea and is usually but not invariably associated with diarrhea. Urgency, tenesmus, cramping abdominal pain in association with bowel movements, and abdominal tenderness may be present.

The intestinal syndromes caused by *E histolytica* form a continuum ranging in severity from mild diarrhea to hemorrhagic dysentery. The span from mild to severe diarrhea is classified as **nondysentery colitis** (Table 79-1). **Amebic dysentery** has a dramatically different clinical presentation. The diarrhea is replaced by dysenteric stools consisting largely of pus and blood without feces. There is evidence of systemic toxicity with fever, dehydration, and electrolyte abnormalities. Tenesmus and abdominal tenderness are regular features. This fulminant presentation may occur suddenly or evolve from less severe, pre-existing disease.

Occasionally, and for no apparent reason, colonic infection with *E histolytica* will evoke a proliferative granulomatous response at an ulcer. This infectious pseudotumor, called an **ameboma,** may become the leading point of an intussusception or may cause intestinal obstruction. However, these complications are uncommon.

Peritonitis as a result of perforation has been reported in connection with severe amebic colitis and, much less often, in patients with few or no symptoms. Other complications of intestinal amebiasis include colocutaneous fistula, perianal ulceration, urogenital infection, colonic stricture, intussusception, and hemorrhage. Most of these complications are uncommon and therefore may prove difficult to diagnose. The term *postamebic colitis* is used for nonspecific colitis following a bout of severe acute amebic colitis. In such cases, the colon is free of parasites and the clinical findings resemble those of chronic ulcerative colitis.

Extraintestinal amebiasis begins with hepatic involvement. Many patients with acute intestinal infection also have hepatomegaly, but in these cases amebas are not demonstrable in the liver and the pathogenesis of the hepatomegaly is not clear. A focal amebic abscess in the liver, on the other hand, represents metastasis of intestinal infection. Symptomatic intestinal infection need not be present. The abscess appears as a slowly enlarging liver mass. Often the patient will have right upper quadrant pain, which may be referred to the right shoulder. If the abscess is located in a palpable portion of the liver, the area will be tender. Occasionally the enlarging abscess presses on the hepatic duct and causes jaundice. If located under the dome of the diaphragm, the abscess may press on the right lung base, causing atelectasis and physical findings of consolidation. As the abscess nears the diaphragm it may stimulate pleural effusion.

Pleural, pulmonary, and pericardial infection occurs as a result of direct extension from the liver. Lung involvement is far more common than pericardial infection. Infection metastatic from the liver can involve other viscera or can give rise to a brain abscess. However, these complications are uncommon.

STRUCTURE

E histolytica has a relatively simple life cycle that consists of trophozoite and cyst stages (Figs. 79-1 and 79-2). The trophozoite is the actively metabolizing, motile stage and the cyst is dormant and environmentally resistant. Diagnostic concern centers on both stages (Fig. 79-3 and Table 79-2). Trophozoites vary remarkably in size — from 10 to 60 μm or more in diameter — and when they are alive they may be actively motile. Amebas are anaerobic organisms and do not have mitochondria. The finely granular endoplasm contains the nucleus and food vacuoles, which in turn may contain bacteria or red blood cells. The parasite is sheathed by a clear outer ectoplasm. Nuclear morphology is best seen in permanent stained preparations. The nucleus has a distinctive central karyosome and a rim of finely beaded chromatin lining the nuclear membrane.

The cyst is a spherical structure, 10-20 μm in diameter, with a thin, transparent wall. Fully mature cysts contain four nuclei with the characteristic amebic morphology. Rod-like structures (*chromatoidal bars*) are variably present but are more common in immature cysts. Inclusions in the form of glycogen masses also may be present.

A number of nonpathogenic amebae can parasi-

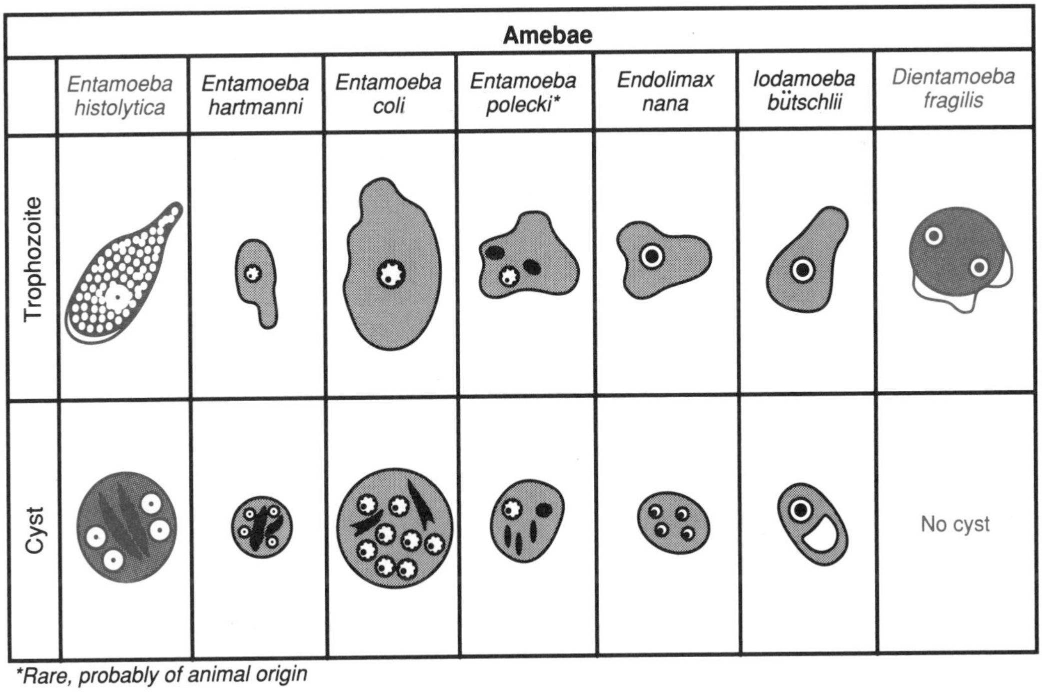

Amebae						
Entamoeba histolytica	*Entamoeba hartmanni*	*Entamoeba coli*	*Entamoeba polecki**	*Endolimax nana*	*Iodamoeba bütschlii*	*Dientamoeba fragilis*

Trophozoite / **Cyst** (No cyst under *Dientamoeba fragilis*)

Rare, probably of animal origin

FIGURE 79-3 Amebas found in stool specimens of humans. (Modified from Brooke MM, Melvin DM: Morphology of diagnostic stages of intestinal parasites of man. Public Health Service Publication No. 1966, 1969.)

Table 79-2   Intestinal Amebas and *Dientamoeba* of Humans

Organism	Size (μm)		Trophozoite		Cyst		
	Trophozoite	Cyst	Motility (Fresh)	Nuclei (Stained)	Nuclei (Numbers)	Chromatoidals	Remarks
Entamoeba histolytica	10–60	10–20 Round	Active	Karyosome small and central; chromatin, fine and peripheral	1–6	Ends rounded or square	Pathogenic
Entamoeba hartmanni	4–12	5–10 Round	Active	Karyosome small and central; chromatin fine and peripheral	1–4	Ends rounded or square	Nonpathogenic
Entamoeba gingivalis	5–35	—	—	Karyosome small and central; chromatin fine and peripheral	—	—	Mouth-dwelling nonpathogenic
Entamoeba polecki	10–20	5–10 Round	Sluggish	Karyosome small and central; chromatin variable	1	Ends pointed	Rare in humans; nonpathogenic
Entamoeba moshkovskii	10–60	5–20 Round	—	Karyosome small and central; chromatin fine and peripheral	1–4	Ends rounded	Nonpathogenic
Entamoeba coli	10–50	10–35	Sluggish	Karyosome large and eccentric; chromatin clumpy and peripheral	1–8	Ends jagged	Nonpathogenic
Endolimax nana	6–15	4–14 Oval	Sluggish	Karyosome large and variable; little or no chromatin	1–4	None	Nonpathogenic
Iodamoeba bütschlii	6–25	6–20	Active	Karyosome large and central; chromatin absent	1	None	Nonpathogenic
Dientamoeba fragilis	3–20	—	Active	Karyosome central; four to eight central chromatin granules	—	—	Pathogenic

tize the human gastrointestinal tract and may cause diagnostic confusion. These include *Entamoeba hartmanni, Entamoeba gingivalis, Entamoeba coli, Endolimax nana,* and *Iodamoeba bütschlii* (Fig. 79-3 and Table 79-2).

CLASSIFICATION

Many infections with *E histolytica* occur without evidence of invasion of the intestinal lining. Virulence in the ameba—the ability to produce intestinal invasion or extraintestinal disease—is a heritable characteristic. Morphologically identical amebas may be identified as pathogenic or nonpathogenic on the basis of size, culture characteristics, virulence in a rat model, selective agglutination by lectins, reaction with monoclonal antibodies, or isoenzyme patterns.

A number of nonpathogenic but apparently genuine *E histolytica* strains have been isolated from human carriers. These amebas can be cultured at room temperature as well as at 37°C and will grow in hypotonic media, whereas pathogenic amebas require isotonic media and 37°C for growth. These low-temperature strains have isoenzyme patterns identical with the sewage-associated, nonpathogenic *Entamoeba moshkovskii.* Two classic tests to identify pathogenic strains are the ability to cause cecal ulceration in weanling rats and agglutination by the lectin concanavalin A. These tests of virulence have been supplanted by isoenzyme analysis. Monoclonal antibodies have recently been used to identify pathogenic strains of *E histolytica,* but the clinical applicability of this technique has not been tested.

Isoenzyme patterns are known for four amebic enzymes: glucose phosphate isomerase (GPI), hexokinase (HK), malate:NADP$^+$ oxidoreductase (ME), and phosphoglucomutase (PGM). The isoenzyme patterns of three of these, GPI, HK, and PGM, can be used to define 20 zymodemes of *E histolytica.* The enzyme markers associated with pathogenicity are the presence of a β band and the absence of an α band for PGM. Zymodemes II, VI, VII, XI, XII, XIII, XIV, XIX, and XX are pathogenic. Zymodemes II and XI are responsible for liver abscesses. There have been several reports of cultured amebas undergoing a change in zymodeme pattern after manipulation of associated bacterial flora. Zymodeme patterns are of epidemiologic and research interest but their limited availability makes them less useful clinically. A number of other factors, primarily environmental, that affect virulence are discussed below.

MULTIPLICATION AND LIFE CYCLE

Amebas multiply in the host by simple binary fission. Most multiplication occurs in the host, and survival outside the host depends on the desiccation-resistant cyst form. Encystment occurs apparently in response to desiccation as the ameba is carried through the colon. After encystment, the nucleus divides twice to produce the quadrinucleate mature cyst. Excystment is followed by rapid cell division to produce four amebas which undergo a second division. Each cyst thus yields eight tiny amebas.

PATHOGENESIS

The fecal-oral transmission of the ameba usually involves contaminated food or water. The parasite can also be transmitted directly by anogenital or oroanal sexual contact. Latent or commensal infections can become invasive in a setting of impaired host immunity.

Ingested cysts of *E histolytica* excyst in the small intestine (Figs. 79-1 and 79-2). Trophozoites are carried to the colon, where they mature and reproduce. The parasite may lead a commensal existence on the mucosal surface and in the crypts of the colon. Successful colonization depends on factors such as inoculum size, intestinal motility, transit time, the presence or absence of specific intestinal flora, and the host's diet. As amebas pass down the colon they encyst under the stimulus of desiccation, and then are evacuated with the stool.

The factors that lead to tissue invasion by *E histolytica* are poorly understood. The genetic virulence factors mentioned above play a major role but several environmental factors are also important. Although the mechanisms of action are not clear, both changes in the intestinal flora and the nature of the host's diet have been implicated. The discovery that the zymodeme pattern of the ameba can be altered in vitro from nonpathogenic to pathogenic by altering the culture conditions or associated bacterial flora may unify the considerations of virulence.

The initial lesion is in colonic mucosa, most often in the cecum or sigmoid colon. The slow transit of the intestinal contents in these two locations seems an important factor in invasion of the mucosa, both because it affords the ameba greater mucosal contact time and because it permits changes in the intestinal milieu that may facilitate invasion. The initial superficial ulcer may deepen into the submucosa and muscularis to become the characteristic flask-shaped, chronic amebic ulcer. Spread may occur by direct extension, by undermining of the surrounding mucosa until it sloughs, or by penetration that can lead to perforation or fistulous communication to other organs or the skin. If the amebas gain access to the vascular or lymphatic circulation, metastases may occur first to the liver and then by direct extension or further metastasis to other organs, including the brain.

Virulent *E histolytica* strains are capable of penetrating intact intestinal mucosa. The infection is not opportunistic and does not require pre-existing mucosal damage. Numerous proteases have been noted in *E histolytica;* however, the mechanism of penetration remains unclear. Metastatic foci present as abscesses with a central zone of lytic necrosis surrounded by a zone of inflammatory cell infiltration. Metastatic abscesses behave as space-occupying lesions unless they become infected or rupture.

The clinical presentation of intestinal infections depends on the extent and anatomic location of the ulceration and mucosal damage. Small, sparse ulcerations may be asymptomatic. As the involved areas of mucosa increase in size, motility disturbances occur, primarily diarrhea with cramping pain. Exudation from the denuded mucosa adds to this problem. When the mucosal involvement becomes extensive, diarrhea is replaced by dysentery, with the passage of exudate, blood, and mucus. Toxic megacolon and perforation are rare complications of extensive involvement. Systemic signs of infection include fever, rigor, and polymorphonuclear leukocytosis.

HOST DEFENSES

The gastric acid "barrier" and the steady movement of food through the intestine are nonspecific defense mechanisms invoked to explain both the experimental observation that large inocula are required to produce consistent infection in animals and the pathologic observation that few lesions are found in the small intestine, a zone of rapid transit. Usually amebas alone stimulate little or no direct cellular response. Primary intestinal lesions elicit little reaction until secondary bacterial infection occurs. Amebic abscesses similarly elicit only a mild leukocytic response, which may be largely a response to the host cellular debris in the abscess. Amebas are antigenic and stimulate an antibody response and cellular sensitivity. In vivo studies have yielded contradictory results regarding the response of amebas to exposure to humoral antibodies. The occurrence of progressive and/or recurrent infection in the face of established immune sensitivity suggest that the host immune response is relatively ineffective against established infections.

EPIDEMIOLOGY

Fecal-oral transmission occurs when food preparation is not sanitary or when the drinking water is contaminated. Contamination may come directly from infected food handlers or indirectly from faulty sewage disposal. Endemic or epidemic disease may result. The prevalence of amebiasis in underdeveloped countries reflects the lack of adequate sanitary systems.

Amebas are found in all climates, arctic to tropical. Symptomatic infections (amebic disease) are far more prevalent in certain geographic foci, and this uneven prevalence of disease, as opposed to infection, is now explained by the variable geographic predominance of pathogenic zymodemes. Similar environments thus are likely to have a comparable infection rate but may have widely different disease prevalence.

DIAGNOSIS

Table 79-1 gives the classification of the clinical syndromes caused by *E histolytica* adopted by the World Health Organization and their related pathophysiologic mechanisms. Amebic infections are diagnosed definitively by identifying the ameba in stool or exudate (see Fig. 79-4). Under some circumstances, however, the physician must settle for a presumptive diagnosis based on serologic or clinical evidence alone. Diagnosis may be difficult if few organisms are shed in the stool. Effective methods exist for concentrating cysts but not trophozoites in stool specimens. Fortunately, a direct relationship is usually seen (although there are exceptions) between the severity of disease and the number of amebas shed in the stool; hence, the more severe the infection the easier the diagnosis. Unfortunately, a number of substances that may be administered to the patient in the course of diagnosis or therapy can impair the ability to make a direct diagnosis. These compounds can suppress the shedding of amebas into the stool but may not interfere with the course of invasive infection.

Such compounds include barium, bismuth, kaolin, soapsuds enemas, and antimicrobials that reach the intestinal lumen. The suppression of shedding may be short-lived (soapsuds enema), or may last weeks or months (broad-spectrum antibiotics). These compounds render direct diagnosis unreliable and often impossible.

Amebas may be identified in direct smears, but specific diagnosis usually depends on obtaining a fixed stained preparation. Trophozoites deteriorate rapidly in stool specimens, and therefore preservatives, either polyvinyl alcohol or the merthiolate-iodine-formaldehyde (MIF) combination, are important diagnostic aids. Finally, it is unrewarding to search for trophozoites in formed stool because most trophozoites encyst as the stool forms. Trophozoites can be found in diarrhea, however. Most infections will be detected by examining three stool specimens passed over a 7- to 10-day period. A negative examination of a single stool specimen does not rule out infection. Trophozoites may be obtained by administering a purgative agent or by scraping suspicious lesions at the time of sigmoidoscopy.

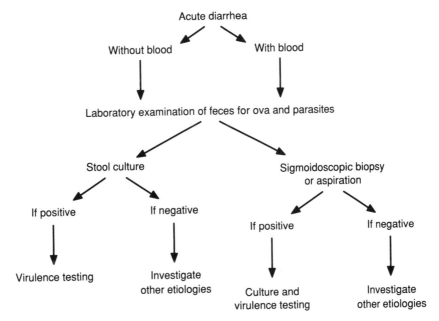

FIGURE 79-4 Evaluation of suspected cases of intestinal amebiasis.

Amebas are difficult to demonstrate in aspirates from extraintestinal abscesses (Fig. 79-5) unless special precautions are taken. The contents of most amebic abscesses are relatively free of the organism. Instead, the organisms concentrate adjacent to the wall of the abscess cavity. If care is taken during aspiration to separate serial aliquots of aspirate, amebas may be found in the last syringe that empties the cavity. Cysts or trophozoites are not found in approximately one-half of patients with amebic liver abscess.

Serologic studies (Fig. 79-5) may be useful, particularly when direct diagnosis is not possible. Such methods include gel diffusion, immunoelectrophoresis, countercurrent electrophoresis, indirect hemagglutination, indirect fluorescent antibody, skin test, enzyme-linked immunosorbent assay (ELISA), and latex agglutination. Many of these techniques are best suited for immunoepidemiology, but gel diffusion, countercurrent electrophoresis, and latex agglutination are available for clinical studies because they are readily run on a single serum sample. A positive result on these tests indicates only prior experience with invasive amebiasis. In environments where the incidence of amebiasis is low, such as in the United States, a positive titer often indicates active disease, particularly if the clinical findings agree. In areas of high prevalence a single elevated antibody titer is less significant. The physician rarely observes the patient long enough to measure a rising titer as evidence of active ongoing invasive infection.

Amebas may be cultured from the stool. However, because the techniques involved are somewhat more cumbersome than those routinely used for bacterial organisms, culturing is not widely used as a diagnostic tool. It is essential for virulence testing.

A number of nonpathogenic amebas that can inhabit the human intestinal tract may confuse di-

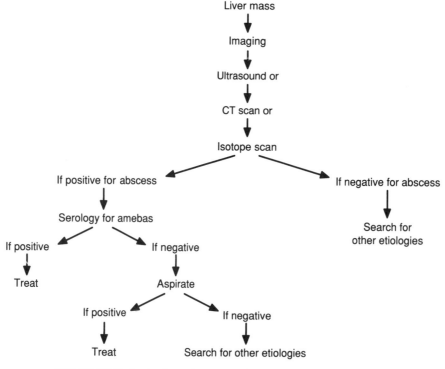

FIGURE 79-5 Evaluation of suspected cases of hepatic amebiasis.

rect diagnosis. These include *Entamoeba hartmanni, Entamoeba gingivalis, Entamoeba coli, Endolimax nana,* and *Iodamoeba bütschlii.* Although these parasites do not cause illness, they indicate that the patient has ingested feces-contaminated food or water, so their presence may prompt careful study of additional specimens (Fig. 79-3).

CONTROL

Preventive measures are limited to environmental and personal hygiene. Treatment depends on drug therapy, which in the case of some abscesses must be supplemented with drainage, either open or by aspiration. Effective drugs are available for liver abscess but intestinal infection is less successfully treated. No single drug is completely effective in eradicating amebas from the gut, so reliance is often placed on combination therapy.

Acute intestinal disease is best treated with metronidazole at a dose of 750 mg three times a day orally for 10 days. In children the dose is 40 mg/kg/day divided into three doses and given orally for 10 days. While this treatment is effective against invasive intestinal disease, it is less effective in clearing amebas from the intestine. Patients unable to take metronidazole may be given a broad-spectrum antibiotic for two weeks. It too is relatively ineffective at clearing the amebas from the gut. There are two choices for a drug to clear amebas from the lumen of the gut: iodoquinol at an adult dose of 650 mg orally three times daily for 20 days or diloxanide furoate at an adult dose of 500 mg orally three times daily for 10 days.

Amebic liver abscess is best treated with metronidazole at several possible dose regimens, but cases of drug failure have been reported. Chloroquine or dehydroemetine are less desirable alternatives. Aspiration of the abscess is not helpful except for diagnostic purposes unless rupture is imminent. Amebic abscesses heal at the same rate with or without aspiration. Abscesses with secondary bacterial infection must be drained surgically. Abscesses involving other organs respond less well to drugs and require drainage.

◁ *DIENTAMOEBA FRAGILIS* ▷

CLINICAL MANIFESTATIONS

Dientamoeba fragilis presents clinically as a nonspecific gastroenteritis. The primary symptom is diarrhea which may alternate with constipation. Other complaints include abdominal pain, nausea, vomiting, and flatus. Findings from studies of several small outbreaks suggest that crampy abdominal pain may be more common than diarrhea, but it is a relatively nonspecific symptom and not helpful for diagnosis. Far less common is the passage of blood-tinged mucus. There is no evidence that *D fragilis* is invasive. Systemic complaints such as fever, headache, and weight loss are reported but are rare. Although at onset the infection may behave as an acute process it can lapse into a chronic diarrheal state.

STRUCTURE

Dientamoeba fragilis is an ameboid parasite of the human large intestine. It has a disputed taxonomic status and is now generally thought to be not an ameba but a flagellate. Under the light microscope it resembles an ameba and it lacks flagella and certain other structures that would be characteristic of a flagellate (Fig. 79-3 and Table 79-2). The trophozoite form is 3 to 20 μm in diameter, ameboid in shape, and actively motile. Ectoplasm and endoplasm are differentiated. In stained preparations the nucleus shows a characteristic clumping of chromatin around the central karyosome with an otherwise clear nucleoplasm.

MULTIPLICATION AND LIFE CYCLE

Dientamoeba fragilis reproduces by binary fission. Binucleate cells, which are common, may represent incomplete reproduction.

PATHOGENESIS

The portal of entry for *D fragilis* is the mouth. Once in the gut, the parasite occupies the crypts of the colon. It is not known to be invasive. The usual target organs are the colon and the appendix, and the organism has been recovered from the biliary tract, where it was also lumen dwelling. The mechanism of disease is largely speculative. Because *D fragilis* infection is not fatal, examination of pathologic material has been limited to tissue obtained at the time of appendectomy. Fibrosis of the appendix is regularly described, but without evidence of mucosal invasion. Irritability coupled with increased mucus production is the suggested mechanism for the diarrhea.

HOST DEFENSES

Dientamoeba fragilis has not been shown to stimulate an immune response, but further research is needed. Antigenic material useful in serologic testing is not readily available. Reinfection can occur after treatment without evidence of development of host resistance. Spontaneous remission of symptoms also occurs.

EPIDEMIOLOGY

Transmission is through ingestion of contaminated food or water, much as with *E histolytica*. Because *D fragilis* lacks a cyst form the opportunities for transmission are limited. It is a hardy organism but cannot survive desiccation or extended exposure to gastric acid. There is epidemiologic evidence that eggs of the pinworm *Enterobius vermicularis* may act as vectors for this organism.

Dientamoeba fragilis is widely distributed in the environment and is found in temperate and tropical zones. The best information suggests it is present in 2 percent or more of United States residents. No nonhuman or reservoir host is known.

DIAGNOSIS

Dientamoeba fragilis infection is diagnosed by identifying the parasite in stools or in tissue. *Dientamoeba fragilis* may be cultured by methods used for *E histolytica*, but culturing is little used for diagnosis. Because it is small, *D fragilis* is easily confused with small nonpathogenic amebas such as *E hartmanni*. The regular occurrence of binucleate forms causes confusion with host cells, particularly

polymorphonuclear leukocytes and macrophages. For this reason permanently stained preparations, like those employed for *E histolytica*, are important. Gastroenteritis caused by *D fragilis* differs from other forms of gastroenteritis only by its chronicity and the occurrence of mild eosinophilia in some patients.

CONTROL

Dientamoeba fragilis infection can be treated effectively with the drugs used for intestinal *E histolytica* infection. There have been no reports on the effectiveness of newer drugs, such as metronidazole or diloxanide furoate. The mainstay of therapy remains broad-spectrum antibiotics such as tetracycline or paramomycin.

REFERENCES

Beaver PC, Jung RC, Cupp EW: Clinical Parasitology. 9th Ed. Lea & Febiger, Philadelphia, 1984

Jackson TFHG, Gathiram V, Simjee AE: Seroepidemiological study of antibody responses to the zymodemes of *Entamoeba histolytica*. Lancet 1:716, 1985

Kean BH: The treatment of amebiasis. JAMA 235:501, 1976

Martinez-Palomo A, Gonzalez-Robles A, de la Torre M: Selective agglutination of pathogenic strains of *Entamoeba histolytica* induced by Con A. Nature 245:186, 1973

Miller V, Spencer MJ, Chapin M, et al: *Dientamoeba fragilis*, a protozoan parasite in adult members of a semicommunal group. Dig Dis Sci 28:335, 1983

Mirelman D, Bracha R, Chayen A, et al: *Entamoeba histolytica:* Effect of growth conditions and bacterial associates on isoenzyme patterns and virulence. Exp Parasitol 62:142, 1986

Mirelman D, Bracha R, Wexler A, et al: Changes in isoenzyme patterns of a cloned culture of nonpathogenic *Entamoeba histolytica* during axenization. Infect Immun 54:827, 1986

Sargeaunt PG, Baveja UK, Nanda R, et al: Influence of geographical factors in the distribution of pathogenic zymodemes of *Entamoeba histolytica:* Identification of zymodeme XIV in India. Trans Soc Trop Med Hyg 78:96, 1984

Sargeaunt PG, Williams JE, Neal RA: A comparative study of *Entamoeba histolytica* (NIH:200, HK9, etc.), "*E histolytica*-like" and other morphologically identical amoebae using isoenzyme electrophoresis. Trans R Soc Trop Med Hyg 74:469, 1980

Strachan WD, Spice WM, Chiodini PL, et al: Immunological differentiation of pathogenic and non-pathogenic isolates of *Entamoeba histolytica*. Lancet 1:561, 1988

World Health Organization: Amoebiasis: Report of a WHO Expert Committee. WHO Tech Rep Ser 1969

Yang J, Scholten T: *Dientamoeba fragilis:* A review with notes on its epidemiology, pathogenicity, mode of transmission, and diagnosis. Am J Trop Med Hyg 26:16, 1977

80 OTHER INTESTINAL PROTOZOA AND *TRICHOMONAS VAGINALIS*

ERNEST A. MEYER

GENERAL CONCEPTS

GIARDIA LAMBLIA

Clinical Manifestations

Giardiasis may be asymptomatic or may cause a variety of intestinal symptoms, including chronic diarrhea, steatorrhea (fatty diarrhea), cramps, bloating, fatigue, and weight loss.

Structure

This parasite is a distinctive flagellate trophozoite with two nuclei and an adhesive disk. Cysts are egg-shaped (6×12 μm).

Multiplication and Life Cycle

Multiplication is by binary fission of trophozoites in the small intestine. Trophozoites begin to encyst as they pass through the lower small intestine; cysts are excreted in formed stool. Ingestion of cysts results in infection.

Pathogenesis

The presence of intestinal trophozoites results in an increased turnover of intestinal epithelium, with replacement of mature cells by immature intestinal cells. The result is a reduced ability to digest and absorb fats and fat-soluble vitamins.

Host Defenses

Cellular and humoral immunity are involved in host defense. Infection does not regularly elicit antibodies.

Epidemiology

Fecal-oral transmission can occur via drinking water and may be a problem wherever sanitation is poor. Many mammalian species harbor *Giardia* indistinguishable from *G lamblia*. There is evidence that some animal *Giardia* strains (e.g., those of beaver) may infect humans.

Diagnosis

Traditionally, *Giardia* is identified by cysts or trophozoites in stool. Some cases are difficult to diagnose. Other methods are to examine duodenal specimens for *Giardia*.

Control

Attention to personal hygiene (e.g., handwashing) will reduce direct transmission. Another method of control is to treat drinking water by disinfection and filtration. In the U.S., infections are treated with quinacrine or furazolidone. Methonidazole is also effective, but not officially approved.

TRICHOMONAS VAGINALIS

Clinical Manifestations

Trichomoniasis is a common urogenital disease in women. Vaginitis, with foul-smelling discharge and small hemorrhagic lesions, may be present; frequency of urination and painful urination are common. This infection is usually asymptomatic in men.

Structure

Trichomonas vaginalis is a pear-shaped trophozoite (7 to 23 µm long) with four anterior flagella and a fifth forming the outer edge of a short undulating membrane. A slender rod, the axostyle, extends the length of the body and protrudes posteriorly.

Multiplication and Life Cycle

The trophozoite, the only form of this organism, divides by binary fission in the urogenital tract. Transfer of the relatively delicate trophozoite is usually directly from person to person.

Pathogenesis

The organism causes low-grade inflammation by mechanisms that are not clear but may involve mechanical irritation.

Host Defenses

Host defenses are poorly understood. A protective antibody response, if present, is short-lived.

Epidemiology

The organisms typically are transferred during sexual intercourse.

Diagnosis

Trichomonas organisms can be demonstrated in vaginal fluid, scrapings, or washings.

Control

The drug of choice for treating trichomoniasis is metronidazole. Male sex partners may be asymptomatic carriers; if they are, both sex partners should be treated simultaneously.

OTHER TRICHOMONADS

Trichomonas tenax in the mouth and *T hominis* in the intestine are considered harmless commensals.

Chilomastix mesnili

This parasite is a nonpathogenic, flagellated intestinal protozoan.

Balantidium coli

The largest human protozoan parasite, this rare intestinal ciliate is an acknowledged pathogen. Transmission is fecal-oral via cysts. The relation between *Balantidium* infections in pigs and human balantidiasis remains to be resolved.

Isospora

Isosporid parasites have a life cycle with alternating sexual and asexual stages. Some *Isospora* species multiply sexually within cells of the human intestinal mucosa. Most infections are asymptomatic or mild and self-limited. Immunodeficient individuals (e.g., those with AIDS) may suffer severe, chronic infections.

CRYPTOSPORIDIUM

Clinical Manifestations

Cryptosporidial diarrhea is mild and self-limited in normal individuals, particularly children, but is severe, unrelenting, and life-threatening in immuno-compromised hosts, including those with AIDS.

Structure

Sexual and asexual stages occur in the vertebrate host intestine. The oocyst, the result of the sexual part of the cycle, is spherical or oval, 4 to 5 µm long, and contains four sporozoites when mature.

Multiplication and Life Cycle

Both sexual and asexual phases of the life cycle occur in association with the brush border of epithelial cells. The excreted oocyst, the end result of the sexual cycle, is infectious when ingested.

Pathogenesis

Although infection alters the architecture of the small intestinal epithelium, the cause of diarrhea is not known.

Host Defenses

Cell-mediated immunity appears to be primary defense mechanism.

Epidemiology

Infection is acquired by ingesting oocysts of human or (possibly) animal origin in food or water. The infectivity for humans of the numerous cryptosporidians that parasitize animals remains to be determined.

Diagnosis

Diagnosis is by detection of characteristic oocysts in feces. This usually requires special stains (e.g., acid-fast, auramine) and stool concentration.

Control

Proper sanitation controls transmission.

INTRODUCTION

This chapter discusses human protozoan parasites belonging to six different genera—*Giardia, Trichomonas, Chilomastix, Balantidium, Isospora,* and *Cryptosporidium. Giardia, Trichomonas,* and *Chilomastix* are flagellates; *Balantidium coli* is a ciliate, and *Isospora* and *Cryptosporidium* are coccidians. All are intestinal parasites that are transmitted by the fecal-oral route, except for *T. vaginalis,* which is usually spread by sexual contact. The most common of these intestinal parasites is *Giardia lamblia.* Of the three trichomonads discussed, only the common genitourinary tract inhabitant *T vaginalis* causes disease. *Chilomastix (C mesnili),* an intestinal flagellate that parasitizes humans, is generally considered nonpathogenic, and representatives of the genera *Balantidium* and *Isospora,* although not commonly encountered in humans, are considered capable of causing disease. Observations indicate that protozoa in the genus *Cryptosporidium* may cause mild or severe gastroenteritis.

GIARDIA LAMBLIA

CLINICAL MANIFESTATIONS

Giardia infection may be asymptomatic or it may cause disease ranging from a self-limiting diarrhea to a severe chronic syndrome. The length of the incubation period, usually 1 to 3 weeks, depends at least partly on the number of cysts ingested.

Most *Giardia* infections are asymptomatic. For this reason, and because these organisms are so widespread, it was earlier believed that *Giardia* was a nonpathogenic commensal. Enough evidence has accumulated, however, to show that *G lamblia* can cause disease. For example, in some cases of diarrheal disease, *Giardia* is the only known pathogen present, and treatment with any of a number of antiprotozoal agents promptly results in the disappearance of both disease and organisms. Rein-

fection is accompanied by return of symptoms. Normal human hosts with giardiasis may have any or all of the following signs and symptoms: diarrhea or loose, foul-smelling stools, steatorrhea (fatty diarrhea), malaise, abdominal cramps, excessive flatulence, fatigue, and weight loss.

Some patients with giardiasis develop a severe disease that is not self-limited. Signs and symptoms may include interference with the absorption of fat and fat-soluble vitamins, retarded growth, weight loss, or a celiac-disease-like syndrome. Although most cases are seen in hosts with some concurrent condition, such as an immune deficiency, protein-calorie malnutrition, or bacterial overgrowth of the small intestine, some cases of severe giardiasis occur in apparently normal hosts. Different strains of *G lamblia* possibly vary in virulence.

STRUCTURE

The *Giardia* life cycle involves two stages: the trophozoite and the cyst. The *G lamblia* trophozoite is easily recognized under a microscope: it is about 12 to 15 µm long, shaped like a pear cut in half lengthwise, and has two nuclei that resemble eyes, structures called **median bodies** that resemble a mouth, and four pairs of flagella that look like hair; these combine to give the stained trophozoite the eerie appearance of a face (Fig. 80-1). The flagella help these organisms to migrate to a given area of the small intestine, where they attach by means of an adhesive disk to epithelial cells and thus maintain their position despite peristalsis. The *Giardia* cyst—the form usually seen in the feces—is ovoid, 6 to 12 µm long, and can often be seen to contain two to four nuclei at one end and prominent diagonal fibrils (Fig. 80-1).

MULTIPLICATION AND LIFE CYCLE

The trophozoite, or actively metabolizing, motile form, lives in the upper two-thirds of the small intestine (duodenum and jejunum) and multiplies

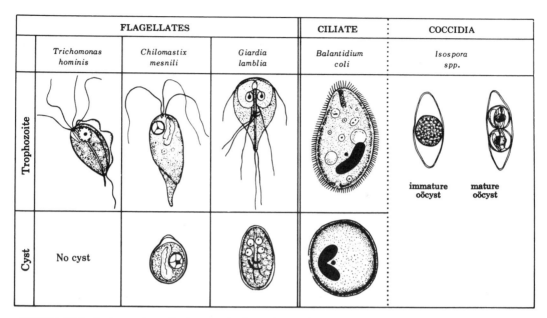

FIGURE 80-1 Protozoa found in human stool specimens. (From Brooke MM, Melvin DM: Morphology of Diagnostic Stages of Intestinal Parasites of Man. Public Health Service Publication No. 1966, 1969.)

by binary fission. Trophozoites that are swept into the fecal stream lose their motility, round up, and are excreted as dormant, resistant cysts (Fig. 80-2).

Excreted trophozoites disintegrate. The cyst, although not as resistant as many bacterial endospores, is sufficiently hardy to survive host-to-host transfer. For example, some *Giardia* cysts excyst successfully after more than 2 months storage in water at refrigerator temperatures.

Giardia infection is acquired by ingesting cysts. The exposure of cysts to host stomach acidity and body temperature triggers excystation, which is completed in the small intestine with the emergence of trophozoites that promptly attach to host intestinal epithelium.

PATHOGENESIS

The mechanisms that cause the signs and symptoms of giardiasis are not known. Ordinarily, the trophozoites remain in the intestinal lumen. It seems unlikely that their mere presence, even in enormous numbers, is sufficient to interfere mechanically with digestion. Rather, the symptoms probably result from inflammation of the mucosal

cells of the small intestine, which *Giardia* is known sometimes to cause. Inflammation results in an increased turnover rate of intestinal mucosal epithelium. The immature replacement cells have less functional surface area and less digestive and absorptive ability. Additional mechanisms of pathogenesis may well exist.

HOST DEFENSES

The fact that many *Giardia* infections in humans and experimental animals resolve spontaneously implies that an effective host immune response develops. There is evidence that both humoral and cellular immune mechanisms are involved. Hosts with gamma globulin deficiencies are prone to severe disease, suggesting that humoral immunity plays a role. Although the fact that milk from immune mothers can prevent infection in suckling mice seems to indicate a role for IgA, the nature of this protection is not clear. Furthermore, experiments with nude (congenitally athymic) mice suggest that the thymus-dependent (T-cell mediated) immune system also plays a role. In these mice, wasting and premature death may result from

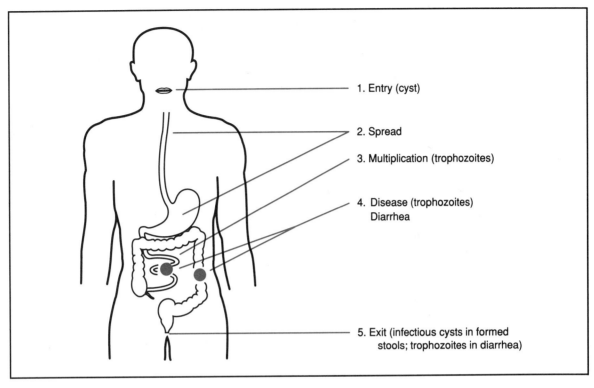

1. Entry (cyst)

2. Spread

3. Multiplication (trophozoites)

4. Disease (trophozoites)
   Diarrhea

5. Exit (infectious cysts in formed
   stools; trophozoites in diarrhea)

FIGURE 80-2   *Giardia* life cycle in humans. A similar life cycle occurs in other mammals, with probable transmission to humans.

Giardia infection, whereas nude mice "reconstituted" with thymus transplants are able to reduce the numbers of infecting *Giardia.*

In vitro studies have found that normal human milk (but not cow's milk or goat's milk) kills trophozoites of both *G lamblia* and *Entamoeba histolytica,* and that this killing does not depend on secreted IgA. This finding raises the possibility that even mother's milk that does not have antiprotozoal antibody may protect infants exposed to these parasites.

EPIDEMIOLOGY

Giardia infection occurs worldwide, with an incidence usually ranging from 1.5 to 20 percent. Higher incidences are likely where sanitary standards are low. Although people of all ages may harbor these organisms, infants and children are more often infected than are adults. Carriers are probably more important in the spread of these organisms than symptomatic patients because cysts are less likely to be present in diarrheic stool. Like other diseases spread by the fecal-oral route, giardiasis can be a problem in institutions, nurseries, and day-care centers.

Recent outbreaks, some of epidemic proportions, have occurred, particularly in North America and the Soviet Union. These outbreaks have been caused by contaminated water drunk from community water supplies or directly from rivers and streams.

Many animals harbor *Giardia* organisms that are indistinguishable from *G lamblia.* In the past, these isolates were assumed to be host-specific. Recent evidence suggests this is not always the case; at least some of the *Giardia* strains that parasitize animals may also infect humans and vice versa. This possibility complicates the problem of defining species in this genus. It also raises the question of the existence of animal reservoirs of *Giardia* from which humans may be infected. The finding of *Giardia*-infected animals in watersheds from which humans acquired giardiasis, and the successful interspecies transfer of these organisms, strengthens the possibility that giardiasis is a zoonotic infection. Infected beaver are believed to be one source of water-borne giardiasis. Beaver *Giardia* isolates were found capable of infecting dogs and humans. Canines thus may be another source of human giardiasis.

It has been recognized only recently that *Giardia* infection may be transmitted by sexual activity, particularly among homosexual men but also heterosexually. Physicians should attempt to determine if giardiasis is being acquired in this way so that they can distinguish between failure of drug treatment and prompt reinfection. Perhaps more important, a *Giardia* infection that may have been acquired in this way should alert the physician to the possible presence of more serious fecal-oral infections, such as amebiasis, syphilis, gonorrhea, or hepatitis.

DIAGNOSIS

The symptoms of giardiasis are not pathognomonic. The patient's history may indicate recent exposure to *Giardia,* but the infection is diagnosed, as in most parasitic infections, by identifying the organism. In the case of giardiasis, cysts are found in formed stool. Diarrheal specimens may also contain trophozoites. If still motile, the trophozoites exhibit a typical "falling leaf" movement.

Because cysts are often shed intermittently, three stool specimens should be obtained at approximately 48-hour intervals. Examination of these specimens permits detection of the organism in most cases. The chance of finding cysts in a light infection increases if the stool specimen is subjected to a concentration method, such as the zinc sulfate centrifugal flotation technique. When stools are negative, giardiasis can be diagnosed by obtaining trophozoites directly from the small intestine by duodenal intubation, by capsule (the Enterotest capsule), or by the use of a long nylon thread. One end of the thread is swallowed. The trophozoites attach to it, and it is then retrieved.

Identification of *Giardia* in a specimen does not necessarily mean that this organism is responsible for the patient's symptoms. *Giardia* should be treated and eliminated when found, but other pathogens should be sought as well.

CONTROL

Attention to personal hygiene is the key to preventing the spread of giardiasis. Controlling the spread of *Giardia* in drinking water should be possible where community water treatment methods (e.g., disinfection and filtration) are available. For example, iodine and chlorine kill *Giardia* cysts under appropriate conditions. Destruction of *Giardia* cysts is more difficult if the water is near freezing or contains considerable organic matter, because under such conditions so much iodine or chlorine must be added that the water is not palatable. Boiling promptly inactivates *Giardia* cysts and is the best solution.

The drug of choice for treating *Giardia* infections is quinacrine hydrochloride. This drug frequently causes dizziness, headache, and vomiting. Metronidazole and furazolidone also may be used. Although metronidazole is highly effective, its use in treating *Giardia* infections has not been officially approved in the United States. One drawback is that it frequently causes headache and nausea; another is that it is believed to be carcinogenic in rodents and mutagenic in bacteria. Its use in pregnant women is generally contraindicated, particularly in the first trimester. Furazolidone is less effective against *Giardia* than the other two drugs, but its availability in liquid form makes it useful for treating young children. None of these drugs can cure all *Giardia* infections, and none is particularly well tolerated. An anti-*Giardia* agent without these drawbacks would be welcome.

◁ *TRICHOMONAS VAGINALIS* ▷

CLINICAL MANIFESTATIONS

Although the incidence of *T vaginalis* infections varies widely, trichomoniasis is one of the commonest, if not the most common, of the sexually transmitted diseases. In some areas of the United States, incidence among women is as high as 50 percent. More women than men are infected with *T vaginalis*. In both sexes, most infections are asymptomatic or mild. Symptomatic infection is common in women, rare in men.

Trichomoniasis in women is frequently chronic and is characterized by vaginitis, a vaginal discharge, and dysuria. The inflammation of the vagina is usually diffuse and is characterized by hyperemia of the vaginal wall (with or without small hemorrhagic lesions) and migration of polymorphonuclear leukocytes into the vaginal lumen.

STRUCTURE

All the trichomonads are morphologically similar, having a pear-shaped body 7 to 23 μm long, a single anterior nucleus, three to five forward-directed flagella, and a single posteriorly directed flagellum that forms the outer border of an undulating membrane. A hyaline rod-like structure, the axostyle, runs through the length of the body and exits at the posterior end (Fig. 80-1).

Of the three trichomonads that commonly colonize humans, only one, *T vaginalis*, causes disease. *T vaginalis* inhabits the vagina in women, the prostate and seminal vesicles in men, and the urethra in both sexes.

MULTIPLICATION AND LIFE CYCLE

Trichomonads have the simplest kind of protozoan life cycle, in which the organism occurs only as a trophozoite. Division is by binary fission. Because there is no resistant cyst, transmission from host to host must be relatively direct.

PATHOGENESIS

Although the cause of the inflammatory response in trichomoniasis is not known, it may be the mechanical irritation resulting from contact between the parasite and vaginal epithelium. However, inflammation can occur in areas where parasites are not found, suggesting that the full explanation may be more complicated.

HOST DEFENSES

Relatively little is known about the human immune response to *T vaginalis* infection. Studies employing experimental animals suggest that antibody

may play a protective role. Whatever protective antibodies are elicited are short-lived, however, and disappear completely in 6 to 16 months.

EPIDEMIOLOGY

Trichomoniasis is a common, worldwide infection. Although sexual intercourse is believed to be the usual means of transfer, some infections probably are acquired through fomites such as towels, toilet seats, and sauna benches; the organisms may spread through mud and water baths as well. Survival studies of *T vaginalis* in vaginal discharges have shown that these trophozoites can be cultured from toilet seats for 30 minutes or more.

It has been suggested that this organism is frequently transmitted from a woman, serving as a reservoir of infection, to a man, the carrier, and subsequently to another woman. Although nonvenereal spread of *T vaginalis* is a subject of conjecture, little evidence exists on the importance of this means of transmission.

DIAGNOSIS

A wet mount preparation of discharge from the patient should be examined microscopically as a first step in diagnosing *T vaginalis* infection. The presence of typical pear-shaped trophozoites, usually 7 to 23 μm in length, with ''bobbling'' motility and, on careful examination, the wavelike movement of the undulating membrane, are usually sufficient to identify *T vaginalis*. Material that is negative by wet mount examination should be cultured because culturing is a considerably more sensitive, although time-consuming, method of diagnosis.

CONTROL

Because of the frequent role of asymptomatic men in spreading trichomoniasis, control of this infection necessitates examination and, if necessary, treatment of male sex partners. Avoidance of sexual intercourse and the use of condoms are effective ways to prevent transmission.

A number of 5-nitroimidazole compounds are effective antitrichomonal agents. The chemical in this group that is approved for treating trichomoniasis in the United States is metronidazole. (The potential drawbacks of this drug are discussed in the section on control of *Giardia*.) Treatment of both sexual partners at the same time is recommended to prevent "ping pong" reinfection.

OTHER TRICHOMONADS

Another trichomonad, *T tenax*, inhabits the human oral cavity, occurring particularly in tartar, cavities, and at the gingival margins. The incidence of infection with this cosmopolitan parasite is inversely proportional to the level of oral hygiene. Because it cannot survive intestinal passage, *T tenax* transfer must be by oral droplets, by kissing, or on fomites such as eating utensils. Although considered nonpathogenic, it has been reported rarely in lung or thoracic abscesses.

The third human trichomonad parasite inhabits the intestinal tract in the area of the cecum. This parasite has been called either *T hominis* or, because most of these organisms in culture have five (rather than four) anterior flagella, *Pentatrichomonas hominis*. There is no evidence that the parasite is pathogenic.

CHILOMASTIX MESNILI

Chilomastix mesnili is a nonpathogenic intestinal commensal of humans. The trophozoite is pear-shaped, usually 10 to 15 μm long, with a large anterior cytostome, three forward-directed flagella, and a sharply pointed posterior end. The organism also occurs as a lemon-shaped, uninucleate cyst 7 to 9 μm long (Fig. 80-1).

BALANTIDIUM COLI

Balantidium coli, the only ciliate and by far the largest organism in this group, is a pathogen. The trophozoites, which are ovoid, 40 to 70 μm or longer, and covered with cilia (Fig. 80-1) live in the large intestine of humans, swine, and perhaps other animals. The trophozoites divide by transverse binary fission. They have a large, kidney-shaped macronucleus and a smaller ovoid micronucleus; conjugation has been described. The cyst form is usually 50 to 55 μm in diameter. Although

the usual diet of *B coli* is believed to be host intestinal contents (hence some infections are asymptomatic), at times these organisms attack the host large intestine (aided apparently by a boring action and the enzyme hyaluronidase) and cause ulcers. In contrast to *E histolytica*, *B coli* does not invade extraintestinal tissues. Balantidiasis often is accompanied by diarrhea or dysentery, abdominal pain, nausea, and vomiting. Diagnosis is made by demonstrating cysts or trophozoites in stools or host tissue.

Balantidium infection is acquired by ingesting cysts in fecal material from another parasitized host; water-borne epidemics have been reported. The precise relationship between human and pig *Balantidium* strains is not clear. The organism is relatively rare in humans and common in pigs. Tetracyclines are the most effective drugs for treating *Balantidium* infections, but their use for this purpose has investigational status in the United States.

ISOSPORA

Organisms in the genus *Isospora* are uncommon intestinal parasites of humans. Like *Cryptosporidium* and *Toxoplasma*, *Isospora* is a coccidian parasite, and hence has a complex life cycle including both sexual and asexual stages occurring within the cells of the host's intestinal mucosa. The *Isospora* life cycle in the human host has been described from intestinal biopsy material from chronically infected patients.

The diagnostic forms of human isosporids are oocysts, inside of which are sporocysts (Fig. 80-1); however, oocysts are transparent and are easily overlooked in stool specimens. The immature oocyst has a single nucleus. Division within the oocyst yields two sporocysts, each with a cyst wall containing four elongate sporozoites. The mature oocyst, usually 28 to 30 μm in length, thus contains two sporocysts, each with four sporozoites.

Most *Isospora* infections are believed to be asymptomatic. Experimental infections are usually mild and self-limited, consisting of diarrhea and abdominal pain. However, this organism causes severe chronic diarrhea in patients with acquired immune deficiency syndrome (AIDS). It has also been reported to be a cause of chronic travelers' diarrhea in the normal host, where it can mimic giardiasis or cryptosporidiosis. Diagnosis is made by demonstrating oocysts in the feces. Although no animal reservoir has been identified, the rarity but wide distribution of human infection raises the possibility that humans are incidental hosts. The treatment of choice is administration of furazolidone; alternatively, trimethoprim-sulfamethoxazole is recommended.

◀ *CRYPTOSPORIDIUM* ▶

CLINICAL MANIFESTATIONS

It is now clear that *Cryptosporidium* species may be pathogenic for humans. Evidence from clinical studies indicates that these organisms can produce illness in some cases. *Cryptosporidium* oocysts—the form excreted in feces and used for diagnosis—were found in some of a series of patients with gastroenteritis, but not in patients without intestinal symptoms. The infection occurs most often in children and is characterized by an incubation period averaging 4 to 12 days and a moderate-to-profuse diarrhea lasting 4 to 30 (average 10) days. Although the disease is self-limiting in normal persons, the diarrhea can be chronic and fatal in immunocompromised individuals.

STRUCTURE

Members of this genus are intracellular parasites, occurring in large numbers in small intestinal mucosal epithelial cells (Fig. 80-3). The oval oocyst (the form passed in the feces) is 4 to 5 μm long and may be seen to contain four sporozoites.

MULTIPLICATION AND LIFE CYCLE

The usual habitat of *Cryptosporidium* is the vertebrate host intestine, in which the protozoa grow attached to the epithelial cell membrane in the brush border. Both sexual and asexual forms are found in this area (Fig. 80-3). Whether this organism should be regarded as an intracellular or an extracellular parasite is not resolved.

Cryptosporidia have been found in a variety of mammals, birds, and reptiles since their discovery in 1907, but they were not reported to be associated with human disease until 1976. Until recently, they received little attention because few diagnosticians were aware of their existence, because they were considered not pathogenic, and because they are not likely to be encountered in routine stool examinations.

PATHOGENESIS

Little is known about the mechanism by which these organisms cause disease. They are believed to be noninvasive. Examination of biopsy material from symptomatic patients has revealed a variety of changes in intestinal mucosa, including partial villous atrophy, crypt lengthening, low cuboidal surface epithelium, cellular infiltration of the jejunal and ileal lamina propria, and inflammation. The cause of one fatal case was probably malabsorption resulting from the intestinal damage caused by prolonged protozoal infection.

Although host cells are damaged in cryptosporidiosis, the means by which the organism causes damage is not known. Mechanical destruction and the effects of toxins, enzymes, or immune-mediated mechanisms, working alone or together, may be instrumental.

HOST DEFENSES

The fact that cryptosporidiosis is self-limiting in normal persons but usually severe and long-lasting in lower animals and immunocompromised humans indicates that host immune mechanisms are probably involved in eliminating the parasite. Cell-mediated immunity appears to be the primary defense mechanism. Neonatal infections of calves and lambs can produce a severe or fatal diarrhea. Serum antibodies to *Cryptosporidium* have been shown to develop during recovery from infection.

The importance of cryptosporidiosis in immunocompromised patients generally, and in AIDS patients in particular, should not be underestimated. In this group, cryptosporidiosis can cause diarrhea that is severe, prolonged, and life-threatening. In cryptosporidiosis patients who are im-

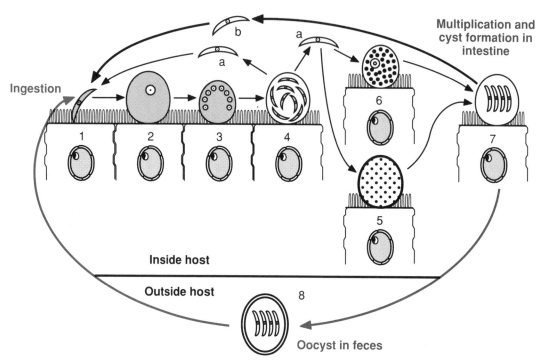

FIGURE 80-3   The life cycle of *Cryptosporidium*. (1–4) Asexual cycle of the endogenous stage: (1) sporozoite or merozoite invading a microvillus of a small intestinal epithelial cell; (2) a fully grown trophozoite; (3) a developing schizont with eight nuclei; (4) a mature schizont with eight merozoites. (5,6) Sexual cycle: (5) microgametocyte with many nuclei; (6) macrogametocyte. (7) A mature oocyst containing four sporozoites without sporocyst. (8) Oocyst discharged in the feces. (a) Merozoite released from mature schizont; (b) sporozoite released from mature oocyst. (Modified from Tzipori S: Cryptosporidiosis in animals and humans. Microbiol Rev 47:84, 1983, with permission.)

munosuppressed because of drug treatment, the disease can be reversed by withdrawing the drug. Unfortunately, this cure cannot be resorted to with AIDS patients.

EPIDEMIOLOGY

Many questions remain about the epidemiology of cryptosporidiosis. These organisms are not highly host specific, and human infections may be acquired from other humans or from animals. Infection probably is by ingestion of oocysts, although the identification of this infection in the upper respiratory tract of at least three animal species, including humans, raises the possibility that the respiratory route also may be involved. The acquisition of this infection via drinking water has also been reported.

DIAGNOSIS

Traditionally, cryptosporidiosis is diagnosed by microscopic observation of development stages of the organism in an intestinal biopsy specimen. Because *Cryptosporidium* oocysts have been found to be shed in feces during infection, many researchers have experimented with techniques for recovering these forms in stool specimens. Several studies have found that formalin concentration techniques and a modified Ziehl-Neelsen acid-fast stain are effective (Fig. 80-4). Routine procedures for diagnosing ova and parasites in stools do not generally detect this organism. The physician who suspects *Cryptosporidium* should so indicate to the laboratory when the specimen is submitted, to ensure appropriate staining. The development of serologic tests employing antibody against these organisms would be a valuable contribution.

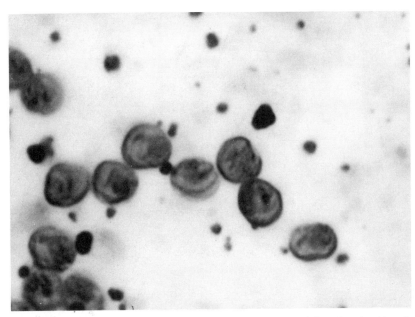

FIGURE 80-4 *Cryptosporidium* oocysts recovered from stool material and stained by the modified acid-fast technique (×2,700). (From Garcia LS, Bruckner DA, Brewer TC, Shimizu RY: *Cryptosporidium* oocysts from stool specimens. J Clin Microbiol 18:185, 1983, with permission.)

CONTROL

Because so much remains to be learned about the epidemiology of cryptosporidiosis, the only recommendations for prevention of this infection are those usually made for avoiding any pathogen transmitted by the fecal-oral route. Most persons with normal immunity recover spontaneously from cryptosporidiosis and thus do not require therapy directed at the parasite, although they may require supportive treatment. Because this infection may be life-threatening in immunocompromised individuals, however, many antimicrobial agents have been tested for anticryptosporidial effects; no safe, effective therapeutic agent has been discovered.

REFERENCES

Beaver EC, Jung, RC, Cupp EW: Clinical Parasitology. 9th Ed. Lea & Febiger, Philadelphia, 1984

Erlandsen SL, Meyer EA (eds): *Giardia* and Giardiasis. Biology, Pathogenesis and Epidemiology. Plenum, New York, 1984

Janoff EN, Reller LB: *Cryptosporidium* species, a protean protozoan. J Clin Microbiol 25:967, 1987

Jarroll EL, Bingham AK, Meyer EA: Effect of chlorine on *Giardia lamblia* cyst viability. Appl Environ Microbiol 41:483, 1978

Kulda J, Cerkasov J (eds): Trichomonads and Trichomoniasis. Proc Int Symp, Charles University, Prague. Acta Univ Carol [Med Monogr] (Paris) 30:178, 1986

Manson-Bahr PEC, Bell DR: Manson's Tropical Diseases. 19th Ed. Bailliere Tindall, London, 1987

Meyer EA (ed): Human Parasitic Diseases. Vol. 3. Giardiasis. Elsevier, New York, 1990

Meyer EA, Radulescu S: *Giardia* and giardiasis. Adv Parasitol (London) 17:1, 1979

Pape JW, Verdier RI, Johnson WD: Treatment and prophylaxis of *Isospora belli* infection in patients with the acquired immunodeficiency syndrome. N Engl J Med 320:1044, 1989

Soave R, Johnson WD: Cryptosporidium and *Isospora belli* infections. J Infect Dis 157:225, 1988

81 FREE-LIVING AMEBAS: NAEGLERIA AND ACANTHAMOEBA

AUGUSTO JULIO MARTINEZ

GENERAL CONCEPTS

NAEGLERIA FOWLERI

Clinical Manifestations

Naegleria fowleri causes primary amebic meningoencephalitis, a rare, rapidly fatal disease with sudden onset of headache, fever, stiff neck, lethargy, and coma in otherwise healthy people.

Structure

The trophozoites are 10 to 15 μm in diameter and produce broadly rounded lobopodia. Cysts are single-walled, spherical, and 8 to 12 μm in diameter. The trophozoites can also transform to a flagellated form.

Multiplication and Life Cycle

The trophozoites are free-living inhabitants of soil and warm fresh water. They reproduce by binary fission.

Pathogenesis

Amebas splashed or inhaled onto the olfactory epithelium migrate up the olfactory nerve to the brain and spread via the subarachnoid space.

Host Defenses

None are known.

Epidemiology

The organism is found worldwide in soil and warm fresh water. Infectious cysts may be carried in dust.

Diagnosis

Diagnosis relies on identifying trophozoites by microscopic examination of fresh cerebrospinal fluid specimens or histologic sections of CNS tissue, and on culturing if necessary.

Control

Early, aggressive treatment with amphotericin B and miconazole may be effective, but almost all patients die.

ACANTHAMOEBA SPECIES

Clinical Manifestations

Acanthamoeba species usually act as opportunistic pathogens in immunocompromised or debilitated individuals, in which they cause pneumonitis or dermal ulcerations. From these lesions the amebas may spread to the brain to cause an insidious, slowly progressive, usually fatal encephalitis called granulomatous amebic encephalitis. In healthy individuals, *Acanthamoeba* spp can cause an ulcerating keratitis, which is often associated with the use of improperly sterilized contact lenses.

Structure

Trophozoites are 25 to 40 μm in diameter with characteristic spine-like pseudopodia. Cysts are double-walled, usually polygonal, and 15 to 20 μm in diameter.

Multiplication and Life Cycle

The trophozoites are free-living inhabitants of soil and fresh and salt water. They reproduce by binary fission.

Pathogenesis

Encephalitis is caused by hematogenous spread from superficial or pulmonary lesions to the brain. Keratitis results from contamination of superficial corneal abrasions.

Host Defenses

Except in the case of keratitis, the defenses of a healthy host seem sufficient to prevent infection.

Epidemiology

Acanthamoeba organisms live worldwide in soil and fresh and salt water. They may contaminate contact lens solution, physiotherapy pools, air-conditioning units, etc.

Diagnosis

Diagnosis is usually by microscopic examination of biopsy specimens from lesions; both trophozoites and cysts may be seen. Amebas may also be cultured.

Control

No effective treatment is known for opportunistic *Acanthamoeba* infections in debilitated and immunosuppressed individuals. The incidence of keratitis may be reduced by properly cleaning and sterilizing contact lenses. Keratitis may respond to treatment with propamidine (often combined with neomycin) followed, if necessary, by keratoplasty.

INTRODUCTION

Two genera of free-living amebas, *Naegleria* and *Acanthamoeba,* are known to infect humans. *Naegleria fowleri* causes an acute and almost invariably fatal encephalitis, which, fortunately, is rare. Several species of *Acanthamoeba* can cause lung and skin infections, as well as an insidious encephalitis, in immunocompromised patients. In addition, amebas of this genus cause an ulcerative keratitis, which is usually associated with improper sterilization of soft contact lenses. Amebas of both genera live free in fresh waters, soil, and coastal waters. The resistant cysts can be transported in dust.

◀ *NAEGLERIA FOWLERI* ▶

CLINICAL MANIFESTATIONS

Naegleria fowleri is the agent of **primary amebic meningoencephalitis,** a fulminating, rapidly fatal disease. A total of about 150 cases of this rare disease have been recorded worldwide (Table 81-1). The disease usually affects children and young adults. In almost all cases, the victims contract the amebas by swimming in infected fresh water. The amebas enter the brain via the olfactory tract after being inhaled or splashed onto the olfactory epithelium. The incubation period ranges from 2 to 3 days to as long as 7 to 15 days, depending partly on the size of the inoculum and the virulence of the strain. The incubation period in animals infected experimentally with *N australiensis* or with a mildly virulent strain of *N fowleri* has been as long as 3 or 4 weeks.

The disease appears with the sudden onset of bifrontal or bitemporal headache, fever, nausea, vomiting, and stiff neck (Table 81-2). Symptoms progress rapidly to lethargy, confusion, and coma. In all but three of the recorded cases, the patient died within 48 to 72 hours.

STRUCTURE

Naegleria fowleri isolated from humans is morphologically identical to the common, nonpathogenic amebas *N gruberi* and *N australiensis.* The trophozoites are active and constantly change size and shape (Fig. 81-1). When rounded, they measure about 10 to 15 μm in diameter. The cytoplasm is finely granular and contains a conspicuous clear

TABLE 81-1   Comparison of Diseases Caused by Free-Living Amebas

Ameba	*Naegleria fowleri*	*Acanthamoeba* spp.
Protozoology	*Trophozoites:* 10–15 µm with broad, blunt pseudopodia. *Cyst:* spherical	*Trophozoites:* 25–40 µm, with slender, tapering pseudopodia. *Cyst:* star shape with double walls.
Disease	Primary amebic meningoencephalitis	Granulomatous amebic encephalitis (GAE); *Acanthamoeba* keratitis
No. of cases reported as of 1990	About 150 cases	GAE: >50 cases; *Acanthamoeba* keratitis: >250 cases
Epidemiology	Good health; recent history of swimming in lake or swimming pool in warm weather	Immunoincompetence (e.g., AIDS)
Incubation (days)	3–7 days	Probably >10 days
Portal of entry	Olfactory neuroepithelium	Skin, lung, olfactory neuroepithelium
Onset	Fast	Slow, insidious
CNS spread	Direct; amyelinic nervous plexus	Probably hematogenous
Organs affected	Brain only	Brain, skin, eyes, lungs
Clinical course	Acute, fulminant; fatal within 10 days	Subacute (8–30 days) or chronic (>32 days)
Signs and symptoms	Headache, anorexia, nausea, vomiting, fever, meningism, mental abnormalities, diplopia, seizures	Mental abnormalities, seizures, fever, hemiparesis, headache, meningism, visual abnormalities
Ocular involvement	None	Keratitis
Laboratory diagnosis & CSF	CSF similar to bacterial meningitis: neutrophilic pleocytosis, high protein, low glucose. Direct examination of fresh CSF shows active trophozoites. Culturing or inoculation into mice also used.	CSF finding similar to those in viral encephalitides. Culturing or inoculation into mice also used.
Host response	Purulent leptomeningitis, hemorrhagic necrotizing meningoencephalitis, brain edema, perivascular collection of amebas	Granulomatous encephalitis with focal necrosis and multinucleated giant cells, necrotizing angiitis
CNS amebic forms	Trophozoites	Trophozoites + cysts
Differential diagnosis	Acute pyogenic (bacterial) leptomeningitis	Tuberculous, viral or fungal encephalitis; brain tumors; brain abscess. *Ocular:* herpes; fungal keratitis
Therapy	Amphotericin B + miconazole + rifampin	?Sulfadiazine, ?ketoconazole, propamidine isethionate (for keratitis)

nuclear halo and a dense central nucleolus. Numerous vacuoles are usually visible in the cytoplasm. The trophozoites travel by producing broadly rounded processes (lobopodia) which are clear initially but fill with granular cytoplasm. Under adverse conditions, the trophozoites encyst. The cysts are spherical, 8 to 12 µm in diameter, with a smooth, single-layered wall. The wall is pierced by one or two flat, mucus-plugged pores

through which the regenerated trophozoite will emerge. The cytoplasm of the cyst is finely granular, with a characteristic central nucleus. When exposed to distilled water, trophozoites can convert within a few minutes to a flagellated form.

The pathogenic species of *Naegleria* was named *N fowleri* after Malcolm Fowler, who first isolated the organism from a patient with primary amebic meningoencephalitis. Previously, these amebas

TABLE 81-2   Signs and Symptoms in Primary Amebic
Meningoencephalitis (PAM) and Granulomatous Amebic Encephalitis (GAE)

Symptoms and Signs	PAM	GAE
Symptoms		
Mental status abnormalities[a]	+	+
Headache	+	+
Fever > 38.2°C		
Nausea and vomiting	+	+
Stiff neck	+	+
Seizures	+	+
Anorexia	+	+
Diplopia and blurred vision	+	+
Photophobia	+	+
Hallucinations	+	+
Sleep disturbances	0	+
Sore throat	+	0
Rhinitis	+	0
Ageusia	+	0
Parosmia	+	0
Hearing difficulties	0	+
Signs	**Early**	**Late**
Coma		
Papilledema	+	+
Cranial nerve palsies (nerves III and VI)	+	0
Nystagmus	+	+
Gait ataxia	+	+
Babinski's sign	+	+
Kernig's sign	+	+
Hemiparesis	0	+
Aphasia	0	+
Anisocoria	+	0
Disconjugate gaze	+	0
Cause of death	Cardiorespiratory arrest, pulmonary edema, brain edema	Bronchopneumonia, liver/kidney failure

[a] Lethargy, drowsiness, stupor, disorientation, confusion, delirium, obtundation, restlessness, irritability, combativeness.

were also called *N aerobia* and *N invadens*. *Naegleria australiensis* and *N australiensis italica* are species that show low virulence in animal experiments. Immunoelectrophoresis is important in identifying free-living amebas. Even though *N fowleri* and other free-living amebas may reliably be differentiated by morphology and immunoperoxidase methods, the use of various zymodemes helps in distinguishing pathogenic from nonpathogenic amebas.

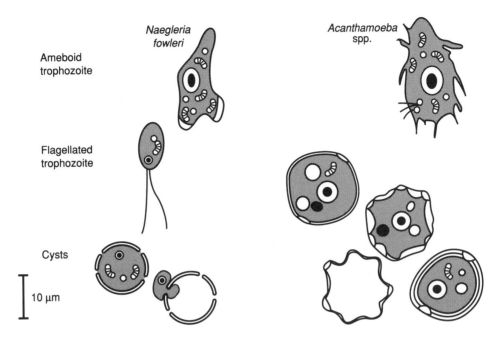

FIGURE 81-1   Comparative morphology of free-living amebas. (Modified from Page F: Redefinition of the genus *Acanthamoeba* with descriptions of three species. J Protozool 14:709, 1967, with permission.)

MULTIPLICATION AND LIFE CYCLE

Naegleria fowleri is a free-living inhabitant of fresh water and soil. The ameboid trophozoite form reproduces by binary fission and also gives rise to the encysted and flagellated forms, which do not reproduce. *Naegleria fowleri* is thermophilic, preferring warm water and reproducing successfully at temperatures up to 46°C. In temperate climates, the amebas overwinter as cysts in bottom sediments of lakes, swimming pools, and rivers.

PATHOGENESIS

In almost all cases, *N fowleri* enters the body by being inhaled or splashed onto the olfactory epithelium (Fig. 81-2). In some cases, however, the patients had had no recent contact with fresh water, and apparently contracted the disease by inhaling cyst-laden dust. The sustentacular cells of the olfactory neuroepithelium are capable of active phagocytosis, and this appears to be the mechanism by which the amebas invade the body. The amebas then travel up the mesaxonal spaces of the unmyelinated olfactory nerve to the brain. The olfactory nerve terminates in the olfactory bulb, which is located in the richly vascularized subarachnoid space and is bathed by cerebrospinal fluid. The subarachnoid space is the route of dissemination to the rest of the central nervous system (CNS). Respiratory symptoms in some patients may be the result of hypersensitivity or allergic reactions or may represent a subclinical infection.

The brain of a patient with primary amebic meningoencephalitis usually shows swollen, edematous, congested cerebral hemispheres and evidence of increased intracranial pressure. Uncal and cerebellar tonsillar hernias may be present. The arachnoid is severely congested, and a scant purulent exudate may be found along the sulci. The olfactory bulbs and orbitofrontal cortices are usually necrotic and hemorrhagic. The leptomeninges show a fibrinous-purulent exudate composed of polymorphonuclear leukocytes, eosinophils, a few monocytes, and some lymphocytes.

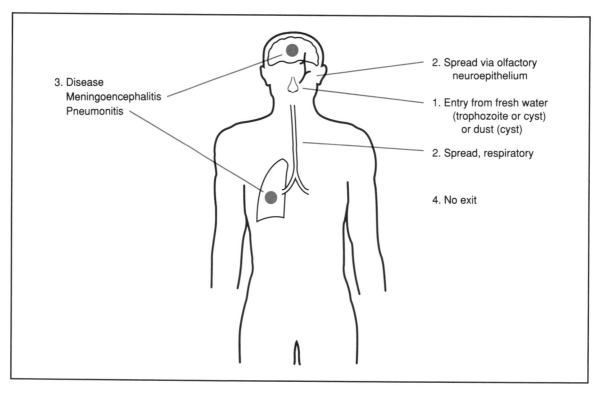

3. Disease
   Meningoencephalitis
   Pneumonitis

2. Spread via olfactory
   neuroepithelium

1. Entry from fresh water
   (trophozoite or cyst)
   or dust (cyst)

2. Spread, respiratory

4. No exit

FIGURE 81-2 Pathogenesis of *Naegleria* infection.

These changes may be present throughout the cerebral hemispheres, brainstem, cerebellum, and upper portion of the spinal cord. Necrotizing angiitis is occasionally seen. A few amebas can be found in the purulent exudate, some in the process of being phagocytosed by polymorphonuclear leukocytes and macrophages.

HOST DEFENSES

It is not yet clear whether *N fowleri* can elicit a protective cellular or humoral immune response.

EPIDEMIOLOGY

Naegleria fowleri is ubiquitous in warm fresh waters. It is clear that the number of infections represents only a minute fraction of the number of exposures. Nevertheless, clusters of cases associated with a given source occur. It is not clear why primary amebic meningoencephalitis is not found predominantly in the tropics, where the ameba flourishes. Most patients with primary amebic meningoencephalitis have been in a swimming pool, freshwater lake, or pond a few days before the onset of symptoms. However, as mentioned above, the disease may also be transmitted by cyst-laden dust. Chlorination of water does not entirely eliminate pathogenic strains. *Naegleria fowleri* has also been isolated from air conditioning units.

DIAGNOSIS

Primary amebic meningoencephalitis cannot be distinguished clinically from acute pyogenic or bacterial meningoencephalitides. The disease usually occurs in children and young adults in good health who have recently swum in warm water. Computed tomography of the brain shows obliteration of the cisternae surrounding the midbrain and of the subarachnoid space over the cerebral hemispheres. The disease may be diagnosed rapidly by examining one or two drops of fresh cerebrospinal fluid under a light microscope for *N fowleri*. The organism may also be cultured from cerebrospinal fluid or brain tissue for a definitive diagnosis. Retrospective diagnoses have been made by examining paraffin-embedded brain tissue sections stained with hematoxylin and eosin.

CONTROL

Only three patients have survived primary amebic meningoencephalitis. In these patients, the disease was diagnosed early and treated aggressively with high doses of amphotericin B. Amphotericin B and miconazole appear to be the drugs of choice. The chance of catching the disease can presumably be reduced by properly chlorinating swimming pools, whirlpools, and Jacuzzis and by not diving or splashing in warm water.

◀ *ACANTHAMOEBA* ▶

Acanthamoeba castellanii, *A culbertsoni*, and other *Acanthamoeba* species can cause opportunistic lung and skin infections in immunocompromised or otherwise debilitated individuals. The amebas may spread hematogenously from such lesions to the brain, where they cause a subacute, slowly progressive, and usually fatal encephalitis. In addition, *Acanthamoeba* can cause an ulcerating keratitis in healthy individuals, usually associated with improperly sterilized contact lenses.

CLINICAL MANIFESTATIONS
Granulomatous Amebic Encephalitis

Granulomatous amebic encephalitis is a multifocal, hemorrhagic, necrotizing encephalitis caused by opportunistic free-living *Acanthamoeba* species, principally *A castellanii* and *A culbertsoni*. The disease usually afflicts debilitated or immunosuppressed individuals. It sets in with insidious focal neurologic changes that mimic the clinical picture of single or multiple space-occupying brain lesions (Table 81-2). Focal neurologic changes, hemiparesis, drowsiness, personality changes, and seizures

are common early symptoms. Headache sets in early and is insidious. Nausea and vomiting may also be early symptoms. Fever is sporadic and generally low. Signs and symptoms of brain parenchymal inflammation develop, such as altered mental status, diplopia, paresis, lethargy, and cerebellar ataxia. The disease progresses over a period of one to several weeks and usually ends in coma and death.

The incubation period is difficult to determine, as pulmonary and skin lesions containing the organisms may be present for months before encephalitis appears. *Acanthamoeba* species apparently multiply more slowly than *Naegleria fowleri*.

Acanthamoeba Infections of the Lungs and Skin

Acanthamoebic pneumonitis and dermatitis, characterized by the presence of cysts and trophozoites in alveoli or in multiple nodules or ulcerations of the skin, are opportunistic diseases that usually affect immunosuppressed or debilitated individuals. In acanthamoebic pneumonitis, chest radiographs may show areas of consolidation. Granulomatous amebic encephalitis usually develops as a result of hematogenous spread from lesions in the lungs, upper respiratory tract, or skin. Multiple skin nodules may represent "terminal" dissemination in cases of granulomatous amebic encephalitis.

Acanthamoeba Keratitis

Painful corneal ulcerations that fail to respond to the usual antibacterial, antiviral, and antifungal treatments may be caused by *Acanthamoeba*. The disease is a nonsuppurative keratitis that characteristically follows a waxing and waning clinical course. The damaged corneal tissue may show a characteristic annular infiltrate and congested conjunctivae or there may be a dendriform epitheliopathy and patchy stromal infiltrate with lacunar areas. If not successfully treated, the disease progresses to corneal perforation and loss of the eye or to a vascularized scar over thinned cornea, with impaired vision. The disease is quite rare. It is usually associated with contaminated contact lenses.

STRUCTURE

Acanthamoeba trophozoites may be recognized by the presence of slender spinelike processes (Fig. 81-1). When rounded, the cells measure 25 to 40 μm in diameter. The finely granular cytoplasm, as a rule, contains a single nucleus with a large, dense central nucleolus surrounded by a nuclear clear zone. Water and digestive vacuoles are usually visible in the cytoplasm. The double-walled cysts are generally polygonal, spherical, or star-shaped, 15 to 20 μm in diameter, with a nucleus containing a large dense central nucleolus surrounded by a clear nuclear halo. The smooth inner wall of the cyst contacts the wrinkled outer wall at a number of points, forming pores, opercula, or ostioles.

MULTIPLICATION AND LIFE CYCLE

Acanthamoeba species are free-living amebas of soil and of fresh and salt water. Reproduction is by binary fission of the trophozoites. Infective cysts can be transmitted in dust and aerosols.

PATHOGENESIS

Free-living amebas have been isolated from human throats, suggesting that they are generally harmless in healthy individuals. *Acanthamoeba* spp usually act as opportunistic pathogens, taking advantage of a loss of metabolic, physiologic, or immunologic integrity by the host. Among the most common factors predisposing an individual to *Acanthamoeba* infection are immunosuppressive therapy, treatment with broad-spectrum antibiotics, diabetes mellitus, various cancers, malnutrition, pregnancy, acquired immune deficiency syndrome (AIDS), and chronic alcoholism. Surgical trauma, burns, wounds, and radiation therapy can also promote infection.

The primary focus of infection for opportunistic *Acanthamoeba* is usually the lower respiratory tract or skin. The amebas may enter the respiratory tract by the inhalation of aerosols or dust containing cysts (Fig. 81-3). Spread to the CNS is apparently hematogenous. The cerebral hemispheres in gran-

ulomatous amebic encephalitis may be edematous, with focal cortical softening, hemorrhage, and abscesses. Uncal notching and cerebellar herniation may be present. Foci of hemorrhagic necrosis may be seen in the basal ganglia, midbrain, brainstem, and cerebellum. The histopathologic changes consist of a chronic granulomatous encephalitis with multinucleated giant cells mainly in the posterior fossa structures, basal ganglia, and cerebellum. Trophozoites and cysts may be found in the lesions.

Acanthamoeba keratitis usually results from direct invasion of ocular tissue by the amebas through a break in the corneal epithelium. In most cases, the portal of entry is a minor corneal lesion, such as those caused by previous herpes simplex or by abrasion from hard or soft contact lenses. The amebas are often introduced in the eye by using contaminated contact-lens cleaning solutions or by swimming in contaminated water. The incubation period is unknown. Amebic trophozoites and cysts are usually located deep in the corneal stroma, with moderate granulomatous inflammation and negligible acute inflammatory response.

HOST DEFENSES

Except in the case of amebic keratitis, the defenses of a healthy host seem sufficient to prevent *Acanthamoeba* infection. Patients who contract granulomatous amebic encephalitis usually have impaired humoral and/or cell-mediated immunity. However, there are reports of patients with no demonstrable underlying disease or predisposing factor.

EPIDEMIOLOGY

Pathogenic *Acanthamoeba* species are ubiquitous in fresh and salt water and in soil. Infective cysts can be carried by water or dust.

DIAGNOSIS

In many cases, granulomatous amebic encephalitis is not diagnosed until after or, at best, shortly before death. Immunosuppression or other predisposing factors may provide important clues. The

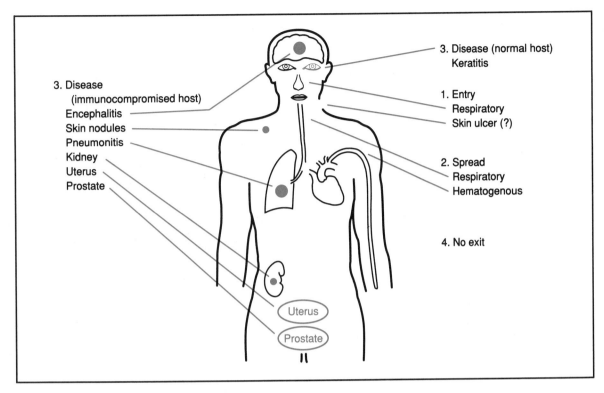

FIGURE 81-3 Pathogenesis of *Acanthamoeba* infection.

differential diagnosis includes space-occupying lesions such as tumors, abscesses, and even infarcts, as well as tuberculoma or fungal infection (Table 81-1). Computed tomography and magnetic resonance imaging of the brain are important diagnostic tests, as is examination of cerebrospinal fluid and brain biopsy specimens. The diagnosis usually is made after examination of brain tissue with a light microscope. Amebic dermatitis is often diagnosed by microscopic examination of a skin biopsy. Both trophozoites and cysts are usually visible.

In the case of amebic keratitis, scrapings of the corneal ulceration and biopsy specimens may contain amebic trophozoites and cysts. Both light and electron microscopy may be useful. Amebic cysts in the corneal stroma may be demonstrated by staining with hematoxylin and eosin, trichrome, calcofluor-white, or immunofluorescence techniques. Alternatively, amebas may be cultured at

37°C on non-nutrient agar with Page's saline containing *Escherichia coli, Enterobacter aerogenes,* or other Gram-negative bacteria. Cysts and trophozoites may be identified on the basis of morphology and locomotion; isoenzyme electrophoresis may be used to further classify species.

CONTROL

There is no effective treatment for lung, skin, or brain *Acanthamoeba* infections. Sulfadiazine is apparently ineffective, perhaps as a result of the host's impaired immune system. Since the amebas are ubiquitous, preventive measures to reduce contact are difficult. The incidence of *Acanthamoeba* keratitis, on the other hand, can be greatly reduced by correctly sterilizing contact lenses. Lenses should be cleaned properly, using commercial rather than homemade saline, and should be disinfected with a chemical or (preferably) a thermal system. Lenses should be removed before swimming.

Drug treatment of *Acanthamoeba* keratitis is sometimes successful. Brolene (propamidine isethionate) and dibromopropamidine have been reported to be effective. Polymyxin B, miconazole, and neomycin also appear to be useful in combination with propamidine. Ketoconazole gives evidence of being effective both in vitro and in vivo. Acridine derivatives and paromomycin are effective in vitro but are still in the experimental stage. Cases that do not respond to drug therapy have been treated with penetrating keratoplasty and corneal grafting. Cysts apparently may occupy the deeper layers of the cornea. These cysts are probably responsible for the resistance of the infection to drugs and for recurrence after corneal transplantation. For this reason, the infection should be controlled before corneal transplantation is performed. Steroids should be used with caution in ophthalmic infections, even though they may reduce or inhibit inflammation and tissue damage and prevent an immune response.

ACKNOWLEDGMENT

This work was supported in part by the Pathology Education and Research Foundation of the Department of Pathology, University of Pittsburgh.

REFERENCES

Binder PS: Cryotherapy for medically unresponsive *Acanthamoeba* keratitis. Cornea 8:106, 1989

Butt CG: Primary amebic meningoencephalitis. N Engl J Med 274:1473, 1966

Carter RF: Primary amebic meningoencephalitis: An appraisal of present knowledge. Trans R Soc Trop Med Hyg 66:193, 1972

Carter RF, Cullity CJ, Ojeda VJ, et al: A fatal case of meningoencephalitis due to a free-living amoeba of uncertain identity—probably *Acanthamoeba* species. Pathology 13:51, 1981

Gonzalez MM, Gould E, Dickinson G, et al: Acquired immunodeficiency syndrome associated with *Acanthamoeba* infection and other opportunistic organisms. Arch Pathol Lab Med 110:749, 1986

Jones DB: *Acanthamoeba*—the ultimate opportunist? Am J Ophthalmol 102:527, 1986

Martinez AJ: Is acanthamoebic encephalitis an opportunistic infection? Neurology (NY) 30:567, 1980

Martinez AJ: Free-living amoebae: Pathogenic aspects. A review. Protozool Abstr 7:293, 1983

Moore MB, McCulley JP, Luckenback M, et al: *Acanthamoeba* keratitis associated with soft contact lenses. Am J Ophthalmol 100:396, 1985

Warhurst DC, Mann PG: *Acanthamoeba* keratitis. Br Med J 296:568, 1988

Wiley CA, Safrin RE, Davis CE, et al: Acanthamoeba meningoencephalitis in a patient with AIDS. J Infect Dis 155:130, 1987

Seidel JS, Harmatz P, Visvesvara GS, et al: Successful treatment of primary amebic meningoencephalitis. N Engl J Med 306:346, 1982

82

HEMOFLAGELLATES

RODRIGO A. ZELEDÓN

GENERAL CONCEPTS

AMERICAN TRYPANOSOMIASIS (CHAGAS DISEASE)

Clinical Manifestations

Symptoms of acute disease may include fever, local or general edema, lymphadenopathy, tachycardia, heart enlargement, and myocarditis. Heart alterations and, occasionally, megaesophagus or megacolon may appear as late sequelae.

Structure

Typical, small trypomastigotes are found in peripheral blood and intracellular amastigotes in tissues.

Classification and Antigenic Types

Strains are differentiated by isoenzyme patterns and DNA sequencing. No antigenic variation is observed.

Multiplication and Life Cycle

Intracellular amastigotes divide to form pseudocysts, which release nondividing trypomastigotes into the blood. Trypomastigotes ingested by a vector bug transform in the insect intestine into epimastigotes, which reproduce to form infective metacyclic trypomastigotes, which are expelled in feces and enter a new host through skin abrasions.

Pathogenesis

Inflammatory reactions around pseudocysts lead to myocarditis and destruction of parasympathetic ganglia (mainly of the heart and myenteric plexus). An autoimmune reaction may develop.

Host Defenses

Inflammatory reactions, antibodies, and cell-mediated responses all develop.

Epidemiology

The disease is vectored by triatomine (cone-nosed) bugs and may also be transmitted congenitally and by transfusion. Animal reservoirs include opossums, armadillos, rodents, dogs, and cats. Outbreaks are associated with mud, thatched, or dirt-floored dwellings that harbor the vector.

Diagnosis

The clinical picture is suggestive; direct demonstration of parasites or serologic tests are definitive.

Control

Insecticides should be used to kill vectors in dwellings. Serologic screening of blood donors is important in endemic regions. Drug treatment is effective only in the acute phase.

AFRICAN TRYPANOSOMIASIS (SLEEPING SICKNESS)

Clinical Manifestations

Early symptoms are an inoculation chancre, fever, headache, and lymphadenopathy. Victims later develop meningoencephalitis, become somnolent, and die unless treated.

Structure

Typical, sometimes pleomorphic trypomastigotes are found in blood and cerebrospinal fluid.

Classification and Antigenic Types

Sleeping sickness is caused by *Trypanosoma brucei* subspp *rhodesiense* and *gambiense*. Frequent variation of surface antigens allows the parasites to evade specific immunity.

Multiplication and Life Cycle

Trypomastigotes multiply in blood. When ingested by a vector tsetse fly, the parasites multiply as epimastigotes in the salivary glands, producing infective trypomastigotes which enter a new host when the fly bites.

Pathogenesis

Inflammatory changes (possibly autoimmune) cause CNS demyelination. Immunosuppression by the parasite facilitates secondary infections.

Host Defenses

Inflammatory responses, high IgM antibody levels, and cell-mediated immunity occur.

Epidemiology

T b rhodesiense is maintained in various mammals of open savannahs; *T b gambiense* is maintained mainly in domestic animals.

Diagnosis

Parasites appear first in the blood and lymph nodes and later in the cerebrospinal fluid. The diagnosis is made by inoculating susceptible laboratory animals or by serologic tests.

Control

Control centers on reducing the population of tsetse flies. Humans are treated with pentamidine and arsenical drugs.

CUTANEOUS AND MUCOCUTANEOUS LEISHMANIASIS

Clinical Manifestations

This form of leishmaniasis consists of skin or mucosal lesions, which are frequently ulcerated. Lesions may be self-healing or chronic; localized or spreading.

Structure

Leishmania occurs as an intracellular amastigote in the mammalian host and as promastigotes in the intestine of the sand fly vector.

Classification and Antigenic Types

Numerous species of *Leishmania* cause forms of leishmaniasis in various geographic areas. Different antigens are recognized by monoclonal antibodies.

Multiplication and Life Cycle

Amastigotes divide in mammalian macrophages and other reticuloendothelial cells. When ingested by a sand fly vector, they multiply in the gut as promastigotes, migrate to the proboscis, and enter a new host when the fly bites.

Pathogenesis

The severity of disease depends on the infecting species and on the host's immune response. There may be lymphatic and hematogenous spread.

Host Defenses

Host defense relies on cell-mediated immunity; antibody titers are low. The response ranges from a local tuberculoid granuloma with few parasites to a histiocytoma with many parasites.

Epidemiology

Some species are zoonotic; others are transmitted in a human-fly-human cycle. Transmission is determined by the range and habits of the vector.

Diagnosis

The diagnosis is confirmed if parasites are seen in scrapings or cultures from the lesion. Serologic and skin tests are also useful.

Control

Control centers on elimination of sand flies whenever possible. Disease is treated with organic antimonials and amphotericin B.

VISCERAL LEISHMANIASIS (KALA-AZAR)

Clinical Manifestations

In visceral leishmaniasis, the parasite infects the entire reticuloendothelial system. Most infections are mild and self-limiting. Classic kala-azar, which is progressive and fatal if not treated, is marked by hepatosplenomegaly, lymphadenopathy, anemia, leukopenia, and emaciation.

Classification and Antigenic Types

Kala-azar is caused by at least three species of *Leishmania*.

Pathogenesis

The parasite invades reticuloendothelial cells of the liver, spleen, bone marrow, and lymph nodes, causing histiocytic hyperplasia and hypertrophy. Hematopoietic tissues are replaced by macrophages.

Host Defenses

Cellular immunity is responsible for resolving mild disease. High levels of antibodies are found.

Epidemiology

Human-sand fly-human cycles occur in some areas (India); in others, rodents or canines serve as reservoirs.

Diagnosis

Parasites are visible in stained or cultured bone marrow and spleen samples. Serologic tests are also necessary.

Control

Control is as with cutaneous leishmaniasis; pentamidine and antimonials are used in treatment.

INTRODUCTION

The family Trypanosomatidae consists of many parasitic flagellate protozoans. Two genera, *Trypanosoma* and *Leishmania,* include important pathogens of humans and domestic animals. The diseases caused by these protozoa are endemic or enzootic in different parts of the world and constitute serious medical and economic problems. Because these protozoans require hematin obtained from blood hemoglobin for aerobic respiration, they are called **hemoflagellates.** The digenetic (two-host) life cycles of both genera involve an insect and a vertebrate. The family also includes the digenetic genus *Phytomonas,* which infects plants, and some monogenetic (one-host) species which infect only invertebrate hosts.

The hemoflagellates have up to eight life cycle stages which differ in the placement and origin of the flagellum. Two stages—the **amastigote** and the **trypomastigote**—may occur in vertebrate hosts, and three stages—the **promastigote, paramastigote,** and **epimastigote**—in invertebrate hosts (Fig. 82-1).

Besides the nucleus and the flagellum, a trypanosomatid cell has a unique organelle called the **kinetoplast.** The kinetoplast appears to be a special part of the mitochondrion. It is rich in DNA and apparently controls certain hereditary functions, particularly those related to morphogenesis. Two types of DNA molecules, *maxicircles* and *mini-*

circles, have been found in the kinetoplast; when Giemsa stained, the kinetoplast is reddish purple and darker than the nucleus, contrasting with the pale blue cytoplasm.

Monogenetic trypanosomatids are more primitive than the digenetic species and grow easily in synthetic culture media. Some digenetic species can be cultivated in complex synthetic media. The medium most commonly used is NNN medium, which has a solid phase of rabbit blood agar and a liquid phase of a physiologic salt solution. Liquid media are also available. Only the invertebrate stages appear in such media, and they may or may not be infectious for the vertebrate hosts, depending on the species.

Replication of trypanosomatids occurs by single or multiple fission, involving first the kinetoplast, then the nucleus, and finally the cytoplasm.

AMERICAN TRYPANOSOMIASIS (CHAGAS DISEASE)

Clinical Manifestations

Chagas disease begins as a localized infection that is followed by parasitemia and colonization of internal organs and tissues. Infection may first be evidenced by a small tumor (**chagoma**) of the skin

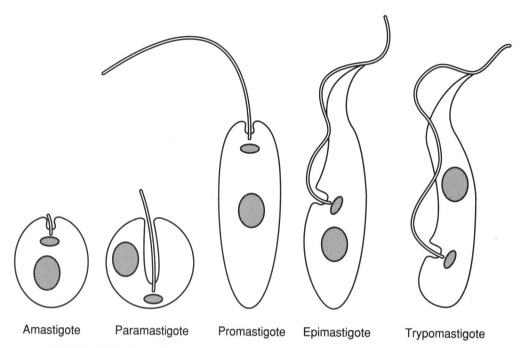

Amastigote   Paramastigote   Promastigote   Epimastigote   Trypomastigote

FIGURE 82–1 Five of the eight morphologic stages of a trypanosomatid flagellate.

or, when the port of entry is the conjunctiva, by Romaña's sign (unilateral bipalpebral edema) (Fig. 82-2). These typical inflammatory reactions are usually accompanied by a swelling of the satellite lymph nodes that persists for 1 to 2 months. Symptoms and signs include fever, general edema, adenopathy, moderate hepatosplenomegaly, myocarditis with or without heart enlargement, and sometimes in children, meningoencephalitis. The acute disease is frequently subclinical and patients may become lifelong asymptomatic carriers. This chronic phase may result after 10 to 20 years in a cardiopathy and, in some geographic areas, in enlargement of parts of the digestive tract (megaesophagus, megacolon).

STRUCTURE

Trypanosoma cruzi is found in the peripheral blood as a 20 μm trypomastigote with a large kinetoplast and a poorly developed undulating membrane. In the tissues (mainly heart, skeletal and smooth muscle, and reticuloendothelial cells) the parasite occurs as a 3 to 5 μm amastigote.

CLASSIFICATION AND ANTIGENIC TYPES

Studies with isolates of *T cruzi* from various hosts have shown intraspecific variation. Biochemical methods such as analysis of isoenzyme patterns (yielding zymodemes) and DNA molecular sequences (yielding schizodemes) are used to group different strains. At least three zymodemes differentiate sylvatic strains from those of domestic origin. Surface membrane glycoproteins specific for different stages of the parasite have been detected, although antigenic variation has not been observed. The glycoprotein detected in blood trypomastigotes can induce partially protective immunity in mice challenged with a virulent strain.

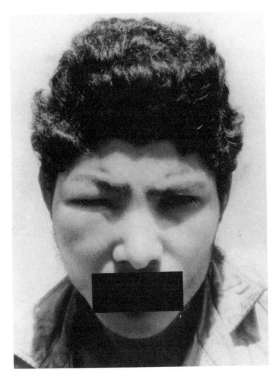

FIGURE 82–2 Romaña's sign in an acute case of Chagas disease.

MULTIPLICATION AND LIFE CYCLE

In the vertebrate host, multiplication is carried out only by the amastigote form, which divides inside cells or muscle fibers to form groups called **pseudocysts.** Trypomastigotes ingested when the insect takes a blood meal from an infected host transform into epimastigotes in the intestine (Fig. 82-3). In the rectal sac these attach by the flagellar sheath mainly to the surface of the epithelium on the rectal gland, where they reproduce actively (Figs. 82-4 and 82-5). In about 8 to 10 days, metacyclic trypomastigote forms appear which are flushed out of the gut with the feces of the insect. These organisms are able to penetrate the vertebrate host only through the mucosa or abrasions of the skin; hence, transmission does not necessarily occur at every blood meal. Within the vertebrate the trypo-mastigotes transform into amastigotes. After a period of intracellular multiplication at the portal of entry, the amastigotes are released into the blood as trypanosomes which may then invade other cells or tissues, becoming amastigotes again.

PATHOGENESIS

Surface glycoproteins and certain serum factors bound to the parasite may be important in adherence to and penetration of cells. Inflammatory reactions at the sites of rupturing pseudocysts can lead to pathologic manifestations, such as acute myocarditis and destruction of parasympathetic ganglia of the heart and myenteric plexus, which can cause the changes observed in the chronic phase of the illness. Destruction of neurons in the central nervous system and in other tissues may be due to an autoimmune process. Antibodies against endocardial-vascular-interstitial tissue (EVI), neurons, striated muscle, and laminin have been demonstrated. The histopathologic changes in chronic myocardiopathy, such as focal myocarditis and extensive fibrosis and myocytolysis, usually occur in the absence of demonstrable parasites and can lead to sudden death. Thromboemboli can be caused by heart damage, and thinning of the apex of the left ventricle is a characteristic lesion.

HOST DEFENSES

The host response includes both inflammatory and immune reactions. During the acute stage, rupture of pseudocysts stimulates an infiltration of polymorphonuclear neutrophils, monocytes, and lymphocytes, accompanied by edema, particularly in the heart. IgM antibodies are produced early and are subsequently replaced by IgG. Apparently only lytic antibodies (detectable by a complement-mediated lysis test using blood stages of the parasite) are involved in host resistance. There is also evidence that cell-mediated immune mechanisms are involved in controlling infection in experimental hosts.

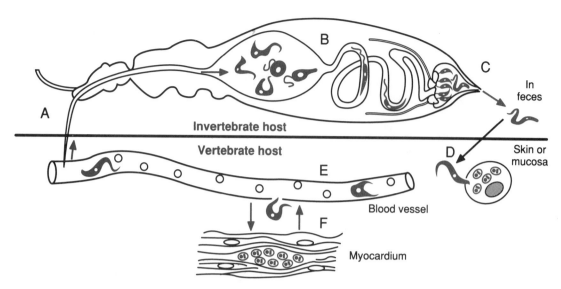

FIGURE 82–3 Life cycle of *T cruzi* in the intestine of a triatomine bug and in the vertebrate host. After entering the bug in infected blood (*A*), the trypanosomes transform to epimastigotes in the stomach and midgut (*B*). Epimastigotes attach to the walls of the rectal sac and produce infective metacyclic trypomastigotes, which are eliminated with feces (*C*) and enter the vertebrate host through breaks in the skin. The parasites transform to amastigotes inside local cells (*D*), and multiply to release blood trypanosomes, which invade other tissues (*E & F*).

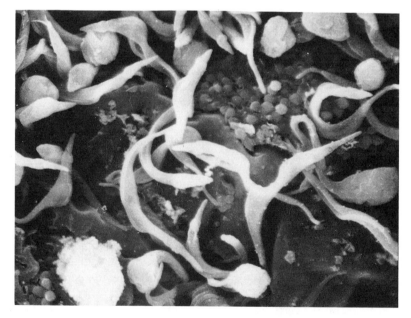

FIGURE 82–4 Metacyclic trypomastigotes and epimastigotes of *T cruzi* attached to the epithelium of the rectal gland of *Triatoma dimidiata*. (From Zeledón R: Life cycle of *Trypanosum cruzi* in the insect vector. In Brenner RR, Stoka Am (eds): Chagas' Disease Vectors. Vol. 2. Anatomic and Physiological Aspects. CRC Press, Boca Raton, FL, 1987, with permission.)

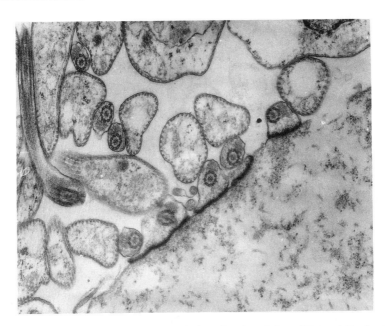

FIGURE 82-5 Transmission electron micrograph showing flagellates of *T cruzi* attached by hemidesmosomes to the epithelium of the rectal gland of *Triatoma dimidiata*. (From Zeledón R: Life cycle of *Trypanosoma cruzi* in the insect vector. In Brenner RR, Stoka Am (eds): Chagas' Disease Vectors. Vol. 2. Anatomic and Physiological Aspects. CRC Press, Boca Raton, FL, 1987, with permission.)

EPIDEMIOLOGY

Chagas disease is transmitted by cone-nosed triatomine bugs of several genera *(Triatoma, Rhodnius, Panstrongylus)*. Congenital and blood transfusion transmission also can occur.

Natural foci of Chagas disease exist among wild mammals and their associated triatomines. Humans and domestic animals became involved in the epidemiologic chain several centuries ago, when insects living under wild conditions began adapting to households. Opossums, armadillos, and wild rodents are reservoirs of the parasite, linking the wild and domestic cycles (Fig. 82-6). Cases of human trypanosomiasis have been reported in almost all countries of the Americas, including the southern United States, but the main foci are in poor rural areas of Latin America.

Different vectors are associated with different types of dwellings: *Rhodnius prolixus* prefers huts with palm-thatch roofs; *Triatoma infestans* is found mainly in houses with mud and cane walls; *T dimidiata* has a preference for dirt floors.

DIAGNOSIS

In the acute phase, the symptoms and signs described above suggest the disease. In the chronic phase electrocardiographic alterations, particularly arrhythmia and right bundle branch block in young adults, are indicative. In the early stages of the disease the parasite is demonstrated relatively easily by direct microscopic blood examination, by xenodiagnosis (allowing clean, laboratory-reared insects to feed on a suspected victim and later examining the insect feces), or by culturing the blood. In the chronic phase, xenodiagnosis and culturing, alone or in combination, reveal the parasite in only 30 to 60 percent of cases, but serologic tests (indirect hemagglutination, indirect immunofluorescence, enzyme-linked immunosorbent assay (ELISA) can be diagnostic.

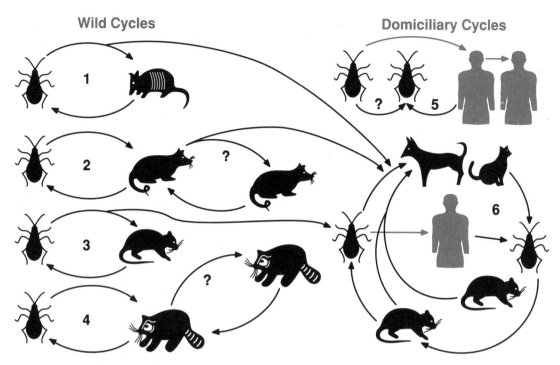

FIGURE 82–6   Wild and domiciliary life cycles of Chagas disease. Some triatomine bugs transmit *T cruzi* to various wild animals (cycles 1 – 4). Other bugs are adapted to houses and transmit the parasite among humans and domestic animals (cycles 5 and 6). (Modified from Zeledón R: Epidemiology: modes of transmission and reservoir hosts of Chagas' disease. In Elliot K, O'Connor M, Wolstenholme GFW (eds): Trypanosomiasis and Leishmaniasis. Ciba Found Symp 20, 1974, with permission.)

CONTROL

The only practical control measures for Chagas disease are the use of insecticides to eliminate the vector bugs from dwellings. Improving the household environment helps considerably by eliminating lodging places for the insects. Vaccination trials in animals have yielded only partial protection. Live attenuated vaccines apparently are most effective but are too risky for use in humans. In endemic areas, serologic screening in blood banks is important to prevent transmission by transfusion.

Nitrofurans (nifurtimox) and benznidazole are used with good or partial success in acute cases, but new drugs effective against both the trypomastigotes and the amastigotes are needed.

AFRICAN TRYPANOSOMIASIS (SLEEPING SICKNESS)

CLINICAL MANIFESTATIONS

Sleeping sickness (African trypanosomiasis) is caused by *Trypanosoma brucei*. An initial chancre with regional lymphadenitis is frequently observed in patients infected by *Trypanosoma brucei rhodesiense* but seldom in patients infected by *T b gambiense*. The lesion persists for several weeks. After a period of local multiplication, the trypanosomes enter the general circulation via the lymphatics, and recurrent fever, headache, lymphadenopathy, and splenomegaly may occur. Later, signs of meningoencephalitis appear, followed by somnolence, cachexia, coma, and death. Enlargement of the posterior cervical chain of lymph nodes (Winterbottom's sign) is more common in *T b gambiense* infection.

STRUCTURE

The two subspecies of *T brucei* are morphologically indistinguishable. They may be pleomorphic, ranging from 12 to 42 μm long (mean, 30 μm), and have a small kinetoplast and a well-developed undulating membrane. The posterior end is more rounded than that of *T cruzi*.

CLASSIFICATION AND ANTIGENIC TYPES

The various subspecies of *T brucei* differ in their capacity to infect mammals other than man. The subspecies that do not infect man are killed by human serum. *Trypanosoma brucei* subspecies also can be separated into zymodemes, schizodemes, and groups based on DNA hybridization. Both metacyclic and blood forms are covered by glycoprotein surface variable (GSV) antigens, which are expressed in certain sequences of variable antigenic types (VAT) by activation of the specific genes. This variability allows the trypanosomes to evade specific antibodies. The so-called common antigens include structural and functional immunogenic components.

MULTIPLICATION AND LIFE CYCLE

Trypanosoma brucei trypanosomes, unlike those of *T cruzi*, multiply while in the blood or cerebrospinal fluid. Trypanosomes ingested by a feeding fly must reach the salivary glands within a few days, where they reproduce actively as epimastigotes attached to the microvilli of the gland until they transform into metacyclic trypomastigotes, which are found free in the lumen. Around 15 to 35 days after infection the fly becomes infective through its bite.

PATHOGENESIS

As the disease progresses, inflammatory changes lead to a demyelinating encephalitis. Antibodies against myelin have been detected, suggesting that this condition may have an autoimmune basis. The immunosuppressive action of components of the parasite's membrane is probably responsible for such concomitant infections as pneumonia. The GSV antigens stimulate high concentrations of IgM antibodies. Periodic changes occur in the surface antigens, thereby circumventing the host's immune responses (see Ch. 78). On the other hand, the common antigens are liberated in every trypanolytic crisis (episode of trypanosome lysis) and lead to antibody and cell-mediated hypersensitivity reactions. It is believed that some cytotoxic and physiopathologic processes are the result of biochemical and immune mechanisms.

HOST DEFENSES

Inflammatory reactions occur initially at the site of inoculation and are accompanied by regional lymphadenitis; inflammation in the heart and brain soon develops. A vasculitis with perivascular infiltration by lymphocytes and plasma cells is the most common lesion. In addition to the high levels of IgM antibody, active cell-mediated immune responses occur.

EPIDEMIOLOGY

Both forms of African trypanosomiasis are transmitted during the daytime by the bite of infected tsetse flies (*Glossina* species), which inhabit the open savannah of eastern Africa (*T b rhodesiense*) or riverine areas in western and central Africa (*T b gambiense*). Wild game mammals (bushbuck, hartebeest, lion, hyena) as well as cattle act as reservoirs of *T b rhodesiense*. This zoonotic subspecies, which is the more virulent of the two, is thus maintained in the most resistant reservoirs, resulting in continuous selection of aggressive strains. *Trypanosoma b gambiense* has been found mostly in domestic pigs, cattle, and dogs, although there is evidence that antelopes in certain areas may also carry the parasite. Man-fly-man transmission is hence more common in West and Central Africa. Asymptomatic persons can carry the parasites in their blood for long periods and could be continuously infective for the vectors (Fig. 82-7).

DIAGNOSIS

The Rhodesian type of sleeping sickness evolves more acutely to death and its neurologic effects are less characteristic. The Gambian form tends to be more chronic and sometimes takes several years to develop central nervous system (CNS) involvement. In the early stages of the disease, the parasites can be demonstrated in lymph nodes and blood; later, they appear in the cerebrospinal fluid. In the Rhodesian type, lumbar puncture is indicated because of early CNS invasion. Culture or laboratory animal inoculations can be useful.

Serologic tests, such as indirect immunofluorescense, direct card agglutination, and indirect hemagglutination, are used successfully for diagnosis.

CONTROL

Tsetse fly populations have been reduced successfully by the use of insecticides or traps with an attractant bait plus insecticide. No reliable vaccine is available, and the variability in antigenic composition of the blood populations makes vaccination a difficult goal. Drugs such as pentamidine and the arsenical suramin, are successful in treatment, particularly in the early phase, and melarsoprol, another arsenical, is used in advanced disease.

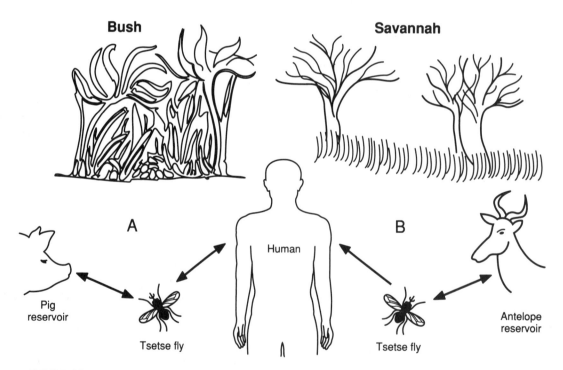

FIGURE 82–7 Domestic and wild cycles of Gambian and Rhodesian types of African sleeping sickness. (A) In West Africa, riverine tsetse flies (*palpalis* group) living in the bush transmit the Gambian form to humans (man-fly-man cycle) and sometimes to domestic animals, particularly pigs. (B) In East Africa, *morsitans* group tsetse flies of the open savannah transmit the Rhodesian form to various mammals, mainly antelopes, and to humans. The Gambian cycle can result in an epidemic.

CUTANEOUS AND MUCOCUTANEOUS LEISHMANIASIS

CLINICAL MANIFESTATIONS

Leishmaniasis is a general term for diseases caused by species of the genus *Leishmania,* which are transmitted by the bite of infected sand flies. The lesions of cutaneous and mucocutaneous leishmaniasis are limited to the skin and mucous membranes. The much more severe disease visceral leishmaniasis, which involves the entire reticuloendothelial system, is discussed in the next section. Cutaneous leishmaniasis appears 2 to 3 weeks after the bite of an infected sand fly as a small cutaneous papule. This lesion slowly grows, becoming indurated and often ulcerated, and develops secondary infection. Secondary or diffuse lesions may develop. The disease is occasionally self-limiting but usually chronic. Leishmaniasis from a primary skin lesion may involve the oral and nasopharyngeal mucosa.

STRUCTURE

All species of *Leishmania* parasitic in man are morphologically similar and appear as intracellular amastigotes 3 to 6 μm long by 1.5 to 3 μm in diameter. Promastigotes develop in the intestine of the sand fly.

CLASSIFICATION AND ANTIGENIC TYPES

The criteria used to differentiate *Leishmania* species are clinical, morphologic, behavioral (vector specificity, laboratory animal patterns, in vitro culture), immunologic (monoclonal antibodies), and biochemical (restriction enzymes, DNA probes, isoenzymes). The main species in the Old World are *Leishmania tropica, L major,* and *L aethiopica* (causing oriental sore); in the New World, *L mexicana* (causing chiclero ulcer), *L amazonensis, L peruviana* (causing uta), *L braziliensis, L panamensis, L guyanensis* (causing dermal leishmaniasis or espundia); other species occur in different geographic areas. Various *Leishmania* cell surface glycopro-

teins and lipopolysaccharides are being studied for possible use in species differentiation.

MULTIPLICATION AND LIFE CYCLE

In mammalian hosts, amastigotes are phagocytosed by macrophages but resist digestion and divide actively in the phagolysosome. Parasites ingested by a female sand fly that sucks the blood of an infected person or animal pass into the stomach, transform into promastigotes, and multiply actively. A paramastigote form also occurs in sand flies. The parasites finally attach by the flagellum to the walls of the esophagus, midgut, and hindgut of the fly, and some eventually reach the proboscis and are inoculated into a new host. Infective sand flies may become so blocked by parasites that probing alone leads to transmission.

PATHOGENESIS

Promastigotes from the proboscis of an infected female sand fly are injected into the skin and taken up by local macrophages. Lesions of oriental sore and chiclero ulcer normally resolve spontaneously after a few months; nevertheless, in the latter, destructive and chronic lesions of the pinna of the ear are observed in 50 to 60 percent of patients. In *L panamensis* and *L guyanensis* infections, lesions usually become chronic, sometimes with lymphatic compromise and hematogenous dissemination (Fig. 82-8). In *L braziliensis* infection, highly destructive spread to the oral or nasal mucosa frequently occurs (Fig. 82-9); in the diffuse type (*L mexicana, L amazonensis, L aethiopica),* there is a disseminated nodular picture similar to lepromatous leprosy (Fig. 82-10).

HOST DEFENSES

The local granuloma consists of lymphocytes, plasma cells, and macrophages containing intracellular parasites. In diffuse cutaneous leishmaniasis, foamy histiocytes filled with parasites are found, a reaction typical of an impaired cell-mediated immune mechanism. In fact, these patients are specifically anergic to the Montenegro skin test (see Diagnosis), and the phenomenon has been at-

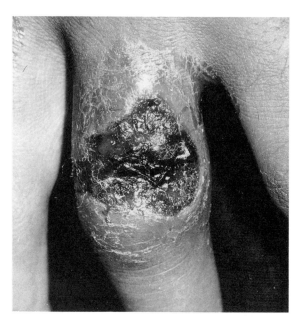

FIGURE 82–8 Ulcerative dermal leishmaniasis of central finger of the right hand produced by *L panamensis.*

tributed to the presence of a specific monocyte suppressor cell. It has also been observed that the lymphocytes fail to express the interleukin-2 receptors. As a result, interferon γ, the major lymphokine mediating macrophage activation to destroy the parasite, is not produced. Chronic lesions of the ear and nose cartilage are due to a poor immune response. When the immune response is normal, a tuberculoid picture develops with epith-

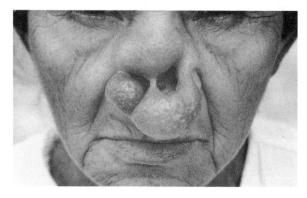

FIGURE 82–9 Mucocutaneous leishmaniasis caused by *L braziliensis.* (Courtesy of Carlos Ponce.)

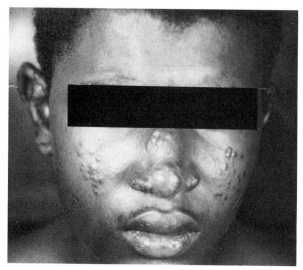

FIGURE 82–10 Diffuse cutaneous leishmaniasis attributed to *L amazonensis.* (Courtesy of Jacinto Convit, M.D.)

elioid and giant cells, lymphocytes, and plasma cells. Cell-mediated immunity is important; relatively low titers of antibodies are produced.

EPIDEMIOLOGY

The vectors of *Leishmania* are sand flies of the genus *Lutzomyia* in the New World and *Phlebotomus* in the Old World. Animal reservoirs are wild rodents, sloths, marsupials, carnivores, and others. In the Old World, anthroponotic urban foci caused by *L tropica* are found, whereas *L major* and *L aethiopica* are typically zoonotic, involving rodents and hyraxes, respectively, as reservoirs. In the New World, with the exception of *L peruviana,* all forms are zoonotic and mainly sylvatic. In the case of *L panamensis* the main reservoir animals are arboreal, as are the various vectors. For *L mexicana,* some rodents serve as reservoir species, and the transmission is accomplished mainly by forest floor sand flies (Fig. 82-11).

DIAGNOSIS

The patient presents single or multiple ulcers or nodules or dry verrucous lesions. Metastatic, granulomatous oral or nasal lesions, with or without

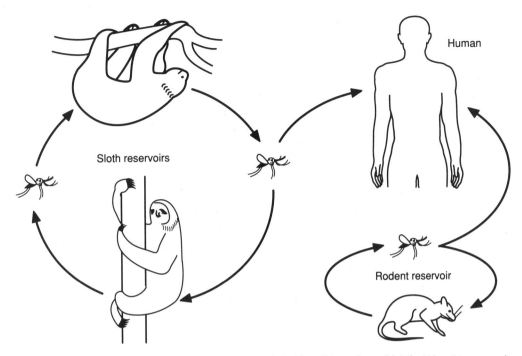

FIGURE 82–11   Simplified life cycles of *L panamensis* (left) and *L mexicana* (right). At least two species of sloths are common reservoirs of *L panamensis;* humans become victims when they enter the tropical forest and are attacked by infected arboreal sand flies. In the same way, *L mexicana* is maintained in rodents and is transmitted to humans by sand flies that live close to the forest floor.

perforation or destruction of the nasal septum, may develop, usually several years after the skin lesions have healed. In the *panamensis* type mucosal lesions are uncommon and are less destructive than in the *braziliensis* type. In the latter, the process sometimes extends from the palate to the pharynx and larynx. These destructive lesions (constituting the condition called espundia) are common in Brazil but are also observed in Sudan, produced there by *L aethiopica,* usually in a less severe form. The diffuse type, characterized by disseminated plaques, papules, or nodules, especially on the face or limbs, is observed in areas where organisms of the *mexicana* and *amazonensis* types exist, as well as in some parts of Africa *(L aethiopica).*

Parasites can be demonstrated in scrapings of the borders of the lesions but they become scarce once ulceration and bacterial contamination occur. Culturing in blood agar media increases markedly the possibility of isolating the parasite; material from direct puncture of the lesions' borders or lymph nodes or triturated biopsy tissue is used. Various serologic tests (ELISA, immunofluorescent antibody) are satisfactory for indirect diagnosis. The Montenegro skin test, in which an indurated area appears at the site of inoculation of the antigen after 48 to 72 hr, is usually positive after 2 to 3 months of infection and remains so throughout the patient's lifetime.

CONTROL

Leishmaniasis transmitted in or near houses can be prevented with insecticides, but this procedure is not practical for the forest tegumentary type. No effective vaccine is yet available. Pentavalent antimonials, such as sodium antimony gluconate (Pentostam) and meglumine antimoniate (Glucantime), are available for treatment, but have some limitations owing to their toxic side effects. Amphoteri-cin B has been used in cases with mucosal involve-ment and in cases of diffuse disease where antimonial therapy fails. Less toxic drugs that can be administered orally and that could used for both prophylaxis and treatment are needed.

VISCERAL LEISHMANIASIS (KALA-AZAR)

CLINICAL MANIFESTATIONS

Like cutaneous leishmaniasis, visceral leishma-niasis begins with a nodule at the site of inocula-tion. This lesion rarely ulcerates and usually disap-pears spontaneously in a few weeks or months. In contrast to cutaneous leishmaniasis, symptoms and signs of systemic disease develop, such as un-dulating fever, malaise, diarrhea, splenomegaly, hepatomegaly, lymphadenopathy, emaciation, anemia, and leukopenia (Fig. 82-12). Infiltrative or nodular lesions of the skin may appear after treatment (post-kala-azar dermal leishmaniasis), a condition seen frequently in India. In some areas of Europe and Latin America, *L infantum* may cause a cutaneous form without apparent visceral involvement (Fig. 82-13). Subclinical cases also occur.

STRUCTURE, MULTIPLICATION, AND LIFE CYCLE

The *Leishmania* species that cause kala-azar are similar in morphology and life cycle to other leish-maniids.

CLASSIFICATION AND ANTIGENIC TYPES

Kala-azar can be caused by at least three *Leish-mania* species, which are differentiated by zymo-deme, serodeme, and DNA hybridization. *Leish-mania donovani* and *L infantum* are responsible for visceral leishmaniasis in the Old World; *L chagasi* and *L infantum* (which may be the same organism) cause the disease in the New World.

PATHOGENESIS

In more serious cases of visceral leishmaniasis the parasites, which can resist the internal body tem-perature, invade internal organs (liver, spleen, bone marrow, and lymph nodes) where they oc-cupy the reticuloendothelial cells. The pathoge-netic mechanisms of the disease are not fully un-derstood, but, clearly, in those organs that exhibit marked cellular alteration, hyperplasia of histio-cytes leads to hypertrophy. Parasitized macro-phages replace hematopoietic tissue in the bone marrow. Patients with advanced disease are prone to superinfection with other organisms.

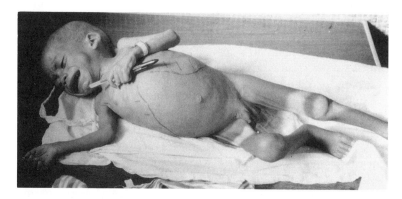

FIGURE 82-12   Visceral leishmaniasis in a child from Honduras with marked emaciation and hepato-splenomegaly. (Courtesy of Carlos Ponce.)

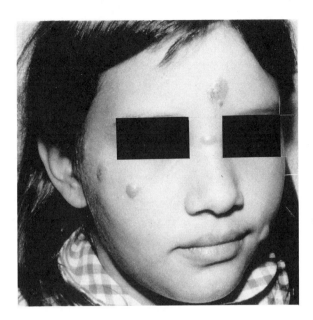

FIGURE 82–13 Nodular cutaneous leishmaniasis produced by *L infantum* in Costa Rica.

HOST DEFENSES

High levels of IgG and other immunoglobulins are common. The Montenegro skin test for delayed hypersensitivity is usually negative during the disease but becomes positive after treatment.

EPIDEMIOLOGY

In India, transmission occurs in villages in an anthroponotic man-sand fly-man cycle without nonhuman reservoir. In Europe and Africa, several rodents may act as reservoirs. In rural semi-arid zones of Latin America, both wild and domestic dogs enter the epidemiologic chain and the vector is a common anthropophilic and zoophilic sand fly, *Lutzomyia longipalpis,* abundant in and around houses. The disease is more common in children in both Latin America and the Mediterranean area.

DIAGNOSIS

The typical symptoms, particularly hepatosplenomegaly and the pancytopenia, strongly suggest visceral leishmaniasis. The parasite usually can be demonstrated in stained or cultured bone marrow or spleen material. Serologic tests (ELISA, immunofluorescent antibody) are useful, particularly in surveys.

CONTROL

The same insecticides and drugs that work for cutaneous leishmaniasis are used for visceral leishmaniasis. Aromatic diamidines are also used.

REFERENCES

Blackwell J, McMahon-Pratt D, Shaw JJ: Molecular biology of *Leishmania.* Parasitol Today 2:45, 1986

Brener Z, Krettli AU: Immunology of Chagas' disease. In Wyler DJ (ed): Modern Parasite Biology: Cellular, Immunological and Molecular Aspects. WH Freeman, New York, 1990

Brenner RR, Stoka AM (eds): Chagas' Disease Vectors. Vols. 1–3. CRC Press, Boca Raton, FL, 1987

Castes M, Cabrera M, Trujillo D, Convit J: T-cell subpopulations, expression of interleukin-2 receptor, and production of interleukin-2 and gamma interferon in human American cutaneous leishmaniasis. J Clin Microbiol 26:1207, 1988

Chang KP, Bray RS (eds): Leishmaniasis. Elsevier Biomedical, Amsterdam, 1985

Kierszenbaum E, Hudson L: Autoimmunity in Chagas' disease: Cause or symptom? Parasitol Today 1:4, 1985

Lumsden WHR, Evans DA, (eds): Biology of the Kinetoplastida. Vols. 1 and 2. Academic Press, London, 1979

Miles MA, Cibulskis RE, Morel CM, et al: The heterogeneity of *Trypanosoma cruzi.* Parasitol Today 2:94, 1986

Molyneaux DH, Ashford RW: The Biology of *Trypanosoma* and *Leishmania* Parasites of Man and Domestic Animals. Taylor and Francis, London, 1983

Pentreath VW: Neurobiology of sleeping sickness. Parasitol Today 5:215, 1989

Peters W, Killick-Kendrick R (eds): The Leishmaniases in Biology and Medicine. Vols. 1 and 2. Academic Press, London, 1987

Petry K, Eisen H: Chagas' disease: A model for the study of autoimmune diseases. Parasitol Today 5:111, 1989

World Health Organization: The Leishmaniases. Report of a WHO Expert Committee. WHO Tech Rep Ser 701, 1984

World Health Organization: Epidemiology and Control of African Trypanosomiasis. Report of a WHO Expert Committee. WHO Tech Rep Ser 739, 1986

Zeledón R, Rabinovich JE: Chagas' disease: An ecological approach with special emphasis on its insect vectors. Ann Rev Entomol 26:101, 1981

83 MALARIA

LELAND S. RICKMAN
STEPHEN L. HOFFMAN

GENERAL CONCEPTS

Clinical Manifestations

Initially patients have fever, chills, sweating, headache, weakness, and other symptoms mimicking a "viral syndrome." Later, severe disease may develop, with abnormal level of consciousness, renal failure, and multisystem failure.

Classification

Plasmodia are protozoa. Only the species *Plasmodium falciparum*, *P vivax*, *P malariae,* and *P ovale* are usually infectious for humans. Of these, *P falciparum* is the most dangerous.

Structure and Life Cycle

Mature, uninucleate sporozoites in the salivary glands of infected mosquitoes are injected into a human host when the mosquito feeds. The sporozoites rapidly invade liver parenchymal cells, where they mature into liver-stage schizonts, which burst to release 2,000 to 50,000 uninucleate merozoites. In *P vivax* and *P ovale* infections, maturation of the schizont may be delayed for 1 to 2 years. Each merozoite can infect a red blood cell. Within the red cell, the merozoite matures either into a uninucleate gametocyte—the sexual stage, infectious for *Anopheles* mosquitoes—or, over 48 to 72 hours, into an erythrocytic-stage schizont containing 10 to 36 merozoites. Rupture of the schizont releases these merozoites, which infect further red cells. If a vector mosquito ingests gametocytes, the gametocytes develop in the mosquito gut to gametes, which undergo fertilization and mature in 2 to 3 weeks to sporozoites.

Pathogenesis

The fever and chills of malaria are associated with the rupture of erythrocytic-stage schizonts. In severe falciparum malaria, parasitized red cells may obstruct capillaries and postcapillary venules, leading to local hypoxia and the release of toxic cellular products. Obstruction of the microcirculation in the brain (cerebral malaria) and in other vital organs is thought to be responsible for severe complications.

Host Defenses

Both innate and acquired immunity occur. Innate immunity consists of various traits of erythrocytes that discourage infection. The sickle-cell trait protects against the development of severe *P falciparum* malaria, and the absence of Duffy antigen prevents infection by *P vivax*. Recurrent infections lead to the development of humoral and cellular immune responses against all plasmodium stages. Acquired immunity does not prevent reinfection but does reduce the severity of disease.

Epidemiology

Malaria is distributed worldwide throughout the tropics and subtropics.

Diagnosis

Diagnosis depends on the identification of plasmodia in thick and thin blood smears.

Control

Treatment: Treatment of falciparum malaria is complicated by the nearly worldwide resistance of *P falciparum*
to chloroquine. Alternative drugs such as mefloquine,
pyrimethamine/sulfadoxine, quinine, and quinidine are
used. Chloroquine has provided virtually 100 percent
clinical cure of *P vivax, P malariae,* and *P ovale* malaria.
Disease caused by *P vivax* and *P ovale* requires primaquine for *radical* cure.

Prevention: Malaria may be prevented by chemoprophylaxis and other measures involving the individual, and by
community-wide measures to control the vector. Exposure to night-feeding anopheles mosquitoes is reduced
by using protective clothing, insect repellents, insecticides, bed nets, etc. The population and life span of the
mosquitoes may be reduced by destroying breeding
places and by application of insecticides. Vaccines are
being developed.

INTRODUCTION

Malaria has been a major disease of humankind for
thousands of years. It is referred to in numerous
biblical passages and in the writings of Hippocra-
tes. Although excellent drug treatments are available, malaria is still considered by many to be the
most important infectious disease of humans:
there are approximately 200 million to 500 million
new cases each year in the world, and the disease is
the direct cause of 1 million to 2.5 million deaths
per year.

Malaria is caused by protozoa of the genus *Plasmodium.* Four species cause disease in humans: *P
falciparum, P vivax, P ovale* and *P malariae.* The
family Plasmodiidae also contains protozoa that
infect other mammals, reptiles, and birds. Malaria
is spread to humans by the bite of female mosquitoes of the genus *Anopheles.*

CLINICAL MANIFESTATIONS

The clinical course of malaria consists of bouts of
fever and other symptoms alternating with symptom-free periods (Fig. 83-1). The classic malaria
paroxysm comprises three successive stages. The
first is a 15- to 60-min **cold stage** characterized by
shivering and a feeling of cold. Next comes the 2-
to 6-hr **hot stage,** in which there is fever, sometimes reaching 41°C; flushed, dry skin; and often
headache, nausea, and vomiting. Finally, there is

the 2- to 4-hr **sweating stage** during which the
fever drops rapidly and the patient sweats. In all
types of malaria the periodic febrile response is
caused by rupture of mature schizonts. In *P vivax*
and *P ovale* malaria, a brood of schizonts matures
every 48 hr, so the periodicity of fever is *tertian*
("tertian malaria"), whereas in *P malariae* disease,
fever occurs every 72 hours ("quartan malaria").
The fever in falciparum malaria may occur every
48 hr, but is usually irregular, showing no distinct
periodicity. These classic fever patterns are usually
not seen early in the course of malaria, and therefore the absence of periodic, synchronized fevers
does not rule out a diagnosis of malaria. In addition to fever, chills, sweats, and headache, individuals with uncomplicated malaria may have symptoms and signs suggesting a respiratory illness,
gastroenteritis, or a "viral syndrome." Physical examination may show splenomegaly or hepatomegaly but equally may reveal no abnormalities.

If the diagnosis of malaria is missed or delayed,
especially with *P falciparum* infection, potentially
fatal **complicated malaria** may develop. The most
frequent and serious complications of malaria are
hyperparasitemia (parasitization of more than 3 to 5
percent of the erythrocytes) and *cerebral malaria.*
Cerebral malaria is defined as any abnormality of
mental status in a person with malaria. As would be
expected, comatose patients with cerebral malaria
are at the highest risk of dying, with a case fatality
rate of 15 to 50 percent.

Typical temperature chart of *P vivax* infection showing tertian periodicity related to the maturation and rupture of erythrocytic schizonts.

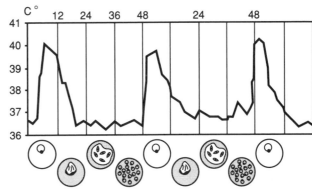

Typical temperature chart of *P malariae* infection showing quartan periodicity

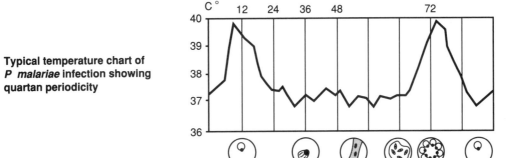

Typical temperature chart of *P falciparum* infection showing irregular tertian periodicity and the influence of successful treatment

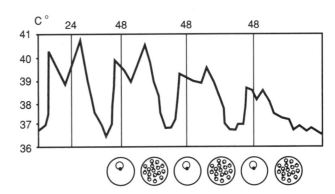

FIGURE 83-1   Typical temperature charts of malarial infections. (Adapted from Bruce-Chwatt LJ: Essential Malariology. 2nd Ed. John Wiley & Sons, New York, 1985, p. 52, with permission.)

Complications can occur in virtually any organ system and include prolonged hyperthermia, seizures, hypoglycemia, renal failure, Gram-negative sepsis and shock, gastrointestinal bleeding, diarrhea, pulmonary edema, and aspiration pneumonia. Rupture of an enlarged spleen occasionally occurs, especially with vivax malaria, and may be life-threatening. The treatment of these and other

complications is discussed below under Ancillary Therapy and Treatment of Complications.

Routine laboratory examinations in a case of uncomplicated malaria may reveal anemia, thrombocytopenia, and leukopenia. Eosinophilia is not seen. Patients with complicated malaria occasionally show evidence of massive intravascular hemolysis with hemoglobinemia and hemoglobinuria, disseminated intravascular hemolysis with thrombocytopenia and prolonged coagulation, and renal failure with or without an active urinary sediment.

CLASSIFICATION

Only four species of the protozoan genus *Plasmodium* usually infect humans: *P falciparum, P vivax, P malariae,* and *P ovale* (Fig. 83-2). Of these, *P falciparum* causes the most severe disease.

STRUCTURE AND LIFE CYCLE

Like many protozoa, plasmodia pass through a number of stages in the course of their two-host

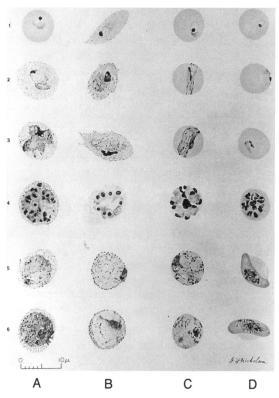

FIGURE 83-2 Blood stages of *Plasmodium.* Column **A,** *Plasmodium vivax;* **B,** *P ovale;* **C,** *P malariae;* **D,** *P falciparum.* Row 1, young trophozoites; 2, growing trophozoites; 3, mature trophozoites; 4, mature schizonts; 5, macrogametocytes; 6, microgametocytes. (From Strickland GT: Hunters Tropical Medicine. 6th Ed. WB Saunders, Philadelphia, 1984, p. 524, with permission.)

life cycle. The stage infective for humans is the uninucleate, lancet-shaped **sporozoite** (approximately 1×7 μm). Sporozoites are produced by sexual reproduction in the midgut of vector anopheline mosquitoes and migrate to the salivary gland. When an infected *Anopheles* mosquito bites a human, she may inject sporozoites along with saliva into small blood vessels (Fig. 83-3). Within 30 min the sporozoites enter liver parenchymal cells. In the liver cell, the parasite develops into a spherical, multinucleate **liver-stage schizont** which contains 2,000 to 50,000 uninucleate **merozoites.** This process of enormous amplification is called **exoerythrocytic schizogny.** This **exoerythrocytic** or **liver phase** of the disease usually takes between 5 and 21 days, depending on the species of plasmodium. However, in *P vivax* and *P ovale* infections, maturation of liver-stage schizonts may be delayed for as long as 1 to 2 years. These quiescent liver-phase parasites are sometimes called **hypnozoites.** Patients infected with *P vivax* or *P ovale* must be treated with a tissue schizonticide to prevent late recurrence of disease (see Control, below).

Regardless of the time required for development, the mature schizonts eventually rupture, releasing thousands of uninucleate merozoites into the bloodstream. Each merozoite can infect a red blood cell. Within the red cell, the merozoite develops to form either an **erythrocytic-stage schizont** (by the process of **erythrocytic schizogony**) or a spherical or cigar-shaped, uninucleate **gametocyte.** The mature erythrocytic-stage schizont contains 10 to 36 merozoites, each 5 to 10 μm long, which are released into the blood when the schizont ruptures. These merozoites proceed to infect another generation of erythrocytes. The time required for erythrocytic schizogony—which determines the interval between the release of successive generations of merozoites—varies with the species of plasmodium and is responsible for the classic periodicity of fever in malaria.

The gametocyte, which is the sexual stage of the plasmodium, is infectious for mosquitoes that ingest it while feeding. Within the mosquito, gametocytes develop into female and male gametes (macrogametes and microgametes, respectively), which undergo fertilization and then develop over

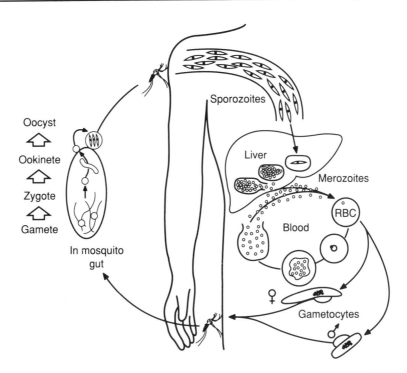

FIGURE 83-3 Life cycle of the malaria parasite. (Adapted from Miller LH, Howard RJ, Carter R et al: Research toward malaria vaccines. Science 234:1350, 1986, with permission.)

2 to 3 weeks into sporozoites that can infect humans. The delay between infection of a mosquito and maturation of sporozoites means that female mosquitoes must live a minimum of 2 to 3 weeks to be able to transmit malaria. This fact is important in malaria control efforts.

PATHOGENESIS

Clinical illness is caused by the erythrocytic stage of the parasite. No disease is associated with sporozoites, the developing liver stage of the parasite, the merozoites released from the liver, or the sexual, gametocyte form of the parasite. The primary clinical manifestations of malaria are the result of the host's response to the systemic and local release of parasite material, on the one hand, and to decreased delivery of oxygen to the tissues because of obstruction of blood flow caused by parasitized erythrocytes, on the other.

The first symptoms and signs of malaria are associated with the rupture of erythrocytes when erythrocytic-stage schizonts mature. This release of parasite material presumably triggers a host immune response. The cytokines, reactive oxygen intermediates, and other cellular products released during the immune response play a prominent role in pathogenesis, and are probably responsible for the fever, chills, sweats, weakness, and other systemic symptoms associated with malaria. In the case of falciparum malaria (the form that causes most deaths), infected erythrocytes adhere to the endothelium of capillaries and postcapillary venules, leading to obstruction of the microcirculation and local tissue anoxia. In the brain this causes cerebral malaria (Fig. 83-4); in the kidney it may cause acute tubular necrosis and renal failure; and in the intestines it can cause ischemia and ulceration, leading to gastrointestinal bleeding and to bacteremia secondary to the entry of intestinal bacteria into the systemic circulation. The severity of malaria-associated anemia tends to be related to the degree of parasitemia. The pathogenesis of this anemia appears to be multifactorial. Hemolysis or

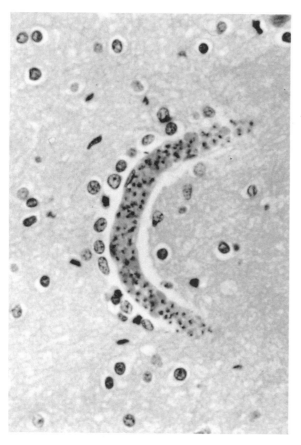

FIGURE 83-4 Light micrograph of a cerebral capillary blocked with parasitized erythrocytes. This specimen is from a patient with cerebral malaria. (From Aikawa M: Morphological changes in erythrocytes induced by malarial parasites. Biol Cell 64:174, 1988, with permission.)

phagocytosis of parasitized erythrocytes and ineffective erythropoiesis are the most important factors, and phagocytosis of uninfected erythrocytes and an autoimmune hemolytic anemia have also been implicated. Massive intravascular hemolysis leading to hemoglobinuria and renal failure, a syndrome called **blackwater fever,** has been associated with the use of quinine. It was described more frequently in the past than currently. Hemolysis may also occur after the use of certain antimalarials in patients with glucose 6-phosphate dehydrogenase deficiency.

HOST DEFENSES

Susceptibility to malaria infection and disease is regulated by hereditary and acquired factors (Fig. 83-5). It now seems clear that the sickle cell trait (which is the cause of sickle-cell anemia) developed as a balanced polymorphism to protect against serious *P falciparum* disease. Although individuals with sickle cell anemia or the sickle cell trait are as easily infected with malaria parasites as normal individuals, they rarely exhibit malaria disease since *P falciparum* develops poorly in their erythrocytes. The virtual absence of *P vivax* infections in many areas of Africa is explained by the fact that most blacks do not have Duffy blood-group antigens, which apparently function as erythrocyte surface receptors for *P vivax* merozoites; without the Duffy antigen, the parasites cannot invade. Malaria parasites do not develop well in ovalocytes, and it has been suggested that ovalocytosis, which is quite common in some malarious areas, such as New Guinea, may reduce the incidence of malaria. Some investigators have suggested that glucose 6-phosphate dehydrogenase deficiency, as well as a number of other hemoglobinopathies (including the thalassemias and hemoglobin E), also protect against malaria infection, but the evidence for these associations is less compelling.

Acquired immunity can also protect against malaria infection and the development of malaria disease. In malarious areas, both the prevalence and the severity of malaria infections decrease with age. However, in contrast to many viral infections, multiple infections with malaria do not confer long-lasting, sterile protective immunity. Virtually all adults in malarious areas suffer repeated malaria infections. Individuals who are repeatedly exposed to malaria develop antibodies against many sporozoite, blood stage, and sexual stage malaria antigens. Since T helper cells are required for the production of antibodies to malarial proteins, these individuals also have T cells that proliferate after stimulation with malarial antigens. It is thought that antibodies, particularly those against blood stages of the parasite, are responsible for the decreased susceptibility to infection and malarial disease seen in adults in malarious areas, and that

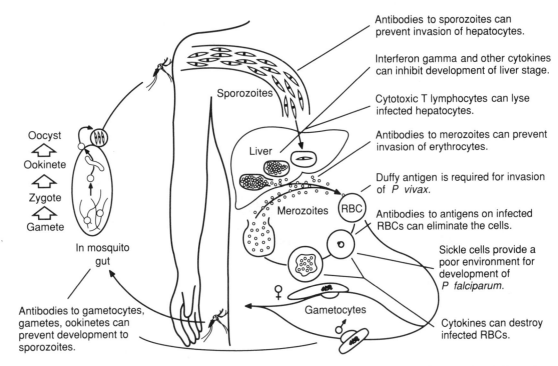

Antibodies to sporozoites can prevent invasion of hepatocytes.

Interferon gamma and other cytokines can inhibit development of liver stage.

Cytotoxic T lymphocytes can lyse infected hepatocytes.

Antibodies to merozoites can prevent invasion of erythrocytes.

Duffy antigen is required for invasion of *P vivax.*

Antibodies to antigens on infected RBCs can eliminate the cells.

Sickle cells provide a poor environment for development of *P falciparum.*

Cytokines can destroy infected RBCs.

Antibodies to gametocytes, gametes, ookinetes can prevent development to sporozoites.

Sporozoites

Liver

Merozoites RBC

Gametocytes

In mosquito gut

Oocyst
Ookinete
Zygote
Gamete

FIGURE 83-5 Host defense against malaria. (Adapted from Miller LH, Howard RJ, Carter R et al: Research toward malaria vaccines. Science 234:1350, 1986, with permission.)

antibodies against the sexual stages of plasmodia may reduce malaria transmission. Recent work also suggests that the naturally acquired immunity includes the release of cytokines that act against all stages of the parasite, and also a cytotoxic T cell response directed at liver stages of the parasite.

Acquired antibody-mediated immunity is apparently transferred from mother to fetus across the placenta. This passively transferred immunity is lost within 6 to 9 months, as is the immunity in adults if they leave a malarious area and are no longer exposed to plasmodia. Pregnant women, particularly primigravidas, are more susceptible to malaria infections and serious malaria disease than their nonpregnant sisters.

EPIDEMIOLOGY

Malaria is transmitted only by anopheline mosquitoes. It was once transmitted in many parts of the world, for example, as far north as North Dakota in the United States. Due both to changes in the environment that made it inhospitable to the mosquito and to eradication campaigns conducted in the years after World War II, endemic malaria transmission has been eliminated from many areas, including the United States and Europe. The disease is still widely transmitted in the tropics and subtropics (Fig. 83-6). In these areas malaria transmission may be *endemic,* occurring predictably every year, or it may be *epidemic,* occurring sporadically when conditions are correct. Endemic transmission of malaria may be year-round or seasonal. In some areas of Africa, 90 to 100 percent of children less than 5 years old have malaria parasites circulating in their blood all the time. Because naturally acquired immunity develops with increasing exposure, in endemic areas malaria disease is primarily found in children. In epidemic areas, on the other hand, naturally acquired immunity falls off between epidemics, and malaria therefore affects all age groups during epidemics.

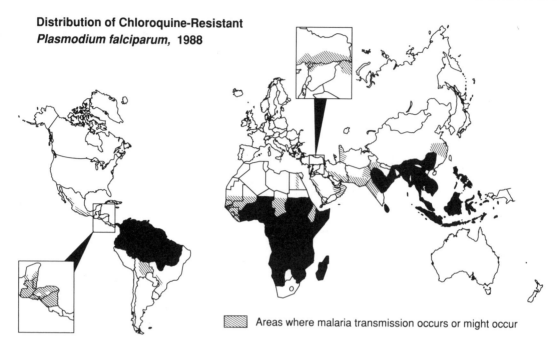

Distribution of Chloroquine-Resistant
Plasmodium falciparum, **1988**

▨ Areas where malaria transmission occurs or might occur

FIGURE 83-6   Epidemiologic assessment of the status of malaria. (From World Health Organization: Health Information for International Travel. WHO, Geneva, 1988, with permission.)

Approximately 1,000 cases of malaria are reported each year in the United States. Most of these cases are acquired abroad. Between 1980 and 1988, 1,534 cases of falciparum malaria in American civilians were reported to the Centers for Disease Control. Of these, 80 percent were acquired in sub-Saharan Africa and 14 percent in Asia, the Caribbean, or South America, despite the fact that only approximately 90,000 Americans travel to sub-Saharan Africa each year and an estimated 900,000 Americans travel to malarious areas of Asia and South America each year. This disparity in the risk of acquiring malaria stems from the fact that travelers to Africa are at risk in most rural and many urban areas, and, moreover, tend to spend evening and nighttime hours in rural areas where malaria risk is highest. In contrast, most travelers to Asia and South America stay in urban or resort areas where there is limited, if any, risk of exposure, and travel to rural areas mainly during daytime hours when there is limited risk of infection.

Because of increased foreign travel and the development of drug-resistant plasmodia, the number of cases of malaria in Americans has increased in recent years. Malaria is sometimes transmitted in the United States by blood transfusions, by needles shared among intravenous drug abusers, and congenitally from infected mothers to their offspring. In addition, since *Anopheles* species are found in a number of areas of the United States, including the Central Valley and San Diego County in California, small epidemics with local transmission have occurred in recent years in these areas when malaria-infected individuals from abroad were bitten by local mosquitoes. In the United States death from malaria is infrequent, but nevertheless occurs every year, usually because of misdiagnosis resulting in late therapy.

In the late 1950s and early 1960s, it appeared that malaria was being adequately controlled by campaigns to eradicate mosquitoes using residual insecticides such as DDT and by treatment of suspected cases with chloroquine. Since then, the mosquitoes have developed high degrees of resistance to DDT, the cost of malaria control has increased dramatically, the organizations required to control malaria have been diminished, and in many regions *P falciparum* has become resistant to chloroquine and other antimalarials (Fig. 83-6). These changes have resulted in a dramatic increase in the incidence of malaria in many parts of the world, and an increase in malaria-related mortality in some of these areas.

DIAGNOSIS

In the United States, many of the deaths from malaria are the result of delayed diagnosis and treatment because the health care provider did not suspect malaria. The diagnosis of malaria requires a high index of suspicion; malaria should be considered in any individual who has a fever and has visited an endemic area for malaria, received a blood transfusion, or used intravenous drugs. Although 95 percent of individuals infected with malaria develop their primary illness within 6 weeks of exposure, some may have primary attacks a year after exposure, and relapses of malaria can occur 1 to 2 years after exposure. Therefore, individuals having a febrile illness and a history of exposure in the last 2 years should be evaluated for malaria.

The laboratory diagnosis of malaria is established by demonstrating malaria parasites in blood smears (Fig. 83-2). Although thick blood smears are more difficult to examine than thin blood smears, they are much more sensitive, as more blood is examined. Thin blood smears, in which parasites are seen within erythrocytes, are used to determine the species of the infecting parasite. Since *P falciparum* may be sequestered in the microcirculation of the deep organs for one-half of the 48 hr life cycle of the parasite, blood smears should be examined every 6 to 12 hr for 48 hr in individuals suspected of having malaria, regardless of whether they are febrile at the time. A new, rapid and sensitive technique for detecting parasitemia using fluorescent staining of centrifuged parasites has been described.

A number of other techniques, including immunologic assays to detect circulating malaria antibodies and antigens, and DNA and RNA probes, have been described. These techniques are rarely used to diagnose acute malaria in individual patients.

CONTROL

Appropriate therapy of malaria requires prompt diagnosis, prompt treatment with a blood schizonticide, recognition and treatment of patients with severe or complicated malaria, recognition of treatment failures, and use of a tissue schizonticide when indicated (Fig. 83-7). All patients with malaria can be cured of the infection with the available antimalarials; the challenge is to recognize the disease and the indicators of its severe forms promptly so that therapy can be initiated and complications and death prevented.

There are two types of cure in malaria therapy. A **clinical cure** is the elimination of the symptoms and signs of an acute malaria attack, whereas a **radical cure** is the eradication of all parasites from the body. Because all the signs and symptoms of malaria are associated with the erythrocytic stage of the parasite, a clinical cure is achieved by using drugs called blood-stage schizonticides that are effective against these. In cases of *P falciparum* and *P malariae* disease, an effective dose of a blood schizonticide to which the parasite is sensitive should lead to radical cure. In cases of *P vivax* and *P ovale* malaria, in which development of liver stage parasites (hypnozoites) may be delayed for as long as 1 to 2 years, radical cure requires therapy against exoerythrocytic or liver stage parasites with drugs called **tissue schizonticides.**

Recurrence of malaria infections after treatment is due either to **recrudescence** or to **relapse.** Recrudescence occurs when the blood schizonticide does not eliminate all parasites from the bloodstream, either because the dose was inadequate or because the parasite is resistant to the drug. *Relapse* occurs in *P vivax* and *P ovale* infections after the delayed development of liver stage parasites that have not been treated adequately with a tissue schizonticide.

Resistance of malaria parasites to antimalarials may be *complete* or *relative;* relative resistance can

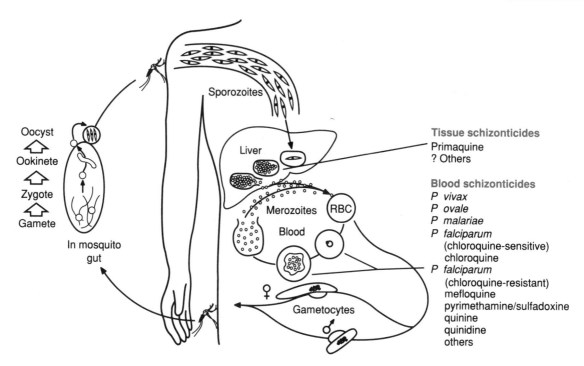

FIGURE 83-7 Treatment of acute malaria. (Adapted from Miller LH, Howard RJ, Carter R et al: Research toward malaria vaccines. Science 234:1350, 1986, with permission.)

be overcome by raising the dosage of the antimalarial.

The clinician, in assessing the patient with malaria, must recognize patients with severe or complicated malaria. Any patient with hyperparasitemia (more than 3 to 5 percent of the erythrocytes parasitized); a history or findings of abnormal level of consciousness (indicating cerebral malaria); prolonged fever; shock; pulmonary, cardiac, hepatic, or renal dysfunction; or high-output diarrhea or vomiting should be considered to have severe malaria and should be treated immediately with intravenous antimalarials and hospitalized in an intensive care unit.

The choice of blood schizonticide depends on the species of plasmodium, the probable drug sensitivity pattern of the parasite based on its geographic origin, and the clinical status of the patient. Parenteral therapy is reserved for patients unable to take medications by mouth and for those with complicated malaria. All patients with un-

complicated *P vivax, P malariae,* and *P ovale* infections should be treated with oral chloroquine. All patients with uncomplicated *P falciparum* infections should receive an antimalarial other than chloroquine, unless the physician knows the origin of the parasite and is confident that it will respond to chloroquine. All patients with complicated malaria, regardless of the plasmodium involved, should be treated as if they had falciparum malaria; the drug of choice is intravenous quinine or quinidine.

The response to antimalarial therapy is monitored both clinically and by examining repeated blood films. The degree of apparent parasitemia may increase during the first 6 to 12 hr after the institution of appropriate therapy, but should drop by more than 75 percent within 48 hr. If this reduction in parasitemia does not occur, drug resistance or inappropriate therapy should be suspected. The patient usually becomes afebrile within 48 to 72 hr after therapy begins. A slow or poor clinical response may indicate drug resistance or inappropriate drug delivery or, alternatively, malaria complications such as anemia, hypoglycemia, recurrent seizures, renal failure, pulmonary edema, aspiration pneumonia, Gram-negative sepsis, and splenic rupture.

When parenteral therapy with either quinine or quinidine is used, the patient must be observed closely for signs of hypotension or myocardial conduction abnormalities. Therapeutic plasma levels are 5 to 15 μg/ml for quinine and 5 to 10 μg/ml for quinidine.

Treatment of Specific Infections

Uncomplicated P falciparum Malaria

Infections acquired in Central America, the Caribbean, and the Middle East are treated with oral chloroquine as shown in Table 83-1. Infections acquired in other areas should be treated with a single dose of mefloquine. Alternative regimens include a single dose of pyrimethamine-sulfadoxine (Fansidar) or oral quinine sulfate and oral doxycycline or oral clindamycin (especially for infections acquired in Southeast Asia, in Oceania including New Guinea, and in the Amazon Basin).

Complicated P falciparum Malaria

Any patient with evidence of complicated malaria should be treated in an intensive care unit using parenteral antimalarials. The drugs of choice are quinine and quinidine. If the disease was acquired in an area where *P falciparum* is known to be chloroquine-sensitive, chloroquine may be given, preferably by continuous infusion, but alternatively by subcutaneous or intramuscular injections. Oral quinine sulfate is substituted as soon as there is evidence of clinical improvement. The addition of a second blood schizonticide such as doxycycline may be required to ensure elimination of infection. Studies from China and Burma indicate that qinghaosu (a drug derived from a medicinal herb used for millennia in China) and its derivatives are more effective than standard antimalarials in rapidly reducing parasitemia in cases of severe malaria.

Uncomplicated P malariae Malaria

Uncomplicated *P malariae* infections are treated with chloroquine alone. Mefloquine is also effective.

Uncomplicated P vivax and P ovale Malaria

Uncomplicated *P vivax* and *P ovale* infections are treated with two drugs: chloroquine to treat the erythrocytic stage parasites and primaquine to treat the persistent liver stage parasites. Some strains of *P vivax*, especially strains from New Guinea and parts of Asia, are relatively resistant to primaquine and may require larger doses for radical cure. Recent reports from these areas indicate that resistance of *p vivax* to chloroquine is emerging. Both Fansidar and mefloquine are also effective against *P vivax*.

Complicated P vivax, P ovale, or P malariae Malaria

Any complicated *P malariae*, *P vivax*, or *P ovale* infection should be treated in the same way as a complicated *P falciparum* infection, since mixed infections are common.

Ancillary Therapy and Treatment of Complications

Supportive therapy and the recognition and treatment of malaria complications may be as critical in treatment as choosing the correct antimalarial. Hyperthermia should be treated with cooling blankets and antipyretics. Fluid and electrolyte balance must be closely monitored so as to maintain adequate cardiac output and renal perfusion and to prevent fluid overload; it may be necessary to monitor right heart or pulmonary artery wedge pressures. The hematocrit must be observed closely, as most individuals with malaria develop anemia. Transfusion of erythrocytes may be necessary. Seizures are frequent in cases of cerebral malaria, and may also be caused by fever or hypoglycemia. Patients with recurrent seizures are treated with standard anticonvulsants, and status epilepticus is treated with diazepam. Hyperparasitemia may be treated with exchange transfusion. Ex-

TABLE 83-1   Treatment of Malaria

Species	Disease Severity	Choice of Drug	Drug	Route of Administration	Initial Dose (mg/kg)	Other Doses (mg/kg)	Interval Between Doses (hr)	Duration of Treatment	Comments
P falciparum	Severe or complicated	Drug of choice:	Quinine dihydroch-loride[a]	IV infusion (2–4 hr)	20 (salt)	10	8	3–10 days	Dosage can be reduced where parasite more sensitive. Oral therapy with quinine sulfate should be started when improvement occurs
		If quinine is not available:	Quinidine gluconate	IV infusion (1–2 hr) followed by continuous infusion	10 (salt)	0.02 mg/kg/min	—	3–10 days	
			Chloroquine sulfate	IV infusion (continuous)	0.83 mg/kg/hr (base)	—	—	30 hr	Oral chloroquine is given to a complete total dose of 25 mg/kg.
			Chloroquine sulfate	IM or SC	3.5 (base)	—	6	>12 hr	Oral chloroquine is given to a complete total dose of 25 mg/kg. The higher dose is for children.

1044

Species	Clinical type		Drug	Route					Comments
P falciparum	Uncomplicated Chloroquine sensitive	Drug of choice:	Chloroquine phosphate	Oral	10 (base)	5–10	6–24	48 hr	Total of 25 mg/kg in 48 hr (see text)
	Chloroquine resistant	Depending on sensitivity:	Mefloquine[c]	Oral	15–25	—	Single dose	Single dose	
			Pyrimethamine/sulfadoxine (PS)[b]	Oral	p = 1.25 s = 25	—		Single dose	3 tablets for adults
			Quinine sulfate[d]	Oral	10	10	8	3–10 days	More effective with doxycycline
			Doxycycline[d]	Oral	1.5–2.0	1.5–2	12	7–10 days	Should be given with quinine
			Clindamycin[d]	Oral	10	10	12	5 days	Should be given with quinine
	Severe	Same as for *P falciparum* (see text), followed by radical cure of *P vivax* and *P ovale* with primaquine (see below).							
P vivax *P ovale* *P malariae*	Uncomplicated	Drug of choice:	Chloroquine		Same regimen as for uncomplicated *P falciparum*				
		Alternatives:	Quinine		Same regimen as for uncomplicated *P falciparum*				
			Mefloquine		Same regimen as for uncomplicated *P falciparum*				
			Pyrimethamine/Sulfadoxine[b]		Same regimen as for uncomplicated *P falciparum*				
		(*P vivax* and *P ovale* require addition of primaquine for radical cure)	Primaquine base[e]	Oral	0.25 or 0.75	0.25 or 0.75	24 or weekly	14 days or 8 weeks	Some strains require twice the dose

---

[a] In the United States, quinine is available from the CDC.
[b] Fansidar should not be given to persons with known allergy to sulfanomides.
[c] Mefloquine (Lariam) is now available in the United States.
[d] Not approved for this indication by the Food and Drug Administration.
[e] Primaquine may cause hemolysis in individuals with glucose 6-phosphate dehydrogenase deficiency.

change transfusion is generally reserved for individuals with more than 15 percent parasitemia or more than 5 percent parasitemia with cerebral malaria or evidence of other organ dysfunction. Hypoglycemia may be seen in cases of severe malaria and is a treatable complication: plasma glucose levels should be monitored every 6 hr, and low levels treated with parenteral glucose infusions. Renal failure in malaria is associated with hyperparasitemia, hypovolemia, and intravascular hemolysis, and may result in acute tubular necrosis. The fluid status of the patient must be monitored and hypovolemia, if present, corrected with fluids. If oliguric renal failure persists after fluid status is corrected, the patient is treated like other patients in the oliguric stage of acute tubular necrosis. Pulmonary edema is an uncommon but frequently fatal complication of severe *P falciparum* infection. It is most often associated with hyperparasitemia and may resemble the adult respiratory distress syndrome (ARDS). It is treated by careful fluid management and application of the principles used in treating ARDS. Aspiration pneumonia occurs often when unconscious cerebral malaria patients suffer seizures and vomiting. Aspiration is prevented by administering anticonvulsants and antiemetics and by attention to general airway management in the unconscious patient. Gram-negative bacteremia is a frequent accompaniment of severe *P falciparum* infection. Gram-negative organisms probably enter the circulation in areas of the bowel wall that are ischemic as a result of microcirculatory obstruction by parasitized erythrocytes. Any patient who is not responding to antimalarial therapy as expected should be investigated for bacteremia, and treatment considered. Hypotension, shock, and myocarditis may complicate severe malaria. If these occur, other treatable causes should be considered, including Gram-negative sepsis, pulmonary edema, metabolic acidosis, gastrointestinal hemorrhage, hypovolemia, and splenic rupture. Splenic rupture is seen infrequently but is one of the few fatal complications of vivax malaria. Diagnosis depends on a high index of suspicion. Disseminated intravascular coagulation (DIC) may be seen with severe malaria and is associated with hyperparasitemia and multiple organ dysfunction. Most authorities treat DIC with fresh frozen plasma and platelets.

Special Conditions

Malaria during pregnancy presents a unique problem. Pregnant women are at higher risk of developing severe and fatal malaria. Hypoglycemia is more common in pregnant women with *P falciparum* infections. Pregnant women should be treated promptly with appropriate doses of antimalarials. Quinine does not appear to induce labor as was once thought. Pregnant women with *P vivax* infections should be treated with chloroquine to eliminate the erythrocytic-stage infection and then placed on weekly chloroquine to prevent relapse, as the safety of primaquine in pregnancy is not known.

Prevention of Malaria

Individuals with little or no previous exposure who develop malaria may rapidly progress to severe, often fatal disease. Most cases of malaria in Americans can be prevented by chemoprophylaxis and by avoiding the mosquito vector. Deaths from malaria can be avoided by these preventive measures and by rapid, appropriate treatment. Most travelers to Asia do not require chemoprophylaxis because, as mentioned above, they do not spend time at night in rural areas and therefore have little exposure to the vector.

The female *Anopheles* mosquito feeds from dusk until dawn. During these hours, individuals should avoid contact with the mosquito by wearing protective clothing, by staying in screened areas and spraying these areas with pyrethrum-containing insecticides, and by using an insect repellent containing *N,N*-diethyl-*m*-toluamide. A 35 percent long-acting cream form of this repellent appears to be efficacious and minimizes systemic absorption of the active ingredient, which can result in a toxic encephalopathy. Systemic absorption is of concern with high-concentration products, particularly in children, and particularly when the repellent is applied to the child's hands (which are likely to touch the eyes or mouth) or to wounds or irritated skin.

Travelers to endemic areas should be advised not only on avoiding the mosquito vector but also on chemoprophylaxis. It must be emphasized that chemoprophylaxis is not one hundred percent effective; regardless of prophylaxis, malaria must be considered in the differential diagnosis of any febrile illness in an individual who has been in an area endemic for malaria within the last 2 years.

Chemoprophylaxis is designed to suppress the development of asexual erythrocytic stage infections. As described above, relapses due to *P vivax* and *P ovale* are prevented with the use of primaquine. Primary infections can be prevented in two ways: by **suppressive chemoprophylaxis** and by **causal prophylaxis.** Suppressive chemoprophylaxis uses blood stage schizonticides to first suppress and then eliminate blood stage infections before the parasites can multiply. Causal prophylaxis is accomplished with tissue schizonticides that prevent the development of mature liver stage parasites.

The choice of a chemoprophylactic regimen depends on several factors: the health of the individual (including factors such as pregnancy, age, and chronic illness); the risk and types of malaria in the areas to be visited; and the presence of drug-resistant *P falciparum.* Prophylaxis with most antimalarials should begin 1 to 2 weeks before entering the malarious area (to ensure tolerance to the drug and to provide adequate blood levels) and should continue throughout the stay in the area and for 4 to 6 weeks after leaving. Doxycycline should be started 1 to 2 days before travel to a malarious area and should be taken daily during the stay in the area and for 4 weeks after leaving. When there has been a significant risk of exposure to *P vivax* or *P ovale*, the tissue schizonticide primaquine should be taken after returning home to eliminate remaining liver stage parasites. See Table 83-2 for dosages of primaquine.

In areas with chloroquine-resistant *P falciparum*, chloroquine or mefloquine is used for suppressive chemoprophylaxis against *P vivax, P malariae,* or *P ovale* infections, and mefloquine or an additional drug is used for chloroquine-resistant *P falciparum* (Table 83-2). Most experts now consider mefloquine to be the single drug of choice for chemoprophylaxis of malaria, since it is useful against all four species. The side effects of mefloquine should not preclude its use.

TABLE 83-2   Drugs Used for Chemoprophylaxis of Malaria

Drug	Adult Dose	Pediatric Dose
Chloroquine phosphate (Aralen)	300 mg base orally, once per week	5 mg/kg base orally, once per week (maximum dose of 300 mg base)
Mefloquine[a] (Lariam)	250 mg salt, orally, once per week	15–19 kg: 1/4 tablet per week 20–30 kg: 1/2 tablet per week 31–45 kg: 3/4 tablet per week >45 kg: 1 tablet per week
Doxycycline	100 mg orally, once/day	>8 years of age: 2 mg/kg/day to maximum adult dose
Primaquine[b]	15 mg base orally, per day for 14 days *or* 45 mg base orally, once per week for 8 weeks	0.3 mg/kg base orally per day for 14 days *or* 0.9 mg/kg base orally per week for 8 weeks

[a] Three weekly doses should be taken after leaving the malarious area.
[b] Primaquine is best taken during the last 2 weeks of prophylaxis.

Control in Populations

Control of malaria is difficult and requires the sustained effort of many individuals from many disciplines (Fig. 83-8). It is much more easily accomplished in some areas of the world than others. Control can be extremely difficult in areas where the *Anopheles* vector is numerous, long-lived, and feeds only on humans.

Transmission of malaria requires the presence of three factors: (1) malaria-infected humans carrying gametocytes that are infective to mosquitoes, (2) anopheles mosquitoes that live long enough for the malaria parasites to develop within them to the infective sporozoite stage, and (3) infected mosquitoes that bite noninfected humans. Malaria control can be applied at each of these points: by reducing or eliminating the number of infected humans that mosquitoes feed on, by eliminating or reducing the numbers of anopheles mosquitoes,

by shortening the life span of mosquitoes to less than that required for the parasite to develop, or by providing alternative hosts for the mosquitoes to feed on.

There have been numerous efforts to reduce transmission by treating infected humans with drugs, especially primaquine, that render gametocytes noninfective to mosquitoes. The success of these efforts is not clear. Major efforts are under way to develop vaccines against malaria. These vaccines could be used to control malaria directly by preventing transmission of infective gametocytes from humans to mosquitoes, or indirectly by preventing human infection. In the direct approach, vaccines are being designed to render gametocytes noninfective to mosquitoes. In the indirect approach, vaccines are being developed that produce immune responses against sporozoites, liver-stage parasites, or erythrocytic-stage parasites that prevent their development to infective

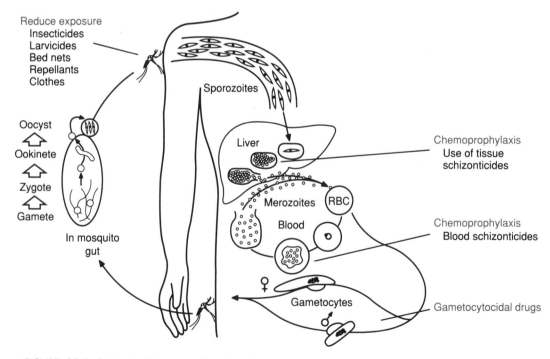

FIGURE 83-8 Strategies for prevention of malaria. (Adapted from Miller LH, Howard RJ, Carter R et al: Research toward malaria vaccines. Science 234:1350, 1986, with permission.)

gametocytes. Vaccines against sporozoites and erythrocytic-stage parasites are currently undergoing evaluation in clinical trials.

The second approach is to reduce transmission by eliminating mosquitoes—primarily by eliminating breeding places such as lagoons and swamps or by killing the larvae in these breeding places. This approach has been quite successful in some parts of the world, particularly in areas where malaria transmission is not intense.

A third approach, and a common one, is to treat dwellings with residual insecticides, such as DDT, that shorten the lifespan of mosquitoes, thereby reducing the chance that they will live long enough to transmit malaria. This approach has been quite successful in some parts of the world, but has had significant problems because of the development of mosquitoes resistant to insecticides.

In some areas of the world where malaria vectors prefer animals, such as cows, to humans, the introduction of these animals has reduced malaria transmission.

REFERENCES

Bruce-Chwatt LJ: Essential Malariology. Wiley, New York, 1985

Centers for Disease Control: Health Information for International Travel 1989. HHS Publication (CDC) 89-8280. Washington, DC, 1989

Centers for Disease Control: Revised Recommendations for the Prevention of Malaria in Travelers. MMWR 39:1–10, 1990

Cook GC: Prevention and treatment of malaria. Lancet 1:32, 1988

Hoffman SL: Treatment of malaria. p. 171. In Strickland GT (ed): Clinics in Tropical Medicine and Communicable Diseases. WB Saunders, London, 1986

Hoffman SL: Malaria. p. 71. In Rakel RE (ed): Conn's Current Therapy. WB Saunders, Philadelphia, 1988

Miller KD, Greenberg AE, Campbell CC: Treatment of severe malaria in the United States with a continuous infusion of quinidine gluconate and exchange transfusion. New Engl J Med 321:65, 1989

Moran JS, Bernard KW: The spread of chloroquine-resistant malaria in Africa. Implications for travelers. JAMA 262:245, 1989

Rickman LS, Long GL, Oberst R et al: Rapid diagnosis of malaria by acridine orange staining of centrifuged parasites. Lancet 1:68, 1989

White NJ, Miller KD, Churchill FC et al: Chloroquine treatment of severe malaria in children. Pharmacokinetics, toxicity, and new dosage recommendations. New Engl J Med 319:493, 1989

84 TOXOPLASMA GONDII

J. P. DUBEY

GENERAL CONCEPTS

Clinical Manifestations

Infection is often asymptomatic. Immunocompetent individuals may present with fever, lymphadenopathy, muscle aches, and headache. Congenitally infected children may suffer impaired vision and mental retardation. Immunosuppressed patients may have central nervous system disease (encephalitis).

Structure and Life Cycle

Members of the cat family (Felidae) are the definitive hosts; many mammals and birds serve as intermediate hosts. Infection is contracted by ingesting either oocysts or meat containing live organisms. Organisms enter the intestinal epithelium and can spread to many host tissues. Individual organisms are lunate, about 6×2 μm, and multiply within host cells. Tissue cysts containing hundreds of quiescent organisms may form as infection wanes. *Toxoplasma* reproduces sexually only in cats: organisms infecting the intestinal epithelium produce oocysts which are shed in the feces. Mature oocysts are 12 μm in diameter and contain eight infective sporozoites.

Classification and Antigenic Types

Toxoplasma gondii, a member of the Apicomplexa, is the sole species.

Multiplication and Life Cycle

Asexual multiplication by cell division can occur in virtually any host cell.

Pathogenesis

Host cells are destroyed by active multiplication of *T gondii*. Necrotic foci may result. Congenital infection often involves the retina and brain; focal chorioretinitis may result in impaired vision. Brain involvement in immunosuppressed patients may lead to large necrotic abscesses. Disease reactivation in immunosuppressed patients may result from the rupture of a tissue cyst.

Host Defenses

Immunocompetent individuals mount an effective cell-mediated immune response that eradicates active infection within weeks or months and results in immunity against reinfection. Tissue cysts are unreactive and may persist for the life of the host.

Epidemiology

Toxoplasmosis shows a nonseasonal worldwide distribution. Most natural infections are acquired by ingesting undercooked meat containing tissue cysts or food contaminated by cat feces.

Diagnosis

Diagnosis is based on serology and on histologic examination of tissues.

Control

Infection may be prevented by thorough cooking of meat and by proper management of cats. Acute cases are treated with sulfadiazine and pyrimethamine.

INTRODUCTION

Toxoplasma gondii is an intestinal coccidium that parasitizes members of the cat family as definitive hosts and has a wide range of intermediate hosts. Infection is common in many warm-blooded animals, including humans. In most cases infection is asymptomatic, but devastating disease can occur.

CLINICAL MANIFESTATIONS

Toxoplasma gondii usually parasitizes both definitive and intermediate hosts without producing clinical signs. In humans, severe disease is usually observed only in congenitally infected children and in immunosuppressed individuals, including patients with acquired immune deficiency syndrome (AIDS). Postnatally acquired infections may be local or generalized and are rarely severe in immunocompetent individuals. Lymphadenitis is the most common manifestation in humans. Any node can be infected, but the deep cervical nodes are the most commonly involved. Infected nodes are tender and discrete but not painful; the infection resolves spontaneously in weeks or months. Lymphadenopathy may be accompanied by fever, malaise, fatigue, muscle pains, sore throat, and headache.

Encephalitis is an important and severe manifestation of toxoplasmosis in immunosuppressed patients including patients with AIDS. Symptoms may include headache, disorientation, drowsiness, hemiparesis, reflex changes, and convulsions. Coma and death may ensue.

Prenatally acquired *Toxoplasma* often infects the brain and retina and can cause a wide spectrum of clinical disease. Mild disease may consist of slightly diminished vision, whereas severely diseased chil-

dren may exhibit a classic tetrad of signs: retinochoroiditis, hydrocephalus, convulsions, and intracerebral calcifications. Hydrocephalus is the least common but most dramatic lesion of congenital toxoplasmosis. Ocular disease is the most common sequela.

Toxoplasma is capable of causing severe disease in animals other than humans. It is one of the major causes of abortion in sheep and goats in many countries, including Australia and the United States. It is important to diagnose toxoplasmic abortion to distinguish it from other causes of abortion, because congenital transmission of *Toxoplasma* occurs only during the initial infection of the mother and the animal is safe for breeding thereafter. Cats, dogs, and many other pets can die of pneumonia, hepatitis, and encephalitis due to toxoplasmosis. In dogs, clinical toxoplasmosis is often associated with concurrent distemper virus infection. Certain species of marsupials and New World monkeys are highly susceptible to toxoplasmosis.

STRUCTURE, MULTIPLICATION, AND LIFE CYCLE

The life cycle of *T gondii* was described only in 1970, when it was discovered that the definitive hosts are members of the family Felidae, including domestic cats. Various warm-blooded animals serve as intermediate hosts. *Toxoplasma* is transmitted by three known modes: congenitally, through the consumption of uncooked infected meat, and via fecal matter. Figure 84-1 shows the life cycle of *T gondii*.

Cats acquire *Toxoplasma* by ingesting any of three infectious stages of the organism: the rapidly multiplying forms called **tachyzoites** (Figs. 84-2

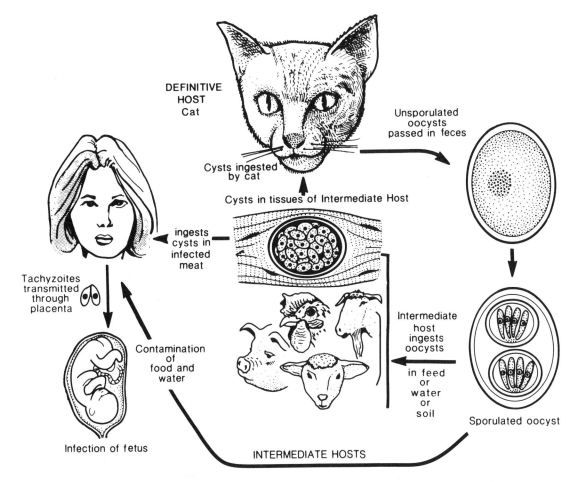

FIGURE 84-1   Life cycle of *Toxoplasma gondii*. Cats, the definitive hosts of *T gondii*, can become infected by ingesting sporulated oocysts or (most often) infected animals. The oocysts are infectious to most mammals and birds. *Toxoplasma* can be transmitted to intermediate hosts through oocysts, by carnivorism, or transplacentally. Transplacental transmission is most important in humans and sheep. (From Dubey JP: Toxoplasmosis. J Am Vet Med Assoc 189:166, 1986.)

and 84-3), the quiescent **bradyzoites** that occupy cysts in infected tissue (Fig. 84-4), and the **oocysts** shed in feces (Fig. 84-5). Successful infection of the cat is revealed by the shedding of oocysts in the feces. The chance of infection and the *prepatent period* (the time between infection and the shedding of oocysts) varies with the stage of *Toxoplasma* ingested. Fewer than 50 percent of cats shed oocysts after ingesting tachyzoites or oocysts, whereas nearly all cats shed oocysts after ingesting

tissue cysts. Only the cyst-induced cycle has been studied in detail.

When a cat ingests meat containing tissue cysts, the cyst wall is dissolved by the proteolytic enzymes in the stomach and small intestine, releasing the bradyzoites. The bradyzoites, which are a slow-multiplying stage, penetrate the epithelial cells of the small intestine and initiate the formation of numerous asexual generations before the sexual cycle (**gametogony,** the production of gametes)

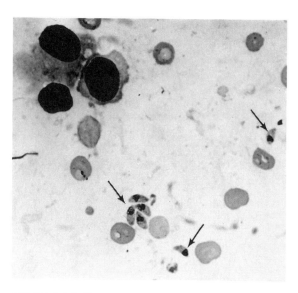

FIGURE 84-2 Tachyzoites (arrows) released after intracellular multiplication in macrophages (impression smear). (Giemsa stain, × 1,250.)

begins. After the male gamete fertilizes the female gamete, two walls are laid down around the fertilized zygote to form the oocyst, which is excreted in the feces in an unsporulated stage. Oocysts measure about 10 by 12 μm. Sporulation occurs outside the body, and the oocyst becomes infectious 1 to 5 days after excretion. Each sporulated oocyst contains two **sporocysts** and each sporocyst contains four **sporozoites.** Sporulated oocysts are remarkably resistant and can survive in soil for several months.

At the same time that some bradyzoites enter the surface epithelial cells of the feline intestine and multiply there to produce oocysts, other bradyzoites penetrate the lamina propria and begin to multiply as tachyzoites (Fig. 84-6). Tachyzoites are about 6 × 2 μm in size and generally lunate. Within a few hours of infection, tachyzoites may disseminate to extraintestinal tissues through the lymph and blood. Tachyzoites can enter almost any type of host cell and multiply until the host cell is filled with parasites and dies. The released tachyzoites enter new host cells and multiply. This cycle may result in microfoci of tissue necrosis. The host

usually overcomes this phase of infection, and the parasite then enters the "resting" stage in which bradyzoites are isolated in tissue cysts. Tissue cysts are formed most commonly in the brain, liver, and muscles. Cysts in neural tissues are up to 50 μm in diameter and contain hundreds of bradyzoites in a thin membrane (Fig. 84-4). Tissue cysts usually cause no host reaction and may remain for the life of the host.

In nonfeline intermediate hosts, such as humans or mice, the extraintestinal cycle of *Toxoplasma* is similar to the cycle in cats. However, sexual stages are produced only in the feline definitive hosts.

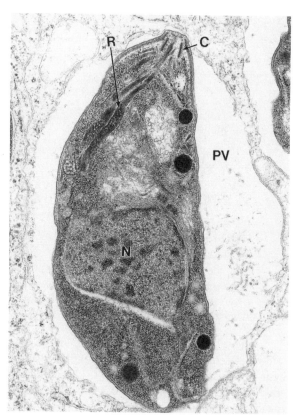

FIGURE 84-3 Transmission electron micrograph of a *T gondii* tachyzoite in a murine macrophage. Note that the tachyzoite is separated from the host cell cytoplasm by a parasitophorous vacuole (PV). C, conoid; R, rhoptries; N, nucleus. (× 20,000.) (Courtesy of Dr. C. A. Speer, Montana State University, Bozeman, MT.)

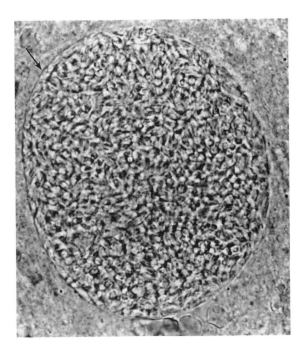

FIGURE 84-4 Tissue cyst with a thin cyst wall (arrow) enclosing hundreds of bradyzoites. (Unstained, ×1,000.)

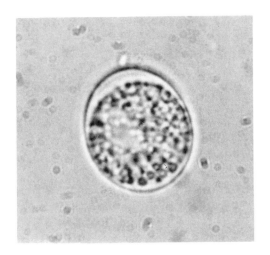

FIGURE 84-5 Unsporulated oocysts in feline feces. (Unstained, ×1,000.) (From Dubey JP: Feline toxoplasmosis and coccidiosis: a survey of domiciled and stray cats. J Am Vet Med Assoc 162:873, 1973.)

PATHOGENESIS

Most cases of toxoplasmosis in humans are probably acquired by the ingestion of either tissue cysts in infected meat or oocysts in food contaminated with cat feces. Bradyzoites from the tissue cysts or sporozoites released from oocysts penetrate the intestinal epithelial cells and multiply in the intestine. *Toxoplasma* may spread both locally to mesenteric lymph nodes and to distant organs by invading the lymphatics and blood. Necrosis in intestinal and mesenteric lymph nodes may occur before other organs become severely damaged (Fig. 84-6). Focal areas of necrosis may develop in many organs. The clinical picture is determined by the extent of injury to these organs, especially to vital and vulnerable organs such as the eye, heart, and adrenals. *Toxoplasma* does not produce a toxin; necrosis is caused by intracellular multiplication of tachyzoites.

The ocular disease characteristic of congenital toxoplasmosis is almost always confined to the posterior chamber but occasionally involves the entire eye. *Toxoplasma* proliferates in the retina, leading to inflammation of the choroid; hence the term *retinochoroiditis*. The lesions of human ocular toxoplasmosis are fairly characteristic. In the acute or subacute stage of inflammation, the lesions appear as yellowish white, cottonlike patches in the fundus. Lesions may be single or multiple and may involve one or both eyes. During the acute stage, inflammatory exudate may cloud the vitreous and may be so dense as to prevent visualization of the fundus by an ophthalmoscope. The vitreous clears as inflammation subsides. Alternatively, retinal lesions may appear as single or multifocal small gray areas of active retinitis with minimal edema and reaction in the vitreous humor. Such punctate lesions are usually harmless unless located in the macula. Although severe infections may be detected at birth, milder infections may not flare up until adulthood.

Opportunistic toxoplasmosis in AIDS patients usually represents reactivation of chronic infection. The predominant lesion of toxoplasmosis encephalitis in these patients is necrosis, which often results in multiple abscesses, some as large as a tennis ball.

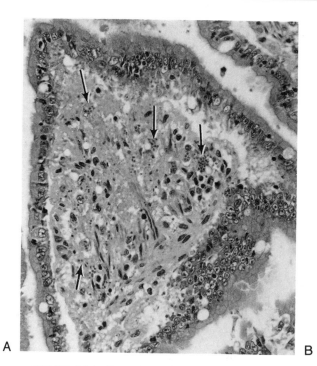
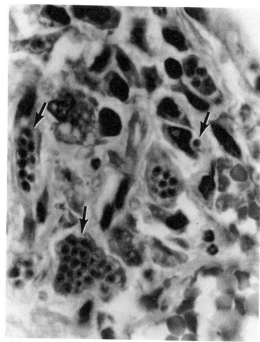

A B

FIGURE 84-6   *Toxoplasma* tachyzoites (arrows) causing necrosis in the intestine of a cat. *(A)* Necrosis of lamina propria. × 300. *(B)* × 1,000.

HOST DEFENSES

The host may die from toxoplasmosis but much more often recovers and acquires immunity. Inflammation usually follows necrosis. By about the third week after infection, *Toxoplasma* tachyzoites begin to disappear from visceral tissues and may localize as tissue cysts in neural and muscular tissues. *Toxoplasma* tachyzoites may persist longer in the spinal cord and brain because immune responses are less effective in these organs. Chronic infections may be reactivated locally (for example, in the eye). Reactivation possibly results from the rupture of a tissue cyst. Probably tissue cysts rupture periodically during the life of the host, and the bradyzoites released are normally destroyed by the host's immune responses. This reaction may cause local necrosis accompanied by inflammation. Hypersensitivity is said to play a major role in such reactions; however, in immunocompetent hosts the infection usually subsides, with no local re-

newed multiplication of *Toxoplasma*. In immunosuppressed patients, rupture of a tissue cyst may result in renewed multiplication of bradyzoites into tachyzoites, and the host may die from toxoplasmosis.

EPIDEMIOLOGY

Toxoplasma infection in humans is widespread throughout the world. Approximately half a billion humans have antibodies to *T gondii*. The incidence of infection in humans and animals may vary in different parts of a country. The cause for these variations is not yet known: environmental conditions, cultural habits, and animal fauna are among factors that may determine the degree of natural spread of *Toxoplasma*. Only a small proportion (less than 0.1 percent) of people acquire infection congenitally. Mothers of congenitally infected children do not give birth to infected children in subsequent pregnancies. However, repeated congenital infection can occur in mice, rats, guinea pigs, and hamsters without reinfection from outside sources.

The relative frequency with which postnatal toxoplasmosis is acquired by eating raw meat and by ingesting food contaminated by oocysts from cat feces is unknown and difficult to investigate. Both modes of infection are reported to cause clinical toxoplasmosis. *Toxoplasma* infection occurs commonly in many animals used for food (for example, sheep, pigs, and rabbits). Infection is less prevalent in cattle than in sheep or pigs.

Oocysts are shed by cats—not only the domestic cat but also other felids such as ocelots, margays, jaguarundi, bobcats, Pallas cats, and Bengal tigers. Oocyst formation is greatest in the domestic cat, however. Widespread natural infection is possible because a cat may excrete millions of oocysts after ingesting few tissue cysts. Oocysts are resistant to most ordinary environmental conditions and can survive in moist conditions for months and even years. Invertebrates such as flies, cockroaches, and earthworms can spread oocysts mechanically.

Only a few cats may be involved at any one time in spreading *Toxoplasma* in an area: at any given time as little as 1 percent of the domestic cat population in the United States is shedding oocysts. It is not known whether cats shed oocysts only once or several times in nature. Under experimental conditions, cats usually did not reshed oocysts after reinoculation with *Toxoplasma* tissue cysts. Immunity to *T gondii* in cats may wane with time, however, and cats may reshed oocysts in nature.

DIAGNOSIS

Diagnosis of toxoplasmosis can be aided by serologic or histocytologic examination. Clinical signs of toxoplasmosis are nonspecific and cannot be depended on for a definite diagnosis; toxoplasmosis clinically mimics several other infectious diseases.

Many serologic tests have been used to detect antibodies to *T gondii*. The most reliable of these is the cytoplasm-modifying or dye test. Live virulent tachyzoites of *Toxoplasma* are used as antigen and are exposed to dilutions of the test serum and to a complement accessory factor resembling complement that is obtained from *Toxoplasma*-antibody-free human serum. This test is sensitive and so far is the most specific test for toxoplasmosis. Its main disadvantages are its high cost and the human hazard of using live organisms. The indirect fluorescent antibody test (IFAT) overcomes some of the disadvantages of the dye test. In IFAT, killed tachyzoites of *Toxoplasma,* which are available commercially, are used as antigen. Titers obtained by IFAT are similar to those from the dye test. Disadvantages of the IFAT are that a microscope with UV light is needed, fluorescent anti-species globulin is required for each species to be tested, and false-positive titers may occur in hosts with anti-nuclear antibodies. The suitability of IFAT in animal diagnostic work is therefore limited, but it has proved useful in diagnosing acquired human toxoplasmosis. Other serologic tests—the indirect hemagglutination test, the agglutination test, the enzyme-linked immunoabsorbent assay (ELISA), and the complement-fixation test—offer some advantages. For example, agglutination tests are easy to perform.

Soluble antigens used for indirect hemagglutination tests are now commercially available in several countries, including the United States. Although this test is easy to perform, it usually does not detect antibodies during the acute phase of toxoplasmosis. In the modified agglutination test, whole killed tachyzoites are used as antigen, and the test serum is treated with 2-mercaptoethanol to eliminate nonspecific agglutinins. The ELISA test using soluble antigens appears to be specific and may become the standard test in the future.

A single positive serum sample proves only that the host has been infected at some time in the past. Serologic evidence for an acute acquired infection is obtained when antibody titers rise by a factor of 4 to 16 in serum taken 2 to 4 weeks after the initial serum collection, or when specific IgM antibody is detected. The finding of antibody in even undiluted serum is useful in the diagnosis of ocular toxoplasmosis because patients with this disorder usually have low *T gondii* antibody titers.

Diagnosis can be made by finding *Toxoplasma* in host tissue removed by biopsy or at necropsy. This procedure is particularly useful in immunosuppressed patients or patients with AIDS, in whom antibody synthesis may be delayed and low. *Toxoplasma* infection can be rapidly diagnosed by making impression smears of lesions on glass slides. After drying for 10 to 30 min, the smears are fixed in methyl alcohol and stained with Giemsa stain. Well-preserved *Toxoplasma* organisms are crescent-shaped and stain well with any of the Romanowsky stains (Fig. 84-2); however, degenerating organisms — common in lesions — usually appear oval and have cytoplasm that stains poorly compared to the nucleus. A diagnosis of toxoplasmosis should not be made unless organisms with the typical structure are seen, as degenerating host cells may resemble degenerating *Toxoplasma* parasites. In thin sections the tachyzoites are oval to round and usually do not stain differently from host cells (Fig. 84-5). In sections stained with hematoxylin and eosin, tachyzoites may be easily located by the deep staining of the host tissue. Tissue cysts are occasionally encountered in areas with lesions. Cysts are usually spherical and have silver-positive walls; the bradyzoites stain strongly with periodic acid–Schiff stain. Immunoperoxidase staining can be used to identify *Toxoplasma* tissue cysts or tachyzoites in fixed impression smears and in tissues fixed in formalin. Electron-micrographic examination can aid in diagnosis (Fig. 84-3). Computed tomography techniques are also useful in the diagnosis of human cerebral toxoplasmosis. Inoculation of biopsy materials into laboratory mice and/or cell cultures can help diagnosis.

CONTROL

Sulfonamides and pyrimethamine (Daraprim) are two drugs widely used to treat toxoplasmosis in humans. They act synergistically by blocking the metabolic pathway involving *p*-aminobenzoic acid and the folic-folinic acid cycle, respectively. These two drugs usually are well tolerated by the patient, but sometimes thrombocytopenia, leukopenia, or both may develop. These effects can be overcome without interrupting treatment by administering folinic acid and yeast because the vertebrate host

can utilize presynthesized folinic acid whereas *Toxoplasma* cannot. The commonly used sulfonamides — sulfadiazine, sulfamethazine, and sulfamerazine — are all effective against toxoplasmosis. Generally, any sulfonamide that diffuses across the host cell membrane is useful in antitoxoplasmid therapy. Although these drugs are helpful when given in the acute stage of the disease, usually they will not eradicate infection when active multiplication of the parasite occurs. Because sulfa compounds are excreted within a few hours of administration they must be administered in daily divided doses. Spiramycin, a drug used in France to treat pregnant women to minimize the effects of congenital toxoplasmosis, is not approved for toxoplasmosis in the United States.

No vaccine is currently available to reduce or prevent congenital infections in humans and animals, but research to develop such an agent is under way. Certain drugs can minimize or prevent oocyst formation in cats.

To prevent *Toxoplasma* infection, several precautions should be taken. Meat should be cooked to 66°C throughout before eating. Hands should be washed with soap and water after handling meat. Raw meat should never be fed to cats; only dry or canned food or cooked meat should be fed. Cats should be kept indoors and litter boxes changed daily. Cat feces should be flushed down the toilet or burned. Litter pans should be cleaned by immersing them in boiling water. Gloves should be used while working in the garden. Children's sandboxes should be covered when not in use.

REFERENCES

Dubey JP, Beattie CP: Toxoplasmosis of Animals and Man. CRC Press, Boca Raton, FL, 1988

Jackson MH, Hutchison WM: The prevalence and source of *Toxoplasma* infection in the environment. Adv Parasitol 28:55, 1989

Koskiniemi M, Lappalainen M, Hedman K: Toxoplasmosis needs evaluation. An overview and proposals. Am J Dis Child 143:724, 1989

Remington JS, Desmonts G: Toxoplasmosis. In Remington JS, Klein J (eds): Infectious Diseases of the Fetus and Newborn. WB Saunders, Philadelphia, 1983

85 PNEUMOCYSTIS CARINII

WALTER T. HUGHES

GENERAL CONCEPTS

Clinical Manifestations

Respiratory manifestations—tachypnea, dyspnea and cough, and fever—are the usual symptoms of *Pneumocystis* pneumonia.

Structure

The spherical, oval, cup-shaped, thick-walled cyst, 6 to 8 μm in diameter, contains up to eight intracystic pleomorphic sporozoites. The extra-cystic trophozoite is thin-walled and varies in size from 2 to 6 μm.

Classification and Antigenic Types

It is not yet established whether *P carinii* is a fungus or a protozoan. Antigenic differences have been found in strains derived from the various mammalian hosts.

Multiplication

Multiplication is by a cyst–trophozoite–cyst cycle within the definitive host.

Pathogenesis

In normal individuals, asymptomatic infection of the lungs occurs in early life. The organism persists in an inactive or latent state unless the host becomes immunocompromised. Organisms attached to the alveolar septal wall replicate resulting in diffuse alveolitis and impaired oxygenation.

Host Defenses

A cell-mediated immune response is the major defense mechanism.

Epidemiology

Pneumocystis carinii infection is nonseasonal and worldwide. The organism is probably acquired by the respiratory route.

Diagnosis

Pneumonitis is diagnosed by radiography plus demonstration of *P carinii* in lung tissue for respiratory tract secretions.

Control

Trimethoprim-sulfamethoxazole or pentamidine is used to treat the disease; chemoprophylaxis with trimethoprim-sulfamethoxazole is effective.

INTRODUCTION

Pneumocystis carinii is a cause of diffuse pneumonia in immunocompromised hosts. Even in fatal cases, the organism and the disease remain localized to the lung. The pneumonia rarely, if ever, occurs in healthy individuals.

Pneumocystis carinii, an extracellular protozoan, has been observed in three forms. Diagnosis requires identification of *P carinii* in lung tissue, obtained by invasive techniques, or in lower airway fluids. Experimental studies have shown that the organism can be transmitted by inhalation.

CLINICAL MANIFESTATIONS

Pneumocystis carinii causes bilateral diffuse pneumonitis in immunocompromised patients and no discernible disease in otherwise healthy individuals. Clinical features are to some extent age-dependent. In premature and debilitated infants, onset is subtle, starting with mild tachypnea. Within a week or so, respiratory distress is apparent, with marked tachypnea, flaring of the nasal alae, retractions, and cyanosis. The illness may last

4 to 6 weeks and has a mortality rate of 25 to 50 percent. In the immunodeficient child or adult, onset is abrupt, with fever, tachypnea, and respiratory distress. Deterioration progresses to death in almost all cases if no treatment is given. In both types of patient, arterial oxygen tension is low, arterial pH usually increased, and carbon dioxide retention usually does not occur.

STRUCTURE

The structural forms of *P carinii* that have been recognized are the cyst, which is thick-walled; the sporozoite, an intracystic structure; and the thin-walled trophozoite (Fig. 85-1). The cyst is a spherical to ovoid structure 4 to 6 μm in diameter (Fig. 85-2). It contains up to eight pleomorphic sporozoites (Fig. 85-3). The trophozoite is a thin-walled extracystic cell representing an excysted sporozoite. Although the mode of replication has not been described, the organism can be briefly propagated in embryonic thick epithelial lung cells, Vero cells, and WI-38 cells. The organism does not enter the host cell, but instead attaches to its surface

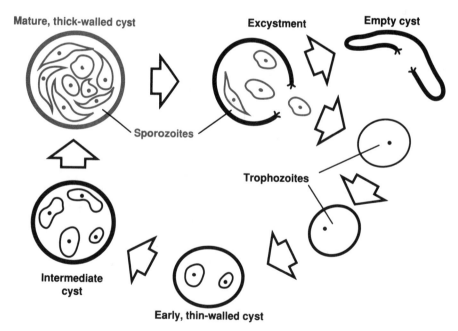

FIGURE 85-1 Stages in the life cycle of *P carinii*. The mode of replication is not known.

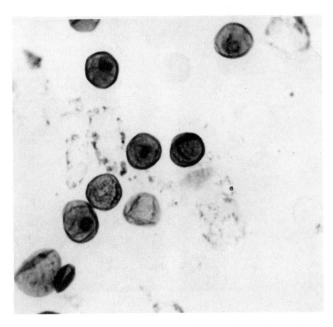

FIGURE 85-2 *Pneumocystis carinii* cysts stained with Gomori's methenamine silver nitrate method. Cysts stain brownish black and measure 4 to 6 μm in diameter. (From Hughes WT: *Pneumocystis carinii* pneumonia. In Kelley VC (ed): Practice of Pediatrics. Vol. 2. JB Lippincott, Philadelphia, 1977, with permission.)

during a phase in the replicative cycle. There is no evidence of toxin production.

CLASSIFICATION AND ANTIGENIC TYPES

Only one species has been identified. However, antigenic differences have been demonstrated between organisms obtained from humans and from lower mammals such as the rat, rabbit, and ferret. The taxonomy of *P carinii* has not been established. It is either a protozoan or a fungus, although membership in a heretofore undescribed category cannot be excluded. Recent studies show close homology of nucleotide sequences of 16S ribosomal RNA of *P carinii* to *Saccharomyces cerevisiae* and *Neurospora crassa*, but this evidence is not sufficient for taxonomic placement.

MULTIPLICATION

The mode of replication of *P carinii* has not been established. However, the stages in its life cycle have been characterized (Fig. 85-1). Sporozoites

excyst through breaks in the cyst wall and then are termed trophozoites. The means by which the trophozoite form progresses to the cyst phase is not known.

PATHOGENESIS

The portal of entry for *P carinii* has not been firmly established; however, because with rare exceptions the organism has been found in only the lung, inhalation is a likely mode of transmission. Airborne transmission has been demonstrated in animals. In most individuals, the organism is dormant and sparsely dispersed in the lung, with no apparent host response (latent infection). In susceptible (immunocompromised) hosts, the organism occurs in massive numbers, filling the alveolar spaces and eliciting an active response of the alveolar macrophages and phagocytosis. In debilitated infants with *Pneumocystis* pneumonia, the alveolar septum is thickened and there is an interstitial plasma cell and lymphocyte infiltration. The infection results in impaired ventilation and severe hypoxia.

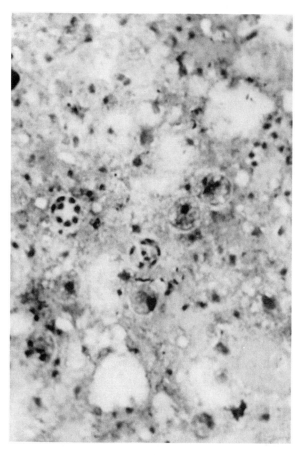

FIGURE 85-3 *Pneumocystis carinii* stained with poly-chrome methylene blue. Intracystic sporozoites are visualized, but the cyst wall is not stained. Sporozoites measure 1 to 2 μm in diameter. (From Hughes WT: *Pneumocystis carinii* pneumonia. In Kelley VC (ed): Practice of Pediatrics. Vol. 2. JB Lippincott, Philadelphia, 1977, with permission.)

HOST DEFENSES

With rare exceptions, *P carinii* causes disease only when natural mechanisms of host defense are compromised. Pneumonitis has occurred in patients with B and/or T cell deficiency, and it is a major infection in patients with the acquired immune deficiency syndrome (AIDS). Severe protein-calorie malnutrition alone may provoke the disease. Immunosuppressive drugs used for cancer or organ transplantation render the indi-

vidual susceptible to *P carinii* pneumonitis. Both IgG and IgM antibody may appear in response to infection or experimental immunization, but humoral antibody does not protect against the disease. Alveolar macrophages actively engulf and digest the parasite. Infected infants show extensive plasma cell infiltration of the alveolar septae, but immunosuppressed children and adults do not.

EPIDEMIOLOGY

Pneumocystis carinii has been found in the lungs of rats, rabbits, mice, dogs, sheep, goats, ferrets, chimpanzees, guinea pigs, horses, and monkeys. The organism has been reported in lower animals and humans from all continents. Animal-to-animal transmission by the airborne route has been demonstrated. Because up to 70 percent of healthy individuals may have humoral antibody to *P carinii*, subclinical infection must be highly prevalent.

DIAGNOSIS

Tachypnea and fever are consistent features of the pneumonitis, and diffuse bilateral alveolar disease can be observed by radiography. Diagnosis requires the identification of *P carinii* in pulmonary tissue or lower airway fluids. Such specimens may be obtained by lung biopsy, inducement of sputum, bronchoalveolar lavage, or needle aspiration of the lung. The Gomori, Giemsa, Gram-Weigert, or toluidine blue O stains may be used to identify the organism. Serologic studies for antibodies and antigen are not helpful in establishing a specific diagnosis.

CONTROL

Experimental studies show that immunization with *P carinii* does not protect the animal from pneumonia; however, the disease can be prevented by prophylactic administration of trimethoprim-sulfamethoxazole or aerosolized pentamidine.

The drugs currently available for therapy of *P carinii* pneumonitis are pentamidine isethionate and trimethoprim-sulfamethoxazole. The two are equally effective, but trimethoprim-sulfamethoxazole is preferred because of its low toxicity. Drugs of promise in clinical trials are dapsone, 566C80 (ahydroxynaphthoquinone) trimetrexate, and aerosolized pentamidine.

REFERENCES

Edman JC, Kovacs JA, Masur H, et al: Ribosomal RNA sequence shows *Pneumocystis carinii* to be a member of the fungi. Nature 334:519, 1988

Fischl MA, Dickinson GM, La Voie L: Safety and efficacy of sulfamethoxazole and trimethoprim chemoprophylaxis for *Pneumocystis carinii* pneumonia in AIDS. JAMA 259:1185, 1988

Gigliotti F, Hughes WT: Passive immunoprophylaxis with specific monoclonal antibody confers partial protection against *Pneumocystis carinii* pneumonitis in animal models. J Clin Invest 81:1666, 1988

Hughes WT: *Pneumocystis carinii* pneumonitis. CRC Press, Boca Raton, FL, 1987

Hughes WT, Rivera GK, Schell MJ, et al: Successful intermittent chemoprophylaxis for *Pneumocystis carinii* pneumonitis. N Engl J Med 316:1627, 1987

Kovacs JA, Halpern JL, Lundgren B, et al: Monoclonal antibodies to *Pneumocystis carinii:* Identification of specific antigens and characterization of antigenic differences between rat and human isolates. J Infect Dis 159:60, 1989

Walzer PD, Cushion MT, Juranek D, et al: Serology and *P. carinii* [letter]. Chest 91:935, 1987

86 HELMINTHS: STRUCTURE, CLASSIFICATION, GROWTH, AND DEVELOPMENT

GILBERT A. CASTRO

GENERAL CONCEPTS

The helminths are worm-like parasites. The clinically relevant groups are separated according to their general external shape and the host organ they inhabit. There are both hermaphroditic and bisexual species. The definitive classification is based on the external and internal morphology of egg, larval, and adult stages.

Flukes (Trematodes)

Adult flukes are leaf-shaped flatworms. Prominent oral and ventral suckers help maintain position in situ. Flukes are hermaphroditic except for blood flukes,

which are bisexual. The life cycle includes a snail intermediate host.

Tapeworms (Cestodes)

Adult tapeworms are elongated, segmented, hermaphroditic flatworms that inhabit the intestinal lumen. Some species have cystic or solid larval forms that inhabit extraintestinal tissues.

Roundworms (Nematodes)

Adult and larval roundworms are bisexual, cylindrical worms. They inhabit intestinal and extraintestinal sites.

INTRODUCTION

Helminth is a general term meaning *worm*. The helminths are invertebrates characterized by elongated, flat or round bodies. In medically oriented schemes the **flatworms** or **platyhelminths** (*platy* from the Greek root meaning "flat") include **flukes** and **tapeworms. Roundworms** are **nematodes** (*nemato* from the Greek root meaning "thread"). These three groups are subdivided for convenience according to the host organ in which

they reside, e.g., lung flukes, extraintestinal tapeworms, and intestinal roundworms. This chapter deals with the structure and development of the three major groups of helminths. Helminths develop through egg, larval (juvenile), and adult stages. Table 86-1 gives the names applied to various larval helminths. Knowledge of the different stages in relation to their growth and development is the basis for understanding the epidemiology and pathogenesis of helminth diseases, as well as for the diagnosis and treatment of patients har-

1065

TABLE 86-1   Common Larval Forms of Helminths Found in Humans

Flukes (Trematodes)	Tapeworms (Cestodes)	Roundworms (Nematodes)
Miracidium[a]	Cysticercus[b,c,d]	Rabditiform[d]
Sporocyst[a]	Cysticercoid[b]	Filariform[b]
Redia[a]	Coenurus[b,d]	Microfilaria[a,d]
	Coracidium[a]	
Cercaria[a,b,c]	Procercoid[a,b]	
Metacercaria[b]	Plerocercoid[a,b,c,d] (sparganum)	
	Hydatid[a,c,d]	

[a] Infective to or develops within intermediate hosts or vectors
[b] Infective stage for humans
[c] Cause of pathogenic changes in humans
[d] Can be isolated from human host and, therefore, is important in definitive diagnosis

boring these parasites. The contributions of various stages to disease are listed in Table 86-2.

Platyhelminths and nematodes that infect humans have similar anatomic features that reflect common physiologic requirements and functions. The outer covering of helminths is the **cuticle** or **tegument.** Prominent external structures of flukes and cestodes are acetabula (suckers) or bothria (false suckers). Male nematodes of several species possess accessory sex organs that are external modifications of the cuticle. Internally, the alimentary, excretory, and reproductive systems can be identified by an experienced observer. Tapeworms are unique in lacking an alimentary canal. This lack means that nutrients must be absorbed through the tegument. The blood flukes and nematodes are bisexual. All other flukes and tapeworm species that infect humans are hermaphroditic.

TABLE 86-2   Stages of Helminths Commonly Responsible for Pathologic Changes in Humans

Helminths	Egg	Larva	Adult
Flukes	+	+[a]	+
Tapeworms	−	+	+
Nematodes	−	+	+

[a] Migrating and developing larval forms may cause transient pathologic responses in the host.

With few exceptions, adult flukes, cestodes, and nematodes produce eggs that are passed in excretions or secretions of the host. The various stages and their unique characteristics will be reviewed in more detail as each major group of helminths is considered.

FLUKES (TREMATODES)

The structure of flukes is summarized in Figures 86-1 and 86-2. A dorsoventrally flattened body, bilateral symmetry, and a definite anterior end are features of platyhelminths in general and of trematodes specifically. Flukes are leaf-shaped, ranging in length from a few millimeters to 7 to 8 cm. The tegument is morphologically and physiologically complex. Flukes possess an oral sucker around the mouth and a ventral sucker or acetabulum that can be used to adhere to host tissues. A body cavity is lacking. Organs are embedded in specialized connective tissue or parenchyma. Layers of somatic muscle permeate the parenchyma and attach to the tegument.

Flukes have a well-developed alimentary canal with a muscular pharynx and esophagus. The intestine is usually a branched tube (secondary and tertiary branches may be present) consisting of a single layer of epithelial cells. The main branches may end blindly or open into an excretory vesicle. The excretory vesicle also accepts the two main lateral collecting ducts of the excretory system, which is of a protonephridial type with flame cells.

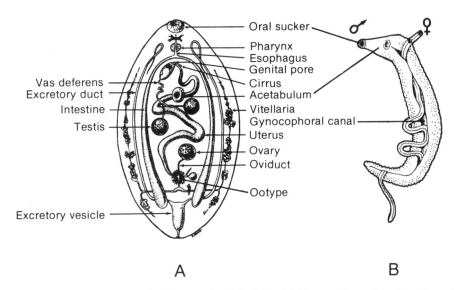

FIGURE 86-1 Structure of flukes. (*A*) Hermaphroditic fluke. (*B*) Bisexual fluke. (Modified from Hunter GW, Swartzwelder JC, Clyde DF: A Manual of Tropical Medicine. 5th Ed. WB Saunders, Philadelphia, 1976, with permission.)

A flame cell is a hollow, terminal excretory cell that contains a beating (flamelike) group of cilia. These cells, anchored in the parenchyma, direct tissue filtrate through canals into the two main collecting ducts.

Except for the blood flukes, trematodes are hermaphroditic, having both male and female reproductive organs in the same individual. The male organ consists usually of two testes with accessory glands and ducts leading to a *cirrus,* or penis equivalent, that extends into the common genital atrium. The female gonad consists of a single ovary with a seminal receptacle and *vitellaria,* or yolk glands, that connect with the oviduct as it expands into an ootype. The tubular uterus extends from the ootype and opens into the genital atrium. Both self- and cross-fertilization occur. The components of the egg are assembled in the ootype. Eggs pass through the uterus into the genital atrium and exit ventrally though the genital pore. Fluke eggs, except for those of schistosomes, are *operculated* (have a lid).

The **blood flukes** or **schistosomes** are the only bisexual flukes that infect humans (Fig. 86-1). Although the sexes are separate, the general body structure is the same as that of hermaphroditic flukes. Within the definitive host, the male and female worms inhabit the lumen of blood vessels and are found in close physical association. The female lies within a tegumental fold, the **gynecophoral canal,** on the ventral surface of the male.

The medically important flukes belong to the taxonomic category Digenea. This group of flukes has a developmental cycle requiring at least two hosts, one being a snail intermediate host. Depending on the species, other intermediate hosts may be involved to perpetuate the larval form that infects the definitive human host.

Flukes go through several larval stages, each with a specific name, before reaching adulthood. Taking into account variations among species (see Fig. 86-2), a generalized life cycle of digenetic flukes runs the following course. Eggs are passed in the feces, urine, or sputum of humans and reach an aquatic environment. The eggs hatch, releasing ciliated larvae, or **miracidia,** which either penetrate or are eaten by a snail intermediate host. In rare instances land snails may serve as intermediate hosts. A saclike **sporocyst** or **redia** stage develops from a miracidium within the tissues of the snail.

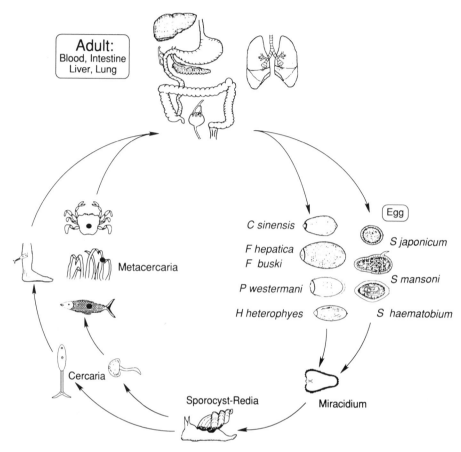

FIGURE 86-2   Generalized life cycle of flukes. All cycles involve snails as intermediate hosts. Hermaphroditic flukes—*Clonorchis sinensis, Fasciola hepatica, Fasiolopsis buski, Paragonimus westermani,* and *Heterophyes heterophyes*. Metacercaria are infective for humans. Bisexual flukes: *Schistosoma japonicum, S mansoni,* and *S hematobium*. Cercariae are infective for humans. (From Castro GA: Trematodes: schistosomiasis. p. 1710. In Kelley WN (ed): Textbook of Internal Medicine. JB Lippincott, Philadelphia, 1989, with permission.)

The sporocyst gives rise either to rediae or to a daughter sporocyst stage. In turn, from the redia or daughter sporocyst, **cercariae** develop asexually and migrate out of the snail tissues to the external environment, which is usually aquatic.

The cercariae, which may possess a tail for swimming, develop further in one of three ways. They either penetrate the definitive host and transform directly into adults, or penetrate a second intermediate host and develop as encysted **metacercariae,** or they encyst on a substrate, such as vegeta-tion, and develop there as metacercariae. When a metacercarial cyst is ingested, digestion of the cyst liberates an immature fluke that migrates to a specific organ site and develops into an adult worm.

TAPEWORMS (CESTODES)

As members of the platyhelminths, the **cestodes, or tapeworms,** possess many basic structural characteristics of flukes, but also show striking differences. Figure 86-3 shows the general features of

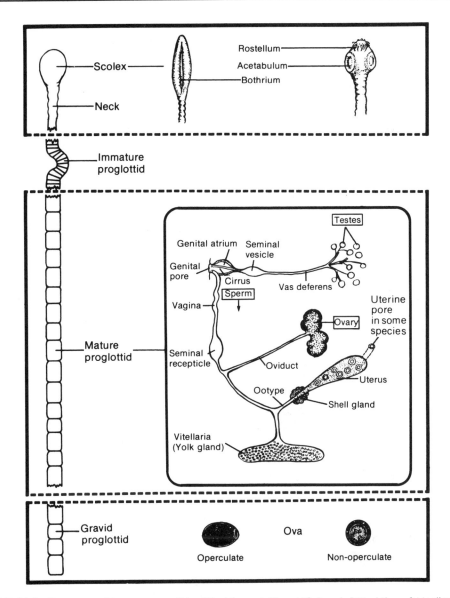

FIGURE 86-3 Structure of tapeworms. (Modified from Jeffrey HC, Leach RM: Atlas of Medical Helminthology and Protozoology. Churchill Livingstone, Edinburgh, 1968, with permission.)

the structure and development of tapeworms. Whereas flukes are flattened and generally leaf-shaped, adult tapeworms are flattened, elongated, and consist of segments called **proglottids.** Tapeworms vary in length from 2 to 3 mm to 10 m, and may have three to several thousand segments.

Anatomically, cestodes are divided into a **scolex,** or head, which bears the organs of attachment, a **neck** that is the region of segment proliferation, and a chain of proglottids called the **strobila.** The strobila elongates as new proglottids form in the neck region. The segments nearest the neck are immature (sex organs not fully developed) and those more posterior are mature. The terminal

TABLE 86-3   Differences between Pseudophyllidean and Cyclophyllidean Tapeworms

Differentiating Feature	Pseudophyllidea	Cyclophyllidea
Scolex	Two sucking grooves (bothria)	Four muscular suckers (acetabula)
Genital pore	Center of each proglottid	Margin(s) of each proglottid [may be located on both sides in an irregular pattern (*Taenia* spp); all on the same side (*Hymenolepis* spp); or each proglottid may have a pore on each side (*Dipylidium caninum*)]
Uterine pore	Center of proglottids on ventral surface	Absent; uterus ends blindly
Uterus (gravid)	Relatively long and coiled	Saclike, highly branched
Eggs	Operculate	Nonoperculate
Oncosphere	Ciliated (coracidium)	Nonciliated
Larvae	Procercoid and plerocercoid; both forms solid	Cysticercoid, cysticercus, hydatid; all forms cystic

segments are gravid, with the egg-filled uterus as the most prominent feature.

The scolex contains the cephalic ganglion, or "brain," of the tapeworm nervous system. Externally, the scolex is characterized by **holdfast organs.** Depending on the species, these organs consist of a **rostellum, bothria,** or **acetabula.** A rostellum is a retractable, conelike structure that is located on the anterior end of the scolex, and in some species is armed with hooks. Bothria are long, narrow, weakly muscular grooves that are characteristic of the pseudophyllidean tapeworms. Acetabula (suckers like those of digenetic trematodes) are characteristic of cyclophyllidean tapeworms. Differential features of pseudophyllidean and cyclophyllidean tapeworms are listed in Table 86-3. Most human tapeworms are cyclophyllideans.

A characteristic feature of adult tapeworms is the absence of an alimentary canal, which is intriguing, since all of these adult worms inhabit the small intestine. The lack of an alimentary tract means that substances enter the tapeworm across the tegument. This structure is well adapted for transport functions, since it is covered with numerous microvilli resembling those lining the lumen of the mammalian intestine. The excretory system is of the flame cell type.

Cestodes are hermaphroditic, each proglottid possessing male and female reproductive systems similar to those of digenetic flukes. However, tapeworms differ from flukes in the mechanism of egg deposition. Eggs of pseudophyllidean tapeworms exit through a **uterine pore** in the center of the ventral surface rather than through a genital atrium, as in flukes. In cyclophyllidean tapeworms, the female system includes a uterus without a uterine pore (Fig. 86-3). Thus, the cyclophyllidean eggs are released only when the tapeworms shed gravid proglottids into the intestine. Some proglottids disintegrate, releasing eggs that are voided in the feces, whereas other proglottids are passed intact.

The eggs of pseudophyllidean tapeworms are operculated, but those of cyclophyllidean species are not. Eggs of all tapeworms, however, contain at some stage of development an embryo with six hooks called a hexacanth embryo or **oncosphere.** The oncosphere of pseudophyllidean tapeworms is ciliated externally and is called a **coracidium.** The coracidium develops into a **procercoid** in its micro-crustacean first immediate host and then into a **plerocercoid** larva in its next intermediate host, which is a vertebrate. The plerocercoid larva develops into an adult worm in the definitive (final) host. The oncosphere of cyclophyllidean tapeworms, depending on the species, develops into a **cysticercus** larva, **cysticercoid** larva, **coenurus** larva, or **hydatid** larva (cyst) in specific intermediate hosts. These larvae, in turn, become adults in

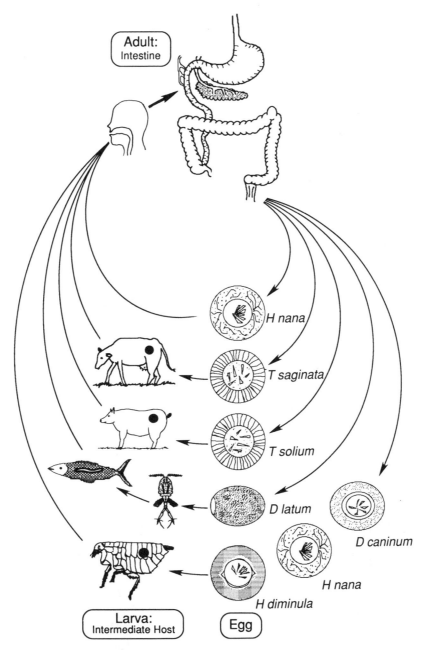

FIGURE 86-4   Generalized life cycle of tapeworms. *Hymenolepsis nana, H diminuta, Taenia saginata, T solium, Diphyllobothrium latum, Dipylidium caninum.* Note hexacanth embryos. Cysticercus larva in cow and pig; procercoid larva in copepod, plerocercoid (sparganum) larva in fish; cysticercoid larva in insect.

the definitive host. Figure 86-4 illustrates these larval forms and representative life cycles.

ROUNDWORMS (NEMATODES)

Figure 86-5 shows the structure of nematodes. In contrast to platyhelminths, nematodes are cylindrical rather than flattened; hence the common name *roundworm.* The body wall is composed of an outer cuticle that has a noncellular, chemically complex structure, a thin hypodermis, and musculature. The cuticle in some species has longitudinal ridges called **alae.** The **bursa,** a flaplike extension of the cuticle on the posterior end of some species of male nematodes, is used to grasp the female during copulation.

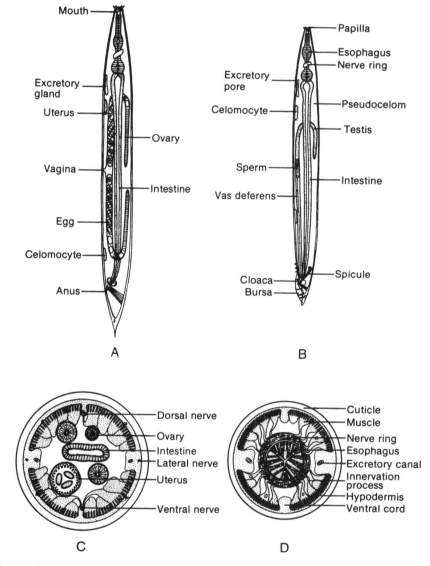

FIGURE 86-5 Structure of nematodes. (*A*) Female. (*B*) Male. Transverse sections through the midregion of the female worm (*C*) and through the esophageal region (*D*). (Modified from Lee DL: The Physiology of Nematodes. Oliver and Boyd, Edinburgh, 1965, with permission.)

The cellular **hypodermis** bulges into the body cavity or **pseudocoelom** to form four longitudinal cords—a dorsal, a ventral, and two lateral cords—which may be seen on the surface as lateral lines. Nuclei of the hypodermis are located in the region of the cords. The somatic musculature lying beneath the hypodermis is a single layer of smooth muscle cells. When viewed in cross-section, this layer can be seen to be separated into four zones by the hypodermal cords. The musculature is innervated by extensions of muscle cells to nerve trunks running anteriorly and posteriorly from ganglion cells that ring the midportion of the esophagus.

The space between the muscle layer and viscera is the **pseudocoelom,** which lacks a mesothelium lining. This cavity contains fluid and two to six fixed cells (celomocytes) which are usually associated with the longitudinal cords. The function of these cells is unknown.

The alimentary canal of roundworms is complete, with both mouth and anus. The mouth is surrounded by lips bearing sensory papillae (bristles). The esophagus, a conspicuous feature of nematodes, is a muscular structure that pumps food into the intestine; it differs in shape in different species. The intestine is a tubular structure composed of a single layer of columnar cells possessing prominent microvilli on their luminal surface.

The excretory system of some nematodes consists of an excretory gland and a pore located ventrally in the midesophageal region. In other nematodes this structure is drawn into extensions that give rise to the more complex tubular excretory system, which is usually H-shaped, with two anterior limbs and two posterior limbs located in the lateral cords. The gland cells and tubes are thought to serve as absorptive bodies, collecting wastes from the pseudocoelom, and to function in osmoregulation.

Nematodes are usually bisexual. Males are usually smaller than females, have a curved posterior

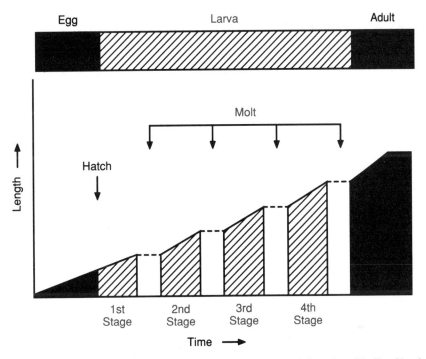

FIGURE 86-6   Stages in the development of nematodes. (Adapted from Lee DL: The Physiology of Nematodes. Oliver and Boyd, Edinburgh, 1965, with permission.)

end, and possess (in some species) copulatory structures, such as spicules (usually two), a bursa, or both. The males have one or (in a few cases) two testes, which lie at the free end of a convoluted or recurved tube leading into a seminal vesicle and eventually into the cloaca.

The female system is tubular also, and usually is made up of reflexed ovaries. Each ovary is continuous, with an oviduct and tubular uterus. The uteri join to form the vagina, which in turn opens to the exterior through the vulva.

Copulation between a female and a male nematode is necessary for fertilization except in the genus *Strongyloides,* in which parthenogenetic development occurs (i.e., the development of an un-

fertilized egg into a new individual). Some evidence indicates that sex attractants (pheromones) play a role in heterosexual mating. During copulation, sperm is transferred into the vulva of the female. The sperm enters the ovum and a **fertilization membrane** is secreted by the zygote. This membrane gradually thickens to form the chitinous shell. A second membrane, below the shell, makes the egg impervious to essentially all substances except carbon dioxide and oxygen. In some species, a third proteinaceous membrane is secreted as the egg passes down the uterus by the uterine wall and is deposited outside the shell. Most nematodes that are parasitic in humans lay eggs that, when voided, contain either an un-

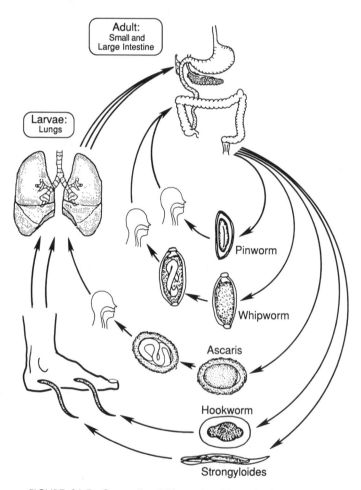

FIGURE 86-7 *Generalized life cycle of intestinal nematodes.*

cleaved zygote, a group of blastomeres, or a completely formed larva. Some nematodes, such as the filariae and *Trichinella spiralis,* produce larvae that are deposited in host tissues.

The developmental process in nematodes involves egg, larval, and adult stages. Each of four larval stages is followed by a molt in which the cuticle is shed. The larvae are called **second-stage larvae** after the first molt, and so on (Fig. 86-6). The nematode formed at the fifth stage is the adult. Figure 86-7 summarizes the life cycles of several intestinal nematodes.

REFERENCES

Ash L, Orihel TC: Parasites: A Guide to Laboratory Procedures and Identification. American Society of Clinical Pathologists, Chicago, 1987

Bogitsh BJ and Cheng TC: Human Parasitology. WB Saunders, Philadelphia, 1990

Castro GA: Trematodes: schistosomiasis. p 1710. In Kelly WN (ed): Textbook of Internal Medicine. JB Lippincott, Philadelphia, 1989

Hunter GW, Swartzwelder JC, Clyde DF: A Manual of Tropical Medicine. 5th Ed. WB Saunders, Philadelphia, 1976

Jeffrey HC, Leach RM: Atlas of Medical Helminthology and Protozoology. Churchill Livingstone, Edinburgh, 1968

Lee DL: The Physiology of Nematodes. Oliver and Boyd, Edinburgh, 1965

Smyth JD: The Physiology of Trematodes. Oliver and Boyd, Edinburgh, 1966

Schmidt GD, Roberts LS: Foundations of Parasitology. 3rd Ed. Times Mirror/Mosby College Publishers, St Louis, 1985

Zamen V: Atlas of Medical Parasitology. Lea & Febiger, Philadelphia, 1979

87 HELMINTHS: PATHOGENESIS AND DEFENSES

DEREK WAKELIN

GENERAL CONCEPTS

Classification
Helminth is a general term for a parasitic worm. The helminths include the Platyhelminthes or flatworms (flukes and tapeworms) and the Nematoda or roundworms.

Characteristics
All helminths are relatively large (> 1 mm long); some are very large (> 1 m long). All have well-developed organ systems and most are active feeders. The body is either flattened and covered with plasma membrane (flatworms) or cylindrical and covered with cuticle (roundworms). Some helminths are hermaphrodites; others have separate sexes.

Epidemiology
Helminths are worldwide in distribution; infection is most common and most serious in poor countries. The

distribution of these diseases is determined by climate, hygiene, diet, and exposure to vectors.

Infection
The mode of transmission varies with the type of worm; it may involve ingestion of eggs or larvae, penetration by larvae, bite of vectors, or ingestion of stages in the meat of intermediate hosts. Worms are often long-lived.

Pathogenesis
Many infections are asymptomatic; pathologic manifestations depend on the size, activity, and metabolism of the worms. Immune and inflammatory responses also cause pathology.

Host Defenses
Nonspecific defense mechanisms limit susceptibility. Antibody- and cell-mediated responses are important, as is inflammation. Parasites survive defenses through many evasion strategies.

INTRODUCTION

Helminths—worms—are some of the world's commonest parasites (see Ch. 86). They belong to two major groups of animals, the flatworms or Platyhelminthes (flukes and tapeworms) and the roundworms or Nematoda. All are relatively large and some are very large, exceeding 1 meter in length. Their bodies have well-developed organ systems, especially reproductive organs, and most helminths are active feeders. The bodies of flat-worms are flattened and covered by a plasma membrane, whereas roundworms are cylindrical and covered by a tough cuticle. Flatworms are usually hermaphroditic whereas roundworms have separate sexes; both have an immense reproductive capacity.

The most serious helminth infections are acquired in poor tropical and subtropical areas, but some also occur in the developed world; other, less serious, infections are worldwide in distribution. Exposure to infection is influenced by climate, hygiene, food preferences, and contact with vectors. Many potential infections are eliminated by host defenses; others become established and may persist for prolonged periods, even years. Although infections are often asymptomatic, severe pathology can occur. Because worms are large and often migrate through the body, they can damage the host's tissues directly by their activity or metabolism. Damage also occurs indirectly as a result of

host defense mechanisms. Almost all organ systems can be affected.

Host defense can act through nonspecific mechanisms of resistance and through specific immune responses. Antibody-mediated, cellular, and inflammatory mechanisms all contribute to resistance. However, many worms successfully avoid host defenses in a variety of ways, and can survive in the face of otherwise effective host responses.

INFECTION

Transmission of Infection

Helminths are transmitted to humans in many different ways (Fig. 87-1). The simplest is by accidental ingestion of infective eggs (*Ascaris, Echinococcus, Enterobius, Trichuris*) or larvae (some hookworms). Other worms have larvae that actively penetrate the skin (hookworms, schistosomes, *Strongyloides*). In several cases, infection requires an intermediate host vector. In some cases the intermediate vector

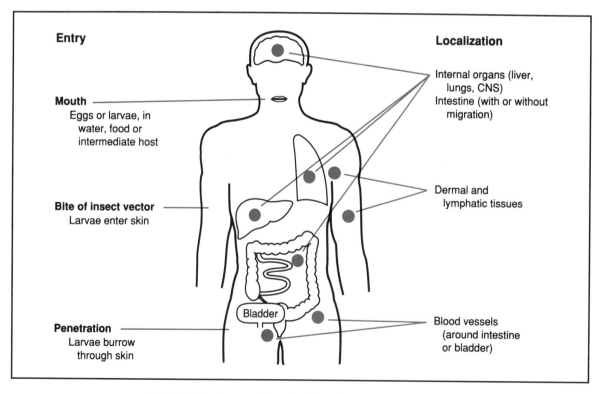

FIGURE 87-1   Entry and localization of pathogenic helminths.

transmits infective stages when it bites the host to take a blood meal (the arthropod vectors of filarial worms); in other cases, the larvae are contained in the tissues of the intermediate host and are taken in when a human eats that host (*Clonorchis* in fish, tapeworms in meat and fish, *Trichinella* in meat). The levels of infection in humans therefore depend on standards of hygiene (as eggs and larvae are often passed in urine or feces), on the climate (which may favor survival of infective stages), on the ways in which food is prepared, and on the degree of exposure to insect vectors.

Host Factors Influencing Susceptibility

Human behavior is a major factor influencing susceptibility to infection. If the infective stages of helminths are present in the environment, then certain ways of behaving, particularly with regard to hygiene and food, will result in greater exposure. Because helminths, with few exceptions (*Strongyloides, Trichinella,* some tapeworm larvae), do not increase their numbers by replication within the same host, the level of infection is directly related to the number of infective stages encountered. Obviously, not every exposure results in the development of a mature infection. Many infective organisms are killed by the host's nonspecific defense mechanisms. Of those that do become established, many are destroyed or eliminated by specific defenses. The number of worms present at any one time therefore represents a dynamic balance between the rate of infection and the efficiency of defense. This balance (which reflects the host's overall susceptibility) is altered by changes in the host's behavior and ability to express forms of defense. Children are more susceptible to many helminths than are adults, and frequently are the most heavily infected members of a community. The waning of immune competence with age may also result in increased levels of infection. Individuals differ genetically in their ability to resist infection, and it is well known that in infected populations, some individuals are predisposed to heavier infections than others. Changes in diet may affect susceptibility, as do the hor-

monal-immune changes accompanying pregnancy and lactation. An important cause of increased susceptibility is the immune suppression that accompanies concurrent infections with some other pathogens (particularly human immunodeficiency virus) and the development of certain tumors. Similarly, immunosuppressive therapies (irradiation, immunosuppressant drugs) may enhance susceptibility to helminth infection. A particular hazard in immunocompromised patients is the development of disseminated strongyloidiasis, in which large numbers of larvae develop in the body by autoinfection from relatively small numbers of adult *Strongyloides stercoralis.*

PARASITE FACTORS INFLUENCING SUSCEPTIBILITY

The ability of hosts to control infection is offset by the ability of parasites to avoid the host's defenses and increase their survival, thus increasing the numbers of organisms in the body. In addition to their ability to evade specific immune defenses (see below), many worms avoid the host's attempts to limit their activities or to destroy them simply by being large and mobile. Many important species measure several centimeters in length or diameter (*Ascaris,* hookworms, hydatid cysts, *Trichuris*) and others may exceed 1 meter in length (tapeworms). Size alone renders many defense mechanisms inoperative, as does the tough cuticle of adult roundworms. The ability of worms to move actively through tissues enables them to escape inflammatory foci. Many of the pathogenic consequences of worm infections are related to the size, movement, and longevity of the parasites, as the host is exposed to long-term damage and immune stimulation, as well as to the sheer physical consequences of being inhabited by large foreign bodies.

PATHOGENESIS
Direct Damage from Worm Activity

The most obvious forms of direct damage are those resulting from the blockage of internal organs or from the effects of pressure exerted by growing parasites (Fig. 87-2). Large *Ascaris* or tapeworms can physically block the intestine, especially after

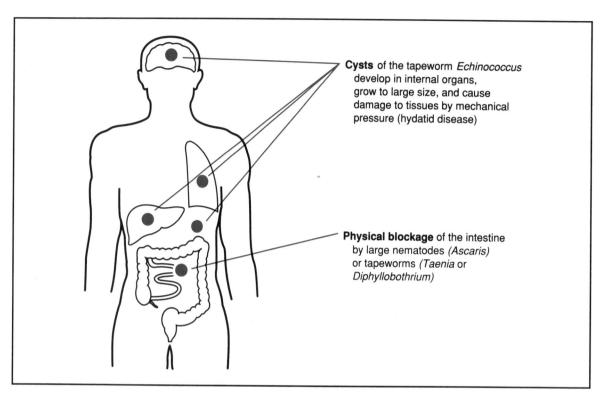

FIGURE 87-2 Pathogenesis: direct damage caused by large helminths.

some forms of chemotherapy. Migrating *Ascaris* may also block the bile duct. Granulomas that form around schistosome eggs may block the flow of blood through the liver, and blockage of lymph flow, leading to elephantiasis, is associated with the presence of adult *Wuchereria* in lymphatics. Pressure atrophy is characteristic of larval tapeworm infections (hydatid cyst, the larva of *Echinococcus granulosus*) where the parasite grows as a large fluid-filled cyst in the liver, brain, lungs, or body cavity. The multilocular hydatid cysts caused by *Echinococcus multilocularis* have a different growth form, metastasizing within organs and causing necrosis. The larvae of *Taenia solium,* the pork tapeworm, frequently develop in the central nervous system (CNS) and eyes. Some of the symptoms of the resulting condition, called *cysticercosis,* are caused by the pressure exerted by the cysts.

Intestinal worms cause a variety of pathologic changes in the mucosa, some reflecting physical and chemical damage to the tissues, others result-ing from immunopathologic responses. Hookworms (*Ancylostoma* and *Necator*) actively suck blood from mucosal capillaries. The anticoagulants secreted by the worms cause the wounds to bleed for prolonged periods, resulting in considerable blood loss. Heavy infections in malnourished hosts are associated with anemia and protein loss. Protein-losing enteropathies may result from the inflammatory changes induced by other intestinal worms. Diversion of host nutrients by competition from worms is probably unimportant, but interference with normal digestion and absorption may well aggravate undernutrition. The tapeworm *Diphyllobothrium latum* can cause vitamin B_{12} deficiency through direct absorption of this factor.

Many helminths undertake extensive migrations through body tissues, which both damage tissues directly and initiate hypersensitivity reactions. The skin, lungs, liver, and intestines are the organs most affected. Petechial hemorrhages, pneumonitis, eosinophilia, urticaria and pruritus, organomegaly, and granulomatous lesions are among the signs and symptoms produced during these migratory phases.

Feeding by worms upon host tissues is an important cause of pathology, particularly when it induces hyperplastic and metaplastic changes in epithelia. For example, liver fluke infections lead to hyperplasia of the bile duct epithelium. Chronic inflammatory changes around parasites (for example, the granulomas around schistosome eggs in the bladder wall) have been linked with neoplasia, but the nature of the link is not known. The continuous release by living worms of excretory-secretory materials, many of which are known to have direct effects upon host cells and tissues, may also contribute to pathology.

Indirect Damage from Host Response

As with all infectious organisms, it is impossible to separate the pathogenic effects caused strictly by mechanical or chemical tissue damage from those caused by the immune response to the parasite. All helminths are "foreign bodies" not only in the sense of being large and invasive but also in the immunologic sense: they are antigenic and therefore stimulate immunity. An excellent illustration of this interrelation between direct and indirect damage is seen in the pathology associated with schistosome infections, especially with *Schistosoma mansoni* (Fig. 87-3). Hypersensitivity-based, granulomatous responses to eggs trapped in the liver cause a physical obstruction to blood flow, which leads to liver pathology. Hypersensitivity-based inflammatory changes probably also contribute to the lymphatic blockage associated with filarial infections (*Brugia, Wuchereria*).

Immune-mediated inflammatory changes occur in the skin, lungs, liver, intestine, CNS, and eyes as worms migrate through these structures. Systemic changes such as eosinophilia, edema, and joint pain reflect local responses to parasites. The pathologic consequences of immune-mediated inflammation are seen clearly in intestinal infections (especially *Strongyloides* and *Trichinella* infections). Structural changes, such as villous atrophy, de-

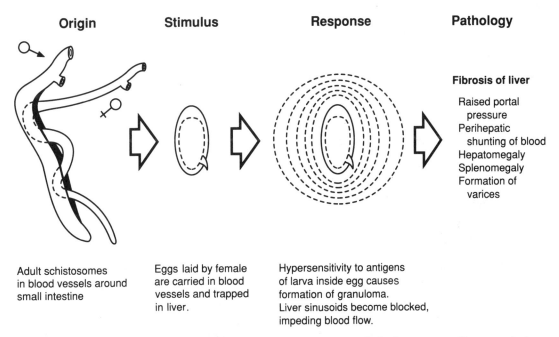

Origin	Stimulus	Response	Pathology

Fibrosis of liver

Raised portal
  pressure
Perihepatic
  shunting of blood
Hepatomegaly
Splenomegaly
Formation of
  varices

Adult schistosomes in blood vessels around small intestine

Eggs laid by female are carried in blood vessels and trapped in liver.

Hypersensitivity to antigens of larva inside egg causes formation of granuloma. Liver sinusoids become blocked, impeding blood flow.

FIGURE 87-3 Pathogenesis: indirect damage caused by immunopathologic responses (for example, in schistosomiasis).

velop. The permeability of the mucosa changes, fluid accumulates in the gut lumen, and intestinal transit time is reduced. Prolonged changes of this type may lead to a protein-losing enteropathy. The inflammatory changes that accompany the passage of schistosome eggs through the intestinal wall also cause severe intestinal pathology. Heavy infections with the whipworm *Trichuris* in the large bowel can lead to inflammatory changes resulting in blood loss and rectal prolapse.

The severity of these indirect changes is a result of the chronic nature of the infection. The fact that many worms are extremely long-lived means that many inflammatory changes become irreversible, producing functional changes in tissues. Three examples are the hyperplasia of bile ducts in long-term liver fluke infections, the extensive fibrosis associated with chronic schistosomiasis, and the skin atrophy associated with onchocerciasis. Severe pathology may also result when worms stray into abnormal body sites.

DEFENSES AGAINST INFECTION
Nonspecific Resistance

Infective stages attempting to enter via the mouth or through the skin are opposed by the same nonspecific defenses that protect humans from invasion of other pathogens. Following oral ingestion, parasites must survive passage through the acid stomach to reach the small bowel. The natural parasites of humans are adapted to do this, but opportunistic parasites may be killed. Similarly, natural parasites are adapted to the environmental conditions of the bowel (and in many cases require them as cues for development), but accidental parasites may find them inappropriate. Penetration into the intestinal wall may trigger inflammatory responses that immobilize and kill the worm. This may itself lead to serious pathology (as in *Anisakis* infection). Worms entering through the skin must survive the skin secretions, penetrate the epidermal layers, and avoid inflammatory trapping in the dermis. Invasion of humans by the larvae of dog and cat hookworms (*Ancylostoma*) results in dermatitis and 'creeping eruption' as the worms

become the focus of inflammatory reactions that form trails in the skin.

Once in the tissues, worms need the correct sequence of environmental signals to mature. Absent or incomplete signals constitute a form of nonspecific resistance that may partially or completely prevent further development. The parasite may not die, however; indeed, prolonged survival at a larval stage may result in pathology from the continuing inflammatory response (e.g., *Toxocara* infection).

Specific Acquired Immunity

There is no doubt that specific immunity is responsible for the most effective forms of host defense, although the dividing line between nonspecific and specific mechanisms is difficult to draw with precision (Fig. 87-4). All helminths stimulate strong immune responses, which can easily be detected by measuring specific antibody or cellular immunity. Although these responses are useful for diagnosing infection, they appear frequently not to be protective. The high prevalence of helminth infection in endemic areas (sometimes approaching 100 percent), and the fact that individuals may remain infected for many years and can easily be reinfected after they are cured by chemotherapy, suggest that protective immunity against helminths is weak or absent in humans. However, some degree of immunity does appear to operate, because the intensity of infection often declines with age, and many individuals in endemic areas remain parasitologically negative and/or clinically normal. Evidence from laboratory studies provides some clues as to the mechanisms involved. Antibodies that bind to surface antigens may focus complement- or cell-mediated effectors that can damage the worm. Macrophages and eosinophils are the prime cytotoxic effector cells, and IgM, IgG, and IgE are the important immunoglobulins. Antibodies may also block enzymes released by the worm, thus interfering with its ability to penetrate tissues or to feed. Inflammatory changes may concentrate effector cells around worms, and the release of cellular mediators may then disable and kill the worm. Encapsulation of trapped worms by in-

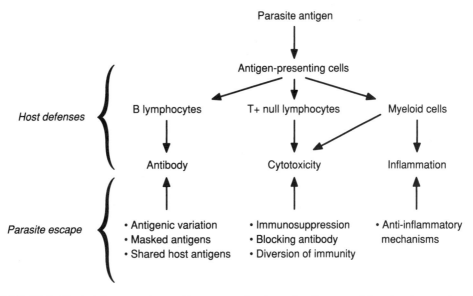

FIGURE 87-4   Host defense and parasite escape. A schematic diagram of the development and expression of acquired immunity to helminths and of the ways in which parasites escape the immune response.

flammatory cells may also result in the death of the worm, although this is not always the case. Intestinal worms can be dislodged by the structural and physiologic changes that occur in the intestine during acute inflammation. It has long been suspected that IgE-mediated hypersensitivity reactions, involving mast cells and basophils, contribute to this process, but the evidence is still circumstantial. Despite the abundance of IgA in the intestinal lumen, there is no conclusive evidence that it is involved in protective immunity in humans, although laboratory data suggest it is.

Avoidance of Host Defenses

Despite their immunogenicity, many helminths survive for extended periods in the bodies of their hosts. Some of the reasons have already been mentioned (size, motility), but we now know that worms employ many sophisticated devices to render host defenses ineffective (Fig. 87-4). Some worms (schistosomes) disguise their outer surface by acquiring host molecules which reduce their antigenicity; intrinsic membrane changes also make these

worms resistant to immune attack. Filarial nematodes acquire serum albumin on their cuticle, which may act as a disguise. Many worms release substances that depress lymphocyte function, inactivate macrophages, or digest antibodies. Larval cestodes appear to prolong their survival by producing anticomplement factors which protect their outer layers from lytic attack. Antigenic variation in the strict sense is not known to occur, but many species show a stage-specific change of antigens as they develop, and this phenomenon may delay the development of effective immune mechanisms. All helminths release relatively large amounts of antigenic materials, and this voluminous production may divert immune responses or even locally exhaust immune potential. Irrelevant antibodies produced by the host may block the activity of potentially protective antibodies, as has been shown to be the case in schistosome infections.

It is striking that many helminth infections are associated with a degree of immune suppression, which may affect specific or general responsiveness. Many explanations have been proposed for this immune suppression, including antigen over-load, antigenic competition, induction of suppressor cells, and production of lymphocyte-specific suppressor factors. Reduced immune responsiveness may not only prolong the survival of the original infecting worm species but increase the host's susceptibility to other pathogens. Epidemiologic evidence also raises the possibility that infections acquired early in life—before or shortly after birth—may induce a form of immune tolerance, allowing heavy worm burdens to accumulate in the body.

The subtlety with which parasitic worms manipulate the host's immune system not only increases their importance as pathogens but also creates formidable problems for their control and eradication.

REFERENCES

Brown HA, Neva, FA: Basic Clinical Parasitology. Appleton-Century-Crofts, East Norwalk, CT, 1983

Crewe W (ed): Blacklock and Southwell's Guide to Human Parasitology. 11th Ed. Chapman and Hall, London, 1990

Despommier DD, Karapelou JW: Parasite Life Cycles. Springer-Verlag, New York, 1988

Katz M, Despommier DD, Gwadz RW: *Parasitic Diseases.* Springer-Verlag, New York, 1982

Manson-Bahr PEC, Bell DR: Manson's Tropical Diseases. 19th Ed. Balliere Tindall, London, 1987

Peters W, Gilles HM: A Colour Atlas of Tropical Medicine and Parasitology. 3rd Ed. Wolfe Medical Publications, London, 1989

Warren KS, Mahmoud AAF: Tropical and Geographical Medicine. McGraw-Hill, New York, 1984

88 SCHISTOSOMES AND OTHER TREMATODES

KENNETH S. WARREN

GENERAL CONCEPTS

Clinical Manifestations

Signs and symptoms are related largely to the location of the adult worms. Infections with *Schistosoma mansoni* and *S japonicum* (mesenteric venules) result in eosinophilia, hepatomegaly, splenomegaly, and hematemesis. *Schistosoma haematobium* (vesical venules) causes dysuria, hematuria, and uremia. *Fasciola hepatica, Clonorchis sinensis,* and *Opisthorchis viverrini* (bile ducts) cause fever, hepatomegaly, abdominal pain, and jaundice. Infections with *Paragonimus westermani* (lungs, brain) result in cough, hemoptysis, chest pain, and epilepsy. *Fasciolopsis buski* (intestines) causes abdominal pain, diarrhea, and edema.

Structure

Trematodes are multicellular eukaryotic helminths.

Multiplication and Life Cycle

Free-swimming larvae (**cercariae**) are given off by infected snails. These either penetrate the skin of the human definitive host (schistosomes) or are ingested after encysting as metacercariae in or on various edible plants or animals (all other trematodes). After entering a human the larvae develop into adult males and females (schistosomes) or hermaphrodites (other flukes), which produce eggs that pass out of the host in excreta. These

eggs hatch in fresh water into **miracidia** which infect snails.

Pathogenesis

In schistosomiasis, eggs trapped in the tissues produce granulomatous inflammatory reactions, fibrosis, and obstruction. The hermaphroditic flukes of the liver, lungs, and intestines induce inflammatory and toxic reactions.

Host Defenses

Host defenses against schistosomiasis include antibody or complement-dependent cellular cytotoxicity and modulation of granulomatous hypersensitivity. The defenses against hermaphroditic flukes are unknown.

Epidemiology

Most infected individuals show no overt disease. In a relatively small proportion of individuals, heavy infections due to repeated exposure to parasitic larvae will lead to the development of clinical manifestations. The distribution of flukes is limited by the distribution of their snail intermediate host. Larvae from snails infect a human by penetrating the skin (schistosomes) or by being eaten (encysted larvae of other trematodes).

Diagnosis

Diagnosis is suggested by clinical manifestations, geographic history, and exposure to infective larvae. The diagnosis is confirmed by the presence of parasite eggs in excreta.

Control

As a control measure, exposure to parasite larvae in water and food should be prevented. Treatment with praziquantel is effective.

INTRODUCTION

Trematodes, or flukes, are parasitic flatworms with unique life cycles involving sexual reproduction in mammalian and other vertebrate definitive hosts and asexual reproduction in snail intermediate hosts. These organisms are divided into four groups on the basis of their final habitats in humans: (1) the hermaphroditic **liver flukes** which reside in the bile ducts and infect humans on ingestion of watercress (*Fasciola*) or raw fish (*Clonorchis* and *Opisthorchis*); (2) the hermaphroditic **intestinal fluke** *(Fasciolopsis)*, which infects humans on ingestion of water chestnuts; (3) the hermaphroditic **lung fluke** *(Paragonimus)*, which infects humans on ingestion of raw crabs or crayfish; and (4) the bisexual **blood flukes** *(Schistosoma)*, which live in the intestinal or vesical (urinary bladder) venules and infect humans by direct penetration through the skin.

Fascioliasis is a cosmopolitan zoonosis; sporadic cases in humans have appeared in most parts of the world. The remaining hermaphroditic fluke infections of humans are confined largely to Asia. Schistosomiasis occurs in South America, the Caribbean, Africa, the Middle East, and Asia, and is spreading in many areas due to the introduction of dams and irrigation systems.

Flukes do not multiply in humans, so the intensity of infection is related to the degree of exposure to the infective larvae. In most endemic areas, the majority of infected individuals have light or moderate worm burdens. Overt disease occurs largely in the relatively small proportion of the population with a heavy worm burden, although genetic predisposition may also play a role. Pathol-

ogy may be caused by the worms themselves (as with liver flukes, which damage the bile ducts) or by their eggs (for example, schistosome eggs, which induce granulomatous inflammation in the venules or tissues). Treatment of all fluke infections has been greatly improved by the introduction of the anthelminthic drug praziquantel.

CLINICAL MANIFESTATIONS

Schistosomiasis

Three major disease syndromes occur in schistosomiasis: **schistosome dermatitis, acute schistosomiasis,** and **chronic schistosomiasis.** The first is a pruritic rash that appears after repeated exposure to cercariae, usually those of birds and small mammals. Acute schistosomiasis (Katayama fever) begins 4 to 8 weeks after primary exposure and may last for a few weeks. It appears most commonly in *Schistosoma japonicum* infection, is much less common in *S mansoni* infections, and is seen rarely in patients infected with *S haematobium*. Acute schistosomiasis is the self-limited febrile illness that occurs on primary exposure to the parasite. It is characterized by cough, hepatosplenomegaly, lymphadenopathy, and eosinophilia. It may be fatal.

A wide variety of symptoms have been associated with chronic schistosomiasis mansoni and japonica, including fatigue, abdominal pain, and intermittent diarrhea or dysentery. Over the past 15 years, however, field studies have demonstrated that few infected individuals—even those with heavy infections—show such symptoms. Similar findings were reported in hospitalized patients in the United Kingdom. In schistosomiasis haematobia, dysuria and hematuria are frequently seen in the early stages of infection. Chronic disease may appear many years later, developing usually in individuals with a heavy worm burden. In schistosomiasis japonica and mansoni, chronic disease is characterized by hepatomegaly, splenomegaly, portal hypertension, and bleeding esophageal varices. In schistosomiasis haematobia, inflammation and fibrosis of the bladder and ureters occur; obstruction of the ureters leads to hydronephrosis and eventually to uremia.

Hermaphroditic Flukes

The signs and symptoms of infection with the hermaphroditic flukes are related largely to the location of the adult worms—the bile ducts (*Fasciola hepatica, Clonorchis sinensis, Opisthorchis viverrini*), the intestines (*Fasciolopsis buski*), or the lungs (*Paragonimus westermani*). *Fasciola hepatica* infection is the one exception, in that the disease has two distinct phases. The first occurs in the initial 6 to 9 weeks of infection when the larvae migrate through the liver; the second begins when they enter the bile ducts. The acute clinical syndrome is characterized by prolonged fever, pain in the right hypochondrium, and sometimes hepatomegaly, asthenia, and urticaria; Marked eosinophilia usually also occurs during this period. Asymptomatic acute infection has been reported in England and seems to be common in Peru. After the flukes enter the bile ducts, the symptoms decline and then disappear completely. Although animals with particularly heavy worm burdens may develop chronic biliary tract disease, this condition is rare in humans, and when reported is usually an incidental finding at surgery or autopsy.

In contrast, an acute syndrome does not occur in clonorchiasis and opisthorchiasis because the larval flukes enter directly into the bile ducts. Most individuals with *Clonorchis* and *Opisthorchis* infections show no significant signs or symptoms of disease. Pathologic studies have revealed no gross changes in the liver in mild, early infections. Despite these generally negative findings, patients with severe chronic disease, manifested by cholangitis, cholangiohepatitis and cholangiocarcinoma, occasionally appear at hospitals.

Fasciolopsiasis caused by the intestinal fluke also appears to be associated with few or no disease manifestations in individuals examined in field environments. In a controlled study involving clinical examination, evaluation of growth and development, hematologic studies, and screening tests for intestinal malabsorption, no significant differences between infected and uninfected subjects were found. However, cases of severe clinical illness characterized by diarrhea, abdominal pain, edema (often facial), and passage of undigested food in the feces have been reported in patients with heavy infections.

Paragonimiasis due to the lung fluke usually comes to the attention of the physician when the patient complains of cough or intermittent hemoptysis. Profuse expectoration and chest pain of a pleuritic type are also found. Nevertheless, clinical studies indicate that in most endemic areas most infections are light or moderate and are associated with few signs or symptoms. Cerebral paragonimiasis is encountered in highly endemic regions and is manifested as Jacksonian epilepsy, tumors, or embolism of the brain.

STRUCTURE AND LIFE CYCLE

The trematodes or flukes are multicellular flatworms. Different species range in length from less than 1 mm to several centimeters. The flukes of medical importance are all digenetic, reproducing sexually in a definitive vertebrate host and asexually in a snail intermediate host. Flukes have a variety of different life cycle stages (Figs. 88-1 and 88-2; also see Ch. 86, Figs. 86-1 and 86-2). Adult male and female or hermaphroditic flukes inhabit the definitive vertebrate host and lay eggs. Free-swimming ciliated miracidia hatch from the eggs and infect snails, in which they give rise to sporocysts and rediae. The snails emit cercariae, which infect the vertebrate host either directly or via an encysted form known as a metacercaria.

Schistosomes

Three major species of schistosomes infect humans: *Schistosoma mansoni, S japonica,* and *S haematobium.* The adult male and female schistosomes

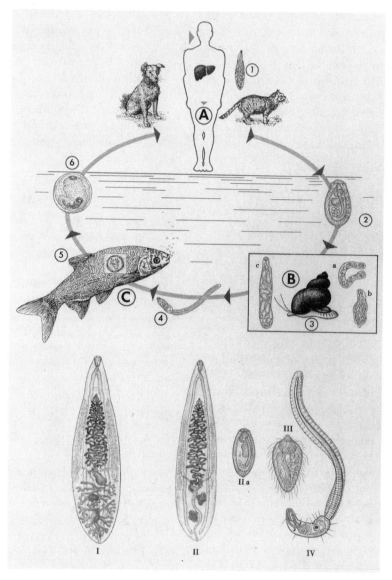

FIGURE 88-1 Life cycle of the liver fluke.

A. Final host: human, cats, dogs, and household and farm animals

   1. Sexually mature liver fluke

   2. Egg (with miracidium) of *Clonorchis sinensis*

B. Intermediate hosts: snails of the genus *Bulimus* (=*Bythinia*) and others

   3. (a) Young sporocyst

     (b) Mother redia

     (c) Daughter redia with rudiments of cercariae

   4. Cercariae that have become free

C. Intermediate host: chiefly fishes of the family Cyprinidae

   5. Fish with cercariae

   6. Metacercariae (greatly magnified)

     I. *Clonorchis sinensis* (magnified about 5:1)

     II. *Opisthorchis felineus* (magnified about 7:1)

     IIa. Egg of *Opisthorchis felineus* with miracidium

     III. Free miracidium from snail

     IV. Cercaria as it typically appears when swimming

(From Piekarski G: Medical Parasitology. Springer-Verlag, Heidelberg, 1989, p. 136, with permission.)

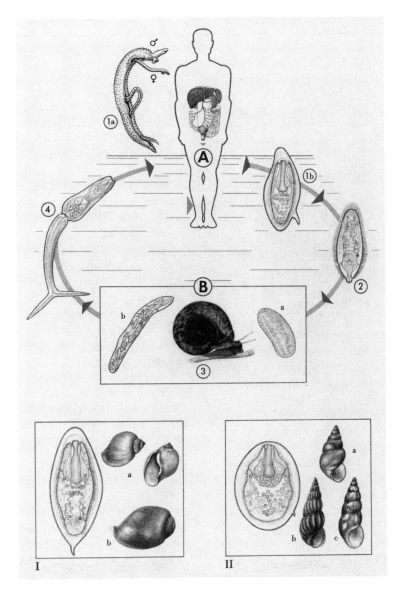

FIGURE 88-2 Life cycle of schistosome.

A. Final host: humans. Site of the worms: the mesenteric vessels
  1. (a) Sexually mature pair of flukes of *Schistosoma mansoni*
     (b) Mature egg of *Schistosoma mansoni* (lateral spine)
  2. Miracidium

B. Intermediate host: aquatic snails (Planorbidae; for example, *Planorbis boissyi, Australorbis glabratus*)
  3. (a) Sporocyst of the first order (mother sporocyst)
     (b) Sporocyst of the second order (daughter sporocyst)

  4. Free cercaria (forked-tail cercaria)
     I. *Schistosoma haematobium:* egg with miracidium (terminal spine); shells of the intermediate hosts of the species:
        a. *Bulinus truncatus* (North Africa)
        b. *Bulinus globosa* (West Africa)
     II. *Schistosoma japonicum:* egg with miracidium (very small lateral spine); shells of intermediate hosts of the genera:
        a. *Schistosomophora*
        b. *Oncomelania*
        c. *Katayama*

(From Piekarski G: Medical Parasitology. Springer-Verlag, Heidelberg, 1989, p. 160, with permission.)

reside in human mesenteric or vesical venules. Fertilized female worms produce large numbers of eggs, which pass out of the blood vessels, through the tissues, and into the lumen of the gut (*S mansoni* and *S japonicum*) or urinary bladder (*S haematobium*), from which they are shed into the environment, where they may infect a snail intermediate host. After a period of asexual multiplication in the snail, the cercariae pass out into water from which they directly penetrate into human skin. The young schistosomes migrate from the skin to the lungs and then to the hepatoportal system, where they mature, mate and pass down into the mesenteric or vesical venules (Fig. 88-1).

Liver Flukes

Fasciola hepatica is a hermaphroditic liver fluke that infects mainly ruminants but may incidentally infect humans. It resides in the bile ducts of the liver, where it produces large numbers of eggs daily for many years. The eggs pass into the lumen of the small intestine and leave the body in the feces. If deposited in fresh water, the eggs hatch into ciliated miracidia, which, upon penetration of the correct species of snail, undergo several developmental stages and produce large numbers of cercariae. These tailed, free-swimming organisms leave the snail and encyst as metacercariae on the leaves of freshwater plants, particularly watercress. When ingested by the definitive host, the larvae excyst, penetrate through the gut wall into the peritoneal cavity, enter the liver capsule, and begin to wander through the hepatic tissues. This migratory phase continues for about 7 weeks. The half-grown flukes then enter the bile ducts, mature, and begin to produce eggs.

Clonorchis sinensis and *Opisthorchis viverrini* are also liver flukes; in the case of these flukes, however, the eggs hatch only after ingestion by certain species of snails, and the cercariae penetrate under the scales or into the flesh of certain freshwater fishes, where they encyst as metacercariae. After they are ingested in raw or inadequately cooked fish, the organisms excyst within the duodenum and, in contrast to *F. hepatica,* pass directly into the bile ducts through the ampulla of Vater (Fig. 88-2).

Intestinal and Lung Flukes

The cercariae of *Fasciolopsis buski,* the intestinal fluke, encyst on certain species of water plants. When ingested, the metacercariae excyst within the duodenum, attach to the nearby intestinal wall, develop into adult worms, and begin egg production. The eggs pass out in the feces into fresh water, where the hatched miracidia penetrate into snails and develop there into cercariae. The eggs of *Paragonimus westermani,* the lung fluke, pass into the bronchioles, are coughed up, and are voided in the sputum or swallowed and passed in the feces. After undergoing a period of embryonation, the eggs hatch and the miracidia penetrate into certain species of fresh water snails. Cercariae develop within the snails and then pass out into the water and penetrate crustaceans, in which they encyst. When inadequately cooked freshwater crayfish and crabs are eaten, the metacercariae excyst in the duodenum, penetrate the intestinal wall, and enter the peritoneal cavity, from which they migrate through the diaphragm and pleural cavity into the lungs and occasionally into the brain.

PATHOGENESIS

The diseases caused by flukes result from the inflammation, and in most cases fibrosis, elicited by the parasites and their products. The severity of disease is clearly related to intensity of infection, as shown in both experimental models and at autopsy. In schistosomiasis, the adult worms reside in the intestinal venules and produce large numbers of eggs. The embryo is enclosed in a semipermeable membrane, which in turn is protected by a tanned protein eggshell pierced by ultramicroscopic pores. The mature embryo (miracidium) secretes a variety of antigenic molecules, including enzymes.

While approximately fifty percent of the eggs pass through the mucosa into the lumen of the intestine, the rest remain within the mammalian host, many breaking free into the mesenteric veins, from which they pass into the liver via the portal venous system and become trapped in the presinusoidal venules. They survive in this milieu for approximately 3 weeks. During that period the host tissues react to the egg secretions by forming a focal granulomatous lesion of the kind seen in tuberculosis (see Ch. 87, Fig. 87-3). This lesion has been shown to be essentially a cell-mediated immunologic reaction of the delayed hypersensitivity type—i.e., based on an anamnestic reaction specific to egg antigens that is transferrable by cells but not by serum. Furthermore, granuloma formation can be suppressed by inhibitors of cell-mediated immune reactivity and do not occur in nude athymic mice. Investigations of granuloma formation around fluke eggs both in vivo and in vitro have demonstrated a high rate of collagen synthesis. That is later balanced by collagen degradation, fibrosis being the net result of both the intensity of infection and an imbalance toward collagen synthesis (see Fig. 87-3). After treatment with drugs that kill the flukes, collagen tends to be resorbed; that occurs at a higher rate in early than in late infections.

Studies of the hepatic microcirculation in experimentally infected animals have revealed that portal venous obstruction is caused not by the eggs alone but by the granulomas around them. Portal vein obstruction leads to portal hypertension, splenomegaly, and the development of esophageal varices. In spite of severe portal venous obstruction, the total liver blood flow remains within normal limits, as there is marked neovascular formation of arterial vessels in the areas of inflammation and fibrosis.

The typical lesions of advanced hepatosplenic schistosomiasis, called "pipestem fibrosis," consist of enlarged, whitish, fibrous triads surrounding portal vein lumina and resembling clay pipestems in cross section. The liver parenchymal cells appear normal. The spleen may become markedly enlarged and is firm in consistency, fibrotic, and congested. Hypersplenism may occur, with attendant anemia and pancytopenia.

The acute clinical syndrome of *Fasciola hepatica* infection occurs during migration of the fluke larvae in the liver parenchyma, with resultant inflammation and localized destruction of liver cells. Once in the bile ducts, liver flukes of all species produce inflammation due to mechanical irritation and toxic secretions. Highly immunogenic predominant antigens have been found in the eggs of *Opisthorchis*. Studies in humans have revealed hyperplasia of the epithelial cells lining the biliary tract, periductal fibrosis, thickening of the duct wall, and dilation and obstruction of the duct lumen. Secondary infection occurs due to biliary stasis, resulting in chronic recurrent, suppurative infections; cholangiocarcinoma also may occur.

The intestinal fluke *Fasciolopsis buski* attaches to the duodenal and jejunal mucosa. Inflammation at the site of attachment may be followed by ulceration and even bleeding. The flukes affect the secretion of intestinal fluids and mucus. The adults of the lung fluke *Paragonimus* are usually found just beneath the pleural surface, where they induce local necrosis, hemorrhage, inflammation and fibrous encapsulation. These flukes may also be found in other tissues including the brain. In heavy infections a syndrome similar to that of chronic bronchitis occurs, with cough and sputum production, sometimes accompanied by intermittent hemoptysis. Cerebral lesions are characterized by necrosis and an eosinophilic granulomatous reaction.

HOST DEFENSES

Schistosomes

Many experimental animals have natural resistance to schistosomiasis; some will essentially not develop an infection on exposure, whereas others kill all but a very small proportion of the parasites. Even in the most susceptible animals, the cercaria-to-worm ratio is well under 50 percent. It is also of interest that nonspecific immunity against schistosomes can be induced with bacille Calmette-Guérin and derivatives. The mechanism of this response apparently involves arginase secreted by mononuclear cells. With respect to specific acquired resistance, delayed hypersensitivity and a wide variety of antibodies have been demonstrated in experimental animals and in humans. Partial immunity has been found in some primates and laboratory animals, and field studies indicate that humans develop some degree of resistance to reinfection. Although various mechanisms of acquired resistance have been seen in experimental animals, antibody-dependent cellular cytotoxicity, mediated principally by eosinophils, has been shown in animals in vivo and humans in vitro. Furthermore, schistosomiasis is an immune disease caused by cell-mediated granulomatous hypersensitivity initiated by the parasite eggs. An ameliorating factor is modulation of granuloma formation, which occurs naturally in chronic infection. This modulation is caused by suppressor cells and antibodies. Recently it has been possible to induce immunity in experimental animals using antigens derived from schistosomes, in many cases through genetic engineering. These antigens include not only molecules on the surface of the organisms, but structural proteins and enzymes as well.

Hermaphroditic Flukes

With respect to the hermaphroditic flukes, studies of *Fasciola hepatica* in experimental animals have revealed resistance to reinfection. Adoptive and passive transfer of resistance has been achieved with cells and serum. Immunity has also been induced by nonliving vaccines. It is of interest that immunization with *Fasciola* antigens will induce resistance to *Schistosoma* infection and vice versa. Relatively little work in this area has been performed with the other trematodes.

EPIDEMIOLOGY

Trematodes do not multiply directly in humans, but instead mate and produce large numbers of eggs that pass out of the body in the feces, urine, or sputum. Thus, the intensity of human infection is related largely to the rate of exposure to infective larvae—i.e., to the frequency and extent of contact with water and of consumption of contaminated foods. Mathematical models suggest that the intensity of infections in mammalian populations follows a negative binomial distribution, with most individuals having light to moderate infections. In recent years, controlled studies have revealed that most infected individuals show no overt signs or symptoms of disease. Significant disease occurs mainly in the few individuals with a heavy burden of flukes.

Three different species of human schistosome parasites are responsible for two hundred million infections. *Schistosoma mansoni* occurs in South America, the Caribbean, and Africa; *S japonicum* in the Far East; and *S haematobium* in Africa and the Middle East. *S japonicum* is the only species that has significant animal reservoirs. The distribution of all the flukes is limited by the distribution of their snail intermediate host.

Fasciola hepatica occurs worldwide in ruminants and causes significant morbidity and mortality in sheep and cattle. For the most part, human infection is sporadic; only a few hundred cases have been reported in the world literature, usually associated with ingestion of wild watercress. Fascioliasis in humans has almost always been identified during the acute migratory stage of infection; occasionally, worms are found in the bile ducts at surgery or autopsy. Foci of chronic human fascioliasis have been found in rural areas of Peru.

Clonorchis sinensis and *O viverrini* are common liver flukes of cats and dogs; they also infect many other mammalian hosts. Although humans are incidental hosts, millions of individuals are infected with these organisms. Clonorchiasis is prevalent in China, Hong Kong, Vietnam, Korea, and Taiwan. *Opisthorchis viverrini* infection is widespread in Thailand. Infection with another species, *O felineus*, has been reported in many parts of Southeast Asia and Asia as well as Eastern Europe and the Soviet Union. Infection occurs after ingestion of raw or inadequately cooked freshwater fish (saltwater fish do not carry these parasites). *Fasciolopsis buski* is a common parasite of humans and pigs in the Far East and Southeast Asia. Infection results from consumption of the raw pods, roots, stems, or bulbs of certain water plants, often water chestnuts, and is related to the habit of peeling the metacercaria-infested hull of these vegetables with the teeth before consumption.

Paragonimus westermani has a cosmopolitan distribution among mammals; human infection is found largely in the Far East. Closely related species have been reported in Africa and in South and Central America. Paragonimiasis is transmitted by eating uncooked freshwater crayfish or crabs.

DIAGNOSIS

The anatomic locations of the symptoms and signs suggest a diagnosis of schistosomiasis or of disease caused by the liver, intestinal, urinary tract, or lung flukes. Except in the case of fascioliasis, the geographic history should be of particular value, because all other fluke infections of humans have relatively specific distributions. A careful dietary history is important in the case of the hermaphroditic flukes and provides relatively clear-cut evidence. In diagnosing schistosomiasis, a history of significant contact with fresh water is of diagnostic value.

Demonstrating the eggs of the parasite in the excreta provides the definitive diagnosis in all cases of fluke infection. A quantitative method is of great importance because of the relationship between the intensity of infection and the development of disease. The best method for doing this, which is equivalent in many ways to a concentration technique, is the Kato thick smear method, in which a 50 mg feces sample is placed on a slide covered with a plastic coverslip soaked in glycerol and is allowed to clear for 24 hr. For *S haematobium* infections, Nucleopore filtration of 10 ml of urine is the simplest and most rapid method. Most immunodiagnostic methods are not specific or sensitive enough to assess these infections.

CONTROL

A key control measure for all fluke infections is preventing egg-containing excreta from contaminating water sources. Another approach is to control snail populations, largely by the use of mollus-cicides. For schistosomiasis, contact with infected water should be minimized. For the hermaphroditic flukes, infection can be avoided by careful preparation and cooking of fresh water fish, crustacea, and vegetables.

Treatment of all fluke infections other than fascioliasis is accomplished by a one-day course of the oral drug praziquantel. For *Fasciola hepatica,* the current drug of choice is bithional, given orally for 15 days.

REFERENCES

Colley D, Newport G: Schistosomiasis and other trematodes. In Warren KS (ed): Immunology and Molecular Biology of Parasitic Infections. Blackwell, Scientific Publications, Oxford, in press

Plaut AG, Kamapanart Sanyakorn C, Manning GS: A clinical study of *Fasciolopsis buski* infection in Thailand. Trans R Soc Trop Med Hyg 63:470, 1969

Siongok TKA, Mahmoud AAF, Ouma JH, et al: Morbidity in schistosomiasis mansoni in relation to intensity of infection: Study of a community in Machakos, Kenya. Am J Trop Med Hyg 25:273, 1976

Soulsby EJL: Immunology of helminths. In Good RA, Day SB (eds): Immunology of Human Infection. Part II: Viruses and Parasites. Plenum, New York, 1982

Upatham ES, Viyanant V, Kurathong S, et al: Morbidity in relation to the intensity of infection of *Opistorchis viverrini:* Study of a community of Khon Kaen, Thailand. Am J Trop Med Hyg 31:1156, 1982

Warren KS: The kinetics of hepatosplenic schistosomiasis. Semin Liver Dis 4:293, 1984

Zhong H, He L, Xu Z, Cao W: Recent progress in studies of *Paragonimus* and paragonimiasis control in China. Chinese Med J 94:483, 1981

89 CESTODES

DONALD HEYNEMAN

GENERAL CONCEPTS

Clinical Manifestations

Adult Tapeworms: Adult worms are found in the small intestine; these infections are usually well tolerated or asymptomatic, but may cause abdominal distress, dyspepsia, anorexia (or increased appetite), nausea, localized pain, and diarrhea.

Larval Tapeworms: Larvae locate in extraintestinal tissues and produce systemic infections with clinical effects related to the size, number, and location of cysts. *Taenia solium* cysticercosis (infection with the cysticercus larval stage) is often asymptomatic and chronic; neurocysticercosis, ophthalmic cysticercosis, and subcutaneous and muscular cysticercosis are reported. *Echinococcus granulosus* hydatid larvae may form massive cysts in liver, lungs, and other organs, including long bones and the central nervous system.

Structure

Adults, which mature sexually in the definitive or final host, are ribbon-shaped, multisegmented, hermaphroditic flatworms; each segment has a complete male and female reproductive system. An anterior holdfast organ (the scolex) is followed by a germinative portion ("neck") and segments at successively later stages of development. Larvae encyst in various tissues of the intermediate host; larval cysts contain one or many scoleces of future adult worms.

Multiplication and Life Cycle

The tapeworm's life cycle involves a definitive and one or more intermediate hosts (except for the one-host cycle of *Hymenolepis nana*). Each type of cycle has specialized larval forms (cysticercus, cysticercoid; coenurus, hydatid; coracidium, procercoid, plerocercoid).

Pathogenesis

Pathology due to adult worms results from the physical presence and activity of the large worms (*Taenia* species), occasional erosive action (causing local inflammation) by scolex hooks (*T solium, H nana),* or reduced host intake of vitamin B_{12} *(Diphyllobothrium latum).* Allergic reactions may also be responsible for symptoms such as headache, dizziness, inanition, and anal and nasal pruritus.

Host Defenses

Adult worms are probably only weakly immunogenic, although some evidence exists for a cell-mediated host response; moderate eosinophilia and increased IgE may occur. Larvae elicit strong immunity against reinfection that is derived from both cell-mediated and humoral responses induced by antigenic stimulation of tissues.

Epidemiology

Infective larvae are acquired by eating contaminated raw or undercooked meat, grains, or fish. *Taenia solium* cysticercosis or *H nana* can be transmitted in a direct cycle via ingestion of eggs from human feces. *Echino-coccus* eggs from dog or fox fur cause human hydatid disease (humans are the intermediate host; canids are the definitive hosts). Reinfection with adult tapeworms is common; second infections with larvae are rare. *T solium* cysticercosis may be acquired by autoinfection; internal autoinfection with *H nana* from a cysticercoid infection is possible.

Diagnosis

Adult Worms: Taenia infections are diagnosed by finding gravid segments in stool specimens; the eggs of these species are indistinguishable. Other species are diagnosed on the basis of eggs in stool specimens.

Larval Worms: Cysts in tissues may be identified in biopsy specimens, by radiography (calcified cysts), and by computed tomography (brain cysts). Serology (indirect hemagglutination, ELISA) is useful but of variable sensitivity and specificity. A history of travel in endemic areas is often of great importance.

Control

Meat should be cooked thoroughly or frozen at −20°C for 10 days; beef and pork should be inspected for *Taenia* ("measly meat"); human feces should not contaminate drinking water; sheepdogs should be treated and should not be fed sheep viscera. Humans may be treated with praziquantel or niclosamide.

INTRODUCTION

Tapeworms are ribbon-shaped multisegmented flatworms that dwell as adults entirely in the human small intestine. The larval forms lodge in skin, liver, muscles, the central nervous system, or any of various other organs. Their life cycles involve a specialized pattern of survival and transfer to specific intermediate hosts, by which they are transferred to another human host. Each pattern is characteristic of a given tapeworm species.

In general, the common gut-dwelling adult cestodes are well adapted to the human host, induce few symptoms, and only rarely cause serious pathology. This reality belies innumerable fearsome and largely apocryphal stories of tapeworms stealing food and causing ravenous hunger (far more commonly, the appetite is depressed). Larval cestodes, however, develop in human organs or somatic tissues outside of the gut and are therefore far more pathogenic.

The adult cestodes elicit little host inflammatory or immune response in contrast to the strong responses elicited by the larval stages in tissues. Adult cestodes are often acquired by ingestion of meat from intermediate hosts. Extraintestinal infection with larvae results from ingestion of eggs of fecal origin. Diagnosis of infection with adult cestodes is based on identification of eggs and segments (proglottids) in feces. Larval infections are more difficult to assess; serology and biopsy are helpful. Control depends on sanitation, personal hygiene, and thorough cooking of meat and fish.

TAENIA SAGINATA, THE BEEF TAPEWORM

CLINICAL MANIFESTATIONS

The clinical manifestations of infection with adult *T saginata* tapeworms are confined to occasional nausea or vomiting, appetite loss, epigastric or umbilical pain, and weight loss. Moderate eosinophilia may develop. A disturbing manifestation of *T saginata* infection is the active crawling of the muscular segments out of the anus. Rarely, intestinal perforation may occur from the scolex of *Taenia,* or proglottids may be vomited and then aspirated.

STRUCTURE

Adults are ribbonlike, flattened, segmented, hermaphroditic flatworms 5 to 10 m long, consisting of scolex, neck, and immature, mature, and ripe segments in linear sequence. The distinctive morphologic and physiologic properties of the adult tapeworm reflect on the one hand their remarkable specialization for survival in the vertebrate intestine, and on the other hand their massive reproductive powers, which are made possible by the multiple sexual units, or segments. This ensures the worm species against the enormous rate of loss of the segments or eggs passed in the feces, with only the most remote probability of any one egg succeeding in reaching an intermediate host and being transferred to another human. The terminal one-third to one-half of the worm's length consists of gravid (egg-filled) segments. These segments are muscular and can crawl caterpillar-fashion through the anal sphincter to the outside environment — which renders them available to their herbivore intermediate hosts.

The larval cyst of *T saginata* — the **cysticercus** — is a pea-sized, fluid-filled cyst, which develops in the muscles of the intermediate host. Within the cyst is a single inverted scolex, formed from a germinative portion of the inner cyst wall (Fig. 89-1).

MULTIPLICATION AND LIFE CYCLE

Figure 89-2 illustrates the life cycle of *T saginata*. Gravid segments break off from the worm and are carried in the fecal bolus or by their own crawling activity to the soil. The segments move away from the bolus and adhere to grass. If ingested by a bovine intermediate host, the segments are digested open in the gut, each releasing 50,000 to 100,000 eggs. The eggs hatch, each releasing a six-hooked larva, the **oncosphere** (also called the **hexacanth**), which penetrates the gut wall and reaches the muscles via the circulation. There the oncosphere fills with fluid and develops into the 8-mm cysticercus. If a human eats raw or undercooked infected beef, the cysticercus is digested free and inverts the scolex, which attaches to the wall of the small intestine and begins to bud off the long chain of segments. In about 3 months the worm reaches 4–5 m in length and gravid segments begin to pass through the anus. The worm is long-lived, surviving 5 to 20 years or more.

PATHOGENESIS

Rare intestinal blockage or penetration have been reported, but pathology is usually inconsequential — although the psychological distress at passing motile segments may be extreme.

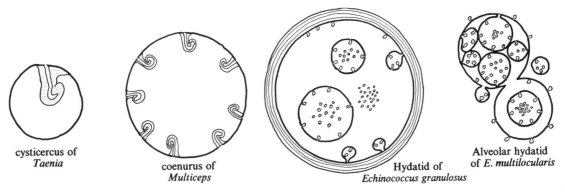

cysticercus of
Taenia

coenurus of
Multiceps

Hydatid of
Echinococcus granulosus

Alveolar hydatid
of *E. multilocularis*

FIGURE 89-1 Larval types found in the taeniid tapeworms. (From Muller R: Worms and Disease: A Manual of Medical Helminthology. William Heinemann Medical Books, London, 1975, with permission.)

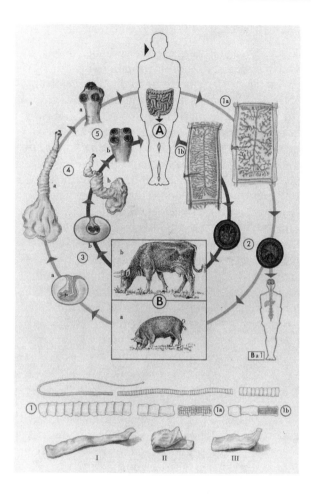

FIGURE 89-2 Life cycles of *Taenia solium* and *T saginata*. (a) The pork (pig) tapeworm (outer developmental cycle); (b) the beef (cattle) tapeworm (inner developmental cycle).

A. Final host: humans only. Tapeworm in the small intestine
    1. Tapeworm with its head (see B-5 below)
    1a. Mature segment of *T solium*
    1b. Mature segment of *T saginata*
    2. Tapeworm egg (=embryophore with six-hooked larva; the eggs of *Taenia* species cannot be morphologically differentiated)
B. Intermediate host
    a. Pig; humans rarely (Ba$_1$) (cysticercosis)
    b. Cattle
    3-4. Cysticercus (measle) in different stages of evagination of the scolex
    3a. *Cysticercus cellulosae* of *T solium* (with its crown of hooklets and four suckers) commencing evagination
    3b. *Cysticercus bovis* of *T saginata* (with four suckers only)
    4. Evaginated cysticercus stage of *T solium* (a) and *T saginata* (b)
    5. Head: a. of the pork tapework (with a crown of hooklets)
             b. of the beef tapeworm (without a crown of hooklets)

I–III. Phases of the movements of freshly detached tapeworm segments
(From Piekarski G: Medical Parasitology. Springer-Verlag, Heidelberg, 1989, with permission.)

HOST DEFENSES

Because of its limited contact with the epithelial lining, the gut-dwelling adult tapeworm induces little host inflammatory, allergic, cell-mediated, or humoral response. The sucking action of the scolex appears to have relatively limited immunogenic effect. The long life span of the worm suggests the absence of an effective inhibitory mechanism.

EPIDEMIOLOGY

Taenia saginata, the commonest large tapeworm of humans, is transmitted as cysticerci in beef ("mea-sly beef"). Partially cooked, smoked, or pickled beef can be infective, although raw beef (steak tartare) is the commonest bearer of infection, as witnessed by the frequency of taeniasis in countries such as Ethiopia and Argentina where raw or undercooked beef is often eaten.

Large worms may grow by 15 to 30 cm a day in the human gut, passing 10 segments daily, which may convey up to a million eggs a day into the environment throughout the long life span of the worm. Eggs may also be found in pastures flooded by human sewage or on which human sewage is used as fertilizer.

DIAGNOSIS

Adult infections can be diagnosed by identifying segments in the feces. The species of *Taenia* can be identified only by the segments, because their eggs are identical. The uterus of *T saginata* usually forms 12 to 20 branches on each side of the main uterine stem, whereas there are 7 to 10 branches in the smaller and relatively wider *T solium* segment (see Fig. 89-2).

CONTROL

Inspection of beef for cysticerci is the best preventive measure. Beef must be thoroughly cooked in endemic areas—to at least 56°C throughout the meat. Freezing at −7 to −10°C for 4 days usually is lethal to *Taenia* cysticerci, but they can withstand 70 days at 0°C.

Treatment is readily available for the intestinal adult worms. Niclosamide, the drug of choice, is a nonabsorbed oxidative phosphorylation inhibitor that kills the scolex and anterior segments on contact, after which the worm is expelled. Praziquantel, a synthetic isoquinoline-pyrazine derivative, is a highly effective and relatively nontoxic cesticidal compound. Since the scolex is usually but not always destroyed, and since a new worm can regenerate if the scolex and a minute portion of the neck survive, the patient should be observed for several months.

TAENIA SOLIUM, THE PORK TAPEWORM

CLINICAL MANIFESTATIONS

The clinical effects of *T solium* infection are similar to those caused by *T saginata*.

STRUCTURE

The scolex of *T solium* differs from that of *T saginata* in possessing an anterior circle of sharply spined hooks arranged in a double row. These are under muscular control and work with the four suckers to adhere to the gut wall. As described above, gravid segments of *T solium* can be distinguished from those of *T saginata* by the number of outpocketing branches of the uterus. The adult worm is usually 3 to 5 m long. Gravid segments tend to be less muscular and more square than those of *T saginata*.

MULTIPLICATION AND LIFE CYCLE

As shown in Figure 89-2, the life cycle of *T solium* is similar to that of *T saginata* except that the pig is the principal intermediate host. Because the gravid segments are less motile than those of *T saginata*, they are usually eliminated in the fecal matter and remain in the fecal bolus (which increases the chance of infecting pigs, which are coprophagous).

Of great clinical importance is the fact that humans who ingest *eggs* from human feces, as distinct from *cysticerci* in undercooked pork, may develop the larval infection just as pigs do, resulting in the serious disease cysticercosis.

PATHOGENESIS

The hooked scolex of *T solium* may cause greater intestinal disturbance, pain, and inflammatory response than that caused by *T saginata*, but symptoms are still generally mild and the pathology minor. However, *T solium* larval infection (cysticercosis) is a potentially dangerous systemic infection, the degree of damage depending on the site and number of cysticerci that develop. Infection most commonly occurs in the central nervous system (CNS); less often in muscles and subcutaneous tissues. The globe of the eye is also a common site. In the CNS, the larvae most often occupy the brain hemispheres. They may also be found in the cisternae and ventricles. Hydrocephalus may result from obstruction of cerebrospinal fluid flow. Infection in specific sites can induce epilepsy, mental disturbances, or a meningeal syndrome. Nevertheless, up to one-half of CNS infections are thought to be asymptomatic. After death of the scolex within the cyst—often years after infection—the capsule becomes fibrosed or calcified.

HOST DEFENSES

Owing to the systemic migration and tissue localization of the cysticerci, cysticercosis elicits considerable host sensitization. This response is usually insufficient to block the initial infection but probably renders the normal host immune to a subsequent one. Much of the damage from cysticercosis is caused by the severe inflammatory host response that occurs after the death and disruption of the parasite.

EPIDEMIOLOGY

A remarkable and tragic aspect of *T solium* infection is the ability of this worm to develop both adult and larval stages in humans. If *T solium* eggs are ingested (from fecally contaminated water or by anus-to-mouth transfer of infective eggs), they may hatch in the gut and spread systemically, causing human cysticercosis. It appears likely (although it is unproven) that human cysticercosis may also be caused when reverse peristalsis induced by adult *T solium* in the gut washes gravid segments into the duodenum, where the eggs hatch and release invasive oncospheres. Cysticerci develop to potency in about 3 months and may live many years. Cysticerci that die may become calcified, rendering them demonstrable by radiography.

Human cysticercosis is a serious and widespread disease, being especially common in Latin America. The disease is frequently found among Mexican agricultural workers in California and other Western states. Human cysticercosis apparently cannot develop from eggs of *T saginata*.

DIAGNOSIS

Diagnosis of adult worm infection is similar to that for *T saginata*. Cysticercosis is difficult to diagnose and usually requires radiologic, serologic, and clinical assessment. Subcutaneous nodules can usually be felt or observed, and can be sampled by biopsy. The enzyme-linked immunosorbent assay (ELISA) is useful, especially with the purified antigens that have been developed recently. Plain radiographs of soft tissues may demonstrate the oval or elongated cysts (4–10 mm × 2–5 mm) if they are wholly or partially calcified. Cysts in muscles are usually aligned with the fibers. Soft tissue or brain calcifications are strongly indicative of cysti-

cercosis. Plain skull films may show cerebral calcifications or indicate intracranial hypertension. Computed tomography is the most useful procedure, as it detects calcified and noncalcified cysts as well as edema or intracranial hypertension.

CONTROL

The control of infection of humans as definitive hosts is the same as that for *T saginata*, except that the control measures apply to pork not beef. In addition, human sewage from infected individuals may contaminate the source of drinking water. The eggs are highly resistant and can withstand many months of environmental exposure over a broad temperature range. Treatment for adult *T solium* is the same as for *T saginata*.

Cysticercosis may require surgery for ophthalmic or brain involvement, but chemotherapy should precede surgery when possible. Tissue infection can be treated with praziquantel (combined with corticosteroids to reduce the inflammatory response to the dead cysticerci). Praziquantel should not be used for ocular or spinal cord infections. The latter have been treated successfully with metrifonate, and albendazole has also been effective against tissue and CNS infections.

◁ ## *TAENIA MULTICEPS,* THE COENURUS TAPEWORM ▷

The adult worm of *Taenia multiceps* is found in dogs or wild canids. The larva is a bladderworm with multiple scoleces—from a few to 100 or more—in an encysted vesicle. This vesicle, usually 2–5 cm in diameter, is called a **coenurus** (Fig. 89-1). The usual intermediate host is the sheep. Human infection can occur from accidental ingestion of dog feces containing the eggs.

Infection in humans usually occurs in the brain in temperate areas, and in the eye or subcutaneous tissues in tropical areas. Diagnosis and treatment are similar to those for *Echinococcus* infection, which may be difficult to distinguish from coenurus infection. Treatment is chiefly surgical, although the drugs used for cysticercosis may also be effective against coenurus infection.

ECHINOCOCCUS GRANULOSUS, THE HYDATID TAPEWORM

CLINICAL MANIFESTATIONS

Echinococcosis (hydatid disease) results from the presence of one or more massive cysts, or **hydatids,** which can develop in any tissue site, including the liver, lungs, heart, brain, kidneys, and long bones. The clinical manifestations of this infection therefore vary greatly, depending on the site and size of the cyst, but resemble those of a slow-growing tumor that causes gradually increasing pressure. Infections in the liver, lungs, or subcutaneous tissue sites may be asymptomatic for many years, but pressure effects eventually develop. In sensitive or vital areas, hydatids produce a panoply of symptoms, chiefly owing to mechanical compression or blocking effects but also include collapse of infected long bones, blindness, and epileptiform seizures. The rupture of a hydatid cyst may induce sudden anaphylactic shock in a previously asymptomatic individual.

STRUCTURE

Adult *E granulosus* tapeworms are relatively minute, consisting of 3 to 5 segments, and usually are less than 1 cm long. Dogs and wild canids are the only final hosts in which the adults are found, often adhering in great numbers to the small intestinal mucosa. The scolex has four suckers and is crowned with a circle of spines as in *T solium*. It is followed by a germinative neck region, one developing segment, and usually one gravid segment containing several hundred eggs.

The hydatid larva is found in sheep, in many other herbivores—and in humans. In humans the cyst is slow-growing, but in a period of years may reach a diameter of 30 cm with a 1 mm thick, laminated sheath surrounded by fibrous reactive host tissue. The cyst is usually fluid-filled and, if viable, has a germinative inner lining from which many thousands of scoleces are budded off into the lumen or remain attached to the germinative wall (Fig. 89-1). The floating scoleces often enlarge, become vesicular, and develop into daughter floating colonies within the parent cyst. These in turn may bud off a third generation of cysts within themselves. The result is an enclosed sac containing myriads of future adult worms ready to infect a dog or other susceptible carnivore that feeds on the hydatid-infected animal and the scolex-filled cyst fluid.

MULTIPLICATION AND LIFE CYCLE

Echinococcus granulosus causes a zoonosis; the adult is a parasite of canids. The dog-sheep cycle (Fig. 89-3) is the one most germane to humans. Wild animal cycles, such as wolf–caribou or coyote–deer, also occur. Eggs passed by the dog can be ingested by sheep or other herbivores, or by humans who have close contact with feces-contaminated dog fur. Within the sheep or human intermediate host, the eggs hatch, the oncospheres penetrate the gut, migrate, and ultimately one or several may form the enormous hydatid cysts. Because the scoleces in the hydatid fluid resemble sand grains, they are called *hydatid sand*. If a cyst bursts within the human body, it can give rise to dozens of new cysts—limited, in most cases, by a strong cellular immune response of the host.

PATHOGENESIS

Jaundice and portal hypertension can result from pressure effects of a cyst in the liver; hemoptysis and dyspnea from a lung cyst; and acute inflammatory effects may follow brain or spinal cord infections.

HOST DEFENSES

The migrating and growing larvae, and antigens that leak from the cyst, induce a strong immune

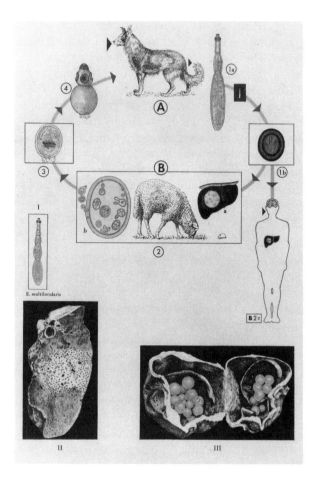

FIGURE 89-3   Life cycles of *Echinococcus granulosus* and *E multilocularis*.

A. Final host: dog (and other canids)
  1a. *Echinococcus granulosus* (beside it, the worm is reproduced in its natural size)
   b. Embryophore, the so-called egg with its six-hooked larva (oncosphere)
B. Intermediate host: sheep (for *E granulosus*); mouse (for *E multilocularis*)
  2a. Liver with *Echinococcus* cyst (hydatid stage)
   b. Diagram of an *Echinococcus* hydatid with daughter cysts and scoleces (compare with III)
   c. Humans as the accidental intermediate host (echinococcosis); the organs most often infected are the liver and brain
  3–4. Isolated scoleces: invaginated (3), and evaginated (4) on which the crown of hooklets and the suckers can be seen
   I. *Echinococcus multilocularis,* sexually mature worm
   II. Human liver infected by the hydatid of *E multilocularis*
   III. Hydatid cyst of *E granulosus* opened up; daughter cysts visible.
(From Piekarski G: Medical Parasitology. Springer-Verlag, Heidelberg, 1989, with permission.)

response—but rarely one capable of penetrating and destroying the cyst. Ruptured cysts may cause anaphylaxis and the appearance of new cysts in other sites, suggesting an active but ineffectual immune response.

EPIDEMIOLOGY

Echinococcus granulosus is most common in temperate sheep-raising areas: southern South America, the southern and central USSR, East Africa, and the western United States. The source of most human infections is sheepdog feces containing *E granulosus* eggs (which often adhere to the fur of dogs petted by humans). Killed sheep fed to dogs maintain the infection; sheep ingest eggs with dog feces in their grazing. Other species of *Echinococcus* are also found in Africa, South America, and else-

where, sustained by similar canid-prey relationships.

DIAGNOSIS

Symptoms of a tumorlike, slowly growing mass with eosinophilia are strongly suggestive—especially in an endemic sheep-raising area. Isolated hooks in the sputum suggest rupture of a lung cyst. The serologic tests that are currently most useful are indirect hemagglutination, latex agglutination, and ELISA. Radioactive uptake tests will show nonreactive ("cold"), cyst-filled areas in the liver or other organs; computed axial tomography scans are of increasing diagnostic value; radiographs are less precise or useful, although they demonstrate the hollow cyst areas.

CONTROL

Effective control is chiefly epidemiologic: denying sheep dogs access to carcasses of infected sheep, obligatory testing and treatment of all sheep dogs, prevention of contact of children with possibly infected sheep dogs, and widespread education on the danger and method of spread of hydatid disease.

Treatment is chiefly by surgical resection (with extreme care to avoid or decontaminate spillage). Recent work suggests that a long course of albendazole may kill the scoleces within the cyst and even reduce the size of the cyst. Long, continued use of mebendazole has also proved effective, although the results are variable.

ECHINOCOCCUS MULTILOCULARIS, THE MULTILOCULATE OR ALVEOLAR HYDATID TAPEWORM

Echinococcus multilocularis, which normally follows a fox-rodent cycle in northern Siberia and North America, is occasionally conveyed to human fur trappers via fox pelts. In humans it causes a frequently fatal form of echinococcosis. The appearance and life cycle of this cestode closely resemble those of *E granulosus,* except for the restricted range and small number of hosts. The cyst, however, is extremely dangerous as it lacks the laminated membrane that confines the cyst of *E granulosus,* and develops an invasive, uncontrolled series of connected chambers (hence the designation "multiloculate" and the alternative name *alveolar hydatid*). It therefore resembles a malignant growth, capable of budding off to cause metastatic spread. The primary cyst usually forms in the liver. The disease is usually diagnosed late, when it is inoperable, and ends fatally. Early diagnosis with ELISA, indirect hemagglutination, or latex agglutination is essential, followed by treatment with mebendazole, albendazole, or praziquantel, and surgery.

HYMENOLEPIS NANA, THE DWARF TAPEWORM

CLINICAL MANIFESTATIONS

Hymenolepis nana infections are often asymptomatic, especially in light cases. Heavy infections can induce enteritis with nausea and vomiting, diarrhea, abdominal pain, and dizziness. Massive infection with several thousand worms may follow autoreinfection.

STRUCTURE

These small worms, 15 to 50 mm long, have minute segments that are wider than long, a four-sucker scolex with a retractable spined anterior rostellum, and terminal gravid segments that break up and release their egg load after they are caught up in the fecal bolus.

The larval form is a **cysticercoid,** a tailed structure that has a withdrawn scolex and lacks a fluid-filled bladder. Typically, *Hymenolepis* larvae are found in insect or crustacean intermediate hosts —with the sole and remarkable exception of *H nana,* whose cysticercoid larvae can develop *either* in an insect or in the small intestinal villi of its human (or rodent) final host.

MULTIPLICATION AND LIFE CYCLE

The life cycle of this parasite is shown in Figure 89-4. Infection is acquired most commonly from eggs in the feces of another infected individual, which are transferred in food, by contaminated fingers, or in sewage-contaminated drinking water.

The ingested eggs hatch in the duodenum, and the oncospheres penetrate only into the villi (Fig. 89-5). There, each oncosphere forms a cysticercoid larva that emerges, 4 to 5 days later, into the gut lumen as a young scolex and neck; the scolex attaches to the mucosa, the neck proceeds to strobilate, and the worm reaches full size in 5 to 10 days. The adult worm sheds gravid terminal segments, which disintegrate in the intestine, releasing eggs that are passed in the feces. When these

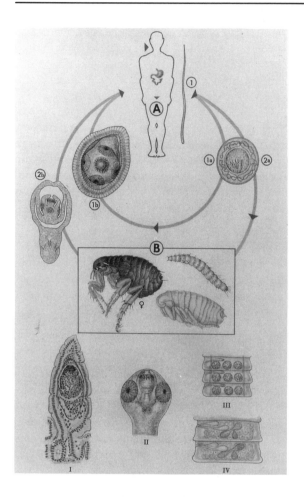

FIGURE 89-4 Life cycle of *Hymenolepis nana.*
A. Final host: humans (also dog, rodents)
    1. *Hymenolepis nana,* sexually mature worm, about natural size
  1a–1b. Development without an intermediate host
    1a. Egg with six-hooked larva (oncosphere)
    1b. Cysticercoid from the intestinal mucosa (compare with I below)
B. Intermediate host: for example, a rodent flea (including larva and pupa)
    2a. Development within intermediate host, in which the flea larva takes up the egg of the tapeworm, to a
    2b. Cysticercoid from the body cavity of the flea (tail appendage with the hooks left in it)—longitudinal section
    I. Villus of the small intestine of a mouse with cysticercoid (transverse section)
    II. Scolex of *Hymenolepis nana*
    III. Immature ⎱
    IV. Mature ⎰ segments of the tapeworm

(From Piekarski G: Medical Parasitology. Springer-Verlag, Heidelberg, 1989, with permission.)

eggs are ingested by another (nonimmune) human, this direct or one-host life cycle begins again. Worms live only a short time, perhaps 4 to 6 weeks. Rodents also can harbor these worms and may serve as reservoir hosts, infecting humans via their pellets.

Remarkably, an indirect, two-host cycle may also occur, involving grain beetles, fleas, or other insects that feed on contaminated rodent droppings. Insects that ingest the *H nana* eggs can serve as hosts for the cysticercoid larvae. Humans who accidentally ingest infected grain beetles (some of which, such as *Tribolium,* are only 2 to 3 mm long) digest the cysticercoid free; digestive enzymes then act on the cysticercoid to release the scolex, which attaches and develops by this indirect cycle into an adult worm identical to that acquired by the direct life cycle.

A third mode of infection is by internal infection or autoreinfection. Eggs from worms acquired in an initial infection—probably via the indirect, insect cycle, which is nonimmunizing (see Host Defenses, below)—can hatch, invade the villi, and produce a second generation of worms. Since many eggs can be involved, this pathway can lead to massive infection with several thousand worms.

PATHOGENESIS

Little or no pathology occurs from development of cysticercoids in the villi, and only after a heavy infection (perhaps produced by autoreinfection) do symptoms develop from the adult worms. Children may be particularly subject to massive worm loads and show the most severe intestinal symptoms.

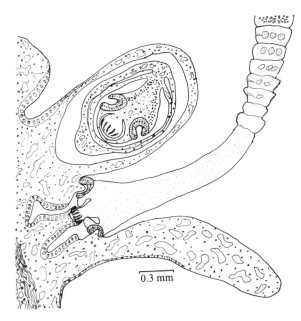

FIGURE 89-5 Diagrammatic section of adult and larval *H nana* in the gut of a mouse. In heavy infections in this host, much of the mucosal lining is abraded. (From Muller R: Worms and Disease: A Manual of Medical Helminthology. William Heinemann Medical Books, 1975, with permission.)

HOST DEFENSES

The tissue phase of the direct cycle of *H nana* infection (Figs. 89-4 and 89-5) initiates a profound cellular and humoral response, rendering most hosts immune to subsequent infection (as demonstrated experimentally in rodents). In contrast, the indirect cycle through infected insects does not involve mucosal embryogenesis in humans and induces little or no immunity, even permitting occasional massive internal reinfection to occur. The immune response is seldom effective against the initial infection because the tissues have already been invaded and a protective cyst formed by the time the response develops.

EPIDEMIOLOGY

Hymenolepis nana is probably the commonest human cestode, owing to its wide distribution, particularly in crowded areas, such as India and China. The direct infectiousness of the eggs frees

the parasite from its former dependence upon an insect intermediate host, making rapid infection and person-to-person spread possible. The short life span and rapid course of development also facilitate the spread and ready availability of this worm. Congested areas, day-care centers, and crowded institutions such as prisons frequently have high levels of infection with *H nana*, despite its strong immunizing capacity and short life span.

DIAGNOSIS

H nana infections can be diagnosed accurately and rapidly by inspecting the stool for eggs.

CONTROL

Preventing fecal contamination of food and water in institutions and crowded areas is of primary importance. General sanitation and rodent and insect control (especially control of fleas and grain insects) are also essential for prevention of *H nana* infection. Treatment with praziquantel or niclosamide is usually effective, and can be repeated if necessary.

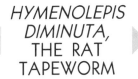

HYMENOLEPIS DIMINUTA, THE RAT TAPEWORM

The rat tapeworm, which is larger than *H nana* (up to 40 cm long), has a life cycle involving grain insects, similar to the indirect cycle of *H nana*. *H diminuta* rarely infects humans, but may do so if a human eats an insect carrying cysticercoids of this worm. The infection is most common in children, causes a mild diarrhea, is diagnosed by finding the characteristic eggs in the stool, and is readily treated with praziquantel.

DIPYLIDIUM CANINUM, THE DOUBLE-PORED TAPEWORM

Dipylidium caninum causes a cosmopolitan infection of dogs and cats. Fleas are the intermediate hosts in which the infective cysticercoids develop. Children in close and continuous contact with pets are occasionally infected as a result of the accidental ingestion of an infected flea. The infection is usually asymptomatic and is self-limited, although praziquantel would probably be an effective treatment. Flea control of pets would largely eliminate the infection from household pets and children.

DIPHYLLOBOTHRIUM LATUM, THE BROAD FISH TAPEWORM

CLINICAL MANIFESTATIONS

Infection with *Diphyllobothrium latum* is usually asymptomatic, although occasional diarrhea, abdominal pain, fatigue, vomiting, dizziness, or numbness of fingers and toes may be present. Eosinophilia develops during the early stages of worm growth.

STRUCTURE

Diphyllobothrium latum is the largest parasite of humans, reaching lengths up to 10 m and consisting of a chain of 3,000 to 4,000 segments, each up to 2 cm wide. The adult worm, a member of the order Pseudophyllidea, is characterized by a scolex with a pair of linear sucking grooves instead of suckers and hooks, and by having a rosette-shaped uterus connected to the outside by a uterine pore through which the eggs are passed. Hence, mature segments produce eggs until they die and are shed, rather than by breaking off as intact egg-filled segments, as in *Taenia*. Up to a million eggs can be produced daily. The developmental stages are (1) the ciliated, swimming **coracidium** that hatches from the egg, (2) the **procercoid** that develops in the copepod primary host, and (3) the **plerocercoid** (or **sparganum**), a nonencysted, nonsegmented larval worm, 20 mm or more in length, found in the fish secondary hosts. The plerocercoid develops into the adult tapeworm in the small intestine of a fish-eating final host, such as a human, cat, dog, or bear.

MULTIPLICATION AND LIFE CYCLE

Diphyllobothrium latum is the only adult cestode of humans that has an aquatic life cycle (Fig. 89-6). Eggs are passed in feces of an infected human (or bear, dog, cat, wolf, raccoon, or other freshwater-fish-eating reservoir host). If passed into lake or pond water, the eggs develop in 2 or more weeks (varying with the temperature) and hatch, releasing the spherical ciliated coracidium that contains the oncosphere. When ingested by an appropriate water flea (copepods such as *Cyclops* or *Diaptomus*), the coracidium sheds the ciliated coat, penetrates into the hemocoel, and changes in 2 to 3 weeks into the 0.5 mm, tailed second-stage embryo, the procercoid. If the infected copepod is then ingested by a minnow or other fish, the procercoid penetrates the fish gut in a few hours and later develops into a third-stage larva, the plerocercoid or sparganum. Usually, these small infected fish are eaten by larger ones; in each new fish host, the plerocercoid penetrates into the fascia or muscles. Eventually, a large game fish, such as a perch or pike, is infected; after being eaten by a human, the fish releases its tapeworm passenger, which attaches and begins adult life. In a few months, the worm is 5 to 10 m long.

PATHOGENESIS

Infection with this tapeworm usually produces no pathology, although the minor symptoms noted above are occasionally present. Megaloblastic anemia ("tapeworm anemia")—which is exacerbated by the worm's uptake of vitamin B_{12}—is now seldom seen, as a result of improved diet, prenatal care, and ready treatment. This condition was formerly most common in Finland.

HOST DEFENSES

Little or no protective immunity develops, owing to the lack of an intimate tissue phase in the human host. Reinfection is common.

FIGURE 89-6 Life cycle of *Diphyllobothrium latum.*
A. Final host: Humans, dogs, cats (and other fish-eating domesticated and wild animals). Site of the tapeworm: small intestine
   1. Egg after it is passed in feces
   2. Ciliated larva, the coracidium, containing the embryo with six hooklets (oncosphere)
B. First intermediate host: small crustacean (copepod such as *Cyclops*)
   3a. Six-hooked larva emerged from coracidium in gut of a *Cyclops*
   3b. Procercoid in body cavity of *Cyclops*
C. Second intermediate host: predatory fish or fish such as the carp
   4. Trout with a plerocercoid (sparganum); final larval stage.
   4a. Isolated plerocercoid
   I. Sexually mature *D latum;* pieces of tapeworm composed of proglottids in different stages of maturity
   Ia. Mature proglottid with rosette-shaped uterus (see III)
   IIa. Scolex, spatula-shaped
   b. Transverse section of a scolex; the suctorial grooves on the two sides are seen clearly
   III. Mature tapeworm segment (proglottid)
   e. Mehlis' gland
   h. Testes
   o. Ovary
   g. Sexual opening
   u. Uterus
   IV. A single egg from the stool
(From Piekarski G: Medical Parasitology. Springer-Verlag, Heidelberg, 1989, with permission.)

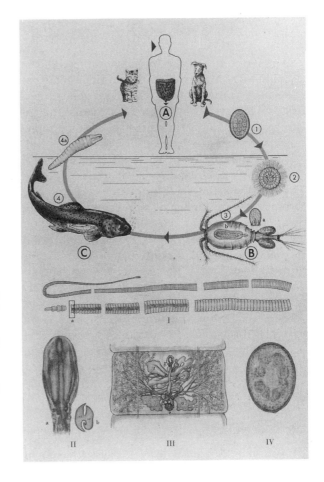

EPIDEMIOLOGY

Infection with the broad fish tapeworm is common in temperate and subarctic regions, wherever freshwater fish are eaten raw — as in Scandinavia, Siberia, the Great Lakes, Japan, Central Europe, and Chile.

DIAGNOSIS

The ovoid, operculated eggs passed in abundance in the human stool are diagnostic. Occasionally, strands of exhausted segments with the characteristic rosette-shaped uteri are also passed.

CONTROL

Plerocercoids in fish are quickly killed by thorough cooking, freezing at −10°C for 15 minutes, or thorough pickling. Treatment of sewage before it enters lakes greatly reduces the prevalence of infection, as has been demonstrated in Finland. Treatment with praziquantel or niclosamide is effective and nontoxic.

◀ *SPIROMETRA* ▶

Sparganosis is a tissue infection with the sparganum (or plerocercoid) of *Spirometra,* a genus related to *Diphyllobothrium.* These two genera have similar life cycles, but *Spirometra* usually utilizes frogs, reptiles, or various small mammals as intermediate hosts, whereas *Diphyllobothrium* uses fish. In the Far East, frog flesh (rather than beef steak) is used as a poultice over a wound or black eye, which allows the sparganum to crawl into the wound or orbit, initiating a severe inflammatory response. Humans can also acquire the infection as a result of drinking water containing infected *Cyclops* and possibly from undercooked snake or other infected meat. The procercoids from *Cyclops* invade the gut wall of the human or animal intermediate host and usually migrate to subcutaneous tissues to form a sparganum, which induces in humans formation of a fibrous 2-cm nodule that encloses and destroys the worm. The nodule can usually be removed surgically or can be treated with praziquantel if the cyst is inaccessible to surgery.

REFERENCES

Arambulo P, Steele JH (eds): Handbook Series in Zoonoses. Section C. Parasitic Zoonoses. CRC Press, Boca Raton, FL, 1982

Arme C, Pappas PW (eds): Biology of the Eucestoda. Academic Press, London, 1983

Barkovitch AJ, Citrin CM, Klara P, et al: Magnetic resonance imaging of cysticercosis. West J Med 145:687, 1986

Desnos M, Brochet E, Cristofini P et al: Polyvisceral echinococcosis with cardiac involvement imaged by two-dimensional echocardiography, computed tomography and nuclear magnetic resonance imaging. Am J Cardiol 59:383, 1987

Gemmell MA, Lawson JR, Roberts MG: Control of echinococcosis/hydatidosis. Present state of worldwide progress. Bull WHO 64:333, 1986

Ito A, Smyth JD: Adult cestodes. In Soulsby EJL (ed): Immune Responses in Parasitic Infections: Immunology, Immunopathology, and Immunoprophylaxis. Vol. 2. Trematodes and Cestodes. CRC Press, Boca Raton, FL, 1987

McCormick GF: cysticercosis — Review of 230 patients. Bull Clin Neurosci 50:76, 1985

Pawlowski ZS: Cestodiases: taeniasis, cysticercosis, diphyllobothriasis, hymenolepiasis, and others. In Warren KS, Mahmoud AAF (eds): Tropical and Geographical Medicine. 2nd Ed. McGraw-Hill Information Services, New York, 1990

Schantz PM: Cestode diseases. In Goldsmith R, Heyneman D (eds): Tropical Medicine and Parasitology. Appleton & Lange, East Norwalk, CT, 1989

Sortelo J, Escobedo F, Penagas P: Albendazole vs. praziquantel for therapy of neurocysticercosis. Arch Neurol 45:532, 1988

90 ENTERIC NEMATODES OF HUMANS

JOHN H. CROSS

GENERAL CONCEPTS

ASCARIS LUMBRICOIDES
Clinical Manifestations
Symptoms correlate with worm load: light loads are asymptomatic; heavier loads cause abdominal symptoms, diarrhea, and sometimes malnutrition. A bolus of worms may obstruct the intestine. Migrating larvae can cause pneumonitis and eosinophilia.

Structure
Ascaris lumbricoides is the largest intestinal nematode of humans. Females are up to 30 cm long; males are smaller. Three types of eggs may appear in feces: fertilized, unfertilized, and decorticated.

Multiplication and Life Cycle
Adults in the small intestines produce eggs that pass in feces, embryonate in soil, are ingested, and hatch; the larvae migrate from the intestine to the lung and back to the intestine, where they mature.

Pathogenesis
Migrating larvae cause eosinophilia and sometimes allergic reactions. Erratic adult worms may invade other organs. Heavy infections can impair nutrition.

Host Defenses
Resistance increases with age; the mechanism is not clear.

Epidemiology
Eggs prefer warm, moist soil. Transmission is favored by unsanitary disposal of feces. Prevalence is highest in children.

Diagnosis
Diagnosis is by identifying eggs in stool; occasionally, erratic adults emerge from body orifices.

Control
Control is by sanitary disposal of feces and by education and treatment.

HOOKWORMS
Clinical Manifestations
Itching may occur where larvae enter skin ("ground itch"). Pneumonitis, cough, dyspnea and hemoptysis may mark the migration of larvae through the lungs. Depending on the worm load, intestinal infection can cause anorexia, fever, diarrhea, weight loss, and anemia.

Structure
Two species of hookworms infect humans: *Ancylostoma duodenale* and *Necator americanus*. They may be distinguished by the morphology of the mouth parts and male bursa. Females are larger. Eggs are oval, thin-shelled, and transparent. Eggs hatch to release rhabditiform larvae, which mature into filariform (infective stage) larvae.

Multiplication and Life Cycle

Adults attach to the mucosa of the small intestine. Eggs passed in feces embryonate and hatch in soil; mature larvae penetrate the skin and migrate first to the lungs and then to the intestine, where they mature.

Pathogenesis

Larvae entering skin often cause an erythematous reaction. Larvae in the lung may cause small hemorrhages, eosinophilic infiltration, and pneumonitis. Blood loss from sites of intestinal attachment may cause iron-deficiency anemia.

Host Defenses

Spontaneous self-cure may represent a hypersensitivity reaction. Infection induces high levels of IgE.

Epidemiology

Transmission is favored by poor sanitation and warm, moist soil. Prevalence rises with age.

Diagnosis

Diagnosis is by detection of eggs and (sometimes) larvae in stool. Low levels of hemoglobin are suggestive.

Control

Control is by sanitary disposal of feces and by education and treatment.

STRONGYLOIDES STERCORALIS

Clinical Manifestations

Ground itch may occur where larvae penetrate the skin. Pneumonitis, epigastric pain, mucous diarrhea, and eosinophilia may occur. In immunocompromised individuals, worms may disseminate to other organs.

Structure

Males are free-living; females may be free-living or parasitic. Eggs develop into rhabditiform and then filariform (infectious) larvae.

Multiplication and Life Cycle

Parasitic females parthenogenetically produce embryonated eggs, which hatch in the intestine. Larvae pass in the feces, mature to the infective form in soil, penetrate the skin, and migrate to the lungs and then intestine. Autoinfection also occurs. Free-living worms reproduce sexually in soil.

Pathogenesis

Worms cause inflammation and ulceration of the intestines. Migrating larvae cause cutaneous pruritus and pneumonitis. Hyperinfection, sloughing of mucosa, and disseminated infection occasionally lead to pulmonary hemorrhage, pneumonia, or meningitis and death.

Host Defenses

Immunity is not well understood. Infection induces elevated IgE and eosinophilia. Impairment of cell-mediated immunity favors disseminated disease and autoinfection.

Epidemiology

Prevalence is usually low; the infection is more common in tropical countries with poor sanitation, especially Southeast Asia and parts of Africa. Dogs occasionally serve as a reservoir.

Diagnosis

Epigastric pain, eosinophilia, and mucous diarrhea are suggestive; diagnosis is confirmed by detecting rhabditiform larvae in feces, duodenal aspirates, or sputum. Fecal cultures and serology may be helpful.

Control

Control is by sanitary disposal of feces and by education and treatment.

TRICHURIS TRICHIURA

Clinical Manifestations

Diarrhea, anemia, weight loss, abdominal pain, nausea, vomiting, eosinophilia, tenesmus, rectal prolapse, stunted growth, and finger clubbing may occur.

Structure

Adults are whip-shaped, slender anteriorly and broader posteriorly. Males are shorter than females and have a coiled posterior. The unembryonated eggs are barrel-shaped with bipolar plugs.

Multiplication and Life Cycle

Adults in the large intestine lay eggs which pass in feces and embryonate in soil. Eggs that are ingested hatch and mature in the gut.

Pathogenesis

Adults prefer the cecum but will also colonize the large intestine. Worms cause mucosal inflammation, eosinophilic infiltration, and minor blood loss; heavy infections may lead to anemia and nutritional deficiency.

Host Defenses

Defenses are little understood; resistance does not increase with age.

Epidemiology

Transmission is favored by poor sanitation and warm soil.

Diagnosis

Diagnosis is by detection of eggs in feces.

Control

Control is by sanitary disposal of feces and by education and treatment.

ENTEROBIUS VERMICULARIS

Clinical Manifestations

Enterobiasis is most common in children, who usually manifest pruritus ani and sometimes insomnia, abdominal pain, anorexia, and pallor. Genitourinary infection may occur in females.

Structure

Worms are white and spindle-shaped with a large, bulbar esophagus. Males are smaller and have a curved posterior. Eggs are ovoid, thin-shelled, and flat on one side.

Multiplication and Life Cycle

Females usually migrate out the anus at night and deposit eggs on the perianal skin. The eggs embryonate quickly and, if ingested, hatch and mature in the intestines.

Pathogenesis

Intestinal lesions are rare; extraintestinal infection may lead to complications.

Host Defenses

The defenses are little known. Most infections occur in children.

Epidemiology

Enterobius vermicularis is the most common helminth in the United States. Household and institutional epidemics occur, usually in children. Transmission is usually from hand to mouth.

Diagnosis

Eggs are rare in feces but are readily collected by Scotch-tape perianal swabs.

Control

Control is by anthelmintic treatment and by improved personal hygiene, including washing the perianal region and changing nightclothes.

INTRODUCTION

Enteric nematodes are among the most common and widely distributed animal parasites of humans. In his classic address to the American Society of Parasitologists in 1946, entitled "This Wormy World," Stoll estimated 2.3 billion helminthic infections in a human population of 2.2 billion. Since 1946, the world population has doubled and, by all indications, enteric nematode infections of humans have kept pace. The most common intestinal roundworms are those transmitted through contact with the soil (for example, *Ascaris lumbricoides, Trichuris trichiura,* the hookworms, and *Strongyloides stercoralis*); in Stoll's estimate, these worms, with *Enterobius vermicularis,* accounted for three-quarters of all helminthic infections.

Most enteric nematodes have established a well-balanced host-parasite relationship with the human host; humans tolerate these parasites well. Little disease is associated with light infection, but when the worm load increases, a corresponding increase in disease usually occurs. The worms may irritate the intestinal mucosa, causing inflammation and ulceration. Some produce toxic substances. The larger worms may become entangled and block the intestinal tract. Larval worms that migrate through the tissue to complete their life cycle may lose their way, end up in the wrong organ, and cause severe disease. Nutritional problems occasionally are associated with the intestinal parasitosis, and persons with deficient diets often suffer from polyparasitism.

Diagnosis usually is based on microscopic examination of feces for eggs and larvae, except in the case of pinworm infections, which are diagnosed by examining samples taken with perianal swabs. Many anthelmintics are available to treat patients with these infections. Control depends largely on proper disposal of human feces and on personal hygiene.

The enteric nematodes discussed in this chapter are *A lumbricoides;* the hookworms *Necator americanus* and *Ancylostoma duodenale; S stercoralis; T trichiura;* and *E vermicularis.*

◀ ASCARIS LUMBRICOIDES ▶

CLINICAL MANIFESTATIONS

Adult *A lumbricoides* infections involving only a few worms are usually asymptomatic, but as the worm load increases, symptoms of abdominal discomfort, nausea, vomiting, weight loss, fever, and diarrhea develop. Allergic manifestations in hypersensitized persons lead to pneumonitis, cough, low-grade fever, and eosinophilia. Large numbers of worms may form a bolus and cause intestinal obstruction. Stimulation causes adult worms to become erratic and invade the appendix and biliary and pancreatic ducts. Worms may enter and block small orifices. Migrating adults have been vomited and passed from the nose and mouth, anus, umbilicus, and lacrimal glands. They can perforate the intestines and enter the peritoneal cavity, the respiratory tract, urethra, and vagina, and even the placenta and fetus. Excessive worm loads, especially among the malnourished, can lead to nutritional impairment because the worms interfere with the absorption of proteins, fats, and carbohydrates.

STRUCTURE

Ascaris lumbricoides is the largest and most common intestinal nematode of humans. Females are approximately 30 cm long; sexually mature males are

smaller. The diameter varies from 2 to 6 mm. Mated females produce fertile eggs that are oval to subspherical, 45 to 75 μm by 35 to 50 μm, and are covered by a thick shell with a light brown, mammillated, albuminous outer coat. Unmated females (for example, in a single-sex infection), produce unfertilized eggs that are thin-shelled, ellipsoidal, and measure 78 to 105 μm by 38 to 55 μm. The mammillated coat of unfertilized eggs is irregular and the contents are granular and disorganized. Some eggs are passed without the outer mammillated coat (decorticated eggs) and can be confused with eggs from hookworms or other worms.

MULTIPLICATION AND LIFE CYCLE

Ascaris lumbricoides is found in the small intestine, particularly the jejunum. Females produce as many as 240,000 eggs per day and as many as 65 million in a lifetime. The eggs are unsegmented and are passed in the feces. In moist, warm, shady soil, the eggs embryonate, and an infective larva develops within the egg in about 3 weeks. After ingestion by a human, the eggs pass to the duodenum where the larvae hatch, penetrate the intestinal mucosa, enter the lymphatics and portal system, and are carried to the liver, heart, and lungs. This migratory phase requires a few days. The larvae then break out of the capillaries into the alveoli, pass up the respiratory tree, and are swallowed. They reach the intestines and continue their development, and 8 to 12 weeks after infection, become sexually mature adults. The adults live for about a year and are subsequently passed in the feces (Fig. 90-1).

PATHOGENESIS

The initial pathology is associated with migrating larvae; the severity depends upon the number of invading organisms, the sensitivity of the host, and the host's nutritional status. Persons repeatedly infected become sensitized, and migrating larvae may cause tissue reactions in the liver and lungs, with eosinophilic infiltration and granuloma formation. The reactions lead to pneumonitis and a condition known as Loeffler's syndrome. Adult

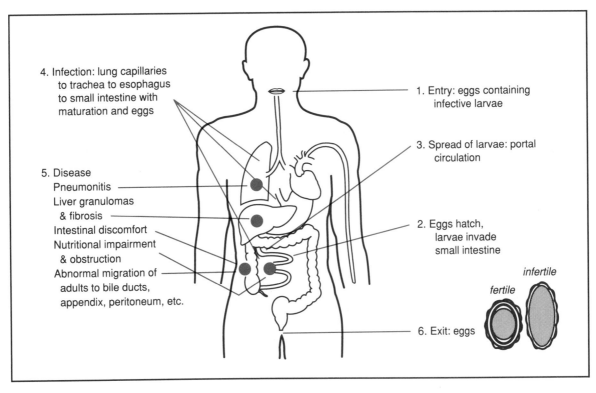

4. Infection: lung capillaries
   to trachea to esophagus
   to small intestine with
   maturation and eggs

5. Disease
   Pneumonitis
   Liver granulomas
     & fibrosis
   Intestinal discomfort
   Nutritional impairment
     & obstruction
   Abnormal migration of
     adults to bile ducts,
     appendix, peritoneum, etc.

1. Entry: eggs containing
   infective larvae

3. Spread of larvae: portal
   circulation

2. Eggs hatch,
   larvae invade
   small intestine

infertile
fertile

6. Exit: eggs

FIGURE 90-1   Life cycle of *Ascaris lumbricoides*.

worms may cause blockage of the intestines, and migrating adults may provoke severe pathology when they wander into other organs. The rare fatalities usually result from intestinal obstruction or biliary ascariasis. Furthermore, the pathogenicity of the worms may vary in different regions of the world.

HOST DEFENSES

The fact that children are more often infected with *A lumbricoides* than adults suggests that resistance develops with age. The mechanisms underlying this resistance are not known. IgE antibodies are present in infected persons, and some persons can develop allergic manifestations such as urticaria, asthma, fever, conjunctivitis, and eosinophilia. Some parasitologists become sensitized and subsequently develop severe reactions when exposed to *A lumbricoides* antigens.

EPIDEMIOLOGY

Ascaris lumbricoides is distributed widely in tropical and subtropical areas, especially in the developing countries of South America, Africa, and Asia. More than one billion infections are estimated to exist at any given time. In rural areas of Asia, it is not unusual to find 85 percent of the population passing eggs. Prevalence rates are much lower in the United States. Some people appear to be predisposed to infection with intestinal helminths, including *A lumbricoides:* in a given community, some individuals are found to be constantly infected and usually have a higher intensity of infections than others.

DIAGNOSIS

Symptomatic ascariasis is rarely diagnosed on clinical grounds alone because the pneumonitis, eosinophilia, and intestinal symptoms are similar to those caused by other helminth infections. Infections before the appearance of eggs in the feces, infections with only male worms, and extraintestinal infections are difficult to diagnose. Radiologic examination may reveal adult worms in the intestine, but definitive diagnosis requires finding characteristic eggs in feces. Eggs are usually so numerous in any infection involving laying females that simple microscopic examination of a fecal smear is all that is necessary. Concentration techniques involving flotation or sedimentation also may be used. Techniques are available to estimate the intensity of an infection on the basis of the number of eggs in a measured stool sample.

CONTROL

The most effective method to control ascariasis, as well as other soil-transmitted helminthiasis, is sanitary disposal of feces. In some areas, this requires changing centuries-old habits and educating the population. Mass treatment programs have been initiated in many parts of the world and, in some Asian countries, efforts are being made to deworm all school children. In a pilot program in the Philippines attempting to eradicate the soil-transmitted helminths by periodic mass treatment of a barrio population, the prevalence of ascariasis decreased from 78 percent to less than 1 percent over 3 years. Mebendazole, the drug used, is effective against numerous intestinal nematode infections and causes few side effects. Levamisole is also useful, as are pyrantel pamoate, piperazine citrate, and thiabendazole. Care must be taken in treating mixed helminthic infections involving *A lumbricoides,* because an ineffective ascaricide may stimulate the parasite to migrate to another location. Persons in whom asymptomatic ascariasis is detected incidentally should be treated to prevent the possibility of a future abnormal migration of these large worms into extraintestinal sites.

◀ HOOKWORMS ▶

CLINICAL MANIFESTATIONS

"Ground itch" (itching at the site of invasion by the larvae), pneumonitis, cough, dyspnea, and, occasionally, hemoptysis are early symptoms of hook-worm infection. Symptoms associated with the intestinal phase of infection include anorexia or a huge appetite with pica (desire to eat unusual substances, such as dirt), fever, diarrhea, abdominal discomfort, weight loss, nausea and vomiting, spleen and liver enlargement, and edema. Children may suffer from mental, physical, and sexual retardation. Eosinophilia is usually marked. Hemoglobin levels as low as 2 percent are common in some endemic areas. Even where hookworm infection is widespread, not all infections lead to hookworm disease.

STRUCTURE

Two major hookworm species infect humans: the Old World hookworm *Ancyclostoma duodenale* and the New World hookworm *Necator americanus.* The worms are cylindrical and grayish white. Females are approximately 1 cm long; males are smaller. The major differentiating characteristics between the two species involve the buccal capsule and the male bursa. The bell-shaped bursa, used for attachment to the female during copulation, is membranous and symmetrical and has finger-like rays that are arranged differently in each species. The most prominent difference in the buccal capsules is that *N americanus* has two ventral semilunar cutting plates, whereas *A duodenale* has four ventral teeth. Female *A duodenale* hookworms produce 10,000 to 20,000 eggs per day, compared to 5,000 to 10,000 for *N americanus.* The eggs of both species are ovoid, thin-shelled, and transparent. Eggs in fresh stools are in the four- or eight-cell stage. The eggs from these species are indistinguishable from each other and measure 55 to 79 μm by 35 to 47 μm. The first-stage (rhabditiform) larva develops within the egg and has a thick-walled, long, narrow buccal cavity. The muscular esophagus is flask-shaped and occupies the anterior one-third of the body. Slender third-stage (filariform) larvae are 500 to 700 μm long. The mouth is closed, and the elongate esophagus occupies one-third of the body. The tail is sharply pointed. The rhabditiform larvae of the two species cannot be differentiated, but the filariform larvae of *N americanus* have dark, prominent buccal spears and a striated cuticle seen more clearly at the posterior end; these characteristics are not seen in *A duodenale.*

MULTIPLICATION AND LIFE CYCLE

Adult hookworms generally attach to the jejunal mucosa, and the females deposit eggs that pass in the feces. In the proper soil, under ideal conditions, the eggs hatch in 1 to 2 days. The rhabditiform larvae that emerge feed on bacteria and organic debris, molt twice, and develop into slender, infective filariform larvae in 5 to 8 days. These larvae do not feed; if they are unable to penetrate a host, they die in a few weeks. Once in the skin, they enter the venules and are carried to the heart and lungs where they grow and eventually break out into the alveoli and pass up the respiratory tree. After they are swallowed, they attach to the intestinal mucosa and become sexually mature in 5 to 6 weeks (Fig. 90-2). Although infections are known to persist for as long as 14 years, most terminate in 2 to 6 years. Infection by ingestion of larvae may also occur; *A duodenale* is well adapted to this route.

PATHOGENESIS

Hookworm larvae usually gain access to the body by penetrating the skin. A local reaction called ground itch may occur at the invasion site (usually the feet or hands), particularly in sensitized individuals. Secondary bacterial infection may also occur at these sites. Large numbers of larvae migrating through the lungs at the same time may cause pneumonitis. In the small intestine, worms attach to the mucosa by the buccal capsule. As the worms feed on the mucosa they cause a considerable amount of blood loss. The worm ingests mucosal tissue with blood; much of the blood is then excreted into the lumen of the host's intestine. Blood also is lost by seepage around the attachment site. When the worm changes attachment sites, the wound oozes blood for several days. One *A duodenale* is estimated to be responsible for the loss of 0.15 to 0.26 ml blood per day, and one *N americanus* for the loss of 0.03 ml per day. An anti-

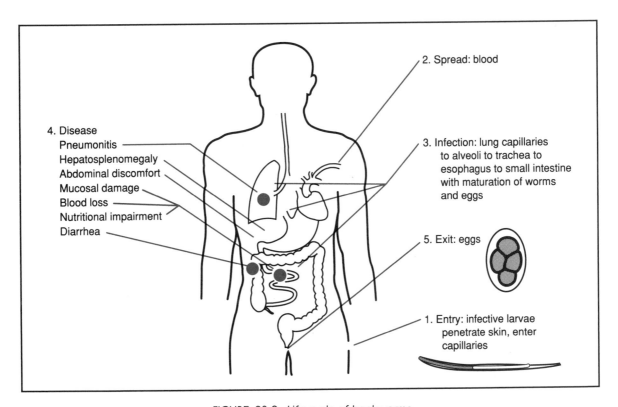

FIGURE 90-2   Life cycle of hookworms.

coagulant secreted in the buccal capsule of these worms also contributes to blood loss. Excessive blood loss can lead to iron deficiency anemia. Infections involving a few worms usually are asymptomatic, but in heavy infections, hookworm disease with hypoproteinemia, hepatosplenomegaly, and hypochromic microcytic anemia results, especially if the hookworm infection is accompanied by other infections and by malnutrition. Infections with *A duodenale* are considered more pathogenic than *N americanus* infections.

HOST DEFENSES

Immunity to hookworm develops in dogs, but no strong evidence suggests that it occurs in humans. Ground itch is thought to be an allergic reaction, but the response is minimal unless accompanied by bacterial infection.

Seasonal fluctuation in hookworm egg production in *A duodenale* has been reported and is thought to be due to host resistance, but may also reflect arrested development of the parasite. In some persons, a 'self-cure' or a spontaneous reduction of worms occurs and may be attributed to immediate hypersensitivity reactions in the intestinal wall. IgE antibody (high in persons with hookworm), mast cells, and worm allergens are thought to provide the necessary ingredients for the reaction.

EPIDEMIOLOGY

Close to one billion infections are estimated to exist at any time. Surveys conducted in Asia often find prevalences as high as 70 percent. Infections are found equally in males and females, with the lowest prevalence rates in children. The incidence of hookworm infection has decreased dramatically in the southern United States, where it was once highly endemic.

Both *N americanus* and *A duodenale* are endemic in warm, moist tropical areas where people defecate in the soil. Places where individuals defecate collectively, such as homes and schools without outhouses and underground mines such as coal mines, are frequent sites of infection. *Necator americanus* is not confined to the Americas, being the most common species in Asia, Central and South Africa, and Central and South America. *Ancyclostoma duodenale* is found in these areas to a lesser degree, but is more prominent in India, China, the Soviet Union, and North Africa. Surveys using Harada-Mori cultures in the Philippines showed 30 percent of the stools positive for *N americanus*, 5 percent for *A duodenale*, and less than 1 percent positive for both. Some individuals apparently have a predisposition to hookworm infection.

Temperatures between 25°C and 35°C and a shady, sandy, or loamy soil with vegetation favor larval development. A population that does not wear shoes also facilitates spread of the parasite.

DIAGNOSIS

Hookworm infection is difficult to differentiate clinically from other parasite infections and certain other diseases. Diagnosis is made by demonstrating eggs in stool specimens. The two species cannot be distinguished on the basis of their eggs. Direct microscopic examination of the stools may suffice in heavy infections, but a concentration method should be used in most cases (e.g., zinc sulfate flotation or formalin–ethylacetate concentration). An estimate of the intensity of infection can be made on the basis of the number of eggs in a measured fecal sample. Specimens should be examined promptly since rhabditiform larvae may develop and hatch from the egg within a few hours. When larvae are present in the feces, they must be differentiated from those of other nematode species.

CONTROL

Hookworm can be controlled in a population by sanitary disposal of feces, treatment of infected persons, wearing of shoes, health education, and improved nutrition. In the Philippines, the prevalence rate was decreased from 33 percent to less than 1 percent in 3 years by a control program of mass treatment with mebendazole.

Mebendazole is an effective treatment. Also effective are thiabendazole, pyrantel pamoate, and levamisole. Anthelmintic treatment should be supplemented with an improved diet, including administration of iron.

STRONGYLOIDES STERCORALIS

CLINICAL MANIFESTATIONS

Most infections with *S stercoralis* are asymptomatic except for the ground itch that may occur when infective larvae from the soil penetrate the skin in large numbers. Pneumonitis can result from larval invasion in the lung. Intestinal invasion may lead to epigastric pain and mucous diarrhea. Eosinophilia is common. Dissemination of strongyloidiasis into extraintestinal organs sometimes occurs in persons receiving immunosuppressive drugs. The infection can be perpetuated by an autoinfection cycle, which can lead to massive infection, especially in the immunocompromised. Linear skin lesions on the lower abdomen and buttocks may also develop in patients with autoinfection due to penetration of the perianal skin by infective larvae; this condition is called *larva currens* (see discussion of the similar conditions called larva migrans in Ch. 91).

STRUCTURE

Strongyloides stercoralis is unique in that adults may be either parasitic or free-living. Parasitic adults are exclusively female (approximately 2 mm by 40 to 50 μm); there are no parasitic males. Very thin-shelled, embryonated eggs (55 to 60 μm by 28 to 32 μm) release rhabditiform larvae, which develop into more slender infective-stage filariform larvae.

Free-living adult males (650 to 950 μm long) and females (0.8 to 1.6 mm long) live in the soil and reproduce sexually.

MULTIPLICATION AND LIFE CYCLE

Parasitic females are found in the epithelium of the duodenum or upper jejunum and reproduce by parthenogenesis. Embryonated eggs are laid in the mucosa. The eggs mature rapidly and hatch in the mucosa. First-stage rhabditiform larvae pass in the feces and develop in the soil into infective-stage filariform larvae. These penetrate the skin of humans, enter cutaneous blood vessels, migrate to the lungs, and finally mature in the small intestines. Females begin to lay eggs about 1 month after infecting the host. In the indirect life cycle, larvae passed in the feces develop in the soil into free-living adult males and females, which mate; the eggs that are laid hatch and give rise to a generation of infective larvae, which can penetrate skin and develop as in the direct life cycle. In autoinfection, first-stage larvae transform into infective larvae while they are in the intestine or on the skin of the perianal region; these larvae penetrate the wall of the intestine or the perianal skin. Some eventually develop into adults in the small intestine after a lung migration. Thus, autoinfection can replace or increase the patient's intestinal worm burden, and accounts for the persistence of this infection in patients who no longer live in endemic areas (Fig. 90-3).

PATHOGENESIS

Light infections elicit only a mild inflammatory response, whereas in heavy infections, damage to the intestines may be severe, with edema, inflammation, ulceration, increased secretion of mucus, and sloughing of the mucosa, as well as functional changes of the gut. A malabsorption syndrome has been reported. In disseminated strongyloidiasis the parasite may be found in any part of the body. In pulmonary infections there may be pneumonia and hemorrhage. Meningitis is also reported. Hyper-disseminated infections may be fatal.

HOST DEFENSES

Immunity in strongyloidiasis is not well understood, but autoinfection generally occurs in persons with suppressed cell-mediated immunity. Most susceptible are patients who have lymphocytic leukemia, malignancy, malnutrition, leprosy, or systemic lupus erythematosus and who are receiving immunosuppressive therapy. Serum IgE levels usually are elevated in persons with this parasite. In severe strongyloidiasis, some patients may have significantly decreased IgG levels and low levels of

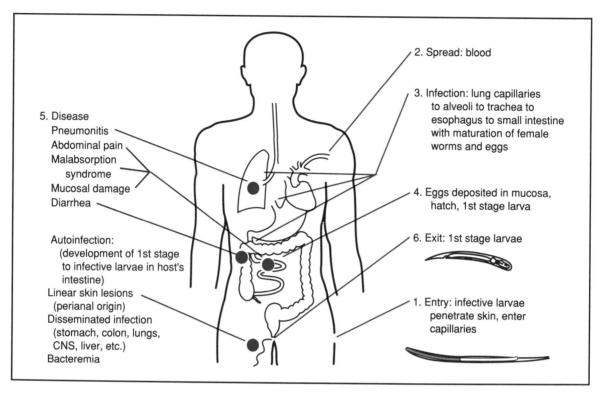

FIGURE 90-3   Life cycle of *Strongyloides stercoralis*.

IgA and IgM. Eosinophil counts also may be depressed in patients with massive infections. These findings indicate that eosinophils and antibodies may be important in the defense against *S stercoralis* larvae.

EPIDEMIOLOGY

Strongyloides stercoralis may coexist with hookworms; both require similar soil and climatic conditions for development. Warm, moist soils that foster reproduction by the free-living stages may become heavily contaminated with *S stercoralis*. Because of autoinfection, persons who have contracted this infection in endemic areas may remain infected for years after leaving such areas.

Strongyloidiasis is most common in tropical and subtropical areas, but is much less prevalent than hookworm infection. Recent surveys in the Philippines and Indonesia rarely found the parasite,

even with the use of filter paper cultures. Other parts of Southeast Asia, however, have a higher prevalence of infection, and parts of Africa report prevalence as high as 21 percent. In the United States, infections are more common in the South and in institutionalized populations.

Dogs are sometimes infected with *S stercoralis*. Although dogs are considered a source of human infections, the primary source continues to be humans.

Cases have been reported in which the infection was transferred to a new host along with a kidney transplant. These patients were immunosuppressed.

DIAGNOSIS

Eosinophilia, epigastric pain, and mucous diarrhea suggest *S stercoralis* infection, but definitive diagnosis requires finding larvae in the stool or, on rare occasions, in sputum or urine. Eggs are not found except in cases of severe dysentery. Direct smear or concentration methods of stool examination usually suffice, but the sample can be cultured in cases where infection is suspected but unconfirmed. Baermanization of charcoal fecal cultures is recommended. (A Baermann apparatus is a funnel with a rubber tube with a pinch-clamp attached to the spout. A sieve is placed in the funnel, gauze is added, and a culture placed on the gauze. Warm water is added to the funnel just above the culture. Larvae will migrate into the water and fall to the bottom. After a few hours, the pinch-clamp is opened and the larvae flushed out into a flask and examined microscopically.) Larval stages of *S stercoralis* must be distinguished from hookworm larvae. The rhabditiform larvae resemble those of hookworms but can be distinguished by the shorter buccal capsule and larger genital primordium. The filariform larvae also resemble those of hookworms, but the tail is notched and the esophagus is about one-half the length of the body.

Duodenal intubation and examination of aspirates, or a string test (Enterotest) and examination of intestinal mucus, is recommended in suspected cases, even when serial stool examinations are negative. A number of reliable serology tests are also available to aid in the diagnosis of strongyloidiasis.

CONTROL

Like other soil-transmitted nematode infections, strongyloidiasis can be controlled by improving sanitary conditions and by proper disposal of feces. Patients with this infection should be treated even if they are asymptomatic to preclude possible onset of autoinfection. Immunosuppressants are contraindicated in these patients. Strongyloidiasis must be ruled out in persons to be given immunosuppressants, especially those with eosinophilia.

Thiabendazole, the most effective therapeutic agent, can cause side effects of vertigo, nausea, and vomiting. Prolonged or repeated treatment may be required in patients receiving immunosuppressive drugs. Ivermectin was recently reported also to be effective.

 ## TRICHURIS TRICHIURA

CLINICAL MANIFESTATIONS

The parasite *T trichiura* lives primarily in the cecum and appendix but can also be found in large numbers in the colon and rectum. Light infections are asymptomatic but heavy infections may cause diarrhea, at times containing mucus and blood. Anemia may develop, along with weight loss, abdominal pain, nausea, vomiting, tenesmus, and rectal prolapse. Nutritional changes can cause stunted growth and clubbing of fingers. Eosinophilia may also develop in response to worms embedded in the mucosa.

STRUCTURE

Trichuris trichiura is known as *whipworm* because the long, narrow anterior end and the shorter, more robust posterior end give the worm the look of a whip. The pinkish-white worms are threaded through the mucosa and attach by their anterior end. Females (approximately 45 mm long) are larger than males; they are bluntly rounded posteriorly, whereas the males have a coiled posterior. The characteristic eggs are brown and barrel-shaped with prominent bipolar blister-like protuberances; they measure 22 μm by 52 μm.

MULTIPLICATION AND LIFE CYCLE

Females produce 2,000 to 10,000 single-celled eggs per day. These pass in the feces and embryonate in the soil. Under favorable conditions, they become infective in about 3 weeks. After being ingested, embryonated infective eggs hatch in the small intestine. The infective larvae penetrate the villi and continue to develop. Young worms move to the cecum, penetrate the mucosa, and complete development. Females begin to lay eggs about 3 months after infecting the host (Fig. 90-4).

PATHOGENESIS

Petechial hemorrhage, edema, inflammation, and mucosal bleeding develop, and heavy infections can cause rectal prolapse. Small amounts of blood

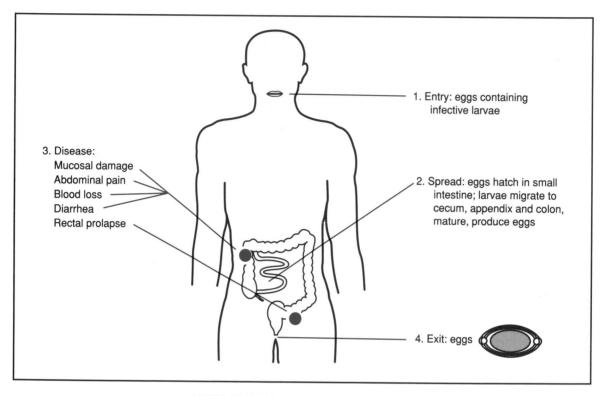

1. Entry: eggs containing infective larvae

3. Disease:
   Mucosal damage
   Abdominal pain
   Blood loss
   Diarrhea
   Rectal prolapse

2. Spread: eggs hatch in small intestine; larvae migrate to cecum, appendix and colon, mature, produce eggs

4. Exit: eggs

FIGURE 90-4 Life cycle of *Trichuris trichiura*.

(0.005 ml per worm) are lost each day by seepage at the attachment site. Colitis/proctitis, anemia, clubbing of fingers, and growth retardation are also reported to be associated with heavy *T trichiura* infections.

HOST DEFENSES

Very little information is available on resistance and immune responses to *T trichiura* infection. In some endemic areas, equal occurrence of infection in all age groups suggests that resistance does not develop with age.

EPIDEMIOLOGY

Whipworm infections are prevalent in tropical and subtropical countries with moist, shaded, warm soil. Up to 800 million infections are estimated to exist. In Asia, some surveys indicate that *T trichiura* is more common than *A lumbricoides*.

No reservoir hosts for *T trichiura* are known to exist. Most infections are acquired by eating contaminated soil, foods, or drink. A single infection may last for several years.

DIAGNOSIS

The symptoms of trichuriasis are nonspecific, but the infection is readily diagnosed by identifying eggs in the feces. In heavy infections, the stools are frequently mucoid and contain Charcot-Leyden crystals. Concentration methods are required for diagnosis in light infections. In heavy infections, the parasite can be seen in the rectal mucosa by sigmoidoscopy.

CONTROL

Sanitary disposal of feces is the best control measure. Mass treatment of populations with mebendazole has shown promise in the Philippines, where administration of the drug periodically over 3 years has reduced the prevalence rate from 88 percent to 2 percent. Mebendazole is presently the drug of choice for treating trichuriasis. Oxantel is also known to be effective.

◁ ENTEROBIUS ▷ VERMICULARIS

CLINICAL MANIFESTATIONS

Enterobiasis, or pinworm infection, usually causes little disease. The most common symptom is pruritus ani, which disturbs sleep and which, in children, may be responsible for loss of appetite. Abdominal pain, irritability, and pallor may also be signs of enterobiasis. The parasite has been suspected as a cause of appendicitis, and gravid female worms have been known to migrate up the vagina and fallopian tubes and into the peritoneal cavity, where they become encapsulated. Recurrent urinary tract infections have been attributed to ectopic pinworm infections.

STRUCTURE

The whitish, spindle-shaped worms have characteristic cephalic swellings (alae) and a large muscular esophagus with a large posterior bulb. Females are approximately 1 cm long and males are half that size. The curved posterior end of male worms has a single copulatory spicule. The males are rarely seen because they die shortly after copulation and are expelled. The eggs are thin-shelled, ovoid, flattened on one side, and measure 50 to 60 μm by 20 to 30 μm.

MULTIPLICATION AND LIFE CYCLE

The parasites mature in the large intestine. When gravid, female worms migrate out the anus at night when the anal sphincter is relaxed and lay eggs that adhere to the perianal skin. The female essentially ruptures, releasing as many as 10,000 eggs. The eggs embryonate and become infective within a few hours after being deposited onto the skin. Infection is transmitted hand-to-mouth. The ingested eggs hatch in the small intestine, each releasing an infective stage larva. The parasite moves to the cecum and matures into an adult 2 to 4 weeks after infecting the host (Fig. 90-5). Infections are self-limited; re-infection can occur.

PATHOGENESIS

Intestinal lesions are reported, but the worms usually cause little intestinal pathology. The parasite has been found in diseased appendices but is not necessarily the cause of the pathology. Pinworms can make their way to extraintestinal locations and cause complications. For example, the parasites may carry bacteria into other organs, resulting in abscess formation.

HOST DEFENSES

Little is known about immune responses to pinworm infection. Infections are more common in children than in adults, suggesting that acquired immunity or some other type of age-related resistance develops. IgE immunoglobulin serum levels in patients are reported to be within normal limits.

EPIDEMIOLOGY

It is safe to say that everyone, at one time or another, has pinworms. It is a cosmopolitan parasite found most often in families and in institutionalized children. The parasite is transmitted hand-to-mouth after scratching the perianal region, by handling contaminated bedding and night clothing, or by inhaling eggs in airborne dust. Eggs will not embryonate at temperatures below 23°C, but embryonated eggs remain viable for several weeks under moist and cool conditions.

Prevalence rates for *E vermicularis* are highest in temperate regions. It is estimated that more than 200 million persons are infected. In the United States, pinworm is considered the most common helminthic infection. No animal reservoir exists for *E vermicularis,* although dogs and cats have been incriminated erroneously.

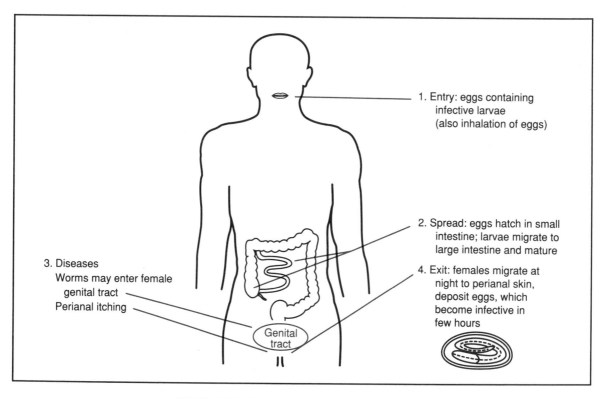

1. Entry: eggs containing
   infective larvae
   (also inhalation of eggs)

2. Spread: eggs hatch in small
   intestine; larvae migrate to
   large intestine and mature

3. Diseases
   Worms may enter female
   genital tract
   Perianal itching

4. Exit: females migrate at
   night to perianal skin,
   deposit eggs, which
   become infective in
   few hours

Genital
tract

FIGURE 90-5 Life cycle of *Enterobius vermicularis.*

DIAGNOSIS

Children suffering sleepless nights because of perianal itching often have pinworms. Eggs are rarely found in the feces, and the diagnosis is made by finding eggs on perianal swabs made of Scotch tape. The tape is pressed first onto the perianal region and then onto a microscope slide, and is examined microscopically. Perianal specimens are best obtained in the morning before bathing or defecation. Three specimens should be taken on consecutive days before pinworm infection is ruled out.

CONTROL

When an infection is recognized, efforts should be made to improve personal hygiene. Fingernails should be cut short, the perianal region washed in the morning, and bedding and sleeping garments

washed daily. Other members of a patient's family should be checked; the entire family may need treatment to eliminate infection. Although several anthelmintics are effective in treating enterobiasis, the drugs presently recommended are pyrvinium pamoate, pyrantel pamoate, and mebendazole. It is advisable to re-treat the patient one month later.

REFERENCES

Baird JK, Mistrey M, Pimsler M, Connor DH: Fatal human ascariasis following secondary massive infection. Am J Trop Med Hyg 35:314, 1986

Cooper ES, Bundy DAP: *Trichuris* is not trivial. Parasitol Today 4:301, 1988

Croll NA: Human behavior, parasites, and infectious diseases. In Croll NA, Cross JH (eds): Human Ecology and Infectious Diseases. Academic Press, San Diego, 1983

Crompton DWT: The prevalence of ascariasis. Parasitol Today, 4:162, 1988

Cross JH, Basaca-Sevilla V: Biomedical Surveys in the Philippines. NAMRU-2 SP-47:1, 1984

Genta RM: Strongyloidosis. p. 979. In Balows A, Hausler WJ, Lennete E (eds): Laboratory Diagnosis of Infectious Diseases: Principles and Practice. Springer-Verlag, New York, 1988

Naquira C, Jimenez G, Guerra JG et al: Ivermectin for human strongyloidiasis and other intestinal worms. Am J Trop Med Hyg 40:304, 1989

Schad GA, Anderson EM: Predisposition to hookworm infection in humans. Science 228:1537, 1985

World Health Organization: Prevention and control of intestinal parasitic infections. WHO Tech Rep Ser 749, 1987

91 ENTERIC NEMATODES OF LOWER ANIMALS: ZOONOSES

DORIS S. KELSEY

GENERAL CONCEPTS

VISCERAL AND OCULAR LARVA MIGRANS

Clinical Manifestations

Visceral Larva Migrans: Symptoms include hepatosplenomegaly, fever, and eosinophilia. The symptoms and duration of the illness depend on the site and extent of larval migration.

Ocular Larva Migrans: Symptoms include leukokoria (white pupillary reflex), loss of vision in the affected eye, eye pain, and strabismus. There are usually no systemic symptoms.

Structure

Toxocara canis is the most frequent cause of these diseases. The larvae are 400 μm $\times$ 20 μm; adult females are 5 to 18 cm long and adult males 4 to 10 cm long. Eggs are about 85 μm $\times$ 75 μm, with a thick brown shell.

Multiplication and Life Cycle

The life cycle of *T canis* in the dog, its natural host, is similar to that of *Ascaris* in humans. Ingested eggs hatch in the intestine. The larvae migrate extraintestinally for a period, and then return to the intestine to mature and lay eggs, which are shed in the feces. In humans, ingested eggs hatch and larvae migrate into the deep tissues, but development proceeds no further.

Pathogenesis

Larvae persisting in either the viscera or the eyes cause granulomatous reactions.

Host Defenses

Leukocytosis and eosinophilia are common. Hypergammaglobulinemia and antibodies against the larvae appear.

Epidemiology

The egg of the parasite is ubiquitous in soil wherever infected dogs defecate. Infection occurs when contaminated soil or fomites are ingested. Visceral larva migrans is most common in preschool children with a history of pica (dirt-eating); ocular disease is more common in school-age children.

Diagnosis

The clinical picture, serologic tests (ELISA), and occasionally biopsy are the chief means of diagnosis.

Control

Larva migrans can be controlled by keeping pets wormed and by sanitary disposal of pet feces.

CUTANEOUS LARVA MIGRANS

Clinical Manifestations

Larvae migrating erratically just below the epidermis cause serpiginous tracks that advance by 1 to 2 cm daily and may be intensely pruritic. Untreated disease resolves in a month or two as the larvae die.

Structure

Ancylostoma braziliense, the common hookworm of dogs and cats, is the usual cause of cutaneous larva migrans. Infective larvae are about $600 \mu m \times 20 \mu m$. Adult males are 5 to 7.5 mm long, and adult females, 6 to 10.5 mm long.

Multiplication and Life Cycle

In the natural hosts, the life cycle is similar to that of *A duodenale* in humans: infective larvae in the soil penetrate the skin, migrate through the tissues, and eventually attach, mature, and lay eggs in the small intestine. In humans, by contrast, larvae penetrate and migrate through the skin (possibly also into deeper tissues), but development proceeds no further.

Pathogenesis

Migrating larvae cause inflammatory responses.

Host Defenses

The host may develop a hypersensitivity reaction, and eosinophilia may occur. No protective immunity develops.

Epidemiology

Cutaneous larva migrans is primarily a disease of the subtropics, including the southern United States, and occurs wherever soil is contaminated by the feces of infected animals.

Diagnosis

The clinical appearance is diagnostic.

Control

Worming of pets and sanitary disposal of pet feces are essential to control. Human skin lesions can be treated topically with 10 percent thiobendazole.

OTHER LARVAL MIGRATORY DISEASES

Several other nematodes of lower animals have larvae that can infect human tissue and cause a visceral larva migrans.

TRICHINOSIS

Clinical Manifestations

Disease manifestations include the classic diagnostic triad of myalgias, periorbital edema, and eosinophilia. The severity of disease depends on the number of larvae ingested.

Structure

The *Trichinella spiralis* adult female is viviparous and measures $4 mm \times 60 \mu m$; males are $1.5 mm \times 40 \mu m$. The infective larvae are about 1 mm long.

Multiplication and Life Cycle

The parasite completes all stages of development in one host. Infective larvae encyst in striated muscles and hatch in the gut of carnivores that eat the infected meat. The worms mature and reproduce in the small intestine; progeny larvae migrate to the muscles to encyst.

Pathogenesis

Symptoms depend on the stage of infection. The intestinal phase may be marked by diarrhea or abdominal pain. Systemic symptoms follow, with myalgias, edema, fever, and eosinophilia as larvae migrate and encyst.

Host Defenses

Immune responses facilitate the expulsion of adult worms from the small intestine and inhibit both migrating larvae and the production of larvae by mature worms.

Epidemiology

Trichinella is acquired by eating undercooked meat (especially pork).

Diagnosis

Diagnosis is made on the basis of the clinical picture, serologic tests (e.g., the bentonite flocculation test), and muscle biopsy.

Control

Trichinosis is prevented by cooking meat to 77°C (170°F). No therapy has been proven effective.

INTRODUCTION

This chapter reviews the more common zoonoses caused by enteric nematodes of lower animals. Humans are not natural hosts for these parasites. Human infections are accidental, and the human disease may or may not resemble that of the animal host. To understand the epidemiology and pathogenesis of these zoonoses, one must understand the life cycle of the involved nematode in its natural animal host and in humans. Some of these nematodes are not able to complete their life cycle in a human as they do in the animal host; the disease process will differ accordingly. For example, in visceral larva migrans, which is caused by the ascarids of dogs and cats, the worms cannot mature in the human host, so development is arrested in the larval stage. Larvae persisting in tissues produce the clinical symptoms associated with this syndrome. Other enteric nematodes such as *Trichinella spiralis* can complete their life cycle in humans and produce disease similar to that in other mammalian hosts.

◄ VISCERAL AND OCULAR ► LARVA MIGRANS

CLINICAL MANIFESTATIONS

Two distinct patterns of larva migrans infection are recognized: **visceral larva migrans** and **ocular larva migrans.** These clinical syndromes result from the systemic migration of the larval forms of animal helminthic parasites. *Toxocara* species, the common roundworms of dogs and cats, are the usual cause. The disease affects mainly children.

The classic visceral larva migrans syndrome usually occurs in preschool children with a history of pica (dirt-eating). Patients who have severe infections often present with eosinophilia, fever, and marked hepatomegaly which may persist for months; there may be associated respiratory symptoms with wheezing and coughing. Pulmonary infiltrates may be seen on chest roentgenograms but are usually transient. Pruritic rashes are common. Neurologic involvement may cause seizures. Death

has been associated with myocarditis, encephalitis, and respiratory syndromes.

The ocular form of the disease usually occurs in children who are between school age and young adulthood. Ocular invasion by the larva may produce retinal granulomas or endophthalmitis, leukokoria (white pupillary reflex), decreased visual acuity, strabismus, and eye pain. The syndrome may resemble retinoblastoma; misdiagnosis has resulted in unnecessary enucleation of the involved eye. The host usually is asymptomatic until ocular involvement becomes apparent. Patients with ocular disease rarely have a history of pica. It has been suggested that ocular larva migrans is associated with fewer larvae than visceral larva migrans. This view is generally supported by the finding of higher serum antibody titers in patients with visceral than with ocular disease. Rarely, the two forms of the disease coexist, presumably as a result of massive infection. Infections not involving the eye that are caused by few parasites may be asymptomatic and hence not recognized.

STRUCTURE

Toxocara canis is the most common cause of visceral and ocular larva migrans. Mature *Toxocara canis* worms are white and live in the small intestine of the dog, their natural host. They have an average life span of about 4 months. The female is 5 to 18 cm long and the male, 4 to 10 cm. A single female may produce 200,000 eggs per day. A heavily infected dog can pass millions of eggs per day in feces. The egg is about 85 μm $\times$ 75 μm with a light brown, thick shell. Under appropriate soil conditions the egg embryonates and develops to the infective stage. The infective larva is approximately 400 μm $\times$ 20 μm and resembles the adult.

MULTIPLICATION AND LIFE CYCLE

When infective eggs of *Toxocara canis* are ingested by a dog, the larvae hatch in the small intestine, invade the intestinal mucosa, and undergo an extraintestinal migratory phase. In older dogs, many larvae remain trapped in body tissues. In puppies, most of the larvae migrate through the bronchioles to the trachea and pharynx, where they are swallowed and complete maturation to the adult form in the intestine. Eggs are shed in the feces and develop into an infective stage in the soil.

Most puppies born of older dogs are infected prenatally with *Toxocara canis*. Presumably, hormonal changes during gestation facilitate transplacental migration of larvae from maternal tissues. Puppies may also be infected by the transmammary route or by ingestion of embryonated eggs.

PATHOGENESIS

Humans contract *Toxocara* infections by ingesting embryonated eggs. The larvae hatch in the small intestine, invade the mucosa, and enter the portal system. Some are trapped in the liver, but others proceed to the lungs and into the systemic circulatory system where they may disseminate to virtually any organ (Fig. 91-1). The parasite cannot complete its life cycle in humans as it does in the animal host. Developmental arrest occurs in the larval stage. The larvae persist in tissues, where they evoke a granulomatous reaction and eventually die. The clinical manifestations depend on the amount of tissue damage caused by the invading larvae and on the associated immune-mediated inflammatory response.

HOST DEFENSES

Visceral larva migrans is associated with a marked hematologic and immune host response, in contrast to the ocular disease, in which, presumably, the small number of parasites cause less host reaction. Serum *Toxocara* antibody titers usually are elevated to diagnostic levels in both syndromes. Leukocytosis with eosinophilia (usually in excess of 30 percent) occurs in visceral disease. Peripheral leukocyte counts exceeding 100,000/mm³ are seen. Hypergammaglobulinemia is common, and IgE is markedly elevated. In addition to antibodies specific for larvae and their secretory-excretory products, a number of nonspecific antibodies may be produced, including rheumatoid factor and

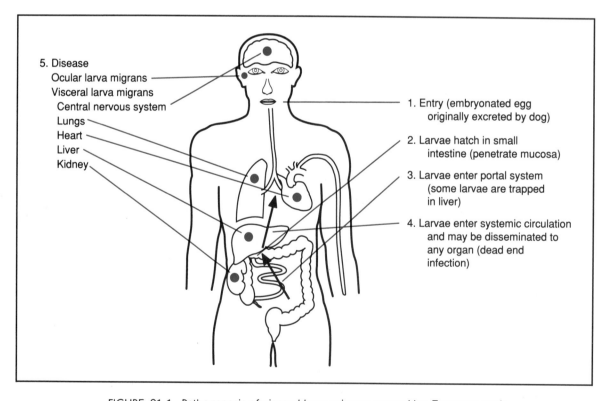

FIGURE 91-1   Pathogenesis of visceral larva migrans caused by *Toxocara canis*.

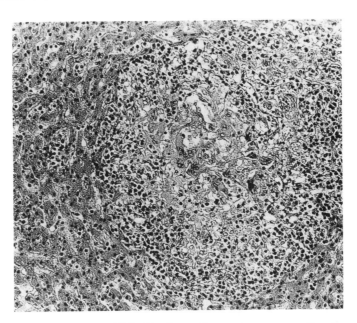

FIGURE 91-2 Liver biopsy from child with visceral larva migrans caused by *Toxocara.* (× 200.)

elevated antibody titers to human A and B blood group substances.

EPIDEMIOLOGY

Most young puppies and approximately 20 percent of adult dogs are actively infected with *Toxocara canis.* Young puppies between 3 weeks and 3 months of age excrete large numbers of eggs and constitute the greatest hazard to the environment. Backyards, children's sandboxes, public parks, and beaches accessible to dogs are often contaminated with *Toxocara* ova, which may remain infective for years. These areas are potential exposure sites for young children or others who accidentally ingest the infective eggs. Children who habitually eat dirt are at particular risk. Direct contact with pets is not a factor in infection because of the incubation period required for the eggs to become infective.

DIAGNOSIS

The diagnosis of visceral larva migrans is usually suggested by the clinical findings of visceral involvement in association with hypergammaglobulinemia, leukocytosis, and eosinophilia. Liver biopsy may be diagnostic, although the larvae are difficult to find even in the presence of eosino-

philic granulomas (Figs. 91-2 and 91-3). Elevated titers of antibodies against the A and B isohemagglutinin *Toxocara* antigens support the diagnosis. The enzyme-linked immunosorbent assay (ELISA) using larva-specific antigen has proven a reliable

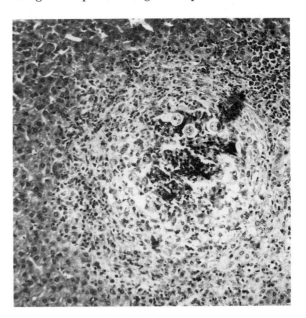

FIGURE 91-3 *Toxocara canis* larva in a liver lesion from an experimental animal. (× 200.)

serologic test. It is especially useful in evaluating ocular infections, which characteristically do not exhibit the peripheral eosinophilia and other evident host responses of visceral disease.

CONTROL

Prevention of human infection centers on the appropriate treatment of *Toxocara* infections in dogs and cats and on sanitary disposal of pet feces. Public education on the necessity of these preventive measures is needed. Many responsible pet owners are unaware of the health hazards imposed on humans by animal roundworm infections. Once the soil has become contaminated, infective eggs persist indefinitely.

There is no treatment of proven efficacy for disease caused by *Toxocara* species in humans. The anthelmintic drugs diethylcarbamazine and thiabendazole are of uncertain benefit. Corticosteroids have been used to decrease the inflammatory response in ocular infections and in severe respiratory or cardiac disease.

◀ CUTANEOUS LARVA MIGRANS ▶

Cutaneous larva migrans (creeping eruption) is a dermatitis caused by the larvae of *Ancylostoma braziliense,* the dog and cat hookworm, which penetrate human skin and migrate in the subepidermal tissue. *Ancylostoma caninum* and other species of hookworms also can cause this infection. A similar cutaneous eruption may occur in patients with intestinal *Strongyloides stercoralis* when the perianal skin is autoinoculated by infective larvae passed in the stool. This syndrome is called **larva currens** (''racing larva'') because of the rapid migration of this larva in the skin (see Ch. 90).

CLINICAL MANIFESTATIONS

As the larvae invade the skin, a tingling sensation may be felt at the site of invasion. An erythematous, pruritic papule usually develops within a few hours. This lesion intensifies over the next few days and develops into a slightly raised, erythematous,

serpiginous track that usually progresses at the rate of 1 to 2 cm/day (Fig. 91-4). The track may be especially pruritic at its advancing edge, over the offending larva. Skin lesions may be single or numerous depending on exposure. The most frequent areas involved are the feet, hands, buttocks, and genital area. The disease is self-limited because the larvae die in a month or two. Secondary bacterial infections may result from frequent scratching of the lesions.

STRUCTURE

Ancylostoma braziliense is the smallest of the common canine and feline hookworms. It has the typical hookworm shape with the anterior end bent dorsally. The adult female is 6 to 10.5 mm long and the smaller male is 5 to 7.5 mm long. The infec-

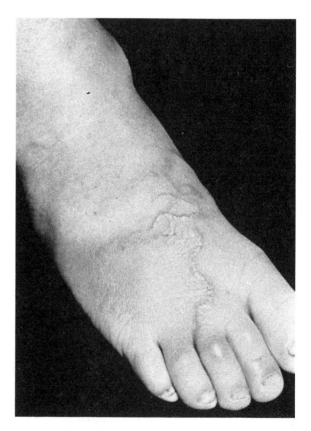

FIGURE 91-4 Cutaneous larva migrans.

tious third-stage filariform larvae are approximately 600 μm $\times$ 20 μm.

MULTIPLICATION AND LIFE CYCLE

The basic life cycle of *Ancylostoma braziliense* in an animal host is similar to that of *A duodenale* in humans (see Ch. 90). In humans, the larvae cannot complete their life cycle, and generally remain trapped in the cutaneous tissues.

PATHOGENESIS

The larvae migrate in the epidermis just above the basal layer, and rarely penetrate into the dermis. Proteolytic enzymes in larval secretions may cause an inflammatory reaction associated with intense pruritus as the lesion progresses. Although in the unnatural human host the larvae cannot reach the intestine to complete their life cycle, they do occasionally migrate to the lungs where they produce pulmonary infiltrates. Both larvae and eosinophils have been demonstrated in the sputum of patients with pulmonary involvement.

HOST DEFENSES

Hypersensitivity to the parasite can occur. Peripheral eosinophilia is common. However, protective immunity does not develop, and repeated infections may occur with subsequent exposure.

EPIDEMIOLOGY

Cutaneous larva migrans is primarily a disease of the southern United States, Central and South America, and other subtropical climates. The major agent, *Ancylostoma braziliense,* is a common enteric parasite of dogs and cats. Humans acquire the infection when infected pets deposit feces containing eggs on the soil. Within a few days under favorable conditions of moisture and temperature, these eggs hatch and develop into rapidly growing rhabditiform larvae, which feed on organic matter in the soil, molt, and develop into nonfeeding infective filariform larvae. These larvae remain in the upper half inch of soil, from which they penetrate the skin of humans and other hosts.

This disease is an occupational hazard for construction workers, plumbers, and electricians who are exposed to contaminated soil under buildings and in crawl spaces. Sunbathers on the beach and children who go barefoot or who play in backyards or sandboxes accessible to infected dogs and cats are other prime candidates. Anyone who has skin contact with damp soil contaminated with the excreta of infected animals is subject to infection, however.

DIAGNOSIS

The classic serpiginous eruption is usually diagnostic (Fig. 91-4). A biopsy specimen taken at the leading edge of the track may contain the larva.

CONTROL

Control of human infections depends on responsible pet ownership. Dogs and cats should be examined periodically for intestinal parasites and wormed as necessary; pet feces should be disposed of in a sanitary way. Topical treatment of cutaneous larva migrans with a 10 percent thiabendazole suspension is usually effective and avoids the side effects of oral therapy. For multiple or persistent infections, a combination of oral and topical thiabendazole may be given.

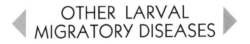

OTHER LARVAL MIGRATORY DISEASES

Several other animal parasites have been associated with visceral larva migrans-like syndromes. These include *Ascaris suum, Capillaria hepatica, Angiostrongylus cantonensis, Angiostrongylus costaricensis,* and *Baylisascaris procyonis.* The tissue phase of such human helminths as *Strongyloides stercoralis* and *Ascaris lumbricoides* can also produce similar clinical syndromes. Larvae of species of *Anisakis* and closely related nematodes of marine mammals have been reported to invade the stomach and other areas of the gastrointestinal tract of humans.

Ascaris suum, the common intestinal roundworm of domestic swine, is morphologically very similar to the human roundworm *Ascaris lumbricoides.*

Human infections with *Ascaris suum* are uncommon, but have been associated with a visceral larva migrans syndrome in children. The larvae invade the liver and lungs but usually do not develop to maturity in the intestine.

Capillaria hepatica is a rat liver parasite. If an infected rat is eaten by a predator, the eggs in the liver are released by the digestive process and passed in feces to the soil. Humans acquire the infection by ingesting the infective eggs in contaminated food or water. The larvae hatch in the intestine and migrate to the liver, where maturation is completed. Clinical manifestations are usually those of an acute or subacute hepatitis. Eosinophilia and massive hepatomegaly may develop. Diagnosis is made by liver biopsy (Fig. 91-5). There is no proven drug therapy.

Gnathostoma spinigerum is a nematode that resides in the stomach wall of dogs and cats. Most human infections occur in Thailand and other Asian countries. Infective larvae develop in copepods and are transferred through the food chain. Human infection results from consumption of improperly cooked fish or other food containing infective larvae. The larvae migrate in the tissues and may invade the eyes, brain, or any organ. They may cause eosinophilic meningitis. The immature worm may be demonstrated in subcutaneous nodules. Surgical removal of the larva from eye lesions may be indicated to prevent migration to the central nervous system, which may result in death. Treatment with mebendazole is recommended.

Angiostrongylus cantonensis, the rat lungworm, causes eosinophilic meningitis and ocular disease in Southeast Asia, the Pacific Islands, and Cuba. Hawaii is the only endemic area in the United States. Human infections are caused by eating infected snails, slugs, or other mollusk intermediate hosts, or other members of the food chain that have acquired infective larvae by eating these hosts. The larvae migrate to the brain, producing an eosinophilic meningitis. Paresthesias and ocular palsies are common. There is no specific treatment, but the prognosis is usually favorable.

Angiostrongylus costaricensis is a parasite of the mesenteric arteries of wild rats. The parasite is widespread from Mexico to Brazil; it is even found in cotton rats in Texas. Most reported cases of

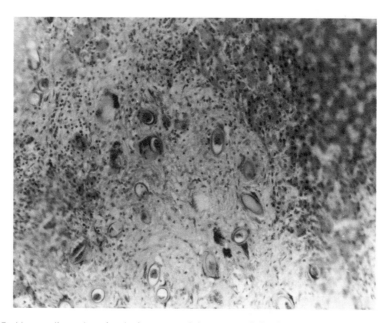

FIGURE 91-5   Human liver showing lesions containing eggs of *Capillaria hepatica.* (Courtesy of G. M. Ewing and I. L. Tilden.)

human disease have occurred in children from Costa Rica. Humans become infected by eating raw vegetables that have been contaminated by a slug intermediate host with infective third-stage larvae. The larvae mature in the mesenteric arteries, producing a granulomatous inflammatory reaction. Abdominal pain and a mass in the right iliac fossa, the usual clinical manifestations, simulate appendicitis. The diagnosis is usually made by surgical exploration. A visceral larva migrans syndrome has been reported, with migration of the parasite to the liver. Thiabendazole has been used for treatment.

Baylisascaris procyonis, the common raccoon ascarid, may cause an especially virulent form of visceral larva migrans. The infection may be acquired by ingestion of the eggs passed in animal feces or by ingestion of paratenic hosts (hosts in which the parasite survives without further development) bearing the encysted larvae. *Baylisascaris procyonis* has a tendency to invade the central nervous system of humans and other animal hosts. In two reported cases, young children died of a visceral larva migrans syndrome and eosinophilic meningoencephalitis. Larvae were demonstrated in brain and other organs at autopsy.

Species of *Anisakis* and certain related genera have been reported in the stomach and other areas of the alimentary tract of humans. Some 25 to 50 cases of infection due to the anisakine species have been recognized in the United States. With the rising popularity of raw fish as a delicacy, the list of parasitic worms and the risk of infection is increasing. Humans acquire this infection by eating raw seafood containing the larvae of these nematodes. The larvae penetrate the gastric mucosa and elicit an intense inflammatory response, gastric pain, vomiting, and diarrhea. Many infections are eliminated by regurgitation of the worm. Diagnosis is by examination of vomitus or by gastroscopic examination and surgery when indicated. In nature, these species develop to adults in the stomach of marine mammals. Eggs passed in the feces hatch and are ingested by crustaceans in which larvae develop into a stage infective for fish. Ingestion of infected fish by marine mammals completes the life cycle.

The risk of infection may be avoided in humans by cooking fish at 65°C for 10 minutes or by freezing fish for at least five days at −20°C.

◀ TRICHINOSIS ▶

Trichinosis is acquired by eating raw or inadequately cooked meat that contains encysted larvae of the nematode *Trichinella spiralis.* Any carnivorous mammal can be infected. *Trichinella* occurs worldwide except for Australia and a few Pacific Islands.

CLINICAL MANIFESTATIONS

The severity of the disease is proportionate to the number of larvae ingested. In heavy infections, the clinical symptoms correlate with the biologic stages of *Trichinella* as it completes its life cycle. During the intestinal phase there may be abdominal discomfort and diarrhea. Within 1 week to 10 days after infection, the larvae begin to migrate, and eosinophilia, periorbital edema, and myalgias usually develop as a result of a diffuse inflammatory and allergic response. A wide range of associated symptoms may appear, because any organ may be invaded in addition to striated muscle. Muscle involvement may be associated with muscle pain and edema, and is indicated by elevated serum levels of muscle enzymes (creatine kinase and serum glutamic oxaloacetic transaminase). The diaphragm, intercostal muscles, tongue, and facial muscles are often involved. Urticaria and conjunctival or subungual splinter hemorrhages are common. Although most infections are self-limited, serious complications or death may result from invasion of the heart, lungs, or central nervous system.

STRUCTURE

Trichinella spiralis is a parasite of carnivorous animals. The adult viviparous female (4 mm × 60 μm) is larger than the male (1.5 mm × 40 μm) and may produce 1,000 to 10,000 larvae during her 6-week life span. The infective larvae (about 1 mm long) become encysted in striated muscle where they may retain their viability and infectivity for years.

MULTIPLICATION AND LIFE CYCLE

Trichinella spiralis completes its life cycle within one animal host. When striated muscle containing encysted infective larvae is ingested, larvae are released from the cyst by gastric acid and peptic enzymes to mature and reproduce in the small intestine of the host (Fig. 91-6).

PATHOGENESIS

Trichinosis is acquired by eating inadequately cooked meat containing the encysted larvae of the nematode *Trinchinella spiralis*. The severity of the disease is proportionate to the number of larvae ingested. The encysted larvae are released in the small intestine, where maturation to the adult stage occurs within a period of 2 to 6 days. The

adult worms burrow into the intestinal mucosa, where the viviparous female gives birth to the larvae. The enteric phase is completed within 1 month. The larvae are disseminated throughout the body via the circulatory system. Any organ may be invaded, with the potential for serious complications, but the larvae survive and encapsulate only in striated muscle. Larval encystment in muscle usually begins at about 3 weeks and is completed by 3 months. Calcification may take place within 6 to 9 months. This completes the life cycle. Humans are usually an end-stage host.

HOST DEFENSES

Many immune responses may play a role in decreasing the severity of *Trichinella* infections. Massive eosinophilia, hypergammaglobulinemia with markedly elevated IgE, and circulating immune complexes may accompany infection. Activated macrophages also appear to be involved in host

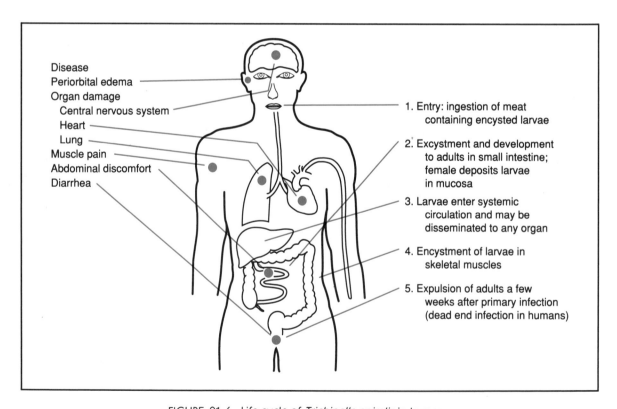

FIGURE 91-6 Life cycle of *Trichinella spiralis* in humans.

defense. Although these responses are poorly understood in humans, animal experiments suggest the rate of expulsion of the adult worms from the intestine depends on B and T lymphocyte function.

Serum antibodies (IgM, IgG, and secretory IgA) have also been shown to inhibit production of larvae by mature worms. Other defenses act against the migrating larvae, which do not possess the thick cuticle of the adult. They may be exposed to or elicit a variety of humoral and cellular effector mechanisms during the migratory phase. Host resistance has been shown to be enhanced by cell-mediated immunity.

EPIDEMIOLOGY

The incidence of *Trichinella* infections has declined in recent years; fewer than 100 cases per year are currently reported in the United States. Most cases are acquired from infected pork that is inadequately cooked. The most common way that pigs become infected is by eating garbage containing meat scraps. Certain ethnic groups whose culinary preferences include raw pork are at special risk. The custom of sampling raw homemade sausage for flavor while adding seasonings and spices is a recognized cause of infection in the Southeastern United States. Inspection for *Trichinella* larvae is not included under the United States Department of Agriculture specifications for pork products. Many consumers are unaware that the stamp "US Inspected and Passed" on raw pork products does not include inspection for *Trichinella*. Although cattle are herbivorous and consequently not a reservoir for *Trichinella,* beef products or horse meat may be contaminated by meat grinders also used for pork. According to USDA specifications, *Trichinella* larvae are eliminated from pork products when the products are heated to an internal temperature of at least 137°F (58.3°C) or when frozen at 5°F (−15°C) for 20 days. Freezing may not be adequate to eliminate cold-resistant strains of *Trichinella,* however. Wild game is another minor source of *Trichinella* infection in humans. *Trichinella spiralis* is maintained in nature by passage among carnivorous or omnivorous animals.

It appears that, in addition to *Trichinella spiralis,* some other *Trichinella* species are of minor epidemiologic importance to humans. These species resemble *T spiralis* in morphology but differ in biologic properties. They include *T nativa,* a variant especially resistant to freezing which is found in Arctic regions and infects humans through ingestion of polar bear meat, and *T nelsoni,* which is found in Africa and tropical regions and infects humans through the ingestion of wild pig meat.

DIAGNOSIS

Trichinosis is suggested by a history of eating undercooked pork and by the distinctive clinical features in association with eosinophilia. Any leftover, suspect meat should be examined for *Trichinella* larvae. Serum antibodies are not usually detectable before 3 weeks. A number of serodiagnostic tests, including the bentonite flocculation test, ELISA latex agglutination, fluorescent antibody, and complement fixation tests can be used. The bentonite flocculation test, a reliable serodiagnostic method, is positive in over 90 percent of cases. Serum specimens may be submitted through State Public Health Departments, which send them to the Center for Disease Control for the test. Definitive diagnosis is by biopsy of striated muscle (Fig. 91-7). The biopsy site should be near a tendinous insertion of an involved muscle, which is the area where the larvae concentrate. Histopathologic examination for larvae should be done. Also, a specimen of muscle should be examined fresh by compressing it between two microscope slides and examining it under a microscope; this simple technique may reveal larvae. Treatment of a portion of the muscle for several hours with pepsin and hydrochloric acid to liberate the encysted larvae, followed by microscopic examination of the concentrated sediment for larvae, may improve the diagnostic yield.

CONTROL

Trichinosis can be prevented by adequately cooking pork or wild game. Freezing of pork at −15°C for 20 days will eliminate the infectivity of most larvae, but not necessarily of cold-resistant *Trichi-*

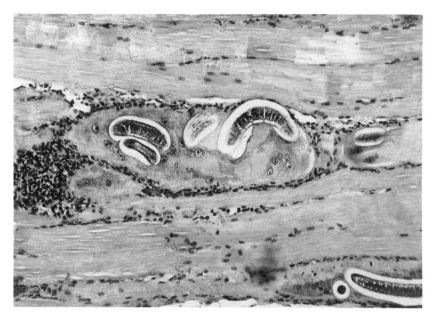

FIGURE 91-7   Encapsulated *Trichinella spiralis* larva in muscle from experimental animal. (X 200.)

nella strains. There is no proven effective therapy for trichinosis, but thiabendazole is thought to be an effective prophylactic agent for persons known to have ingested infected meat. Thiabendazole and corticosteroids have been used in serious infections. It has been suggested that some of the benefits of thiabendazole may result from its anti-inflammatory effects.

REFERENCES

Bathrick ME, Mango CA, Mueller JF: Intraocular gnathostomiasis. Ophthalmology 99:1293, 1981

Cypess RH, Karol MH, Zidian JL et al: Larva-specific antibodies in patients with visceral larva migrans. J Infect Dis 135:633, 1977

Edelgass JW, Douglass MC, Stiefler R, Tessler M: Cutaneous larva migrans in northern climates: A souvenir of your dream vacation. J Am Acad Dermatol 7:353, 1982

Fox A, Kazacos KR, Gould NS et al: Fatal eosinophilic meningoencephalitis and visceral larva migrans caused by the raccoon ascarid *Baylisascaris procyonis*. New Engl J Med 312:1619, 1988

Glickman LT, Schantz PM: Epidemiology and pathogenesis of zoonotic toxocariasis. Epidemiol Rev 3:230, 1981

Huntley CC, Costas MC, Lyerly AD: Visceral larva migrans syndrome: Clinical characteristics and immunologic studies in 51 patients. Pediatrics 36:523, 1966

Kazura JW: Host defense mechanisms against nematode parasites: Destruction of newborn *Trichinella spiralis* larvae by human antibodies and granulocytes. J Infect Dis 143:712, 1981

Levine ND: Nematode Parasites of Domestic Animals and of Man. 2nd Ed. Burgess Publishing, Minneapolis, MO, 1980

Morera P, Perez F, Mora F, Castro L: Visceral larva migrans-like syndrome caused by *Angiostrongylus costaricensis*. Am J Trop Med Hyg 31:67, 1982

Nelson GS: More than a hundred years of parasitic zoonoses: With special reference to trichinosis and hydatid disease. J Comp Pathol 98:135, 1988

Schantz PM: The dangers of eating raw fish. New Engl J Med 320:1143, 1989

92 FILARIAL NEMATODES

ADAM EWERT

GENERAL CONCEPTS

LYMPHATIC FILARIAE

Clinical Manifestations

Disease manifestations include inflammation of lymph nodes (lymphadenitis), irregular fevers, and lymphedema. Repeated, chronic infection may result in elephantiasis.

Structure

Adults are elongate and threadlike. Microfilariae are 250 to 300 μm long, equal in diameter to a red blood cell, and sheathed.

Classification

Filariae are nematodes (roundworms). They are vectored by arthropods; mature and mate in specific host tissues; and produce microfilariae. The lymphatic filariae *Wuchereria bancrofti* and *Brugia malayi* reside in lymphatics.

Multiplication and Life Cycle

Adult female worms produce microfilariae. Feeding vector mosquitoes ingest microfilariae from the bloodstream. In the mosquito the microfilariae mature to infective larvae, which migrate to the mosquito's mouthparts, enter a new host via the vector's puncture wound, migrate to the lymphatics, mature, and mate.

Pathogenesis

Disease manifestations are due to lymphatic dysfunction resulting from the presence of living and dead worms, lymph thrombi, inflammation, and immune reactions to worms and worm products.

Host Defenses

Inflammatory reactions result in cellular infiltration and fibrosis of lymphatics. Damage to vessel walls result in endothelial cell proliferation. It is not yet clear to what extent circulating antibodies to filariae are protective.

Epidemiology

Lymphatic filariasis is prevalent in many tropical and subtropical countries where the vector mosquitoes are common.

Diagnosis

Diagnosis is suggested clinically by lymphangitis and irregular fever; definitive diagnosis depends on demonstrating microfilariae in thick blood smears.

Control

There is no consistently effective treatment to kill adult worms. Control is by avoiding or reducing vector mosquitoes and by treating individuals with microfilariacides.

ONCHOCERCA VOLVULUS

Clinical Manifestations

Patients present with subcutaneous nodules, dermatitis, and eye lesions.

Structure

Long, thread-like adult worms live coiled in subcutaneous nodules and produce microfilariae that are slightly smaller than those of lymphatic filariae and are not sheathed.

Classification

Onchocerca volvulus is a typical filarial nematode that is primarily a parasite of humans.

Multiplication and Life Cycle

Adult worms live in subcutaneous nodules. Microfilariae wander through the skin, where they may be picked up by a feeding vector blackfly. In the blackfly they mature to infective larvae, which may enter a new host when the blackfly feeds. The larvae then move to the subcutaneous tissues, mature, mate, and produce microfilariae.

Pathogenesis

Reaction to worms and microfilariae causes dermatitis with loss of skin elasticity and the formation of fibrotic subcutaneous nodules. Living and dead microfilariae in the eye cause trauma and reactions that can result in blindness.

Host Defenses

There is an inflammatory and immune response to living and dead parasites and to antigen-antibody complexes. Adult worms are localized in the subcutaneous tissues, surrounded by fibrotic nodules and ultimately calcify.

Epidemiology

Onchocerciasis is common in Africa; foci also occur in South and Central America and Mexico. The blackfly vectors breed in oxygen-rich water; thus, the disease characteristically is associated with fast-flowing streams.

Diagnosis

The clinical picture is indicative; final diagnosis is made by identifying microfilariae in skin snips.

Control

Individuals may be treated by removal of nodules and by administering microfilariacides that kill microfilariae. Control of vector blackflies minimizes reinfection.

Minor Filariae

Several other minor filarial nematodes parasitize humans; the pathology depends on the tissues preferred by the worms. In addition, humans occasionally are infected with dog heartworm larvae, which are unable to mature in human tissues but can cause lesions.

INTRODUCTION

The filariae are thread-like parasitic nematodes (roundworms) that are transmitted by arthropod vectors. The adult worms inhabit specific tissue locations, where they mate and produce **microfilariae,** the characteristic tiny, thread-like larvae. The microfilariae infect vector arthropods, in which they mature to infective larvae. Filarial diseases are a major health problem in many tropical and subtropical areas. The disease produced by a filarial worm depends on the tissue locations preferred by adults and microfilariae. The adults of the lymphatic filariae inhabit lymph vessels, where blockage and host reaction can result in lymphatic inflammation and dysfunction, and eventually in lymphedema and fibrosis. Repeated, prolonged infection with these worms can lead to **elephantia-sis,** a buildup of excess tissue in the affected area. Other filariae mature in the skin and subcutaneous tissues, where they induce nodule formation and dermatitis; migrating filariae of these species can cause ocular damage. Table 92-1 summarizes the filarial infections of humans.

LYMPHATIC FILARIAE: *WUCHERERIA BANCROFTI* AND *BRUGIA MALAYI*

CLINICAL MANIFESTATIONS

In lymphatic filariasis, disease is caused by the presence of worms in the regional lymphatic ves-

TABLE 92-1   Summary of Filarial Nematodes that Infect Humans

Species	Location of Adults	Major Pathology	Location of Microfilariae	Major Vectors	Geographic Distribution
Major filariae					
Wuchereria bancrofti	Lymphatics	Lymphangitis, elephantiasis	Blood; may exhibit nocturnal periodicity	Species of *Culex, Aedes,* and *Anopheles* mosquitoes	Widespread in tropical and subtropical countries
Brugia malayi	Lymphatics	Lymphangitis, elephantiasis	Blood	Species of *Mansonia* mosquitoes	Southeast Asia
Onchocerca volvulus	Subcutaneous nodules	Loss of vision, dermatitis	Tissue fluid in the skin	*Simulium* spp (blackflies)	Africa, Mexico, Guatemala, foci in Central and South America
Minor filariae					
Loa loa	Subcutaneous nodules	Transient swelling, temporary loss of vision	Blood; exhibit diurnal periodicity	*Chrysops* spp (deer flies)	Tropical Africa
Mansonella streptocerca	Skin	Dermatitis	Skin	Small biting flies	West Africa
Mansonella perstans	Body cavities	Not well defined	Blood	Small biting flies	Africa and South America
Mansonella ozzardi	Subcutaneous and connective tissue (based on experimental animal studies)	Not well defined	Blood	Small biting flies in the genera *Simulium* and *Culicoides*	West Indies, Central and South America
Dirofilaria spp	None in humans	Subcutaneous nodules, lung lesions	None in humans	Many species of mosquitoes	Cosmopolitan

sels and, particularly, by the host response to the worms and worm products. The microfilariae are released into the blood. Infections involving small numbers of worms are often asymptomatic. Early symptoms of lymphatic filariasis consist of intermittent fever and enlarged, tender lymph nodes. The inguinal lymph nodes are very often involved. The lymphatic vessels that drain into the lymph nodes and that harbor the developing and adult worms also become inflamed and painful. In more chronic infections, there may be pain also in the epididymis and testes. Swollen lymphatics may burst and drain into the genitourinary system; the resulting chyluria is sometimes the symptom that brings the patient to a doctor. In a small number of chronic cases, permanent lymphatic dysfunction caused by repeated exposure to infection over a number of years results in the massive lymphedema and accumulation of excess tissue known as elephantiasis.

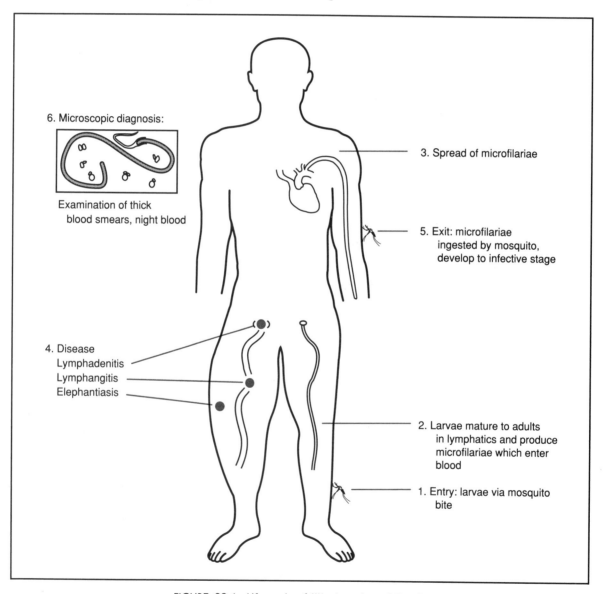

FIGURE 92-1 Life cycle of *Wuchereria* and *Brugia*.

STRUCTURE AND CLASSIFICATION

Adult *Wuchereria* and *Brugia* are elongated and slender (30 to 100 mm by 100 to 300 *μ*m); males are about half the size of females. Microfilariae are the diameter of a red blood cell and 250 to 300 *μ*m long. They are enclosed in a characteristic sheath. In addition to *B malayi*, some other, related *Brugia* species can infect humans or animals; they resemble *B malayi* in structure and life cycle, and are not discussed here.

MULTIPLICATION AND LIFE CYCLE

The filariae require an intermediate arthropod host to complete their life cycle (Fig. 92-1). However, no multiplication takes place in the intermediate host. Adult male and female worms live in regional lymphatic vessels, where the female produces a large number of microfilariae, which circulate in the blood and may be ingested by a feeding vector mosquito. The female worms show a circadian periodicity in microfilaria production. The time of peak production varies among the species and geographic strains of worms and usually corresponds to the peak feeding period of the vector mosquitoes. Microfilariae ingested by a vector mosquito migrate out of the midgut to the thoracic muscles, where they develop, molt several times, and finally migrate to the mouthparts of the mosquito as infective larvae. As the infective mosquito feeds on another host, the larvae leave the proboscis and enter the puncture wound made by the mosquito. Larvae quickly migrate to the lymphatics, where they mature, mate, and produce microfilariae in the new host. The time from infection until microfilariae can be detected in the blood varies from 3 to many months. There is no reliable information on the average life span of adult worms; however, humans who leave endemic areas have been observed to have circulating microfilaria for several years.

PATHOGENESIS

Infective larvae from a feeding vector mosquito migrate to the regional lymphatic vessels and by inducing a host inflammatory reaction cause the eventual blockage and edema characteristic of *W bancrofti* and *B malayi* infections (Fig. 92-1). The pathology varies greatly from one individual to another, and the exact mechanisms are not completely understood. The host reaction to the parasite is considerable and worsens when the worms molt, when the females first begin to produce microfilariae, and when the worms die and degenerate. Lymphatic vessels are often partially or completely blocked by lymph thrombi, by masses of dead worms, or by endothelial proliferation, fibrin deposition, and granulomatous reactions. Lymph stasis favors secondary bacterial and mycotic infection. The initial inflammation of regional lymph nodes and major lymphatic vessels may be followed by a prolonged asymptomatic period and then by recurring attacks of lymphangitis and "filarial fever" over a period of years. Figure 92-2 shows an example of elephantiasis, a grotesque enlargement of the infected area that develops when recurring attacks of lymphangitis result in permanent lymphatic blockage and lymphedema. The exact cause of elephantiasis is not understood; however, repeated exposure appears to lead to production of

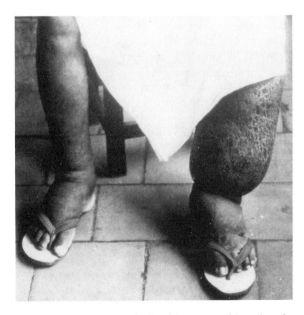

FIGURE 92-2 Elephantiasis of leg caused by chronic infection with the filarial nematode *Wuchereria bancrofti*. (Courtesy of Shoyei Yamauchi, Honolulu, HI.)

abnormally large amounts of collagenous material and to fibrosis of the tissue around the affected lymphatics.

HOST DEFENSES

The reaction to developing and adult worms results in endothelial cell proliferation and thrombus formation within the lymphatic vessels. Some aspects of the wide disease spectrum seen in lymphatic filariasis can be correlated with host immune responses. Individuals living in endemic areas and frequently bitten by infective mosquito vectors vary in clinical manifestations. Patients with characteristic symptoms such as recurring fever and regional lymphangitis may or may not have microfilariae in peripheral blood. Although antibodies to microfilariae and adult worms may be present, they do not seem to prevent reinfection or disease, since in endemic areas the proportion of exposed individuals who have microfilariae or clinical symptoms may increase until middle age. As a general rule, adults not previously infected with lymphatic filariae will show symptoms, but not circulating microfilariae, following infection with large numbers of infective larvae. Patients with elephantiasis also usually do not have circulating microfilariae. They do, however, have high levels of antibody to microfilariae and increased lymphocyte proliferative responses to adult worm antigens.

EPIDEMIOLOGY

Wuchereria bancrofti is prevalent in many parts of the tropics and subtropics. Species from three major genera of mosquitoes that serve as vectors are the common house mosquito *Culex pipiens quinquefasciatus (C fatigans)* in many urban centers, *Aedes* species in the South Pacific islands, and *Anopheles* species in more isolated rural areas. The relation between the degree and frequency of infection and the development of the disease is still not fully understood; severe disease such as elephantiasis develops gradually as a result of repeated exposure. Circulating microfilariae may persist for many years in the absence of specific symptoms.

Humans previously were assumed to be the only

hosts for *W bancrofti;* however, studies have shown that several species of monkeys can be infected experimentally with *W bancrofti* larvae recovered from mosquitoes allowed to feed on infected human volunteers. No naturally infected reservoirs other than humans have been identified.

Brugia malayi differs somewhat from *W bancrofti* in epidemiology. Whereas *W bancrofti* is prevalent in tropical areas all over the world, *B malayi* is found mainly in Southeast Asia. In contrast to *W bancrofti,* which is transmitted by mosquitoes of the three major genera, the principal mosquito vectors of *B malayi* belong to the genus *Mansonia. B malayi* is less host-specific than *W bancrofti;* it has been recovered from naturally infected monkeys, cats, and dogs, and has been maintained in several laboratory animals.

DIAGNOSIS

Enlarged and tender lymph nodes, especially in the inguinal region, or inflammation of lymphatic vessels in the extremities should alert physicians in an endemic area to filariasis. Definitive diagnosis may be accomplished by identifying microfilariae in thick blood smears (Fig. 92-1). Species identification is based on the presence of a sheath and the position of terminal nuclei. Because of the nocturnal periodicity of microfilariae, blood smears are better made at night when microfilaria levels are usually higher. Light infections may be detected by using one of several concentration methods.

Unfortunately, microfilariae may not be present in the blood during the early and late stages of the disease. When microfilariae are not detectable, a history of recurrent episodes of lymphangitis and lymphadenitis may form the basis for a presumptive diagnosis. Skin tests have been largely unsatisfactory, and commercial antigen is not widely available. Serologic tests are useful in epidemiologic studies, but to date have had limited value in the management of individual cases.

CONTROL

Attempts to reduce the prevalence of lymphatic filariae include vector control and mass treatment campaigns using diethylcarbamazine citrate. This drug significantly reduces the level of microfilariae in the blood. However, it must be given over a prolonged period, and frequent side effects, such as fever, vertigo, headaches, nausea, and lymphatic inflammation, discourage patient cooperation. Ivermectin, a drug that has recently been shown to be effective in the treatment of onchocerciasis, is being evaluated for use in lymphatic filariasis. Neither drug is very effective at killing adult worms.

◄ *ONCHOCERCA VOLVULUS* ►

Onchocerca volvulus is a filarial worm that is transmitted to humans by blackflies *(Simulium)*. Mature worms live in the subcutaneous tissues and produce microfilariae that migrate through the skin and connective tissues.

CLINICAL MANIFESTATIONS

Changes in skin pigmentation are often the first obvious signs of *Onchocerca* infection. Later stages of dermatitis present as atrophy and loss of skin elasticity. Although lymph nodes may become involved in onchocerciasis, involvement is not as prominent as with the lymphatic filariae. The subcutaneous nodules that harbor adult *Onchocerca* are usually firm and nontender. They vary in size and location but usually are easily recognized when they occur in geographic areas where the disease is endemic. However, in some geographic regions, nodules may be in deeper tissue, and thus not easily palpable.

The most serious clinical manifestation of onchocerciasis is blindness, caused by microfilariae that wander into the eye. In endemic areas, corneal opacities resulting from the reaction to dying microfilariae often suggest onchocercal infection. Alternatively, active living microfilariae may be seen when the eye is examined with a slit lamp.

STRUCTURE

Adult *Onchocerca* may be up to 60 cm long but are usually coiled in subcutaneous nodules. The microfilariae are slightly smaller than those of *W bancrofti* and *B malayi* and differ from them in lacking a sheath, having a different nuclear arrangement, and not usually being found in the blood.

MULTIPLICATION AND LIFE CYCLE

Figure 92-3 shows the life cycle of *Onchocerca*. The microfilariae produced by adult female worms in subcutaneous nodules migrate into the skin and connective tissue; they do not generally enter the circulatory system. Microfilariae are ingested by vector blackflies, develop to the infective stage in the muscles of the flies, and then migrate to the mouth parts. When the infected flies feed on a new host, the larvae leave the mouth parts and enter the wound produced by the biting fly. Developing male and female worms congregate in subcutaneous tissue where they usually induce formation of a nodule.

PATHOGENESIS

Adult worms in the subcutaneous tissues cause varying degrees of inflammation and may induce subcutaneous nodules. Nodules appear 3 to 4 months after infection, but microfilariae are not generally detectable until 1 year after infection. Adult worms may be surrounded by an inflammatory response that progresses to granuloma formation and fibrosis or calcification, depending on the condition of the worm and age of the nodule (Fig. 92-3).

Microfilariae appear to move upward, and in chronic heavy infections may be seen in the eye. Ocular damage is thought to be due both to the trauma caused by living microfilariae and to a hypersensitivity reaction to dead ones. A major problem in the management of onchocerciasis patients is the acute inflammatory response to dying microfilariae in the eye during treatment. Antigen-antibody complexes probably play a role in the development of eye lesions resulting from microfilariae.

HOST DEFENSES

Nodules containing adult worms are surrounded by inflammatory cells that are replaced by collagen and fibrotic tissue, thereby localizing the worms. A study of nodules has shown that they are areas of high cellular activity. Some microfilariae appear to be killed before they ever leave the nodules where they are produced by the female worm. Obviously

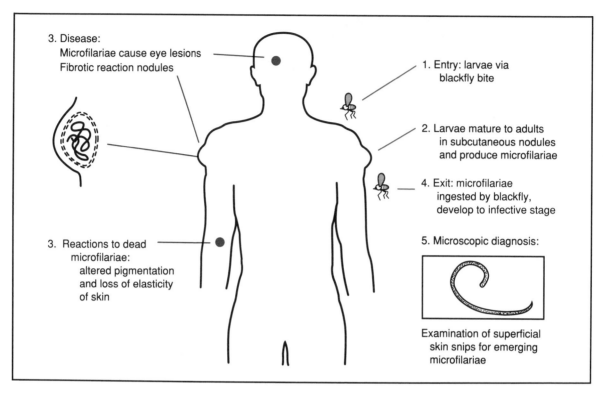

FIGURE 92-3 Life cycle of *Onchocerca*.

many others escape the chronic inflammatory responses and the granulomas commonly seen surrounding nematodes in tissue. The exact composition of the nodules varies depending on the distance from the adult worms and the age of the nodule. In general, neutrophils are followed by eosinophils and macrophages. The involvement of eosinophils in killing microfilariae in untreated patients suggests specific immune reactions similar to those reported in other helminth infections. The fibrous outer layer of the nodule contains blood vessels which may be surrounded in older nodules by cellular infiltrates that include plasma cells and eosinophils.

EPIDEMIOLOGY

Transmission occurs through bites of vector blackflies in the family Simuliidae. Although a few vector species breed in slow-moving streams, most require fast-flowing, highly oxygenated streams. For

this reason, ocular onchocerciasis is often called "river blindness."

Onchocerciasis is prevalent in many parts of tropical Africa and has been reported in a few places in the Middle East. In the Western hemisphere, it is an important and widespread infection in Guatemala and the southern states of Mexico. It also appears in other areas of Central America, and a few foci have been found in Venezuela, Colombia, Surinam, Brazil, and Ecuador.

DIAGNOSIS

Onchocerciasis is suggested by subcutaneous nodules or by the characteristic scaly dermatitis in individuals living in endemic areas. Positive diagnosis is usually made by identifying microfilariae in a superficial skin biopsy made with a scalpel or an appropriate punch. The skin samples, which are usually taken from the shoulder, are placed in a drop of saline or distilled water on a microscope slide, incubated for 30 minutes, and examined (Fig. 92-3). The diagnosis may also be made by finding adult worms in nodules or by observing microfilariae in the eye. Serologic tests are being developed to aid in diagnosis when microfilariae cannot be detected but onchocerciasis is suspected.

CONTROL

Three main measures — vector control, nodule removal, and drug treatment — provide limited control of onchocerciasis. Control of blackfly vectors is difficult because most species breed in fast-flowing streams to which insecticides cannot easily be applied. Nodules harboring adult worms are usually removed, which presumably reduces the rate at which microfilariae are produced and thus the risk to the eyes (as well as the number of microfilariae available to vectors). Mass treatment poses difficulties, because suramin, the drug of choice for killing adult worms, must be given intravenously and is toxic. Diethylcarbamazine kills microfilariae but has limited efficacy against adult worms and has the disadvantage that some patients experience a severe reaction, which may exacerbate eye damage, to dying microfilariae. Ivermectin, a semisynthetic macrolide antibiotic, has recently been shown to be more effective and to produce fewer side effects than diethylcarbamazine.

◄ MINOR FILARIAL INFECTIONS ►

Human filarial parasites of minor importance include the following (Table 92-1):

Loa loa, limited in distribution to tropical Africa, best known for its superficial migration under the conjunctiva of the eye and for the presence of "fugitive" or "calabar" temporary swellings

Mansonella (syn. *Dipetalonema* or *Acanthoceilonema*) *streptocerca,* also limited to tropical Africa and frequently presenting as a chronic itching dermatitis; both adult worms and microfilariae are present in the skin

Mansonella (syn. *Dipetalonema* or *Acanthoceilonema*) *perstans,* found in Africa and South America

Mansonella ozzardi, restricted to the western hemisphere

DIROFILARIA SPECIES

Dirofilaria immitis (the dog heartworm) is a worldwide filarial parasite of dogs; adult worms (up to 30 cm long) usually are located in the dog's heart. In heavy infections, or when adult worms die, the parasites may be carried to the pulmonary vessels where they may produce emboli. The worms do not mature to adulthood in humans, but larval stages have been reported in cutaneous nodules (which may be confused with tumors) and have sometimes produced lesions in the lungs (coin lesions) or in breast tissue. Pulmonary lesions may be asymptomatic or may cause coughing or chest pains. Roentgenograms frequently show a discrete mass suggestive of a tumor. Larvae of other *Dirofilaria* spp. that parasitize lower animals occasionally may be found in the skin or eyes of humans.

DRACUNCULUS MEDINENSIS

Dracunculus medinensis, the guinea worm, is not a true filarial worm, but is often grouped with the filariae. It is one of the oldest known parasitic diseases of man. Some authors suggest that the ancient technique of removing the adult female worm, which may be more than 1 meter long, by winding it on a stick, may be the origin of the medical emblem, the caduceus.

Dracunuliasis is still quite common in parts of Africa and Asia. Humans acquire the infection when they swallow infected copepods (genus *Cyclops*) in drinking water. Often, the first sign of infection is the formation of a blister when the adult female worm migrates to the subcutaneous tissue. On contact with water, the blister breaks and the worm ruptures and discharges larvae into the water. The larvae are ingested by *Cyclops,* in which they develop to the infective stage.

The ultimate location of the adult worm determines the pathology, since lesions develop in response to the worms. Frequent sites of inflammation and abscess include knee and ankle joints, as well as the subcutaneous tissues of the extremities.

REFERENCES

Beaver PC, Jung RC, Cupp EW: Clinical Parasitology. 9th Ed. Lea & Febiger, Philadelphia, 1984

Palmieri JR, Connor DH, Marwoto HA: Animal model of human disease: Bancrofti filariasis. *Wuchereria bancrofti* infection in the silvered leaf monkey *(Prebytis cristatus)*. Am J Pathol 112:383, 1983

Sasa M: Human Filariasis. A Global Survey of Epidemiology and Control. University Park Press, Baltimore, MD, 1976

Strickland GT: Hunter's Tropical Medicine. 6th Ed. WB Saunders, Philadelphia, 1984

Taylor HR, Greene BM: The status of ivermectin in the treatment of human onchocerciasis. Am J Trop Med Hyg 41:460, 1989

World Health Organization: Control of Lymphatic Filariasis: A Manual for Health Personnel. WHO, Geneva, 1987

V

INTRODUCTION TO INFECTIOUS DISEASES

The record of human suffering and death caused by smallpox, cholera, typhus, dysentery, malaria, etc. establishes the eminence of the infectious diseases. Despite the outstanding successes in control afforded by improved sanitation, immunization, and antimicrobial therapy, the infectious diseases continue to be a common and significant problem of modern medicine. The most common disease of mankind, the common cold, is an infectious disease, as is the feared modern disease AIDS. Some chronic neurological diseases that were thought formerly to be degenerative diseases have proven to be infectious. There is little doubt that the future will continue to reveal the infectious diseases as major medical problems.

In the study and care of patients with infectious disease, physicians use some terms that are not easy to define precisely. A definition of **infection** as growth of a microorganism in an animal with any resulting host response will include essentially all of the infectious diseases of humans. Many of the body surfaces of humans that communicate with the external environment (e.g., the skin and the gastrointestinal and respiratory tracts) support a normal flora, but these microorganisms usually do not invade and cause disease. Under the right circumstances, however, elements of the flora can invade and produce an infection.

A number of other terms are commonly used in describing the infectious diseases. **Pathology** refers to the abnormality induced by an infection, and **pathogenesis** to the events producing the pathology. A pathogenic microorganism is a microbe that can cause pathology. **Disease** refers to the existence of pathology and an **infectious disease** is a disease caused by a microorganism. **Virulence** is a term referring to the power of a microbe to produce disease in a particular host. For example, a microorganism may be avirulent for a normal host and highly virulent for an immunosuppressed host. **Immunity** refers to the degree of resistance of the host for a particular microbe. Finally, it must be appreciated that the occurrence of an infectious disease in a human is a dynamic process that represents a **host-parasite interaction.** The parasite attempts to multiply and the host defenses seek to control this effort. The task of the physician is to recognize that such a process accounts for the patient's problem and to intervene for the benefit of the patient.

The infectious diseases are usually characterized by the dominant organ system involved. This classification is useful as a guide in approaching patients. For example, patients do not present complaining of pneumococcal pneumonia; patients present complaining of fever, cough, and chest pain. The physician localizes the disease to the chest (respiratory infection) and then proceeds to develop data proving the presence of a pneumonia caused by the pneumococcus. Thus, we classify infections as respiratory infections, gastrointestinal infections, genitourinary infections, nervous system infections, skin and soft tissue infections, bone and joint infections, cardiovascular infections, and generalized (disseminated) infections. The chapters in this section are organized according to this scheme. The section is intended primarily to help the student begin to integrate the knowledge of microbiology and immunology into a framework useful for the practice of medicine. The diagnosis, prevention, and treatment of the infectious diseases is a stimulating and gratifying process.

Robert B. Couch

93 INFECTIONS OF THE RESPIRATORY SYSTEM

MARY C. O'CONNOR
CHIEN LIU

GENERAL CONCEPTS

UPPER RESPIRATORY INFECTIONS: COMMON COLD, PHARYNGITIS, EPIGLOTTITIS, AND LARYNGOTRACHEITIS

Etiology

Most upper respiratory infections are viral. Epiglottitis and laryngotracheitis are exceptions: most of the severe cases are caused by *Haemophilus influenzae*. Pharyngitis is often caused by *Streptococcus pyogenes*.

Pathogenesis

Organisms gain entry by inhalation or inoculation and invade the mucosa. Epithelial destruction may ensue, along with redness, edema, hemorrhage, and sometimes an exudate.

Clinical Manifestations

Initial symptoms of a cold are a runny, stuffy nose, sneezing, and a sore throat. Colds do not usually cause a fever, but other upper respiratory infections may. Children with epiglottitis may have difficulty breathing, muffled speech, drooling, and stridor, and children with serious laryngotracheitis (croup) may also have tachypnea and stridor.

Microbial Diagnosis

Common colds can usually be recognized clinically. Bacterial and viral cultures of throat swab specimens are used for pharyngitis, epiglottitis, and laryngotracheitis. Blood cultures are also obtained in cases of epiglottitis.

Prevention and Treatment

Viral infections are treated symptomatically. Streptococcal pharyngitis and epiglottitis caused by *H influenzae* are treated with antibacterials. *Haemophilus* type b vaccine is recommended for children.

LOWER RESPIRATORY INFECTIONS: BRONCHITIS, BRONCHIOLITIS, AND PNEUMONIA

Etiology

Most lower respiratory infections are viral or bacterial. Viruses cause most cases of bronchitis and bronchiolitis. Most community-acquired infectious pneumonias are bacterial; *Streptococcus pneumoniae*, *H influenzae*, and *Legionella* spp are common agents. Atypical pneumonias are caused by such agents as *Mycoplasma pneumoniae*, *Chlamydia* spp, and viruses. Nosocomial pneumonias and pneumonias in immunosuppressed patients have a protean etiology.

Pathogenesis

Organisms enter the distal airway by inhalation, aspiration, or hematogenous seeding. The pathogen multiplies in or on the epithelium, causing inflammation, increased mucus secretion, and impaired mucociliary function; other lung functions may be affected. In severe bronchiolitis, inflammation and necrosis of the epithelium may block small airways.

Clinical Manifestations

Symptoms include cough, fever, chest pain, tachypnea, wheezing (sometimes), and sputum production. Patients with pneumonia may also exhibit nonrespiratory symptoms such as confusion, headache, myalgias, abdominal pain, nausea, vomiting, and diarrhea.

Microbial Diagnosis

Sputum specimens are cultured for bacteria, fungi, and viruses. Culturing of nasal washings is usually sufficient in infants with bronchiolitis. A fluorescent-antibody stain is used for *Legionella* spp, and the Quellung test for *S pneumoniae*. Blood cultures and/or serologic methods are used for viruses, rickettsiae, fungi, and many bacteria.

Prevention and Treatment

Symptomatic treatment is used for most viral infections; bacterial pneumonias are treated with antibacterials. A vaccine against *S pneumoniae* is available for individuals at high risk.

UPPER RESPIRATORY INFECTIONS

Infections of the respiratory tract are grouped according to their symptomatology and anatomic involvement. Acute upper respiratory infections include the common cold, pharyngitis, epiglottitis, and laryngotracheitis (Fig. 93-1). These infections are usually benign, transitory, and self-limited, although epiglottitis and laryngotracheitis may be severe diseases in children and small neonates. Etiologic agents associated with upper respiratory infections include viruses, bacteria, mycoplasma, and fungi (Table 93-1).

COMMON COLD

ETIOLOGY

Common colds are the most prevalent of all respiratory infections and are the leading cause of visits to the physician, as well as work and school absenteeism. Most colds are caused by viruses. Rhinoviruses are the most common pathogens, causing approximately 25 percent of colds in adults. Coronaviruses may be responsible for more than 10 percent of cases. Parainfluenzaviruses, respiratory syncytial virus, adenoviruses, and influenza viruses have all been linked to the common cold syndrome. All of these organisms show seasonal variations in incidence. The cause of 30 to 40 percent of cold syndromes has not been determined.

PATHOGENESIS

The viruses appear to act through direct invasion of epithelial cells of the respiratory mucosa, but whether there is actual destruction and sloughing of these cells or loss of ciliary activity seems to depend on the specific organism involved. There is an increase in both leukocyte infiltration and nasal secretions, including large amounts of protein and immunoglobulins, suggesting that immune mechanisms may be responsible for some manifestation of the common cold.

CLINICAL MANIFESTATIONS

The classic symptoms of nasal discharge and obstruction, sneezing, sore throat, and cough occur in both adults and children. Fever is rare. The duration of symptoms and of viral shedding varies with the pathogen and the age of the patient.

MICROBIOLOGIC DIAGNOSIS

The diagnosis of a common cold is usually based on the symptoms (lack of fever combined with symptoms localized to the nasopharynx). Unlike allergic rhinitis, eosinophils are absent in nasal secretions.

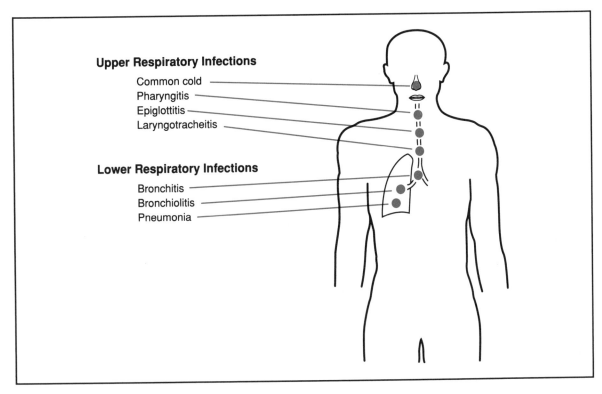

Upper Respiratory Infections

Common cold
Pharyngitis
Epiglottitis
Laryngotracheitis

Lower Respiratory Infections

Bronchitis
Bronchiolitis
Pneumonia

FIGURE 93-1 Upper and lower respiratory tract infections.

Although it is possible to isolate the viruses for definitive diagnosis, that is rarely warranted.

PREVENTION AND TREATMENT

Treatment of the uncomplicated common cold is generally symptomatic. Decongestants, antipyretics, fluids, and bed rest usually suffice. Restriction of activities to avoid infecting others, along with good hand washing, are the best measures to prevent spread of the disease. No vaccine is commercially available for cold prophylaxis.

◄ PHARYNGITIS ►

ETIOLOGY

Pharyngitis is an inflammatory syndrome of the pharynx and is caused by bacterial, viral, and fungal agents, as well as noninfectious etiologies such

as smoking. Most cases are due to viral infections and accompany a common cold or influenza. Type A coxsackievirus can cause severe ulcerative pharyngitis in children (herpangina), and adenovirus and herpes simplex virus, although less common, also can cause severe pharyngitis. Pharyngitis is a common symptom of Epstein-Barr virus and cytomegalovirus infections.

Group A β-hemolytic streptococci or *Streptococcus pyogenes* account for up to 50 percent of pharyngitis cases in children during certain periods of the year. *Corynebacterium diphtheriae* causes occasional cases of acute pharyngitis, as do mixed anaerobic infections (Vincent's angina), *Corynebacterium haemolyticum*, *Neisseria gonorrhoeae*, and *Chlamydia trachomatis*. Outbreaks of *Chlamydia pneumoniae* (TWAR agent) causing pharyngitis or pneumonitis have occurred in military recruits. *Mycoplasma pneumoniae* and *Mycoplasma hominis* have been associated with acute pharyngitis. *Can-*

TABLE 93-1   Common Agents of Respiratory Infections

Clinical Illness	Bacteria	Viruses	Fungi	Other
Common cold (rhinitis, coryza)	Rare	Rhinoviruses Coronavirus Parainfluenza viruses Adenoviruses Respiratory syncytial virus Influenza viruses	Rare	Rare
Pharyngitis and tonsillitis (tonsillopharyngitis)	Group A β-hemolytic streptococci *Corynebacterium diphtheriae* *Neisseria gonorrhoeae* *Mycoplasma pneumoniae* *Mycoplasma hominis* (type 1) Mixed anaerobes	Adenoviruses Coxsackieviruses A Influenza viruses Rhinovirus, coronavirus Parainfluenza viruses Epstein-Barr virus, cytomegalovirus Herpes simplex virus	*Candida albicans*	Rare
Epiglottitis and laryngotracheitis (croup)	*Haemophilus influenzae* type b *Corynebacterium diphtheriae*	Respiratory syncytial virus Parainfluenza viruses	Rare	Rare
Bronchitis and bronchiolitis	*Haemophilus influenzae* *Streptococcus pneumoniae* *Mycoplasma pneumoniae*	Parainfluenza viruses Respiratory syncytial virus Adenoviruses Herpes simplex virus	Rare	Rare
Pneumonia	*Streptococcus pneumoniae* *Staphylococcus aureus* *Streptococcus pyogenes* *Haemophilus influenzae* *Klebsiella pneumoniae* *Escherichia coli* *Pseudomonas aeruginosa* *Mycoplasma pneumoniae* *Legionella* spp Anaerobic bacteria *Mycobacterium tuberculosis* and other *Mycoplasma* spp *Coxiella burnetii* *Chlamydia psittaci* *Chlamydia trachomatis* *Chlamydia pneumoniae*	Adenoviruses Parainfluenza viruses Respiratory syncytial virus Influenza viruses Varicella-zoster virus Measles virus Cytomegalovirus Herpes simplex virus	*Histoplasma capsulatum* *Blastomyces dermitidis* *Paracoccidioides brasiliensis* *Coccidioides immitis* *Candida albicans* *Filobasidiella* (*Cryptococcus*) *neoformans* *Aspergillus fumigatus* and other *Aspergillus* spp	*Pneumocystis carinii*

dida albicans, which causes oral candidiasis or thrush, can involve the pharynx, leading to inflammation and pain.

PATHOGENESIS

As with the common cold, viral pathogens in pharyngitis appear to invade the mucosal cells of the nasopharynx and oral cavity, resulting in edema and hyperemia of the mucous membranes and tonsils (Fig. 93-2). Bacteria attach to and, in the case of group A β-hemolytic streptococci, invade the mucosa of the upper respiratory tract. Many clinical manifestations of infection appear to be due to the immune reaction to products of the bacterial cell. In diphtheria, a potent bacterial exotoxin causes local inflammation and cell necrosis.

CLINICAL MANIFESTATIONS

Pharyngitis usually presents with a red, sore, or "scratchy" throat (Fig. 93-3). An inflammatory exudate or membranes may cover the tonsils and tonsillar pillars. Vesicles or ulcers may also be seen on the pharyngeal walls. Depending on the pathogen, fever and systemic manifestations such as malaise, myalgias, or headache may be present.

MICROBIOLOGIC DIAGNOSIS

The goal in the diagnosis of pharyngitis is to identify cases that are due to group A β-hemolytic streptococci, as well as the more unusual and potentially serious infections. The various forms of pharyngitis cannot be distinguished on clinical grounds. Routine throat cultures for bacteria are inoculated onto sheep blood and chocolate agars. Thayer-Martin medium is used if *N gonorrhoeae* is suspected. Viral cultures are not routinely obtained for most cases of pharyngitis. Serologic studies may be used to confirm the diagnosis of pharyngitis due to viral, mycoplasmal, or chlamydial pathogens. Rapid diagnostic tests with fluorescent antibody or latex agglutination to identify group A streptococci from pharyngeal swabs are now available.

PREVENTION AND TREATMENT

Symptomatic treatment is recommended for viral pharyngitis. The exception is herpes simplex virus infection, which may be treated with acyclovir if clinically warranted or if diagnosed in immunocompromised patients. The specific antibacterial agents will depend on the causative organism, but penicillin G is the therapy of choice for streptococcal pharyngitis.

EPIGLOTTITIS AND LARYNGOTRACHEITIS

ETIOLOGY

Inflammation of the upper airway is classified as epiglottitis or laryngotracheitis (croup) on the basis of the location, clinical manifestations, and usual pathogens of the infection. *Haemophilus influenzae* type b is most commonly identified as the cause of epiglottitis, particularly in children aged 2 to 5 years. Epiglottitis is less common in adults. Some cases in adults may be of viral origin. Most cases of laryngotracheitis are due to viruses, but more serious, bacterial infections have been associated with *H influenzae* type b, group A β-hemolytic streptococcus, and *C diphtheriae*. Parainfluenza viruses, respiratory syncytial virus, adenoviruses, influenza viruses, enteroviruses, and *M pneumoniae* have been implicated.

PATHOGENESIS

A viral upper respiratory infection may precede infection with *H influenzae* in episodes of epiglottitis. However, once *H influenzae* type b infection starts, there is rapidly progressive erythema and swelling of the epiglottis, and bacteremia is usually present. The viral infection of laryngotracheitis commonly begins in the nasopharynx and eventually moves into the larynx and trachea. Inflammation and edema involve the epithelium, mucosa, and submucosa of the subglottis and can lead to airway obstruction.

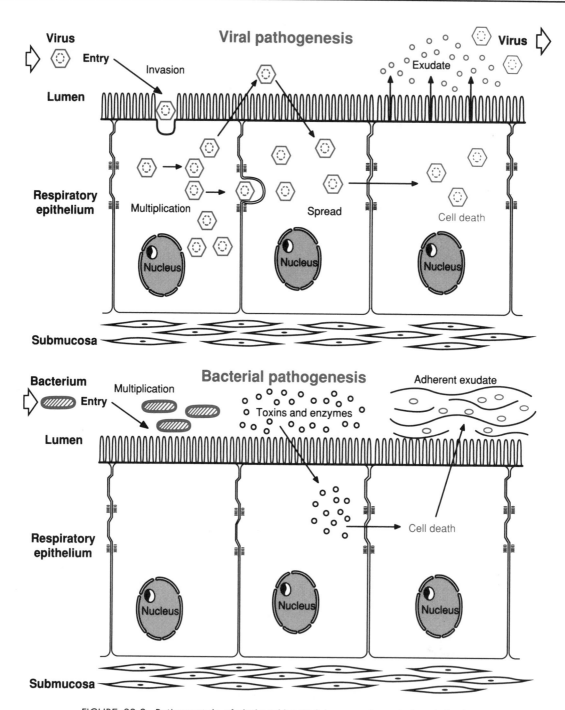

FIGURE 93-2 Pathogenesis of viral and bacterial mucosal respiratory infections.

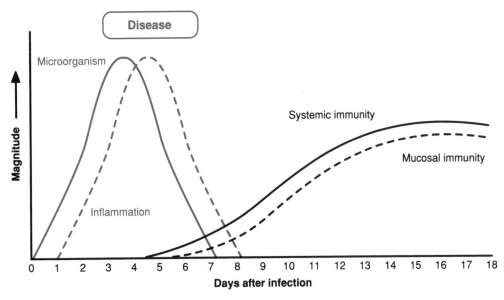

FIGURE 93-3 Pathogenesis of upper respiratory tract infections.

CLINICAL MANIFESTATIONS

The syndrome of epiglottitis begins with the acute onset of fever, sore throat, hoarseness, drooling, and dysphagia and progresses within a few hours to severe respiratory distress and prostration. The clinical course can be fulminant and fatal. The pharynx may be inflamed, but the diagnostic finding is a "cherry-red" epiglottis.

A history of preceding coldlike symptoms is typical of laryngotracheitis, with rhinorrhea, fever, sore throat, and a mild cough. Tachypnea, a deep barking cough, and inspiratory stridor eventually develop. Children with bacterial tracheitis appear more ill than adults and are at greater risk of developing airway obstruction.

Haemophilus influenzae type b is isolated from the blood or epiglottis in most patients with epiglottitis; therefore, a blood culture is always indicated. Sputum cultures or cultures from pharyngeal swabs may be used to isolate bacterial and viral pathogens in patients with laryngotracheitis. Serologic studies to detect a rise in antibody titers to various viruses are helpful for retrospective diagnosis. Newer, rapid diagnostic techniques, using indirect or direct immunofluorescent-antibody staining to detect virus in sputum, pharyngeal swabs, or nasal washings, have been successfully used, as has enzyme-linked immunosorbent assay (ELISA) for detection of viral antibody or antigens.

PREVENTION AND TREATMENT

Epiglottitis is a medical emergency, especially in children. All children with this diagnosis should be observed carefully and be intubated to maintain an open airway as soon as the first sign of respiratory distress is detected. Antibacterial therapy should be directed at *H influenzae*. Patients with croup are usually successfully managed with close observation and supportive care, such as fluids, humidified air, and racemic epinephrine. *Haemophilus influenzae* type b polysaccharide vaccine or conjugated vaccine is recommended for all pediatric patients, as is immunization against diphtheria. However, children under 2 years of age do not respond well to polysaccharide vaccines. The true value of *H influenzae* type b vaccination in this age group is unsettled.

LOWER RESPIRATORY INFECTIONS

Infections of the lower respiratory tract include bronchitis, bronchiolitis, and pneumonia (Fig. 93-1). These syndromes, especially pneumonia, can be severe or fatal. Although viruses, mycoplasma, rickettsiae, and fungi can all cause lower respiratory tract infections, bacteria are the dominant pathogens, accounting for a much higher percentage of lower than of upper respiratory tract infections.

BRONCHITIS AND BRONCHIOLITIS

ETIOLOGY

Bronchitis and bronchiolitis involve inflammation of the bronchial tree. Bronchitis is usually preceded by an upper respiratory tract infection or forms part of a clinical syndrome in diseases such as influenza, rubeola, rubella, pertussis, scarlet fever, and typhoid fever. Chronic bronchitis with a persistent cough and sputum production appears to be caused by a combination of environmental factors, such as smoking, and bacterial infection with pathogens such as *H influenzae* and *S pneumoniae*. Bronchiolitis is a viral respiratory disease of infants and is caused primarily by respiratory syncytial viruses. Other viruses, including parainfluenza viruses, influenza viruses, and adenoviruses (as well as occasionally *M pneumoniae*) are also known to cause bronchiolitis.

PATHOGENESIS

When the bronchial tree is infected, the mucosa becomes hyperemic and edematous and produces copious bronchial secretions. The damage to the mucosa can range from simple loss of mucociliary function to actual destruction of the respiratory epithelium, depending on the organism(s) in-

volved. Patients with chronic bronchitis have an increase in the number of mucus-producing cells in their airways, as well as inflammation and loss of bronchial epithelium. Infants with bronchiolitis initially have inflammation and sometimes necrosis of the respiratory epithelium, with eventual sloughing. Bronchial and bronchiolar walls are thickened. Exudate made up of necrotic material and respiratory secretions and the narrowing of the bronchial lumen lead to airway obstruction. Areas of air trapping and atelectasis develop and may eventually contribute to respiratory failure.

CLINICAL MANIFESTATIONS

Symptoms of an upper respiratory tract infection with a cough is the typical presentation in acute bronchitis. Mucopurulent sputum may be present, and moderate temperature elevations occur. Typical findings in chronic bronchitis are an incessant cough and production of large amounts of sputum, particularly in the morning. Development of respiratory infections can lead to acute exacerbations of symptoms with possibly severe respiratory distress.

Coryza and cough usually precede the onset of bronchiolitis. Fever is common. A deepening cough, increased respiratory rate, and restlessness follow. Retractions of the chest wall, nasal flaring, and grunting are prominent findings. Wheezing or an actual lack of breath sounds may be noted. Respiratory failure and death may result.

MICROBIOLOGIC DIAGNOSIS

Bacteriologic examination and culture of purulent respiratory secretions should always be performed for cases of acute bronchitis not associated with a common cold. Patients with chronic bronchitis should have their sputum cultured for bacteria initially and during acute exacerbations. Aspirations of nasopharyngeal secretions or swabs are sufficient to obtain specimens for viral culture in infants with bronchiolitis. Serologic tests demonstrating a rise in antibody titer to specific viruses can also be performed. Rapid diagnostic tests for antibody or viral antigen may be performed on nasopharyngeal secretions by using fluorescent-antibody staining or ELISA.

PREVENTION AND TREATMENT

With only a few exceptions, viral infections are treated with supportive measures. Respiratory syncytial virus infections in infants may be treated with ribavirin. Amantadine is available for patients with influenza type A; it is effective if given early in the course of the disease. Selected groups of patients with chronic bronchitis receive benefit from corticosteroids, bronchodilators, or prophylactic antibiotics.

◀ PNEUMONIA ▶

Pneumonia is an inflammation of the lung parenchyma (Fig. 93-4). Consolidation of the lung tissue may be identified by physical examination and chest x-ray. Numerous factors, including environmental contaminants and autoimmune diseases, as well as infection, may cause pneumonia. The various infectious agents that cause pneumonia are categorized in many ways for purposes of laboratory testing, epidemiologic study, and choice of therapy. A common system groups organisms by the environment the patient occupied or the physical condition of the patient at the time pneumonia is diagnosed. Thus, infections which arise while a patient is hospitalized or living in an institution such as a nursing home or in any chronically debilitated patient are called **hospital-acquired** or **nosocomial pneumonias.** Infections that appear in usually healthy persons not confined to an institution are classified as **community-acquired pneumonias.** Many organisms cause both types of infection.

ETIOLOGY

Bacterial Pneumonias

Streptococcus pneumoniae is the most common agent of community-acquired acute bacterial pneumonia. More than 80 serotypes, as determined by

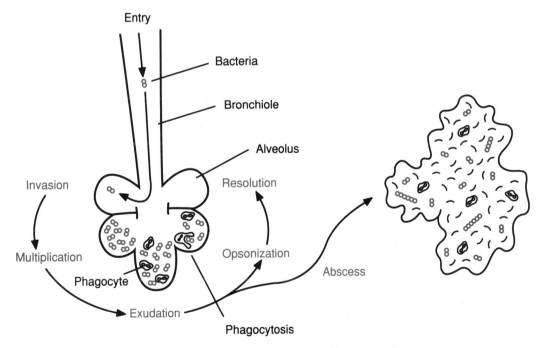

FIGURE 93-4 Pathogenesis of bacterial pneumonias.

capsular polysaccharides, are known, but 23 serotypes account for 90 percent of all pneumococcal pneumonias in the United States. Pneumonia from other streptococci are uncommon. *Streptococcus pyogenes* pneumonia is often associated with a hemorrhagic pneumonitis and empyema. Community-acquired pneumonias caused by *Staphylococcus aureus* are also uncommon and usually occur after influenza or from staphylococcal bacteremia. Infections due to *Haemophilus influenzae* (usually nontypeable) and *Klebsiella pneumoniae* are more common among patients over 50 years old who have chronic obstructive lung disease or alcoholism.

The most common agents of nosocomial pneumonias are aerobic Gram-negative bacilli that rarely cause pneumonia in healthy individuals. *Pseudomonas, Escherichia coli, Enterobacter, Proteus,* and *Klebsiella* species are often identified. Less common agents of pneumonias include *Francisella tularensis,* the agent of tularemia; *Yersinia pestis,* the agent of plague; and *Neisseria meningitidis,* which usually causes meningitis but can cause pneumonia, especially among military recruits. *Xanthomonas pseudomallei* causes melioidosis, a chronic pneumonia in Southeast Asia.

Mycobacterium tuberculosis typically causes pneumonia. Although the incidence of tuberculosis is lowest in industrialized countries, *M tuberculosis* infections still continue to be a significant public health problem in the United States, particularly among immigrants from developing countries, intravenous drug abusers, patients infected with human immunodeficiency virus (HIV), and the institutionalized elderly. Atypical *Mycobacterium* species can cause lung disease indistinguishable from tuberculosis.

Aspiration Pneumonia

Aspiration pneumonia from anaerobic organisms usually occurs in patients with periodontal disease or depressed consciousness. The bacteria involved are usually part of the oral flora, and cultures are generally mixed. *Actinomyces, Bacteroides, Peptostreptococcus, Veillonella, Propionibacterium, Eubacterium,* and *Fusobacterium* spp are often isolated.

Atypical Pneumonias

Atypical pneumonias are those that are not typical pneumococcal lobar pneumonias. *Mycoplasma pneumoniae* produces pneumonia most commonly in young people between 5 and 19 years of age. Outbreaks have been reported among military recruits and college students.

Legionella species, including *L pneumophila,* can cause a wide range of clinical manifestations. The 1976 outbreak in Philadelphia was manifested as a typical serious pneumonia in affected individuals, with a mortality of 17 percent (see Ch. 40). These organisms can survive in water and cause pneumonia by inhalation from aerosolized tap water, respiratory devices, air conditioners, and showers. They also have been reported to cause nosocomial pneumonias.

Chlamydia spp noted to cause pneumonitis are *C trachomatis, C psittaci,* and *C pneumoniae. Chlamydia trachomatis* causes pneumonia in neonates and young infants. Various subtypes of *C psittaci* cause occupational pneumonitis in bird handlers such as turkey farmers. *Chlamydia pneumoniae* has been associated with outbreaks of pneumonia in military recruits and on college campuses.

Coxiella burnetii, the rickettsia responsible for Q fever, is acquired by inhalation of aerosols from infected animal placentas and feces. Pneumonitis is one of the major manifestations of this systemic infection.

Most viral pneumonias are rare in healthy civilian adults. An exception is the viral pneumonia caused by influenza viruses, which can have a high mortality in the elderly and in patients with underlying disease. A serious complication following influenza virus infection is a secondary bacterial pneumonia, particularly *Staphylococcus* pneumonia. Respiratory syncytial virus can cause serious pneumonia among infants as well as outbreaks among institutionalized adults. Adenoviruses may also cause pneumonia. Serotypes 1, 2, 3, 7, and 7a have been associated with a severe, fatal pneumonia in infants. Although varicella-zoster virus pneumonitis is rare in children, it is probably common in individuals over 19 years old. Mortality can be as high as 10 to 30 percent. Measles pneumonia may occur in adults.

Other Pneumonias and Immunosuppression

Cytomegalovirus is well known for causing congenital infection in neonates, as well as the mononucleosislike illness seen in adults. However, among its manifestations in immunocompromised individuals is a severe and often fatal pneumonitis. Herpes simplex virus also causes a pneumonia in this population. Giant-cell pneumonia is a serious complication of measles and has been found in children with immunodeficiency disorders or underlying cancers who receive live attenuated measles vaccine. *Actinomyces* and *Nocardia* spp can cause pneumonitis, particularly in immunocompromised hosts.

Among the fungi, *Cryptococcus neoformans* and *Sporothrix schenckii* are found worldwide, whereas *Blastomyces dermatitidis, Coccidioides immitis, Histoplasma capsulatum,* and *Paracoccidioides brasiliensis* have specific geographic distributions. All can cause pneumonias, which are usually chronic and possibly clinically inapparent in normal hosts, but are manifested as more serious disease in immunocompromised patients. Other fungi, such as *Aspergillus* and *Candida* spp, occasionally are responsible for pneumonias in severely ill or immunosuppressed patients and neonates.

Pneumocystis carinii, a protozoan-like organism, produces a life-threatening pneumonia among patients immunosuppressed by acquired immune deficiency syndrome (AIDS), hematologic cancers, or medical therapy. It is the most common cause of pneumonia among patients with AIDS.

PATHOGENESIS AND CLINICAL MANIFESTATIONS

Infectious agents gain access to the lower respiratory tract by the inhalation of aerosolized material, by aspiration of upper airway flora, or by hematogenous seeding. Pneumonia occurs when lung defense mechanisms are diminished or overwhelmed. The major symptoms of pneumonia are cough, chest pain, fever, shortness of breath, and sputum production. Patients are tachycardiac. Headache, confusion, abdominal pain, nausea, vomiting, and diarrhea may be present, depending on the age of the patient and the organism involved.

MICROBIOLOGIC DIAGNOSIS

Etiologic diagnosis of pneumonia on clinical grounds alone is almost impossible. Sputum should be examined for a predominant organism in any patient suspected to have a bacterial pneumonia, and blood and pleural fluid (if present) should be cultured. A sputum specimen with fewer than 10 white blood cells or with more than 25 epithelial cells per high-power field under a microscope is considered to be contaminated with oral secretions and is unsatisfactory for diagnosis. Acid-fast stains and cultures are used to identify *Mycobacterium* and *Nocardia* spp. Most fungal pneumonias are diagnosed on the basis of culture of sputum or lung tissue. Viral infection may be diagnosed by demonstration of antigen in secretions or cultures or by an antibody response. Serologic studies can be used to identify viruses, *M pneumoniae, C burnetii, Chlamydia* species, *Legionella, Francisella,* and *Yersinia.* A rise in serum cold agglutinins may be associated with *M pneumoniae* infection, but the test is positive in only 60 to 70 percent of patients with this pathogen.

Rapid diagnostic tests, as described in previous sections, are available to identify respiratory viruses; the direct fluorescent-antibody test is used for *Legionella* species. A sputum quellung test can specify *S pneumoniae* by serotype.

Some organisms that may colonize the respiratory tract are considered to be pathogens only when they are shown to be invading the parenchyma. Diagnosis of pneumonia due to cytomegalovirus, herpes simplex virus, *Aspergillus* spp, or *Candida* spp require specimens obtained by transbronchial or open-lung biopsy. *Pneumocystis carinii* can be found by silver stain of expectorated sputum. However, if the sputum is negative, deeper specimens from the respiratory tract obtained by bronchoscopy or by lung biopsy are needed for confirmatory diagnosis.

PREVENTION AND TREATMENT

Until the organism causing the infection is identified, decisions on therapy are based upon clinical history, including history of exposure, age, underlying disease and therapies, past pneumonias, geographic location, severity of illness, clinical symptoms, and sputum examination. Once a diagnosis is made, therapy is directed at the specific organism responsible.

The pneumococcal vaccine should be given to any patient at high risk for developing pneumococcal infections, including asplenic patients, the elderly, and any patients immunocompromised through disease or medical therapy. Yearly influenza vaccinations should also be provided for these particular groups. An enteric-coated vaccine prepared from certain serotypes of adenoviruses is available, but is used mainly in military recruits.

REFERENCES

Beneson AS (ed): Control of Communicable Diseases in Man. 14th Ed. American Public Health Association, 1985

Cates KL: Clinical considerations in the diagnosis of viral respiratory infections. Diagn Microbiol Infect Dis 4:235, 1986

Donowitz CR, Mandell GL: Acute pneumonia. p. 540. In Mandell GL, Douglas RG, Bennett JE (eds): Principles and Practice of Infectious Diseases. 3rd Ed. Churchill Livingstone, New York, 1990

Gwaltney JM, Jr: Virology and immunology of the common cold. Rhinology 23:265, 1985

Hedges JR, Lowe RA: Approach to acute pharyngitis. Emerg Med Clin North Am 5:335, 1987

Liu C: Epiglottitis, laryngitis, and laryngotracheobronchitis. p. 328. In Hoeprich PD, Jordan MC (eds): Infectious diseases. JB Lippincott, Philadelphia, 1989

McMillan JA et al: Viral and bacterial organisms associated with acute pharyngitis in a school-aged population. J Pediat 109:747, 1986

Rubin RH, Greene R: Etiology and management of the compromised patient with fever and pulmonary infiltrates. p. 131. In Rubin RH, Young LS (eds): Clinical Approach to Infection in the Compromised Host. 2nd Ed. Plenum, New York, 1988

Steele RW: Antiviral agents for respiratory infections. Pediat Infect Dis J 7:457, 1988

94 MICROBIOLOGY OF THE CIRCULATORY SYSTEM

LAWRENCE L. PELLETIER, JR.

GENERAL CONCEPTS

MICROBEMIA

Etiology

Gram-negative enteric bacilli, *Staphylococcus aureus,* and *Streptococcus pneumoniae* are the most common pathogens in the United States. Of these, the most likely agent of a given case of microbemia depends on host characteristics (age, granulocyte count, associated conditions, prior antimicrobial therapy) and epidemiologic setting (community vs. hospital-acquired, travel, animal exposure, etc.).

Pathogenesis

Microbes generally enter the circulatory system via the lymphatics from areas of localized infection or from diseased skin and mucous membranes colonized by members of the normal bacterial flora.

Clinical Manifestations

Microbemias may be asymptomatic, symptomatic, transient, continuous, or intermittent. Microbemias due to small numbers of relatively nonpathogenic microorganisms are usually asymptomatic. Larger inocula or more pathogenic organisms may produce **systemic** signs and symptoms: fever, chills, rigors, sweating, malaise, sleepiness, and fatigue.

Microbiologic Diagnosis

Techniques used in diagnosis include cultures of localized sites of infection, multiple blood cultures, and (rarely) blood serology.

Prevention and Treatment

Prevention in hospitals consists of hand-washing by personnel in contact with patients and avoidance of unnecessary urinary and intravenous catheterization. After samples are taken for culturing, treatment with intravenous broad-spectrum antimicrobial agents is usually begun, based on an estimate of the most likely organisms and their usual antimicrobial susceptibility patterns. This empirical therapy is modified if necessary when the pathogen and its susceptibility pattern are identified.

SEPTIC SHOCK

Etiology

Gram-negative enteric bacilli are the most common causes of septic shock, but the syndrome may be produced by a wide range of microorganisms.

Pathogenesis

Vascular injury from the microbes and release of inflammatory mediators cause local circulatory failure and multiorgan failure.

Clinical Manifestations

Manifestations of septic shock are widespread; they include hypotension, hypoxia, respiratory failure, lactic acidosis, renal failure, disseminated intravascular coagulation, and bleeding.

Microbiologic Diagnosis

Diagnosis is made by culturing local infections thought to be the source of microbemia and by culturing the blood.

Prevention and Treatment

Preventive measures are the same as for microbemia. Treatment consists of high-dose intravenous broad-spectrum antimicrobial agents, intravenous fluids, supplemental oxygen therapy, mechanical ventilation, hemodialysis, and transfusions of blood products and clotting factors, as needed.

INFECTIVE ENDOCARDITIS

Etiology

Staphylococcus aureus, viridans streptococci, and enterococci are the most common causes of endocarditis.

Pathogenesis

Microbes that enter the blood lodge on heart valves. Previously damaged heart valves are more susceptible. Bacterial colonies become covered with fibrin and plate-lets, which protect the organisms from phagocytes and complement. Clots may dislodge as infected emboli.

Clinical Manifestations

Infective endocarditis may affect native or abnormal cardiac valves, prosthetic valves, and, secondarily, other intravascular sites. Manifestations include fever, malaise, fatigue, weight loss, skin petechiae, embolic infarction of vital organs, and valve dysfunction with congestive failure. Metastatic infection in acute endocarditis is caused by virulent organisms.

Microbiologic Diagnosis

Infective endocarditis is diagnosed through blood cultures.

Prevention and Treatment

Antimicrobial prophylaxis is administered to patients with defective heart valves who are undergoing dental and other procedures known to produce bacteremia. Therapy consists of prolonged intravenous treatment with bactericidal antibiotics to eradicate bacteria within the protective clot. Surgical replacement of infected valves may be required to cure prosthetic valve infections.

INTRODUCTION

The circulatory system, consisting of the blood, blood vessels, and the heart, is normally free of microbial organisms. Isolation of bacteria or fungi from the blood of ill patients usually signifies serious and uncontrolled infection that may result in death. The presence of bacteria (**bacteremia**) and fungi (**fungemia**) in the blood occurs in more than 250,000 individuals per year in the United States and causes at least 50,000 deaths annually. Because rapid isolation, identification, and performance of antimicrobial susceptibility tests may lead to initiation of lifesaving measures, the culturing of blood to detect microbemia is one of the most important clinical microbiology laboratory procedures. Bacteremia may be prevented in some instances by the early recognition of localized in-fection and initiation of appropriate treatment with antimicrobial agents and surgical drainage of abscesses.

CLINICAL SYNDROMES

Microbemia

Asymptomatic Microbemia

Microbes enter the circulatory system via lymphatic drainage from localized sites of infection or mucosal surfaces that are subject to trauma and are colonized with members of the normal bacterial flora. Organisms may also be introduced directly into the bloodstream by infected intravenous needles or catheters or contaminated intravenous infusions. A number of disseminated viral infections are also spread through the body via the bloodstream. Viremias are discussed in Chapter 45. Small numbers of organisms or non-virulent microbes are removed from the circulation by fixed macrophages in the liver, spleen, and lymph nodes. The phagocytes are assisted by circulating antibodies and complement factors present in serum. Under certain conditions, antibodies and complement factors may kill Gram-negative bacteria by lysis of the cell wall. Also, they may promote phagocytosis by coating bacteria (opsonization) with antibody and complement factors that have receptor sites for neutrophils and macrophages.

When defense mechanisms effectively remove small numbers of organisms, clinical signs or symptoms of microbemia may not occur (asymptomatic microbemia). Asymptomatic bacteremias caused by members of the endogenous bacterial flora have been observed in normal individuals after vigorous chewing, dental cleaning or tooth extraction, insertion of urinary bladder catheters, colon surgery, and other manipulative procedures. Asymptomatic bacteremias may occur if localized infections are subjected to trauma or surgery.

Most asymptomatic bacteremias are of no consequence; however, occasionally, virulent organisms that cause a localized infection (such as a *Staphylococcus aureus* skin boil) may produce infection at a distant site (e.g., bone infection) by means of asymptomatic bacteremia. Similarly, artificial or damaged heart valves may be colonized by viridans streptococci during asymptomatic bacteremia induced by dental manipulation. Infection of the heart valve (infective endocarditis) is fatal if not treated. Therefore, individuals with known valvular heart disease who undergo dental work or other procedures that produce asymptomatic bacteremias are given antibiotics to prevent colonization of the heart.

Symptomatic Microbemia

When a sufficient number of organisms are introduced into the bloodstream, an individual will develop fever, chills, shivering (rigors), and sweating (diaphoresis). Patients with symptomatic microbe-mias usually look and feel ill. As macrophages and polymorphonuclear leukocytes phagocytose microbes, they synthesize and release interleukin-1 into the circulation. This small protein acts on the temperature-regulatory center in the brain and sets the body thermostat at a higher level. The thermoregulatory center acts to decrease heat loss by reducing peripheral blood flow to the skin (pale appearance) and increases heat production by muscular activity (shivering), resulting in a rise in body temperature. When either a high body temperature level is attained or the microbemia terminates, the central nervous system thermostat becomes reset at a lower level and acts to reduce body temperature by increased peripheral blood flow to the skin (flushed appearance) and by sweating.

Symptomatic microbemias are most commonly caused by the organisms listed in Figure 94-1. In recent years, the incidence of Gram-positive coccal bacteremias resulting from intravascular access infections in debilitated patients with serious underlying conditions has increased steadily, but Gram-negative bacillary infection still predominates. Hospitalized patients frequently have had surgery, severe trauma, or neoplasms that predispose to complicated local infections; also, these individuals' host defenses have been compromised by malnutrition, age, or corticosteroid or cancer chemotherapy. Granulocytopenia due to leukemia, cancer, or cancer chemotherapy is a frequent predisposing cause of microbemia and a reason for poor response to antimicrobial therapy. Gram-negative bacteremia is frequently due to pulmonary infections in intubated patients receiving ventilator therapy or to urinary tract infections caused by indwelling urinary catheters. Table 94-1 lists a number of conditions predisposing to symptomatic microbemia and the organisms most commonly associated with those conditions. Organisms other than those listed in Table 94-1 may produce microbemia in severely compromised hosts. Skin contaminants, such as *Staphylococcus epidermidis* and diphtheroid species, may cause significant microbemias (indicated by isolation from multiple blood cultures). Bacteremias of this type are associated with intravenous catheters or prosthetic heart valves.

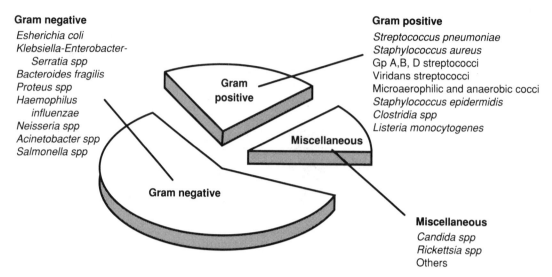

FIGURE 94-1   Common causes of symptomatic microbemia.

Transient microbemias are self-limited and often due to manipulation of infected tissues, such as incision and drainage of an abscess; early phases of localized infection, such as pneumococcal bacteremia in pneumococcal pneumonias; or bacteremias associated with trauma to mucosal surfaces colonized by the normal host flora. When multiple blood cultures are positive over a period of 12 hours or more, a continuous microbemia is present. The presence of continuous microbemia suggests a severe spreading infection that has overwhelmed host defenses. A continuous microbemia may originate from an intravascular site of infection in which organisms are shed directly into the bloodstream (e.g., infective endocarditis or an infected intravascular catheter), or from an early phase of a specific infection characterized by a continuous microbemia (e.g., typhoid fever).

Microbemias may persist despite treatment with antimicrobial agents to which the organisms are susceptible. Therefore, repeated blood cultures should be performed in patients who do not appear to respond to sustained antimicrobial treatment. During the first 3 days of treatment, positive blood cultures often are associated with inadequate antimicrobial dosage. Microbemias that persist longer than 3 days may be caused by organisms resistant to multiple antimicrobial agents, by undrained abscesses, or by intravascular foci of infec-

tion. When positive blood cultures with the same organism are separated by negative cultures, an **intermittent microbemia** is present.

Septic Shock

Septic shock occurs in approximately 40 percent of patients with Gram-negative bacillary bacteremia and 5 percent of patients with Gram-positive bacteremia. The septic shock syndrome consists of a fall in systemic arterial blood pressure with resultant decreased effective blood flow to vital organs. Septic shock patients frequently develop renal and pulmonary insufficiency and coma as part of a generalized metabolic failure caused by inadequate blood flow. Survival depends on rapid institution of broad-spectrum antimicrobial therapy, intravenous fluids, and other supportive measures. Elderly patients and those with severe underlying surgical or medical diseases are less likely to survive. Mortality from Gram-negative septic shock ranges from 40 to 70 percent. Septic shock may also occur with rickettsial, viral, and fungal infections.

Septic shock due to Gram-negative bacillary bacteremias constitutes the most common serious infectious disease problem in hospitalized patients. The high frequency of septic shock in Gram-negative bacillary infection is attributed to

TABLE 94-1 Conditions Predisposing to Symptomatic Microbemia

Condition	Mechanism	Organisms
Urinary tract catheter	Microbial colonization of urinary tract	Gram-negative enteric bacilli, *P aeruginosa*, *Serratia* spp, enterococci
Intravenous catheter	Direct access of skin flora to circulatory system	*S aureus*, *S epidermidis*, Gram-negative bacilli, *Candida* spp
Endotracheal intubation or tracheotomy	Microbial colonization of lower respiratory tract	*S aureus*, Gram-negative enteric bacilli, *P aeruginosa*
Extensive burns	Loss of skin barrier function with burn wound infection	Group A streptococci, *P aeruginosa*, Gram-negative enteric bacilli, *Candida* spp
Granulocytopenia	Loss of polymorphonuclear leukocyte phagocyte function	*P aeruginosa*, *Klebsiella* spp, other Gram-negative enteric bacilli, *Candida* spp, *S aureus*
Hypogammaglobulinemia	Loss of opsonization of microbes by antibodies	Pneumococci, *H influenzae*, meningococci
Splenectomy	Loss of fixed macrophages and antibody-producing lymphocytes	Pneumococci, *H influenzae*, meningococci
Newborns	Immature host defense mechanisms; colonization by maternal and hospital-acquired organisms	Group B streptococci, *E coli*, other Gram-negative enteric bacilli, *S aureus*, *L monocytogenes*
Acquired immune deficiency syndrome (HIV infection)	Impaired helper T-cell function	*Mycobacterium avium-intracellulare*
Contaminated intravenous infusions	Direct intravascular infusion of microbes that grow at or below room temperature	*Klebsiella-Enterobacter* spp, *Candida* spp
Abnormal heart valve	Increased likelihood of colonization of heart valve during transient bacteremias	Viridans streptococci, enterococci, nonenterococcal group D streptococci, *S aureus*, microaerophilic streptococci, *Haemophilus* spp
Prosthetic heart valve (within 2 months of surgery)	Foreign body providing site of intravascular colonization at or after surgery	*S aureus*, *S epidermidis*, Gram-negative bacilli, *Candida* spp, group D streptococci, diphtheroids
Prosthetic heart valve (more than 2 months after surgery)	Focus of colonization for transient bacteremias	Streptococci, enterococci, *S aureus*, *S epidermidis*, *Haemophilus* spp

the toxic effect on the circulatory system of lipo-polysaccharides (endotoxin) found in the cell wall of Gram-negative organisms (Fig. 94-2). Endo-toxin within the circulatory system has multiple and complex effects on neutrophils, platelets, complement, clotting factors, and inflammatory mediators in the blood. The symptoms of bacteremia and septic shock are reproduced when purified cell wall endotoxin is injected into the circulation.

Infective Endocarditis

Heart valve infections generally are classified as acute endocarditis, subacute endocarditis, and prosthetic valve endocarditis. If they are untreated, these infections are fatal. With treatment, mortality averages 30 percent; it is higher in acute and prosthetic valve infections.

Acute endocarditis usually occurs when heart valves are colonized by virulent bacteria in the course of microbemia (Fig. 94-3). The most common cause of acute endocarditis is *Staphylococcus aureus;* other less common causes are *Streptococcus pneumoniae, Neisseria gonorrhoeae, Streptococcus pyogenes,* and *Streptococcus faecalis* (enterococcus). Pa-tients with acute endocarditis usually have fever, marked prostration, and signs of infection at other sites. Infected heart valves may be destroyed rapidly, leading to heart failure from valve leaflet perforation and acute valvular insufficiency. Infected pieces of fibrin and platelet vegetations on the valves may break loose into the circulation and lodge at distant sites, producing damage to target organs. Metastatic infection due to emboli may involve arterial walls (mycotic aneurysm) or produce abscesses.

Patients with **subacute endocarditis** usually have underlying valvular heart disease and are infected by less virulent organisms such as viridans streptococci, enterococci, nonenterococcal group D streptococci, microaerophilic streptococci, and *Haemophilus* species. Frequently, the source and onset of infection are not clear, and patients consult physicians with complaints of fever, weight loss, or symptoms related to embolic phenomenon and congestive heart failure.

Prosthetic valvular endocarditis may present either acute or subacute in onset, and the infecting organisms differ, depending on whether endocarditis develops within 2 months of surgery or later (Table 94-1). Whereas infections on nonprosthetic

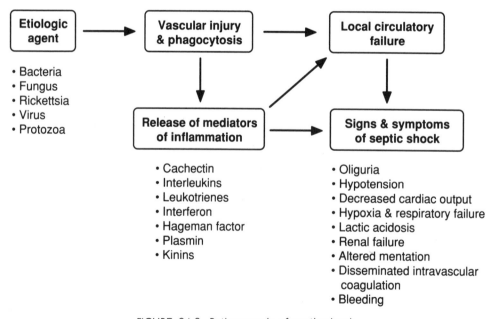

FIGURE 94-2 Pathogenesis of septic shock.

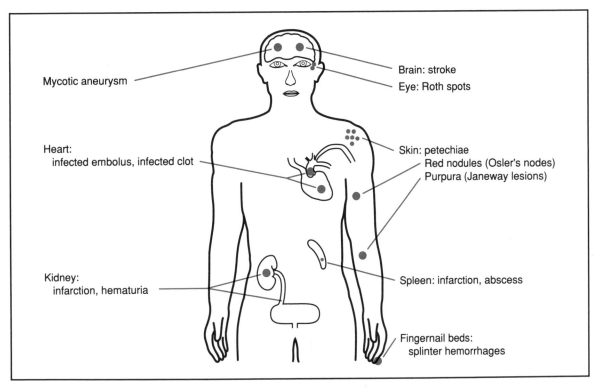

FIGURE 94-3 Infective endocarditis: metastatic infections due to emboli.

valves usually are eradicated by antimicrobial therapy alone, prosthetic valve infections frequently require surgical removal of the infected valve before the infection is eliminated. Antimicrobial therapy of endocarditis is prolonged and should be guided by susceptibility studies. Fungal endocarditis is rare, but *Candida* infections occur in those with prosthetic valves and in drug addicts. *Aspergillus* endocarditis may occur after cardiac valve surgery.

BLOOD CULTURES

Because several commercial blood culture systems are used by clinical microbiology laboratories, blood culture specimens may be processed differently by different laboratories. Most clinical laboratories will give a preliminary report of a negative culture if no growth is detected after 4 days of incubation. A final negative report is made if there is no growth after 7 days of incubation.

Clinicians should know when it is necessary for

the laboratory to use special or nonroutine blood culture techniques to detect microorganisms. Failure to tell the clinical laboratory about the need for special culture conditions may result in false-negative blood culture reports.

If the patient has received antimicrobial agents before the blood specimen was obtained, the clinical laboratory can add penicillinase to remove β-lactam antibiotics, use an antimicrobial removal device or special resin bottle to remove or inactivate the antimicrobial agent, or prolong blood incubation for 2 weeks to improve the chances of obtaining a positive culture. If infective endocarditis is suspected, the blood culture bottles should be incubated for 2 weeks to allow growth of slow-growing or fastidious microorganisms. When fungemia is suspected, special media and techniques are used to grow fungi. When *Mycobacterium avium-intracellulare* bacteremia is suspected in patients with human immunodeficiency virus (HIV) infection, the laboratory must be alerted to use special mycobacterium culture bottles and media.

Special culture techniques or media are required for the isolation of brucellae, *Listeria monocytogenes,* leptospires, *Francisella tularensis,* and *Mycoplasma hominis.*

If a central venous catheter infection is suspected, blood should be drawn both from the line and from a peripheral vein, and the results of quantitative cultures compared. If the catheter blood culture has a 10-fold greater count than the peripheral blood culture or has more than 100 CFU/ml, the catheter is probably infected. Semiquantitative culture of peripheral intravenous catheters may also help establish whether they are the portal of entry for bacteremia. When the results of blood cultures do not fit with the clinical condition of an infected patient, the clinician should review the situation with the clinical microbiology laboratory director or an infectious diseases specialist.

REFERENCES

Benezra D, Kiehn TE, Gold JWM et al: Prospective study of infections in indwelling central venous catheters using quantitative blood cultures. Am J Med 85:495, 1988

Bisno AL, Dismukes WE, Durack DT et al: Antimicrobial treatment of infective endocarditis due to viridans streptococci, enterococci, and staphylococci. J Am Med Assoc 261:1471, 1989

Bryan CS, Reynolds KL, Brenner ER: Analysis of 1,186 episodes of gram-negative bacteremia in non-university hospitals: the effects of antimicrobial therapy. Rev Infect Dis 5:629, 1983

Harris RL, Musher DM, Bloom K et al: Manifestations of sepsis. Arch Intern Med 147:1895, 1987

Meyers BR, Sherman E, Mendelson MH et al: Bloodstream infections in the elderly. Am J Med 86:379, 1989

Reuben AG, Musher DM, Hamill RJ et al: Polymicrobial bacteremia: clinical and microbiologic patterns. Rev Infect Dis 11:161, 1989

Scheld WM, Sande MA: Endocarditis and intravascular infections. p. 670. In Mandell GL, Douglas RG, Bennett JE (eds): Principles and Practice of Infectious Diseases. 3rd Ed. Churchill Livingstone, New York, 1990

Weinstein MP, Reller LB, Murphy JR et al: The clinical significance of positive blood cultures: a comprehensive analysis of 500 episodes of bacteremia and fungemia in adults. I. Laboratory and epidemiologic observations. Rev Infect Dis 5:35, 1983

95 MICROBIOLOGY OF THE GASTROINTESTINAL TRACT

SHERWOOD L. GORBACH

GENERAL CONCEPTS

Composition and Distribution of the Intestinal Microflora

The intestinal microflora is a complex ecosystem containing over 400 bacterial species. Anaerobes outnumber facultative anaerobes. The flora is sparse in the stomach and upper intestine, but luxuriant in the lower bowel. Bacteria occur both in the lumen and attached to the mucosa, but do not normally penetrate the bowel wall.

Metabolic Activities

Intestinal bacteria are a crucial component of the enterohepatic circulation, in which metabolites that are conjugated in the liver and excreted in the bile are deconjugated in the intestine by bacterial enzymes, then absorbed across the mucosa and returned to the liver in the portal circulation. Many drugs and endogenous compounds undergo enterohepatic circulation. Antibiotics that suppress the flora can alter the fecal excretion and hence the blood levels of these compounds. The flora also plays a role in fiber digestion and synthesizes certain vitamins.

The Intestinal Microflora

The intestinal microflora may prevent infection by interfering with pathogens. The flora includes low populations of potentially pathogenic organisms such as *Clostridium difficile*. Antibiotics that upset the balance of the normal flora can favor both infection by exogenous pathogens and overgrowth by endogenous pathogens. If the bowel wall is breached, enteric bacteria can escape into the peritoneum and cause peritonitis and abscesses.

Bacterial Diarrheas

Enterotoxin-Mediated Diarrheas: Enterotoxigenic bacteria, such as *Vibrio cholerae* and enterotoxigenic *Escherichia coli* strains, colonize the upper bowel and cause watery diarrhea by producing an enterotoxin that stimulates mucosal cells to secrete fluid via an increase in intracellular AMP.

Invasive Diarrheas: Invasive bacteria, such as *Shigella* and *Salmonella*, penetrate the intestinal mucosa. A bloody, mucoid diarrheal stool with inflammatory exudate is produced.

Viral Diarrheas

Rotavirus and Norwalk virus are major causes of diarrheal disease. Rotavirus diarrhea affects mostly young children; Norwalk virus causes disease in all age groups.

Parasitic Diarrheas

Some protozoa (especially *Entamoeba histolytica* and *Giardia lamblia*) as well as some intestinal helminths can cause diarrheal disease.

Clinical Diagnosis

In general, enterotoxigenic bacteria and viruses affect the upper bowel, causing watery diarrhea and periumbilical pain. The invasive bacteria act primarily in the colon (*Shigella*) or lower ileum (*Salmonella*). The stool in these diseases may contain blood. Colitis is marked by painful straining at stool (tenesmus).

COMPOSITION AND DISTRIBUTION OF THE MICROFLORA

The bacterial inhabitants of the human gastrointestinal tract constitute a complex ecosystem. More than 400 bacterial species have been identified in the feces of a single person. Anaerobic bacteria predominate. The upper gastrointestinal tract (the stomach, duodenum, jejunum, and upper ileum) normally contains a sparse microflora; the bacterial concentrations is less than 10^4 organisms/ml of intestinal secretions (Fig. 95-1). Most of these organisms are derived from the oropharynx and pass through the gut with each meal. Colonization of the upper intestine by coliform organisms is an abnormal event and is characteristic of certain infectious pathogens such as *Vibrio cholerae* and enterotoxigenic *Escherichia coli*. In contrast, the large intestine normally contains a luxuriant microflora with total concentrations of 10^{11} bacteria/g of stool (Fig. 95-1). Anaerobes

such as *Bacteroides,* anaerobic streptococci, and clostridia outnumber facultative anaerobes such as *E coli* by a factor of 1,000.

The character of the bacterial flora changes not only along the length of the gastrointestinal tract but also cross-sectionally with regard to the mucosal surface. Bacteria occupy the lumen, overlie the epithelial cells, and occasionally adhere to the mucosa. Penetration of bacteria through the mucosal surface is an abnormal event; pathogens such as *Shigella, Salmonella,* and *Yersinia* invade in this way.

The same mechanisms that control the normal flora also protect the bowel from invasion by pathogens. Gastric acid in the stomach kills most organisms that are swallowed. Individuals with reduced or absent gastric acid have a high incidence of bacterial colonization in the upper small bowel and are more susceptible to bacterial diarrheal disease. Bile has antibacterial properties and thus may be another factor in controlling the flora. Forward

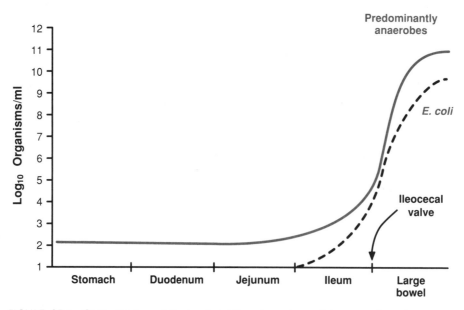

FIGURE 95-1 Concentration of the bacterial flora in regions of the gastrointestinal tract.

propulsive motility (peristalsis) is a key element in suppressing the flora of the upper bowel. Finally, the microflora itself, by producing its own antibacterial substances (e.g., bacteriocins and fatty acids), stabilizes the normal populations and prevents implantation of pathogens.

METABOLIC ACTIVITIES OF THE MICROFLORA

The metabolic capacities of the intestinal bacteria are extremely diverse. Bacterial enzymes can use as substrate virtually any compound in the intestinal lumen, whether taken orally or entering the intestine by secretion through the biliary tract or directly across the mucosa.

The Enterohepatic Circulation

Enzymes produced by intestinal bacteria play a central role in the **enterohepatic circulation.** Substances that undergo enterohepatic circulation are metabolized in the liver, excreted in the bile, and passed into the intestinal lumen, where they are reabsorbed across the intestinal mucosa and returned to the liver via the portal circulation. The enterohepatic circulation generally involves compounds that are conjugated in the liver to a polar group such as glucuronic acid, sulfate, taurine, glycine, or glutathione. Conjugation increases the solubility of the metabolite in bile, but the conjugated compounds are poorly absorbed by the intestinal mucosa. Enzymes produced by intestinal bacteria—such as β-glucuronidase, sulfatase, and various glycosidases—deconjugate these compounds, releasing the parent compounds, which are readily absorbed across the intestinal wall. Many endogenous compounds undergo enterohepatic circulation, including bilirubin, bile acids, cholesterol, estrogens, and metabolites of vitamin D. In addition, many drugs that are excreted by the liver, including digitalis, diethylstilbestrol, morphine, cholchicine, rifampin, and chloramphenicol, enter this pathway.

Many antibiotics block the enterohepatic circulation by suppressing the intestinal flora and thereby reducing the levels of deconjugating enzymes. If an antibiotic is given to a patient who is also taking a drug that undergoes enterohepatic circulation, the resulting depression of the enterohepatic circulation will increase the fecal excretion of the drug and thereby lower its plasma level and half life. For example, the blood levels and half life of the estrogen in birth control pills decrease when antibiotics are administered.

The Microflora and Nutrition

Enzymes produced by intestinal bacteria are important in the metabolism of several vitamins. The intestinal microflora synthesizes vitamin K, which is a necessary cofactor in the production of prothrombin and other blood clotting factors. Treatment with antibiotics, particularly in individuals eating a diet low in vitamin K, can result in low plasma prothrombin levels and a tendency to bleed. Intestinal bacteria also synthesize biotin, vitamin B_{12}, folic acid, and thiamine.

The intestinal flora is capable of fermenting indigestible carbohydrates (dietary fiber) to short-chain fatty acids such as acetate, propionate, and butyrate. The major source of such fermentable carbohydrate in the human colon is plant cell wall polysaccharides such as pectins, cellulose, and hemicellulose. The acids produced from these fiber substrates by bacteria can be an important energy source for the host.

Some people are deficient in intestinal lactase, the mucosal enzyme responsible for hydrolyzing the disaccharide lactose in milk. In these individuals, lactose is not adequately digested and absorbed in the intestine. Lactose that reaches the large bowel undergoes vigorous bacterial fermentation. The result can be distention, flatus, and diarrhea.

THE INTESTINAL MICROFLORA AND INFECTION
Protective Activities of the Flora

Like other complex ecosystems, the intestinal microflora is relatively stable over time, maintaining roughly constant numbers and types of bacteria in each area of the bowel. The stability of normal flora both discourages infection by exogenous pathogens and prevents overgrowth of potentially pathogenic members. New organisms that enter the system in contaminated food or water generally are suppressed by the established flora. This suppression is related to production by members of the resident flora of antimicrobial substances such as bacteriocins or short-chain fatty acids, which inhibit the growth of alien microorganisms. Antibiotics that kill off part of the intestinal flora can upset its balance and may open the door to infection or pathologic overgrowth. The pathogenesis of *Salmonella* food poisoning illustrates this phenomenon. Normal individuals are quite resistant to *Salmonella,* and a large oral inoculum is required to initiate infection. If the intestinal flora is suppressed by antibiotics, however, the individual becomes much more susceptible and can be infected by a relatively small inoculum.

Diseases Caused by Overgrowth of Potential Pathogens

The normal intestinal flora includes small populations of organisms that cause disease if they overgrow. For example, overgrowth of *Clostridium difficile* produces severe inflammation of the colon with diarrhea (pseudomembranous colitis). Administration of antibiotics initiates the process by suppressing the normal flora.

Peritonitis

Bacteria from the intestinal flora are the prime cause of infection in the peritoneal cavity when the normal barriers of the intestinal wall are violated. The intestinal wall can be perforated by trauma (knife wounds, gunshot wounds, blunt trauma), by disease (appendicitis, penetrating intestinal cancers), or by surgical procedures. Once the mucosal barrier is breached, bacteria penetrate through the intestinal wall into the normally sterile peritoneal cavity and its surrounding structures. Poor circulation, reduced oxygen supply, and dead tissue in the vicinity of the perforation promote the formation of an abscess and particularly favor the growth of anaerobic bacteria. Cultures of a peritoneal abscess generally yield several types of bacteria from the intestinal microflora, particu-

larly species of *Bacteroides, Clostridium,* and *Peptostreptococcus* and *E coli.*

BACTERIAL DIARRHEAS

Enterotoxin-Mediated Diarrheal Diseases

Several enterotoxin-producing bacteria cause diarrheal diseases (Table 95-1). The diarrheal disease caused by *Vibrio cholerae* and enterotoxigenic strains of *E coli* has three main characteristics. First, there is intestinal fluid loss that is related to the action of an enterotoxin on the small bowel epithelial cells. Second, the organism itself does not invade the mucosal surface; rather, it colonizes the upper small bowel, adhering to the epithelial cells and elaborating the enterotoxin. The mucosal architecture remains intact, with no evidence of cellular destruction. Bacteremia does not occur. Third, the fecal effluent is watery and often voluminous, so that the diarrhea can result in clinical dehydration. The fluid originates in the upper small bowel, where the enterotoxin is most active.

Cholera

The paradigm of the enterotoxigenic diarrheal diseases is cholera (see Ch. 24), in which stool volume can exceed 1 L/h, with daily fecal outputs of 15 to 20 L if the patient is kept hydrated. Cholera is caused by *V cholerae,* which is usually ingested in contaminated water. Vibrios that survive passage through the stomach colonize the surface of the small intestine, proliferate, and elaborate the enterotoxin. Cholera toxin acts via adenylate cyclase to stimulate secretion of water and electrolytes from the epithelial cells into the lumen of the gut. The duodenum and upper jejunum are more sensitive to the toxin than the ileum is. The colon is insensitive to the toxin and continues to absorb water and electrolytes normally. Thus, cholera is an "overflow diarrhea," in which the large volumes of fluid produced in the upper intestine overwhelm the resorptive capacity of the lower bowel.

Cholera stool is described as resembling rice water—a clear fluid flecked with mucus—and is

TABLE 95-1   Toxin-Producing Bacteria Associated with Diarrheal Disease

Microorganism	Action of Toxin		
	Adenylate Cyclase	Cytotoxic	Guanylate Cyclase
Vibrio cholerae	+		
E coli (heat-labile toxin)	+		
E coli (heat-stable toxin)			+
Shigella		+	
Staphylococcus aureus		+	
Clostridium perfringens		+	

isotonic with plasma. Microscopy reveals no in-flammatory cells in the fecal effluent; all that can be seen are small numbers of shed mucosal cells.

Enterotoxigenic E coli Diarrhea

Certain strains of *E coli* cause diarrheal disease by elaborating enterotoxins (see Ch. 25). These strains produce two types of enterotoxin. One, called heat-labile toxin, is similar in structure and in its mechanism of action to cholera toxin. The other, called heat-stable toxin, appears to act via guanylate cyclase. Enterotoxigenic *E coli* strains are by far the most common cause of travelers' diarrhea.

Other Diarrhea-Causing Toxins

Many strains of *Shigella* produce an enterotoxin, called Shiga toxin, that causes secretion of fluid from the small intestine (see Ch. 22). Shiga toxin has a destructive, cytotoxic effect on the small-bowel epithelium, causing gross injury to the bowel surface. It does not activate adenylate cy-clase. Another organism that produces a cytotoxin is *Vibrio parahaemolyticus,* a bacterium associated with seafood. Food-poisoning strains of *Staphylo-coccus aureus* and *Clostridium perfringens* both pro-duce enterotoxins that are directly cytotoxic. The staphylococcal enterotoxin also has a direct effect on the vomiting center in the brain.

Gastrointestinal Disease Caused by Invasive Bacteria

Unlike the enterotoxigenic organisms, invasive bacteria exert their main impact on the host by causing gross destruction of the epithelial archi-tecture; histologic findings include mucosal ulcer-ation and an inflammatory reaction in the lamina propria. The principal pathogens in this group are *Salmonella, Shigella, Campylobacter,* invasive *E coli,* and *Yersinia.* The enteric viruses also invade intes-tinal epithelial cells, but the extent of mucosal de-struction is considerably less than that caused by invasive bacterial pathogens.

Salmonella Enteritis

Salmonella species are a common cause of food poisoning. The main site of attack is the lower ileum, where the salmonellae cause mucosal ulcer-ation. They rapidly make their way through the epithelial surface into the lamina propria and enter the lymphatics and bloodstream. At least two virulence factors are associated with intestinal in-fection: one responsible for mucosal invasion, and the other causing secretion of fluid and electro-lytes into the bowel.

Shigella Dysentery

Shigella organisms cause **bacillary dysentery,** an invasive diarrheal disease of the lower bowel in which the stool contains an inflammatory exudate composed of polymorphonuclear leukocytes. The bacilli invade the epithelium of the colon and cause superficial ulceration. This invasive process de-pends on the presence of two virulence factors. The first mediates the initial penetration of the mucosal surface by destroying the brush border;

the bacteria are subsequently engulfed by invagination of the plasma membrane. The second virulence factor allows the organism to multiply within the mucosal tissue. Mucosal ulceration results, accompanied by an intense inflammatory response in the lamina propria. The infection is usually restricted to the mucosa; lymph node involvement and bacteremia are uncommon.

Fluid Production in Invasive Diarrheal Diseases

The mechanism(s) by which the fluid that causes watery diarrhea is produced in the invasive diarrheal diseases is under debate. Three mechanisms have been proposed. First, *Shigella* and possibly *Salmonella* strains apparently produce an enterotoxin that stimulates the mucosa to secrete water and electrolytes. Second, there is evidence that invasive organisms stimulate prostaglandin synthesis at the site of inflammation and that the prostaglandins induce fluid secretion. In experimental animals, fluid secretion can be blocked by prostaglandin inhibitors such as indomethacin and aspirin. Third, some evidence suggests that damage to the colonic epithelium causes diarrhea by prevention of normal resorption of fluid.

VIRAL DIARRHEAS

Two viruses—rotavirus (see Ch. 63) and Norwalk virus (see Ch. 65)—have been identified as major enteric pathogens in humans. The rotaviruses are a very important cause of infantile diarrhea, which in undeveloped countries can be fatal. Adults may be infected and shed virus, but clinical disease appears almost exclusively in children younger than 2 years. Norwalk virus, in contrast, can produce gastroenteritis in all age groups and is a cause of major epidemics. The initial lesion forms in the proximal small bowel. The mucosal architecture is damaged, with shortening of the villi and hyperplasia of the crypts. An inflammatory exudate then appears in the lamina propria.

The mechanisms responsible for fluid secretion in viral diarrheas have not been elucidated. It is

known that infection with Norwalk virus can produce steatorrhea and xylose malabsorption and causes direct damage to brush border enzymes. The activity of adenylate cyclase in the epithelial cells is not altered in the acute illness.

PARASITIC DIARRHEAS

Several species of protozoa and helminths can cause diarrheal disease. Some of these infections can be acquired in the United States, although exposure to most enteric parasites is far more common in tropical and developing countries. Some of the more common causes of parasitic diarrhea are *Entamoeba histolytica, Giardia lamblia, Strongyloides stercoralis,* and the intestinal flukes.

CLINICAL DIAGNOSIS OF DIARRHEAL DISEASE

An understanding of pathophysiology can be used to make a presumptive diagnosis in patients with infectious diarrhea (Table 95-2). Perhaps the most convenient approach is to separate pathogens that involve the small intestine from those that attack the large bowel. Enterotoxigenic bacteria *(E coli, V cholerae)*, viruses, and the parasite *Giardia* are examples of small-bowel pathogens. These organisms produce watery diarrhea, which may lead to dehydration. Abdominal pain, although often diffuse and poorly defined, is generally periumbilical. Microscopic examination of the stool fails to reveal formed cellular elements such as erythrocytes and leukocytes.

The large-bowel pathogens (the major ones being *Shigella* and *Campylobacter*) are invasive organisms and cause the clinical syndrome known as dysentery. Involvement of the colon is strongly suggested by the characteristic rectal pain known as **tenesmus.** Although the fecal effluent may be watery at first, by the second or third day of illness the stool is scanty and often bloody or mucoid. Microscopic examination almost invariably reveals abundant erythrocytes and leukocytes. Proctoscopy shows a diffusely ulcerated, hemorrhagic, and friable colonic mucosa.

Salmonella food poisoning does not fit into this simple scheme, because the disease can display

TABLE 95-2   Clinical Features of Diarrheal Diseases

	Location of Infection	
	Small Bowel	Large Bowel
Pathogens	*V Cholerae* *E coli* (LT/ST)[a] Reovirus Parovirus *Giardia*	*Shigella* *Campylobacter* *E coli* (invasive) *Entamoeba histolytica*
Location of pain	Midabdomen	Lower abdomen, rectum
Volume of stool	Large	Small
Type of stool	Watery	Mucoid
Blood in stool	Rare	Common
Leukocytes in stool	Rare	Common (except in amebiasis)
Proctoscopy	Normal	Mucosal ulcers, hemorrhagic, friable mucosa

[a] LT/ST, Heat-labile and heat-stable toxins.

features typical of both small- and large-bowel disease. The organism is invasive for the mucosa of the small intestine, particularly the lower ileum, and can cause voluminous fluid secretion. In additional, septicemia and metastatic spread of the pathogen to other organs sometimes occur.

REFERENCES

Goldin BR, Lichtenstein AH, Gorbach SL: The role of the intestinal flora. p. 500. In Shils ME, Young VR (eds): Modern Nutrition in Health and Disease. Lea & Febriger, Philadelphia, 1988

Gorbach SL: Bacterial diarrhea and its treatment. Lancet 2:1738, 1987

Gorbach SL (ed): Infectious diarrhea. Infect Dis Clin North Am 2:557, 1988

Kasper DL, Onderdouk AB (eds): International Symposium on Anaerobic Bacteria and Bacterial Infections. Rev Infect Dis 12:5121, 1990

96

MICROBIOLOGY OF THE NERVOUS SYSTEM

RICHARD T. JOHNSON

GENERAL CONCEPTS

The anatomy of the brain and meninges determines the special character of central nervous system (CNS) infections. Epidural abscesses remain localized, whereas subdural abscesses spread over a hemisphere. Subarachnoid space infections spread widely over the brain and spinal cord. The **blood-brain barrier** formed by the tight junctions between cells of the cerebral capillaries, choroid plexus, and arachnoid largely prevents macromolecules from entering the brain parenchyma. As a result, immunoglobulins and immune-competent cells are scarce in the brain except at foci of inflammation. The space between cells in the brain parenchyma is too small to permit passage even of a virus. However, tetanus toxin and some viruses travel through the CNS by axoplasmic flow.

MENINGITIS
Etiology
Major bacterial causes are *Haemophilus influenzae, Streptococcus pneumoniae,* and *Neisseria meningitidis.* Major viral causes are enteroviruses, mumps virus, and lymphocytic choriomeningitis virus.

Pathogenesis
Most agents invade from the blood. Bacteria grow rapidly in cerebrospinal fluid; viruses infect meningeal and ependymal cells.

Clinical Manifestations
Headache, fever, and stiff neck are the symptoms of meningitis. Untreated bacterial meningitis is fatal; viral meningitis is benign. Cerebrospinal fluid findings are critical in differential diagnosis.

Treatment
Antibiotics are used to treat bacterial and fungal meningitis. Viral meningitis is treated symptomatically.

BRAIN ABSCESS
Etiology
Brain abscesses usually contain a mixed flora of aerobic and anaerobic bacteria. Fungi are uncommon.

Pathogenesis
Abscesses begin when bacteria seed sites of necrosis, caused usually by infarction.

Clinical Manifestations
Headache, focal signs, and seizures indicate a brain abscess. There are also characteristic computed tomography and magnetic resonance imaging findings.

Treatment
Treatment consists of surgical drainage and appropriate antibiotics.

ENCEPHALITIS

Etiology

Many viruses cause mild meningoencephalitis; herpes simplex viruses and arboviruses are the major causes of potentially fatal disease.

Pathogenesis

Herpes simplex virus type 2 causes acute diffuse encephalitis in neonates. Herpes simplex virus type 1 causes focal temporal and frontal encephalitis in children and adults, probably owing to invasion along olfactory or sensory nerves in the immune host. Arboviruses invade from the blood and cause diffuse, predominantly neuronal infection. Rabies virus invades along peripheral nerves.

Clinical Manifestations

Encephalitis is marked by headache, fever, CNS depression, seizures, and mononuclear cells in cerebrospinal fluid. Focal temporal lobe signs occur in herpes simplex virus encephalitis.

Treatment

Acyclovir is used to treat herpes simplex virus encephalitis. Some arbovirus infections can be prevented by mosquito control or vaccines.

SLOW AND CHRONIC CNS INFECTIONS

Spirochetes

Untreated syphilis and Lyme disease can cause varied late CNS disease.

Retroviruses

Human immunodeficiency virus can cause acute and progressive CNS disease. HTLV-1 occasionally causes chronic spastic paraparesis.

Conventional Viruses

Persistent measles and rubella virus infections can cause subacute encephalitis with dementia. JC virus, a papovavirus, can cause progressive demyelinating disease in immunodeficient patients.

Unconventional Agents

Kuru and Creutzfeldt-Jakob disease are chronic, noninflammatory, degenerative diseases of the brain that are caused by unconventional agents.

Parasites

Parasites may cause acute meningitis or encephalitis, chronic encephalopathy, and cerebral granulomas. Cysticercosis is the most common parasitic neurologic disease.

INTRODUCTION

Infections of the nervous system are rare but life-threatening complications of systemic infections. The central nervous system (CNS) presents a special milieu for bacterial, fungal, viral, and parasitic infections: the brain and spinal cord are protected by bone and meningeal coverings that compartmentalize infection; they are divided by barriers from the systemic circulation; they lack an intrinsic immune system; and they have a unique compact structure.

Gross Anatomy

The brain is protected by the bony calvaria. The outer meningeal covering, the dura, is tightly bound to the bone. Epidural infections usually arise from bone infection (osteomyelitis) and remain localized (Fig. 96-1). At the foramen magnum the dura becomes free, forming a true epidural space around the spinal cord. The dura and arachnoid do not adhere to each other. Consequently, when bacteria penetrate the dura into the subdural space, infection can spread rapidly over a cerebral hemisphere. However, subdural empyema is usually confined to one hemisphere by the dural reflexions along the falx and tentorium. The subarachnoid space is a true space, containing cerebrospinal fluid (CSF) that flows from the ventricles to the basilar cisternae over the convexities of the hemispheres and through the spinal subarachnoid space. The CSF contains little antibody or complement and few phagocytic cells. Therefore, bacteria that enter this space undergo an ini-

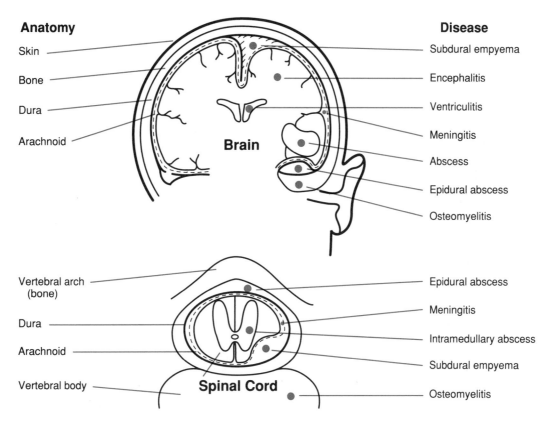

FIGURE 96-1   Anatomy and site of infection of the brain and spinal cord. (Modified from Butler IJ, Johnson RT: Central nervous system infections. Pediatr Clin N Am 21:650, 1974, with permission.)

tial phase of logarithmic growth, accounting for the often explosive onset of acute bacterial meningitis.

Blood-Brain Barrier

Dyes such as trypan blue injected into the systemic circulation stain virtually all tissues, with the exception of the brain and spinal cord. The **blood-brain barrier** demonstrated by such experiments, which excludes most macromolecules and microorganisms, is due to the cellular configuration in the cerebral capillaries, the choroid plexus, and arachnoid cells (Fig. 96-2). This barrier excludes not only most microbes, but also most immunocompetent cells and antibodies. Therefore, although the barrier deters invasion of infectious agents, it hampers their clearance once it is penetrated.

Immune System

Antibodies found in the normal CNS are derived from the serum. Levels of IgG and IgA in the CNS are approximately 0.2 to 0.4 percent of the levels in serum. Since diffusion of macromolecules across the barrier is largely size dependent, IgM is present at even lower levels. There is also no lymphatic system in the usual sense, and there are few, if any, phagocytic cells. Complement is also largely excluded.

When trauma or inflammation disrupts the blood-brain barrier, antibody molecules passively leak into the CNS along with other serum proteins. When an inflammatory reaction has been mounted against an infection, B cells from the peripheral circulation can move into the perivascular spaces of the CNS and generate immunoglobulins intrathecally.

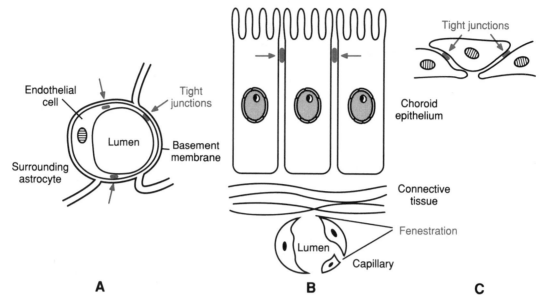

FIGURE 96-2 Blood-brain barrier. Tight junctions envelop the CNS between capillary endothelial cells, choroid plexus epithelial cells, and arachnoid cells. The cerebral capillaries (*A*) lack fenestrations, have a dense basement membrane, and have tightly apposed footplates of astrocytes. The capillaries in the choroid plexus (*B*) are fenestrated, lack tight junctions, and have loose surrounding connective tissue. The choroid epithelial cells are joined by tight junctions at their apices. Tight junctions join arachnoid cells (*C*).

Polymorphonuclear cells are usually the dominant inflammatory cells in acute bacterial infections of the CNS; they are attracted by chemotactic factors mediated primarily by components of complement activated by antibody-antigen reactions. Mononuclear cells are the dominant inflammatory cells in viral infections and in subacute infections such as tuberculosis and fungal infections. In viral infections, specifically sensitized T cells cross the blood-brain barrier into the CNS first, and lymphokines released by these cells probably recruit the entry of B cells and macrophages.

Cellular Structure

There is no brain-CSF barrier. The ependymal cells have no tight junctions, so the CSF in the ventricles and extracellular fluid in the brain are in direct contact. However, the cellular gap between neural cells measures only about 10 to 15 nm, less than the diameter of even the smallest virus, and so movement of inflammatory cells or microorganisms within the extracellular space of the brain and spinal cord is restricted.

The highly specialized nature of neural cells is important in the pathogenesis of CNS infection. Different subpopulations of neurons have different surface receptors, which have been usurped by viruses to permit entry into cells. Furthermore, both bacterial toxins and viruses can be carried by axoplasmic flow either into the CNS or within the CNS along the long axonal processes to distant but functionally linked neurons. Tetanus toxin, for example, is picked up in vesicles at peripheral axon terminals and is carried to the neuron cell body within the CNS; viruses such as rabies virus are also moved within the axon transport system (Table 96-1).

TABLE 96-1   Pathways of Spread to the Central
Nervous System

Pathway	Predominant Pathogens
Direct	
Craniotomy and skull fracture	*Staphylococcus aureus* and members of the Enterobacteriaceae
Spread from adjacent sinus	
Congenital ectodermal defect	
Via surgical shunt	*Staphylococcus epidermidis*
Neural (via axon transport)	Tetanus toxin, rabies virus, *herpesvirus simiae* (rare)
Olfactory	Herpes simplex viruses, *Naegleria fowleri*
Hematogenous	*Haemophilus influenzae, Streptococcus pneumoniae, Neisseria meningitidis, Mycobacterium tuberculosis*
	Fungi (cryptococci, coccidioides)
	Rickettsiae
	Enteroviruses, arboviruses, mumps virus, HIV, lymphocytic choriomeningitis virus
	Plasmodium falciparum, trypanosomes, tapeworm embryos

(Modified from Johnson RT: Response of the nervous system to infection. p. 1406. In Asbury AK, McKhann GM, MacDonald WI (eds): Diseases of the Nervous System. WB Saunders, Philadelphia, 1986, with permission.)

◀ MENINGITIS ▶

Meningitis is an inflammation of the pia-arachnoid meninges. It is caused by growth of bacteria, fungi, or parasites within the subarachnoid space or by growth of intracellular bacteria or viruses within the arachnoid or ependymal cells. It is therefore a diffuse infection with a variety of different agents (Fig. 96-3).

ETIOLOGY

Approximately 20,000 cases of bacterial meningitis occur in the United States each year. Seventy percent of these are in children younger than ten years. Infants are particularly susceptible because of their predisposition to bacterial infection, possible lower integrity of barriers, and immature defense mechanisms. In neonates younger than 28 days, meningitis is usually due to enteric bacilli (especially *Escherichia coli*), group B streptococci, or *Listeria* species. Neonatal meningitis represents fewer than 10 percent of cases of meningitis, but more than 50 percent of meningitis deaths. In the postnatal period, *Haemophilus influenzae* is the most common cause of bacterial meningitis, but this infection is largely limited to childhood. Adult bacterial meningitis is predominantly due to *Neisseria meningitidis* and *Streptococcus pneumoniae*, except when there has been a penetrating wound to the skull, surgery, or immunosuppression in the host. *Neisseria meningitidis* causes epidemic disease; all other forms of pyogenic meningitis are sporadic. Tuberculosis and fungi usually cause subacute meningitis. *Cryptococcus neoformans* often causes meningitis in immunosuppressed patients, but can cause indolent meningitis in immunocompetent individuals. *Coccidioides immitis* and, rarely, other fungi also cause a subacute meningitis.

Viral meningitis is even more frequent than bacterial meningitis, with probably more than 50,000 cases each year in the United States. The disease is benign and tends to be seasonal. Enteroviruses (echoviruses and coxsackieviruses) cause disease primarily in the late summer and early fall; mumps virus spreads predominantly in the spring; and lymphocytic choriomeningitis virus is more common in winter, since it is acquired from mice, which move indoors during cold weather and increase human exposure.

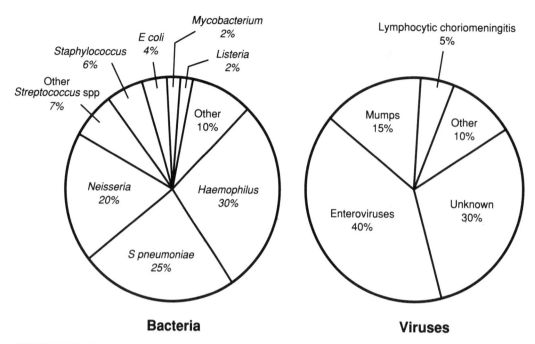

Bacteria   **Viruses**

FIGURE 96-3 Major causes of acute meningitis (all ages, worldwide). "Other viruses" include herpes simplex virus type 2, arthropod-borne viruses, Epstein-Barr virus, influenza virus, and measles virus, as well as infections caused by *Mycoplasma pneumoniae, M tuberculosis, Leptospira,* fungi and rickettsiae that may be difficult to differentiate from viral meningitis.

PATHOGENESIS

Most bacteria and viruses invade the CNS from the blood (Table 96-1), and the risk of CNS invasion is related to the magnitude and duration of bacteremia or viremia. Particles in the blood, including bacteria or viruses, are normally cleared by the reticuloendothelial system, and speed of removal is proportional to size. The bacteria that maintain a bacteremia (and incidentally cause meningitis) are largely those that elaborate capsid polysaccharides that increase their resistance to phagocytosis. Intracellular bacteria and a variety of viruses elude clearance by growing within blood cells. Enteroviruses and some arthropod-borne viruses (arboviruses) are cleared less effectively from serum because of their small size. Some viruses enter the CNS by infecting endothelial cells or choroid plexus epithelium. Indeed, in mumps virus meningitis, choroid plexus cells containing viral nucleocapsids are frequently found within the CSF.

CLINICAL MANIFESTATIONS

The primary clinical manifestations of meningitis are headache, fever, and nuchal rigidity (stiffness of the neck on passive forward flexion as a result of stretching of the inflamed meninges). Flexion of the neck may also cause reflex flexion of the legs (Brudzinski sign), and meningeal irritation may limit extension of the leg when flexed at the knee (Kernig sign). Meningeal inflammation may also be associated with some degree of obtundation (reduced consciousness), and seizures are common in children. If bacterial meningitis is not promptly treated, purulent material collecting around the base of the brain can cause cranial nerve palsies and obstruct the flow of CSF, resulting in hydrocephalus. Vasculitis develops, with infarction of the brain and multifocal neurologic deficits. Untreated bacterial meningitis is uniformly fatal. Viral meningitis, on the other hand, is benign and self-limited.

Systemic clinical signs sometimes suggest the agent (e.g., the rash or herpangina of enterovirus infections, the parotitis of mumps, or the multiple petechiae of meningococcemia). Examination of the CSF provides the most important diagnostic information (Table 96-2). Acute bacterial infections evoke a polymorphonuclear cell response in the CSF and profound reduction of CSF sugar content. Bacteria are usually visible on smears of the CSF and can be cultured if antibiotics have not been given. Subacute tuberculous or fungal meningitis is more difficult to diagnose. The inflammatory response is usually composed of mononuclear cells, and the reduction of CSF sugar content evolves slowly. Organisms are difficult to see on direct smears, although cryptococci may be identified by mixing India ink with the CSF to outline the capsule of the organism and differentiate it from mononuclear inflammatory cells. In general, viruses produce a modest mononuclear cell response, and although the CSF protein level may be elevated, the CSF sugar level is normal or only mildly depressed. Viruses such as enteroviruses and mumps virus can be grown from the CSF, but this requires special viral cultures. A rapid diagnosis may be made by demonstrating antigens of various bacterial and fungal agents or the presence of IgM against specific viral agents.

TREATMENT

Early diagnosis of bacterial and fungal meningitis and treatment with appropriate antimicrobial

agents are crucial. The mortality of untreated disease approaches 100 percent. Even with treatment, the mortality of acute bacterial meningitis remains approximately 15 percent; it is as high as 30 percent for pneumococcal meningitis. Sequelae are frequent in survivors. The mortality and morbidity have remained relatively unchanged since the introduction of antibiotics. Further reduction of death and disability rests primarily on the physician's early suspicion, diagnosis, and treatment of the disease. Viral meningitis requires only symptomatic treatment since the disease is self-limited. The prime management problem is to rule out nonviral, treatable illnesses that can mimic acute viral meningitis (partially treatable bacterial meningitis, tuberculous or fungal meningitis, syphilis, Lyme disease, etc.).

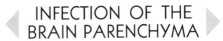

INFECTION OF THE BRAIN PARENCHYMA

ABSCESS

An **abscess** is a focus of purulent infection and is usually due to bacteria. Brain abscesses develop from either spread from a contiguous focus of infection (such as the ears, the sinuses, or the teeth) or hematogenous spread from a distant focus (such as the lungs or heart, particularly in chronic purulent pulmonary disease, subacute bacterial endocarditis, or cyanotic congenital heart disease). In many cases the source is not detected.

TABLE 96-2   CSF Findings in Nervous System Infections

Infection	Pressure	Type (Number) of Cells	Protein	Sugar	Culture
Meningitis					
Viral	Normal	Mononuclear (10–1,000)	↑	Normal	Special tests
Bacterial	Normal or ↑	Polymorphonuclear (>100)	↑↑	↓↓↓	+++
Subacute	Normal	Mononuclear	↑↑	Normal to ↓	±
Brain abscess	↑	Polymorphonuclear (small numbers)	↑	Normal	0
Encephalitis	↑	Mononuclear	↑	Normal	Special tests in some forms only

Etiology

Many brain abscesses have a mixed flora of aerobic and anaerobic bacteria. Approximately 60 to 70 percent contain streptococci; and *Staphylococcus aureus*, enterobacteria, and *Bacteroides* species are frequently present. Fungi cause fewer than ten percent of brain abscesses.

Pathogenesis

Abscesses in the brain parenchyma are thought to result from bacterial seeding of already devitalized tissue. In experimental animals, direct injection of bacteria into the carotid arteries does not lead to brain abscess, whereas injection of microspheres that occlude small vessels, followed by injection of bacteria, does lead to abscess formation. With chronic purulent ear or sinus infection, infection extending along the veins may cause infarction of brain tissue; a bacterial abscess may then evolve. In cyanotic congenital heart disease (right-to-left shunt), emboli cause small infarcts of the brain, which are then seeded by bacteria from the blood.

Clinical Manifestations

The primary clinical manifestations of abscess are headache, focal signs, and seizures. The headache may not be severe, however, and the development of signs may be insidious. There may be no fever. If focal signs are present, computed tomography or magnetic resonance imaging is performed rather than CSF examination. An abscess is identified by a hypodense area, representing pus, surrounded by an enhancing area, representing the neovascularization and edema around the fibrous abscess wall. The CSF is usually sterile, and bacteriologic diagnosis is made only by culturing an aspirate of the abscess cavity.

Treatment

If a poorly defined area of cerebritis is found, treatment is begun with multiple antibiotics to cover all common organisms. If there is encapsulation, the abscess should be drained to determine specific bacterial flora and prevent catastrophic rupture of the abscess into the ventricles.

In contrast, epidural abscesses usually cause local pain and tenderness. Pressure against a localized area of the brain may lead to focal signs. Spinal epidural abscesses and cerebral or spinal subdural abscesses are surgical emergencies. Spinal epidural abscesses have a rapid course if not diagnosed and surgically drained: symptoms start with segmental pain along nerve roots, followed by paresthesias of the body below the abscess level, and finally irreversible paraplegia. Subdural abscesses (subdural empyema) spread rapidly over a wider area. Subdural empyema causes septic thrombosis of bridging veins, leading to hemiplegia and seizures (Fig. 96-1).

ENCEPHALITIS

Encephalitis is defined as inflammation of the brain. Unlike an abscess, which is a localized area of bacterial or fungal growth, encephalitis is usually due to viruses that produce more widespread intracellular infections.

Etiology

Many viruses, including enteroviruses, mumps virus, and lymphocytic choriomeningitis virus, cause mild forms of encephalitis. Life-threatening viral encephalitis is due primarily to herpes simplex virus and arboviruses. Rabies virus causes uniformly fatal infection, but fewer than five cases occur per year in the United States.

Pathogenesis

The pathogenesis of encephalitis due to herpes simplex virus, arboviruses, and rabies virus is different for each virus. Herpes simplex virus types 1 and 2 (HSV-1 and HSV-2) both cause encephalitis. In neonates, the disease is predominantly due to type 2 virus, and irrespective of serotype the acute generalized necrotizing encephalitis is often accompanied by evidence of systemic infection of the liver, adrenals, and other organs. In children and adults, however, encephalitis is caused by type 1 virus and is usually localized. This virus, which is acquired in childhood, remains latent within the trigeminal and other ganglia. It may reactivate to cause cold sores. Encephalitis in an immune host results either from the entry of a new virus, possibly across the olfactory mucosa, or from reactivation of latent virus in the trigeminal ganglia, which spread along fibers to the base of the anterior and middle fossa. In either case, infection is localized to the orbital frontal and medial temporal lobes. Because the host is immune, virus presumably spreads from cell to cell over a contiguous localized area, infecting neurons and glial cells.

In contrast, arboviruses (mainly togaviruses, flaviviruses, and bunyaviruses) spread to the brain from the blood. The systemic infection causes few, if any, symptoms. Depending on the virus, between 1 in 20 and 1 in 1,000 infections are complicated by CNS infection. The encephalitis is diffuse, but is localized largely to neurons.

Rabies virus, in contrast, is usually acquired through the bite of a rabid warm-blooded animal. This virus spreads by axonal transport from the inoculated skin or muscle to the corresponding dorsal root ganglion or anterior horn cells and then to populations of neurons throughout the CNS. The early involvement of neurons of the limbic system causes the typical behavioral changes of clinical rabies. Polioviruses also show a selective infection of specific neuron populations, which explains the asymmetric flaccid motor paralysis of poliomyelitis.

Clinical Manifestations

Herpes simplex virus encephalitis in the non-neonate typically causes focal signs that may evolve over a period of 1 or 2 weeks. In addition to headache and fever, hallucinations and bizarre behavior are common and are sometimes confused with psychiatric illness. Focal seizures and hemiparesis are frequent, and aphasia develops if the disease is localized to the dominant temporal lobe.

Arbovirus infections cause a more diffuse and acute disease, with a rapid depression of consciousness, greater frequency of generalized seizures, and multifocal signs. At times, however, this, or any other form of encephalitis, may localize to the temporal areas, producing signs very similar to those of herpes simplex virus encephalitis.

The CSF examination for acute encephalitis may or may not show an increase in pressure, but usually reveals an inflammatory response of mononuclear cells. Examination early in disease may show no cellular response or a predominance of polymorphonuclear cells. Red blood cells are frequently found in herpes simplex virus encephalitis because of the necrotizing pathology of the disease, but they are not universally present, nor are they specific to the disease. The CSF protein level is usually elevated, and the CSF sugar level remains normal. Cultures for herpes simplex virus are usually negative. Intrathecal anti-herpesvirus antibody may be detected late in the course of disease, but too late to instigate therapy. In many of the arbovirus infections, virus-specific IgM is present in CSF even at the time of initial presentation, so rapid diagnosis is feasible.

The electroencephalogram (EEG) is helpful in the diagnosis of herpes simplex virus encephalitis because periodic spikes and slow waves often localize to the infected temporal lobe. In other forms of encephalitis, slowing is more diffuse. Computed tomography in herpes simplex virus encephalitis usually shows an attenuated area in the medial temporal lobes and sometimes a mass effect, but these findings, like the CSF and EEG changes, are not diagnostic. A prompt, definitive diagnosis of herpes simplex virus encephalitis requires brain biopsy of the area where typical encephalitis with inclusion bodies is seen, and the diagnosis is confirmed by immunocytochemical staining of herpes simplex virus antigens in brain cells or by virus isolation.

Treatment

Rapid diagnosis of herpes simplex virus encephalitis is important because a specific antiviral therapy, acyclovir (acycloguanosine), reduces the mortality from 70 percent without treatment to 25 percent if treatment is initiated prior to the onset of coma. Other forms of viral encephalitis are treated primarily with supportive care, although some arboviral encephalitides, such as Japanese encephalitis, can be prevented by vaccines and others can be reduced by mosquito control.

SLOW AND CHRONIC INFECTION AND CHRONIC NEUROLOGIC DISEASE

Chronic nervous system infections, such as those that occur during syphilis, run over many years with the unpredictable appearance of various neurologic complications. In contrast, slow infections (see Ch. 71), such as Creutzfeldt-Jakob disease, have more predictable incubation periods with a progressive buildup of infectivity followed by a disease with a predictable course lasting months or years. The slow infections resemble acute infections, with a predictable incubation period and disease course, but extend over time into months or years. Chronic or slow neurologic diseases due to persistent infection must be differentiated from chronic diseases that represent the static sequelae of acute bacterial meningitis or viral encephalitis; the former are progressive and depend on the ongoing replication of the infectious agent in the nervous system (Table 96-3).

TABLE 96-3   Slow and Chronic Infections of the Nervous System

Agent	Disease	Nature of Disease
Spirochetes		
Treponema pallidum	Neurosyphilis Meningovascular General paresis Tabes dorsalis	Acute meningitis with initial infection; chronic vasculitis, meningitis, and arachnoiditis years later
Borrelia burgdorferi	Lyme disease Primary Secondary Tertiary	Acute encephalomyelitis and/or facial palsy at time of rash; chronic encephalitis and neuropathies months or years later
Retroviruses		
HIV-1	HIV meningitis	Acute at time of seroconversion, chronic asymptomatic incubation period
	HIV encephalopathy Vacuolar myelopathy	Chronic dementia or paraparesis late in infection
	HIV neuropathy	Demyelinating (acute or chronic) during asymptomatic seropositive period or axonal neuropathy during AIDS
HTLV-I	Tropical spastic paraparesis	Chronic inflammatory myelopathy
Conventional viruses		
Measles virus	Subacute sclerosing panencephalitis (SSPE)	Progressive dementia with myoclonus years after measles
Papovavirus, JC virus	Progressive multifocal leukoencephalopathy	Progressive demyelinating disease in immunosuppressed patients
Rubella virus	Congenital rubella encephalitis and rubella panencephalitis	Progressive neonatal encephalopathy and adolescent disease resembling SSPE
Unconventional agents		
Kuru agent	Kuru	Progressive degenerative disease with ataxia
Creutzfeldt-Jakob agent	Creutzfeldt-Jakob disease	Presenile dementia with myoclonus

SPIROCHETES

Syphilis can cause varied neurologic disease over the lifetime of the untreated patient. During secondary syphilis, which sets in 6 weeks to 3 months after primary infection, a benign, mild meningitis may accompany the primary CNS invasion that occurs in approximately 25 percent of untreated patients. Later complications include acute meningovascular inflammatory disease leading to stroke (meningovascular syphilis) 3 to 5 years after the primary infection, progressive dementia (general paresis) 8 to 10 years after infection, or a chronic arachnoiditis involving primarily the posterior roots of the spinal cord (tabes dorsalis) 10 to 20 years after infection. This development of vasculitis, parenchymal involvement, and chronic arachnoiditis resembles the complications that occur over weeks during untreated bacterial meningitis. Lyme disease also may be complicated by early and late neurologic involvement. Mild meningitis may accompany the initial rash and systemic symptoms following the tick bite. In 15 percent of untreated patients, subacute or recurrent meningitis, encephalitis, cranial nerve palsies, and peripheral neuropathies develop 1 to 9 months later, and, rarely, a chronic meningoencephalitis has been described years later.

RETROVIRUSES

Two human retroviruses cause chronic diseases. Human immunodeficiency virus (HIV) infects the CNS soon after systemic infection in most patients. An acute meningitis occasionally occurs at the time of seroconversion: a variety of complications such as Guillain-Barré syndrome can occur during the long, otherwise asymptomatic seropositive period; and years later, at the time of clinical acquired immune deficiency syndrome (AIDS), dementia and myelopathy are frequent. In contrast, most persons infected with human T-cell leukemia virus type 1 (HTLV-1) suffer no neurologic disease. Rarely, a slowly progressive spastic paraparesis with inflammation of the spinal cord develops, usually during the fourth or fifth decade of life. This may follow a perinatal infection, thus having an incubation period of some 40 to 50 years.

In chronic spirochetal and retroviral infections, the CSF often has a mild mononuclear cell inflammatory response, mild elevation of protein levels, and elevated IgG levels in an oligoclonal pattern indicating the ongoing infection.

CONVENTIONAL VIRUSES

Some conventional viruses occasionally produce chronic disease: this outcome may result from a mutation of the virus or a defect in the host. Following uncomplicated measles, approximately 1 in 10^6 children develops a chronic dementia, subacute sclerosing panencephalitis (SSPE), 6 to 8 years later as a result of a defective measles virus in the CNS. Progressive multifocal leukoencephalopathy, in contrast, is due to a ubiquitous papovavirus, JC virus, which infects almost all children without recognized symptoms. In immunodeficient patients, this virus may cause a subacute or chronic demyelinating disease of the brain with multifocal signs, leading to death in usually less than 6 months. Rubella virus has also been associated with chronic encephalitis after congenital infection, and in very rare cases there has been a relapse of a disease in adolescence that resembles subacute sclerosing panencephalitis. In these infections the precise location of virus and the virus-host relationship during the long incubation period are not known.

UNCONVENTIONAL AGENTS

The unconventional agents, or **prions** (see Ch. 71), are transmissible agents in which no nucleic acid has been identified. Kuru, the first prion-mediated disease to be described, has been limited to an isolated population in New Guinea. Creutzfeldt-Jakob disease, however, occurs worldwide. It is a presenile dementia with histopathologic abnormalities limited to the CNS; the brain shows vacuolization of neurons and glia, but no inflammatory response. The disease has a course of gradually increasing severity until death, usually in less than 6 months. In experimental infection with these agents, infectivity in the brain and extraneural tissues slowly accumulates during the long incubation period, but no immune response to the agent is found in natural or experimental infection.

PARASITES

Parasitic infections such as malaria, amebiasis with free-swimming amoebae, and trichinosis can produce acute encephalopathy or meningitis. Others are associated with chronic disease, such as the chronic sleeping sickness of African trypanosomiasis, the chronic cerebral granulomas caused by *Schistosoma japonicum,* or abscesses caused by *Toxoplasma gondii* in immunodeficient patients. The commonest parasitic neurologic disease is cysticercosis caused by the larvae of *Taenia solium;* the parasitic cysts and resulting basilar arachnoiditis are the commonest causes of epilepsy and hydrocephalus in many areas of South America and Asia.

REFERENCES

Chun CH, Johnson JD, Hofstetter M et al: Brain abscess: a study of 45 consecutive cases. Medicine 65:415, 1986

Gabuzda DH, Johnson RT: Nervous system infection with human immunodeficiency virus biology and pathogenesis. Curr Aspects Neurosci 1:285, 1990

Johnson RT: Viral Infections of the Nervous System. Raven Press, New York, 1982

Kennedy PGE, Johnson RT (eds): Infections of the Nervous System. Butterworth (Publishers), London, 1987

Quagliarello VJ, Scheld WM: Review: recent advances in the pathogenesis and pathophysiology of bacterial meningitis. Am J Med Sci 292:306, 1986

Spanos A, Harrell FE, Durack DT: Differential diagnosis of acute meningitis. J Am Med Assoc 262:2700, 1989

97 MICROBIOLOGY OF THE GENITOURINARY SYSTEM

ALLAN R. RONALD
MICHELLE J. ALFA

GENERAL CONCEPTS

GENITAL INFECTIONS
Clinical Manifestations

In women, genital infections may cause a vaginal discharge, mucosal ulceration producing local discomfort and pain on intercourse, or pelvic inflammatory disease. Ongoing infection of the upper genital tract leads to infertility, ectopic pregnancies and chronic pelvic pain. In men, genital infection may cause urethral discharge, pain on voiding, and painful scrotal swellings. Genital ulcers are usually painful. Some diseases cause enlarged inguinal lymph nodes.

Etiology

Primary genitourinary infections are usually sexually transmitted; common pathogens include parasites (*Trichomonas vaginalis*), bacteria (*Treponema pallidum, Neisseria gonorrhoeae, Chlamydia trachomatis, Haemophilus ducreyi*), and viruses (herpes simplex virus, human papillomavirus, human immunodeficiency virus). Members of the normal flora, such as the fungus *Candida albicans,* may cause opportunistic infections.

Pathogenesis

Pathogens may enter the genital tract by local invasion or ascending infection. *Treponema pallidum, H ducreyi,* herpes simplex virus, etc., locally invade the skin and mucous membranes. They may also disseminate via the bloodstream to distant sites. Other pathogens such as *N gonorrhoeae* ascend through the urethra and cervix. Infants born through a genital tract infected with some of these pathogens may become infected.

Microbiologic Diagnosis

The organisms responsible for genital infections are generally fastidious and are often difficult to culture. Specimens must be correctly collected and transported. Dark-field examination and serologic studies are necessary to diagnose syphilis; specialized tissue culture or antigen detection techniques are used for *C trachomatis,* viral culture for herpes simplex virus, and specialized media for *N gonorrhoeae* and *H ducreyi*.

Prevention and Treatment

Education to modify sexual behavior and use of condoms are essential. Screening asymptomatic individuals in some populations and case contact tracing are also effective measures. Effective drug therapies exist for all bacterial genital infections and for herpes simplex.

URINARY TRACT INFECTIONS
Clinical Manifestations

Urinary tract infections in adults may cause painful, frequent urination with a feeling of incomplete emptying of the bladder, perineal pain, fever, chills, and back pain. Most elderly patients are asymptomatic, and in small children, the symptoms are nonspecific.

1189

Etiology

Most urinary tract infections are caused by bacteria from the intestinal flora. *Eschericia coli* causes about 70 percent of all infections. *Staphylococcus saprophyticus* causes about 15 percent of infections in girls. *Pseudomonas aeruginosa, Serratia marcescens,* and *Staphylococcus epidermidis* are common hospital-acquired pathogens. Yeasts, and in some parts of the world protozoa, are occasional pathogens.

Pathogenesis

Organisms can ascend through the urethra to infect the bladder and renal pelvis. Occasionally, they interfere with renal function or produce abscesses within renal tissue. Intercourse often promotes urinary tract infections in women. Pyuria is almost always present. Hydrolysis of urea by bacteria (e.g., *Proteus mirabilis*) can cause the formation of struvite stones.

Microbiologic Diagnosis

Presumptive diagnosis can be made by demonstrating pyuria. Quantitative urine culture is essential for diagnosis. Properly submitted urine that contains $> 10^5$ organisms/ml indicates significant infection. However, in urethral syndrome, bacteria are sparser. Blood cultures may be positive in patients with pyelonephritis.

Prevention and Treatment

Antimicrobial agents cure most urinary tract infections. Recurrence is common, and may be prevented by prolonged therapy. Prolonged use of a urinary catheter greatly increases the likelihood of a urinary tract infection.

INTRODUCTION

Genitourinary infections fall into two main categories: (1) primary infections due to sexually transmitted pathogenic microorganisms and (2) infections due to members of the resident flora. Genital infections are relatively uncommon in children and increase dramatically in sexually active adults, in whom sexually transmitted diseases are the second most prevalent group of reportable communicable illness in North America. Sexually transmitted pathogens include parasites *(Trichomonas vaginalis),* bacteria *(Treponema pallidum, Neisseria gonorrhoeae, Chlamydia trachomatis, Haemophilus ducreyi),* and viruses (herpes simplex virus, human papillomavirus, human immunodeficiency virus). Genital infections due to the fungus *Candida albicans* or to members of the endogenous bacterial flora *(Bacteroides fragilis* and members of the family Enterobacteriaceae) are not known to be sexually transmitted.

The urinary tract and urine are normally sterile. Numerous mechanical and biologic processes ensure that microorganisms normally do not enter the urinary tract. Women are more susceptible to urinary infections because the female urethra is short and because the area around the urethral opening is densely colonized with potential pathogens.

URETHRITIS AND EPIDIDYMITIS

CLINICAL MANIFESTATIONS

Urethritis (inflammatory disease of the urethra) is characterized by urethral discharge (Table 97-1). The incubation time varies, averaging 3 days for gonococcal urethritis and 7 days for nongonococcal urethritis. The clinical symptoms range from mild to severe. In both men and women, dysuria is common. Both discharge and dysuria are seen in 70 percent of patients with gonococcal urethritis, whereas patients with nongonococcal urethritis are more likely to have one or the other but not both. Other symptoms include itching, frequency, urgency, or a feeling of heaviness in the genitals. Polyarthralgia involving large joints, characteristic

TABLE 97-1 Genital Infections in Males

	Urethritis		Genital Ulcers		
	Gonococcal	Nongonococcal	Herpes Simplex	Chancroid	Syphilis
Incubation time (days)	2–5	5–10	3–10	3–10	21
Ulcer	—	—	Vesicle or ulcer	Deeply eroded, purulent	Painless, papule/ulcer
Urethral discharge	+++	++	+	+	+
Microscopy	Gram stain (Intracellular Gram-negative diplococci)	Gram stain (PMN, no intracellular Gram-negative diplococci)	N[a]	Gram stain insensitive (Gram-negative rod "school of fish")	Dark-field (spirochetes)
Culture	y[b]	y[c]	y	y	n[b]
Antigen detection	n	y (C trachomatis)	n	n	n
Serology	n	n	n	n	y

[a] N, Test not used for diagnosing this disease.

[b] y, Test routinely performed; n, test can be done but not routine.

[c] Culture is the "gold standard" for C trachomatis but, because of the length of time required, direct fluorescent-antibody or antigen detection methods are usually used.

rash, and low-grade fever is typically present in patients with disseminated gonococcal infection.

Orchitis and epididymitis are complications of both *N gonorrhoeae* and *C trachomatis* infections. These involvements present as a painful, swollen mass in the scrotum. Testicular atrophy follows in approximately one-half of cases of orchitis.

ETIOLOGY

Neisseria gonorrhoeae and *C trachomatis* account for most cases of urethritis in men. *Chlamydia trachomatis* is responsible for 40 to 60 percent of cases of nongonococcal urethritis (Fig. 97-1). The etiology of *Chlamydia*-negative nongonococcal urethritis is uncertain. *Ureaplasma urealyticum* can cause nongonococcal urethritis; however, the high incidence of this organism in the normal flora makes it difficult to interpret its role in nongonococcal urethritis. Less common agents isolated from nongonococcal urethritis include herpes simplex virus and *Trichomonas vaginalis*. Although gonococcal ure-

thritis is more acute than nongonococcal urethritis, overlap in the symptoms mandates laboratory confirmation. Patients often have multiple sexually transmitted pathogens. Approximately one-third of heterosexual men infected with *Neisseria gonorrhoeae* are concurrently infected with *Chlamydia trachomatis*. If only the gonococci are treated, these patients develop a nongonococcal urethritis called **postgonococcal urethritis.** Therefore, patients with gonorrhea should also be treated with agents that will effectively eradicate *C trachomatis*.

PATHOGENESIS

Neisseria gonorrhoeae and *C trachomatis* are transmitted by sexual intercourse (Fig. 97-2). *Neisseria gonorrhoeae* attaches to mucosal cells via pili and other surface proteins. The organism then is phagocytosed and passes through the mucosal epithelium. Proliferation occurs with subsequent influx of polymorphonuclear neutrophils (PMN), which

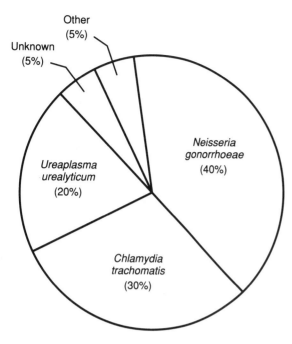

FIGURE 97-1   Major causes of urethritis.

produce the exudate that is the hallmark of gonorrhea. *Neisseria gonorrhoeae* spreads to cause disseminated gonococcal infection in approximately 1 to 3 percent of patients with gonorrhea. Disseminated gonococcal infection is more prevalent in women than in men. Up to 80 percent of patients with disseminated gonococcal infection have had an asymptomatic local infection for 7 to 30 days prior to dissemination.

Chlamydia trachomatis is an obligate intracellular parasite with a dimorphic life cycle (Fig. 97-3). Urethral infection is asymptomatic in about 30 percent of men. If left untreated, the infection can progress to cause epididymitis. Proctitis also can occur in homosexual males.

MICROBIOLOGIC DIAGNOSIS

Neisseria gonorrhoeae

Diagnosis of gonorrhea is based on microscopic examination of exudate and culturing of the organism. Urethral exudates should be examined by

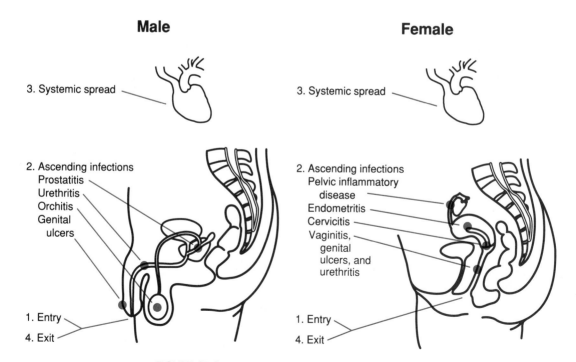

FIGURE 97-2   Pathogenesis of genital tract infections.

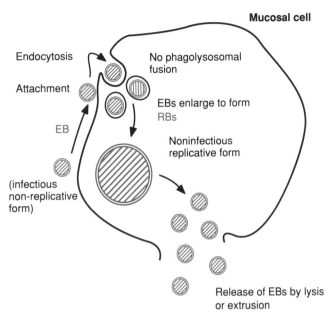

FIGURE 97-3 Replication cycle of *Chlamydia* (EB, elementary body; RB, reticulate body).

Gram stain for leukocytes and Gram-negative intracellular diplococci. The Gram stain has good sensitivity (90 percent) and specificity (95 percent) in males. Ideally, urethral exudate should be plated directly onto a split plate containing modified Thayer-Martin and chocolate agar. The Thayer-Martin agar contains vancomycin, colistin, nalidixic acid, and trimethoprim. Approximately 5 percent of strains of *N gonorrhoeae* are susceptible to vancomycin, thus necessitating the use of a noninhibitory medium such as chocolate agar. The medium is incubated in 5 percent CO_2 in a moist environment for 48 hours. *Neisseria gonorrhoeae* grows as translucent gray colonies that are oxidase positive. The identity of the cultures is confirmed by carbohydrate utilization: glucose is fermented, but lactose, maltose, and sucrose are negative. Fluorescent-antibody analysis with monoclonal antibodies may also be used to confirm the identity of cultures.

Chlamydia trachomatis

Diagnosis of *C trachomatis* infection involves growing the organism in tissue culture or using direct bacterial antigen detection techniques. Since the organism is an intracellular parasite, infected urethral cells must be collected on the swab sample. The best transport media are 2-sucrose-phosphate and sucrose-glutamate-phosphate. If swab specimens are not processed immediately, they should be stored at $-70\,°C$ prior to culturing. The swabs are then used to inoculate cell culture lines that have been treated with cycloheximide. After 48 to 72 hours, the monolayer is fixed and, after staining, is examined for chlamydial inclusion bodies. Because of the labor intensiveness of tissue culture, direct antigen detection methods have been developed for *C trachomatis*. These include either direct visualization of the organism by using fluorescein-conjugated antibodies or enzyme-linked immunosorbent assay (ELISA) methods which detect solubilized chlamydial components. Serologic tests based on either complement fixation or microimmunofluorescence are available in specialized laboratories.

PREVENTION AND TREATMENT

No vaccines exist for *N gonorrhoeae* or *C trachomatis*. Control requires modification of sexual behavior and cure of patients and their contacts.

For gonorrhea, ceftriaxone is the drug of choice. Resistance to penicillin by β-lactamase has been increasing; therefore, all isolates of *N gonorrhoeae* should be tested for β-lactamase production and susceptibility testing performed if the strain is β-lactamase positive. Gonorrhea is a reportable disease, and contact tracing is one of the prime methods of containing the spread of infection. As mentioned above, all patients being treated for gonorrhea should be concomitantly treated for the agents of nongonococcal urethritis such as *C trachomatis*. Thus, ceftriaxone combined with tetracycline is an optimal regime.

VAGINITIS, CERVICITIS, ENDOMETRITIS, AND PELVIC INFLAMMATORY DISEASE

CLINICAL MANIFESTATIONS

Endometritis and pelvic inflammatory disease usually result from ascending vaginal or cervical infections (Table 97-2). Vaginal infections seldom have systemic manifestations; they present as an abnormal vaginal discharge that may have an unusual

TABLE 97-2   Genital Infections in Females

	Vaginosis	Vaginitis	Cervicitis	Genital Ulcer	Pelvic Inflammatory Disease
Discharge	+ (pH >4.5, foul smell)	+ (thin, watery, green, frothy)	+ (purulent, yellow)	−	+ (when due to ascending infection)
Symptoms	Vaginal discomfort	Itching, discomfort	Localized vaginal discomfort	Localized vaginal discomfort	Abdominal discomfort
Microscopy	Gram stain (No lactobacilli, curved Gram-negative rods, miscellaneous other organisms)	Wet mount (*T vaginalis, Candida*)	Gram stain (for gonococcal cervicitis, Gram-negative intracellular diplococci) direct fluorescent antibody (*C trachomatis*)	Gram stain (High-level normal flora, therefore not very useful); Dark-field (spirochetes)	Gram stain (on aspirated material)
Culture	n[a,b]	y[a] (for yeasts)	y (*N gonorrhoeae*)	y (Chancroid and herpes simplex)	y (*N gonorrhoeae* or other bacteria)
Antigen detection	n	n	y (*C trachomatis*)	n	n
Serology	n	n	n	y (Syphilis)	n

[a] y, Test routinely performed; n, Can be done, but not routine.
[b] Can culture for *G vaginalis*, but not routinely done.

odor. Pruritus may also be present. The consistency of the discharge often reflects the nature of the disease. A thin, watery discharge that sticks to the anterior and lateral vaginal walls is seen in bacterial or nonspecific vaginosis; the vaginal walls appear normal. In candidiasis the vaginal walls are erythematous, and in trichomoniasis they have a strawberry appearance and the vaginal discharge is green and frothy. A yellow, purulent discharge suggests cervicitis or other forms of vaginitis. In prepubertal girls, gonorrhea causes an inflammatory response in the vagina, whereas following puberty, the infection is primarily a cervicitis. Mucosal ulceration of the vagina results in local discomfort and pain on intercourse. Abdominal discomfort is rare in vaginitis, and is more suggestive of cystitis or pelvic inflammatory disease.

ETIOLOGY

About one-half of the cases of vaginitis are due to *Candida albicans* or *Trichomonas vaginalis* (Fig. 97-4). The rest are classified as bacterial vaginosis or nonspecific vaginitis, an entity of uncertain eti-

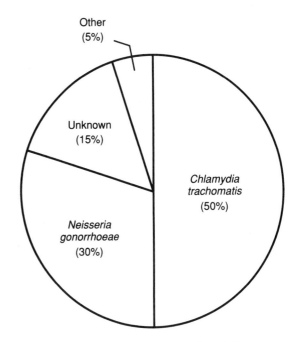

FIGURE 97-5   Major causes of cervicitis.

ology. Nonspecific vaginitis involves an upset in the distribution of the normal flora that is associated with an increase in the numbers of *Gardnerella vaginalis* and anaerobes of the *Bacteroides* group. Since 40 to 50 percent of normal individuals may carry *Gardnerella vaginalis,* isolation of the organism does not reliably predict nonspecific vaginitis; however, the absence of this organism almost rules out nonspecific vaginitis.

Neisseria gonorrhoeae and *C trachomatis* are responsible for the majority of cervical infections (Fig. 97-5). Sexually transmitted infections with more than one pathogen are common; because of the overlap in clinical features, accurate diagnosis requires laboratory confirmation. About two-thirds of women infected with *N gonorrhoeae* or *C trachomatis* do not exhibit purulent cervical discharge. Therefore, for both gonococcal and chlamydial cervicitis, physical examination is not adequate to exclude these infections. Herpes simplex virus is an occasional cause of cervicitis in women and can be isolated from approximately 90 percent

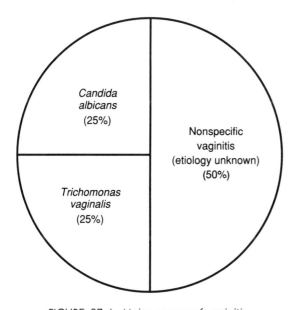

FIGURE 97-4   Major causes of vaginitis.

of women with primary herpes simplex virus infection.

PATHOGENESIS

Vaginitis due to *T vaginalis* and *C albicans* remains localized, producing vaginal discharge and itching. Yeasts are part of the normal flora in 50 percent of adult women of childbearing age. Antibiotics such as tetracyclines disturb the balance of the flora and cause overgrowth by *C albicans*, with resulting vulvovaginal candidiasis.

Trichomonas vaginalis infection is superficial; penetration of the vaginal epithelial cells has not been described. Inflammation of the vaginal walls and exocervix includes erythema, punctate hemorrhages, and small ulcerations. The pH of the vaginal discharge is often higher than 4.5.

Ascending infection may take the form of salpingo-oophoritis or pelvic inflammatory disease. The onset of ascending infection frequently coincides with menses. Ascending genital infection occurs in approximately 10 to 20 percent of women with *N gonorrhoeae* endocervical infection.

Gonococcal ophthalmia neonatorum occurs as a result of the passage of the newborn through the birth canal of infected mothers.

The infective life cycle of *C trachomatis* is summarized in Figure 97-2. The organism spreads by ascending infection from the vagina and endocervix to the endometrium, fallopian tubes, and other contiguous structures. Pelvic inflammatory disease can be an acute or a chronic complication of endocervicitis. Infection results in scarring of the fallopian tubes; this accounts for the 10-fold increase in risk of ectopic pregnancies in women with a history of pelvic inflammatory disease. Each episode of pelvic inflammatory disease also increases the chance of sterility.

MICROBIOLOGIC DIAGNOSIS

A wet mount is the optimal method of detecting *T vaginalis* or *C albicans* in patients with vaginitis. However, the wet mount is negative in 30 percent of symptomatic women with trichomoniasis and therefore does not rule out this infection. Active vaginal candidiasis is characterized by many yeast cells with active budding. Small numbers of *Gardnerella vaginalis* are often present in women who do not have nonspecific vaginitis. Gram-stained smears that contain no lactobacilli but many curved, Gram-negative rods are very suggestive of nonspecific vaginitis. According to current recommendations, a diagnosis of nonspecific vaginitis should be based on a positive Gram-stained smear in conjunction with a vaginal pH higher than 4.5 and a positive "whiff test."

Microbiologic diagnosis of *N gonorrhoeae* involves examining Gram-stained cervical exudate, as well as culturing the organism on selected media such as modified Thayer-Martin agar. The sensitivity of the Gram stain is substantially lower for exudates from women than from men: it is positive in only about 80 percent of women with cervical gonorrhea. If pelvic inflammatory disease or pelvic abscesses are suspected, material should, if possible, be aspirated from the infected site, smeared, and cultured.

Microbiologic diagnosis for *C trachomatis* is performed by either tissue culture or antigen detection techniques. Cervical mucus should be cleared and a second sample taken by vigorously rubbing the cervical orifice to ensure that cervical cells are sampled, since *C trachomatis* is an intracellular parasite. The methods used for culturing and antigen detection are described above.

PREVENTION AND TREATMENT

There are no vaccines for any of these sexually transmitted diseases. Preventive measures are directed at education with emphasis on safe sexual behavior. Barrier methods such as condoms are essential in decreasing the spread of genital infections. Contact tracing of the reportable infections has also been invaluable. *Trichomonas* infection is treated with metronidazole either as a single oral dose of 2 g or as 250 mg orally three times a day for 7 days. Treatment of candidal infection requires local application of an antifungal agent. The imadiazoles (e.g., clotrimazole or miconazole) are usually more effective than the polyenes (e.g., nystatin). The length of treatment varies from 3 to 7 days.

GENITAL ULCER DISEASE

CLINICAL MANIFESTATIONS

Genital ulcers are transmitted by sexual intercourse and can be caused by a variety of microorganisms. However, some clinical features are more common with a particular etiologic agent. Up to one-third of the episodes of genital ulceration have a clinical diagnosis that does not agree with the microbiologic diagnosis. This indicates the importance of microbiologic confirmation of diagnosis for genital ulcers. In developed countries, the most common genital ulcer diseases are herpes simplex, followed by syphilis. In developing countries, the most common causes of genital ulceration are chancroid, followed by syphilis, lymphogranuloma venereum, and granuloma inguinale. The reason for this difference in prevalence between different geographic locations is not understood. The variable incubation period for genital ulcers and the fact that initial lesions are often overlooked are two factors that lead to the increased dissemination of these diseases. Genital ulcers increase the risk of heterosexual transmission of acquired immune deficiency syndrome (AIDS).

The incubation period for chancroid ranges from 3 to 10 days. The ulcers begin as small, inflammatory papules that develop into ulcers that have an undermined edge, contain purulent exudate, and bleed easily. Chancroid is a sexually transmitted disease that is more prevalent in males than females, with a ratio of approximately 8 : 1. In men, the ulcer is located primarily on the prepuce and around the coronal sulcus. In women, the fourchette, labia, and perianal area can be involved. Multiple "kissing" ulcers (ulcers in direct opposition to each other) are common. Approximately one-third of patients with chancroid also have enlarged inguinal lymph nodes that are ex-

tremely tender. These lymph nodes may coalesce, rupture, and drain, forming buboes.

Syphilis usually presents as a small papule that develops into a painless, eroded, indurated ulcer. The mean incubation period is 21 days. If untreated, the genital ulcer disappears, and after a variable length of time, the patient may develop secondary syphilis with widespread, protean symptoms usually involving the skin with disseminated diffuse papules. The final stage of the disease, tertiary syphilis, can remain latent or appear as late syphilis consisting of neurosyphilis, cardiovascular syphilis, or gummatous syphilis.

Lymphogranuloma venereum, a disease due to restricted types of *C trachomatis,* usually begins as a painless papule that frequently goes unnoticed. The second stage of the disease involves enlargement of regional lymph nodes, and the third stage manifests as perirectal abscesses.

Granuloma inguinale also begins as a painless papule that ultimately develops into a painless, raised, beefy-red lesion.

The lesions of herpes simplex initially begin as small papules that develop into extremely painful vesicles or ulcers.

ETIOLOGY

Haemophilus ducreyi is the etiologic agent of chancroid (Fig. 97-6). This organism is a fastidious, Gram-negative rod that requires hemin. The incidence of chancroid has been increasing in the United States. Detailed information about herpes simplex virus is provided in Chapter 68. *Treponema pallidum,* a spirochete, is the agent of syphilis. *Chlamydia trachomatis* serovars L1, L2, and L3 are the agents of lymphogranuloma venereum. These strains of *C trachomatis* differ from strains that cause ocular infections and nongonococcal urethritis in being more invasive in a mouse model and more resistant to trypsin treatment. Granuloma inguinale is caused by *Calymmatobacterium granulomatis,* which is usually demonstrated as intracellular Donovan bodies visualized by Warthin-Starry silver stain or Giemsa stain of histologic sections. The disease is most prevalent in India, Papua-New Guinea, and the Caribbean.

A. Europe & North America

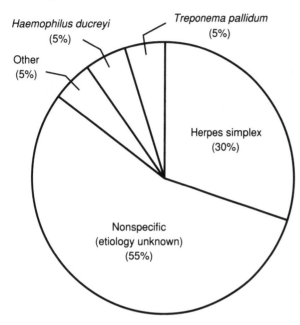

B. Africa & Asia

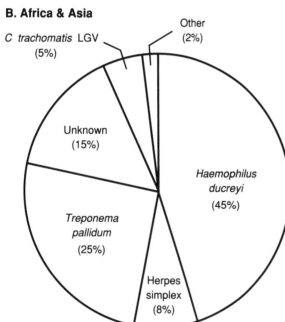

FIGURE 97-6 Major causes of genital ulcers.

PATHOGENESIS

Treponema pallidum invades intact mucosa and, after entering the lymphatics, can disseminate throughout the body to almost any organ. Obliterative endarteritis is the pathologic hallmark of syphilis and is found in all stages of the disease. *Treponema pallidum* can infect the fetus of a syphilitic mother, producing congenital syphilis.

The pathogenesis of chancroid is poorly understood, but the organism is thought to gain access through minute breaks in the mucosal epithelium. The organism is drained to the regional lymph nodes but does not disseminate further in the body. The organisms remain localized in the superficial layers of the ulcer.

Chlamydia trachomatis serovars L1, L2, and L3 and *Calymmatobacterium granulomatis* both remain localized at the site of ulceration but sometimes may show contiguous spread.

MICROBIOLOGIC DIAGNOSIS

Because the clinical symptoms of the genital ulcer diseases overlap, and because two or more pathogens may be present simultaneously, culture is critical to confirming the diagnosis. Chancroid is diagnosed by culturing either ulcer or bubo exudate. The organism is fastidious but can be grown in 48 hours by culturing on Mueller-Hinton or GC medium enriched with IsoVitaleX, fetal bovine serum, and vancomycin. The cultures grow best in a water-saturated environment at 37°C with 5 percent CO_2. Even under optimal culture conditions, the isolation rates are between 50 and 80 percent. The organism is identified by hemin requirement, alkaline phosphatase production, ability to reduce nitrate, and a positive oxidase test.

Treponema pallidum cannot be grown in vitro. Diagnosis is made by dark-field examination of ulcer material for spirochetes and by serologic detection of an antibody response. Herpes simplex is diagnosed by submitting appropriate vesicular fluid for a viral culture or antigen detection. Lymphogranuloma venereum is usually diagnosed by culturing *C trachomatis* and by examination for inclusion bodies in the inoculated cell line. Antigen detection methods using fluorescein-conjugated antibody have also proved useful. *Calymmatobacterium granulomatis* is usually detected by staining histologic sections with Warthin-Starry silver stain and observing Donovan bodies within the host cells.

PREVENTION AND TREATMENT

As with other sexually transmitted diseases, rapid diagnosis, treatment, and contact tracing help contain the spread of disease. Use of condoms and modification of sexual behavior are important preventive measures. Effective treatment is available for all the genital ulcer diseases. Chancroid is treated with a single injection of ceftriaxone. Other useful antibiotics include erythromycin, trimethoprim either with or without sulfonamides, and ciprofloxacin. Syphilis is treated with penicillin. If the patient is allergic to penicillin, tetracycline is an effective alternative. Early treatment of pregnant women with syphilis is crucial to prevent congenital syphilis. The susceptibility profiles of lymphogranuloma venereum strains are similar to those of other *C trachomatis* serovars. Tetracyclines, erythromycin, and sulfonamides are all effective. Granuloma inguinale has been successfully treated with trimethoprim-sulfamethoxazole, tetracycline, and erythromycin. Treatment should be continued for 3 weeks.

URINARY TRACT INFECTIONS: CYSTITIS, PYELONEPHRITIS, ASYMPTOMATIC BACTERIURIA, RENAL ABSCESS

CLINICAL MANIFESTATIONS

Acute cystitis is a superficial inflammation of the bladder and urethra that leads to urinary frequency, painful urination, a feeling of fullness following voiding, and suprapubic discomfort. Acute pyelonephritis is due to bacterial invasion of the renal tissue with inflammation and swelling, leading to fever, back pain, and sometimes renal dys-

function. Acute cystitis occurs together with acute pyelonephritis in about one-third of patients. Acute prostatitis occurs when bacteria invade the prostate, causing perineal pain and fever.

Infection can spread within the urinary tract, and patients often have recurrences of cystitis, sometimes interspersed with episodes of pyelonephritis. Symptoms that persist and recur are often referred to as chronic cystitis, chronic pyelonephritis, or chronic prostatitis. However, these chronic conditions are much more difficult to define. Recurring kidney infection in childhood sometimes leads to renal damage and ultimate kidney failure. Hypertension is also an occasional outcome of chronic renal infection.

Asymptomatic infections of the urinary tract—asymptomatic bacteriuria—are common. In childhood, about 1 percent of girls have asymptomatic bacteriuria. The prevalence increases to 3 to 5 percent in adult women and 10 to 50 percent in elderly men and women. Occasionally, individuals do have symptoms such as incontinence or ongoing malaise that are not associated with asymptomatic bacteriuria until it is diagnosed and treated.

Some patients have what are called "complicated urinary tract infections." These patients include individuals who have congenital or acquired anatomic abnormalities of the urinary tract. Obstruction of the urinary tract as a result of either a stone or a malfunctioning bladder secondary to a neural injury also predisposes to infection and makes infections more difficult to treat. Kidney and bladder stones can be the consequence of infection, and management of the infection is usually successful only if the stone is also removed. Many individuals cared for by urologists have underlying abnormalities of the urinary tract that make infections complicated and difficult to cure without surgical restoration of normal urine flow. Urinary catheters, used to drain the urinary tract in cases of obstruction or incontinence, bypass normal host defenses, and individuals with indwelling catheters are very prone to infections. Nosocomial urinary infections due to catheterization account for almost one-half of all infections acquired in hospitals and can lead to invasive, life-threatening sepsis.

Urinary tract infections are the most common

type of bacterial infection that causes women to seek medical care. In a given year, about 1 in 20 women have acute cystitis. Acute pyelonephritis is one of the most common infections that require hospital admission for intravenous antibacterial therapy.

Urinary tract infections are recurrent in about 5 percent of women, and the recurring cystitis and pyelonephritis cause substantial morbidity. Recurrent urinary infection in women can be due to a number of underlying causes. Sexual intercourse, the syndrome referred to as "honeymoon cystitis," is responsible for about one-half of urinary infections in sexually active adult women. These infections are not acquired from the sexual partner but rather are due to the mechanical irritation associated with intercourse. Unfortunately, women who acquire frequent infections that are associated with intercourse often have difficulty in developing healthy, normal sexual relations, and this may require special attention. The use of a diaphragm for contraception is also a major risk factor, increasing the risk of cystitis threefold.

ETIOLOGY

Organisms normally present in the intestinal tract cause most urinary tract infections. The most common of these by far is *Escherichia coli*, which is responsible for 80 percent of infections that are acquired outside of hospitals (Fig. 97-7). Other Gram-negative rods such as *Klebsiella, Enterobacter,* and *Proteus* spp are relatively common, each accounting for 3 to 5 percent of infections. Within the hospital environment, *Pseudomonas aeruginosa, Serratia marscesens,* and other, more resistant, hospital-associated pathogens account for many infections.

Gram-positive organisms, particularly coagulase-negative staphylococci and enterococci, cause some infections. *Staphylococcus saprophyticus* causes about 15 percent of urinary tract infections in young women. *Candida albicans* is also a frequent pathogen in hospitalized patients, particularly those with diabetes.

Anaerobes and fastidious organisms rarely cause urinary tract infections. A number of vi-

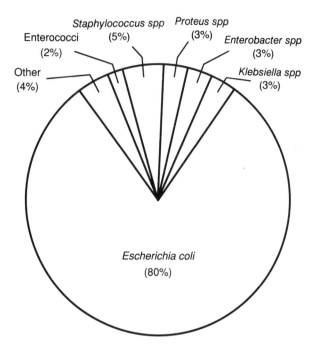

FIGURE 97-7   Major causes of urinary tract infections.

ruses, particularly mumps virus, cytomegalovirus, and coxsackieviruses, can be present in the kidneys and urine, but rarely cause symptoms or any consequences.

A number of sexually transmitted pathogens (e.g., *Neisseria gonorrhoeae*) may invade the urethra. *Chlamydia trachomatis* and herpes simplex virus can cause symptoms that mimic acute cystitis in both men and women.

PATHOGENESIS

Bacteria invade the urinary tract by ascending or hematogenous routes (Fig. 97-8). The ascending route is the more common, with hematogenous spread causing kidney abscesses.

Escherichia coli serogroups O1, O2, O4, O6, O7, and O75 are the most common agents of urinary tract infections. The most important virulence factor for these bacteria is the enhanced ability to adhere to uroepithelial cells. This attachment is mediated by specific pilus adhesins on the surface of *E coli*. The mucosal epithelial cells of women and children with recurrent urinary tract infections

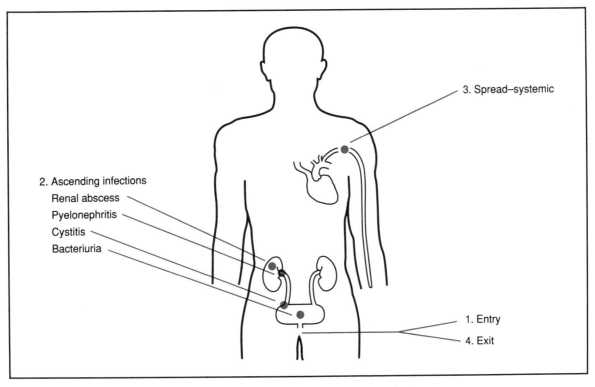

FIGURE 97-8 Pathogenesis of urinary tract infections.

have an increased avidity for attachment of *E coli*. However, phasic variation (Fig. 97-9) occurs after the organism ascends to the kidney or pelvis, and pili are no longer produced. Motility facilitates ascending infection, and bacterial endotoxins can decrease urethral peristalsis.

Alterations of urine flow by scarring, obstruction due to stones, or catheterization greatly enhances the risk of acquiring a urinary tract infection.

MICROBIOLOGIC DIAGNOSIS

The diagnosis of a urinary tract infection is confirmed by culturing the organism from urine. Most bacteria that cause urinary infection grow readily, and the clinical diagnosis of urinary tract infection is usually confirmed within 24 hours. Because urine is an excellent culture medium for a variety of microorganisms, considerable effort must be made to ensure that a urine sample is not contami-

nated during collection and that organisms are not permitted to grow before the urine is cultured. Patients suspected of urinary infection are usually asked to collect a midstream sample after cleaning the perineum or glans penis with soap and water. An early-morning collection is best because the concentration of bacteria in the urine is greatest prior to the morning voiding. The urine is then refrigerated or taken to the laboratory for immediate culture. Urine can be stored in a refrigerator for up to 24 hours without any loss of bacterial viability.

In the laboratory, a quantitative loop that samples 0.001 ml is usually used to inoculate both a nonselective medium (blood agar) and a selective medium (MacConkey agar). The cultures are incubated at 37°C. By the following day, the organism can be identified and quantitated. Cultures that represent true infection, rather than specimen contamination, are identified quantitatively. Approximately 65 percent of patients with acute cys-

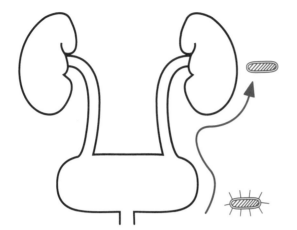

2. *E coli* isolates, non-fimbriated

Fimbriae production turned off to
decrease uptake by phagocytes

Fimbriated strains of *E coli* attach
and ascend better

1. *E coli*, fimbriated

FIGURE 97-9   Phasic variation of *E coli* in urinary tract infections.

titis have $> 10^5$ organisms/ml of urine and almost
90 percent of patients with acute pyelonephritis
and asymptomatic bacteriuria also have counts in
excess of 10^5 organisms/ml. Unless contaminated
or overgrown, most negative urine specimens have
$< 10^4$ organisms/ml. Antibacterial susceptibility
profiles of the pathogens are also analyzed. Examination of urine to demonstrate the presence of pus
cells is important. Most infections of the urinary
tract are associated with an inflammatory response. Thus, quantitative urine culture and the
presence of pyuria are straightforward, reliable
means of confirming the clinical diagnosis of urinary tract infection.

PREVENTION AND TREATMENT

Most antimicrobial agents are excreted in the
urine, and therefore many different treatment
regimens can be used to cure urinary tract infections. The most commonly prescribed agents for
acute cystitis are oral regimens of nitrofurantoin, a
sulfonamide-trimethoprim combination, amoxicillin, cephalexin, and norfloxacin. Each of these
regimens cures 90 to 95 percent of females with
acute cystitis. Long courses are not necessary, and
many studies have shown that single-dose therapy
or therapy prescribed for 3 days is as effective as
longer courses. Intravenous antimicrobial agents
are usually prescribed for patients acutely ill with
pyelonephritis or prostatitis. Aminoglycosides and

cephalosporins are frequently chosen. Longer
courses of oral antibacterial agents are useful to
prevent recurring infections in women who are
susceptible to frequent reinfections; women need
not live in fear of their next infection. If they
prefer not to take continuous preventive therapy,
the next treatment regimens should be carried for
self-initiation with the onset of acute symptoms.

REFERENCES

Barnes RC: Laboratory diagnosis of human chlamydial
    infections. Clin Microbiol Rev 2:119, 1989
Cameron DW, Simonsen JN, D'Costa LJ et al: Female to
    male transmission of human immunodeficiency virus
    type 1: risk factors for seroconversion in men. Lancet
    2:403, 1989
Holmgren K, Danielson BG, Fellstrom B et al: The rela-
    tion between urinary tract infections and stone com-
    position in renal stone formers. Scand J Urol Nephrol
    23:131, 1989
Johnson JR, Stamm WE: Urinary tract infections in
    women: diagnosis and treatment. Ann Intern Med
    111:906, 1989
Jordan PA, Iravani RA, Richard GA et al: Urinary tract
    infections caused by *S. saprophyticus.* J Infect Dis
    142:510, 1980
Kellogg JA, Manzella JP, Shaffer SN, Schwartz BB:
    Clinical relevance of culture versus screens for the
    detection of microbial pathogens in urine specimens.
    Am J Med 83:739, 1987
Krockta WP, Barnes RC: Genital ulceration with re-
    gional adenopathy. Sex Transm Dis 1:217, 1987

Lisby SM, Nahata MC: Therapy review: recognition and treatment of chlamydial infections. Clin Pharm 6:25, 1987

Meares EM: Prostatitis: a review. Urol Clin North Am 2:3, 1975

Meares EM: Long-term therapy of chronic bacterial prostatitis with TMP-SMX. Can Med Assoc J 112:225, 1975

Morse SA: Chancroid and *Haemophilus ducreyi*. Clin Microbiol Rev 2:137, 1989

Nicolle LE, Harding GKM, Preiksaitis J et al: The association of urinary tract infection with sexual intercourse. J Infect Dis 146:579, 1982

Osterberg E, Aberg H, Hallander HO et al: Efficacy of single-dose versus seven-day trimethoprim treatment of cystitis in women: a randomized double-blind study. J Infect Dis 161:942, 1990

Spence MR: The treatment of gonorrhea, syphilis, chancroid, lymphogranuloma venereum, and granuloma inguinale. Clin Obstet Gynecol 31:453, 1988

Sturm AW, Stolting GJ, Cormane RH, Zanen HC: Clinical and microbiological evaluation of 46 episodes of genital ulceration. Genitourin Med 63:98, 1987

Upchurch DM, Brady WE, Reichart CA, Hook EW III: Behavioral contributions to acquisition of gonorrhea in patients attending an inner city sexually transmitted disease clinic. J Infect Dis, 161:938, 1990

98 MICROBIAL INFECTIONS OF SKIN AND NAILS

RAZA ALY

GENERAL CONCEPTS

Etiology

Skin diseases can be caused by viruses, bacteria, fungi, or parasites. The most common bacterial skin pathogens are *Staphylococcus aureus* and group A β-hemolytic streptococci. Herpes simplex is the most common viral skin disease. Of the dermatophytic fungi, *Trichophyton rubrum* is the most prevalent cause of skin and nail infections.

Pathogenesis

Primary Infections: Primary skin infections have a characteristic clinical picture and disease course, are caused by a single pathogen, and usually affect normal skin. Impetigo, folliculitis, and boils are common types. The most common primary skin pathogens are *S aureus*, β-hemolytic streptococci, and coryneform bacteria. These organisms usually enter through a break in the skin such as an insect bite. Many systemic infections involve skin symptoms caused either by the pathogen or by toxins; examples are measles, varicella, gonococcemia, and staphylococcal scalded skin syndrome. Dermatophytic fungi have a strong affinity for keratin and therefore invade keratinized tissue of the nails, hair, and skin.

Secondary Infections: Secondary infections occur in skin that is already diseased. Because of the underlying disease, the clinical picture and course of these infections vary. Intertrigo and toe web infection are examples.

Clinical Manifestations

Most skin infections cause erythema, edema, and other signs of inflammation. Focal accumulations of pus (furuncles) or fluid (vesicles, bullae) may form. Alternatively, lesions may be scaling with no obvious inflammation. Nail infections cause discoloration of the nail and thickening of the nail plate.

Microbiologic Diagnosis

Clinical examination and staining and/or culturing of a specimen of pus or exudate are often adequate for diagnosis. Ultraviolet light (Wood's lamp) is helpful in diagnosing erythrasma and some toe web and fungal infections. Microscopic examination of a KOH preparation of skin scales, nail scrapings, or loose hair is useful for fungal infections. For viral infections, stained smears of vesicle fluid are examined under the microscope for typical cytopathology.

Prevention and Treatment

Cleansing and degerming the skin with a soap or detergent containing an antimicrobial agent may be useful. Drying agents, such as aluminum chloride, and keratinolytic agents, such as topical salicylate, are also helpful. Topical antimicrobial agents can be used for some infections, but systemic therapy may be necessary for patients with extensive disease.

INTRODUCTION

Skin diseases are caused by viruses, rickettsiae, other bacteria, fungi, and parasites. This chapter focuses on the common bacterial diseases of skin. Viral infections are also described, but of the cutaneous fungal diseases, only nail infections are included. The other fungal diseases are described in the Mycology section.

SKIN INFECTIONS

Skin infections may be either primary or secondary (Fig. 98-1). Primary infections have characteristic morphologies and courses, are initiated by single organisms, and usually occur in normal skin. They are most frequently caused by *Staphylococcus aureus, Streptococcus pyogenes,* and coryneform bacteria. Impetigo, folliculitis, boils, and erythrasma are common examples. Systemic infections may also have skin manifestations. Secondary infections originate in diseased skin as a superimposed condition. Intertrigo and toe web infections are examples of secondary infections.

Clinical manifestations vary from disease to disease. Most skin diseases involve erythema, edema, and other signs of inflammation. Focal accumulations of pus (**furuncles**) or fluid (**vesicles and bullae**) may form, but lesions may also be scaling without obvious inflammation.

METHODS FOR LABORATORY DIAGNOSIS

Specimen Collection

Bacteria

Specimens are collected with a blade or by swabbing the involved areas of the skin. When pustules or vesicles are present, the roof or crust is removed with a sterile surgical blade. The pus or exudate is spread as thinly as possible on a clear glass slide for Gram staining.

For actinomycetes, pus is collected from closed lesions by aspirations with a sterile needle and syringe. Material is collected from draining sinuses by holding a sterile test tube at the edge of the lesion and allowing the pus and granules to run into the tube. Granules are aggregates of inflammatory cells, debris, proteinaceous material, and delicate branching filaments. Pus and other exudates are examined microscopically for the presence of granules.

Viruses

Vesicles are cleaned with 70 percent alcohol followed by sterile saline. Viruses are obtained by unroofing a vesicle with a needle or a scalpel blade. The fluid is collected with a swab or with a tuberculin syringe with a 26- to 27-gauge needle. The fluid obtained from fresh vesicles may contain enough viruses for culture. Direct smears are prepared by scraping cells from the base of the lesions. The cells are smeared on a slide, fixed, and stained with Giemsa or Wright stain or with specific antibodies conjugated to fluorescein or peroxidase.

Fungi

Cutaneous samples are obtained by scraping skin scales or infected nails into a sterile Petri dish or a clean envelope. For suppurative lesions of deep skin and subcutaneous tissues, aspiration with a sterile needle and syringe is recommended. Direct mounts are made by mixing a small portion of the sample in two or three drops of physiologic saline or KOH on a microscopic slide. A glass coverslip is placed over the preparation before microscopic examination.

Cultures

Most pathogenic skin bacteria grow on artificial media, and selection of the medium is important. For general use, blood agar plates (preferably 5

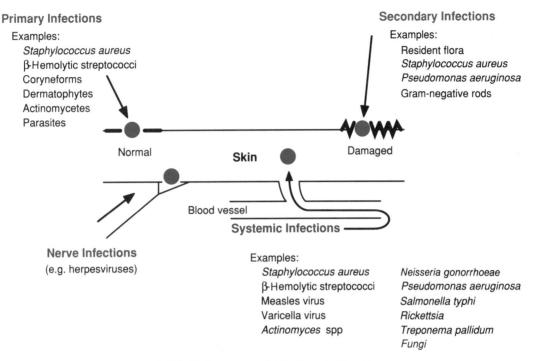

FIGURE 98-1 Spread of infections to the skin.

percent defibrinated sheep blood) are recommended. In many situations, a selective medium combined with a general-purpose medium is recommended. For example, *Staphylococcus aureus* may overgrow *Streptococcus pyogenes* in blood agar medium when both organisms are present. When crystal violet (1 μg/ml) is added to blood agar, *S pyogenes* is selected over *S aureus.* Cultures for meningococci, gonocci, and brucellae must be incubated in a CO_2 atmosphere. If tuberculosis or fungal infection is suspected, specimens are collected on appropriate media and incubated aerobically. Viruses are cultured on tissue cultures selected for the virus that may be contained in the specimen.

BACTERIAL SKIN INFECTIONS

The classification of bacterial skin infections (**pyodermas**) is an attempt to integrate various clinical entities in an organized manner. An arbitrary but useful classification for primary and secondary bacterial infections is presented in Table 98-1. The

list is not complete and includes only the more common skin diseases.

Primary Infections

Impetigo

Three forms of impetigo are recognized on the basis of clinical, bacteriologic, and histologic findings. The lesions of common or superficial impetigo may contain group A β-hemolytic streptococci, *S aureus,* or both, and controversy exists about which of these organisms is the primary pathogen. The lesions have a thick, adherent, recurrent, dirty yellow crust with an erythematous margin. This form of impetigo is the most common skin infection in children. Impetigo in infants is highly contagious and requires prompt treatment.

The lesions in **bullous (staphylococcal) impetigo,** which are always caused by *S aureus,* are superficial, thin-walled, and bullous. When a lesion ruptures, a thin, transparent, varnishlike crust appears, which can be distinguished from the stuck-on crust of common impetigo. This distinctive ap-

TABLE 98-1   Classification of Selected Bacterial
Skin Infections

Disease	Common agents
Primary	
Impetigo	*Staphylococcus aureus, Streptococcus pyogenes*
Cellulitis and erysipelas	Group A streptococci
Staphylococcal scalded skin syndrome	*S aureus*
Folliculitis	*S aureus*
Superficial folliculitis	
Staphylococcal folliculitis	*S aureus*
Gram-negative folliculitis	*Klebsiella pneumoniae, Enterobacter aerogenes, Proteus vulgaris*
Propionibacterium acnes folliculitis	*Propionibacterium acnes*
Deep folliculitis	
Sycosis barbae	*S aureus*
Furuncles or carbuncles	*S aureus*
Pitted keratolysis	Gram-positive coryneforms
Erysipeliod	*Erysipelothrix rhusiopathiae*
Erythrasma	*Corynebacterium minutissimum*
Trichomycosis	*Corynebacterium tenuis,* bacteria resembling *C minutissimum,* and lipophilic coryneforms
Secondary	
Intertrigo	Overgrowth of resident and transient bacteria
Acute infectious eczematoid dermatitis	*S aureus*
Pseudofolliculitis of the beard	Resident flora (Gram-positive cocci)
Toe web infection	Fungi, coryneform bacteria, *Brevibacterium,* and Gram-negative rods
Other diseases	
Mycobacterial infection	*Mycobacterium tuberculosis, M marinum, M ulcerans*
Actinomycete infection	*Actinomyces israelii*

pearance of bullous impetigo results from the local action of the epidermolytic toxin (exfoliation). The lesions most often are found in groups in a single region.

Ecthyma is a deeper form of impetigo. Lesions usually occur on the legs and other areas of the body that are generally covered, and they often occur as a complication of debility and infestation. The ulcers have a punched-out appearance when the crust or purulent materials are removed. The lesions heal slowly and leave scars.

Cellulitis and Erysipelas

Streptococcus pyogenes is the most common agent of **cellulitis,** a diffuse inflammation of loose connective tissue, particularly subcutaneous tissue. The pathogen generally invades through a breach in the skin surface, and infection is fostered by the presence of tissue edema. Cellulitis may arise in normal skin. However, the lesion of cellulitis is erythematous, edematous, brawny, and tender, with borders that are poorly defined.

No absolute distinction can be made between streptococcal cellulitis and **erysipelas.** Clinically, erysipelas is more superficial, with a sharp margin as opposed to the undefined border of cellulitis. Lesions usually occur on the cheeks.

Staphylococcal Scalded Skin Syndrome

Staphylococcal scalded skin syndrome (SSSS), also called Lyell's disease or toxic epidermal necrolysis, starts as a localized lesion, followed by widespread erythema and exfoliation of the skin. This disorder is caused by phage group II staphylococci, which elaborate an epidermolytic toxin. The disease is more common in infants than in adults.

Folliculitis

Folliculitis can be divided into two major categories on the basis of histologic location: superficial and deep.

The most superficial form of skin infection is **staphylococcal folliculitis,** manifested by minute erythematous follicular pustules without involvement of the surrounding skin. The scalp and extremities are favorite sites. Gram-negative folliculitis occurs mainly as a superinfection in acne vulgaris patients receiving long-term, systemic antibiotic therapy. These pustules are often clustered around the nose. The agent is found in the nostril and the pustules. *Propionibacterium acnes* folliculitis has been misdiagnosed as staphylococcal folliculitis. The primary lesion is a white to yellow follicular pustule, flat or domed. Gram stain of pus reveals numerous intracellular and extracellular Gram-positive pleomorphic rods. The lesions are more common in men than in women. The process may start at the age when acne usually appears, yet most cases occur years later.

In deep folliculitis, infection extends deeply into the follicle, and the resulting perifolliculitis causes a more marked inflammatory response than that seen in superficial folliculitis. In sycosis barbae (barber's itch), the primary lesion is a follicular pustule pierced by a hair. Bearded men may be more prone to this infection than shaven men.

A furuncle (boil) is a staphylococcal infection of a follicle with involvement of subcutaneous tissue. The preferred sites of furuncles are the hairy parts or areas that are exposed to friction and macerations. A carbuncle is a confluence of boils, a large indurated painful lesion with multiple draining sites.

Erysipeloid

Erysipeloid, a benign infection that occurs most often in fishermen and meat handlers, is characterized by redness of the skin (usually on a finger or the back of a hand), which persists for several days. The infection is caused by *Erysipelothrix rhusiopathiae.*

Pitted Keratolysis

Pitted keratolysis is a superficial infection of the plantar surface, producing a punched-out appearance. The pits may coalesce into irregularly shaped areas of superficial erosion. The pits are produced by a lytic process that spreads peripherally. The areas most often infected are the heels, the ball of the foot, the volar pads, and the toes. Humidity and high temperature are frequent aggravating factors. Gram-positive coryneform bacteria have been isolated from the lesions.

Erythrasma

Erythrasma is a chronic, superficial infection of the pubis, toe web, groin, axilla, and inframammary folds. Most lesions are asymptomatic, but some are mildly symptomatic with burning and itching. The patches are irregular, dry and scaly; initially pink and later turning brown. The widespread, generalized form is more common in warmer climates. *Corynebacterium minutissimum* is the agent. Because of its small size, the organism is difficult to observe in KOH preparations of infected scales; however, it is readily demonstrable by Gram staining of the stratum corneum. Coral-red fluorescence of the infected scales under Wood's light is diagnostic.

Trichomycosis

Trichomycosis involves the hair in the axillary and pubic regions and is characterized by development of nodules of varying consistency and color. The condition is generally asymptomatic and not contagious. Underlying skin is normal. Infected hairs obtained for microscopic examination are placed on a slide in a drop of 10 percent KOH under a coverslip. The nodules on the hairs are composed of short bacillary forms. Three types of coryneforms are associated with trichomycosis; one resembles *C minutissimum,* one is lipolytic, and the third is *C tenuis.*

Secondary Infections

Intertrigo

Intertrigo is most commonly seen in chubby infants or obese adults. In the skin fold, heat, moisture, and rubbing produce erythema, maceration, or even erosions. Overgrowth of resident or transient flora may produce this problem.

Acute Infectious Eczematoid Dermatitis

Acute infectious eczematoid dermatitis arises from a primary lesion such as a boil or a draining ear or nose, which are sources of infectious exudate. A hallmark of this disease is a streak of dermatitis along the path of flow of the discharge material. Coagulase-positive staphylococci are the organisms most frequently isolated.

Pseudofolliculitis of the Beard

Pseudofolliculitis of the beard, a common disorder, occurs most often in the beard area of black people who shave. The characteristic lesions are usually erythematous papules or, less commonly, pustules containing buried hairs. This occurs when a strongly curved hair emerging from curved hair follicles reenters the skin to produce an ingrown hair. Gram-positive microorganisms that belong to the resident flora are associated with this disorder —a clear illustration of the opportunism of nonpathogenic bacteria when the host defense is impaired.

Toe Web Infection

The disease commonly referred to as **athlete's foot** has traditionally been regarded as strictly a fungal infection. This assumption has been revised, however, because fungi often cannot be recovered from the lesions throughout the disease course. Researchers now believe that the dermatophytes, the first invaders, cause skin damage that allows bacterial overgrowth, which promotes maceration and hyperkeratosis. The fungi, through the production of antibiotics, then create an environment that favors the growth of certain coryneform bac-

teria and *Brevibacterium*. Proteolytic enzymes, which are produced by some of these bacteria, may aggravate the condition. If the feet become superhydrated, resident Gram-negative rods become the predominant flora, and the toe webs incur further damage. The fungi are then eliminated either by the action of antifungal substances of bacterial origin or by their own inability to compete for nutrients with the vigorously growing bacteria.

Other Bacterial Skin Diseases

Skin Tuberculosis (Localized Form)

Localized skin tuberculosis may follow inoculation of *Mycobacterium tuberculosis* into a wound in individuals with no previous immunologic experience with the disease. The course starts as an inflammatory nodule (**chancre**) and is accompanied by regional lymphangitis and lymphadenitis. The course of the disease depends on the patient's resistance and the effectiveness of treatment. In an immune or partially immune host, two major groups of skin lesions are distinguished: **tuberculosis verrucosa** and **lupus vulgaris.**

Mycobacterium marinum Skin Disease

Many cases of *M marinum* skin disease occur in children and adolescents who have a history of using swimming pools or cleaning fish tanks. Often, there is a history of trauma, but even in the absence of trauma the lesions appear frequently on the sites most exposed to injury. The usually solitary lesions are tuberculoid granulomata that rarely show acid-fast organisms. The skin tuberculin test is positive.

Mycobacterium ulcerans Skin Disease

Lesions in *M ulcerans* skin disease occur most often on the arms or legs and occasionally elsewhere, but not on the palms or soles. Most patients have a single, painless cutaneous ulcer with characteristic undermined edges. Geographic association of the disease with swamps and watercourses has been reported. In some tropical areas, chronic ulcers caused by this organism are common.

In **scrofuloderma,** tuberculosis of lymph nodes or bones is extended into the skin, resulting in the development of ulcers.

A disseminated form of the disease occurs when bacteria are spread through the bloodstream in patients who have fulminating tuberculosis of the skin. When hypersensitivity to tubercle bacilli is present, hematogenously disseminated antigen produces uninfected tuberculous skin lesions, such as lichen scrofulosus.

Actinomycetoma

There are several agents of actinomycetoma. About half of the cases are due to actinomycetes (**actinomycetoma**); the rest are due to fungi (**eumycetoma**). The most common causes of mycetoma in the United States are *Pseudallescheria (Petriellidium) boydii* (a fungus) and *Actinomyces israelii* (a bacterium). Regardless of the organism involved, the clinical picture is the same. Causative organisms are introduced into the skin by trauma. The disease is characterized by cutaneous swelling that slowly enlarges and becomes softer. Tunnel-like sinus tracts form in the deeper tissues, producing swelling and distortion, usually of the foot. The draining material contains granules of various sizes and colors, depending on the agent.

Actinomycosis

Actinomyces israelii usually is the agent of human **actinomycosis;** *Arachnia propionica (Actinomyces propinicus)* is the second most common cause. The characteristic appearance of the lesion is a hard, red, slowly developing swelling. The hard masses soften and eventually drain, forming chronic sinus tracts with little tendency to heal. The sinus tracts discharge purulent material containing "sulfur" granules. In about 50 percent of cases, the initial lesion is cervicofacial, involving the tissues of the face, neck, tongue, and mandible. About 20 percent of cases show thoracic actinomycosis, which may result from direct extension of the disease from the neck or from the abdomen or as a primary infection from oral aspiration of the organism. In abdominal actinomycosis, the primary lesion is in the cecum, the appendix, or the pelvic organs.

TREATMENT OF THE PYODERMAS
General Considerations

Debriding superficial pyoderma and then repeatedly cleansing the exposed lesions with topical antiseptics such as chlorhexidine removes the source of infection and minimizes its spread to adjacent skin sites or to other patients. Many secondary superficial skin infections, such as the web infections, will clear with simple twice-daily cleansing. For foot infections, the patient should wear open shoes or sandals, which permit air circulation. Aluminum chloride, a drying agent, inhibits overgrowth of opportunistic bacteria in foot, perineal, and axillary areas. Keratolytic agents (e.g., topical salicylates) remove hyperkeratotic lesions that harbor pathogens, improving the exposure of the infected skin surface to other topical treatments.

Topical Treatment

Topical antibiotics contain a combination of neomycin, bacitracin, and polymyxin. Some newer preparations contain mupirocin, gramicidin, or erythromycin, and others combine these antibiotics with steroids. For an informed, cooperative patient suffering only minimal disease, topical antibiotics are often preferred to oral antibiotics because of the adverse reactions associated with systemic therapy.

Systemic Therapy

Systemic treatment with antibiotics is mandatory for extensive pyoderma. Systemic antibiotics can be administered orally or parenterally. Oral therapy is sufficient for most extensive dermal infections, but the parenteral route is preferred for severe infections.

A wide range of antibiotics for systemic therapy of pyoderma is available (Table 98-2). The choice of a specific antibiotic should be based on two factors: isolation and identification of the pathogen, and the depth and extent of infection. In this cost-conscious world, one must also relate efficacy to consumer cost. Many less expensive antibiotics are just as effective against a given pathogen as the most expensive drugs with wider spectra.

TABLE 98-2   Acceptable Antibacterial Agents for
Treatment of Bacterial Skin Infections

Disease	Antibiotic
Staphylococcal folliculitis	Cloxacillin, dicloxacillin, erythromycin
Furuncles[a]	Cloxacillin, dicloxacillin, erythromycin, nafcillin, methicillin, cephalexin
Carbuncles	As for furuncles
Superificial impetigo	Erythromycin, penicillin, mupirocin (topical only)
Bullous impetigo	Erythromycin, cloxacillin, dicloxacillin, mupirocin (topical only)
Ecthyma	Erythromycin, penicillin
Staphylococcal scalded skin syndrome	Oxacillin, methicillin, nafcillin
Cellulitis	Penicillin, cephalosporin
Erysipelas	Penicillin, erythromycin
Erysipeloid	Penicillin, tetracycline
Erythrasma	Erythromycin
Pitted keratolysis	Topical erythromycin solution or Whitfield ointment
Actinomycosis	Penicillin
Skin tuberculosis, localized form (lupus vulgaris, lupus verrucosus)	Isoniazid
Mycobacterium marinum infection	Rifampin, minocycline
Mycobacterium ulcerans infection	Streptomycin and rifampin

[a] Most furuncles resolve with supportive therapy and do not require systemic antibiotics.

VIRAL SKIN DISEASES

Viral skin diseases can produce both localized and generalized skin infections (Table 98-3). Viruses from several major groups cause skin lesions.

Herpes Simplex Virus

Herpes simplex virus infection is probably the most common viral skin disease (see Ch. 68). Almost the entire adult population has had herpes simplex at one time or another. Herpes simplex virus, a DNA virus, is the agent. There are two types of herpes simplex virus. Type 1 is usually associated with nongenital lesions, whereas type 2 is recovered from genital lesions. The incidence of type 1 genital infections in young patients has recently increased.

Poxviruses

The viruses that cause **smallpox, vaccinia,** and **cowpox** are closely related; all are large DNA viruses (see Ch. 69). The smallpox virus is now extinct. Cowpox virus causes an infection of cattle that is acquired by handling infected animals. Vac-cinia viruses are vaccine strains developed in the laboratory and adapted to grow in the skin of humans, rabbits, and calves. Several clinical manifestations may occur in individuals who were vaccinated against smallpox with vaccinia virus. The main problem with vaccinia virus arose when it became desirable to vaccinate a person already suffering from eczema or other skin diseases; vaccination may produce eczema vaccinatum. **Molluscum contagiosum** also is caused by a poxvirus and is characterized by numerous small, pink nodules, most often on the face, genitalia, or the rectal area. Lesions also occur on the back, arms, buttocks, and inner thighs. The disease is generally harmless and self-limiting.

Papillomaviruses

Human papillomaviruses cause **warts** (see Ch. 66). **Verruca vulgaris** occurs commonly on hands and fingers as single or multiple lesions. These warts are generally painless, firm, dry, and rough. They may remain stable or regress spontaneously. **Verruca plantaris (plantar wart)** is a clinical variety of verruca vulgaris that occurs on the sole of the foot.

TABLE 98-3 Viruses Associated with Skin Infections

Disease	Virus
Localized disease	
Herpes labialis and herpes genitalis	Herpes simplex virus
Herpes zoster	Varicella-zoster virus
Vaccinia	Vaccinia virus
Molluscum contagiosum	Molluscum contagiosum virus
Warts	Papillomavirus
Generalized disease	
Measles	Measles virus
Rubella	Rubella virus
Enteroviral exanthems and enanthems	Several enteroviruses
Erythema infectiosum	Parvovirus
Roseola	Human herpesvirus 6
Hemorrhagic fevers	Several togaviruses, flaviviruses, bunyaviruses, and arenaviruses
Smallpox (extinct)	Variola virus

During standing, walking, and running, these warts push into the skin and may be painful. **Genital warts** appear as large lesions of red, soft masses that may coalesce. **Verruca plana juvenilis** (also known as juvenile flat warts) occurs most commonly in children. The lesions are in groups and may appear on the face, neck, back of the hands, and arms. These warts may also occur in adults.

Treatment

Because of the limited number of effective antiviral agents, prevention is important. Oral and intravenous acyclovir is effective for treatment of primary herpesvirus infection and for recurrent genital herpes and herpes zoster in immunosuppressed persons.

FUNGAL SKIN DISEASES

Several genera of fungi are responsible for diseases of the skin. This group of fungi, known collectively as **dermatophytes**, is discussed in the chapters on mycology. Some nondermatophytes, including yeasts, can also cause skin infections.

NAIL

The nail consists of four epidermal components: the matrix, proximal nailfold, nailbed, and hyponychium (Fig. 98-2). The matrix is close to the bony

phalanx. The horny end product of the matrix is the nail plate, which migrates distally over the nailbed. The distal portion of the matrix, the lunula, is visible as a white, crescent-shaped structure. The proximal nailfold is a modified extension of the epidermis of the dorsum of the finger, which forms a fold over the matrix; its horny end product is the cuticle. The nailbed is an epidermal structure that begins at the distal margin of the lunula and terminates in the hyponychium, which is the extension of the volar epidermis under the nail plate; it ends adjacent to the nailbed.

Fungal Infections of the Nails

Onychomycoses are infections of the nails by fungi. Universally recognized agents of these diseases are species of *Trichophyton, Microsporum* (rarely), and *Epidermophyton* (Table 98-4). These dermatophytes are commonly called **ringworm fungi**. Nondermatophytic fungi also occasionally cause onychomycoses, but usually cause only toenail problems; they rarely affect the fingernails.

Conventionally, onychomycosis is classified into four types:

1. *Distal subungual onychomycosis* primarily involves the distal nailbed and hyponychium, with secondary involvement of the underside of the nail plate. *Trichophtyton rubrum* is one

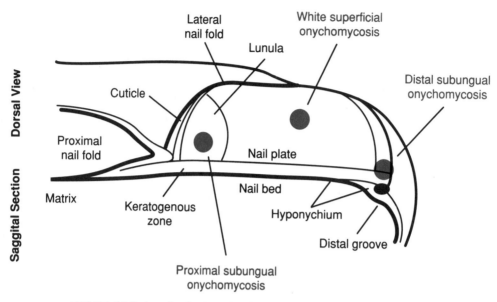

FIGURE 98-2   Longitudinal section (diagrammatic sketch) of fingernail.

of the organisms that cause this clinical type.

2. *White superficial onychomycosis* involves the toenail plate on the surface of the nail. It is caused by *T mentagrophytes* and by species of *Cephalosporium, Aspergillus,* and *Fusarium.*

3. *Proximal subungual onychomycosis* is an invasion of the nail plate from the proximal nailfold producing a specific nail condition. It is caused by *T rubrum* and *T megninii.* This is a rare type of onychomycosis.

4. *Candida onychomycosis* involves all of the nail plate. It is caused by *C albicans* and is seen in patients who have chronic cutaneous candidiasis, a syndrome associated with cellular and humoral immune abnormalities.

TREATMENT OF NAIL DISEASES
Onychomycosis

Superficial types of onychomycosis may be successfully treated. Mechanical scraping of the chalky white material on the nail plate and application of topical antifungal agents such as miconazole, ciclopirox olamine, or clotrimazole, are rec-

ommended. Newer therapeutic nail lacquers are being tested in the United States. Distal subungual and proximal subungual onychomycosis infections are much more difficult to treat. Oral griseofulvin may be required to bring about clearing of the fingernail. For toenails with extensive involvement, no treatment may be the best decision. Avulsion (removal of nail from skin) of the involved nail(s) combined with topical antifungal treatment and oral griseofulvin is another choice. No oral or topical medication is effective in eliminating nondermatophyte mold infection of the nails.

Bacterial Nail Infections

Pseudomonas aeruginosa is associated with green nail syndrome, which is essentially a greenish discoloration of the nail plate. Attempts to culture *Pseudomonas* from the deep section of the nail have not been successful; however, *P aeruginosa* has been isolated on cultures of specimens from the paronychia (inflammatory lesion around the margin of a nail). Whether there is true invasion of the nail plate by the bacteria or just diffusion of the pigment into the nail plate is not certain. Black paronychia is associated with *Proteus* species.

TABLE 98-4   Fungi Associated with Onychomycosis

Dermatophytes	Nondermatophytes
Trichophyton rubrum	*Aspergillus* spp
T mentagrophytes	*Cephalosporium* spp
T violaceum	*Fusarium oxysporum*
T schoenleinii	*Scopulariopsis brevicaulis*
T tonsurans	*Hendersonula toruloidea*
T megninii	*Scytalidium hyalinum*
T concentricrum (rare)	
T soudanense (rare)	
T gourvilii (rare)	
Epidermophyton floccosum	
Microsporum gypseum (rare)	
M audouinii (rare)	
M canis (rare)	

Staphylococci and streptococci may be found as secondary invaders.

REFERENCES

Aly R, Maibach HI: Clinical Skin Microbiology. Charles C Thomas, Springfield, IL, 1978

Aly R, Maibach HI: Susceptibility to skin infection. p. 75. In Rook AJ, Maibach HI (eds): Recent Advances in Dermatology. Churchill Livingstone, Edinburgh, 1983

Elewski BE, Hazen PG: The superficial mycoses and the dermatophytes. J Am Acad Dermatol 21:655, 1989

Maibach HI, Aly R: Bacterial infections of the skin. In Moshella S, Hurley HJ (eds): Dermatology. 3rd Ed. WB Saunders, Philadelphia, 1991 (in press)

Maibach HI, Aly R (eds): Skin Microbiology: Relevance to Clinical Infection. Springer-Verlag, New York, 1981

Noble WC: Microbiology of Human Skin. Lloyd-Luke, London, 1981

Schaffner W, Lowy DR: Rickettsial and viral diseases with cutaneous involvement. In Fitzpatrick TB, Eisen AZ, Wolff K et al (eds): Dermatology in General Medicine. 3rd Ed. McGraw-Hill, New York, 1987

99 MICROBIOLOGY OF DENTAL DECAY AND PERIODONTAL DISEASE

WALTER J. LOESCHE

GENERAL CONCEPTS

BACTERIOLOGY OF DENTAL INFECTIONS

The mouth is colonized by 200 to 300 bacterial species, but only a limited number of these species participate in dental decay (caries) or periodontal disease.

DENTAL DECAY

Dental decay is due to the irreversible solubilization of tooth mineral by acid produced by certain bacteria that adhere to the tooth surface in bacterial communities known as dental plaque.

Etiology

Streptococcus mutans is the main cause of dental decay. Various lactobacilli are associated with progression of the lesion.

Pathogenesis

The tooth surface normally loses some tooth mineral from the action of the acid formed by plaque bacteria after ingestion of foods containing fermentable carbohydrates. This mineral is normally replenished by the saliva between meals. However, when fermentable foods are eaten frequently, the low pH in the plaque is sustained and a net loss of mineral from the tooth occurs. This low pH selects for aciduric organisms, such as *S mutans* and lactobacilli, which (especially *S mutans*) store polysaccharide and continue to secrete acid long after the food has been swallowed.

Clinical Manifestations

Caries become intensely painful when the lesion approaches the tooth pulp.

Microbiologic Diagnosis

New, chair-side culture procedures allow for an estimate of the number of *S mutans* organisms in saliva.

Prevention and Treatment

The widespread use of fluoride in the water supply, in dentifrices, and in local applications by the dentist has reduced the prevalence of caries by 30 to 50 percent among young people in many industrialized countries. In clinical trials, the use of topical antimicrobial agents to eradicate diagnosed *S mutans* infections usually significantly reduces decay.

PERIODONTAL DISEASE

Definition

Periodontal disease can establish itself when the gums detach from the teeth as a result of an inflammatory response to plaque.

Etiology

Periodontal infections are usually mixed, most often involving anaerobes such as *Treponema denticola* and *Bacteroides gingivalis*. The microaerophile *Actinobacillus actinomy-cetemcomitans* causes a rare form known as localized juvenile periodontitis.

Pathogenesis

Plaque bacteria elaborate various compounds (H_2S, NH_3, amines, toxins, enzymes, antigens, etc.) that elicit an inflammatory response that is protective but also is responsible for loss of periodontal tissue, pocket formation, and loosening and loss of teeth.

Clinical Manifestations

There is no apparent pain until very late when abscesses may occur. Bleeding gums and bad breath may occur.

Microbiologic Diagnosis

Microbiologic diagnosis is usually not sought. Spirochetes and other motile organisms are found upon dark-field microscopic examination. Cultural, immunologic, and DNA probes are being developed for *B gingivalis, A actinomycetemcomitans, T denticola,* and other organisms.

Prevention and Treatment

Daily toothbrushing and regular professional cleanings by the dentist appear to be adequate to prevent periodontal disease. Rigorous debridement of tooth surfaces is the standard treatment. Often, some form of surgery is used to improve access to root surfaces. Recent studies suggest that short-term use of antimicrobial agents, especially metronidazole and tetracyclines, is beneficial.

INTRODUCTION

The tooth surfaces are unique in that they are the only body part not subject to metabolic turnover. Once formed, the teeth are, under the correct conditions, essentially indestructible, as witnessed by their importance in fossil records and forensic medicine. Yet in the living individual, the integrity of the teeth is assaulted by a microbial challenge so great that dental infections rank as the most universal affliction of humankind. The discomfort caused by these infections and their enormous cost (dental infections rank third in medical costs, behind heart disease and cancer, in the United States) give dental diseases prominence despite their non-life-threatening nature.

This chapter reviews the bacterial aspects of dental caries and periodontal disease and suggests that, in the future, treatment will be directed toward eliminating or suppressing certain bacterial species that appear to be overt pathogens in the dental plaque.

◁ DENTAL DECAY ▷ (CARIES)

Dental decay (caries) is due to the dissolution of tooth mineral [primarily hydroxyapatite, $Ca_{10}(PO_4)_6(OH)_2$] by acids derived from bacterial fermentation of sucrose and other dietary carbohydrates. These bacteria live in bacterial communities known as dental plaque, which accumulates on the tooth surface. For almost a century it was believed that any bacterial community on the tooth surface could cause decay, and treatment was almost exclusively the mechanical cleaning of these surfaces by toothbrushing with some type of mild abrasive. Such treatments based upon debridement and, in extreme cases, upon dietary carbohydrate restriction, were singularly unsuccessful in reducing dental decay. In fact, the prevalence of dental decay was so high among young men that it was the major cause of rejection from military service in World Wars I and II and the Korean war. This staggering amount of dental morbidity led to the formation of dentistry as a separate health profession in the late 19th century; to the expectation that all people would, if they lived long enough, be edentulous (toothless); and to a dental health bill to the public of approximately 25 billion dollars per year in the 1980s.

There is a happy ending. Water fluoridation has proven to be a most cost-effective way of reducing decay. Fluoride dentifrices were even more effective than initially projected. Research findings indicate that most carious lesions actually reflect a sucrose-dependent *Streptococcus mutans* infection. Individuals at risk for this infection can be diag-

nosed and treated by frequent mechanical intervention, by intensive application of prescription
levels of fluorides or other antimicrobial agents
(such as chlorhexidine), by restriction of sucrose
ingestion between meals, or by use of products
that contain sucrose substitutes (such as xylitol).
The net result is that dental decay in the late 20th
century is a controllable infection and should be
preventable in many individuals.

ETIOLOGY

Dental decay has been known throughout history,
but was not an important health problem until sucrose became a major component of the human
diet. When sucrose is consumed frequently, *S
mutans* emerges as the predominant agent and has
been uniquely associated with dental decay.

In 1924 Clarke isolated *S mutans* from human
carious lesions, but subsequent investigators were
unable to find *S mutans*, leading to its neglect as a
putative dental pathogen. It was rediscovered in
the 1960s, when it was identified as the agent of a
transmissible caries infection in rodent models. In
these studies, performed by Keyes and Fitzgerald,
all of Koch's postulates for infectivity were fulfilled
in animal models. However, it proved difficult to
show that *S mutans* was a human dental pathogen
because it appears to be a member of the normal
flora on the teeth, and it was difficult to show that
an increase in the *S mutans* level actually preceded
and/or coincided with the earliest clinical lesion.

Dental decay is measured clinically as a cavitation on the tooth surface (Fig. 99-1). However,
cavitation is a late event in the pathogenesis of
decay, being preceded by a clinically detectable
subsurface lesion known as a white spot (Fig. 99-1)
and prior to that by subsurface demineralization
that can be detected only microscopically. From a
diagnostic and treatment perspective, the lesion
should be detected at the white spot stage. This
usually cannot be done without rigorous descriptive criteria (not all white spots are due to the decay
process) and because the white spot stage in the
caries-prone fissures and approximal surfaces of
the tooth cannot be directly visualized during a

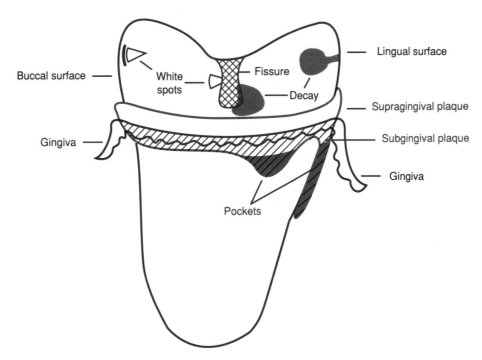

FIGURE 99-1   Schematic drawing of a cross-section of tooth showing decay and white spot lesions.

dental examination. Therefore, results of some bacteriologic studies point to the possibility that the flora associated with the decay was the result, not the cause, of the cavitation.

The prevalence of dental morbidity is documented in terms of the number of teeth (T) or tooth surfaces (S) that have obvious decay (D), contain a dental restoration or filling (F), or are missing (M). These scores of DMF teeth (DMFT) and DMF surfaces (DMFS) do not record the relative proportions of the score due to decay, versus fillings and extractions. This insensitivity of the DMFT and DMFS scores in quantitating the actual decay, independent of morbidity, led to unimpressive associations between S mutans and DMFT or DMFS scores in early studies. However, when the comparison was limited to individuals with decayed teeth or when the plaque samples were taken from a decayed tooth site, a significant association between S mutans and decay was evident.

This association is clearly seen in individuals who developed xerostomia secondary to radiation treatment of head and neck cancer. *Streptococcus*

mutans and lactobacilli are normally present in small numbers in the plaque of these individuals. When the salivary flow decreases, part of the patient's adjustment to a dry mouth is to change his/her dietary habits to a soft, sucrose-containing diet. New decayed lesions become obvious within 3 months after radiotherapy, and the patient may average one or more new decayed surfaces per post-radiation month. During the development of decay, the proportions of S mutans and then of lactobacilli increased significantly. This sequence of events indicated that S mutans was involved with the initiation of decay, whereas the lactobacilli were associated with the progression of the lesion.

This bacterial succession is illustrated in Figure 99-2, which shows the sequence of events occurring on the surface of a caries-free tooth that either becomes carious or remains caries free. In either case, the tooth surface initially represents a carrier state relative to harboring a primary cariogen, such as S mutans, in the plaque on a smooth surface. The proportion of the cariogen in the flora is similar in both cases, but its location differs within

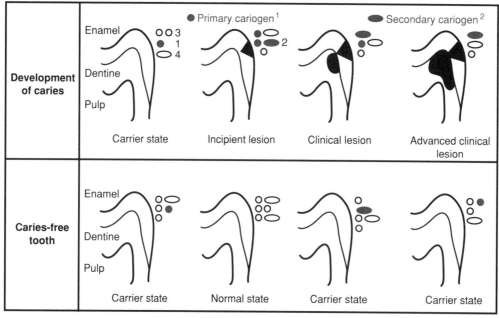

FIGURE 99-2 Relationship between location of cariogenic bacteria and development of dental caries.

the plaques. In the tooth destined to develop decay, *S mutans* is located on the enamel surface, whereas in the tooth destined to remain caries free, *S mutans* is confined to the saliva-plaque interface. Debriding procedures, such as toothbrushing and flossing, might remove most plaque organisms, but could leave untouched those bacteria either firmly attached to the enamel surface or sequestered in defects in the enamel surface. In surfaces destined to become carious, the residual organisms would include *S mutans*, whereas in surfaces destined to remain caries free, *S mutans* would be absent. Over time these caries-free surfaces might alternately acquire and lose *S mutans*, thereby having an intermittent carrier-state status. However, *S mutans* becomes a dominant member of the flora, undoubtedly secondary to frequent sucrose ingestion, on surfaces that will eventually develop caries.

The incipient or white spot lesion occurs when the acidogenic activity of the cariogen causes tooth mineral to be mobilized from the subsurface enamel to buffer the pH at the plaque-enamel interface. Bacteriologic sampling at this stage should reveal both a proportional and an absolute increase in the levels of *S mutans*. When the lesion progresses to the stage of cavitation, the organisms penetrate into the enamel crystals (Fig. 99-2). Also, secondary cariogens, such as the lactobacilli, appear as a result of the selection for aciduric organisms in the plaque. When the lesion reaches the advanced clinical stage, conditions may be such that *S mutans* can no longer survive, and only secondary cariogens such as the lactobacilli and opportunistic organisms can be found.

This model predicts that a bacterial succession occurs during the progression of a carious lesion and that the flora of the advanced lesion may not resemble the flora of the incipient lesion. Thus, it was necessary to sample the plaque during the initial lesion or white spot stage to find the agents of decay. When this was done, *S mutans* dominated in the flora. However, for the lesion to progress to the stage of cavitation, lactobacilli seemed necessary, since *S mutans* were isolated from both progressive and nonprogressive lesions, but *L casei* were isolated only from progressive lesions.

PATHOGENESIS

These clinical studies indicated that of the 200 to 300 species in plaque, only *S mutans* and, to a lesser extent, the lactobacilli can be consistently associated with dental decay. What makes these organisms cariogenic relative to all other bacterial types found in the plaque?

Miller, in the later 19th century, linked microbial acid production from dietary substrates to the etiology of dental decay in what he called the chemoparasitic theory of decay. However, Miller and his followers were not able to associate any single acidogenic species with decay, and they concluded that decay was bacteriologically nonspecific and due to the increased amounts of acid formed when bacteria accumulated in plaque on the tooth surfaces. Miller noted that decay occurred at retentive sites on the teeth and recommended mechanical and chemical debridement of these sites as the best method of reducing decay. Although Miller's clinical observations were correct, he had no way of determining that the retentive sites were caries prone because they provide the microenvironment that selects for *S mutans* and lactobacilli. This section examines the attributes of *S mutans* and the lactobacilli that enable them to be successful on retentive sites and shows that these attributes constitute the virulence factors that make these organisms specific odontopathogens.

Sucrose in the Diet

Considerable evidence from epidemiologic observations and animal experiments indicates that shortly after sucrose is introduced into the diet, a notably higher incidence of decay occurs. The relationship between sucrose ingestion and dental caries is reasonably well understood. The supragingival plaque flora derives its nutrients from various sources, including food, saliva, sloughed epithelial cells, dead microbes, and gingival crevice fluid or exudate. All sources, except the foods in the diet, provide only small amounts of nutrients. Dietary components are normally high-molecular-weight polymers (such as starch and proteins) that are in the mouth for short periods. They have a minimal effect on plaque growth except when food is retained between and on the teeth. Sucrose changes this pattern, however, because it is a low-molecular-weight disaccharide that can be rapidly sequestered and utilized by the plaque flora. Plaque organisms capable of fermenting sucrose have a decided advantage over the sucrose nonfermenters in that they can proliferate during periods of sucrose ingestion and thereby become the dominant plaque organisms.

Sucrose fermentation produces a rapid drop in the pH, to 5.0 or lower, at the point of interface between plaque and enamel. When sucrose is ingested during meals, sufficient saliva is secreted to buffer the plaque pH and decay does not occur. In fact, studies show that as much as one-half pound of sucrose consumed daily at meals for 2 years was not associated with an increase in dental decay. However, when the same or lesser amounts of sucrose were ingested between meals, subjects developed new decay at the rate of about three to four tooth surfaces per year. Frequent ingestion of sucrose increases the lengths of time that it is detected in the saliva. This means that if this sucrose were available for microbial fermentation in the plaque, low plaque pHs would be present for long periods each day. When the plaque pH falls below 5.0 to 5.2, the salivary buffers are overwhelmed and, as lactic acid diffuses into the tooth, enamel begins to dissolve, releasing Ca^{2+} and PO_4^{3-} ions from sites beneath the surface enamel (Fig. 99-3). Normally, the bathing saliva replenishes these minerals, but if the length of the flux from the enamel is great, repair does not occur and cavitation results. Therefore, sucrose consumption per se does not cause decay, but frequent ingestion of sucrose is cariogenic because it prolongs the period when the plaque is acidic.

Plaque bacteria that ferment sucrose produce acids, which lower the pH to below 5.0 in vitro. However, of all these species, only *S mutans* reliably caused decay in germ-free animals fed a high-sucrose diet. This suggested that microbial acid production was not the exclusive determinant of decay and that *S mutans* had to possess other attributes that were responsible for its virulence. *Streptococcus mutans* was subsequently shown to metabolize sucrose in a remarkably diverse fashion that is not matched by any other known plaque organism.

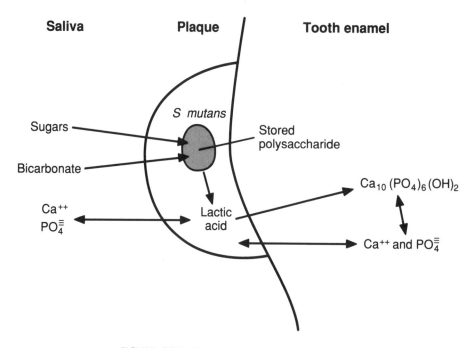

FIGURE 99-3 Pathogenesis of dental decay.

The major pathway is concerned with energy metabolism. In this process, the enzyme **invertase** splits sucrose into its component glucose and fructose molecules, which are then converted to lactic acid by the glycolytic pathway. Other enzymes, called **glucosyltransferases,** split sucrose but transfer the glucose moiety to a glucose polymer known as a **glucan.** *Streptococcus mutans* forms several complex glucans that differ in their core linkage, degree of branching, and molecular weight. The first glucan identified had a core linkage consisting of an α1-6 bond that classified it as a dextran. Later, a unique glucan with an α1-3 core linkage was identified and given the name **mutan.** *Streptococcus mutans* also has enzymes that split sucrose and transfer the fructose moiety to a fructose polymer known as a **fructan.** Other plaque bacteria can use sucrose to synthesize one or more of these polymers, with the exception of mutan. Only *S mutans* can form all of them, however. This fact led to an inquiry into the relationship between polymer production and caries formation.

A series of in vitro experiments showed that the glucans enable *S mutans* to adhere to surfaces. This suggested that in vivo these adhesive polymers would enable *S mutans* to adhere tenaciously to and accumulate on tooth surfaces, thereby causing decay in the underlying surface. Animal experiments have shown that treatment with the enzymes **dextranase** or **mutanase,** or both, which degrade the extracellular polymers, reduces the incidence of caries. Other investigations, in which rodents were infected with mutants of *S mutans* that lacked the ability to form either of these two glucans, indicated that the absence of mutan was associated with a greater reduction in smooth surface decay than was the absence of dextran. In each instance, the amount of pit and fissure decay was not significantly affected by these mutations. Decay on smooth surfaces seems to depend on the retentive polymers formed by *S mutans,* whereas in sites where retention is provided by the anatomy of the teeth (pits, fissures, and contact points between teeth), these polymers are not as important. Accordingly, pit and fissure decay may be caused simply by any acidogenic organism that happens to colonize these retentive sites.

This nonspecific explanation does not seem completely satisfactory, because in animal models and in human caries, *S mutans,* again, is the dominant organism involved or associated with pit and fissure decay. A few other organisms, such as *Lactobacillus casei* and *Streptococcus faecalis,* can cause fissure decay in germ-free rats. These three organisms are all more aciduric than other plaque bacteria (i.e., they not only produce acids, but are also relatively resistant to the resulting low pH caused by acid accumulation). Lactobacilli are the most aciduric of the plaque bacteria, but predominate only by the time the carious lesion has extended into the dentin. At the time the earliest carious lesion is detected, only *S mutans* has reached significant levels and proportions (Fig. 99-2). When *S mutans,* lactobacilli, and other plaque species were compared in vitro for their ability to ferment sucrose at different pH values, *S mutans* was found to be more active than the other bacteria at pH 5.0, and so it is probably most active in vivo at the very pH at which the teeth begin to demineralize.

This aciduricity best explains the involvement of both *S mutans* and lactobacilli in human tooth decay. A retentive site is colonized by organisms present in saliva. *Streptococcus mutans,* although scarce in the initial inoculum (fewer than 0.1 percent of the initial colonizers), is selected for if the average pH value in the site is not well buffered by saliva. Frequent ingestion of sucrose-containing products predisposes toward lower pH values and thus selects for *S mutans.* When the pH remains in the vicinity of 5.0 to 5.5, tooth mineral is solubilized, thereby buffering the plaque and maintaining an environment suitable for growth of *S mutans.* Eventually, enough mineral is lost that cavitation occurs in the enamel, and if this enlarges so that it extends into the dentin, a semiclosed system is formed in which the pH value drops below 5.0. Under these acidic conditions, growth of lactobacilli is favored, and these organisms succeed as the predominant flora in the carious lesion.

CLINICAL MANIFESTATIONS

Dental decay occurs at discrete sites on the surface of the enamel. Progress through the enamel is usually slow, because of the remineralizing action of the saliva, and is asymptomatic. When decay spreads into the dentin the process accelerates, probably because the very low pH that can arise in this semiclosed environment denatures the collagen scaffold that holds the hydroxyapatite salts in place and rapidly solubilizes them. When the dentinal decay approaches the innervated tooth pulp, the pain can be intermittent or continuous, and dull or excruciating. Pain is the chief complaint of patients with advanced dental decay.

MICROBIOLOGIC DIAGNOSIS

A microbiologic diagnosis for an *S mutans/lactobacillus* infection is rarely sought, primarily because the acute pain that brings the patient to the dentist is almost always relieved by dental restoration or extraction. Therefore, knowledge of an underlying *S mutans* infection would not change the treatment. However, microbiologic diagnosis would be advantageous in management of the patient to prevent or minimize future decay. Such situations would occur whenever an expensive treatment is planned, such as orthodontic treatment or the placement of dental crowns and bridges to replace missing teeth. Microbiologic examination would also be useful at the end of any restorative treatment to determine the residual level of *S mutans* and lactobacilli colonization on the teeth.

Scandinavian investigators have empirically determined that 10^6 CFU of *S mutans*/ml of stimulated saliva can be associated with future caries activity. Accordingly, they have recommended active intervention with fluoride, dietary counseling, and antimicrobial agents in infected individuals. They have designed simple chair-side tests that can, in a semiquantitated manner, provide information on the salivary levels of *S mutans*. All of these tests rely on the fact that *S mutans* is resistant to 5 μg of bacitracin/ml and will grow in the presence of 20 percent sucrose. In liquid media containing these additives, *S mutans* will form adherent colonies on the side of glass, plastic strips, or any other solid surfaces that are present.

In a practical application of these tests, the clinician would not place orthodontic bands on an individual with 10^6 CFU of *S mutans,* because this individual would tend to develop decay around the margins of the bands. Likewise, an individual who is having extensive bridgework (the placing of dental restorations across an edentulous space) would be at risk of developing new decay around the margins of these restorations. In both instances, the patient must be treated for *S mutans* infection prior to the placement of the dental devices or restorations.

PREVENTION AND TREATMENT

Conventional dental therapy has not yet incorporated any microbiologically based strategy into its armamentarium. Instead, a treatment based on response to symptoms has prevailed. The bankruptcy of this approach, which depends on a turn-of-the-century biologic base, has been demonstrated in the Scandinavian countries, where a socialized dental delivery system has made high-quality dentistry available to everyone. Because of the emphasis on treatment rather than prevention, the results have prolonged the life span of the tooth by only about 10 years, a rather poor therapeutic result. In England, where the health care system also emphasized treatment rather than prevention, half of the population over 35 years of age were edentulous in the 1970s. The Scandinavians, especially in Sweden, have changed their approach and have instituted plaque prophylactic programs for children and adults. Thorough dental cleaning with a 5 percent fluoride paste given at 2- to 4-week intervals, combined with oral hygiene education, has lowered dental decay in children by about 80 to 90 percent, compared with youngsters receiving symptomatic treatment (i.e., placing dental restorations in an obviously carious tooth, and pulling teeth). Similar success has been achieved in adults with and without periodontal disease.

Thorough cleaning with fluoride apparently selects for the more desirable bacterial types, such as *S sanguis* and *S mitis,* which are capable of rapidly colonizing the tooth surfaces. *Streptococcus mutans* presumably does not have an opportunity to become dominant, because the frequent debridement neutralizes its ability to be selected for by the low pH values that characterize an undisturbed plaque. Also, the 5 percent fluoride paste has an immediate bacteriostatic effect on the plaque organisms.

Fluoride as an Antimicrobial Agent in Plaque

The mechanisms by which fluoride prevents decay are multiple, and the relative contributions of each mechanism are not fully understood. The 30 to 50 percent reduction in decay that follows water fluoridation is generally attributed to replacement of hydroxyl groups in the tooth crystal by fluoride, thereby forming fluorapatite (Fig. 99-4). Fluorapatite is less acid soluble than hydroxyapatite, which means that a tooth containing fluorapatite dissolves slowly in the low pH value found in plaque and, accordingly, remineralizes faster in the intervals between sugar ingestion. These explanations do not completely account for the proven efficacy of topically applied fluorides and raises questions about other modes of fluoride action.

The fluoride ion (F^-) inhibits the bacterial enzyme enolase, thereby interfering with the production of **phosphoenolpyruvate (PEP)**. Phosphoenolpyruvate is a key intermediate of the glycolytic pathway and, in many bacteria, is the source of energy and phosphate needed for sugar uptake.

The presence of 10 to 100 ppm of F^- inhibits acid production by most plaque bacteria (Fig. 99-4). These levels are delivered easily by most prescription fluoride preparations, such as were used in the Swedish studies. Of equal interest is the finding that at low pH values (5.5 or below), low levels of F^- (1 to 5 ppm) inhibit the oral streptococci. These levels are found in plaque, especially in individuals who drink fluoridated water or who have been treated with topical fluorides. If this plaque fluoride is derived from the tooth, an antibacterial mode of action, which involves a depot effect, can be postulated for systemic (water) and topical fluoride administration.

The depot effect comes about in this manner. Water fluoridation promotes the formation of fluorapatite, whereas topical fluorides cause a net retention by the enamel of fluoride as fluorapatite or as more labile calcium salts. Microbial acid production in the plaque may solubilize this enamel-bound fluoride, which, at the prevailing low pH in the plaque microenvironment, could become lethal for the acid-producing microbes. Such a sequence would discriminate against *S mutans* and

1. Tooth mineral is made less soluble by the formation of fluorapatite during development

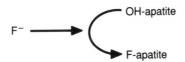

2. Fluoride in saliva and plaque promotes remineralization of tooth surface after tooth eruption

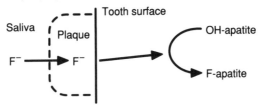

3. Fluoride in plaque enters bacterial cells, especially at low pH, and inhibits enolase, thereby reducing acid production in plaque

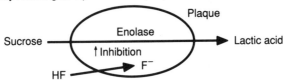

FIGURE 99-4   Anti-caries mechanisms of fluoride.

TABLE 99-1 Effect of Various Regimens on the
Incidence of Dental Caries in Patients with
Radiation Xerostomia

Treatment Regimen	No. of Patients	Increase in Caries Score[a] per Post-radiation Month	
		DMFT	DMFS
Oral hygiene	14	1.2	2.5
Oral hygiene + fluoride[b]	13	0.06	0.1
Oral hygiene + fluoride + daily sucrose restriction	11	0.04	0.05

[a] DMFT, Number of decayed, missing, or filled teeth; DMFS, number of tooth surfaces that are decayed, missing because of extraction, or filled.
[b] Topical fluoride (1 percent NaF).
(Adapted from Dreizen S, Brown LR: Effects of selected caries preventive regiments on microbial change following irradiation-induced xerostomia in cancer patients. p. 275. In Stiles M, Loesche WJ, O'Brien JJ (eds): Microbial Aspects of Dental Caries. Vol. 1. Information Retrieval, Arlington, VA, 1976, with permission.)

lactobacilli because they, as a result of their aciduric nature, are most probably the numerically dominant acid producers at the plaque-enamel interface. The fluoridated tooth thus contains a depot of a potent antimicrobial agent that not only is released at a low pH value but also is most active at this pH value. This hypothesis, then, attributes some of the success of water fluoridation and topical fluorides to an antimicrobial effect. It further suggests that judicious use of topical fluorides would be effective in patients with highly active caries.

The most effective dose schedule and fluoride preparation have not been determined. When neutral 1.0 percent sodium fluoride was given daily to adults who normally would experience rampant caries secondary to a xerostomia following irradiation for jaw cancer, the recipients experienced few or no caries. Controls, who were given a placebo as well as the best available hygiene instruction, averaged more than two new decayed surfaces per post-radiation month (Table 99-1). When the control patients were placed on the daily

fluoride regimen, their decay rate dropped almost to zero. In another study, 5- to 6-year-old children, who had 10 or more carious tooth surfaces, were given the necessary dental restorations and either 1.2 percent F^- as a neutral sodium fluoride gel or a placebo gel. The gels were taken unsupervised at home, twice a day for 1 week. After 2 years, the fluoride group had about 40 percent less decay than the placebo group. Of 20 of these children with formerly rampant caries, 11 had no new decay in their permanent teeth. In these xerostomia and pediatric patients, the initially high proportions of S mutans were decreased by the fluoride treatments, and this resulted in reduced decay.

Sucrose Substitutes That Aid in Caries Control

Eating sucrose-containing foods between meals is highly cariogenic. Dietary counseling that instructs patients to avoid between-meal snacks will help to decrease the incidence of dental decay if the patients are compliant. Another dietary approach to caries control is to recommend that patients eat snack foods that contain compounds that provide the hedonistic appeal of sucrose, but are not fermented by the plaque flora to the low pH levels associated with enamel demineralization.

The least acidogenic sucrose substitutes are the polyols, such as sorbitol, mannitol, and xylitol. Few plaque bacteria can ferment these substances, and those that can (*S mutans* and *L casei* ferment sorbitol and mannitol) exhibit a slow fermentation, because glucose catabolite repression keeps the necessary degradative enzymes at minimum levels. Xylitol, the only polyol with a sweet taste comparable to that of sucrose, and the only one that cannot be fermented by *S mutans,* is noncariogenic, and possibly anticariogenic, when substituted for sucrose in either foods or chewing gum. In a chewing-gum study, young adults who consumed about 6 to 7 g of xylitol gum per day had, after 1 year, an 80 percent reduction in caries increment compared with a control group who consumed 6 to 7 g of sucrose gum per day. In later studies, this type of intensive use of a xylitol chewing gum was shown to decrease salivary and plaque levels of *S mutans*. When the between-meal sucrose supply is reduced, the levels of *S mutans* organisms will decline, as the low plaque pH values that selected for them are not as dominant a factor in the plaque microecology. Thus, xylitol can satisfy the craving for sweets and discriminate against *S mutans.*

◀ PERIODONTAL DISEASE ▶

Periodontal disease is the general description applied to the inflammatory response of the gingiva and surrounding connective tissue to the bacterial or plaque accumulations on the teeth. These inflammatory responses are divided into two general groupings: **gingivitis** and **periodontitis.** Gingivitis is extremely common and is manifested clinically as bleeding of the gingival or gum tissues without evidence of bone loss or deep periodontal pockets. **Pocketing** is the term given to the pathologic loss of tissue between the tooth and the gingiva, creating spaces that are filled by the subgingival plaque (Fig. 99-1). Periodontitis occurs when the plaque-induced inflammatory response in the tissue results in actual loss of collagen attachment of the

tooth to the bone, to loss of bone, and to deep periodontal pockets, which, in some cases, can extend the entire length of the tooth root (15 to 20 mm).

Periodontitis is usually graded according to the severity of the tissue loss and the number of teeth involved. It is not as prevalent as once thought. A recent survey of American adults revealed that only 8 percent of the population surveyed had one tooth site with attachment loss measuring 6 mm or more. This finding was surprising, given past surveys that indicated that almost everyone would experience advanced forms of periodontal disease as they aged, but is in agreement with recent population surveys in other countries, which show that 5 to 15 percent of the population has periodontitis.

ETIOLOGY AND PATHOGENESIS

The most important new finding concerning periodontal disease is the realization that it is really an array of infections. These infections are unusual in that massive or even obvious bacterial invasion of the tissues is rarely encountered. Rather, bacteria in the plaque touching the tissue elaborate various compounds, such as H_2S, NH_3, amines, endotoxins, enzymes (such as collagenases), and antigens, all of which penetrate the gingiva and elicit an inflammatory response. This inflammatory response, although overwhelmingly protective, appears to be responsible for a net loss of periodontal supporting tissue and leads to periodontal pocket formation, loosening of the teeth, and eventual tooth loss. Neutrophils are extremely important in this inflammatory response (see below). If they are absent, as in various neutropenias, or compromised as a result of chemotherapy, an aggressive form of periodontitis occurs. Helper T4 cells play a role in this defense, as witnessed by the periodontitis in patients with acquired immune deficiency syndrome (AIDS).

Gingivitis

The simplest form of gingivitis is associated with the accumulation of supragingival plaque along the gingival margins of the teeth. This form of gingivitis has been extensively studied in human volunteers, and the sequence of events is well known. In these studies, individuals are brought to a state of health and then refrain from all forms of oral hygiene for a 3- to 4-week period. The initial colonizers of the teeth are streptococci, which in turn are replaced by other bacteria present in saliva, such as various *Actinomyces* and *Veillonella* spp. The greatest growth of plaque occurs at the gingival margin, where plaque accumulations usually are visible after several days. This plaque may provoke a bleeding gingivitis in which spirochetes and *Actinomyces viscosus* are prominent members of the plaque flora. If this plaque remains undisturbed, the flora gradually shifts toward an anaerobic, Gram-negative flora that includes black-pigmented *Bacteroides* spp and several types of spirochetes. The increase in these organisms is caused by the low oxidation-reduction potential of the aged plaque and by nutrients derived from the inflammatory exudate at the site.

The gingivitis may resolve or may fester subclinically for an indeterminate period; however, the potential for the formation of a periodontal pocket (periodontitis) exists at any time. When pockets are detected clinically, they usually are associated with calcified plaque deposits, called **calculus,** on the tooth surfaces. For many years, calculus was thought to be the agent of periodontitis because inflammation usually subsided when it was removed and the tooth surfaces mechanically cleaned. However, calculus is always colonized by plaque, and removal of calculus would be synonymous with debridement of plaque. The subgingival plaque flora associated with periodontitis is dominated by an anaerobic, Gram-negative flora in all cases but one, and that is a unique clinical entity formerly known as **periodontosis** and now as **localized juvenile periodontitis (LJP).** Localized juvenile periodontitis is clinically important because of the understanding it has provided of the complex and dynamic interactions between the host and the flora in the pocket ecosystem.

Localized Juvenile Periodontitis

Localized juvenile periodontitis is different from all other periodontal infections as it is not associated with plaque accumulations or calculus (in fact, the absence of these led early investigators to consider it a degenerative condition), is localized to certain anterior or front teeth and first molars, and is seen following puberty. It is rather rare, occurring in about 0.1 to 0.5 percent of teenagers, but is often clustered within families. This familial background suggested a genetic predisposition, which subsequently has been identified as a neutrophil defect associated with reduced chemotaxis. Bacterial examinations of subgingival plaque from affected teeth and adjacent healthy teeth revealed that the diseased teeth were colonized by an essentially Gram-negative flora dominated by organisms subsequently identified as various *Capnocytophaga* and *Wolinella* spp and *Actinobacillus actinomycetemcomitans*. It is *A actinomycetemcomitans* that appears to be the agent of localized juvenile periodontitis, and the arguments for its involvement reflect the arguments made to implicate other species in other forms of periodontitis.

Once localized juvenile periodontitis has been recognized clinically, most of the tissue damage has already occurred, thereby permitting only a retrospective diagnosis of an *A actinomycetemcomitans* infection. *Actinobacillus actinomycetemcomitans* is found primarily but not exclusively in tooth sites associated with localized juvenile periodontitis and is rarely seen at healthy sites in the same mouth or at any sites in periodontally healthy individuals. In older individuals it is usually associated with clinical signs of periodontitis. It is often found in other family members sharing a household with an individual with localized juvenile periodontitis. There are data to suggest that colonization by *A actinomycetemcomitans* in at-risk siblings precedes the development of a pocket and subsequent bone loss. However, the most important reason for implicating *A actinomycetemcomitans* as a periodontopathogen is its killing effect on neutrophils.

Actinobacillus actinomycetemcomitans produces a leukotoxin that kills neutrophils in vitro. It is clear that this leukotoxin is expressed in vivo because patients with localized juvenile periodontitis have developed circulating antibodies that can neutralize this toxin in vitro. From this finding, a scenario can be developed that explains the localized nature of the disease. Children with a neutrophil chemotactic defect become colonized by *A actinomycetem-comitans* in early life, presumably by contact with infected household members. The colonization spreads to permanent teeth that erupted at ages 5 to 7, but remains quiescent as an infection during the time that the primary (or baby) teeth are lost and new permanent teeth appear at about ages 11 to 13. The individual entering puberty has a dentition composed of first molars and incisors that are colonized by *A actinomycetemcomitans* and newly erupted teeth that either are not colonized or are only minimally colonized.

Something then triggers the relative overgrowth of *A actinomycetemcomitans* in the subgingival plaque, and these organisms invade the gingival tissue and cause attachment and bone loss in the absence of an obvious inflammatory response. The latter can be explained by the leukotoxin's inhibiting the neutrophils and thereby preventing a protective host response in the pocket microenvironment. The leukotoxin is antigenic and elicits an antibody response that may neutralize the leukotoxin at other tooth sites, thereby limiting the infection to the originally colonized molars and incisors.

This scenario is incomplete, but does explain the localized nature of the disease, partially explains the absence of an inflammatory response in the tissue, and demonstrates the dynamic role of neutrophils and circulating antibodies in defending the periodontium. Presumably these mechanisms are operating in the more common adult periodontitis. Certainly, the central role of the neutrophils in host defense is unquestioned, as individuals with neutropenias, chronic granulomatous disease, and various leukemias often present with advanced forms of periodontal disease.

Early-Onset Periodontitis and Adult Periodontitis

The more common forms of periodontitis include at least two clinical entities, an early-onset form occurring mainly in young individuals and a chronic form seen in older adults. **Early-onset periodontitis (EOP)** looks more aggressive and may coincide with active tissue loss, whereas **adult periodontitis (AP)** may reflect a stable but tenuous stand-off between the host defensive systems and the plaque bacteria. It is not clear whether these entities represent multiple types of infections with two clinical manifestations or a single mixed infection with different levels of host containment.

The inability to distinguish between these two general patterns reflects methodologic procedures relating to the sampling of the subgingival plaque and the inability of any one culture medium and/or technique to give the total picture of the 200 to 300 bacterial species found in the plaque flora. For example, the spirochetes cannot be quantitatively cultured and may account for more than 40 percent of the flora in both forms of the disease. They can be enumerated by microscopic examination of the plaque but would be ignored in culture studies. These culture studies, in turn, reveal a bewildering array of species, many of them either newly described or as yet unidentified at the species level. None of these cultivable species predominates in all disease-associated plaques. For example, *Bacteroides forsythus*, a nonpigmenting fusiform organism, has been associated with the active periodontal lesion. It is present in 13 percent of the active sites and 8 percent of the inactive sites, a difference that is hardly indicative of etiologic association. However, the authors concluded that *B forsythus* is a probable periodontal pathogen because its levels, when present, were on the average six times higher in the active sites than in the inactive sites (i.e., 2.5 versus 0.6 percent). This difference is well within the error of the methods used to isolate the organisms.

Despite these problems in assigning virulence to any one species, it is clear that the bacterial communities at disease sites are different from the communities at healthy and successfully treated periodontal sites (Table 99-2). The diseased sites are dominated by anaerobes, in particular by spirochetes and black-pigmented *Bacteroides* spp, such as *B gingivalis* and *B intermedius*. Among the latter, *B gingivalis* most often is associated with early-onset periodontitis, whereas *B intermedius* is found in both types. No species, except the ubiquitous spirochetes, are consistently found in all lesions.

TABLE 99-2   Bacterial Profiles of Subgingival Plaques
Isolated from Various Clinical Forms of Periodontitis
and from Periodontally Healthy Sites

Pathogen	Healthy Sites[a]	Periodontitis[b]			
		EOP	AP	LJP	ANUG[c]
Facultative species					
Streptococcus spp	+++	+	+	+	+
Actinomyces spp	+++	+	+	+	+
Veillonella spp	+	+	+	+	+
Microaerophilic species					
A actinomycetemcomitans	−	− to +	±	++	?
Capnocytophaga spp	±	±	±	±	±
Anaerobic species					
Spirochetes	±	+++	+++	±	+++
B gingivalis	−	− to ++	− to ++	−	±
B intermedius	±	− to ++	− to ++	±	++
B forsythus	±	− to ++	− to ++	−	?
Wolinella spp	−	− to ++	− to ++	−	?
Fusobacterium spp	+	+ to ++	+ to ++	±	++

[a] Symbols: −, not present; ±, may be present; +, usually present at levels < 10 percent of flora;
++, levels < 20 percent of flora; +++, levels > 20 percent of flora; ?, not known.
[b] Abbreviations: EOP, early onset periodontitis; AP, adult periodontitis; LJP, localized juvenile
periodontitis.
[c] ANUG, acute necrotizing ulcerative gingivitis.

Treponema denticola is the only spirochete that can be reliably cultured. It possesses a wide array of enzymes, such as a collagenase, peptidases, hyaluronidase, and a keratinolytic enzyme, and to produce noxious end products, such as butyrate, NH_3, H_2S, and endotoxin, that could cause an inflammatory response if they entered the periodontal tissue. However, comparable enzymes occur in *B gingivalis* and other anaerobic species found in the plaque, so that it would be difficult to assign etiologic significance to any one of these organisms on the basis of production of these enzymes. Therefore, it may be best to consider that the collective overgrowth of all these anaerobic species in the plaque causes a mixed infection that is responsible for tissue loss in both types of periodontitis.

CLINICAL MANIFESTATIONS

Periodontal disease is usually painless until late in the disease process, when the teeth are so loose that some discomfort may appear upon chewing.

Retention of food in a pocket site may provoke a sudden burst of microbial growth, which could result in a painful abscess. At other times, the anterior teeth may become so loose that they separate and the patient visits a dentist because of the resulting poor aesthetics. However, under ordinary circumstances, bleeding upon brushing and/or concern over halitosis brings the patient to the dentist. A thorough dental examination should find any pockets. If these pockets bleed upon probing, such bleeding is synonymous with tissue inflammation and warrants therapeutic intervention.

MICROBIOLOGIC DIAGNOSIS

Microbiologic diagnosis is not much used in the management of periodontal disease, but it will probably become common in 5 to 10 years. Several methods are, or soon will be, available to permit identification and quantification of the periodontopathogens listed in Table 99-2. The oldest method is the use of dark-field and phase-contrast microscopy to identify spirochetes and other motile organisms in plaque samples. However, as spirochetes are detectable in most plaques, it is necessary to establish some critical value above which a spirochetal infection can be diagnosed. Our experience suggests that ≥ 20 percent of spirochetes in any plaque sample permits the diagnosis of an anaerobic infection.

A microscopic examination cannot distinguish the species of bacteria present unless an immunologic staining reagent specific for the organism in question is used. Such immunodiagnostic reagents have been used to detect and quantitate the levels of *B gingivalis*, *B intermedius*, *T denticola*, and *A actinomycetemcomitans* in the plaque. Culture methods can, if the appropriate nonselective and selective media are used, provide information on the levels of *A actinomycetemcomitans*, black-pigmented *Bacteroides* spp, *Wolinella* spp, and other periodontopathogens. Also, because viable organisms are available, antibiotic sensitivities of the isolated organisms can be determined; this may be useful in certain instances.

Other diagnostic reagents are being developed to detect the presence in plaque of specific microbes, metabolites, or enzymes unique to inflammation or infection. For example, specific microbes can be demonstrated by the use of DNA probes. Probes for *A actinomycetemcomitans*, *B intermedius*, and *B gingivalis* are commercially available for testing via a reference laboratory. Future diagnostic procedures may rely on the detection of hydroxyproline (a collagen degradation product), prostaglandin (an inflammatory mediator), and enzymes derived from either the host or the microbes. A trypsinlike enzyme is present in *T denticola*, *B gingivalis*, and *B forsythus* and absent from at least 20 other subgingival plaque organisms. This enzyme can be detected by the hydrolysis of the trypsin substrate benzoyl-DL-arginine naphthylamide. The ability of subgingival plaque to hydrolyze benzoyl-DL-arginine naphthylamide was associated with elevated levels and proportions of spirochetes and with probing depths greater than 6 mm. Benzoyl-DL-arginine naphthylamide hydrolysis was later shown to be related to the *T denticola* and *B gingivalis* content of the plaque and to the clinical diagnosis of health or disease. As *T denticola*, *B gingivalis*, and *B forsythus* are anaerobes, a positive benzoyl-DL-arginine naphthylamide test may be useful in the diagnosis of an anaerobic plaque infection.

PREVENTION AND TREATMENT

Gingivitis can be reduced, if not prevented, by good oral hygiene and professional surveillance. Gingivitis is usually effectively treated by tooth debridement and supplemented, if needed, by short-term use of products containing chlorhexidine, stannous fluoride, or other antimicrobial agents. Mouth rinses, gels, and toothpastes, when used in conjunction with toothbrushing and flossing, are probably adequate to deliver any antimicrobial agents to subgingival sites that are 1 to 3 mm in depth. At probing depths greater than 3 mm, there may not be sufficient penetration of the agent to the bottom of the pocket, and infection may persist. Subgingival scaling (debridement) by a professional is indicated, and the use of irrigating devices containing an antimicrobial agent is usually beneficial.

There is rarely any need to use systemic antimicrobial agents to treat gingivitis associated with pocket depths of 1 to 4 mm, with the exception of an increasingly rare and painful condition known today as **acute necrotizing ulcerative gingivitis (ANUG)** and formerly as trench mouth. Cases of acute necrotizing ulcerative gingivitis that are refractory to mechanical debridement and topical antimicrobial agents respond quickly and dramatically to systemic metronidazole. Recognition of the efficacy of metronidazole led to the discovery that it has bactericidal activity against anaerobes. Acute necrotizing ulcerative gingivitis is characterized by tissue invasion by spirochetes and possibly other anaerobes and by elevated plaque levels of spirochetes and *B intermedius* (Table 99-2). It thus resembles periodontitis in being an anaerobic infection.

This brings us to the choice of an antimicrobial agent for the treatment of periodontitis. Clinical dentistry has been successful in treating periodontitis without systemic antimicrobial agents, even though systemic pain relievers, anti-inflammatory agents, and occasionally antibiotics have been used to manage the patient during periodontal surgery. Therefore, there is no tradition for antibiotic use prior to surgical intervention. However, given the recent and convincing evidence that periodontitis is an infection, this tradition may well have to be modified. It would seem that the crucial determination for the clinician's treatment plan will be the diagnosis of either a microaerophilic infection due to *A actinomycetemcomitans* or an anaerobic infection characterized by the overgrowth of spirochetes and black-pigmented *Bacteroides* spp.

Actinobacillus actinomycetemcomitans is susceptible to tetracycline. Early studies showed that tetracycline, scaling and root planing, periodontal flap surgery, and topical treatment with chlorhexidine were able to save hopeless teeth in patients with localized juvenile periodontitis. Additional studies, but none of a double-blind nature, confirm the usefulness of tetracycline in the treatment of this infection. Subsequently it was shown that tetracycline is concentrated in the fluid that seeps out of the periodontium into the pocket microenvironment. This fact, combined with the demonstration that *A actinomycetemcomitans* is present in plaques associated with early-onset periodontitis and adult periodontitis (Table 99-2), has led to the use of tetracycline to treat those infections. Results have been equivocal, but this has not detracted from the popularity of tetracycline as a treatment for periodontitis.

Most bacteriologic studies implicate anaerobes as the agent(s) of early-onset periodontitis and adult periodontitis, and this would point to the use of a drug such as metronidazole. However, early animal studies that used lifetime feeding of extremely high dosages of metronidazole suggested that the drug might be tumorigenic. These studies have not been confirmed, and, indeed, in 1981 the U.S. Food and Drug Administration (FDA) approved metronidazole for treatment of anaerobic infections. In dentistry, this concern has led to a reluctance to use metronidazole, but has also allowed time for well-controlled clinical trials of metronidazole.

Six double-blind studies have demonstrated that metronidazole, given for periods as short as 1 week, can significantly improve periodontal health. In all cases the metronidazole was given in conjunction with professional debriding of the teeth. Maximal benefits were obtained when the metronidazole was given after the debridement. The best clinical response often occurred in patients with more advanced disease, in which the pocket depths were ≥ 6 mm, whereas there was only a moderate benefit when the pocket depths were 4 to 6 mm. In these advanced cases some teeth that were initially scheduled for extraction were found on reexamination not to need extraction and thus, in a sense, were saved.

These data from the double-blind metronidazole studies indicate that early-onset peritonitis and adult peritonitis respond to treatment as if they were anaerobic infections and would seem to presage the more frequent usage of anti-anaerobic agents, such as metronidazole, in future treatment of periodontal disease.

REFERENCES

Baehni P, Tsai CC, McArthur W et al: Interaction of inflammatory cells and oral microorganisms. Infect Immun 24:233, 1979

Dzink JL, Socransky SS, Haffajee AD: The predominant cultivable microbiota of active and inactive lesions of destructive periodontal disease. J Clin Periodontol 15:316, 1988

Genco RJ, VanDyke TE, Levine MJ et al: Molecular factors influencing neutrophil defects in periodontal disease. J Dent Res 65:1379, 1986

Keyes PH: The infectious and transmissible nature of experimental dental caries. Findings and implications. Arch Oral Biol 1:304, 1960

Krasse B: Caries Risk: A Practical Guide for Assessment and Control. Quintessence, Chicago, 1985

Loesche WJ: Role of *Streptococcus mutans* in human dental decay. Microbiol Rev 50:353, 1986

Loesche WJ: The role of spirochetes in periodontal disease. Adv Dent Res 2:275, 1988

Loesche WJ, Schmidt E, Smith BA et al: Metronidazole therapy for periodontitis. J Periodontal Res 22:224, 1987

Miller WD: The Microorganisms of the Human Mouth. SS White Manufacturing, Philadelphia, 1890

National Institute of Dental Research: Oral Health of United States Adults. NIH publication no. 87-2868. National Institute of Health, Washington, DC, 1987

Zambon JJ: *Actinobacillus actinomycetemcomitans* in human periodontal disease. J Clin Periodontol 12:1, 1985

100 BONE, JOINT, AND NECROTIZING SOFT TISSUE INFECTIONS

JON T. MADER
WILLIAM WALLACE

GENERAL CONCEPTS

NECROTIZING SOFT TISSUE INFECTIONS

Etiology

Anaerobic microorganisms such as *Bacteroides* species, *Peptostreptococcus* species, and *Clostridium* species are largely responsible for these infections. Mixed infections by aerobic and facultative anaerobic organisms are common.

Pathogenesis

Susceptible persons have experienced trauma or surgery and frequently have diabetes and/or vascular insufficiency. Organisms gain entry via direct inoculation. Local hypoxia and decreased oxygen-reduction potentials favor anaerobic growth.

Clinical Manifestations

The signs of disease include production of tissue gas, a putrid discharge, tissue necrosis, fever, (occasionally) systemic toxicity, and absence of classic signs of inflammation.

Microbiologic Diagnosis

These infections are usually diagnosed by clinical presentation. Aerobic and anaerobic wound cultures help identify the major pathogens.

Prevention and Treatment

Immediate surgical debridement of all necrotic tissue is vital. High-dose parenteral antibiotic therapy should be started immediately. Hyperbaric oxygen therapy may be indicated.

JOINT INFECTIONS

Etiology

Neisseria gonorrhoeae and *Staphylococcus aureus* are responsible for most cases of bacterial arthritis.

Pathogenesis

Joint infections are usually a result of hematogenous spread, but may also arise from traumatic inoculation or by extension from an adjacent focus of infection. Proteolytic enzymes of polymorphonuclear leukocytes, bacterial toxins, and pressure from joint swelling all contribute to the damage of articular surfaces.

Clinical Manifestations

Joint swelling, pain, warmth (inflammation), decreased range of motion, and fever are the classic symptoms. Disseminated gonococcal infections may also cause migratory polyarthritis, dermatitis, and tenosynovitis.

Microbiologic Diagnosis

Aspiration and culture of synovial fluid usually provides the definite diagnosis.

Prevention and Treatment

Gonococcal arthritis may be prevented by techniques used to decrease the risk for sexually transmitted disease. The treatment for all septic arthritides is administration of parenteral antibiotics. Some cases may require incision and drainage and/or surgical debridement.

BONE INFECTIONS

Etiology

Staphylococcus aureus is the most commonly isolated pathogen. Polymicrobic infections are frequent in contiguous-focus osteomyelitis.

Pathogenesis

Organisms may reach the bones by hematogenous spread, by direct extension from a contiguous focus of infection, or as a result of trauma. A cycle of increased pressure from infection, inflammation, local ischemia, and bone necrosis may establish itself and lead to a chronic infection.

Clinical Manifestations

Hematogenous osteomyelitis classically presents with high fever and pain around the involved bone. Sinus tracts and purulent drainage are evidence of chronic osteomyelitis.

Microbiologic Diagnosis

Bone biopsy cultures are mandatory with rare exceptions. Sinus tract cultures are unreliable.

Prevention and Treatment

Treatment consists of surgical debridement and long-term, culture-directed antimicrobial therapy. Hematogenous osteomyelitis in children may be treated with antibiotics alone.

INTRODUCTION

Necrotizing infections of the soft tissues are characterized by extensive tissue necrosis and production of tissue gas. These infections may extend through tissue planes and are not well contained by the usual inflammatory mechanisms. They may develop and progress with dramatic speed, and extensive surgery and systemic antibiotic therapy are required to eradicate them.

Arthritis or inflammation of a joint space may be caused by a wide variety of infectious or noninfectious processes. **Noninfectious arthritis** is the more common type of arthritis and is usually secondary to degenerative, rheumatoid, or posttraumatic changes within the joint. **Infectious arthritis,** although less common, is often accompanied by a striking polymorphonuclear inflammatory response and can cause severe destruction of the articular cartilage if not properly diagnosed and treated.

Bone infections are called **osteomyelitis** (from *osteo* [bone], plus *myelitis* [inflammation of the marrow]). **Hematogenous osteomyelitis** and **con-**

tiguous-focus osteomyelitis are the two major types of bone infections. Both types can progress to a chronic bone infection characterized by large areas of dead bone.

Bone, joint, and soft tissues, with the exception of the skin, are normally sterile areas. Bacteria may reach these sites by either hematogenous spread or spread from an exogenous or endogenous contiguous focus of infection (Fig. 100-1). Host defenses are important in containing necrotizing soft tissue infections. A systemically or locally compromised host (Table 100-1) is more likely to develop these types of infections and to be unable to overcome them.

NECROTIZING SOFT TISSUE INFECTIONS

An exact classification of necrotizing subcutaneous, fascial, and muscle infections is difficult because the distinctions between many of the clinical entities are blurred. Clinical classification is as fol-

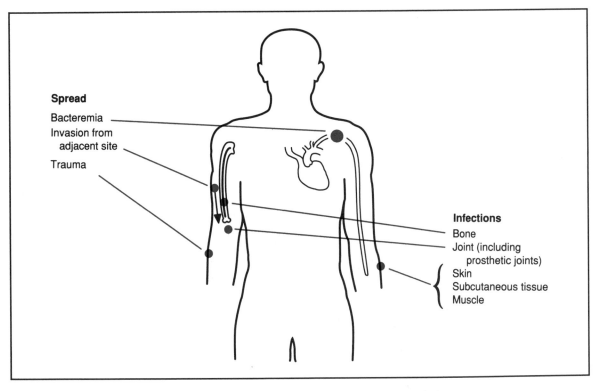

FIGURE 100-1   Bacterial spread to bone, joints, and soft tissue.

lows: (1) crepitant anaerobic cellulitis, (2) necrotizing fasciitis, (3) nonclostridial myonecrosis, (4) clostridial myonecrosis, (5) fungal necrotizing cellulitis, and (6) miscellaneous necrotizing infections in the immunocompromised host. These types of

TABLE 100-1   Systemic and Local Factors That Adversely Affect the Host Response

Systemic Factors	Local Factors
Malnutrition	Major vessel compromise
Renal and hepatic failure	Chronic lymphedema
Diabetes mellitus	Arteritis
Cancer	Extensive scarring
Immunosuppressive	
therapy	Radiation fibrosis
Chronic hypoxia	Small vessel disease
Immune deficiency	Venous stasis
Extremes of age	Insensate region
Alcohol abuse	
Active cigarette abuse	

infections usually occur in traumatic or surgical wounds or around foreign bodies and in patients who are medically compromised by diabetes mellitus, vascular insufficiency, or both. In the traumatically, surgically, or medically compromised patient, local tissue conditions, hypoxia, and decreased oxidation-reduction potential (E_h) promote the growth of anaerobes. Most necrotizing soft tissue infections have an endogenous anaerobic component. Since anaerobes are the predominant members of the microflora on most mucous membranes, there are many potential pathogens. Hypoxic conditions also allow proliferation of facultative aerobic organisms, since polymorphonuclear leukocytes function poorly under decreased oxygen tensions. The growth of aerobic organisms further lowers the E_h, more fastidious anaerobes become established, and the disease process rapidly accelerates.

Discernible quantities of tissue gas are present in most of these infections. Carbon dioxide and water are the natural end products of aerobic metabolism. Carbon dioxide rapidly dissolves in aqueous media and rarely accumulates in tissues. Incomplete oxidation of energy sources by anaerobic and facultative aerobic bacteria can result in the production of gases that are less water soluble and therefore accumulate in tissues. Hydrogen is presumably the major tissue gas in mixed aerobic-anaerobic soft tissue infections. Its presence indicates rapid bacterial multiplication at a low E_h.

Clinically, the hallmarks of mixed aerobic-anaerobic soft tissue infections are tissue necrosis, a putrid discharge, gas production, the tendency to burrow through soft tissue and fascial planes, and the absence of classic signs of tissue inflammation. Table 100-2 shows the differentiation between the common bacterial necrotizing soft tissue infections.

CREPITANT ANAEROBIC CELLULITIS

Nonclostridial and clostridial cellulitides have a similar clinical picture and are discussed together under the term **crepitant anaerobic cellulitis.** Crepitant anaerobic cellulitis appears as a necrotic soft tissue infection with abundant connective tissue gas. The condition usually occurs after local trauma in patients with vascular insufficiency of

the lower extremities. Multiple aerobic and anaerobic organisms have been isolated, including *Bacteroides* species, *Peptostreptococcus* species, *Clostridium* species, and members of the family Enterobacteriaceae. Crepitant anaerobic cellulitis can be differentiated from more serious soft tissue infections by the abundance of soft tissue gas, lack of marked systemic toxicity, gradual onset, less severe pain, and absence of muscle involvement.

NECROTIZING FASCIITIS

Necrotizing fasciitis is a relatively rare infection with a high mortality (40 percent). The infection was originally called **hemolytic streptococcal gangrene** by Meleney in 1924. Although his clinical description was accurate, better culture techniques have demonstrated that organisms other than *Streptococcus pyogenes* more commonly cause these infections. Clinical manifestations include extensive dissection and necrosis of the superficial and often the deep fascia. The infection undermines adjacent tissue and leads to marked systemic toxicity. Thrombosis of subcutaneous blood vessels leads to necrosis of the overlying skin. Initial local pain is replaced by numbness or analgesia as the infection involves the cutaneous nerves. Most cases of fasciitis follow surgery or minor trauma.

TABLE 100-2   Differentiation of the Common
Necrotizing Bacterial Soft Tissue Infections

Variable	Crepitant Anaerobic Cellulitis	Necrotizing Fasciitis	Non-Clostridial Myonecrosis	Clostridial Myonecrosis
Incubation	More than 3 days	1–4 days	Variable (3–14 days)	Under 3 days
Onset	Gradual	Acute	Acute	Acute
Toxemia	None or slight	Moderate to marked	Marked	Marked
Pain	Absent	Moderate to severe	Severe	Severe
Exudate	None or slight	Serosanguinous	"Dishwater pus"	Serosanguinous Profuse
Odor of exudate	Possibly foul	Foul	Possibly foul	Sweet
Gas	Abundant	Usually not present	Not pronounced (≈25%)	Not pronounced (≈25%)
Muscle	No change	Viable	Marked change	Marked change
Skin	Little change	Pale red cellulitis	Minimal change	Tense, dusky, bullous lesions
Mortality	5–10%	30%	75%	15–30%

The highest incidence is seen in patients with small vessel diseases such as diabetes mellitus. When careful bacteriologic techniques are used, anaerobes, particularly *Peptostreptococcus, Bacteroides,* and *Fusobacterium* species, are found in 50 to 60 percent of cases. Aerobic organisms, especially *Streptococcus pyogenes, Staphylococcus aureus,* and members of the Enterobacteriaceae have also been isolated. Most infections are mixed aerobic-anaerobic infections, but a type of necrotizing fasciitis caused solely by *Streptococcus pyogenes* has been reported.

NONCLOSTRIDIAL MYONECROSIS

Nonclostridial myonecrosis, called **synergistic necrotizing cellulitis** by Stone and Martin, is a particularly aggressive soft tissue infection. It is similar to clostridial myonecrosis in that there is widespread involvement of soft tissue with necrosis of muscle tissue and fascia. The prominent involvement of muscle tissue differentiates this infection from necrotizing fasciitis. Subcutaneous tissue and skin are secondarily involved. Clinically, there are exquisite local tenderness, with minimal skin changes, and drainage of foul-smelling "dishwater" pus from small skin surface ulcers. Severe systemic toxicity is found in most patients. Nonclostridial myonecrosis occurs most frequently in the perineal area, as a result of an extension of a perirectal abscess, and in the lower extremities of patients with vascular insufficiency. Multiple organisms have been isolated, including *Peptostreptococcus* and *Bacteroides* species and members of the Enterobacteriaceae. Mortality approaches 75 percent.

CLOSTRIDIAL MYONECROSIS

Clostridial myonecrosis, or **gas gangrene,** is a clostridial infection primarily of muscle tissue. *Clostridium perfringens* is isolated in 90 percent of these infections. Other clostridial species frequently isolated are *C novyi* (4 percent), *C septicum* (2 percent), *C histolyticum, C fallax,* and *C bifermentans.* Classically, clostridial myonecrosis has an acute presentation and a fulminant clinical course. The infection usually occurs in areas of major trauma or surgery or as a complication of thermal burns. However, it also has been reported following minor trauma, including intravenous administration of drugs, intramuscular injections of epinephrine, insect bites, and nail punctures. Moreover, it may occur in the absence of recent trauma, by activation of dormant clostridial spores in old scar tissue.

Clostridial myonecrosis is diagnosed mainly on a clinical basis. The infection may be so rapidly progressive that any delay in recognition or treatment may be fatal. The onset is sudden, often within 4 to 6 hours after an injury. Sudden, severe pain in the area of infection is an early clinical finding. Early in the course of infection, the skin overlying the wound appears shiny and tense and then becomes dusky. Within hours, the skin color may progress from dusky to a bronze discoloration, which can advance at a rate of 1 inch per hour. Vesicles or hemorrhagic bullae appear near the wound. A thin, brownish, often copious fluid exudes from the wound. Bubbles occasionally appear in the drainage. This exudate has often been described as having a sweet "mousy" odor. Swelling and edema in the area of infection is pronounced. Within hours the skin overlying the lesion can rupture and the muscle herniate. At surgery, the infected muscle is dark red to black, is noncontractile, and does not bleed when cut. Crepitus, although not prominent, is sometimes detected. Radiographs may show tissue gas outlining fascial planes and muscle bundles.

The rapid tissue necrosis in clostridial myonecrosis is caused by the clostridial toxins. Clostridial species are capable of producing multiple toxins, each with its own mode of action. *Clostridium perfringens* produces at least 12 different extracellular toxins. The most common of these, a lecithinase called **alpha toxin,** is hemolytic, histotoxic, and necrotizing. Other toxins act as collagenases, proteinases, deoxyribonucleases (DNases), fibrinolysins, and hyaluronidases. The systemic toxic reaction cannot be fully explained by a single circulating exotoxin. The "toxic factor" may be produced by interaction of the clostridial toxins with infected tissue. The mortality from clostridial myonecrosis ranges from 15 to 30 percent.

FUNGAL NECROTIZING CELLULITIS

Phycomyces and *Aspergillus* species may cause a gangrenous cellulitis in compromised hosts. The hallmark of these infections is the invasion of blood vessels by hyphae, followed by thrombosis and subsequent necrosis extending to all soft tissue compartments. Spores from these fungi are ubiquitous.

The *Phycomyces* species are characterized by broad-based nonseptate hyphae. *Rhizopus, Mucor,* and *Absidia* are the major pathogenic genera within the family Mucoraceae. Serious pulmonary, rhinocerebral, or disseminated infections have been found in patient with diabetes, lymphoma, or leukemia. Phycomycotic gangrenous cellulitis usually occurs in patients with severe burns or diabetes. The characteristic dermal lesion is a black, anesthetic ulcer or an area of necrosis with a purple edematous margin. There is no gas or exudate, and the infection may progress rapidly.

Aspergillus species are characterized histologically by branched, septate hyphae. These fungi can cause serious pulmonary or disseminated infections in compromised hosts. *Aspergillus* gangrenous cellulitis may be primary or from a disseminated infection. The dermal lesion is an indurated plaque that leads to a necrotic ulcer. Gas and exudate are not present.

◀ JOINT INFECTIONS ▶

Infectious arthritis may arise either from hematogenous spread or by direct extension from an adjacent bone or soft tissue infection. The infection is usually a localized suppurative process. Although any joint can become infected, the knee is most commonly involved (53 percent), followed by the hip (20 percent), shoulder (11 percent), wrist (9 percent), ankle (8 percent), and elbow (7 percent). The infection is monoarticular almost 90 percent of the time. However, a bacterial polyarthritis may be seen.

In the normal host, polymorphonuclear leukocytes respond rapidly to the infection and release proteolytic enzymes, which can cause extensive destruction of the articular cartilage within 3 days. The joint may also be damaged directly by the release of bacterial toxins and lysosomal enzymes. Furthermore, an effusion is almost always present and is confined within the joint capsule; this increases intra-articular pressure and interferes with blood supply and nutrition. These complications may occur with almost any type of septic arthritis, but are most common in nongonococcal bacterial infections. Children are especially vulnerable since extension to the epiphyseal growth plate may stunt bone growth.

Several conditions are known to predispose joints to the development of septic arthritis. Corticosteroid therapy, rheumatoid arthritis, and degenerative joint disease are the most common underlying factors. Total joint arthroplasties are susceptible to hematogenous infections. Patients with diabetes mellitus, leukemia, cancer, cirrhosis, chronic granulomatous diseases, or hypogammaglobulinemia or those undergoing cytotoxic chemotherapy or practicing substance abuse also have an increased incidence of infectious arthritis.

GONOCOCCAL ARTHRITIS

The most common cause of bacterial arthritis in healthy young adults in North America is *Neisseria gonorrhoeae*. **Gonococcal arthritis** typically follows primary infection of a mucosal site and is thought to spread hematogenously to the joint. Females are affected four times as often as males, and about one-half of all affected females are either pregnant or menstruating. This association supports the theory that endocrine factors play a role in gonococcal arthritis, although the exact mechanism has not been elucidated. Strains of *N gonorrhoeae* that cause disseminated gonococcal infections differ phenotypically from those that cause simple mucosal infections and are thought to be more virulent.

The disease may manifest itself as part of a disseminated gonococcal infection or as a monoarticular joint infection. The presenting symptoms in disseminated gonococcal infections may be mixed, with migratory polyarthralgias, fever, chills, dermatitis, and tenosynovitis. Most of these patients have asymptomatic genital, anal, or pharyngeal gonococcal infections. Skin lesions, when present, begin as small erythematous papules but usually progress to vesicular or pustular stages. Tenosynovitis is characterized by pain, swelling, and periarticular redness. Patients with monoarticular disease often have a history of polyarthralgias, and some authorities believe that this represents a continuum from disseminated gonococcal infection.

NONGONOCOCCAL BACTERIAL ARTHRITIS

Nongonococcal bacterial arthritis is a serious infection with significant sequelae. Mortality as high as 12 percent has been reported, and up to 75 percent of survivors suffer some type of functional loss in the involved joint. Classically, patients present with fever and pain, swelling, warmth, and decreased range of motion in the involved joint. The joint effusion should be aspirated and cultured to determine the exact etiologic agent. There are variations among age groups, but the most common cause of nongonococcal bacterial arthritis is *Staphylococcus aureus*. In adults, all Gram-negative bacilli together account for about 20 percent of cases. It is generally accepted that Gram-negative infections are the most virulent, with *Pseudomonas aeruginosa* and *Escherichia coli* being the most common. Intravenous drug abusers have a significant incidence of infection with Gram-negative organisms. Streptococcal species engender a small but significant proportion of infections (10 to 15 percent). About 10 percent of patients with nongoncoccal arthritis have polymicrobial infections. In addition, there are frequent microbiologic associations with concomitant disease states. For example, bacterial arthritis following infectious diarrhea may be caused by *Shigella, Salmonella, Campylobacter,* or *Yersinia* species. *Streptobacillus moniliformis* may cause a migrating polyarthritis; however, this is rare. In children, *Haemophilus influenzae* is an important cause of septic arthritis.

DIAGNOSIS OF BACTERIAL ARTHRITIS

Several laboratory tests are used to diagnose infectious arthritis. The definitive test involves culturing the fluid from the involved joint after aspiration or incision and drainage. Gram stains are often unreliable, although they may provide initial clues. Synovial fluid analysis usually reveals a turbid fluid with leukocyte counts greater than $100,000/mm^3$ in 30 to 50 percent of cases. In bacterial arthritis, the level of polymorphonuclear leukocytes often approaches 90 percent. Low joint fluid glucose levels and high lactate levels are indicative of septic arthritis, but are nonspecific. Peripheral blood leukocyte counts are usually elevated in children, but are often within normal limits in adults. Finally, radiography may show joint space widening and soft tissue swelling in infections more than 2 weeks old.

GRANULOMATOUS ARTHRITIS

Infectious arthritis may be caused by mycobacteria and certain fungi. This disease may be very insidious and may progress for several months before infection is even considered. These organisms usually produce a chronic monoarticular arthritis with a granulomatous inflammatory response. *Mycobacterium tuberculosis* infections of the musculoskeletal system are the most common extrapulmonary manifestation of tuberculosis and result from hematogenous dissemination. Atypical mycobacteria, especially *M fortuitum, M chelonae,* and *M marinum,* may cause septic arthritis by inoculation or extension from a contiguous focus of infection. The most common cause of fungal arthritis is *Sporothrix schenckii*. This infection usually follows traumatic inoculation, but may also result from pulmonary dissemination. Because of its relative rarity and indolent course, the diagnosis is often missed or delayed. Coccidiomycosis, histoplasmosis, and blastomycosis may all affect the joint. In addition, *Cryptococcus, Aspergillus,* and *Candida* species may cause infectious arthritis in the immunocompromised host. Diagnosis of all the granulomatous arthritides usually involves a high index of suspicion and appropriate fungal or mycobacterial cultures.

BONE INFECTIONS

On the basis of clinical and pathologic considerations, **osteomyelitis** may be classified as either hematogenous or secondary to a contiguous focus of infection. **Contiguous-focus osteomyelitis** can be further subdivided into bone infection with relatively normal vascularity and bone infection with generalized vascular insufficiency. Either major type of osteomyelitis may progress to a chronic bone infection.

HEMATOGENOUS OSTEOMYELITIS

Hematogenous osteomyelitis occurs mainly in infants and children but has recently been found with increasing frequency in the adult population. In infants and children the metaphysis of long bones (tibia, femur) is most frequently involved. The anatomy in the metaphyseal region of long bones seems to explain this clinical finding. Non-anastomosing capillary ends of the nutrient artery make sharp loops under the growth plate and enter a system of large venous sinusoids where the blood flow becomes slow and turbulent. Any obstruction of the capillary ends lead to an area of avascular necrosis. Minor trauma probably predisposes the infant or child to infection by producing a small hematoma and subsequent bone necrosis, both of which can be infected by a transient bacteremia.

The infection produces a local cellulitis, which results in increased bone pressure, decreased pH, and a breakdown of leukocytes. All of these factors contribute to necrosis of bone. The infection may proceed laterally through the haversian and Volkmann canal system, perforate the cortex, and lift the periosteum. It may also extend into the intramedullary canal. Extension leads to further vascular compromise and bone necrosis. In infants, some capillaries still penetrate the growth plate. Therefore, the infection may also spread to the epiphysis and into the joint space. In children over 1 year old, the growth plate is not penetrated by capillaries, and the epiphysis and joint space are protected from infection. In adults, the growth plate has been resorbed and joint extension of a metaphyseal infection can recur. However, in adults, the diaphysis of the long bones and the lumbar and thoracic vertebral bodies of the axial skeleton are most frequently involved. Adults with axial skeletal osteomyelitis often have a history of preceding urinary tract infection or intravenous drug abuse.

A single pathogenic organism is usually responsible for hematogenous osteomyelitis (Table 100-3). Polymicrobic hematogenous osteomyelitis is rare. *Staphylococcus aureus* is the most frequent organism isolated, but *Streptococcus pyogenes* and *Streptococcus agalactiae* are responsible for a significant number of bone infections, especially in infants. Aerobic Gram-negative organisms are responsible for an increasing number of bone infections. *Pseudomonas aeruginosa* is often isolated

TABLE 100-3　Commonly Isolated Organisms
in Osteomyelitis

Hematogenous Osteomyelitis (Monomicrobic Infection)			Contiguous-Focus Osteomyelitis (Polymicrobic Infection)
Infants (1 year)	**Children (1–16 years)**	**Adults (>16 years)**	**All ages**
Group B streptococci	*Staphylococcus aureus*	*Staphylococcus aureus*	*Staphylococcus aureus*
Staphylococcus aureus	Group A streptococci	*Staphylococcus epidermidis*	*Staphylococcus epidermidis*
Escherichia coli	*Haemophilus influenzae*	Gram-negative bacilli	Group A streptococci
		Pseudomonas aeruginosa	*Enterococcus* spp
		Serratia marcescens	Gram-negative bacilli
		Escherichia coli	Anaerobes

from intravenous drug abusers with vertebral osteomyelitis.

Patients with hematogenous osteomyelitis usually have normal soft tissue around the infected bone. If antimicrobial therapy directed at the pathogen is begun prior to extensive bone necrosis, the patient has an excellent chance of cure.

CONTIGUOUS-FOCUS OSTEOMYELITIS

Osteomyelitis Secondary to a Contiguous Infection with No Generalized Vascular Insufficiency

In contiguous-focus osteomyelitis, the organism either is directly inoculated into the bone by trauma or surgery or reaches the bone from adjacent infected soft tissue. Common predisposing conditions include open fractures, surgical reduction and internal fixation of fractures, and wound infections. In contrast to hematogenous osteomyelitis, multiple bacteria are isolated from the infected bone. The bacteriology is diverse (Table 100-3), but *S aureus* remains the most commonly isolated pathogen. In addition, aerobic Gram-negative bacilli and anaerobic organisms are frequently isolated. Bone necrosis, soft tissue damage, and loss of bone stability are all common, making this form of osteomyelitis difficult to manage.

Osteomyelitis Secondary to a Contiguous Infection with Generalized Vascular Insufficiency

The small bones of the feet (principally the metatarsal bones and phalanges) are commonly involved in osteomyelitis secondary to a contiguous infection in patients with generalized vascular insufficiency. Most commonly, the infection develops as an extension of a local infection, either cellulitis or a trophic skin ulcer. The inadequate tissue perfusion favors the infection by blunting the local inflammatory response. Multiple aerobic and anaerobic bacteria are usually isolated from the infected bone. Although cure is desirable, a more attainable goal of therapy is to suppress the infection and maintain functional integrity of the involved limb. Recurrent or new bone infections occur in many patients. In time, amputation of the infected area is almost always necessary.

CHRONIC OSTEOMYELITIS

Both hematogenous osteomyelitis and contiguous-focus osteomyelitis can progress to a chronic bone infection. No exact criteria separate acute from chronic osteomyelitis. Clinically, newly recognized bone infections are considered acute, whereas a relapse of the infection represents chronic disease. However, this simplistic classification is clearly inadequate. The hallmark of chronic osteomyelitis is the presence of large areas of dead bone or sequestra. An involucrum (a reactive bony encasement around the sequestrum) and persistent drainage via one or more sinus tracts are usually present. In chronic osteomyelitis, multiple species of bacteria are usually isolated from the necrotic infected bone (Table 100-3), except in cases of chronic hematogenous osteomyelitis, which usually yield a single organism. Unless the necrotic infected bone can be removed, antibiotic therapy is usually unsuccessful. The prognosis for arresting the infection is worse if there is poor soft tissue integrity surrounding the infection, sclerosis of the involved bone, or bone instability.

DIAGNOSIS OF BACTERIAL OSTEOMYELITIS

The bacteriologic diagnosis of bacterial osteomyelitis rests on isolation of the agent from the bone or the blood. In hematogenous osteomyelitis, positive blood cultures often obviate the need for a bone biopsy when there is associated radiographic or radionuclide scan evidence of osteomyelitis. In chronic osteomyelitis, sinus tract cultures are not reliable for predicting which organism(s) will be isolated from the infected bone. Antibiotic treatment of osteomyelitis should not be based on the results of sinus tract cultures. In most instances, bone biopsy cultures are mandatory to guide specific antimicrobial therapy.

SKELETAL TUBERCULOSIS

Skeletal tuberculosis is the result of hematogenous spread of the tuberculosis bacillus early in the course of a primary infection. Rarely, skeletal tuberculosis develops as a contiguous infection from an adjacent caseating lymph node. Either the primary bone infection or a reactivated quiescent primary bone infection elicits an inflammatory reaction, followed by the development granulation tissue. The granulation tissue erodes and destroys the cartilage and cancellous bone. Eventually the infection causes bone demineralization and necrosis. Proteolytic enzymes that can destroy cartilage are not produced in skeletal tuberculosis. Cartilage is destroyed slowly by granulation tissue, and the joint or disc space is preserved for considerable periods. Healing involves deposition of fibrous tissue. Pain is the most frequent clinical complaint.

Any bone may be involved by skeletal tuberculosis, but the infection usually involves one site. In children and adolescents, the metaphyses of the long bones are most frequently infected. In adults, the axial skeleton, followed by the proximal femur, knee, and small bones of the hands and feet, are most often involved. In the axial skeleton, the thoracic vertebral bodies are most frequently infected, followed by the lumbar and cervical vertebral bodies. Vertebral infection usually begins in the anterior portion of a vertebral body adjacent to an intervertebral disc. The infection destroys nearby bone and the intervertebral disc. Adjacent vertebral bodies may become involved, and a paravertebral abscess may develop. Sixty percent of patients with skeletal tuberculosis have evidence of extraosseous tuberculosis.

Tissue for culture and histology is almost always required for the diagnosis of skeletal tuberculosis. Cultures for *Mycobacterium tuberculosis* are positive in approximately 60 percent of the cases, but 6 weeks may be required for growth and identification of the organism. Histology showing granulomatous tissue compatible with tuberculosis and a positive tuberculin test are sufficient to begin tuberculosis therapy. However, a negative skin test does not rule out skeletal tuberculosis. Therapy for skeletal tuberculosis involves prolonged chemotherapy and in some cases surgical debridement.

FUNGAL OSTEOMYELITIS

Bone infections may be caused by a variety of fungal organisms including *Coccidioides, Blastomyces, Cryptococcus,* and *Sporothrix* species. The lesion most often appears as a cold abscess overlying an osteolytic lesion. Joint space extension may occur in coccidioidomycosis and blastomycosis. Therapy for fungal osteomyelitis involves surgical debridement and antifungal chemotherapy.

REFERENCES

Cierny G, Mader JT: Management of adult osteomyelitis. p. 10, 15. In Evarts CM (ed): Surgery of the Musculoskeletal Systems. Churchill Livingstone, New York, 1983

Finegold SM, Bartlett JG, Chow AK et al: Management of anaerobic infections. Ann Intern Med 83:375, 1975

Mackowiak PA, Jones SR, Smith JW: Diagnostic value of sinus tract cultures in chronic osteomyelitis. J Am Med Assoc 239:2772, 1978

Martin DH: Gonococcal arthritis and Reiter's syndrome. p. 233. In D'ambrosia RD, Marier RL (eds): Orthopaedic Infections. Slack, Thorofare, NJ, 1989

Meijers KA, Dijkmans BA, Hermans J et al: Non-gonococcal infectious arthritis: a retrospective study. J Infect Dis 14:13, 1987

Meleney FL: Hemolytic streptococcal gangrene. Arch Surg 9:317, 1924

Ruthbery AD, Ho G: Nongonococcal bacterial arthritis. p. 213. In D'ambrosia RD, Marier RL (eds): Orthopaedic Infections. Slack, Thorofare, NJ, 1989

Smith JW: Infectious arthritis. p. 697. In Mandell GL, Douglas RG, Bennett JE (eds): Principles and Practice of Infectious Diseases. 2nd Ed. Churchill Livingstone, New York, 1985

Stone HH, Martin JD, Jr: Synergistic necrotizing cellulitis. Ann Surg 175:702, 1972

Waldvogel FA, Medoff G, Swartz MN: 1970. Osteomyelitis: a review of clinical features, therapeutic considerations, and unusual aspects. N Engl J Med 282:198, 260, 316, 1970

INDEX

Page numbers followed by f indicate figures; page numbers followed by t indicate tables. Numbers in boldface indicate boldface text terms.

ALD J. BRENNER ◆ JANET S. BUTEL ◆ GILBERT A. CASTRO ◆ JAN CERNY ◆ JAY O. COHEN ◆ GAR
LE ◆ FRANK M. COLLINS ◆ ROBERT B. COUCH ◆ JOHN P. CRAIG ◆ JOHN H. CROSS ◆ CHARL
CK DAVIS ◆ ERIK DE CLERCQ ◆ FERDINANDO DIANZANI ◆ DENNIS M. DIXON ◆ WALTER DOERFLER
UBEY ◆ GISELA ENDERS ◆ DOLORES G. EVANS ◆ DOYLE J. EVANS, JR. ◆ ADAM EWERT ◆ ANTHO
CI ◆ FRANK FENNER ◆ SYDNEY M. FINEGOLD ◆ HORST FINGER ◆ RICHARD A. FINKELSTEIN ◆ DAN
HBEIN ◆ THOMAS J. FITZGERALD ◆ W. ROBERT FLEISCHMANN, JR. ◆ MICHAEL FONS ◆ SAMUEL
AL ◆ J. R. L. FORSYTH ◆ MARY ANN GERENCSER ◆ RALPH A. GIANNELLA ◆ CLARENCE J. GIBBS, JR.
ND S. GOLDMAN ◆ SHERWOOD L. GORBACH ◆ M. NEAL GUENTZEL ◆ THOMAS L. HALE ◆ DEBORA
IDERSON ◆ DAVID J. HENTGES ◆ DONALD HEYNEMAN ◆ HERBERT HOF ◆ STEPHEN L. HOFFMAN
ALL K. HOLMES ◆ WALTER T. HUGHES ◆ BARBARA H. IGLEWSKI ◆ MICHAEL G. JOBLING ◆ RICHAR
NSON ◆ RUSSELL C. JOHNSON ◆ PETER JURTSHUK, JR. ◆ ALBERT Z. KAPIKIAN ◆ DORIS S. KELSEY
LD T. KEUSCH ◆ KWANG-SHIN KIM ◆ GARY R. KLIMPEL ◆ GEORGE S. KOBAYASHI ◆ CHIEN LIU ◆ WA
LOESCHE ◆ JOAN C. M. MACNAB ◆ JON T. MADER ◆ AUGUSTO JULIO MARTINEZ ◆ CARL F. T. MA
◆ MICHAEL R. McGINNIS ◆ DAVID N. McMURRAY ◆ ERNEST A. MEYER ◆ HARRY M. MEYER, JR. ◆ MA
EBROOKS ◆ STEPHEN A. MORSE ◆ JOHN R. MURPHY ◆ DANIEL M. MUSHER ◆ HAROLD C. NEU
C. O'CONNOR ◆ LEROY J. OLSON ◆ DAVID ONIONS ◆ PAUL D. PARKMAN ◆ GARY PATOU ◆ MAR
PATTERSON ◆ JOHN R. PATTISON ◆ LAWRENCE L. PELLETIER, JR. ◆ GUILLERMO I. PEREZ-PEREZ
NY W. PETERSON ◆ CHARLES J. PFAU ◆ DAVID D. PORTER ◆ ALAN S. RABSON ◆ SHMUEL RAZIN
CES L. REID-SANDEN ◆ LELAND S. RICKMAN ◆ BERNARD ROIZMAN ◆ ALLAN R. RONALD ◆ ZEDA
NBERG ◆ PHILIP K. RUSSELL ◆ MILTON R. J. SALTON ◆ ALAN L. SCHMALJOHN ◆ JOHN RICHARD SEE
ERT E. SHOPE ◆ WILLIAM A. SODEMAN, JR. ◆ PETER C. B. TURNBULL ◆ DAVID A. J. TYRRELL ◆ DERE
LIN ◆ DAVID H. WALKER ◆ WILLIAM WALLACE ◆ THOMAS J. WALSH ◆ KENNETH S. WARREN ◆ JOH
SHINGTON ◆ CAROL L. WELLS ◆ RICHARD J. WHITLEY ◆ TRACY D. WILKINS ◆ WASHINGTON
JR. ◆ ROBERT G. YAEGER ◆ MARGUERITE YIN-MURPHY ◆ RODRIGO A. ZELEDÓN ◆ ARIE J. ZUCKE
◆ THOMAS ALBRECHT ◆ MICHELLE J. ALFA ◆ G. G. ALTON ◆ RAZA ALY ◆ SAMUEL BARON ◆ DERRIC
◆ YECHIEL BECKER ◆ NEIL R. BLACKLOW ◆ MARTIN J. BLASER ◆ ISTVAN BOLDOGH ◆ PHILIP
HMAN ◆ DONALD J. BRENNER ◆ JANET S. BUTEL ◆ GILBERT A. CASTRO ◆ JAN CERNY ◆ JAY C
N ◆ GARRY T. COLE ◆ FRANK M. COLLINS ◆ ROBERT B. COUCH ◆ JOHN P. CRAIG ◆ JOHN H. CROS
ARLES PATRICK DAVIS ◆ ERIK DE CLERCQ ◆ FERDINANDO DIANZANI ◆ DENNIS M. DIXON ◆ WALTE
LER ◆ J. P. DUBEY ◆ GISELA ENDERS ◆ DOLORES G. EVANS ◆ DOYLE J. EVANS, JR. ◆ ADAM EWERT
ONY S. FAUCI ◆ FRANK FENNER ◆ SYDNEY M. FINEGOLD ◆ HORST FINGER ◆ RICHARD A. FINKE
◆ DANIEL B. FISHBEIN ◆ THOMAS J. FITZGERALD ◆ W. ROBERT FLEISCHMANN, JR. ◆ MICHAEL FON
UEL B. FORMAL ◆ J. R. L. FORSYTH ◆ MARY ANN GERENCSER ◆ RALPH A. GIANNELLA ◆ CLAREN
BS, JR. ◆ ARMOND S. GOLDMAN ◆ SHERWOOD L. GORBACH ◆ M. NEAL GUENTZEL ◆ THOMAS
◆ DEBORAH J. HENDERSON ◆ DAVID J. HENTGES ◆ DONALD HEYNEMAN ◆ HERBERT HOF
EN L. HOFFMAN ◆ RANDALL K. HOLMES ◆ WALTER T. HUGHES ◆ BARBARA H. IGLEWSKI ◆ MICHAE
BLING ◆ RICHARD T. JOHNSON ◆ RUSSELL C. JOHNSON ◆ PETER JURTSHUK, JR. ◆ ALBERT
AN ◆ DORIS S. KELSEY ◆ GERALD T. KEUSCH ◆ KWANG-SHIN KIM ◆ GARY R. KLIMPEL ◆ GEORGE
ASHI ◆ CHIEN LIU ◆ WALTER J. LOESCHE ◆ JOAN C. M. MACNAB ◆ JON T. MADER ◆ AUGUSTO
MARTINEZ ◆ CARL F. T. MATTERN ◆ MICHAEL R. McGINNIS ◆ DAVID N. McMURRAY ◆ ERNEST A
◆ HARRY M. MEYER, JR. ◆ MARK MIDDLEBROOKS ◆ STEPHEN A. MORSE ◆ JOHN R. MURPHY
L M. MUSHER ◆ HAROLD C. NEU ◆ MARY C. O'CONNOR ◆ LEROY J. OLSON ◆ DAVID ONIONS
D. PARKMAN ◆ GARY PATOU ◆ MARIA JEVITZ PATTERSON ◆ JOHN R. PATTISON ◆ LAWRENCE L. PE
JR. ◆ GUILLERMO I. PEREZ-PEREZ ◆ JOHNNY W. PETERSON ◆ CHARLES J. PFAU ◆ DAVID D. PORTE
N S. RABSON ◆ SHMUEL RAZIN ◆ FRANCES L. REID-SANDEN ◆ LELAND S. RICKMAN ◆ BERNAR
AN ◆ ALLAN R. RONALD ◆ ZEDA F. ROSENBERG ◆ PHILIP K. RUSSELL ◆ MILTON R. J. SALTON
L. SCHMALJOHN ◆ JOHN RICHARD SEED ◆ ROBERT E. SHOPE ◆ WILLIAM A. SODEMAN, JR. ◆ PETE
TURNBULL ◆ DAVID A. J. TYRRELL ◆ DEREK WAKELIN ◆ DAVID H. WALKER ◆ WILLIAM WALLACE